Treatment of Cancer

Treatment of Cancer

Seventh Edition

Edited by

Pat Price

MA, MD, FRCP, FRCR
Visiting Professor
Department of Surgery and Cancer

Imperial College London, UK

Karol Sikora

MA, MB BChir, PhD, FRCR, FRCP, FFPM
Medical Director
Rutherford Health
and Professor of Medicine
University of Buckingham, UK

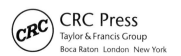

CRC Press
Taylor & Francis Group
Boca Raton London New York

CRC Press is an imprint of the
Taylor & Francis Group, an **informa** business

First edition published 2021
by CRC Press
6000 Broken Sound Parkway NW, Suite 300, Boca Raton, FL 33487-2742

and by CRC Press
2 Park Square, Milton Park, Abingdon, Oxon, OX14 4RN

First issued in paperback 2022

© 2021 Taylor & Francis Group, LLC

CRC Press is an imprint of Taylor & Francis Group, an Informa business

Publisher's Note
The publisher has gone to great lengths to ensure the quality of this reprint but points out that some imperfections in the original copies may be apparent.

ISBN 13: 978-0-367-56002-7 (pbk)
ISBN 13: 978-0-367-13465-5 (hbk)
ISBN 13: 978-0-429-02663-8 (ebk)

Typeset in Warnock Pro
by Deanta Global Publishing Services, Chennai, India

Printed in the UK by Severn, Gloucester on responsibly sourced paper

 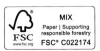

CONTENTS

PREFACE

Welcome to the seventh edition of *Treatment of Cancer*. Since the previous edition, there have been such a lot of advances in oncology understanding and treatment—it is a very exciting time. Sadly, it has also been the time of the Covid-19 pandemic with cancer diagnosis and treatments affected across the world. This has brought together the international cancer community and has reinforced the need for smart solutions to cancer treatment to help our patients. Treatment can now be far more targeted to an individual's tumor biology, technical advances in radiotherapy have meant more precise and effective treatments, and immunotherapy is producing real improvements in survival. The choice and menu for treatments are vast and the nuances to gain improvements are significant. While oncologists are getting more and more sub-specialized, we hope this book provides an up-to-date overview of all the main tumors, useful to both the specialist and the generalist or trainee.

Patients have become increasingly involved in the choice of their own treatment, while cancer lobby groups and charities have driven new patient-directed information networks. The fully engaged cancer patient understands his/her disease, the pros and cons of different therapies, and the concept of risk assessment in differing clinical situations. The chapters here provide a framework on which to base discussions with patients.

Cancer is becoming more prevalent across the world, its incidence rising as the world's population ages and obesity rates increase. The increase in life expectancy is something we should celebrate but it brings challenges to health care systems. There is now a continuous flow of new, very expensive therapies bringing double-digit inflation to cancer care costs. Understanding the cost–benefit equation for any intervention has become an essential component of clinical decision-making in all health care systems.

Oncology has seen many developments, even in the short period since the publishing of the sixth edition in 2015, and the contributing authors have included these by completely updating the chapters, many being completely rewritten and refreshed. We are most grateful to all of our talented and expert contributors for sharing their expertise. We are also responding to a need for a useful, practical guide to the management of cancer and so this version has concentrated solely on the management of individual tumor types. The basic building blocks of surgery, radiotherapy, chemotherapy, and immunotherapy are best obtained from specialist text or current literature, and we have included available treatment guidelines that people may find useful. This is an international textbook written from a UK perspective, and we trust our international colleagues will appreciate seeing how the United Kingdom's evidence-based guidance on the treatment of cancer is implemented in a predominantly single-payer health system.

Our title, *Treatment of Cancer*, has certainly changed to reflect these developments and is now almost unrecognizable from the first edition of 1980. It is shorter, presenting critical reviews of cancer management strategies for different tumor types. In revising this edition, we have tried to retain the characteristic didactic approach to patient care but perhaps with much greater consideration of the options available. This seventh edition is available as both hard copy and an eBook, and we hope you will use both media platforms for different purposes.

We warmly thank all those who have contributed to this edition for sharing their expertise and hope you will find it a helpful contribution to aid excellence in cancer patient care.

Pat Price and Karol Sikora, London

CANCER CARE: TODAY AND TOMORROW

Karol Sikora

This book is written by many authors around one common theme—the optimal treatment of cancer. The problem at first seems relatively simple. There are about 10^{13} cells in the human body. From the fertilized egg to death in old age, a human being is the product of 10^{16} cell divisions. Like all complex systems, growth control can go wrong, resulting in the loss of normal territorial restraint, producing a family of cells that can multiply indefinitely. But it is not just the local growth of tumor cells that makes them so lethal. It is their spread, directly through invasion and by metastases, to other sites of the body. Tumors that remain localized can usually be cured by surgery or radiotherapy, even when enormous. Patients with large, eroding basal cell skin cancers, for example, can be treated successfully, as these tumors seldom invade deep into the skin or spread to lymph nodes. Yet, a breast lump less than 1 cm in diameter, which causes the patient no problems and is picked up in a screening clinic, can be lethal if metastases have already arisen from the primary site. It is this spread that provides the plethora of clinical problems. Just as no two individuals are alike, no two tumors behave in exactly the same way, although we can make some broad generalizations from clinical experience. Much recent emphasis has been on understanding the molecular phenotype of cancers, so leading to the concept of personalized or stratified medicine. A major, and often overlooked, phenomenon is that individual metastases evolve in different ways—a form of somatic Darwinian selection of those cells best able to adapt to their new environment. The ensuing diversity could thwart the simplistic view of determining the right treatment based on a single biopsy. The physical and psychological interactions of a patient with a growing cancer require careful analysis and action by those involved in the patient's care.

Cancer is not universally fatal despite much public misconception. Tremendous advances have been made in the treatment of leukemia, lymphoma, testicular cancer, choriocarcinoma, and several other rare tumors, and cure of even widespread disease is now common. Even with lung cancer, the most common single tumor type throughout the world, about 8% of patients survive for many years and die of other causes. However, although there are some pointers, we do not understand why this 8% should be spared. If they can be cured, why not the rest? What makes these patients so different? For some reason, studying long-term survivors—the outliers of the normal distribution—has not really been helpful for any cancer.

Vast sums of money are currently spent worldwide on research, and yet for most common tumors, there have been only small improvements in overall cure rates over the last 30 years. The recent dramatic inflation in the costs of providing optimal care, by using drugs costing several thousand pounds a month to provide survival gains measured in weeks, is clearly not sustainable in any health economy. Better ways of predicting their efficacy are urgently needed to individualize therapy.

As an intellectual problem to the scientist, malignant disease has always appeared eminently soluble. After all, it would seem a relatively straightforward task to identify the differences between normal and malignant cells and devise a selective destruction process. Yet, we still do not know precisely the first biochemical step that takes a cell down the road to neoplasia. The recent advances in molecular biology seem poised to rectify this and to give us new avenues for clinical exploitation, but we have to treat our patients now—providing for them the best of today's technology with the skill of the caring physician.

Cancer's Timeline

The first recorded reference to cancer was in the Edwin Smith Papyrus of 3000 BC, in which eight women with breast cancer are described. The writings of Hippocrates in 400 BC contain several descriptions of cancer in different sites. But our understanding of the disease really began in the nineteenth century with the advent of cellular pathology.

Successful treatment by radical surgery became possible in the latter part of that century, thanks to advances in anesthetics and antiseptics. Radical surgery involved the removal of the tumor-containing organ and draining its lymph nodes in one block. Within a short timeframe, similar procedures were devised for different parts of the body. Halsted at Johns Hopkins was the main protagonist of the radical mastectomy, Wertheim in Vienna of the hysterectomy, Trotter in London of the pharyngectomy, Whipple in New York of the pancreatico-duodenectomy, and Miles in London of the abdomino-perineal resection of the rectum. These diverse surgical procedures all followed the same principle of removing the cancer in contiguity with the lymph node drainage pathways.

Following such massively destructive surgical approaches, the twentieth century ended with the conservation of organs by minimizing the destruction caused by surgery and replacing it with radiotherapy and, for some sites, effective adjuvant therapy with drugs and radiotherapy (Table 1).

Radiotherapy has come a long way since the first patient with a nasal tumor was treated in 1899, only a year after the discovery of radium by Marie Curie. Although radiobiology developed as a research discipline, it has really contributed little to clinical practice. The rationale behind modern fractionated radiotherapy comes as much from empirical trial and error as from experimental results. Radiotherapy is remarkably successful for certain areas of the body. Increasing sophistication in equipment coupled with dramatic strides in imaging have led to great precision in the planning and execution of treatment, thus sparing critical normal tissues and increasing the dose to the tumor.

The sinking of the US Liberty ship *SS John Harvey* in Bari Harbour in Italy by the Germans in 1942 led to the development of effective chemotherapy. The warship was carrying canisters of mustard gas for use in chemical warfare. Survivors developed leukopenia and this led the naval physicians back in the United States to experiment with halogenated alkylamines in patients with high white cell counts—lymphomas, leukemias, and Hodgkin disease. From the first publication in 1946, the field has blossomed, with more than 200 drugs now available in our global pharmacopeia. But as with radiotherapy, our clinical practice is based mainly on empiricism. Most currently used drugs were found serendipitously from plants or fungi—paclitaxel, vincristine, doxorubicin—and not by rational drug design. Although very successfully used in combination for lymphoma, leukemia, choriocarcinoma, testicular cancer, and several childhood cancers, results in metastatic common solid tumors have been disappointing, with little more than palliative benefit. The advent of molecularly targeted drugs promises to change this, at least for certain patients.

TABLE 1   Cancer's Timeline

3000 BC	Breast cancer described in Edwin Smith Papyrus
400 BC	Hippocrates describes six cancer types
1880	Radical mastectomy
1896	Oophorectomy for breast cancer
1898	Discovery of radium
1899	Discovery of X-rays
1942	Bombing of Bari Harbour leads to discovery of alkylating agents
1946	First publication on nitrogen mustard in lymphoma
1958	Successful use of combination chemotherapy
1999	First molecularly targeted therapy licensed
2008	IMRT/IGRT for radiotherapy become routine
2014	Personalized medicine becomes a reality

Epidemiology

The global incidence of cancer is soaring due to the rapid increase in the number of elderly people in most countries. By the year 2030, there will be 25 million new cancer patients each year, and 70% of them will live in countries that collectively will have less than 5% of the world's resources for cancer control. We have seen an explosion in our understanding of the disease at a molecular level and are now poised to see some very significant advances in prevention, screening, and treatment.

Dramatic technological change is likely in surgery, radiotherapy, and chemotherapy, leading to increased cure rates, but this comes at a price. The Human Genome Project and the development of sophisticated bioinformatic networks will almost certainly bring sophisticated genetic risk assessment methods requiring careful integration into existing screening programs. Preventive strategies could considerably reduce the global disease burden at low cost, and palliative care to relieve pain and suffering should be a basic right of all cancer patients. The next 25 years will be a time of unprecedented change in the way in which we will control cancer. However, the optimal organization of prevention and detection programs as well as of treatment services is a universal problem in all economic environments.

The world is in a health transition. Infection, a major cause of suffering and death, is giving way to new epidemics of non-communicable disorders such as cardiovascular disease, diabetes, and cancer. Different countries are in different stages of this transition depending on their age structure and economy. Some countries are faced with a double burden, with increasing infection problems compounded by surging cancer rates. This is fueled in part by the globalization of unhealthy lifestyles driven by profit-seeking commercial organizations.

Prevention

Tobacco

Optimal use of current knowledge could reduce the overall cancer incidence by at least 3 million cases. Tobacco control is the most urgent need. We need to look for long-term solutions here. The politics of tobacco is a complex conspiratorial web of industrialists, farmers, manufacturers, politicians, and the pensions business, all looking after their own interests. Reduce cigarette consumption in many countries and the economy simply collapses. Governments are naturally cautious. In democracies, they are subject to intense lobbying. In less democratic societies, corruption, using the massive profits generated by the industry,

usually achieves the desired endpoint. Advertising blatantly exploits the young of the developing world, associating images of sex, success, and wealth with cigarettes as a lifestyle marker. The solutions are complex and require considerable political will. But with forceful and concerted international action against cigarette promotion, we could reduce lung cancer incidence by 20% by the year 2030. The use of vaping systems is not without hazard but almost certainly will reduce the cancer risk considerably.

Diet

Dietary modification could result in a further 30% reduction across the board. The problem is refining the educational message and getting it right in different communities. Changing our current high-fat, low-fiber diet with a low fruit and vegetable intake is a common theme for cancer prevention. But many features of the modern Western diet are now being adapted globally as branded fast-food makers seek out new markets. Again, political will is necessary to reduce the costs to the public of healthy foods. We need to obtain more data so that we can make firmer recommendations. The European Prospective Investigation into Cancer and Nutrition study currently in progress is a good example of how painstaking data and serum collection from 400,000 Europeans could, over the years, provide a vast resource for investigating prospectively the complex inter-relationships between diet and cancer. Cancer incidence varies enormously across Europe, providing an excellent natural laboratory for such studies. Interventional epidemiology using rigorously controlled studies could produce the evidence that could lead to major changes. The current problem is the difficulty in making dietary advice specific and, in some countries, affordable. Although several groups have produced guidelines, there are so far few data about their uptake or significance in large populations. Table 2 provides a summary of the main consensus from several sources.

Infection

Infection causes around 15% of cancer worldwide and is potentially preventable. This proportion is greater in the developing world, where an estimated 22% of cancer has an infectious cause. Hepatitis B immunization in children has significantly reduced the incidence of infection in China, Korea, and West Africa. Shortly, we will see if it has reduced the incidence of hepatoma, which begins in endemic regions by the third decade of life. The unconfirmed trends are already encouraging. Cancer of the cervix, the most common women's cancer in parts of India and South America, is clearly associated with certain subtypes of human papilloma virus. Vaccines are now available and entering routine use in both girls and boys. *Helicobacter pylori* is associated with stomach cancer. Here, without any intervention, there has been a remarkable downward trend in incidence worldwide. Dissecting out the complex factors involved, including food storage, contamination, preparation, and content, is a considerable challenge. Other cancer-causing infections include schistosomiasis, the

TABLE 2   Common Dietary Guidelines for Cancer Prevention

Avoid animal fat
Increase fiber intake
Reduce red meat consumption
Increase fruit and vegetable intake
Avoid obesity and stay fit
Avoid excess alcohol

liver fluke, the human T-cell leukemia virus, and the ubiquitous hepatitis B virus. Although geographically localized, their prevention by lifestyle changes and vaccination programs is a realistic short-term goal. Clearly, the effectiveness of any infection control or immunization program at reducing the cancer burden will depend on many factors and require careful research and field evaluation.

Targeting

The key to success in cancer prevention is careful targeting. Targeted prevention programs are very cost-effective and can be shared by different countries with similar cancer patterns, and therefore countries with limited resources need not keep reinventing the wheel. Prevention packages can be tailored and adapted widely. To do this, we need good data of incidence in relation to geography. Descriptive epidemiology provides a fertile hunting ground for patterns of carcinogenesis. Relating genetic changes in cancer to their cause and geography—the emerging discipline of molecular epidemiology—will complete the circle and point the way to specific interventions. The future of prevention will almost certainly be about using such techniques carefully to target preventive strategies to those who would benefit most. In the post-genomic era, it is likely that cancer prevention programs, at least in developed countries, will be completely individualized: a combination of environmental and lifestyle data will be used to construct very specific personalized messages.

Screening

Cancer screening is one of the great controversies of modern medicine. At the interface between public health and specialist care, economics creates tension between professional groups, politicians, and the public: a screening test may be cheap, but applying it to a population (with rigorous quality control and effective processing of patients with abnormal results) creates a huge workload and, therefore, cost. Screening can also have psychological effects on individuals with false-positive results who require investigation but are eventually found not to have cancer.

Unless screening can be shown to reduce the mortality from a specific cancer, the money used is better spent on improving care, and this has led to a disparity in screening recommendations among countries. Large-scale tumor banking and subsequent bioinformatic analysis are likely to provide new approaches to cancer risk assessment and will bring challenges to this complex area. Cancer screening is defined as the systematic application of a test to individuals who have not sought medical attention. It may be opportunistic (offered to patients consulting their doctors for other reasons) or population-based (covering a predefined age range, with elaborate call and recall systems). The risk of dying from cancer increases with its degree of spread or stage; thus, the aim of screening is to detect cancer in its early, asymptomatic phase. The problem is that many screening tests are relatively crude, and cancers may have metastasized before they are detected.

Sensitivity varies between tests. A 100% sensitive test detects all cancers in the screened population. The most rigorous means of calculating sensitivity is to determine the proportion of expected cancers not presenting as interval cases between screens. Good cancer registration is essential when making this calculation. *Specificity* is the proportion of negative results produced by a test in individuals without neoplasia. A 100% specific test gives no false-positive results. Investigation of patients without cancer is a major factor in the cost of screening.

Advantages and disadvantages of screening

The advantages and disadvantages of screening must be considered carefully; they vary between cancers and tests. The three main problems in assessing the benefit of any screening test for cancer are lead-time bias, length bias, and selection bias, all of which impair the effectiveness of screening as a method of reducing cancer mortality. *Lead-time bias* advances the diagnosis but does not prolong survival, as occurs when the disease has already metastasized even though the primary tumor is still small. These patients die at the same time as they would have done if the disease had not been detected early.

Length bias results in the diagnosis of less aggressive tumors. Rapidly growing cancers with a poorer prognosis present in the screening interval, reducing the value of the screening process. *Selection bias* occurs even in the best organized health care systems. Worried but healthy individuals (who would present with cancer symptoms early) comply with screening, whereas less well-educated and socially disadvantaged individuals do not. In the United Kingdom, National Health Service (NHS) breast cancer screening program compliance rates vary between communities depending on their relative deprivation.

Developing a screening program

Rational decision-making about cancer screening requires a detailed analysis of factors that may vary between populations. The cancer should be common, and its natural history should be properly understood. This allows a realistic prediction of the probable value of the proposed test. The test should be effective (high sensitivity and specificity) and acceptable to the population. Cervical smears, for example, are difficult to perform in many Islamic countries, where women prefer not to undergo vaginal examination, and the take-up rate for colonoscopy is low in asymptomatic individuals because it is uncomfortable and sometimes unpleasant. The health care system must be able to cope with patients who produce positive results and require investigation. This may be a particular problem at the start of a population-based study. Ultimately, screening must improve the survival rate in a randomized controlled setting. The natural history of many cancers (including incidence and mortality) may change over time for reasons that are poorly understood. In Europe, the incidence of stomach cancer has decreased dramatically over the last few decades, whereas breast cancer deaths reached a peak in the United Kingdom in 1989 and have decreased slightly each year since then.

Lobby groups often exercise political pressure to implement screening programs (even when their effectiveness is undemonstrated), and manufacturers of equipment or suppliers of reagents may exercise commercial pressure. In fee-for-service-based provider systems, there is a financial inducement for doctors to investigate because doing nothing earns no money. The launch of the NHS breast screening service by the UK government in 1989 was viewed by many as a pre-election vote-winning exercise rather than a rational public health intervention, and there are now similar pressures to introduce prostate cancer screening, though uncertainty remains about the management of men with slightly elevated prostate-specific antigen (PSA).

Many groups (e.g. governmental organizations, medical charities, health maintenance organizations, professional bodies) have produced guidelines on cancer screening. These guidelines vary widely between countries, reflecting bias in the interpretation of evidence and cultural values in the practice of medicine. For example, annual PSA testing and digital rectal examination in men over 50 years of age are recommended by the American Cancer Society, but are not advocated in most other countries. The incidence of a particular cancer in a particular country and the economics of screening must be considered carefully—the cost of the technology required must correspond with the gain. Low-cost, direct-inspection techniques for oral and cervical cancer by non-professional health workers seem attractive in achieving tumor downstaging and hence better survival results, but cervicoscopy programs in India and China have shown surprisingly poor overall effectiveness. It is unclear whether intravital staining with acetic acid can enhance specificity at little extra cost.

A major cost in instituting any screening procedure is informing the public and then developing the logistics, often under difficult geographical conditions. Cultural barriers may be insurmountable without better education, particularly of girls, who as mothers will become responsible for family health.

Low-technology tests have low specificity; as a result, hard-pressed secondary care facilities are inundated with patients with non-life-threatening abnormalities. Detailed field assessment, preferably in a randomized setting, is essential before firm recommendations can be made, but political factors often interfere with this process. The well-meaning charitable donation of second-hand mammography units to some African countries has led to haphazard introduction of breast screening in populations in which the incidence of breast cancer is low and where there are few resources to deal with abnormal results.

Assessing the benefits of screening programs

The ultimate measure of success in a screening program is a demonstrable reduction in mortality in the screened population. This needs large numbers of individuals, however, and at least 10 years' assessment for most of the common cancers. Although randomized studies may show conclusive benefit, it must be remembered that the expertise and professional enthusiasm available to a study population may be considerably greater than those achievable under subsequent field conditions. Quality of mammography interpretation and investigation of breast abnormalities are good examples of this, and may explain the relatively disappointing results of breast screening in practice. Case-control studies using age-matched individuals from the same population and non-randomized comparison between areas providing and not providing screening may provide useful indicators, but are not as conclusive as randomized trials.

Surrogate measures of effectiveness can be used to assess a program with relatively small numbers of patients soon after its implementation, but are insufficient to prove that screening saves lives. When a population is first screened, a higher-than-expected incidence of cancer should be seen because screening is detecting cancer that would not present with symptoms for several years. Subsequent rounds of screening are less productive. Tumor downstaging is a second measure of impact. An increase in early-stage cancer detection and, consequently, reduction in advanced disease are expected over 3–5 years. The third, short-term evaluation is a comparison of the survival of screen-detected patients with that of patients presenting symptomatically. Success in terms of these three indices may not necessarily be translated into a useful screening program. In the 1970s, a study of routine chest radiography and sputum cytology to detect lung cancer showed a 5-year survival of 40% in screen-detected patients compared with an overall figure of 5%, but a reduction in mortality from lung cancer in large populations has not been seen.

Diagnosis

Cancer presents with myriad symptoms depending on the site, size, and growth pattern of the tumor. Although some symptoms alarm patients more than others, there is tremendous variability in the speed at which cancer can be diagnosed. A lump can be biopsied, but many deep-seated tumors present late, long after they have already spread: most patients have actually been harboring the cancer for several years before it becomes apparent.

Trying to speed up the diagnostic process and to get on with definitive treatment makes good sense. But delays plague all health care systems. In the UK, the current obsession is for all patients with cancer-related symptoms to be seen within 2 weeks. This was politically inspired to show something could be achieved quickly. The problem is defining what constitutes a cancer-related symptom—there are just so many. Studies show that having two queues for entry into the hospital system—one urgent and one not—leads to either excess system capacity or serious delays in the slow queue. Forming a unified entry system and shortening it make more sense. A far bigger problem is getting a complex series of investigations performed within a reasonable start time for definitive therapy. Attempts to do this have been hampered by poor information technology systems, which are fragmented, non-communicative, and primitive. In an age when a cell phone can be used to book a complex travel itinerary instantly including hotels and opera tickets, it is a huge indictment that general practitioners (GPs) in many parts of the world cannot fix a hospital appointment for a potential cancer patient without posting a letter.

The two drivers of the improvement of cancer diagnosis are imaging and biomarkers. The last two decades have seen a massive rise in the use of computed tomography (CT) and magnetic resonance imaging (MRI) scans to outline beautifully and in great detail the anatomy of a cancer and its surrounding normal structures. Positron emission tomography (PET), in which a molecule is labeled with a radioactive marker, allows us to examine the living biochemistry of the body. The future of imaging is coupling high-definition structural information with real-time functional change. In this way, the precise effects of drug or other treatment can be monitored in three dimensions. It is also likely that the telecom revolution will produce new devices for examining the interior compartments of the body without causing distress to the patient.

Biomarkers are biochemical changes produced by the presence of a cancer. They may be synthesized directly by the cancer, such as PSA, or represent a complex change in an organ system, such as abnormal liver function tests caused by liver metastases. As we understand more about the molecular abnormalities that lead to cancer through the science of genomics and proteomics, novel biomarkers will be identified. These will give us the ability not only to diagnose cancer at an earlier stage but also to predict the probable natural history of the cancer—whether it will spread rapidly or invade neighboring structures. This information will be essential for planning optimal care. The basic tests are likely to be converted to kits sold in pharmacies. It is possible that cancer screening kits for the four major cancers will be on sale within the next decade. There is great variation in the practice of cancer screening in different countries, and it is likely that the availability of commercial kits will increase consumerism. There will be a rise in cancer screening and prevention clinics in the private sector, almost certainly attached to the "cancer hotels" of the future.

Looking further forward, it is likely that continuous monitoring for potentially dangerous mutations will be possible. Up-market car engines have systems to measure performance against baseline, sending a signal to the driver if a problem arises. Implanted devices to identify genomic change and signal abnormalities to a home computer may allow the detection of cancer well before any metastasis. Just as we now have cheap non-invasive wearable devices to monitor pulse blood pressure and oxygen saturation, it is likely that new methods to monitor for abnormal circulating DNA will provide a new era of early diagnostic tools for cancer. It will be essential to carry out careful outcome research on any such new diagnostic and screening techniques to validate their benefits.

Surgery

Cancer surgery has been a dramatic success. Effective cancer surgery began in the late nineteenth century on the realization that tumors could be removed along with their regional lymph nodes. This enhanced the chances of complete cure, as it had the greatest possibility of avoiding any spread of the cancer. Surgery still remains the single most effective modality for cancer treatment. Increasingly, it has become far more conservative, able to retain organs and structures and, in turn, to maintain good function in many parts of the body. Breast cancer is an excellent example. The radical mastectomy performed up until 30 years ago left women with severe deformity of the chest wall. This was replaced first by the less mutilating simple mastectomy and now by simple excision followed by radiotherapy, the breast remaining fully intact. New technology permits minimally invasive (keyhole) surgery for many cancer types. The science of robotics allows completely automated surgical approaches with enhanced effects and minimal damage to surrounding structures. Ultimately, it is likely that surgery will disappear as an important treatment and become confined simply to biopsy performed under local anesthetic with image guidance to check that the correct sites are biopsied (Table 3). The surgeon of the future will be a combination of a robotic engineer with well-honed information technology (IT) skills and an interventional radiologist.

Radiotherapy

Radiotherapy was first used for cancer treatment over 100 years ago. Originally, crude radium was used as the radiation source, but we now have a variety of sophisticated techniques available. Modern linear accelerators—the workhorses for radiotherapy—allow precise dose delivery to the shape of the tumor. Conformal therapy aims to deliver a high dose just to the tumor volume in three dimensions, killing the cancer cells and avoiding sensitive normal surrounding tissue. Novel computer-based imaging techniques have revolutionized our ability to understand the precise anatomy of cancer in a patient and therefore to deliver far more effective radiotherapy. The future of radiotherapy is about further computerization with multimedia imaging and optimized conformal planning. We have also learned to understand the biological differences between different tumors in patients and

TABLE 3 Future of Surgery

Organ conservation
Minimally invasive surgery
Robotic surgery
Distance surgery
Tailored adjuvant approaches
Biopsy only for many cancers
All fast tracked—next-day service

TABLE 4 Future of Radiotherapy

Multi-media imaging
Robotic set-up
Intensity-modulated radiotherapy (IMRT)
Image-guided radiotherapy (IGRT)
Proton beam therapy
Adaptive RT with MR-LINAC
Biological optimization
Designer fractionation

can begin to plan individualized treatment courses to optimize selective destruction. With remarkable technological changes in imaging and computerization, continued development is essential (Table 4). Radiotherapy, in many parts of the world, is the Cinderella of cancer care.

Radiotherapy works by destroying cancer cells and—as far as possible—leaving normal tissue undamaged. This selectivity is the key to the efficacy of radiotherapy. This is enhanced by fractionating treatments making radiation more damaging to cancer cells as they have limited DNA repair capacity and by the geographical limitation of the deposited energy. The challenge therefore comes in targeting the diseased tissue with the required radiation and leaving as much healthy tissue as possible untouched.

Radiation is delivered to the patient via a linear accelerator (LINAC), which generates beams of ionizing radiation by accelerating electrons in an electrical gradient initially and then using microwave radiation down a linear wave-guide (1 to 2 m long). The electrons, which by then are moving close to the speed of light, hit a tungsten target that converts their energy into heat and high-energy, deeply penetrating X-rays. As they emerge from the LINAC, they can be collimated using specially cut metal-alloy blocks or more recently by a computer-controlled, dynamic collimator consisting of small interweaving tungsten leaves—a multileaf collimator (MLC).

The treating clinicians have to carefully plan the delivery of radiotherapy, breaking treatments down into fractions—which are given to the patient over a number of weeks. The oncologist—working with a dosimetrist who may be a physicist or radiographer—calculates how to deliver a geographically precise deposition of radiation energy to the tumor. Good radiotherapy planning involves the careful assessment of risk to surrounding normal tissues and the subsequent modification of the plan to design the optimal balance of benefit versus collateral damage. The concepts of a planning target volume (PTV), gross tumor volume (GTV), and clinical target volume (CTV) in conjunction with organs at risk (OAR) are used to optimize the risk–benefit ratio of any planned treatment.

The potential sources of error in radiation delivery are listed in Table 5. Image-guided radiotherapy (IGRT) with immediate corrective action before treatment reduces the risk of the

TABLE 5 Errors in Delivering Radiotherapy

Uncertainties in target delineation
Poor treatment planning
Calibration of hardware and software
Errors in delivery of treatment—human and machine
Movement of patient or target—intra- and inter-fraction, poor
  immobilization, patient discomfort, patient anxiety
Physiological shifts—lung, heart, intestine
Tumor shrinkage during fractionated treatment
Movement of the tumor between treatments

last four having a major impact on the precision of treatment. Delivering radiotherapy without continual imaging can be compared to firing a gun blindfolded. Technological advances such as four-dimensional (4D) radiotherapy and new image comparison software are likely to further refine the accuracy of the delivery process.

Image-guided radiotherapy

Traditionally, tattoos or painted ink marks on the skin have been used to position a patient on the LINAC couch for every treatment. X-ray films taken on a treatment simulator at right angles (orthogonal films) were used before treatment to verify the plan. Subsequently, the megavoltage treatment beam has been used to produce planar images, on film or digital detectors, to image the bony anatomy and so verify the position of the treatment fields. This assumes the position and shape of the tumor and critical surrounding normal tissues are fixed with respect to the bony anatomy, which is often not the case, and relies on planar megavoltage images, which are often not very clear.

Both of these problems have been solved by the advent of IGRT in which kilovoltage (kV) imaging equipment, as used in diagnostic radiology, has been attached to the LINAC to produce high-quality 2D planar images (superior to traditional MV images) and 3D cone-beam CT data at the time of treatment. The IGRT process begins on the treatment planning computer where the clinician delineates, on the patient 3D CT dataset, the target volumes and organs at risk (OAR), which the dosimetrist uses in generating an optimal 3D radiation dose distribution and treatment plan. IGRT images are obtained before or during the treatment delivery process on the LINAC. In 2D IGRT, planar images are taken and compared with digitally reconstructed radiographs, while in 3D IGRT, a full cone-beam CT dataset is taken at treatment and compared to the CT dataset used on the treatment planning system. The patient's position is then adjusted based on the congruence of these image datasets such that the images align to within some predetermined localization criteria. In this way, the treatment is delivered precisely and accurately according to the treatment plan approved by the oncologist.

For many years, the only means of verifying the proper orientation of treatment beams during radiotherapy was the use of megavoltage port films obtained periodically during the course of treatment. Such images can indicate that the location of a beam iso-center and field edges agree reasonably well relative to bony landmarks. However, the tumor being treated is often a mobile soft-tissue mass within the body and patient repositioning based on bony landmarks alone is subject to error. One solution to address this problem would be to expand the radiation field sizes adequately to cover the entire range of potential tumor positions within the body. This approach by default incorporates a large volume of normal tissue that might receive unnecessary radiation in the process. Therefore, it would be preferable to limit the radiation field size, if possible.

Radiotherapy equipment and techniques have evolved in recent years so that methods of imaging a tumor or target volume within a patient have been coupled with treatment delivery technology that allows near-simultaneous localization of the tumor and repositioning of the patient. Cone-beam CT, in particular, enables soft tissues to be imaged so that tumor position and shape as well as organs at risk can be visualized before and during treatment. The goal is to direct the radiation beam towards the true location of the tumor volume within the patient, allowing for more tightly focused treatment fields, and avoiding organs at risk as far as possible. In this manner, the images are used to guide the radiotherapy, hence the term image-guided radiation therapy.

Guidelines for the use of IGRT have recently been published by the American Society for Therapeutic Radiology and Oncology (ASTRO) and are in widespread use in the United States. Critical to their implementation are the governance arrangements and the division of responsibilities between the health care professionals involved in adjustment of the beam after each image.

Proton beam therapy

Proton beam therapy (PBT) allows the more precise delivery of radiotherapy and reduces long-term damage to normal tissues surrounding a cancer. But it is expensive, costing two to ten times more than conventional radiotherapy, depending on the system type. Meaningful, large-scale, randomized trials with protons versus photons are unlikely for all clinical indications. Instead, the pre-treatment comparison of proton beam therapy (PBT) versus state-of-the-art intensity-modulated radiotherapy (IMRT) in individual patients using pre-set metrics of plan quality will be used for deciding whether PBT has significant advantages. This assessment can be made objectively by treatment planning software systems. Payers, government, and insurers will use set criteria to assess the value of PBT in an individual using a comparative equation incorporating tumor control, early and late toxicity, and overall lifetime costs of care. Such analyses will determine the level of the therapeutic plateau in the relationship of cost to gain in clinical outcome. The range of published estimates for the utilization of protons in radical radiotherapy ranges from 1% (UK, NHS) to 20% in the US. Recent policy studies in several European countries indicate a 10–15% conversion of photons to protons for optimal care. That would mean nearly 20 proton centers in the UK.

Absolute indications for PBT include children and young adults with spinal cord and base of brain tumors. Cancer types where a significant proportion of patients are likely to benefit include lung, left breast, head and neck, and esophageal through reduced long-term side effects. There are also patients where the anatomy of the tumor and critical normal tissues favors a dose distribution with protons. This could be of any cancer type and at any site where radical radiotherapy—meaning that the radiation is being given with the aim of eradicating the cancer and so curing the patient—is being proposed.

To determine whether protons will be indicated, it will be necessary to construct the proton and photon plans and conduct a comparative analysis of the dose volume histogram carried out manually or by computer scoring. This will require the development of normal tissue complication probability (NTCP) models which are applied to each patient to calculate their individual change in NTCP (ΔNTCP). This represents the difference between proton and photon treatments to different organs at risk. Purchasers of care can set the threshold for proton therapy based on a percentage of ΔNTCP above which protons are preferred for different organs at risk.

It is likely that the European consensus of 10–15% of radical radiotherapy delivered by protons will emerge as the most realistic future scenario and this is now the basis of health department strategic planning in Holland, Germany, France, Italy, and Scandinavia.

Toxicity of radiotherapy

The side effects of radiotherapy are classified into those occurring within weeks to months of treatment and those occurring later—often many years after successful treatment. The late side effects are particularly difficult to manage and can result in considerable reduction in the quality of life for a patient. They may also require costly interventions to attempt to palliate the symptoms caused by fistulae, fibrosis, and obstruction. Optimal radiotherapy planning is a balance between ensuring an adequate tumor dose and the avoidance of as much normal tissue as possible. Different normal tissues have different susceptibility to radiation damage. IGRT systems include software with the capacity to accomplish an automated fusion of the acquired images with the expected image appearance. The software then calculates the vector displacement in 3D space of the actual target location from the expected location. In some cases, rotational distortion is calculated in addition to linear misalignment. The x-, y-, and z-axis displacements and sometimes rotational error are then corrected by moving the couch on which the patient is immobilized.

Although not all cancers require such targeting radiation, IMRT/IGRT is now standard practice internationally. In countries with sophisticated radiotherapy services, such as the United States, a wide range of tumor types—including lung, prostate, breast, head and neck, and gynecological cancers—are now routinely treated with IMRT/IGRT. As outcomes improve, patients are increasingly likely to live for many years after treatment, and so strategies to reduce the potential for long-term collateral damage are essential.

Chemotherapy

The current position of chemotherapy for advanced cancer is shown in Table 1. Essentially, there are three groups of cancers and in the first of these we can achieve a high complete response rate and cure rate. This includes diseases such as Hodgkin disease, childhood leukemia, and testicular cancer. Unfortunately, this group of treatable cancers represents less than 5% of the global cancer burden. At the other end of the spectrum, we have a group with low complete response and cure rates, such as lung, colon, and stomach cancers. So far, chemotherapy has made few inroads into their treatment, although some useful palliation and prolongation of survival, sometimes for months, can be achieved. In the middle, we have a group of diseases with a high complete response but a low cure rate. These cause problems to those involved in rationing cancer care. The use of taxanes in breast and ovarian cancers is a classic example. High-cost drugs can achieve extension of life by several months for many patients, and when deciding on priorities, we have to assess how much we are willing to pay for a month of reasonable quality of life.

We are at the beginning of a revolution in cancer care. The pharmaceutical industry has taken on the new challenge, and is now going through a massive transition from an era of classical chemotherapy drugs (not too dissimilar to nitrogen mustard) that were discovered by screening programs for their potential to destroy cells, to a molecular, targeted approach. Currently, there are 770 molecules in clinical development by 49 pharmaceutical companies. It is likely that fewer than 30 will actually make it to the marketplace, and fewer than 5 will make a really significant impact on cancer care. Increasing consolidation in the industry has resulted in a shrinking of the total number of key players in cancer drug development. However, there has been a dramatic increase in research into molecular therapies. The Human Genome Project has created a dictionary of the genome, and we can now interrogate it through sophisticated bioinformatic systems. Not only do we have the library but we also have the search tools. We can now predict the 3D structural biology of many proteins and create images of drugs in silico using computers to design small molecules that can then be synthesized in the laboratory to check their activity. A platform approach to drug discovery is creating a massive increase in new candidate molecules for cancer therapy.

One of the problems currently is the large number of cellular targets that have been identified and to which new drugs can be developed. These targets include growth factors, cell-surface receptors, signal transduction cog molecules, transcription factors, apoptosis-stimulating proteins, and cell-cycle-control proteins. Deciding which one to target and invest research funds into is difficult. The total cost of bringing an anti-cancer drug to market exceeds £600 million. Well-defined targets are the starting point on the road to our future treatments. It is likely that classical cytotoxic drugs will continue to be used for the next 25 years, although they will have a declining share of the total marketplace. By 2020, it is likely that successful molecular targeted approaches will overtake cytotoxics and transform cancer medicine. These new drugs will be individualized, chosen on the basis of molecular measurements of the patient's tumor and normal cells, and taken orally for long periods.

The classical way in which we develop cancer drugs is split into three phases. In phase I, maximally tolerable doses are determined by gradually escalating the dose in patients with cancer. From this, we can determine a workable dose that patients can tolerate and yet is likely to have a therapeutic effect based on animal studies. We then carry out phase II studies, in which a series of patients with cancers that can be easily measured by X-rays or photographs is given the drug to see what effect it has on their cancer. This allows us to determine the response rate. Phase III is the last and longest phase, in which patients are randomized to receive either the new drug or the best available treatment and their long-term survival is determined.

This traditional approach may not be appropriate for many of our new agents. Toxicity may be minimal and effectiveness may be greatest well below the maximally tolerated dose. Furthermore, tumors may not actually shrink but just become static, so no responses are seen. As the new agents have been discovered by measuring their effect on specific molecular targets in the laboratory, it should be feasible to develop the same assay for use in patients. This gives us a short-term pharmacodynamic endpoint and tells us that we are achieving our molecular goals in a patient. Genomic technology has come to our aid. Gene chips allow us to examine the expression of thousands of genes simultaneously before and after administration of the drug. If a second biopsy can be obtained for the tumor, we can compare gene expression patterns in both tumor and normal cells in the same patient after exposure to a new drug. This enables us to get the drug to work in the most effective way. A particularly intriguing approach for the future is to use gene constructs, which signal tiny light pulses when their molecular switches are affected by a drug.

We would also like to obtain information about how a drug distributes itself within the body, and ideally to get a picture of the changes it causes in a tumor. Functional imaging allows us to do just this. The aim is to understand the living biochemistry of a drug in the body: we label the drug with a radioactive tracer and then image using PET. Such techniques promise to revolutionize our ability to understand drug activity and to select and improve the way in which we choose anti-cancer drugs for further development.

The next decade is likely to be a new golden age for cancer drug discovery, with many novel targeted molecules coming into the clinic. These agents will eventually transform cancer care forever.

Immunotherapy

Immunotherapy, also called biological therapy, is a type of cancer treatment designed to boost the body's natural defenses to fight the cancer. We've known that the immune system can recognize cancer cells as different to those of the rest of the body for many years. But harnessing this recognition to bring about targeted destruction resulting in cancer cell death has been much more challenging. Thousands of mice have been cured of cancer by using simple immunization techniques. But these experiments have been set up to favor the side of the immune system—after all if it were that powerful why would cancer ever arise at all? It should simply be wiped out in its infancy.

There are several ways the science of immunology has been used to target cancer. Until 2019 it was thought that only a limited range of tumor types were susceptible. Melanoma, kidney cancer, and lymphoma were always top of the list. But currently we are seeing a remarkable change in direction with immune approaches being applied apparently successfully in lung, brain, colon, and even breast cancer. The principle is to use materials either made by the body or in the laboratory to improve, target, or restore immune system function by removing its brakes. It is not entirely clear how immunotherapy treats cancer. However, it may work by stopping or slowing the growth of cancer cells, stopping cancer cells from spreading to other parts of the body, or helping the immune system work better to kill cancer cells more effectively. There are several types of immunotherapy, including:

- Non-specific immunotherapies
- Cancer vaccines
- Monoclonal antibodies
- Oncolytic virus therapies

Non-specific immunotherapies

Most non-specific immunotherapies are given after or at the same time as another cancer treatment, such as surgery, radiotherapy, or chemotherapy. However, some non-specific immunotherapies can also be given as the main cancer treatment. The two commonest non-specific immunotherapies are:

Interferon

Interferons help to stimulate the immune system to fight cancer and may slow the growth of cancer cells. An interferon made in a laboratory using recombinant pieces of human DNA is the most common type of interferon used in cancer treatment. Side effects of interferon treatment may include flu-like symptoms, an increased risk of infection, rashes, thinning hair, and tiredness, which can be debilitating.

Interleukin

Interleukins help the immune system produce cells that destroy cancer. An interleukin made in a laboratory, called interleukin-2 (IL-2) is used to treat kidney and skin cancers, including melanoma. Common side effects of IL-2 treatment include weight gain and low blood pressure, which can both be treated with other medication. Some people may also experience flu-like symptoms, which may be severe.

Cancer vaccines

A vaccine is another method used to help the body fight disease. A vaccine exposes the cancer antigen to the immune system and triggers the immune system to recognize and destroy that protein or related materials including the cell on which it is displayed. There are two types of cancer vaccines: prevention vaccines and treatment vaccines.

Prevention vaccines

A prevention vaccine is given to a person with no symptoms of cancer. It is used to keep a person from developing a specific type of cancer or another cancer-related disease. For example, human papillomavirus 9-valent vaccine recombinant *Gardasil* (italics indicate brand name) and human papillomavirus bivalent vaccine, recombinant *Cervarix* vaccines prevent a person from being infected with the human papillomavirus (HPV). HPV is a virus known to cause cervical cancer and some other types of cancer. In many poorer countries all children receive a vaccine that prevents infection with the hepatitis B virus. Long-term, chronic hepatitis B infection is known to be the main cause of liver cancer in later life.

Treatment vaccines

A treatment vaccine helps the body's immune system fight cancer by training it to recognize and destroy cancer cells. It may prevent cancer from coming back, eliminating any remaining cancer cells after other types of treatment, or stop cancer cell growth. A treatment vaccine is designed to be specific, which means it should target the cancerous cells without affecting healthy cells. Currently the only treatment vaccine licensed for cancer is sipuleucel-T *Provenge* designed for treating metastatic prostate cancer. Many additional cancer treatment vaccines are still in development and only available to patients through clinical trials.

Monoclonal antibodies

When the body's immune system detects something harmful, it produces antibodies—proteins that fight infection. Monoclonal antibodies are a specific type of therapy made in a laboratory. They are designed to attach to specific proteins in a cancer cell. These therapies are highly specific, so they do not affect cells that do not have that protein. Monoclonal antibodies are used as cancer treatments in various ways:

- To allow the immune system to destroy the cancer cell

The immune system doesn't always recognize cancer cells as being harmful. This is one of the ways that cancer can grow and spread. Researchers have identified the Programmed Death 1 (PD-1) pathway as being critical to the immune system's ability to control cancer growth. Blocking this pathway with PD-1 and Programmed Death Ligand 1 (PD-L1) antibodies can stop or slow cancer growth. These immunotherapy drugs may be referred to as checkpoint inhibitors because they interrupt an important part of the immune system process. Examples of checkpoint inhibitors include pembrolizumab, *Keytruda*; ipilimumab, *Yervoy*; and nivolumab, *Opdivo*.

- To deliver radiation directly to cancer cells

This treatment, often called *radio-immunotherapy*, uses monoclonal antibodies to deliver radiation directly to cancer cells. By attaching radioactive molecules to monoclonal antibodies in a laboratory, they can deliver low doses of radiation specifically to the tumor while leaving healthy cells alone. Examples of these radioactive molecules include ibritumomab, *Zevalin* and tositumomab, *Bexxar*.

• To carry drugs directly to cancer cell

Some monoclonal antibodies carry other cancer drugs directly to cancer cells. Once the monoclonal antibody attaches to the cancer cell, the treatment it is carrying is delivered inside the cell. This causes the cancer cell to die without damaging other healthy cells. One example is brentuximab, *Adcetris*, a treatment for certain types of Hodgkin and non-Hodgkin lymphoma. Another example is trastuzumab emtansine, *Kadcyla*, which is a treatment for certain types of breast cancer that initially respond to the well-known monoclonal antibody Herceptin.

Clinical trials of monoclonal antibodies are ongoing for several types of cancers. Side effects of monoclonal antibody treatment are usually mild and are often similar to an allergic reaction. Possible side effects include rashes, low blood pressure, and flu-like symptoms, such as fever, chills, headache, weakness, extreme tiredness, loss of appetite, upset stomach, or vomiting.

Future: Getting innovation into practice

Over the last 20 years, a huge amount of fine detail of the basic biological processes that become disturbed in cancer has been amassed. We now know the key elements of growth-factor binding, signal transduction, gene transcription control, cell-cycle checkpoints, apoptosis, and angiogenesis. These have become fertile areas to hunt for rationally based anti-cancer drugs. This approach has already led to a record number of novel compounds currently being in trials. Indeed, targeted drugs such as rituximab *Rituxan*, trastuzumab, imatinib *Gleevec*, sunitinib *Sutent*, sorafenib *Nexavar*, bevacizumab *Avastin*, and cetuximab *Erbitux* are now all in routine clinical use. Over the next decade, there will clearly be a marked shift in the types of agents used in the systemic treatment of cancer.

Because we know the precise targets of these new agents, there will be a revolution in how we prescribe cancer therapy. Instead of defining drugs for use empirically and relatively ineffectively for different types of cancer, we will identify a series of molecular lesions in tumor biopsies. Future patients will receive drugs that target these lesions directly. The Human Genome Project provides a vast repository of comparative information about normal and malignant cells. The new therapies will be more selective, less toxic, and given for prolonged periods, in some cases for the rest of the patient's life. This will lead to a radical overhaul of how we provide cancer care.

Investment in more sophisticated diagnostics is now required (Table 6). Holistic systems such as genomics, proteomics, metabolomics, and methylomics provide fascinating clues as to where needles can be found in the haystack of disturbed growth. By developing simple, reproducible, and cheap assays for specific biomarkers, a battery of companion diagnostics will emerge. It is

likely that for the next decade these will be firmly rooted in tissue pathology, making today's histopathologists essential in moving this exciting field forward. Ultimately, the fusion of tissue analysis with imaging technologies may make virtual biopsies of any part of the body—normal and diseased—a possibility.

Individual cancer risk assessment will lead to tailored prevention messages and a specific screening program to pick up early cancer that will have far-reaching public health consequences. Cancer preventive drugs will be developed that will reduce the risk of further genetic deterioration. The use of gene arrays to monitor serum for fragments of DNA containing defined mutations could ultimately develop into an implanted gene chip. When a significant mutation is detected, the chip would signal the holder's home computer and set in motion a series of investigations based on the most likely type and site of the primary tumor.

There will be an increase in the total prevalence of cancer as a result of improved survival, as well as change in cancer types in those of older age groups, such as prostate cancer which has a longer survival. This will create new challenges in terms of assessing risks of recurrence, designing care pathways, use of IT, and improving access to services. There will be new opportunities for further targeting and development of existing therapies as experience grows with risk factors over the longer term. Careful monitoring of patient experiences could help in improving results. Cancer could soon be a long-term management issue for many patients who would enjoy a high quality of life even with a degree of chronic illness.

The funding of cancer care will become a significant problem. Already we are seeing inequity in access to the taxanes for breast and ovarian cancers and gemcitabine *Gemzar* for lung and pancreatic cancers. These drugs are only palliative, adding just a few months to life. The emerging compounds are likely to be far more successful and their long-term administration considerably more expensive. Increased consumerism in medicine will lead to increasingly informed and assertive patients seeking out novel therapies and bypassing traditional referral pathways through global information networks. It is likely that integrated molecular solutions for cancer will develop, leading to far greater inequity than at present. Cost-effectiveness analyses will be used to scrutinize novel diagnostic technology as well as therapies.

Within the next 10 years, cancer will be considered a chronic disease, joining conditions such as diabetes, heart disease, and asthma—conditions that impact on the way people live but will not inexorably lead to death. The model of prostate cancer—many men dying *with* it rather than *from* it—will be more usual. Progress will be made in preventing cancers. Even greater progress will be made in understanding the myriad causes of cancer. Our concepts will be different to those of today, and the new ways in which cancer will be detected, diagnosed, and treated will be crucial to understanding in the future.

When a cancer does develop, refinements of current technologies and techniques—in imaging, radiotherapy, and surgery—together with the availability of targeted drugs will make it controllable. Cure will still be sought, but will not be the only satisfactory outcome. Patients will be closely monitored after treatment, but the fear that cancer will definitely kill, which is still prevalent in the early years of the twenty-first century, will be replaced by an acceptance that many forms of cancer are a consequence of old age.

Looking into the future is fraught with difficulties. Who could have imagined in the 1980s the impact of mobile phones, the Internet, and low-cost airlines on global communication? Medicine will be overtaken by similarly unexpected step changes in innovation.

TABLE 6   Innovation in Diagnostics

Radiology and pathology will merge into cancer imaging.
Dynamic imaging will create a changing image of biochemical abnormalities.
Cancer changes will be detected prior to disease spread from primary site.
Greater precision in surgery and radiotherapy will be used for pre-cancer.
Molecular signatures will determine treatment choice.
Cost control will be essential for health care payers to avoid inefficient diagnostics.

For this reason, economic analysis of the impact of developments in cancer care is difficult. The greatest benefit will be achieved simply by assuring that the best care possible is on offer to most patients, irrespective of their socioeconomic circumstances and of any scientific developments. But this is unrealistic. Technologies are developing fast, particularly in imaging and the exploitation of the human genome. Well-informed patients, with adequate funds, will ensure that they have rapid access to the newest and the best—wherever it is in the world. More patients will benefit from better diagnosis and newer treatments, with greater emphasis on quality of life. Innovation will bring more inequality to health. The outcome of the same quality of care differs today between socioeconomic groups and will continue to do so.

Clinicians in Europe will continue to be dependent on technologies primarily designed for the major health market in the world—the United States, which currently consumes nearly 65% of the cancer drugs budget but contains less than 5% of the world's population. European legislation covering clinical trials could bring research in the UK to a grinding halt, while ethicists—zealously interpreting privacy legislation—could impose restrictions on the use of tissue. Targeted niche drugs will be less appealing to industry, as the costs of bringing each new generation of drugs to market will not be matched by the returns from current blockbusters. The delivery of innovation will be underpinned by patient expectation. The well-informed will be equal partners in deciding the health care they will receive, much of which will take place close to their homes using mechanisms devised by innovative service providers.

This has huge implications for the training of health professionals and the demarcations between specialties. Emerging technologies will drive the change. Intra-professional boundaries will blur—doctors from traditionally quite distinct specialties may find themselves doing the same job—and clinical responsibilities will be taken up by health professionals who will not be medically qualified. All professionals are likely to find challenges to their territory hard to accept. Table 6 shows the challenges that need to be addressed to deliver most health benefit.

Prevention and screening

At the beginning of the twenty-first century, 10 million people in the world develop cancer each year. The cause of these cancers is known in roughly 75% of cases: 3 million are tobacco-related; 3 million are a result of diet; and 1.5 million are caused by infection. In the UK, 120,000 people die from cancer each year, even though many of these cancers are preventable, a third being related to smoking. But cancer prevention absorbs only 2% of the total funding of cancer care and research. Anti-smoking initiatives are considered to be successful, although it has been 50 years since the association between smoking and cancer was first identified. In the 1960s, 80% of the population smoked; by 2014 the average was under 30%. This masks real health inequality: the percentage of smokers in the higher socioeconomic classes is in low single figures, whereas the percentage among socioeconomically deprived classes is still about 50% in parts of the country. Despite the known risks, if friends and family smoked and there was no social pressure to stop, there was no incentive to do so. Increases in tax were a powerful disincentive to smoke, but the price of a packet of cigarettes is so high that smokers turn to the black market: as many as one in five cigarettes smoked is smuggled into the country. Lung cancer, for example, is a rare disease in higher socioeconomic groups—it is therefore a disease of poverty.

Lessons from anti-smoking initiatives will be instructive for prevention in the future. Although the link between poor diet, obesity and lack of exercise, and cancer has not been confirmed, there is sufficient circumstantial evidence to suggest that strong associations will be found. There will be bans on advertising for crisps, sweets, and soft drinks on television, the introduction of a health tax on these products, and a ban on the sponsorship of any public event by manufacturers of these products. By 2025, obesity among the middle classes will be socially unacceptable, but it will remain common among the economically disadvantaged. Creating meaningful, imaginative incentives for people to adopt healthy lifestyles will be a major challenge.

The future prevention picture will be colored by post-genomic research. In 2020, it is accepted that about 200 genes are associated with the development of a whole range of cancers. The detection of polymorphisms in low-penetrance cancer-related genes—or a combination of changed genes—will identify people at increased risk. Within 10 years, most people will be genetically mapped and the information—gained from a simple blood test—will be easily stored on a smart-card. Legislation will be required to prevent this information being used to determine an individual's future health status for mortgage, insurance, and employment purposes. However, the process of mapping will reveal that every person who has been screened will carry a predisposition to certain diseases—and people will learn to live with risk.

Today, the average age of diagnosis of cancer is 68. Improvements in screening, detection, and diagnosis will reduce this. A predisposition for some cancers that manifests itself in a patient's 70s or 80s will be found in young adult life and detected and corrected successfully in the patient's 30s. Increasing age will remain the strongest risk predictor. Little of what has been described is not happening already in some form, but the computing power of the future will bring accurate calculation of risk, and predictions will take place on an unimaginable scale. Screening programs will be developed on a national basis if they are simple, robust, and cheap. Patients will expect the screening to take place at a venue that is convenient for them—for example in shopping malls—and not be painful or overly time consuming. Health professionals will demand that any program is accurate and does not give misleading results, and governments will demand that its costs will lead to the more effective use of other resources. Novel providers of risk assessment services are likely to emerge.

Detecting cancer

Cancers are fundamentally somatic genetic diseases that result from several causes: physical, viral, radiation, and chemical damage. There are other processes implicated, for example chronic inflammatory change, immunosurveillance, and failure of apoptosis. In the future, cancer will no longer be understood as a single entity; it will be considered to be a cellular process that changes over time. Many diseases labeled as cancer today will be renamed, as their development will not reflect the new paradigm. Patients will accept that cancer is not a single disease and will increasingly understand it as a cellular process. Many more old people will have increased risk or a pre-cancer. This has huge implications for cancer services. Today, most diagnoses of cancer depend on human interpretation of changes in cell structures seen down a microscope. Microscopes will be superseded by a new generation of scanners to detect molecular changes. These scanners will build up a picture of change over time, imaging cellular activity rather than just a single snapshot. We will have the ability to probe molecular events that are markers for early malignant change. This dynamic imaging will lead to more sensitive screening and treatments: imaging agents that accumulate in cells exhibiting tell-tale signs of pre-cancer activity will be used to introduce treatment agents directly.

Imaging and diagnosis will be minimally invasive and enable the selection of the best and most effective targeted treatment. Even better imaging will be able to pick up pre-disease phases and deal with them at a stage long before they are currently detectable. These techniques will also be crucial in successful follow-up. A patient who has a predisposition to a certain cancer process will be monitored regularly and treatment offered when necessary. However, not all cancers will be diagnosed in these earliest of stages—some patients will inevitably fall through the screening net. Nevertheless, there will be opportunities to offer less invasive treatment than at present. Surgery and radiotherapy will continue, but in greatly modified form as a result of developments in imaging. Most significantly, surgery will become part of integrated care. The removal of tumors or even whole organs will remain necessary on occasion. However, the surgeon will be supported by 3D imaging, by radiolabeling techniques to guide incisions, and by robotic instruments. Although many of the new treatments made possible by improved imaging will be biologically driven, there will still be a role for radiotherapy—the most potent DNA-damaging agent—to treat cancer with great geographical accuracy. The targeting of radiotherapy will be greatly enhanced, enabling treatment to be more precise.

In addition to the reconfiguration and merging of the skills of clinicians, the delivery of care will also change. Minimally invasive treatments will reduce the need for long stays in hospital. As more patients are diagnosed with cancer, the provision of care close to where patients live will be both desirable and possible and, as this book will show later, expected. The prospect of highly sophisticated scanning equipment and mobile surgical units being transported to where they are required is not unrealistic. Technicians, surgical assistants, and nurses would provide the hands-on care, while technical support would be provided by the new breed of clinician—a disease-specific imaging specialist working from a remote site. Cost control will be an essential component of the diagnostic phase. Health care payers will create sophisticated systems to evaluate the economic benefits of innovative imaging and tissue analysis technology.

New treatment approaches

Future cancer care will be driven by the least invasive therapy consistent with long-term survival. Eradication, although still desirable, will no longer be the primary aim of treatment. Cancers will be identified earlier and the disease process regulated in a way similar to that for chronic diseases such as diabetes. Surgery and radiotherapy will still have a role, but the extent of their role will depend on the type of cancer a patient has and the stage at which the disease is identified, as well as on how well the drugs being developed today perform in the future.

Cancer treatment will be shaped by a new generation of drugs. What this new generation will look like will critically depend on the relative success of agents currently in development. Over the next 3–5 years, we will understand more fully what benefits compounds such as kinase inhibitors are likely to provide. It is estimated that there are about 700 drugs currently being tested in clinical trials. Of these, around 500 inhibit specific molecular targets. But this number is set to rise dramatically: 2000 compounds will be available to enter clinical trials by 2020 and 5000 by 2022. Many of these drug candidates will be directed at the same molecular targets, and industry is racing to screen those most likely to make it through to the development process.

Tremendous commercial pressures are coming from the loss of patent protection of the majority of high-cost chemotherapy drugs by 2020. Unless new premium-priced innovative drugs are available, cancer drug provision will come from global generic manufacturers currently gearing up for this change.

So what will these drug candidates look like? Small molecules are the main focus of current research, most of which are designed to target specific gene products that control the biological processes associated with cancer such as signal transduction, angiogenesis, cell-cycle control, apoptosis, inflammation, invasion, and differentiation. Treatment strategies involving monoclonal antibodies, cancer vaccines, and gene therapy are also being explored. Although we do not know exactly what these targeted agents will look like, there is growing confidence that they will work. More uncertain is their potential overall efficacy at prolonging survival. Many could just be expensive palliatives. In the future, advances will be driven by a better biological understanding of the disease process.

Already we are seeing the emergence of drugs targeted at a molecular level: trastuzumab, directed at the HER2 protein; imatinib, which targets the Bcr-Abl tyrosine kinase; gefitinib *Iressa* and erlotinib *Tarceva* directed at epidermal growth factor receptor (EGFR) tyrosine kinase; and crizotinib *Xalkori* at the ALK mutation. These therapies will be used across a range of cancers. What will be important in the future is whether a person's cancer has particular biological or genetic characteristics. Traditional categories will continue to be broken down, and genetic profiling will enable treatment to be targeted at the right patients. Patients will understand that treatment options are dependent on their genetic profile, and the risks and benefits of treatment will be much more predictable than today.

Therapies will emerge through our knowledge of the human genome and the use of sophisticated bio-informatics. Targeted imaging agents will be used to deliver therapy at screening or diagnosis. Monitoring cancer patients will also change as technology allows the disease process to be tracked much more closely. Treatment strategies will reflect this, and drug resistance will become much more predictable. Biomarkers will allow those treating people with cancer to assess whether a drug is working on its target. If it is not, an alternative treatment strategy will be sought. Tumor regression will become less important as clinicians look for molecular patterns of disease and its treatment response.

There will be more of a focus on therapies designed to prevent cancer. A tangible risk indicator and risk-reducing therapy along the lines of cholesterol and statins would allow people to monitor their risk and seek intervention. Delivering treatment early in the disease process will also be possible because subtle changes in cellular activity will be detectable. This will lead to less aggressive treatment. The role of industry in the development of new therapies will continue to change. Smaller, more specialized companies linked to universities will increasingly deliver drug candidates and innovative diagnostics to the large commercially driven multinational pharmaceutical companies who will market them globally.

People will be used to living with risk and will have much more knowledge about their propensity for disease. Programs will enable them to determine their own predisposition to cancer. This in turn will encourage health-changing behavior and will lead people to seek out information about the treatment options available to them. Patients will also be more involved in decision-making as medicine becomes more personalized. Indeed, doctors may find themselves directed by well-informed patients. This, and an environment in which patients are able to demonstrate choice, will help drive innovation towards those who will benefit. However, inequity based on education, wealth, and access will continue.

Barriers to innovation

Innovation in cancer treatment is inevitable. However, there are certain prerequisites for the introduction of new therapies. First, innovation has to be translated into usable therapies. These therapies must be deliverable, to the right biological target, and to the right patient in a way that is acceptable to the patient, health care professional, and society. Innovation must also be marketed successfully so that professionals, patients, and those picking up the cost understand the potential benefits. Those making the investment in research will inevitably create a market for innovation even if the benefits achieved are minimal. The explosion of new therapies in cancer care is going to continue, and pricing of these drugs will remain high. The cost of cancer drugs in 2014 was estimated to be $84 billion globally, of which $70 billion was spent in the United States. If effective drugs emerge from the research and development pipeline, the cancer drug market could reach $300 billion globally by 2025, with this cost spreading more widely around the world.

But parallel to this explosion in therapies and increase in costs, a number of confounding factors will make markets smaller. The technology will be available to reveal which patients will not respond to therapy, so making blockbuster drugs history. Doctors will know the precise stage of the disease process at which treatment is necessary, and as cancer transforms into a chronic disease, people will have more co-morbidities, which will bring associated drug–drug interactions and an increase in care requirements.

Patient's experience

Two separate developments will determine the patient's experience of cancer care in future. Increasing expectations of patients as consumers will lead health services to become much more responsive to the individual, in the way that other service industries have already become. Targeted approaches to diagnosis and treatment will also individualize care. People will have higher personal expectations, be less deferential to professionals, and be more willing to seek alternative care providers if dissatisfied. As a result, patients will be more involved in their care; they will take more responsibility for decisions rather than accepting a paternalistic "doctor knows best" approach. This will be fueled partly by the Internet and competitive provider systems. By 2025, the overwhelming majority of people in their 70s and 80s will be familiar with using the Internet to access information through the massive computing power that they will carry personally.

With patients having access to so much health information, they will need someone to interpret the huge volumes available and to help them assess the risks and benefits as well as to determine what is relevant to them. These patient brokers will be compassionate but independent advocates who will act as patients' champions, guiding them through the system. They will be helped by intelligent algorithms to ensure patients understand screening and the implications of early diagnosis, and they will spell out what genetic susceptibility means and guide patients through the treatment options. Patients and health professionals will have confidence in computer-aided decision-making because they will have evidence that the programs work.

How the service will be designed around patients' needs and expectations will be determined by the improved treatments available and their individualization. When cancer centers

developed in the mid-twentieth century, the diseases were relatively rare, and survival was low. Although distressing for patients when they were referred to a center, their existence concentrated expertise. Cancers will be commonly accepted chronic conditions and therefore even when inpatient care is required, patients will be able to choose from many places in the world where they will receive care at a "cancer hotel." But for many patients even that option will not be necessary: most new drugs will be given orally, so patients will be treated in their communities. However, this approach to cancer and other concomitant chronic conditions will place a huge burden on social services and families. Systems will be put in place to manage the ongoing control of these diseases and conditions—psychologically as well as physically. Pain relief and the control of other symptoms associated with cancer treatment will be much improved.

Today, 70% of the cancer budget in the United States is spent on care associated with the last 6 months of people's lives. Although many recognize that such treatment has more to do with the management of fear than with the management of cancer, medical professionals have relatively few treatment options available and there has been limited awareness of which patients would benefit. There is also an institutional reluctance to destroy patients' hopes, which led to confusion between the limits of conventional medicines, and a reluctance to face the inevitable—by patients and their families and doctors. There is a widespread perception that if patients are continuing to be offered anti-cancer treatment, there is a possibility that their health might be restored.

With better treatments, consumers of services will be able to focus on quality of life, and much of the fear now associated with cancer will be mitigated. Demand for treatments with few side effects or lower toxicity will be high, even if there are only quite modest survival gains. The transition between active and palliative care is often sudden, but in the future, because patients will be in much greater control of their situation, the change in gear will not be as apparent.

Professional reconfiguration

One of the greatest challenges to providing the best cancer care in future will be having the right people in the right jobs. It will be essential not to continue to train people for jobs that will no longer exist. Policy makers have begun to grasp some of the workforce difficulties that lie ahead, and there are moves to ensure that health care professionals have responsibilities commensurate with their level of education and professional skills. Nurses and pharmacists are being encouraged to take over some responsibilities that have been held firmly by doctors, such as prescribing, while their traditional roles have been handed on to technicians and other support staff.

The appropriate skill mix will become even more critical. Barriers between health care professions will have to be broken down in order for the new approaches to the care of patients with cancer and many other diseases to be delivered. The work of pathologists and radiologists will become one, as their traditional skills are augmented by the new generation of diagnostic and treatment devices. Oncologists will find that many forms of chemotherapy will be delivered with the aid of the new technology, and surgeons will be using robots to enable them to operate. Fewer of the most highly trained specialists will be required, since much of their responsibility will be delegated to specialist technicians and nurses working to protocols. In addition, the most highly trained individuals will be able to work at a number of sites on the same day, since the technology will be mobile and skills will be used remotely. The balance between skills will be driven by a number of factors: the size of the medical workforce and the capacity of the system to provide care, as well as the availability of trained support staff.

The impact of Covid-19 on cancer care

Globally, the pandemic caused by CoV-2 has impacted severely on cancer diagnosis and care. As infection and mortality rates start to decline, cancer services need to be restored and backlogs addressed. Countries have been affected differently and are recovering at distinct rates. Cancer services must be restored to pre-pandemic levels as soon as possible to minimize the potential harm caused by the Covid-19-induced disruption. Additional capacity will be needed to handle the backlog of patients and restore services, and there should be consideration of ensuring greater resilience in cancer services.

There are a broad range of issues to be addressed in all countries:

- *Referrals*
  Patients are choosing not to present to primary care due to a fear of exposure to infection. This will result in a delay to patients entering the system for diagnosis. They need to be assured that their concerns about symptoms should be acted upon and will be managed in a safe environment.
- *Diagnosis*
  Screening programs have either been interrupted or the availability of, and attendance at, screening programs has significantly slowed down.
- *Surgery*
  Cancer surgery needs to continue. Some countries have designated Covid-19 free hubs to increase the throughput of patients, but there are backlogs to address.
- *Treatment*
  About 70% of post-surgical cancer treatments have continued. However, for some vulnerable patients, protection from Covid-19 took priority over starting or continuing cancer treatment. Taken together with patients not yet referred or diagnosed, there is now a significant backlog to address with a surge in demand anticipated.
- *Post-treatment services*
  Some patients will require ongoing support, and the services are already anticipating additional pressure on primary and community care following discharge from treatment.
- *Workforce*
  The workforce has been depleted during the pandemic through staff being ill or self-isolating with symptomatic family members. This is likely to continue and directly affect health systems' ability to recover levels of service. In Britain, the NHS recognizes that staff are exhausted and stressed, which may also impact the pace of service recovery.

Effect of delay on outcome

- A continued delay in the diagnostic pathways for cancer leading to significant upward stage migration of most solid tumors.
- Difficulties in scheduling primary surgical intervention, especially in the chest and abdominal, sites that require complex excision procedures only possible under general anesthesia.
- Delays will inevitably cause upward stage migration in many patients so reducing overall 5-year survival

significantly in many patients. The timing of this upstaging is very variable and depends on both tumor and host factors. Delays in the diagnosis and treatment of cancer is the commonest cause for litigation.

- The upstaging means that effective treatment will require more complex surgery and require more medical intervention—chemotherapy, immunotherapy, and radiotherapy to achieve optimal outcome.
- There will be serious emotional difficulties for cancer patients and their families who will have to be informed of the effects of delay and the possible consequences on their long-term survival.

Protecting patients and the system from Covid-19

Practical measures include:

- *Infection control*: Patient treatment must be undertaken in a controlled safe environment, minimizing unnecessary exposure to patients who have low immunity. Services must be segregated to protect the most vulnerable.
- *Testing*: A "first line of defense" approach to the physical locations, through the introduction of Pre-Entry Assessment prior to entering facilities. These risk-assess the likely presence of any infection, through temperature checks and brief questioning. Where risks are identified, a swift process is implemented to clinically assess the suitability of treatment continuing that day and any necessary additional precautions to enable treatment to continue.
- *Safe staffing*: Ensuring all staff and consultants undergo the daily Pre-Entry Assessments and strictly adhere to isolation requirements. This must be supported by a networked and flexible workforce to ensure treatments can continue without interruption whilst still adhering to safe practices.
- *PPE*: Access to adequate consumables and adherence to strict PPE requirements in line with government directives.

Conclusion

Cancer will become incidental to day-to-day living. Cancers will not necessarily be eradicated, but that will not cause patients the anxiety that it does today. People will have far greater control over their medical destinies. Patients in all socioeconomic groups will be better informed. In addition, surgery and chemotherapy will not be rationed on grounds of age, since all interventions will be less damaging—psychologically as well as physically.

How true this picture will be will depend on whether the technological innovations emerge. Will people, for example, really live in "smart houses" where their televisions play a critical role in monitoring their health and well-being? It is also dependent on health care professionals working alongside each other, valuing the input of carers who, even more than today, will provide voluntary support because of the number of people in older age groups compared with those of working age. The reality for cancer care may be rather different: the ideal may exist for a minority of patients, but the majority may not have access to the full range of services. Some older people having been relatively poor all their lives may suffer from cancer and a huge range of co-morbidities that will limit their quality of life. Looking after them all—rich and poor—will place great strains on younger people: will there be enough of them to provide the care? As with all health issues, the question of access will be determined by cost and political will. In 2005, a cancer patient consumed about £25,000 worth of direct medical care costs, with 70% being spent in the last 6 months of life. Conservatively, with patients living with cancer, rather than dying from it, and with access to new technologies, this could reach £200,000 per patient per year by 2025. In theory, cancer care could absorb an ever-increasing proportion of the health care budget. Would this be a reflection of what patients want? Probably "yes." Surveys reveal that three-quarters of the UK population believe cancer care should be the NHS priority, with no other disease area coming even a close second.

But to achieve that expenditure—and assuming that part of the health service will be funded from taxation—the tax rate might have to rise to 60%. Inevitably, there will be conflicting demands on resources: the choice may be drugs or care costs. How are the costs computed? Although the technology will be expensive, it will be used more judiciously since it will be better targeted. Another argument suggests that when patients are empowered they use less and fewer expensive medicines, in effect lowering the overall costs. An extension of that argument is that although costs will increase for treating each individual patient, the overall costs will decrease because more care will be delivered at home. But because people will live longer, the lifetime costs of cancer care will rise along with co-morbidity costs. Politicians will be faced with a real dilemma: if the prevalence of cancer increases, the cost of delivering innovative care could be massive. Will cancer care need to be rationed in a draconian way?

One dilemma for the future will be the political power of old people. More will be living longer and their chronic problems will not necessarily incapacitate them physically or mentally. This educated gerontocracy will have high expectations that are being sharpened through the first two decades of the twenty-first century and they will not tolerate the standards of care now offered to many old people. They will wield considerable influence. Will a tax-based health system be able to fund their expectations? Politicians will have to consider the alignment between patients' requirements and the wishes of taxpayers and voters. Fewer than 50% of voters now pay tax, and the percentage of tax-paying voters is set to fall as the population ages. Will the younger taxpayers of the future tolerate the expensive wishes of non-taxpayers? The interests of voters may be very different from the interests of taxpayers. It seems likely, therefore, that the days of an exclusively tax-funded health service are numbered. Co-payments and deductibles will be an inevitable part of the new financial vocabulary for cancer.

Whatever system is put in place, there is the prospect of a major socio-economic division in cancer care. A small percentage of the elderly population will have made suitable provision for their retirement, in terms of both health and welfare, but the vast majority will not be properly prepared. Policy-makers need to start planning now, as they are doing for the looming pensions crisis. The most productive way forward is to start involving cancer patient and health advocacy groups in the debate, to ensure that difficult decisions are reached by consensus. Societal change will create new challenges in the provision of care. A decline in hierarchical religious structures, a reduction in family integrity through increasing divorce, greater international mobility, and the increased selfishness of a consumer-driven culture will leave many lonely and with no psychological crutch to lean on at the onset of serious illness. There will be a global shortage of carers—the unskilled, low-paid, but essential component of any health delivery system. The richer parts of the world are now harnessing

TABLE 7   The Challenges of Cancer Care

Increasing the focus on prevention.
Improving screening and diagnosis and the impact of this on treatment.
New targeted treatments—how effective and affordable will they be?
How expectations of patients and their carers will translate into care delivery.
Reconfiguration of health services to deliver optimal care.
The impact of reconfiguration on professional territories.
Will society accept the financial burden of these opportunities?

this from the poorer, but eventually the supply of this precious human capital will evaporate.

New financial structures will emerge with novel consortia from the pharmaceutical, financial, and health care sectors enabling people to buy into the level of care they wish to pay for. Cancer, cardiovascular disease, and dementia will be controlled and will join today's list of chronic diseases such as diabetes, asthma, and hypertension. Hospitals will become attractive health hotels run by competing private sector providers. Global franchises will provide specialty therapies through these structures similar to the internationally branded shops in today's malls. Governments will have long ceased to deliver care. Britain's NHS, one of the last centralized systems to disappear, will convert to UK Health—a regulator and safety net insurer—by the end of the next decade.

The ability of technology to improve cancer care is assured. But this will come at a price: the direct costs of providing it and the costs of looking after the increasingly elderly population it will produce. We will eventually simply run out of things to die from. New ethical and moral dilemmas will arise as we seek the holy grail of compressed morbidity. Living long and dying fast will become the mantra of twenty-first-century medicine. Our cancer future will emerge from the interaction of four factors: the success of new technology, society's willingness to pay, future health care delivery systems, and the financial mechanisms that underpin them (Table 7).

General guidelines and information

www.nice.org.uk/GuidanceMenu/Conditions-and-diseases/Cancer Practice Guidelines NICE.
www.esmo.org/Guidelines-Practice/Clinical-Practice-Guidelines Practice Guidelines Europe.
www.nccn.org
A superb set of clinical care guidelines for all major cancers. Created by 21 leading cancer centers in the United States, it represents the gold standard of cancer care globally.
http://seer.cancer.gov/statfacts/html/all.html
Cancer outcomes in the United States.
www.cancer.gov
The National Cancer Institute's website.
www.cancerresearchuk.org
Very good, easy to read information on staging systems for each cancer and details of outcomes. The most informative site on the technical aspects of cancer care.
www.macmillan.org.uk
The most informative UK site about services on offer to cancer patients in the UK and the softer elements of care.
www.cancer.org
A useful site from the American Cancer Society brimming with information on how to get better cancer care.

CONTRIBUTORS

Ajit T. Abraham
Barts Health NHS Trust
London, UK

Richard Adams
Velindre Cancer Centre
Cardiff, Wales

Mahbubl Ahmed
University College Hospital
London, UK

Claudia von Arx
Imperial College London
London, UK

Mark A. Baxter
Ninewells Hospital and Medical School
Dundee, Scotland

Piers Blombery
Peter MacCallum Cancer Centre
Melbourne, Australia

Mark Bower
National Centre for HIV Malignancy
Chelsea & Westminster Hospital
London, UK

James D. Brierley
Princess Margaret Cancer Centre
Toronto, Canada

Amy Case
Velindre Cancer Centre
Cardiff, Wales

Andrew R. Clamp
The Christie Hospital
Manchester, UK

Rachel Cox
Bristol Royal Hospital for Children
Bristol, UK

Thomas Crosby
Velindre Cancer Centre
Cardiff, Wales

Bernard J. Cummings
Princess Margaret Cancer Centre
Toronto, Canada

Alessia Dalla Pria
National Centre for HIV Malignancy
Chelsea & Westminster Hospital
London, UK

Irene De Francesco
Guy's Hospital
London, UK

Thomas F. DeLaney
Massachussetts General Hospital
Boston, MA

Gwenllian Edwards
Velindre Cancer Centre
Cardiff, Wales

Rosalind A. Eeles
Institute of Cancer Research
London, UK

Dennis A. Eichenauer
University Hospital Cologne
Cologne, Germany

Sarah Ellis
Queen Alexandra Hospital
Portsmouth, UK

Andreas Engert
University Hospital Cologne
Cologne, Germany

Michael Flynn
Royal Marsden Hospital
London, UK

Kieran Foley
Velindre Cancer Centre
Cardiff, Wales

Christina Fotopoulou
Imperial College London
London, UK

Hani Gabra
Imperial College London
London, UK

Elena Gervasi
ASST Papa Giovanni XXIII
Bergamo, Italy

Sadaf Ghaem-Maghami
Imperial College London
London, UK

Paula Ghaneh
University of Liverpool
Liverpool, UK

Ashley B. Grossman
University of Oxford
Oxford, UK

Joanna Hack
Queen Alexandra Hospital
Portsmouth, UK

Clive Harmer
Royal Marsden Hospital
London, UK

David C. Harmon
Massachussetts General Hospital
Boston, MA

Francis J. Hornicek
Massachussetts General Hospital
Boston, MA

Robert Huddart
Institute of Cancer Research
Sutton, UK

J.L. Hungerford
Moorfields Eye Hospital
London, UK

Georgios Imseeh
Royal Marsden Hospital
London, UK

Gordon C. Jayson
The Christie Hospital
Manchester, UK

Philip J. Johnson
University of Liverpool
Liverpool, UK

Jennifer Kahan
Velindre Cancer Centre
Cardiff, Wales

Hemant M. Kocher
Queen Mary University of London
and
Barts Health NHS Trust
London, UK

Márta Korbonits
St Bartholomew's Hospital
London, UK

Pradeep Kumar
Royal Marsden Hospital
London, UK

Amy Kwan
Weston Park Hospital
Sheffield, UK

Howard Kynaston
Cardiff University
Cardiff, Wales

Contributors

James Larkin
Royal Marsden Hospital
London, UK

Kostas Lathouras
Imperial College London
London, UK

David C. Linch
University College Hospital
London, UK

Rachel Lewis
St Bartholomew's Hospital
London, UK

Stephen Lowis
Bristol Royal Hospital for Children
Bristol, UK

Kulbir Mann
University of Liverpool
Liverpool, UK

Malcolm Mason
Cardiff University
Cardiff, Wales

Danish Mazhar
Cambridge University Hospitals
Cambridge, UK

John Moppett
Bristol Royal Hospital for Children
Bristol, UK

Carys Morgan
Velindre Cancer Centre
Cardiff, Wales

Robert D. Morgan
The Christie Hospital
Manchester, UK

Stephen L. Morris
Guy's Hospital
London, UK

Tariq I. Mughal
Tufts University School of Medicine
Boston, MA

Louise Murray
St James's University Hospital
Leeds, UK

Kate Newbold
Royal Marsden Hospital
London, UK

Lorcan O'Toole
Castle Hill Hospital
Hull, UK

Daniel H. Palmer
Clatterbridge Cancer Centre
and
University of Liverpool
Liverpool, UK

Catherine Pembroke
Velindre Cancer Centre
Cardiff, Wales

Russell D. Petty
Ninewells Hospital and Medical School
Dundee, Scotland

Lisa Pickering
Royal Marsden Hospital
London, UK

P.N. Plowman
St Bartholomew's Hospital
London, UK

Rob C. Pollock
Royal National Orthopaedic Hospital
London, UK

Guy Pratt
Queen Elizabeth Hospital
Birmingham, UK

Helen Rees
Bristol Royal Hospital for Children
Bristol, UK

Michael J. Seckl
Charring Cross Hospital
London, UK

Andrea Sheel
University of Liverpool
Liverpool, UK

Susan Short
St James's University Hospital
Leeds, UK

Natasha Shrikrishnapalasuriyar
Morriston Hospital
Swansea, Wales

Karol Sikora
Rutherford Cancer Centres
London, UK

Nicholas D. Stafford
Castle Hill Hospital
Hull, UK

Alexandra Taylor
Royal Marsden Hospital
London, UK

Robert Thomas
Addenbrooke's and Bedford Hospitals
Cambridge, UK

Lisa J. Walker
Oxford University Hospital
Oxford, UK

Harpreet Wasan
Imperial College London
London, UK

Jeremy S. Whelan
University College Hospital
London, UK

Sean Whittaker
Guy's and St Thomas' Hospitals
London, UK

Rachael E. Windsor
University College Hospital
London, UK

Vincent S. Yip
Barts Health NHS Trust
London, UK

Nadia Yousaf
Royal Marsden Hospital
London, UK

1 CENTRAL NERVOUS SYSTEM

Susan Short and Louise Murray

Central nervous system (CNS) tumors include a broad variety of pathologies associated with a wide range of prognoses. Although presenting symptoms due to any space-occupying lesion in the CNS may be similar, the management approach is dependent on detailed histopathological and molecular classification. Some of the commonest malignant CNS tumors are associated with a particularly poor prognosis, and ongoing research to better understand their biology in order to define new treatment approaches is crucial. For many other patients, treatment including surgery, radiotherapy, and systemic agents can lead to significant prolongation of survival. CNS tumors also include categories that do not require immediate intervention. Important advances in neuro-imaging, neurosurgical technique, and radiotherapy and chemotherapy approaches have improved the outlook for many patients, and selection based on molecular pathology is an important component of optimized management.

Pathology

Incidence

The overall incidence (see also Table 1.1) of primary CNS tumors in the United Kingdom is around 15 per 100,000, of which around half are malignant. In 2015, there were 11,400 new cases in the United Kingdom, with equal numbers in men and women.

Brain tumors account for approximately 1.6% of all primary tumors, but they account for nearly 7% of the number of years of life lost from cancer before the age of 70 years. The incidence of some common types of brain tumor appears to be rising, including an increased diagnosis of glioblastoma across all age groups in the last two decades, with 2531 cases diagnosed in the UK in 2015.[1]

Age

CNS tumors affect all age groups. The age-specific incidence is shown in Figure 1.1 and demonstrates a peak in early childhood and a second peak at around 65 years. Overall, CNS is the most common site for solid tumors in childhood, and due to an over-representation of poor-prognosis entities, brain tumors are also the leading cause of cancer deaths in children.

The tumor subtypes and treatment approaches vary significantly across the age range. In children, most tumors are infratentorial or in the midline, and low-grade glial tumors are common, including pilocytic astrocytoma. In adults, the majority are supratentorial, and the commonest diagnoses are brain metastases, primary gliomas, and meningiomas.

Sex

Most brain tumors occur more commonly in males than in females, particularly medulloblastomas, germ cell tumors, astrocytomas, and oligodendrogliomas, and this difference is more marked above the age of 60 years. Some tumors, such as ependymomas and nerve sheath tumors, are equally distributed, and meningiomas are more common in females.

Etiology

The underlying cause of the majority of CNS tumors is unknown. The only environmental factor that is clearly associated with an increased risk of developing a brain tumor is exposure to ionizing radiation, particularly at a young age. Radiation-induced tumors include astrocytomas of all grades, benign and malignant meningiomas, sarcomas, and nerve sheath tumors. A genetic contribution to etiology is also becoming better understood. In addition to a small number of rare syndromes associated with an increased risk of brain tumor (Table 1.2), genome wide association studies (GWAS) have defined at least 10 risk loci for glioblastoma (GBM) and non-GBM tumors.[2] These do not increase the risk enough to merit screening approaches (relative risks 1.2–1.4) and are of variable penetrance; nevertheless, identifying them contributes important information in the understanding of gliomagenesis. The immune environment also contributes to tumor promotion, as evidenced by the fact that systemic immunosuppression due to a variety of causes (e.g., immunosuppression following transplant or human immunodeficiency virus [HIV] infection) predisposes to CNS tumors, including primary CNS lymphoma (PCNSL). Current evidence examining lifestyle or environmental exposure has not suggested a specific contribution to etiology.

Tumor types

Classification of CNS tumors is by reference to the World Health Organization (WHO) classification for CNS tumors and was updated in 2016.[3] An important aspect of this update was a significant shift towards a unified diagnosis that takes account of molecular pathology as well as conventional histopathological features using light microscopy and immunohistochemistry. This has altered the classification of specific tumor types substantially and implies that in these diagnostic categories, management decisions cannot be made without full molecular characterization. It is also becoming apparent that in some circumstances, traditional prognostic features, including grade, are less important than the molecular features, which strongly govern tumor behavior. This is particularly the case in medulloblastoma and in adult diffuse gliomas. An important issue arising from this new approach is that there has been a change in diagnostic categories compared with historical series, meaning that data from older clinical studies may not be directly relevant to outcomes using current classifications.

Molecular biology of brain tumors

The understanding of the genomic, epi-genomic, and proteomic characteristics of CNS tumors has increased significantly in the last few years. The work from the Cancer Genome Atlas, among others, has defined the genomic landscape across adult and pediatric diagnoses and has suggested important approaches to sub-classification dependent on common biology and/or cell of origin. These data have had an important impact on how these tumors are defined and classified, and identifying tumors with different mutational drivers has also led to novel treatment approaches.[4]

TABLE 1.1 Incidence Figures for Brain, CNS and Other Intracranial Tumors, U.K. Data 2015

	Rate per 100,000	Age standardized rate (95% CI)	Cases per annum
Male	17.0	18.7(18.2-19.2)	5,466
Female	18.1	18.4(18.0-18.9)	5,966
Persons	17.6	18.6(18.2-18.90)	11,432

Source: CRUK CancerStats. www.cancerresearchuk.org/cancer-info/cancerstats/. With permission.

An overview of the updated WHO 2016 diagnostic categories incorporating molecular pathology in common adult tumor types is shown in Figure 1.2 (adult diffuse glioma). In the context of clinical studies, it has also become mandatory to select and/ or stratify patients based on this information. This is a rapidly evolving field in line with developments in technologies that permit characterization at whole genome and epigenome level, and it is expected that the understanding of how best to define tumor sub-groups will continue to evolve in the coming years. Importantly, there is now an effort to provide real time updates as new data become available, notably through the c-IMPACT-NOW consortium.[5]

BRAF mutations in pilocytic astrocytomas and other gliomas

BRAFV600 mutations have been identified in a variety of glioma subtypes. The most comprehensive analysis to date of BRAF mutations in glioma sequenced 1320 primary pediatric and adult brain tumors and identified BRAFV600 mutations in 7%, most frequently in pleomorphic xanthoastrocytoma (PXA) (42/64, 66%) (WHO Grade II) and anaplastic PXA (15/23, 65%) (Grade III), with mutations frequently identified in gangliogliomas (14/77,

18%) (Grade I), anaplastic gangliogliomas (3/6, 50%) (Grade III), and pilocytic astrocytomas (9/97, 9%) (Grade I). Other smaller series have shown broadly similar mutation frequencies. A provisional new variant of isocitrate dehydrogenase (IDH)-wildtype glioblastoma, epithelioid glioblastoma, harbors a BRAFV600 mutation in over 50% of cases.[6-8] The development of inhibitors of the V600-mutant BRAF kinase has dramatically improved treatment options for patients with BRAFV600 mutant tumors. A "basket" phase II study of vemurafenib in multiple non-melanoma cancers with BRAF mutations enrolled four patients with PXA with one (25%) radiological response and six patients with unspecified gliomas with one (17%) radiological response.[9] Taken together, these early data suggest that BRAF will be an important druggable target in a subset of glioma patients.

IDH mutation in primary gliomas

IDH1 and 2 are metabolic enzymes that are mutated in >80% of low-grade gliomas, causing a shift in catalytic activity of the enzyme and accumulation of D-2-hydroxyglutarate (2-HG) in place of α-ketoglutarate, the former of which is thought to act as an onco-metabolite. The commonest mutation in *IDH1* is R132H and in *IDH2*, R172G, R172K, and R172M. This alteration is an early oncogenic event, and 2-HG has an important influence on tumor metabolism as well as the epigenome. *IDH1* mutation is tightly associated with alteration in histone marks and shift in the methylome with coordinated extensive CpG island methylation (DNA hypermethylation, Glioma-CIMP). In turn, this causes changes in the transcriptome and is thought to inhibit normal cellular differentiation, promoting tumorigenesis.[10] The presence of IDH mutation is most common in low-grade gliomas and forms the basis of an important dichotomy in current diagnosis associated with improved prognosis (see Figure 1.2). Its presence in glioblastoma denotes transformation from lower-grade disease and is also associated with better outcome. Research

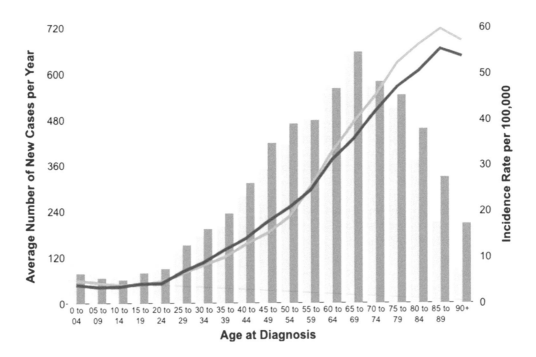

FIGURE 1.1 Age-specific incidence of brain, CNS, and other intracranial tumors. Average number of new cases per year and age-specific incidence rates. U.K. data, 2013–2015. Blue bars = male cases, pink bars = female cases. (From CRUK CancerStats. https://www.cancerresearchuk.org/health-professional/cancer-statistics-for-the-uk#heading-Zero/. With permission.)

TABLE 1.2   Genetic Syndromes Associated with Brain and CNS Tumors

Syndrome	Inheritance pattern	Mutation profile	Prevalence	Tumor type
Li Fraumeni	Autosomal dominant	*TP53*	1/10,000-1/25,000 (UK)	Glioma, Glioblastoma
Neurofibromatosis 1	Autosomal dominant	*NF1*	1/3,000	Neurofibroma Schwannoma Optic glioma Astrocytoma
Neurofibromatosis 2	Autosomal dominant	*NF2*	1/60,000	Acoustic Neuroma Meningioma Neurofibroma Ependymoma
Turcot	Autosomal dominant	*MMR genes APC*	*ND	Glioblastoma Medulloblastoma
Tuberose sclerosis	Autosomal dominant	*TSC1, TSC2*	1/6000	Giant cell astrocytoma
Maffuci syndrome	Somatic mosaicism	*IDH1/IDH2*	< 200 worldwide	Glioma
Lynch syndrome	Autosomal dominant	*MSH2, MLH1, MSH6, PMS2*	1/300	Gioma, Glioblastoma
Melanoma- neural system tumor	NK	*P16/CDKN2A*	< 20 affected families reported	Glioma

*Turcot syndrome now more correctly defined as variant of Lynch syndrome/APC.

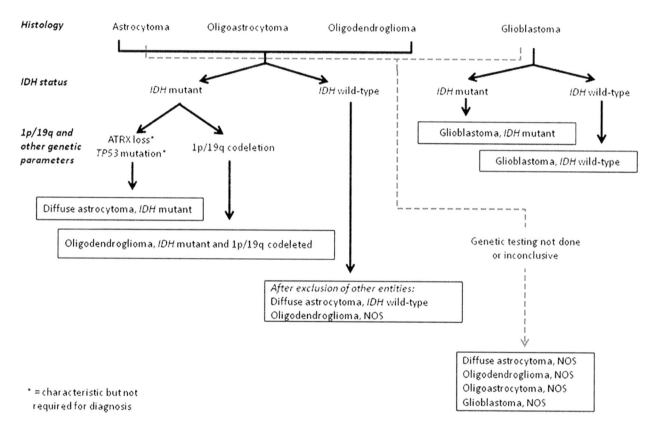

FIGURE 1.2   Molecular classification of diffuse glioma in adults according to WHO 2016. (From Louis et al., 2016. With permission.)

into the influence of IDH mutations on other aspects of tumor biology continue. IDH mutations are also being exploited in new approaches in tumor imaging, for example through radiolabeled probes. Targeting IDH to treat gliomas is currently being actively explored through identifying specific metabolic vulnerabilities in IDH-mutated cells as well as directly targeting the mutation. Specific inhibitors of IDH mutant proteins are now in early phase clinical studies.

The 1p/19q co-deletion in diffuse gliomas

Complete deletion of both the short arm of chromosome 1 (1p) and the long arm of chromosome 19 (19q) (1p/19q co-deletion) is the molecular genetic signature of oligodendrogliomas and

occurs in 10–15% of all gliomas. Based on molecular pathology, as defined in WHO 2016, all diffuse gliomas are divided using integrated histology and molecular pathology into: astrocytoma (non-1p/19q co-deleted) and oligodendroglioma (with co-deletion). Combining additional molecular features, including IDH1 mutation (which is almost universally associated with 1p/19q) loss of heterozygosity [LOH]), O⁶-methylguanine-DNA methyltransferase (MGMT) methylation, and telomerase reverse transcriptase (TERT) promoter mutation, allows a new definition of prognostic groups in these tumors. Notably, the outlook varies from an expected survival of around a year in astrocytomas with poor-risk high-grade features to predicted survivals of more than 10 years in patients with 1p/19q co-deleted tumors.[11]

The 1p/19q co-deletion is also a predictive biomarker and selects for a sub-group of treatment-sensitive tumors, as demonstrated in a series of clinical studies assessing the impact of chemotherapy. The European Organisation for Research and Treatment of Cancer (EORTC) 26951 study included 368 patients allocated to radiotherapy or radiotherapy followed by procarbazine, lomustine, and vincristine (PCV) and demonstrated that median survival for patients with 1p/19q-co-deleted tumors was 9.3 years for those treated with radiotherapy alone but had not yet been reached in those who received radiotherapy plus PCV.[12] In the RTOG 9402 trial, 289 patients received radiotherapy or PCV followed by radiotherapy, and median overall survival doubled from 7.3 to 14.7 years in patients with 1p/19q-co-deleted tumors who received PCV.[13]

MGMT methylation in glioblastoma

The most clinically applicable biomarker to emerge in recent years for GBM relates to the DNA repair enzyme MGMT. This repair enzyme is directly involved in reversing the toxic O^6-methylguanine DNA methylation event, which is the main cytotoxic action of the commonly used CNS penetrant drug temozolomide. Expression of the enzyme is controlled by the methylation status of the gene promoter, and methylation is associated with reduced protein levels in around 40% of glioblastoma cases. As predicted by the drug's mechanism of action, it is patients with MGMT promoter methylation who gain significant benefit from treatment with temozolomide. This was first demonstrated in analysis of tumor material from patients in the landmark EORTC study, which defined the role of temozolomide chemotherapy with radiotherapy in glioblastoma and has since been confirmed in several other studies, suggesting that this is a robust predictive marker.[14] MGMT status is now part of standard histopathology assessment in GBM. Its utility is compromised due to lack of standard analysis methods, and lack of clarity in definition of a threshold level of methylation that is associated with drug sensitivity and better outcomes.

Epidermal growth factor receptor (EGFR) mutation and over-expression in glioblastoma

Another emerging biomarker and potential therapeutic target is a specific mutation in the *EGFR* gene that encodes a constitutively active form of this key growth factor receptor. Known as *EGFRvIII*, this mutation is detected in about 25% of GBMs and appears to be associated with poor prognosis, although the evidence for this

is not entirely consistent. This mutation is invariably associated with over-expression of EGFR, and various strategies targeting the abnormal receptor and/or over-expression of the wild type receptor have shown promise, with randomized phase III studies ongoing.[15]

Wingless-related integration site (Wnt) signaling in medulloblastomas

Extensive transcriptomic analysis and international collaboration through clinical trials and laboratory investigation have resulted in consensus classification and the delineation of four molecular sub-groups of medulloblastoma.[3] The key features are listed in Table 1.3. The Wnt sub-group has the best prognosis, is characterized by defects in the Wnt signaling pathway that can be detected by nuclear staining for β-catenin, and often features monosomy of chromosome 6. The sonic hedgehog (SHH) sub-type occurs across all age groups, has intermediate prognosis, and features abnormal signaling in the SHH pathway. Group 3 tumors have the worst prognosis with high risk of metastases and very high levels of MYC expression, sometimes associated with *MYC* amplification, whereas Group 4 tumors over-express MYCN. Characterization of Groups 3 and 4 is still underway, and further subcategories may yet emerge, for example based on methylome profiling. Important outstanding questions being addressed in current trials are whether new treatment approaches will improve the outcomes in Group 3 and 4 tumors and whether treatment de-intensification is possible in low-risk groups.

Molecular classification of meningiomas

For the majority of patients, challenges remain in defining and managing sub-groups of these patients with higher risk and multiple recurrent disease. The majority of meningiomas incur genetic loss at chromosome 22q12, within which is the locus of the *NF2* gene. Mutations in this gene are observed in nearly all meningiomas associated with the hereditary syndrome neurofibromatosis type 2 (NF2) and also in about half of sporadic meningiomas. Atypical meningiomas exhibit a variety of additional chromosomal aberrations and mutations, but the key mechanisms underlying tumor progression remain under investigation. Recent investigations have suggested that DNA methylation–based classification in meningioma may improve prognostic accuracy compared with standard histopathology.[16]

TABLE 1.3   **Molecular Classification of Medulloblastoma According to WHO 2016**

Genetic profile	Histology	Prognosis
Medulloblastoma. WNT-activated	Classic	Low-nsk tumor, classic morphology found in almost all WNT-activated tumours
	Large cell/anaplastic (very rare)	Tumor of uncertain dinicopathological significance
Medulioblastoma. SHH-activated. TP53-mutant	Classic	Uncommon high-risk tumor
	Large cell/anaplastic	High-risk tumor; prevalent in children aged 7-17 years
	Desmoplastic/nodular (very rare)	Tumour of uncertain dinicopathological significance
Medulloblasloma. SHH-activated. 7P53-wildtype	Classic	Standard-nsk tumor
	Large cell/anaplastic	Tumor of uncertain dinicopathological significance
	Desmoplastic/nodular	Low-nsk tumor in infants; prevalent in infants and adults
	Extensive nodularity	Low-risk tumor of infancy
Medulloblastoma. non-WNT/non-SHH. group 3	Classic	Standard-nsk tumor
	Large cell/anaplastic	High-risk tumor
Medulloblastoma, non-WNT/non-SHH. group 4	Classic	Standard-nsk tumor; dassic morphology found in almost all group 4 tumours
	Large cell/anaplastic (rare)	Tumor of uncertain dinicopathological significance

Source: Louis et al., 2016. With permission.

Histone mutations in diffuse midline gliomas

High-grade gliomas in children have confirmed distinct biology compared with adult cases, with mutations in histone genes being unique drivers of pediatric glioblastoma and diffuse intrinsic pontine glioma (DIPG). A somatic gain-of-function mutation in histone 3 (p.Lys27Met, K27M) occurs in more than 85% of DIPG, in addition to other common mutations in *TP53*, *ATRX*, *ACVR1*, and *PPM1D*. The mutation also occurs in a subset of posterior fossa ependymomas and, in rare incidences, in gangliogliomas and pilocytic astrocytomas. Based on these data, "diffuse midline glioma, H3 K27M-mutant" is a new entity in WHO 2016 classification, which is associated with aggressive behavior. Emerging data from early phase studies in this defined patient population already suggest that novel approaches could transform the outlook for many young patients with this poor-prognosis disease.[17]

Local environment

There is increasing awareness that brain tumors exist within a distinct microenvironment that influences tumorigenesis, tumor biology, and treatment response. GBMs, in particular, exhibit a range of abnormal features, including hypoxia, fluctuating pH, aberrant extracellular matrix, and infiltrating cells of host origin, including immune cells. Perhaps the most striking feature is the heterogeneity that exists within and between tumors of this type. Large regions of most GBMs are markedly hypoxic, which has implications for the delivery of systemic agents and also for response to radiotherapy, because hypoxic cells are intrinsically resistant to radiation. The immune environment of brain tumors has also been re-examined recently. While in non-pathological conditions, the CNS is thought of as an immune privileged site, it is becoming clear that the immune environment of CNS tumors is dynamic and potentially open to manipulation. This field has also been opened up by the remarkable demonstration of the presence of lymphatics in major vessels (dural sinuses) in the CNS, suggesting a non-vascular route for immune cell passage into the brain.[18] The characterization of infiltrating, mainly myeloid, cells in brain tumors, particularly glioblastoma, has also suggested novel treatment approaches focusing on local activation of an anti-tumor immune response.

Imaging

The mainstay of brain tumor diagnosis is MRI, which provides highly sensitive anatomical imaging in the CNS. The use of contrast (gadolinium) enhancement is standard, and tumor characteristics following contrast can provide important diagnostic information.

Standard imaging sequences include T1 pre and post contrast, T2, and fluid-attenuated inversion recovery (FLAIR) imaging. These define active tumor volume reflected in blood–brain barrier breakdown, increased water content, and increased cellularity, respectively. The utility of additional sequences is under active investigation. These include the use of methods that highlight normal and abnormal white matter tract structure (diffusion tensor imaging [DTI]), which may be used to delineate the extent of tumor infiltration and to aid the planning of radiotherapy. Advanced imaging also has an increased role in neuro-surgical planning, particularly the use of functional imaging to map areas of specific activity prior to planned resection.

Typical imaging findings in brain tumors are of space-occupying lesions that infiltrate and/or displace normal brain structures.

In general, benign tumors such as meningioma and neuromas do not infiltrate normal brain, they are present as homogeneously enhancing lesions that have well-defined borders. By contrast, malignant lesions typically show brain invasion, destruction of normal structures, and poorly defined borders. Some subtypes of glioma are particularly prone to widespread microscopic invasion, including low-grade astrocytic tumors in adults and the descriptively named diffuse pontine glioma in children; the extent of these tumors can be challenging to define and is often best delineated using T2 or FLAIR signal abnormalities (Figure 1.3).

Imaging appearances are an essential part of diagnostic work-up but rarely permit a firm diagnosis to be made.

Recent intervention, with either surgery or radiotherapy, can also produce diagnostic problems. Post-operative imaging for residual tumor assessment should ideally be done within 72 hours of the operation, since at later time points, appearances can be misleading due to the presence of altered blood. In the early weeks after radiotherapy, magnetic resonance imaging (MRI) also commonly shows non-specific signal abnormalities that can mimic tumor progression (termed pseudo-progression). Interpretation depends on input from specialist radiologists with reference to standard reporting guidelines, for example the Response Assessment in Neuro-Oncology (RANO) Group Guidelines.[19]

Other imaging modalities may provide complementary information. Positron emission tomography (PET) scanning has been widely assessed in the CNS. The commonly used ^{18}F-glucose tracer has not proven useful in CNS tumors due to significant background activity in normal brain. Alternative tracers that may be more specific to tumor biology, including amino acid tracers, are under investigation, and useful guidelines to implementation in clinical practice are available.[20]

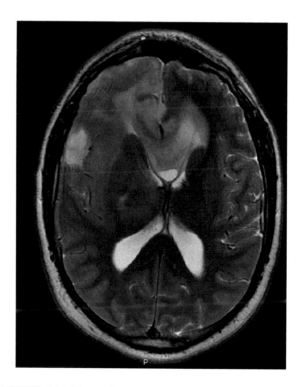

FIGURE 1.3 T2 axial MRI scan showing a typically widely infiltrative low-grade glioma defined by high T2 signal in bilateral frontal regions and corpus callosum.

Treatment of CNS tumors

All patients with known or suspected brain tumors should have access to expertise within a multi-disciplinary team. Initial review of imaging and subsequent histology, including molecular pathology, is mandated in current practice guidelines. Particularly for patients with rare and/or poor prognosis tumors, a joint approach to decision-making with input from specialist neuro-pathology and radiology, is critical in making management decisions as well as accessing appropriate allied health care support.

Surgery

Primary disease

The main aims of surgery in CNS tumors are to establish a tissue diagnosis, palliate symptoms, and improve survival. For many tumors, these goals are best achieved by maximal tumor removal. However, because tumors frequently infiltrate normal brain, an increased resection may be accompanied by an increased risk of morbidity or mortality. This conflict generates the concept of "maximal surgical resection" (MSR). There is no strict definition of MSR; rather, it reflects the balance between extent of tumor removal and procedural risk, as judged by the clinicians involved.

As an example, most convexity meningiomas are cured by gross total resection with minimal accompanying risk. In contrast, most intrinsic tumors are not surgically curable, although there is extensive evidence correlating extent of surgery with duration of survival in high-grade gliomas[21] and low-grade gliomas (LGGs).[22]

The concept of MSR is increasingly accepted in spite of the lack of randomized evidence supporting its benefit in improving survival.[23] In medulloblastoma, residual disease >2 cm^2 in cross section is included in the staging system to indicate higher-risk disease,[24] and multiple attempts at surgery may be recommended to lower the final stage for the patient. For GBM, the association of more complete removal with better outcome has prompted the increased use of resection-enhancing techniques. Even where nearly complete resection is not possible, patients suffering from significant pressure symptoms such as headache and nausea due to tumor volume may benefit from neurosurgical decompression. Likewise, surgery may reduce the frequency and severity of tumor-associated seizure in patients with LGG. At the opposite end of the spectrum, surgery beyond an adequate biopsy has been shown to carry no therapeutic advantage in patients with PCNSL.

Image-guided surgery is an accepted method to facilitate tumor removal. However, powerful new techniques are now available to assist the surgeon in achieving MSR. Intra-operative MRI is available in many units and has been shown to lead to more complete resections. Direct demonstration of improved patient outcome is awaited.[25] 5-Aminolaevulinic acid (5-ALA) is a prodrug of a fluorescent porphyrin that accumulates preferentially in malignant glioma cells after intravenous injection. Using a modified neurosurgical microscope, these cells can be intra-operatively visualized and selectively removed. The rationale that this technique leads to more complete resections and longer progression-free survival compared with standard image-guided surgery was proved in a randomized trial.[26] Improvements in intra-operative technology and neuro-anesthesia have led to the increasing popularity of awake craniotomy and cortical mapping as an aid to tumor surgery. The technique has been shown to decrease iatrogenic neurological deficits and permit earlier discharge as well as improving the extent of resection.[27]

Gliadel is a system comprising a biodegradable polymer wafer impregnated with BCNU (carmustine). The wafers are used to line the cavity after resection, whereupon the polymer slowly disintegrates, delivering the carmustine in a more concentrated and protracted fashion than is possible by systemic delivery. As a single agent, Gliadel has been shown in prospective randomized clinical trials to modestly improve the survival of patients undergoing surgery for newly diagnosed (and recurrent) high-grade glioma.[28] Other surgical strategies explore the delivery of therapeutic agents through catheters implanted at the time of surgery or intra-operative radiotherapy. None has yet confirmed survival advantage.

Recurrent disease

Surgery has no well-defined role in recurrent malignant conditions. For low-grade indolent lesions, a second therapeutic operation can be justified if the first surgery produced a good progression-free interval. In these circumstances, a second review of histology can also be valuable to confirm whether progression to higher-grade disease has taken place. For high-grade tumors, surgery to relieve pressure symptoms can be valuable if the result can be consolidated with additional therapy. There is no evidence of a survival gain with repeated surgical intervention in recurrent glioma.

Radiotherapy

The value of radiation in the treatment of CNS tumors largely depends on their intrinsic radiosensitivity. In rare diagnoses like medulloblastoma or germ cell tumors, it may be curative, and it is an important part of combination treatment in good-prognosis oligodendroglioma, whereas in most conditions, it results in only a modest improvement in survival. Post-operative external beam x-ray therapy remains the dominant treatment technique, although some centers continue to explore less commonly used techniques such as intra-operative radiotherapy, brachytherapy, and particle treatments.

As with any cancer, the underlying radiotherapeutic principle is to maximize dose to the target tissue while optimally sparing the surrounding non-involved (normal) tissue. Precise immobilization during treatment is mandatory and is almost universally achieved using a thermoplastic immobilization system, usually with the patient in a supine position (Figure 1.4). Importantly, the spatial relationship of the brain to bony landmarks is thereby

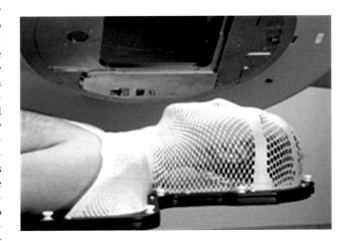

FIGURE 1.4 A patient set up for fractionated radiotherapy for a brain tumor wearing an immobilization mask. The head of the linear accelerator can be seen in the background.

fixed, particularly around the base of the skull. Orthogonal x-rays or cone beam computed tomography (CT) techniques can therefore be used to image the brain and bone during treatment delivery to facilitate inter-fraction re-localization.

Conforming the high-dose radiation region to the selected tumor shape is achieved most commonly using intensity modulation (intensity-modulated radiotherapy [IMRT]) or volumetric modulated arc therapy (VMAT). These techniques improve sparing of sensitive structures (e.g., the chiasm) while maintaining the full dose to adjacent tumor compared with older three-dimensional (3-D) conformal techniques. A challenge in many invasive tumors is that the tumor edge is not well defined. Tumor cells will be found well beyond the edge defined by the T2 abnormality or contrast enhancement limit seen on MRI, which is normally used to delimit the tumor. How the target tumor volume is defined is addressed under the heading for each tumor type later in this chapter.

Delivering dose in a course of small daily fractions spares normal structures from radiation-induced toxicity without adversely affecting tumor control due to their differential repair capacities. It is common, therefore, in delivering a radical treatment, to fractionate as much as possible to improve the therapeutic ratio. Fraction sizes of 1.8–2 Gy are most commonly used.

Whole-brain irradiation

Whole-brain irradiation is a simple technique usually reserved for highly palliative situations such as multiple sites of metastatic disease. Parallel-opposed radiation beams are applied to the immobilized, supine patient. The lower border is defined by Reid's line—a straight line drawn from the tragus to the supra-orbital ridge. The remaining borders enclose the entire brain and its meningeal coverings. Where more accurate definition is needed (e.g., as part of a prophylaxis protocol), the outline can be defined using a planning CT scan and the treatment field more accurately shaped using collimation in the head of the delivery machine (linear accelerator [LinAc]).

Conformal/partial brain irradiation

Radical treatment for CNS tumors is based on CT planning. The post-operative planning CT scan is performed with the patient immobilized in the treatment position. A post-operative MRI scan fused (co-registered) with the CT enhances the ability to delineate tumors. The optimal MRI sequence and contrast requirement will vary according to tumor type. The tumor, at-risk marginal tissues, and organs at risk (OARs) are outlined on the co-registered images, usually on axial slices. Modern planning systems also allow volumes to be defined in multiple planes.

In conventional conformal treatment, planning may be achieved using multiple (typically three) fixed, static beams that are shaped (collimated) to conform to the tumor outline. The beam's central axes are coincident at the isocenter (Figure 1.5a). This usually produces an acceptable tumor dose distribution but may deliver significant doses to large volumes of normal brain in the beam entry and exit paths. Maintaining the OARs within tolerance limits may be difficult and may require compromise of dose to the target. Treatment delivery relies on a LinAc with a multi-leaf collimator (MLC) to define the fields.

External beam IMRT is a more versatile approach to beam shaping, which uses a greater number of static beams (typically between five and nine) with the aperture, and thus the x-ray fluence, modulated across each one. By using inverse planning techniques, the doses to the target and OARs can be predetermined and optimized. The result is a much more highly conformal treatment with a more satisfactory dose distribution outside the target, including any concavities in the tumor volume (Figure 1.5b). VMAT takes the process of conformity one step further by rotating the gantry of the LinAc through one or more arcs with the radiation delivered continuously. During the rotation, the MLC aperture shape and orientation, output rate, and gantry rotation speed can all be varied. These techniques are particularly suited to brain treatments due to the lack of internal organ motion, which makes intra-fraction changes minimal.

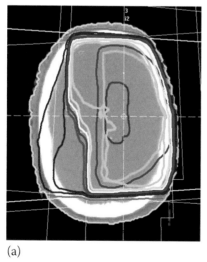   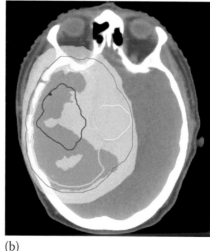

(a)   (b)

FIGURE 1.5 (a) 3D conformal radiotherapy plan for a patient with a high-grade glioma. The tumor volume is shown in red and intended high-dose treatment volume in dark blue. Isodose lines are shown in different colors, green = high dose (95% of prescribed dose) to deep purple = low dose. Note large volume of normal brain on contralateral side receiving high doses. (b) VMAT plan for a patient with a high-grade glioma. The tumor volume is shown in red and intended high-dose treatment volume in green. Brain stem is outlined in light blue as an avoidance structure. Brown color wash denotes high dose volume (95% of prescribed dose) and blue color wash denotes low dose. Note much smaller volumes of contralateral brain receiving high doses.

In addition to reducing the total dose to the uninvolved normal brain and other OARs, the daily dose per fraction to these structures is also reduced. Improvements in survival and reduction in late effects, particularly neuro-cognition, are expected from the implementation of these techniques. The reduction in alopecia, made possible by using VMAT, is also welcome. With appropriate hardware and software implementation, these benefits can be obtained with no increase in treatment planning or delivery times compared with conventionally delivered conformal therapy. These techniques are now the standard approach to partial brain radiotherapy.

Whole-neuraxis radiotherapy (craniospinal irradiation)

This is a highly complex technique used in specific, rare conditions to treat the entire meningeal content when it is at risk from tumor dissemination. The difficulties of the technique arise from the need to cover the whole of the brain (best approached with lateral fields) in continuity with the spinal canal, which requires posteriorly placed fields (see Figure 1.6).

The standard technique uses a 4–6 MV LinAc with the patient immobilized in a prone or supine cast encompassing the head and shoulders. A post-operative CT of brain and spine is used for planning. A co-registered MRI is useful for further defining structures, particularly the lower limit of the thecal sac. The whole of the meningeal surface and content is outlined, with particular care being paid to the cribriform plate, the lower limit of the temporal lobes, and the sacral sac. A pair of lateral fields is used to irradiate the head and upper (cervical) spine with individually shaped fields to define the meningeal surfaces. In children, it is important to ensure that entire vertebral bodies are treated to prevent differential growth. Some units will use compensators or advanced planning techniques to achieve a uniform dose in spite of differences in head width. A collimator rotation on the head fields matches the divergence of the spine field (typically 7°).

The rest of the spine is treated using a direct posterior field. An additional lower spinal field, matched for divergence, may be needed in an adult. Techniques such as field-in-field are used to produce a uniform dose to the cord. The lower border is defined to cover the apex of the sacral sac (normally, at least to the bottom of S2).

The uncertainty of dose to structures at the junction of the spinal fields has classically been addressed by moving the junction at least twice during the treatment program. More recently, IMRT has been used to "feather" the junction over a number of centimeters and eliminate this need. Modern on-treatment imaging has allowed patients to be planned and treated in a supine position with advantages in comfort and reliability of setup. The rarity of the need for craniospinal irradiation (CSI) and the complexity of the techniques suggest that such treatments in future may best be managed in a few highly specialized centers. The use of proton beam radiotherapy also has some advantages in this situation, since exit dose, particularly from spinal fields, is significantly reduced.

Stereotactic radiotherapy (SRT)

Stereotaxy relates to the method of localization in which the target is defined in relation to an external coordinate system. This has the potential for a greater degree of accuracy but implies the need for rigid immobilization. The fixation may be "internal," using pins screwed into the skull and suitable only for one-off treatments, or "external," based on an accurate, re-locatable anterior and posterior, individualized immobilization mask (or beam direction shell), usually in association with a dental mouth-bite. Externally fixated shells can be used for the delivery of single or multiple fractions of SRT. Accuracies of 1–2 mm are standard.

One of the most commonly used systems is the Gamma Knife™ system, in which treatment is delivered using multiple radiation sources collimated to the same circular cross section. Although the resulting isodose volumes are spherical, more complex shapes can be formed using multiple overlapping spheres. Alternatively, multiple fixed beams or arcs can be used from an adapted LinAc or more specialized units (e.g., CyberKnife™).

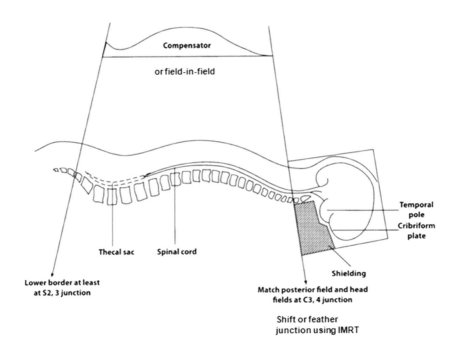

FIGURE 1.6   Radiotherapy field set up for craniospinal radiotherapy in a young patient.

Stereotactic radiosurgery (SRS) refers to the delivery of a single, very high radiation dose. SRS is well-established in the treatment of small metastatic deposits and acoustic neuromas. Multiple fraction treatment is referred to as SRT and may be used to treat tumors in close proximity to OARs (e.g., acoustic neuromas and skull-base tumors). It is also possible to combine the techniques of SRT or SRS with VMAT to deliver extremely accurate, irregularly shaped dose distributions with optimal sparing of surrounding structures. It is important to note that the radiobiologies relating to SRS and SRT are quite different.

Proton therapy

Unlike high-energy photons used in conventional radiotherapy, protons deposit a large proportion of their energy in the final few millimeters of their path—the Bragg peak—leaving no deposition beyond this point and therefore, no exit dose (Figure 1.7). This property can be used to deliver highly localized, three-dimensionally conformed dose distributions close to radiosensitive organs that need to be spared. Protons are therefore used in tumors requiring high doses to be delivered close to vital structures. In the CNS, this mainly applies to tumors close to the spinal cord, optic apparatus, and brain stem. The most common application in the CNS has been to base-of-skull tumors in adults, including chordoma and chondrosarcoma. In younger patients, protons have a specific appeal, since they can reduce exit dose to radiosensitive and developing organs, particularly in the abdomen and chest when treating spinal disease and to developing normal brain when treating brain tumors. There is therefore a relatively strong case for use in many of the common pediatric tumors. Due to the expense of the infrastructure required to deliver high-quality proton beam treatment, this is delivered in specialized centers through national referral pathways in the United Kingdom.

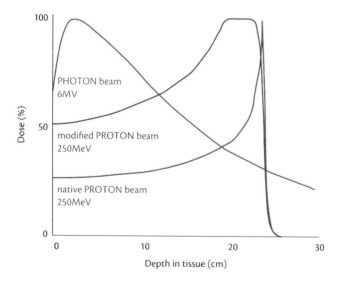

FIGURE 1.7 Energy deposition profile for a high-energy proton beam in tissue. The photon beam (purple) deposits dose a few centimeters below the surface and falls away slowly at depths >10 cm. The native proton beam (red) deposits dose at depth, depending on beam energy, with a very steep dose falloff beyond the peak, known as the Bragg peak. The modified proton beam has a spread-out peak, depositing dose across a broader depth but also falling off steeply beyond a specific tissue penetration.

Re-irradiation

It is clear that over time, there is recovery from radiation effects in normal tissue and that in specific circumstances, additional treatment can be tolerated. Most evidence supporting re-irradiation is in the form of heterogeneous retrospective and single institution studies. In pediatric intracranial ependymoma, re-irradiation is increasingly employed, with encouraging results. In the setting of recurrent GBM, where effective treatment options at relapse are limited, the evidence suggests that conventionally fractionated or hypofractionated external beam re-irradiation results in a median survival in the order of 10 months.[29] Furthermore, one small, non-randomized analysis demonstrated improved outcomes from re-irradiation in comparison to a retrospective series of historical patients treated with nitrosourea-based chemotherapy (median survival [MS] 7 months with chemotherapy and 11 months with re-irradiation).[30] As well as promising survival outcomes, a recent systematic review of more than 3000 re-irradiated GBM patients concluded that re-irradiation also resulted in low incidence of radionecrosis (<10%).[31]

Radiotherapy morbidity in the CNS

As in other sites, radiation injury in the CNS depends on a number of factors that may be patient-related (age, vasculopathy, and intercurrent infection or inflammation) or treatment-related (total dose, dose per fraction, and volume irradiated). In general, the CNS is a late-responding tissue; however, both early and intermediate effects also occur.

Acute effects

Acute effects of radiation begin within days or even hours and are probably an inflammatory response. The acute tolerance of the brain is higher in terms of both total dose (up to 80 Gy in standard 2 Gy fractions) and single doses (6–8 Gy for whole-brain treatments) than is acceptable for late effects. The symptoms are generally those of raised intracranial pressure or a worsening of tumor-induced neurological symptoms. They usually respond well to relatively low doses of steroid therapy.

Early-delayed effects

An intermediate radiation reaction can begin within weeks of completing radiotherapy to the brain. Typically, it results in a feeling of somnolence, lethargy, and sometimes recurrence of presenting symptoms and signs. It lasts between 6 and 10 weeks. It is usually self-limiting, and there is no highly effective intervention, although treatment with steroids is often recommended particularly in the presence of neurological deterioration. The pathogenesis is unknown but is believed to correlate with interruption to myelin synthesis secondary to damage to oligodendroglial cells. A corresponding condition occurs after spinal irradiation and presents with Lhermitte's sign. Neither is believed to indicate an increased risk of developing late effects. Patients with an underlying demyelinating condition such as multiple sclerosis have a relative contraindication for radiotherapy to the brain.

Radiotherapy alone, and more commonly combination chemoradiotherapy, for brain tumors produces, in some patients, the condition known as pseudo-progression. Radiologically, it can be indistinguishable from recurrent or progressive disease on MRI. Clinically, it may be asymptomatic or mimic recurrence. The pathogenesis is unknown, but it probably represents an inflammatory response to tumor cell kill. The condition is self-limiting but may necessitate high-dose corticosteroid treatment. It can make decisions about treatment and prognosis extremely difficult at a critical time in the patient's disease.[32]

Delayed effects

Delayed radiation damage can occur from a few months to many years after radiation exposure and is currently irreversible. Injury is predominantly to the white matter and depends on dose and volume. The clinical manifestations are diverse and may vary from subtle deterioration in higher cognitive function and behavioral changes to gross neurological deficit associated with a space-occupying lesion. The latter may be difficult to differentiate from a recurrent tumor.

Radiation necrosis is the most severe form of damage, often appearing as an expansile mass within the white matter. Radiologically, it can mimic tumor recurrence, since both processes may demonstrate areas of necrosis, contrast enhancement, and associated edema. Functional imaging (e.g., thallium-201 single-photon emission computed tomography [SPECT] or fluorodeoxyglucose [FDG]-PET) might be helpful in differentiating between the two. The risk of radionecrosis is low with doses of radiation below 65 Gy delivered in standard fractionation but rises steeply at higher doses.

The rate of onset and the severity of late radiation damage in the brain depend strongly on fraction size and total dose. However, the dependence on overall treatment time is weak for treatments delivered more than 12 hours apart. A dose of 72 Gy in 36 fractions to partial brain is reported to be associated with an approximate 5% incidence of late radiation necrosis.[33] Currently, the recommended dose for treating high-grade tumors is a relatively conservative 60 Gy in 30 fractions, although both total dose and fraction size are reduced in situations with better prognosis (e.g. 50.4 Gy in 28 fractions or 54 Gy in 30 fractions). To minimize late damage, fraction sizes for radical brain treatments should not exceed 2 Gy, and modern complex delivery techniques such as VMAT should be used to reduce normal brain exposure in radically treated patients.

Other late complications of brain irradiation include hormonal (pituitary) failure and radiation-induced tumors (10% risk at 30 years of principally benign meningiomas). Although it is rare, damage to the optic nerve or chiasm can occur, and the risk increases with doses above 55 Gy to these regions. No late events were reported after doses of 50 Gy or lower in the quantitative analysis of normal tissue effects in the clinic (QUANTEC) study of radiation tolerances.[34]

Late radiation damage to the cord may be sudden or insidious in onset, with sensory or motor abnormalities, bowel and bladder disturbance, and diaphragm dysfunction in higher cord lesions. The most severe form is complete transection of the cord at the affected level. As in the brain, the pathogenesis remains obscure, with both vasculature and oligodendrocytes identified as principal targets and the damage occurring in the white matter.[35] There is no evidence that either the level or the length of the cord irradiated materially affects the incidence of myelitis in patients receiving standard doses of radiotherapy. Most recent evidence suggests that the cord is substantially more resistant to damage than it was previously thought to be, with the estimated risk of myelopathy being <1% and <10% at 54 and 61 Gy, respectively, using standard fractionation.[36] Re-irradiation data in both animals and humans suggest that partial repair of damage is evident from about 6 months post treatment and further repair occurs over the next 2 years.[36]

Some chemotherapeutic drugs, such as methotrexate (MTX) and nitrosoureas, can enhance radiation damage. These are drugs with measurable CNS penetration that can produce toxic damage in their own right. Others, such as doxorubicin, become toxic following disruption of the blood–brain barrier (BBB) after radiation exposure.

Other radiation morbidity resulting from irradiation of the CNS

Radiation side effects from brain treatments can include deafness, cataracts, endocrine dysfunction, skin erythema, and desquamation. Alopecia, which commonly occurs at doses above 30 Gy, can be permanent, and this may be particularly distressing. It should be emphasized that with sophisticated radiotherapy techniques, many of these effects can be avoided or minimized through dose reduction to the relevant organs. Lethargy following brain irradiation is very common, often reaching its peak a few weeks after the completion of treatment. It can be profound, especially in the elderly.

Chemotherapy

For a drug to be effective in brain tumors, it must be able to penetrate the protective BBB to reach the target. Drugs with a high partition coefficient (e.g., nitrosoureas) or that are small (temozolomide) can circumvent this barrier. Although in the vicinity of tumors the barrier is partially defective (as illustrated by the leakage of contrast scanning agents), large hydrophilic molecules remain largely excluded from the tumor and are not useful for therapy. However, some agents thought to be only modestly penetrating can be very effective, for example, platinum compounds in germ cell tumors and medulloblastomas.

Chemotherapy can be given as part of primary treatment in an attempt to influence disease behavior and survival (neoadjuvant, concomitant, or adjuvant) or for recurrent disease, essentially in a palliative setting. The common primary brain tumors are relatively chemo-resistant (astrocytoma) or highly so (meningioma). However, some rarer diseases show marked chemosensitivity. Thus, in medulloblastoma, germ cell cancer, CNS lymphoma, and oligodendrogliomas, systemic treatment contributes effectively to primary treatment and also can be very effective in prolonging and maintaining quality of life (QOL) at recurrence.

Active single agents

The majority of active agents are alkylating agents, principally nitrosoureas, temozolomide, and procarbazine.

The chloroethyl nitrosoureas, for example carmustine (BCNU) and lomustine (CCNU), are highly lipid-soluble, non-ionized drugs that rapidly cross the BBB. Adverse effects include gastrointestinal (GI) toxicity, lung fibrosis, and delayed myelosuppression, which restricts the administration interval to 6 weeks. Permanent myelofibrosis is a feature of these agents, which restricts the total amount of drug that can be given. The Gliadel system is discussed under surgery (see the section "Primary disease").

Procarbazine is a prodrug activated in the liver to an alkylating agent. It has a low single-agent response rate in glioma therapy and is usually used in combination with nitrosourea. It causes nausea, vomiting, and myelosuppression and interacts adversely with alcohol and some smoked and preserved foods.

Temozolomide acts as an alkylating agent by adding methyl groups to sites on DNA bases, most importantly the O^6 position of guanine. It has high oral bioavailability and is converted spontaneously into the active compound at physiological pH on entering the bloodstream. It penetrates readily into brain tumors. The O^6-methylguanine lesion is efficiently repaired by MGMT, a suicide enzyme that removes the methyl adducts. Tumors with methylated *MGMT* gene promoter regions have lower levels of MGMT expression and are therefore less able to repair temozolomide-induced damage. Conversely, tumor cells with unmethylated *MGMT* gene promoter regions that express high levels of MGMT protein are relatively resistant to temozolomide. Temozolomide is active against astrocytic and oligodendroglial tumors and has a predictable and modest toxicity, principally myelosuppression.

Epidophyllotoxins and platinum compounds, including VP-16, cisplatin, and carboplatin, are valuable for treating non-glial brain tumors such as medulloblastoma and germ cell tumors. However, they have only minor activity against gliomas. Topoisomerase inhibitors such as irinotecan have shown activity against glial tumors, including GBM, both as single agents and in combination. All these drugs require intravenous administration and have substantial adverse effect profiles. They are generally reserved for second- or third-line treatments.

Combination chemotherapy

Only a few effective combinations are available. Combination building follows the same rules as those for extra-cranial cancer. A standard treatment has been the combination PCV, comprising procarbazine (100 mg/m^2 po days 1–10), lomustine (100 mg/m^2 po day 1), and vincristine (2 mg iv day 1) repeated 6-weekly. This has been shown to be efficacious as adjuvant treatment in oligodendrogliomas and is also used in relapsed astrocytic tumors. However, evidence that it is superior to single-agent nitrosourea is very sparse, and it is equally acceptable to use single-agent nitrosourea in relapsed GBM. Combinations may be more successful for some less common tumors (see under medulloblastoma, germ cell tumor, and lymphoma).

Combined chemo-radiotherapy

The combination of PCV and radiation has improved outcome in oligodendroglial tumors, as has concomitant/adjuvant treatment with temozolomide and radiation in GBM. Integration of combination chemotherapy with radiation is standard treatment in medulloblastoma and germ cell tumors. All are discussed in later sections under the relevant tumor type.

Novel applications of chemotherapy

Because many agents find access to the brain difficult, alternative strategies have been tried to increase the concentration of drug in the tumor. Arterial catheterization has been used to deliver agents such as the nitrosoureas directly into the tumor. Results have been disappointing and the complication rates high. Global BBB disruption has been achieved with high-dose mannitol prior to infusion of hydrophilic drugs. Again, this approach has proved to be unacceptably toxic.

Convection-enhanced delivery[37] is a surgical technique in which a thin catheter is placed into the brain and connected to an extra-cranial, pump-driven syringe containing a compatible medium. By selecting an appropriate delivery rate, the medium can be made to "flow" into the brain or tumor. The medium can be used to carry a variety of cytotoxic agents, including large molecules or even small viruses, to regions in the brain remote from the catheter tip. Randomized trials have failed to establish a role for this technique in glioma management, and it remains experimental.

Targeted biological therapies

As with other cancers, a number of key proliferation and survival signaling pathways are identified as being important to the growth of brain tumors. For example, abnormal epidermal growth factor (EGF), platelet-derived growth factor (PDGF), hepatocyte growth factor (HGF), insulin-like growth factor (IGF), and vascular endothelial growth factor (VEGF) signaling has been demonstrated in GBMs. Excess activity through over-expression, mutation, or over-stimulation of receptors has been identified to lead to uncontrolled cellular proliferation, survival, and invasion. In spite of intense exploration of these processes, inhibitors of these pathways have yet to find a place in standard management.

Targeting the vasculature

Gliomas are highly vascular tumors that rely on an enhanced blood supply for their rapid growth. Stimulation of the vascular endothelial growth factor receptor (VEGFR) by VEGF underpins this angiogenesis, promoting endothelial cell migration and proliferation and leading to the formation of new vessels. The vessels are abnormal, having large diameters, tortuous routes, decreased pericyte coverage, increased thickness of basement membrane, and altered transport properties. Anti-VEGF agents induce endothelial cell apoptosis and inhibition of new vessel formation while normalizing existing tumor vessels and decreasing permeability.

Bevacizumab is a lead anti-angiogenic compound; it is a humanized monoclonal antibody that binds to and inhibits the activity of VEGF. When given to patients with relapsed GBM, it often produces rapid improvements in imaging appearances by abolishing contrast leakage and enhancing patient well-being by reducing vasogenic edema. On the basis of two small studies, it was given accelerated Food and Drug Administration approval for use in recurrent GBM. However, improved survival has not been demonstrated when it was used either alone or in combination with cytotoxic drugs (commonly irinotecan) in relapsed disease or with standard chemo-radiotherapy in newly diagnosed GBMs.[38,39] It has not found a place in standard of care but is approved for use in relapse settings in some countries.

Bevacizumab is, however, an effective agent in patients with benign tumors (schwannoma or meningioma) associated with NF2 for whom surgery is not an option, when it reduces growth rates and increases neurologic function in up to 50% of patients.

Targeting oncogenic growth factors

EGFR is amplified in nearly half of all patients with GBM. Of these, approximately 30% demonstrate a mutant receptor (EGFRvIII) that has a deletion of exons 2–7. This defect results in constitutive, ligand-independent activation. Attempts to treat GBMs using direct EGFR blockade have not met with any success. However, over-expression and presence of the mutant EGFRvIII is a target for alternative approaches, including immunotherapy and antibody-drug conjugates, that are the subjects of ongoing studies. Other targets under investigation include integrins, protein kinase C, and histone deacetylase. None has shown any benefit to date.[40]

Everolimus is an inhibitor of the mammalian target of rapamycin (m-TOR), a serine-threonine kinase downstream of the PI3K/AKT pathway. This pathway is dysregulated in tuberose sclerosis and in some patients leads to the formation of subependymal giant-cell astrocytomas. It has been shown that treatment with everolimus can produce shrinkage of these tumors, which are otherwise resistant to any form of therapy except surgery. Recent data from a phase II study in newly diagnosed GBM, however, did not suggest an impact on survival in the general glioma population.[41]

Since one of the limiting factors in successful targeting may be redundancy within these complex signaling pathways, an alternative approach of using less specific multiple kinase inhibitors is also being explored. Initial promising data using agents including Regorafenib are the subject of ongoing late-phase studies.

Targeting immune cells

An improved understanding of the immune environment in brain tumors and the observation that 30–40% of cells in gliomas can be accounted for by microglia or macrophages have led to significant interest in manipulation of the immune environment to enhance tumor control. An over-arching principle is the use of therapies that promote an immune stimulatory environment to promote infiltration of cytotoxic T cells into glioma. A variety of approaches are under current investigation, including CAR T-cell therapy, immune checkpoint inhibition using antibodies and small molecules, and immune stimulation using oncolytic viruses that can be delivered to the CNS directly or systemically.

Adjunctive treatments

Corticosteroids produce symptomatic benefit in patients with brain tumors, although the physiological basis for this is not clear. Dexamethasone is most frequently used, typically at doses of 16 mg or lower, which should be titrated down to the minimum needed to control symptoms. This will minimize the impact of severe side effects, which in the elderly are particularly proximal myopathy, diabetes, and osteoporosis and in the young, acne and appetite stimulation. All patients may suffer from weight gain, sleep disturbance, and disorders of mood and perception.

Epilepsy is common in patients with brain tumors. Anticonvulsants should be given in doses determined by the efficacy and toxicity of a drug in a particular patient and not by the measured plasma level. The established agents carbamazepine, phenytoin, and sodium valproate have been largely replaced by a newer generation of drugs including lamotrigine and leveteracetam. The latter have the added advantage that they do not induce hepatic enzymes to the extent of some of the older drugs and thus do not interfere with the metabolism of other therapeutic agents, particularly chemotherapy and the newer small molecule agents.

Although headache is a common presenting symptom, severe pain is fortunately unusual in patients with treated brain tumors, even following recurrence. When pain is a problem, the same analgesic ladder should be used as for other malignant conditions. Dexamethasone is an effective treatment for headache caused by raised intracranial pressure.

Nausea can be a particularly troublesome symptom and may have a variety of causes, such as being a part of posterior fossa syndrome or secondary to raised intracranial pressure. It is also associated with seizure, drug toxicity (particularly anticonvulsants), and peptic pathology. Limited-field brain irradiation uncommonly causes nausea, although this should be a diagnosis of exclusion. Clearly, the cause of the toxicity should be sought and where possible, treated. When the usual anti-emetics fail to control nausea of intracranial origin, subcutaneous delivery of agents such as major tranquillizers or anti-histamines may be useful.

Additional support

Brain tumors are rare, but their effects can be devastating. Cognitive decline and major physical disability often accompany the late stages of malignant tumor progression. Patients may require input from physiotherapists, speech therapists, social workers, palliative care workers, the general practitioner (GP), and the district nurse. The specialist "brain tumor support nurse," who has knowledge of the patient's current condition, needs, and likely prognosis as well as the facilities available in a particular area, can provide invaluable support to all workers involved in care, particularly the GP. Attention needs to be given to the often devastating functional and social consequences of CNS disease, including loss of driving license, reduced employment prospects, loss of status in society and family, behavioral and personality change, and the prospect of limited life expectancy. Clinical depression is more common in these patients than is generally recognized and merits early recognition and treatment.[42] The introduction of counselling and psychiatric, psychological, and social work support at an early stage is important for affected patients.

Individual tumors

Glial tumors can be conceptually divided into those that grow in a relatively circumscribed way, largely represented by pilocytic astrocytoma and ganglioglioma (regarded as Grade 1), and those that infiltrate diffusely into cerebral tissue (Grade 2 and above). However, this distinction does not hold true for all cases.

Grade 1: Pilocytic astrocytoma

These are primarily tumors of children and young adults. They most commonly arise in the posterior fossa but are also found in the cerebral hemispheres, optic nerve and chiasm, thalamus and basal ganglia, brain stem, and spinal cord. There is a strong association with neurofibromatosis type I.

On imaging, they appear as hyper-dense, well-delineated, solid or solid/cystic tumors. They break the rule for low-grade tumors in that they frequently enhance with contrast. They are characterized by slow growth and may, without intervention, stop growing or even regress. Rarely, they progress relentlessly without change in low-grade histology or may seed in the CNS. Very rarely, pilocytic astrocytomas progress to a more malignant phenotype.

The histology is characterized by the presence of bipolar, glial fibrillary acidic protein (GFAP)-positive "pilocytes" and eosinophilic hyaline masses known as Rosenthal fibers. They are often highly vascularized and may show endothelial hyperplasia identical to GBM. They do not demonstrate inactivation of p53. Abnormalities in the mitogen-activated protein kinase (MAPK) pathway have been reported in up to 90% of pilocytic astrocytomas.[6] Unlike higher-grade gliomas, these abnormalities tend to occur in isolation. The most common abnormality is a gene fusion event between *KIAA1549* (a gene with as yet unknown function) and the *BRAF* oncogene, which constitutively activates MAPK signaling and hence promotes cellular proliferation and oncogenesis. This rearrangement is highly specific to pilocytic astrocytomas. The next most common event is an activating mutation in the *BRAF* gene, which, in contrast to the fusion event, is also observed in many different solid tumors. Although pilocytic astrocytomas are often cured by surgery, the aforementioned new understanding of the biology of the disease opens the door to a wide range of potential therapies that target MAPK signaling.

The treatment of pilocytic astrocytoma is surgical and MSR should be performed. Even if this is incomplete, further tumor progression may not occur. There is no evidence that post-operative radiation improves on surgery alone. If re-growth occurs, the treatment is again surgical. Should the second resection be incomplete, adjuvant radiotherapy can be tried (45–50 Gy), but there is no clear documentation that this is beneficial.

Overall, the prognosis for pilocytic astrocytoma is very good, with long-term control or cure rates of 80%–90%. The achievement of a complete resection is an important prognostic factor.[43]

Diffuse gliomas

Diffuse gliomas are most common in the cerebral hemispheres. Irrespective of their histological grade, they infiltrate diffusely into adjacent and distant brain. Tumor grade is based on cytological features, mitotic activity, and features of the microenvironment. The grade allocated is the highest seen in any part of the specimen. Appropriate treatment and prognosis depend not only on grade but also on the molecular pathology of the specimen and clinical factors such as the patient's age, performance status, and mental status. These tumors in adults are sub-classified in the current WHO system, principally depending on IDH status, then further, depending on 1p/19q and ATRX status, into astrocytoma or oligodendroglioma subtypes (see Figure 1.2). In children, diagnosis is also now reliant on molecular pathology to distinguish subtypes, as described later.

Lower grades of diffuse glioma progress to more malignant phenotypes. The rate of progression is very variable. Transformation from astrocytoma to GBM may be complete within 1 year or may not begin for 20 years or more.

Grade 2: (Diffuse) astrocytoma

Low-grade diffuse astrocytomas (LGAs) are well-differentiated, slow-growing tumors that are more frequent in young adults, although they can occur at any age. They most commonly present with seizure. LGAs are best seen on T2-weighted (or FLAIR) MRI sequences, where they appear as infiltrating hyper-intense lesions. They are typically hypo-intense, non-contrast enhancing on T1-weighted MRI sequences and CT.

Histologically, they are recognized to contain abnormal numbers of astrocytes, which show monotonous, minor degrees of anaplasia (nuclear pleomorphism and cytoplasmic changes). Mitoses are uncommon. The background may contain increased numbers of cellular processes and microcysts, which aid diagnosis. GFAP positivity is common. Somatic mutations of isocitrate dehydrogenase *IDH* genes 1 and 2 are common in LGA, particularly the *IDH1 R132* mutation (see the section "Molecular biology of brain tumors"). These tumors also typically harbor ATRX loss and TP53 mutation and by definition, do not have co-deletion of 1p/19q. Recent studies suggest that a sub-group of these tumors without IDH mutation have molecular features in keeping with GBM, including TERT mutations, which predict a poorer outcome.

The management of low-grade astrocytoma without adverse features remains controversial. In many units, if a firm diagnosis is made on scanning, biopsy is delayed until the clinical situation demands it. Other units believe that an upfront biopsy is necessary for adequate management. Some surgeons believe that immediate surgical removal of all imaged tumor is associated with longer survival; however, data supporting this approach are not generalizable to the whole patient population.[44]

LGG patients presenting with controllable seizures as their only symptom and who show non-distorting, non-enhancing lesions on scanning may remain well for many years without active intervention. Adverse prognostic clinical factors for patients with

these tumors have been defined[45] and include tumor size (>6 cm), lesions crossing the midline, presence of neurological symptoms, and age above 40 years. There is no evidence that early radiotherapy intervention in good-prognosis patients improves survival compared with treatment that is delayed until required, in spite of there being an improvement in time to progression. Nor is it clear whether radiotherapy or chemotherapy represents the best choice of initial treatment. The EORTC trial 22033-26033 suggested that primary chemotherapy and radiotherapy were equally effective in terms of subsequent progression-free survival in patients who were deemed to require treatment based on high-risk features.[46]

Patients who require treatment include those with poor prognostic features, those whose tumors show significant progression on serial scanning, and those who develop neurological deficit or possibly loss of seizure control. If most of the tumor mass is accessible, MSR is usually recommended. If minimal tumor remains and the entire resected tumor is low grade with no adverse features, an observation policy can be reinstated. Otherwise, radiotherapy is recommended usually within 4–8 weeks of surgery. Patients are planned using CT/MRI fusion. The tumor is defined as the high signal region on the T2 or FLAIR sequences. This is expanded by 1 to 2 cm to create the clinical target volume (CTV) to encompass microscopic disease beyond the visible tumor edge. The additional margin required to create the planning target volume (to account for uncertainties in set up) is determined by local facilities and techniques. Conformation of the treatment volume to the target is essential, and the condition lends itself well to IMRT or VMAT techniques. A total of 45–50 Gy is delivered in 1.8 Gy fractions, depending on the size of the irradiated volume. Two randomized trials inform us that doses beyond 45–50 Gy do not improve outcomes.[47,48] If resective surgery is not thought to be useful, then radiotherapy as described can be used as primary treatment.

The outcome of this management approach is variable. The majority of patients will relapse, with ultimate tumor transformation, progression, and death. Overall, the median survival is about 5–8 years. However, a sub-group of patients with favorable molecular biology may remain well for up to 20 years from diagnosis. Salvage treatment at relapse can be performed with any of the aforementioned modalities and is individualized.

Grade 3: Anaplastic astrocytoma

Anaplastic astrocytoma (AA) is a diffusely infiltrating, astrocytic tumor typified by increasing cellularity, increasing nuclear size and variation, and the presence of mitoses (growth fraction around 5%–10%). In the WHO classification, tumor necrosis must not be present. Tumors in this category that carry co-deletions on chromosomes 1p and 19q are diagnosed and treated as anaplastic oligodendroglioma (AO). AA is primarily a tumor appearing during middle age. It appears with variable density on CT or signal on MRI. There is usually enhancement with contrast, but this may be diffuse or patchy and is rarely of the classical "ring" type seen in GBM. Unlike LGA, rapid growth in AA is the rule. Treatment must include maximal safe surgery and high-dose radiotherapy as for GBMs, leading to a median survival of 2–5 years. The CATNON Intergroup trial is examining the role of concurrent and/or adjuvant temozolomide in patients with non-1p/19q-deleted anaplastic glioma.[49]

Virtually all patients with AA will recur following treatment and should be actively treated. Chemotherapy with or without prior surgery is the usual approach, although repeat, highly conformed radiotherapy (re-irradiation) is an option in selected cases.

Grade 4: Glioblastoma

GBMs appear to arise *de novo* in older patients with no prior history of glioma and have a particularly poor prognosis. They are characterized by oncogene amplification (particularly *EGFR*), *CDKN2A* deletions, and *PTEN* mutations. Recent work by the Cancer Genome Atlas Research Network has begun to reveal the extent of the genetic and chromosomal abnormalities that contribute to the aggressive and treatment-resistant nature of this tumor and demonstrates remarkable heterogeneity across the tumors studied.[50] Although specific mutations, deletions, and amplifications varied widely, common themes emerged. It was shown that 87% of tumors exhibited abnormalities in the retinoblastoma (Rb) signaling pathway that modulates cell cycle progression, 78% had defects in the p53 pathway (cell cycle and apoptosis), and 88% showed alterations in the EGFR/PI3 kinase network (proliferation and cell survival).

GBM is a poorly differentiated, extensively invasive, highly mitotic, and pathologically heterogeneous astrocytic tumor. It can arise at any age but is most common in the sixth and seventh decades. It occurs preferentially in the cerebral hemispheres, from where it extends into adjacent structures such as basal ganglia and across the corpus callosum to form the classic butterfly tumor. It can arise, rarely, in the cerebellum, brain stem, and spinal cord. It is almost universally fatal.

Macroscopically, the tumors appear as grey masses with areas of hemorrhage, yellow necrosis, and sometimes cysts. Any apparent capsule is always an artefact of rapidly growing tumor and compressed brain. Peri-tumoral edema is common and tends to spread along the white matter tracts to form a conduit for clonogenic, migratory tumor cells, which can be found many centimeters from the main tumor. These cells may form secondary masses, giving the appearance of multifocality.

GBM is highly heterogeneous at the cellular level, with almost any size and shape of cell being seen, including multi-nucleated giant cells, which are a hallmark. A sub-group of GBM arising from lower-grade tumor (Secondary GBM) is more likely to have areas comprising lower-grade astrocytoma. Immunohistochemical staining with GFAP, S-100, and vimentin is also heterogeneous. Recognized GBM variants are giant-cell GBM and gliosarcoma, the natural histories of which are similar to that of classical GBM.

Micro-vascular proliferation and tumor necrosis are histological characteristics of GBM. Angiogenic tyrosine receptors (e.g., VEGFR-1 and 2) are up-regulated in proliferating tumor vessels, and the ligands (e.g., VEGF) are found in the GBM cells themselves, leading to paracrine stimulation of angiogenesis. There are two types of tumor necrosis: large-scale coagulation necrosis, which is usually visible on imaging studies, and microscopic serpiginous foci of necrosis, which form the pseudo-palisading pattern typical of GBMs. The typical imaging appearance of a GBM is a rim-enhancing, irregular tumor with a low-density (necrotic/cystic) center and surrounding low-density edematous brain sited in the deep white matter. The brain is often distorted, with evidence of raised intracranial pressure.

The overall strategy of management will depend on the likely prognosis, and several published guidelines are available.[51] A diagnosis of GBM will be suspected from the imaging in the majority of cases. The very elderly, or patients with severe, steroid-resistant symptoms, may be appropriately managed with symptomatic care alone, as their outlook will be little changed by provision of the precise diagnosis and treatment. All other patients need a minimum of biopsy proof of diagnosis, and in many patients, an attempt at resection is appropriate (see the section "Primary disease"). It is common clinical experience that

patients tolerate subsequent treatment, particularly radiotherapy, better when their tumors have been decompressed. MSR for patients with resectable tumors is now the standard of care, even in older patients.

The use of Gliadel (BCNU-impregnated biodegradable) wafers is supported by the National Institute for Health and Care Excellence (NICE) in newly diagnosed patients whose tumors have had at least 90% resection (2007 guidance, reviewed 2016). Unfortunately, the combination of Gliadel and chemo-radiotherapy has not been adequately evaluated in clinical studies and therefore was not assessed by NICE. A recent study examining the value of Gliadel following 5-ALA-guided resection showed no additional benefit in newly diagnosed GBM.[52]

Multiple studies have shown that treatment with radiation improves survival in patients with malignant glioma compared with best supportive care alone.[53] Surgery followed by limited-volume radiation therapy is established in the standard treatment for this disease. The choice of treatment volume recognizes that when GBMs relapse, they do so within 2 cm of the original enhancing rim in 85% of cases. The treatment volume is defined on a post-operative MRI scan, which is fused with the planning CT scan. The gross tumor volume (GTV) comprises the enhancing tumor margin or the resection margin, whichever is greater. The CTV increases the GTV by 2 to 3 cm but must take natural boundaries into account.[54] Planning should use conformal techniques.

The standard dose for a radical treatment is 60 Gy in 30 fractions over 6 weeks or the equivalent in 1.8 Gy fractions. Not all patients merit a radical approach with radiotherapy. For those with a poor performance status (e.g., WHO 2 or greater) or for the elderly, shorter courses of radiotherapy (40 Gy in 15 fractions or 30 Gy in six fractions on alternate days) are recommended, since these produce less impact on QOL.

Patients thought suitable for radical radiotherapy following surgery should also be treated with concomitant/adjuvant chemo-radiotherapy as the standard of care, unless there is a specific contraindication, as established in the landmark EORTC/NCIC (National Cancer Institute of Canada) randomized trial in which a regime of standard radiotherapy with concomitant daily temozolomide (75 mg/m^2) followed by monthly temozolomide (200 mg/m^2 × 6) produced a survival advantage of 16% (from 10% to 26%) at 2 years.[55] Furthermore, QOL was maintained, and the toxicity was modest. Benefit was greatest in well-resected patients with a WHO performance status of 0 or 1. These results have been reproduced many times since the publication of this study. Further follow-up to 5 years has demonstrated an ongoing survival advantage from combined chemo-radiotherapy (Figure 1.8).[55] Further intensification of the chemotherapy regime has not improved outcome. Benefit from the addition of chemotherapy was most evident in patients whose tumor demonstrated methylation of the *MGMT* gene;[14] however, combined chemo-radiotherapy remains the standard of care in all patients eligible for radical treatment irrespective of *MGMT* status.

The optimal management of elderly patients is a specific challenge, since it is predicted that up to 50% of all GBM cases will be over the age of 65 within the next few years. Patients with poor performance require only supportive care. In contrast, fit patients merit active management with radiotherapy, chemotherapy, or a combination of the two following surgery. Randomized studies show no benefit of 6 weeks of radiotherapy over shorter hypo-fractionated treatments. Also, in some patients, particularly those with *MGMT* methylated tumors, primary chemotherapy may be an option. Data from an NCIC/EORTC trial demonstrated the efficacy of short course

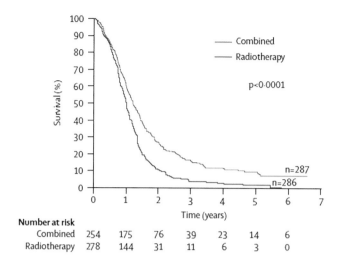

FIGURE 1.8 Combination treatment is effective in glioma subtypes. Survival data from the EORTC-NCIC study demonstrating the significant advantage of adding temozolomide chemotherapy to radiotherapy for patients with glioblastoma. (From Stupp et al., 2009. With permission.)

radiotherapy (40 Gy in 15 fractions) with temozolomide in patients 65 years or older. As predicted from data in younger cohorts, MGMT methylation predicted an enhanced benefit from the addition of temozolomide.[56]

When patients relapse, around 30% of those with good prognostic factors may enjoy a further brief improvement with chemotherapy. Single-agent CCNU (or other nitrosourea), PCV, and temozolomide can all be given as outpatient treatment and produce about the same level of response in chemo-naive patients with only modest acute toxicity.[57] Patients previously exposed to temozolomide can be re-challenged or treated with alternative chemotherapy. Carboplatin with or without etoposide can be used as second-line chemotherapy.

The use of bevacizumab in the relapsed setting, either alone or in combination with irinotecan, remains controversial. Although its use does appear to improve symptoms and scan appearance, survival is unaffected. In Europe, it is not recommended as routine practice but may be applicable in selected cases.[58]

Oligodendrogliomas

Oligodendrogliomas are classed with diffusely infiltrating glial tumors, believed to arise from oligodendrocytes or their progenitor cells. They account for around 5%–10% of gliomas and have a peak age incidence between 30 and 50 years. They arise in white matter, with a predilection for the frontal and parietal lobes.

Low-grade oligodendrogliomas (LGOs) are WHO Grade 2, slow-growing tumors that most commonly present with seizure. Their imaging characteristics are similar to those of LGA, but calcification is more frequent (approximately 50%). Long-standing tumors in the frontal brain may extend across the corpus callosum to affect the contralateral lobe, even when the tumor is low grade.

Macroscopically, the tumors usually appear as grey/pink masses, often well demarcated and with calcium frequently evident to the naked eye. Microscopically, the tumor comprises abundant uniform, small cells with round nuclei and a fine chromatin pattern—often referred to as "chicken wire."

Although the majority of oligodendrogliomas are low grade, a substantial minority are higher-grade histologically with features of increased cellularity, mitotic activity, pleomorphism, and vascular proliferation.

As described earlier, the current WHO definition of these tumors requires loss of heterozygosity on one or both chromosomes 1p and 19q, and this is frequently associated with other good prognostic molecular markers, including IDH mutation and MGMT methylation. In these tumors, TERT mutation is also a good prognostic indicator (see the section "Molecular biology of brain tumors").

The importance of the 1p/19q co-deleted genotype in AO was shown by analysis of two trials begun in the 1990s.[12,13] Both demonstrated that adding PCV chemotherapy to initial treatment with surgery and radiotherapy prolonged survival in co-deleted patients only (Figure 1.8). As a result, the standard treatment for 1p/19q co-deleted oligodendrogliomas comprises maximal surgical resection followed by conformal radiotherapy and adjuvant PCV chemotherapy. There is now also evidence that low-grade tumors with high-risk features and molecular pathology consistent with oligodendroglioma benefit from the same approach.[59]

Ependymoma

Ependymoma is a glioma arising from the ependymal cells that normally line the cerebral ventricles and the central canal of the spinal cord. They can arise at any site, usually in association with the ventricular system, but are most common in the posterior fossa, where they present with obstruction or with posterior fossa syndrome. The incidence of intracranial tumors is greatest in young children. Imaging usually shows a well-circumscribed tumor with variable contrast enhancement in the characteristic location. They comprise fewer than 2% of all primary CNS tumors. In adults, most are located in the spine, whereas in children, the majority are in the brain, most commonly posterior fossa. Survival is worse in younger patients and with supratentorial location and high-grade disease.

Ependymomas are soft, grey/pink tumors that often show their ependymal origin. Histologically, perivascular pseudo-rosettes and ependymal rosettes interrupt a monotonous cellular background. Anaplastic tumors may also show pleomorphism, disorganized cyto-architecture, increased mitosis, and necrosis. The 2016 WHO classification recognizes four variants of ependymoma: subependymoma (Grade I), myxopapillary (Grade I), classic (Grade II with variants papillary, clear cell, and tanycytic), and anaplastic (Grade III). It also includes a molecular sub-group defined by *RELA* fusions in supratentorial Grade II or III tumors in children, which is associated with high risk of recurrence and poor prognosis. The issue of high inter-observer variability in grade assignation is widely recognized, and recent data suggest that a methylome-based classification may be a more robust approach to defining risk groups and aiding management decisions, which is reflected in current consensus guidelines.[60,61]

Ependymomas spread via the cerebrospinal fluid (CSF), but the influence of spinal seeding on outcome has probably been overestimated. Although post-mortem series have shown up to 30% spinal seeding, in practice, it is detected in around only 10% and is symptomatic in fewer than 5%. Spread is more likely with infratentorial high-grade tumors.

All patients should be staged with neuraxis imaging. Maximal tumor resection should be attempted regardless of site, as extent of resection is a major predictor of outcome.[58] Gross total removal of posterior fossa tumors is achieved in only around 50% of cases. Post-operative imaging is strongly recommended, and the option of a second operation for incompletely resected tumors is considered.

The role of radiotherapy is more controversial; it is usually reserved for Grade III or incompletely resected Grade II tumors. A reasonable policy is to deliver post-operative irradiation (54 Gy in 1.8 Gy fractions) to the tumor site using a modest margin (~2 cm). Radiotherapy is generally avoided in children below 12 months of age. Whole-neuraxis treatment may be necessary in disseminated disease, although its value in prolonging survival is not established. Where the surgeon believes a macroscopic complete removal of a low-grade tumor has been achieved, and this is confirmed on MRI, there is a case for a careful observation policy with radiation if recurrence is identified.

The 5-year survival for patients with low-grade tumors is greater than 50%, although it is worse for young children. Most series show lower survival for patients with high-grade tumors. Treatment failure is most commonly due to local recurrence. Chemotherapy is of minimal value for low- or high-grade tumors in the newly diagnosed or relapsed setting. There is therefore interest in the use of re-irradiation at relapse. Ongoing studies are evaluating the role of chemotherapy as adjuvant or neo-adjuvant treatment prior to second look surgery.

Myxopapillary ependymoma is a variant most commonly found in the sacral region. It is of low grade (Grade 1) and may often be watched following resection even if removal is incomplete. The rare subependymoma is a very low-grade lesion that should be treated with surgery alone.

Rare neuro-epithelial tumors

Astroblastoma

This unusual, probably astrocytic, tumor is regarded by some as a growth pattern rather than a separate pathological entity. The lesion comprises prominent elongated tumor cells that form pseudo-rosettes around blood vessels. The tumors are often superficial, well circumscribed, and amenable to surgical resection. The role of radiation and chemotherapy is not established, but they may be appropriate for patients with poorly resected or recurrent tumors. Like other rare glioma types, they frequently harbor *BRAF* mutations (around 40%), suggesting that targeted treatment may be valuable in these cases.[62]

Pleomorphic xanthoastrocytoma

This is usually a cystic and peripherally located tumor in children and young adults, characterized by a mixture of spindle-like cells and mono-nucleated or multi-nucleated giant cells. There is often intracellular lipid accumulation and the marked presence of reticulin fibers. It is normally a low-grade tumor. The major treatment modality is surgery, and complete excision is associated with the best outcome. However, higher-grade tumors are found, and an anaplastic variant is included in WHO 2016 classification. Radiation treatment may be of value in the management of more aggressive tumors or those that recur after surgery.[63] Up to 60% of tumors may harbor BRAFV600E mutations.

Subependymal giant-cell astrocytoma

This very-slow-growing tumor is frequently associated with tuberose sclerosis. Treatment is with surgery or observation only. There is no role for either radiotherapy or chemotherapy in this condition, although recently, the m-TOR inhibitor everolimus was licensed for use in difficult circumstances (see the section "Targeting oncogenic growth factors").

Brain-stem glioma

Gliomas of all types may arise in the brain stem, most commonly in the pons. Biopsy can be associated with a high risk of morbidity, and it may be acceptable to treat on the basis of imaging appearances and clinical features alone. Treatment is usually with radiotherapy (54 Gy for high-grade and 45–50 Gy for low-grade tumors). Studies of hyper-fractionation and adjuvant chemotherapy have not improved outcome. The majority of patients have high-grade tumors, and their outlook is very poor. Patients with lower-grade gliomas may survive for years after treatment. Chemotherapy can produce a further response in patients with low-grade tumors who relapse after radiotherapy. As discussed earlier, new insights into the molecular biology of high-grade gliomas in children, including common histone mutations, may allow better stratification and novel treatment approaches.

Optic nerve glioma

This tumor, which is most common in children and young adults, is usually low grade and very slow growing. Because of its position, it may cause devastating symptoms of visual and hormonal disturbance. Management is controversial. Surgery (for unilateral disease), radiotherapy, and sometimes chemotherapy have been advocated, but the timing is crucial, and some tumors will spontaneously stabilize. Simple guidelines to management cannot be offered, and the reader is referred to more detailed approaches.[64]

Gliomatosis cerebri

This is a pattern of presentation for a variety of glial tumors in which the brain is diffusely affected. Although it was previously considered a separate clinical entity, the WHO 2016 classification no longer includes this diagnosis, limiting the terminology to a radiological description, formal diagnosis depending on histopathology and molecular features. Surgery has almost no therapeutic role in this condition. Chemotherapy or whole-brain radiotherapy (WBRT) may delay the disease process and prolong survival in some patients, particularly those with molecular features suggesting treatment sensitivity. For most, however, the outlook is dismal; many patients die within months of presentation.

Dysembryoplastic neuro-epithelial tumor

This is a benign tumor that arises predominantly in the temporal lobes of children and young adults and is often associated with seizure. Histopathologically, these tumors are characterized by a specific glioneuronal element, often with a nodular component and associated cortical dysplasia. Treatment is by surgical excision; there is no evidence for the value of either radiotherapy or chemotherapy.

Gangliocytoma and ganglioglioma

These tumors comprise neoplastic ganglion cells alone (gangliocytoma) or in association with neoplastic glial cells (ganglioglioma). Most patients are under 30 years of age, and a great majority present with seizure. The primary treatment for both tumors is surgery. Radiotherapy is now usually withheld from these lesions, which are regarded as WHO Class 1, even if resection is incomplete. However, anaplastic transformation may occur in the glial component, when the outcome becomes much more sinister and treatment more aggressive. As described earlier, a significant proportion of these tumors harbor *BRAF* mutations and/or other mutations that activate MAPK signaling. The response to targeting this pathway in these patients is under investigation, with initial promising data.[65, 66]

Central neurocytoma

This is a rare tumor that arises within the ventricles of young adults. Histological features are of small round cells with neuronal differentiation. Treatment is mainly surgical, and the outcome, even after incomplete resection, can be good. However, troublesome recurrence can occur; at that time, radiotherapy and even chemotherapy may be of value. Rare extraventricular tumors occur and may represent a separate biological entity with frequent FGFR1-TACC1 fusion events suggesting a potential response to FGFR targeting.[67]

Choroid-plexus tumors

Choroid-plexus papillomas are rare intra-ventricular tumors derived from the choroid-plexus epithelium. They are predominantly found in children. The malignant choroid-plexus carcinoma is even less common. Treatment is surgical, and the outcome is highly dependent on the completeness of resection. Radiotherapy is reserved for incompletely removed tumors and malignant lesions. CSF spread can occur even in low-grade lesions.

Embryonal tumors

Embryonal tumors are the largest group of malignant pediatric brain tumors. They include medulloblastoma, atypical teratoid/rhabdoid tumors (AT/RT), and CNS primitive neuroectodermal tumors (PNETs). Despite a superficial resemblance to medulloblastoma, patients with CNS PNET and AT/RT fare poorly in comparison.

Medulloblastoma

Medulloblastomas are malignant tumors arising in the posterior fossa, usually in the midline (vermis). They spread by local invasion into the cerebellar hemispheres and rostrally into the fourth ventricle and project into the brain stem. They readily spread via CSF to produce metastases on the leptomeninges of the brain and cord, a process that defines their treatment.

It is found that 70% of medulloblastomas occur in children under the age of 16 years (peak 7 years), and they are rare after the age of 40 years. The European annual incidence rate is approximately 6.5 per million in children aged under 14 years. There is a slight male predominance. Clinically, medulloblastoma presents with a cerebellar syndrome or with raised intracranial pressure due to CSF outflow obstruction. The diagnosis will usually be suspected from the clinical presentation and the imaging appearances. Hydrocephalus might constitute an emergency and require prompt ventricular drainage and steroids prior to a definitive, operative procedure, although some surgeons undertake both the drainage and the tumor decompression simultaneously. Full neuraxis imaging (gadolinium-MRI) should be done pre-operatively to look for metastatic spread before blood is introduced into the CSF at operation. If this is not possible, the investigation should be done within 48 hours following surgery. The CSF should be sampled and examined for malignant cells before manipulation of the tumor. Complete tumor removal is associated with a better prognosis and should be attempted wherever possible. In some situations, for example involvement of the brain stem, total excision may not be possible. Post-operative imaging should be done within 48 hours of surgery to assess the amount of residual disease.

The characteristic imaging appearance is of a solid, often uniformly enhancing mass with a discrete edge (Figure 1.9). Sometimes, the tumor is more irregular, inhomogeneous, and occasionally cystic.

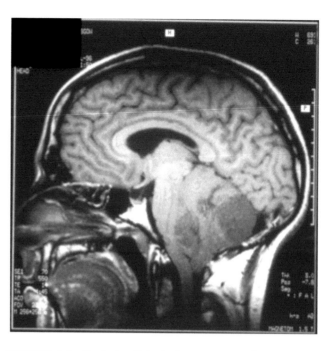

FIGURE 1.9 Typical radiological appearances of medulloblastoma (classical subtype) on MRI showing a relatively well-defined, midline mass in the posterior fossa.

Risk stratification in medulloblastoma was previously based on age, metastatic status, extent of surgical resection, and histopathology; however, our biologic understanding of this disease has been transformed in the last few years, and current (WHO 2016) classification is based on four genetically defined, clinically and prognostically relevant subtypes: WNT-activated, sonic hedgehog (SHH) activated, Group 3, and Group 4. Details are shown in Table 1.3 with associated clinical features. WNT-activated medulloblastomas occur mainly in older children and young adults and are typified by an origin close to the brain stem and a predisposition to hemorrhage. They can be identified by nuclear expression of beta-catenin on immunohistochemistry. These patients have an extremely good prognosis when treated with standard doses of craniospinal radiotherapy and chemotherapy following surgery and may be candidates for treatment de-intensification. SHH-activated medulloblastomas occur mainly in children younger than 3 years and in young adults, accounting for around 30% of diagnoses and have a more variable outlook. Agents targeting smoothened (an upstream target in the SHH signaling pathway) are under investigation in these patients. Group 3 medulloblastomas have the poorest prognosis and account for 25% of cases; the biology is less well understood, although activation of MYC is a recurrent abnormality. Group 4 has an intermediate prognosis despite commonly presenting with metastatic disease and more heterogeneous biology. Overall, although 5-year survival for older children (≥5 years of age at diagnosis) with medulloblastoma is over 75%, new strategies are badly needed for several subsets of patients, including those with metastatic *MYC*-amplified Group 3 or SHH-driven *TP53*-mutated *MYCN*-amplified tumors or those younger than 3 years with Group 3 medulloblastoma, who continue to have poor outlooks. The prognosis is also poor for children with recurrent medulloblastoma, of whom very few can be cured even with the use of multimodal therapies such as high-dose chemotherapy; however, patients who have not undergone upfront radiotherapy, particularly younger children, may still be cured using this treatment modality with or without chemotherapy.[68]

CSI remains standard of care for all patients with medulloblastoma aged over 3 years (see the section "Whole-neuraxis radiotherapy (craniospinal irradiation)"). In children with standard-risk disease, 23.4 Gy is delivered to the entire craniospinal axis (brain and spinal cord with the meningeal coverings) with a further 30.6 Gy (total 54 Gy) delivered to the whole posterior fossa in 30 daily fractions over 6 weeks. The radiotherapy is accompanied by eight weekly doses of concomitant vincristine (1.5 mg/m²: maximum 2 mg). Adjuvant chemotherapy begins 6 weeks after the end of radiotherapy and comprises eight cycles of cisplatin 70 mg/m² i.v. and lomustine 75 mg/m² p.o. on day 1, and vincristine 1.5 mg/m² i.v. on days 1, 8, and 15, with a 6-week interval between cycles. For adults with medulloblastoma, because they tolerate the extensive myelosuppressive and neurotoxic chemotherapy less well and the late consequences of CSI are less severe than for children who are still growing, this "standard" chemo-radiation regime has not been adopted. Rather, full-dose CSI comprising 35 Gy in 20 fractions, with a posterior fossa boost of 19.8 Gy in 11 fractions, is given. Modified adjuvant chemotherapy has been explored, but its value has not been established in randomized studies.

CSI is accompanied by acute and late toxic effects. Acute toxicity includes nausea and vomiting, requiring anti-emetics, and the exit dose from a spinal x-ray field may produce radiation esophagitis. Myelosuppression is common but rarely requires support or interruption of treatment. Some degree of alopecia is universal. Later consequences are ongoing nausea (especially in teenagers), deafness, loss of intelligence quotient, hormonal deficits, loss of height due to direct and indirect (growth-hormone) effects on bone, second cancers (including thyroid cancers and meningiomas), and cataracts from scattered radiation dose. The principal toxic effects of the chemotherapy are myelosuppression, GI upset, and neurotoxicity. Because of the severe physical and psychological effects caused by the disease and its treatment, young people who develop the condition need extensive support during treatment and for many years following its completion.

Atypical teratoid rhabdoid tumor (ATRT)

ATRTs are rare, malignant embryonal tumors, usually arising in the posterior fossa of children, especially infants less than 3 years, accounting for 1–2% of brain tumors in children. Histopathologically, they show rhabdoid cells, often together with cells resembling medulloblastoma. In the great majority of cases, alteration of the locus of the tumor suppressor gene *SMARCB1* (a member of a chromosome remodeling complex) on the chromosome band 22q11.2 is a hallmark genetic aberration. A significant proportion of these patients have germline mutations in SMARCB1 or SMARCA4, associated with a potentially aggressive disease course. Recent analysis of genomic data has suggested three sub-groups of ATRT based on methylation profiles.

The standard approach to treatment is not well-defined in this rare entity. Maximal resection followed by intensive chemotherapy has been suggested. The role of irradiation is unclear, and it is often deferred in younger children. However, the outcome is very poor, particularly in patients aged less than 3 years, where the 2-year survival is under 20%. Exploration of targeting the epigenetic alterations common in this tumor is ongoing.

Embryonal tumor with multilayered rosettes

This is a recently recognized aggressive tumor that occurs mainly in younger children under the age of 4 at a variety of CNS sites, including spinal cord, although the majority are supra-tentorial. Most are localized at diagnosis, but rapid progression is the rule. Pathologically, it resembles a PNET with rosettes of ependymoblastic cells. Three histological patterns are defined: embryonal tumors with abundant neuropil and true rosettes (ETANTR), ependymoblastoma (EBL), and medulloepithelioma (MEPL); however, all histological subtypes carry amplification of C19MC, suggesting biological concordance. Due to the rarity of this entity, no standard treatment recommendations are available, although limited available data support maximal resection, intensive chemotherapy, and radiotherapy.

Tumors of the meninges

Meningiomas

A variety of tumors develop in the meninges, but the most common by far are meningiomas, which arise from the meningothelial cells themselves. They are usually benign. They occur most commonly on the convexity or falcine brain regions, but they may arise anywhere that meninges are present and cause particular difficulties in sites around the base of the skull. Spinal meningiomas are most common in the thoracic region.

Meningiomas present most commonly in middle age, more often in women (female:male = 3:2). They rarely occur in children, when they tend to be more aggressive. They can be induced by radiation and are associated with some genetic syndromes, particularly NF2. A majority of tumors show the presence of progesterone receptors, and a minority are estrogen receptor positive. Whether this is important in the etiology is not established. Loss of chromosome 22 and NF2 mutation or inactivation are common findings in sporadic meningioma. Next-generation sequencing has also demonstrated somatic mutations in *TRAF7*, *KLF4*, *AKT1*, *SMO*, and *PIK3CA*, which are mutually exclusive to NF2/Chr22 loss and align with histological subtypes and anatomical location. For example, meningothelial meningiomas are characterized by *AKT1* mutations, and mutations in *SMO* and *AKT1/TRAF7* are associated with anterior skull-base location.[69]

Most meningiomas are round or lobulated, smooth, firm, and well-delineated tumors, often indenting and compressing the brain but rarely attached to or invading it. More commonly, they invade into or through the dura and induce hyperostosis in the overlying skull. In the base of the skull, they may grow as plaque-like tumors. Meningiomas derive their blood supply from the adjacent meningeal artery and are highly vascular. Identification and embolization of this artery can be therapeutic in its own right and can aid surgical removal.

WHO Grade 1 tumors comprise nine histological variants, all with similar behavior. Atypical meningioma (WHO Grade 2) is identified when tumors show increased cellularity, a sheet-like growth pattern, increased mitosis, high nuclear: cytoplasmic ratio, geographic necrosis, and brain invasion. WHO 2016 specifically allocates any case with brain invasion to this category. Malignant meningioma (WHO Grade 3) is said to be present when these features become increasingly prominent (very high mitotic rates). The rare chordoid subtype represents <1% of meningiomas and is always regarded as WHO Grade 2, since there is a high risk of recurrence. It is clear that these definitions are not precise, and they are subject to variation between pathologists. The combination of histology with genomic and epigenomic data promises a new approach to diagnosis and management in these patients.

Patients with meningioma have diverse presentations. Although headache is very common, seizure and functional deficit are also frequent. CT or MRI usually reveals an iso- to

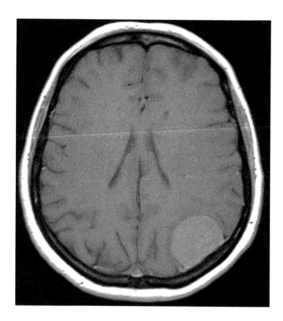

FIGURE 1.10 Typical radiological appearance of a meningioma on contrast enhanced MRI scan, showing a uniformly enhancing lesion with a broad base arising from the dura. (By courtesy of Dr Stuart Currie, Leeds Teaching Hospitals NHS Trust.)

hyper-dense/intense lesion, with a meningeal base, enhancing strongly with contrast (Figure 1.10). Angiography may add further diagnostic information. Increasingly, these tumors are diagnosed incidentally when patients in middle age or older are scanned for unrelated symptoms. Small incidental lesions do not require intervention, but a follow-up protocol should be advised to establish growth patterns, since grade cannot be established on imaging alone.

Surgery dominates the treatment of meningioma. The aim is to remove the entire tumor and any involved adjacent structure (dura, soft tissue, and bone) to maximize the prospect for enduring local control. Pre-operative embolization of the main feeder vessel is often performed as an aid to surgical removal. The site of the tumor determines the surgical procedure. Convexity meningiomas have the best chance of total excision. Removal of parasagittal tumors risks damage to the sagittal sinus and its draining veins. Tumors of the base of the skull are particularly problematic because of the difficult access and the proximity of sensitive structures.

The outcome following surgery strongly depends on the extent of resection. Re-growth varies from less than 10% for patients with complete excision to over 40% for patients undergoing partial resection. It follows that patients with tumors in the most accessible regions have better prospects than patients with tumors in difficult areas such as the sphenoid ridge. A second operation for recurrence is possible in the majority of patients.

Radiotherapy is effective in the management of meningioma. It is usually given in the adjuvant setting following an incomplete resection where further surgery might prove to be difficult, after multiple relapses following surgery, or when the histology is unfavorable.[70]

The GTV will include any visible residual or recurrent tumor. The CTV will include a margin for spread into adjacent structures. Some recommend treating the entire dural base along with the tumor, whereas others recommend treating just the imaged tumor. Neither approach has been demonstrated to be superior.

For malignant tumors, the brain and overlying bone must also be considered at risk. Typically, doses between 50 and 55 Gy in 1.8 Gy fractions are used for Grade 1 lesions, whereas 60 Gy in 30 fractions is recommended where possible for higher-grade tumors. Sophisticated immobilization, localization, and beam-conforming techniques should be used to minimize the irradiated normal tissue, especially in sensitive areas around the skull base where SRS can be used to advantage. SRS has also been used to treat meningiomas, but the tendency for dural spread and the damaging effect of large single doses may limit the success of this approach.

Chemotherapy is of no proven value in benign meningioma, although sarcoma regimes may be tried for palliation of the malignant form. The identification of hormone receptors in the majority of meningiomas has led to the use of anti-androgen hormone therapy, but with little success. Recent guidelines to management include those published by the European Association of Neuro-Oncology (EANO).[71]

Hemangiopericytoma (solitary fibrous tumor)

Previously thought of as a variant of meningioma, this tumor is now believed to be indistinguishable from hemangiopericytoma in other sites, where it is usually designated as solitary fibrous tumor. It has been thought to derive from the meningeal capillary pericyte, although the true histogenesis remains uncertain. It is a rare tumor that tends to arise in a younger age group than meningioma and is more common in men. These tumors arise in the dura as highly vascular, lobulated masses. They are densely cellular and often highly mitotic and may be graded WHO 2 or 3 on this basis. These tumors carry fusions of *NAB2* and *STAT6*, and staining for *STAT6* to identify the fusion event is recommended to confirm diagnosis. Hemangiopericytomas have a marked tendency to recur after surgery alone and to metastasize within and outside the CNS, particularly to bone. Maximal surgery is essential treatment, but post-operative high-dose radiotherapy (55–60 Gy) is often recommended to reduce local recurrence and metastasis. Median survival is around 5 years.

Primary central nervous system lymphoma (PCNSL)

PCNSL is defined as lymphoma arising in the CNS (including the eyes) in the absence of obvious lymphoma elsewhere at the time of diagnosis. Its development is strongly related to immunosuppression due to either disease or therapy. There is a high incidence of PCNSL in patients with AIDS, following organ transplantation, and possibly in rheumatoid disease. The incidence in both immune-competent and immune-compromised patients appears to be rising. PCNSL may occur at any age, but in immune-competent patients, it is most common in middle age. It is slightly more common in men.

PCNSL arises preferentially in peri-ventricular regions of the brain. On imaging, they appear as iso- or hyper-dense lesions that usually enhance uniformly (Figure 1.11). About 20%–60% are multiple at presentation. Characteristically, they respond rapidly to treatment with steroids and may "disappear" within 48 hours of starting treatment, leading to PCNSLs being described as "ghost tumors." Ocular disease is present in 15%–20% of cases. Clinically, they usually present as mass lesions, although more subtle symptoms, such as personality change, are not uncommon. CSF cytology is positive in 10%–20%. Primary spinal lymphoma is extremely rare.

The pathology is much the same as for systemic extra-nodal lymphomas. The great majority of PCNSLs are diffuse large B-cell tumors that express the usual pan B markers (e.g., CD20). Only

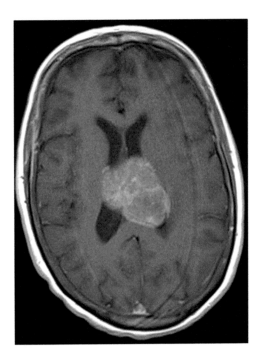

FIGURE 1.11 Typical MRI scan of a patient with primary CNS lymphoma, showing an avidly enhancing mass close to the ventricular system on axial T1 image with gadolinium. (By courtesy of Dr Stuart Currie, Leeds Teaching Hospitals NHS Trust.)

2% are T-cell tumors. A striking feature is the extremely high proliferative activity.

When primary Hodgkin's disease and plasmacytoma occur in the CNS, they are usually dural based. Both are extremely rare.

Although imaging may suggest PCNSL, histological proof is essential for adequate management. Surgical resection does not improve outcome, and a biopsy alone is needed. Steroids should be avoided prior to biopsy, as this can impair diagnostic yield. Whether these patients need full lymphoma staging is controversial, as the pickup for systemic disease is low. However, most agree that a full ophthalmologic examination; a lumbar puncture with cytological evaluation and flow cytometry (where possible); whole-neuraxis MRI; CT of chest abdomen and pelvis; bone-marrow examination; and an immunological screen, including an HIV test, are important.

The chemotherapeutic treatment of PCNSLs is dominated by high-dose methotrexate (HDMTX). A dose of at least 3 g/m² by rapid infusion (~3 hours) is considered necessary to achieve adequate levels in the CNS. Other agents that have been shown to improve outcome in combination with HDMTX include cytarabine, rituximab, and thiotepa. A four-drug regime methotrexate, cytarabine (Ara-C), thiotepa, and rituximab (MATRix) gave impressive improvements in overall survival,[72,73] although this intensive treatment may not be suitable for all patients. Alternative combination regimes with promising outcomes include HDMTX, procarbazine, vincristine, and rituximab or HDMTX, BCNU, rituximab, prednisolone, and etoposide; however, no international standard exists. There are currently no data supporting the use of intrathecal chemotherapy. Treating elderly patients with this disease is a specific challenge, since they tolerate intensive treatments less well, and an effective regime that improves outcome in patients over 60 remains to be defined.

Current guidelines delineate three groups of patients depending on fitness for treatment. These are those eligible for intensive combination immuno-chemotherapy incorporating high-dose methotrexate (HDMTX), those eligible for HDMTX-based immuno-chemotherapy but not intensive combination chemotherapy, and those ineligible for HDMTX-based therapy, i.e., those suitable for palliative treatment.[74] Category 1 patients should be offered MATRix combination chemotherapy for induction with consideration of stem cell transplant or WBRT consolidation for residual disease. Recent data suggest efficacy of both consolidation approaches, although they confirm the risks of neuro-cognitive impairment with WBRT, suggesting that chemotherapy approaches may be preferred.[75] WBRT doses of 36 Gy in 20 fractions are standard but should be reduced for patients with high risk of neurotoxicity. A boost dose to residual enhancing disease (9 Gy) is also recommended. For less fit patients, a treatment regime including HDMTX, rituximab, and an oral alkylating agent is suggested as first-line treatment, while for patients unsuitable for HDMTX, options include oral chemotherapy such as temozolomide, WBRT 20–30 Gy, and corticosteroids.

Treatment of relapsed disease remains challenging, and prognosis is poor, in the region of a few months. No standard approach exists, and management should be individualized with reference to patient performance status and previous treatment. Options include re-challenge with MTX-based regimes for patients with a long interval since previous exposure and ifosfamide-based immuno-chemotherapy.

The treatment of HIV-positive patients is less well-defined. If their condition allows it, an aggressive approach, as for the immune-competent patient, can be followed. For patients who are less well, radiotherapy alone can be given. It is important to continue antiviral therapy. Very elderly patients or those not fit for other approaches can do quite well with an initial course of high-dose steroid alone, which can be tapered down as the tumor responds.

Tumors of the pineal region

Whereas pineal cell and germ cell tumors are particularly associated with the pineal region of the brain, other tumor types, including gliomas, meningiomas, benign tumors, and metastases, also occur. Presentation is most commonly with hydrocephalus and is often accompanied by complete or partial Parinaud's syndrome.

Pineal parenchymal tumors

These are uncommon tumors of the pineocytes. They always arise in the pineal gland but may disseminate in the CSF. They occur in children and adults and show no gender preference. On imaging, they most commonly show as uniform, well-delineated, isodense or hypo-dense lesions that enhance uniformly. Cysts or calcifications may be present.

Classification of pineal parenchymal tumors (PPTs) includes four entities: pineocytoma (Grade 1), pineal parenchymal tumor of intermediate differentiation, papillary tumor of the pineal region (both Grade 2 and Grade 3), and pineoblastoma (Grade 4). These tumors cover a range of outcomes: Pineocytoma is associated with an excellent prognosis following surgical resection, whereas pineoblastomas carry a poor prognosis with a high propensity to disseminate despite combined modality treatment, and intermediate differentiation tumors sit in between. Pineoblastomas have been found to carry frequent mutations of genes that encode microRNA processing enzymes (*DICER1* and *DROSHA*). In contrast, intermediate-grade tumors have recently been found to carry KBTBD4 mutations, thus implying a biologic and potentially diagnostic division between these entities.

The management of pineal tumors includes imaging the entire neuraxis, immediate decompression of hydrocephalus, and establishing a tissue diagnosis. Pineocytoma is a surgical disease and may be cured by total resection. Pineoblastoma is less likely to be cured by surgery, although complete resection should be attempted where possible. There is evidence that whole-neuraxis radiotherapy with the boost directed at the tumor improves outcome, particularly if resection is incomplete. Chemotherapy responses can also be seen. Intermediate (Grade 2/3) tumors present particular difficulties in management. Again, complete surgical excision should be attempted where possible. The need for radiotherapy will depend on the completeness of resection, the mitotic rate, and evidence of dissemination away from the primary.

The outcome in these rare tumors is difficult to estimate. Older children do better than those under 5 years of age, and it appears that avoiding radiotherapy impacts negatively on outcomes in higher-grade tumors. Complete surgical resection is generally associated with better outcome in all grades. Pineoblastoma has a sinister reputation, although failure to recognize and treat it adequately has probably contributed to this.

Germ cell tumors

CNS germ cell tumors are rare, with an estimated incidence of 1 per million per year in Europe. They can be divided into two broad groups: germinomas and non-germinomatous germ cell tumors (NGGCTs). NGGCTs can be further classified into teratomas (mature and malignant forms) and other malignant germ cell tumors, including choriocarcinoma, yolk sac tumor and embryonal carcinoma. It is not infrequent to see mixed histology in NGGCTs. They are tumors of the young; approximately 90% occur before the age of 20 years. The male:female ratio is >2:1. They are predominantly midline tumors, most common around the pineal region and third ventricle (80%), although supra-sellar presentation is not uncommon. Tumors arising elsewhere tend to be non-germinomatous. There is marked geographical variation, with a higher incidence in the Far East, particularly Japan.

The pathology of primary intracranial germ cell tumors is identical to that of their systemic counterparts and is reviewed in Chapter 17.

Germ cell tumors may grow locally, producing potentially reversible effects of pressure and obstruction. Local infiltration of adjacent brain with irreversible destruction may also occur. They tend to spread along the ventricular linings and have a tendency to disseminate via the CSF to affect other areas of the brain and spinal cord. The incidence of this is variably reported, but it is probably around 15%. Systemic spread, either blood borne or via ventriculo-peritoneal shunts, can also occur. Presentation is as for other mass lesions in the pineal region (or other sites).

The testicular tumor markers human chorionic gonadotropin (hCG) (indicating choriocarcinoma) and alpha-fetoprotein (AFP) (indicating yolk sac elements) can often be detected in the serum and CSF of these patients and can be a useful guide to response to treatment as well as aiding diagnosis. Decay of the markers may be delayed by the presence of cysts, which act as reservoirs. The CSF to serum marker ratio in patients with CNS tumors is usually >1. If the ratio is reversed, systemic disease is more likely. The detection of serum AFP is diagnostic of teratoma and may obviate the need for biopsy.

Gadolinium-enhanced MRI is the imaging modality of choice and is essential for planning surgery. Germinomas tend to be homogeneous and enhance uniformly with contrast. Calcification is common, and cystic areas may be present. Teratomas, both benign and malignant, are notably heterogeneous with variable signal characteristics and irregular contrast enhancement. The whole neuraxis should be imaged. All patients presenting with a suspicion of a germ cell tumor require serum estimation for AFP and hCG. The CSF levels should also be evaluated.

The management of germ cell tumors is complex and dependent on the precise histology of the lesion. Tissue (or marker) diagnosis is essential, and high serum or CSF levels may also indicate high risk, for example AFP >1000 kU/L in NGGCT; however, the extent of surgery required is a matter of debate. Biopsy of this region using stereotaxy, although it is possible, may be hazardous. An open procedure may be considered the safest and also provides the opportunity for therapeutic resection. Ventriculoscopy and biopsy can be valuable in difficult cases. Surgical excision is usually curative for differentiated teratoma but offers no advantage over biopsy alone in germinoma. Surgical resection of NGGCTs may be valuable, but with the increasing success of non-surgical treatment, the risk of complications should be considered in each case. In situations where CSF marker levels may determine management, lumbar samples are preferable to ventricular samples.

It is difficult to give simple guidelines for the treatment of these diseases. In the past, the standard treatment for localized germinoma was whole-neuraxis radiotherapy with a boost to the primary lesion. Although the cure rate was very high (>90%), the treatment was associated with substantial early and late toxicity. Most practitioners now advocate initial treatment with a combination of carboplatin and etoposide (two to four cycles) followed by radiation limited to the primary site plus the whole of the ventricular system (24 Gy in 15 fractions) and a boost to the primary site (16 Gy in 10 fractions). The cure rate is much the same but with reduced toxicity.

Although a standard management for patients with poor-prognosis, malignant NGGCT has not been established, it is agreed that they require aggressive multimodality treatment. Chemotherapy regimes may be up to six cycles and are usually platinum based (cisplatin or carboplatin) combined with agents such as etoposide, bleomycin, and ifosfamide. Radiotherapy is an accepted element of management, but there is disagreement as to whether this should be craniospinal[76] or localized, based on a sound knowledge of the disease distribution. Craniospinal treatment is indicated for metastatic CNS disease. Higher doses (>45 Gy) to the primary site are required in all cases. Surgery also has a more prominent role in this disease, as more extensive removal is associated with better outcome. Some recommendations also suggest that residual disease should be resected if feasible as part of planned initial treatment. Recent clinical study data suggest a role for neoadjuvant chemotherapy prior to second-look surgery and craniospinal radiotherapy.[77]

The outcome following these approaches is varied. In pure germinoma, 5-year disease-free survivals of 85%–100% can be expected. Radiotherapy alone for NGGCT produces only around 20% long-term survivors, but the introduction of platinum-based chemotherapy has improved this to around 50% or better, although radiation remains an important element of treatment in all patients. As in gonadal germ cell tumors, it is not uncommon to image residual abnormality in the tumor site following treatment. In the absence of evidence of progression, this may just need observation. However, if there is doubt concerning the completeness of treatment, surgery may be indicated. The treatment options for relapsed disease include chemotherapy for germinoma and high-dose chemotherapy with stem cell rescue for NGGCT.

The functional outcome following treatment is often good, although the same complications of treatment experienced by medulloblastoma survivors occur. Patients presenting with severe Parinaud's syndrome often suffer from persistence of deficit and require the input of a neuro-ophthalmologist. Patients with supra-sellar tumors may suffer from long-term endocrine problems. Recent consensus statements are available.[78]

Other tumors

Craniopharyngioma

Craniopharyngioma is a benign epithelial tumor of the sellar region, thought to arise from a remnant of Rathke's pouch. It is most common in children and young adults. It grows slowly and presents with pressure symptoms and endocrine and visual disturbances. Hydrocephalus may be present. The typical imaging properties of an enhancing solid and cystic lesion, often with calcification in a supra-sellar site, strongly suggest the diagnosis.

Two forms are recognized histologically, papillary and adamantinomatous. Both are slow-growing and excite intense gliosis in neighboring brain. Tongues of the tumor also extend into adjacent brain tissue and may be very difficult to remove surgically. Single or multiple cysts are very common and contain a thick, cholesterol-rich fluid. The fluid in the adamantinomatous tumor is often oilier than that in the papillary type, and calcification is much more common. Papillary tumors occur predominantly in adults, while adamantinomatous tumors have a bimodal age distribution. The latter are characterized by alterations in wnt signaling, while the former commonly harbor *BRAF* mutations.

Optimal management of these tumors is controversial. A common approach in the United Kingdom is to attempt MSR. If this is shown to be complete, routine follow-up with interval imaging is sufficient. Because of the growth pattern, however, total excision may not be possible, and the recurrence rate then is higher. In these cases, radiotherapy can be given. The volume should be minimized using accurate CT localization and conforming techniques, as a dose of 50–54 Gy in 1.8 Gy fractions is needed. This treatment restores the level of tumor control to that of complete excision. In very young children, in whom radiotherapy might produce high levels of morbidity, observation may be appropriate even after partial resection. Follow-up in all cases includes endocrine assessment, neuro-ophthalmology, and neuro-psychology as well as tumor surveillance. Although the 10-year survival is around 90%, fewer patients are free from disease. Ongoing clinical studies are assessing the effect of *BRAF* inhibition in papillary tumors as an alternative to conventional management. Treatment of recurrence is difficult, as re-operation is hazardous. Radiotherapy-naive patients can be irradiated, and re-irradiation is possible in some situations if stereotactic techniques (SRS or SRT) are used.

Chordoma

Chordomas are malignant, embryonal tumors that arise from the notochordal remnant. They are found predominantly in the region of the clivus and at the sacrococcygeous, in the extradural space, but they grow slowly and may invade the dura as they do so (Figure 1.12). Histologically, the identifying features are "physaliferous" cells, which contain large mucus-filled vacuoles, show immunoreactivity for S-100 and epithelial markers such as the epithelial membrane antigen (MUC1) and cytokeratins, and are arranged in lobules, usually surrounded by extracellular mucus. These tumor cells typically express high levels of the notochord transcription factor brachyury, driven by gains of the *TBXT* gene.

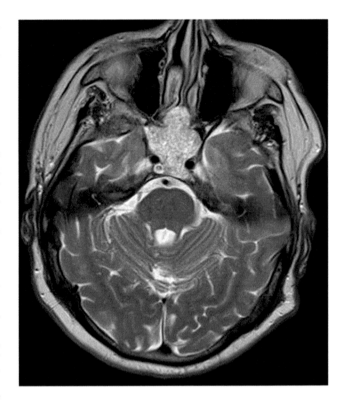

FIGURE 1.12 Base of skull chordoma invading into the clivus and central skull base, shown as expansile lesion with high signal on axial T2 MRI. (By courtesy of Dr Stuart Currie, Leeds Teaching Hospitals NHS Trust.)

The management of these tumors is complex. The best possibility for cure probably results from aggressive surgical resection within the constraint of preserved neurological function. However, even after apparent complete resection, local recurrence occurs in up to 50% of cases. Unfortunately, there is no evidence of response to conventional chemotherapy. High-dose radiotherapy is recommended in the post-operative setting. Dose escalation to highly conformed target volumes using proton beam facilities or intensity-modulated x-ray techniques appears to produce better results. Median survival is around 6 years, and 20-year survival is just 13%.[79] Treatment of recurrence remains challenging, but further surgery is often considered.[80]

Spinal tumors

A similar spectrum of tumors arises in the spine as in the brain, although the frequency of occurrence is different, and some types are absent. Tumors may be grouped according to their site of occurrence into extra-dural (metastasis, chordoma, and sarcoma), intra-dural/extra-medullary (meningioma and neurofibroma), and intra-medullary (astrocytomas, ependymomas, and benign tumors).

For all sites, the commonest presentation is with pain and/or loss of function at and below the level of the lesion. Tumors cause functional loss by direct pressure, generation of spinal edema, spinal infarction, invasion into spinal tissue, and growth along nerve roots. Almost any pattern of motor deficit may occur. Combinations of complete and partial upper and lower motor neuron lesions arise as the tumor develops. Likewise, sensory deficits may be complex.

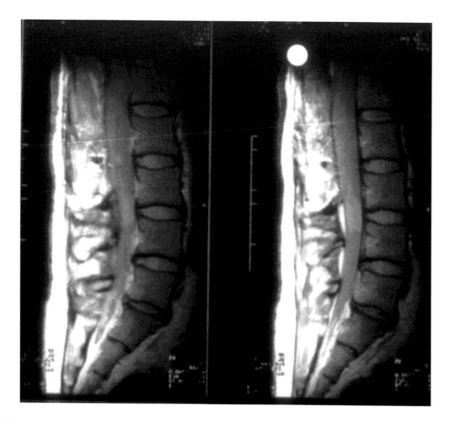

FIGURE 1.13 Radiological appearance of a spinal ependymoma on contrast enhanced MRI, showing a well-circumscribed lesion in the cauda equina.

Plain spinal x-rays still play an important role in the early evaluation of a patient suspected of having metastatic disease, but MRI is the definitive investigation for delineating tumors of the cord and dura (Figure 1.13).

Surgery is the mainstay of treatment for many low-grade spinal tumors. Good results can be expected from the complete excision of meningiomas, neurofibromas, pilocytic astrocytomas, and ependymomas. However, surgical decompression of spinal metastases, fibrillary astrocytomas and AAs, and high-grade ependymomas should usually be followed by post-operative radiotherapy. Spinal cord compression due to an intra-medullary tumor nearly always requires urgent decompression.

Radiotherapy may be given with palliative or radical intent. For palliation, either direct posterior or opposed fields are used to deliver short courses of treatment. Doses of 30 Gy in 10 fractions and 20 Gy in five fractions are common in metastatic disease. Higher doses for radical treatments are often delivered using a technique based on a wedged pair of fields, or more complex delivery techniques such as IMRT can be used. For treatments to low-grade tumors, doses of 45–50 Gy in 1.8 Gy fractions are usual, but for highly malignant tumors, doses up to 60 Gy may be appropriate. Although the risk to the spinal cord from the radiation is increased at these doses, it may not be as high as previously thought, provided megavoltage x-rays are used and the dose per fraction is kept below 2 Gy. This risk must be balanced against the risk of under-treating the tumor and the consequences of early re-growth.

Spinal astrocytomas

The majority of spinal astrocytomas are low grade, but the precise histology is important. If the tumor is pilocytic, the outcome following surgery is usually good, and the value of adjuvant radiotherapy is doubtful. Diffuse astrocytoma, usually fibrillary, has a less good prospect. It is difficult for the surgeon to find any plane between tumor and normal tissue, and there is less argument about the need for additional radiotherapy. Most patients do not survive more than 5 years.[81] AAs and GBMs occur rarely in the spine, but when they do, they should be treated as their cerebral counterparts with surgery and radiotherapy. The prognosis is very poor.

Spinal ependymomas

Ependymomas may arise anywhere in the spine but have a predilection for the lower end around the conus. Ectopic extra-spinal tumors may develop in the pre-sacral region. Most are low grade. A clear operative plane is often found, and complete excision may be possible. In this situation, only follow-up is required. If complete excision is not obtained, adjuvant radiotherapy is often given, but clear evidence of its value is lacking. For low-grade tumors, this would comprise local radiotherapy only. High-grade tumors can rarely be excised completely, and post-operative radiotherapy is required.

The variant myxopapillary ependymoma is found almost exclusively in the conus/cauda equina region. It is treated surgically and has a particularly favorable prognosis.

Malignancy metastatic to the brain

Metastasis to the brain from systemic malignancy is common, occurring in at least 10% of cancer patients. Further, the incidence appears to be increasing, not only from common primaries such as breast,[82] lung, kidney, and melanoma but also from those thought rarely to give rise to brain metastasis, such as prostate.

The outlook for most patients remains poor, and treatment is symptomatic and palliative, with a significant proportion of patients dying a neurologic death. However a minority, although still rarely curable, has a better outlook and merits a more aggressive approach to management. The principal prognostic factors are age; performance status; presence of uncontrolled systemic disease; primary histology; and importantly, the number of metastases present. Scoring systems to aid decision-making and trial stratification such as the graded prognostic assessment tool are available.[83] In general, only those with small-volume oligometastatic disease, or those with chemo-sensitive disease, are likely to benefit from aggressive treatment.

The majority of patients will present with symptomatic disease, and the first step in management is to offer symptomatic care, which usually includes corticosteroids. Thereafter, the patient should be assessed for possible further treatment.

Whole-brain radiotherapy

Until recently, WBRT was the standard of care for the great majority of patients with brain metastasis and was given with palliative intent. However, its role in palliation is now being questioned. Much of the literature claiming a survival advantage is flawed, with selection bias being a common problem. Symptomatic improvement and reduced steroid requirement may be observed clinically following irradiation, but this is at the expense of hair loss and frequently, debilitating lethargy. Overall, the benefit is unclear. The QUARTZ trial in the United Kingdom compared best standard of care (BSC) with BSC plus WBRT for patients with brain metastases from non-small-cell lung cancer. These data have shown no difference in either survival or QOL between the two arms, with the expected toxicities of hair loss, drowsiness, and scalp changes experienced after WBRT.[84] For patients with large-volume disease or multiple metastases and poor performance status after steroid use, there is little to be gained from WBRT. For those with Karnofsky performance status (KPS) 70 or greater, it is reasonable to discuss WBRT and the possibility of some degree of tumor control, but with the aforementioned drawbacks. There is little to suggest that regimes other than 20 Gy in five fractions to opposed fields have any worthwhile advantage. Entry into clinical trials, where available, is probably the best option, and with the development of more novel systemic treatments for common cancers that metastasize to brain, including brain penetrant agents, more studies are becoming available.

Management of oligo-metastatic disease

Oligo-metastatic disease is defined as one to three metastases in the brain. Microsurgery and SRS have become standard tools in this condition. Both techniques have demonstrated a survival advantage for patients with single metastases.[85,86] Where more than one metastasis is present, a survival advantage has not been demonstrated, but focal therapy can still achieve symptomatic control with less morbidity compared with WBRT. Not all patients are suitable for this, and selection for treatment should include recognition of other prognostic factors, including age and performance status.

Pragmatism determines the choice of treatment modality. Larger lesions associated with brain distortion are best treated with surgery to relieve pressure, particularly for example in the posterior fossa. Smaller lesions, multiple lesions, and lesions in inaccessible sites or adjacent to eloquent regions are best treated with SRS, which is also likely to be the less expensive option.

The value of adjuvant WBRT after localized treatment remains controversial. Although studies consistently demonstrate an improvement in local control, and small series suggest an impact on survival in patients with solitary lesions, paradoxically, there is no measurable impact on either survival or (surrogate) measures of QOL.[87] In addition, some data suggest a significant incidence of cognitive decline after WBRT. Hence, it is unclear whether patients should be offered immediate WBRT or surveillance, with WBRT or radiosurgery at relapse. Following surgery, there is a relatively high incidence of early relapse at the resection site; hence, a further option might be to offer radiosurgery following surgical excision to reduce this phenomenon while still avoiding the ill effects of WBRT. Recent data from a study comparing surgery with WBRT versus surgery and salvage radiosurgery to sites of residual disease suggested no difference in overall survival outcomes, although progression-free survival was longer in the WBRT group.[88]

Role of chemotherapy

There is increasing awareness that for patients with chemo-sensitive disease, systemic therapy might offer a reasonable first-line option for intracranial metastases. Small-cell lung cancer, ovarian cancer, germ cell tumors, and even breast cancer can respond well to regimens containing agents possessing some degree of BBB penetration, such as platinum. Although this offers an alternative to WBRT, it must be remembered that most patients have a poor prognosis, and best supportive care may remain the optimal care for them.

Chemotherapy, given as an adjunct to WBRT, has been disappointing and is not currently recommended outside clinical trials.

Prophylactic cranial irradiation

Some cancers have a marked predisposition to produce intracerebral metastases. It has been demonstrated in small-cell lung cancer that prophylactic cranial irradiation (PCI) can reduce the incidence of cerebral metastases and improve survival,[89] and this principle is now being explored in other high-risk diseases such as her-2 positive breast cancer and non-small-cell lung cancer. The drawback of this approach is the risk of radiation-induced neuro-cognitive damage following PCI. The use of complex radiotherapy delivery systems (IMRT and VMAT) to spare the limbic system, where the incidence of metastases is low, while maintaining radiation dose to the rest of the brain may help to reduce this side effect.

Key learning points

- CNS tumors encompass a very broad range of histologies with huge variation in expected outcomes.
- Brain tumors account for a significant proportion of lives lost to cancer, since the commonest diagnoses in adults and children can be associated with a very poor prognosis.
- Diagnosis is increasingly reliant on molecular pathology alongside conventional histology to define sub-groups of patients who may benefit from specific treatments.
- Combination therapy of maximal safe debulking surgery, radiation, and chemotherapy is used for the majority of malignant tumors.
- Diagnosis, surgery, radiotherapy planning, and follow-up rely on MRI imaging in most cases. Novel imaging approaches, to better monitor treatment response and early progression, are under investigation.
- All tumor types require multi-disciplinary management, and holistic support for patients with poor-prognosis tumors is crucial in maintaining QOL.

Useful websites

Specific guidance documents

www.esmo.org/Guidelines/Neuro-Oncology/High-Grade-
Malignant-Glioma
www.eano.eu/publications/eano-guidelines/
https://seer.cancer.gov/statfacts/html/brain.html
www.nice.org.uk/guidance/csg10
www.nice.org.uk/guidance/NG99
https://www.rcpath.org/uploads/assets/abc54563-f574-
40a0-6b9a9a2cfbaa89d/g069-dataset-forhistopatholog-
cal-reportingof-tumours-ofthe-central-nervous-system-
inadults-includingthe-pituitarygland.pdf

Patient and carer support

www.cancer.gov/types/brain
www.cancerresearchuk.org/about-cancer/brain-tumours
www.thebraintumourcharity.org/brain-tumour-diagnosis-tr
eatment/how-brain-tumours-are-diagnosed/brain-tumo
ur-biology/what-is-a-brain-tumour/
http://braintumouraction.org.uk/

References

1. CRUK. CancerStats. https://www.cancerresearchuk.org/health-professional/cancer-statistics-for-the-uk#heading-Zero/.
2. Rice T, Lachance DH, Molinaro AM et al. Understanding inherited genetic risk in adult glioma. A review. *Neurooncol Pract.* 2016; 3(1):10–16.
3. Louis DN, Perry A, Reifenberger G et al. The 2016 World Health Organisation classification of tumours of the central nervous system: a summary. *Acta Neuropathol.* 2016; 131(6):803–20.
4. Kristensen BW, Priesterbach-Ackley LP, Petersen JK, Wesseling P. Molecular pathology of tumours of the central nervous system. *Ann Oncol.* 2019 Aug 1;30(8):1265–78.
5. Louis DN, Aldape K, Brat DJ et al. Announcing c-IMPACT-NOW: the consortium to inform molecular and practical approaches to CNS tumour taxonomy. *Acta Neuropathol.* 2017;133(1):1–3.
6. Dias-Santagata D, Lam Q, Vernovsky K et al. BRAF V600E mutations are common in pleomorphic xanthoastrocytoma: diagnostic and therapeutic implications. *PLoS One.* 2011;6(3):e17948.
7. Lassaletta A, Zapotocky M, Mistry M et al. Therapeutic and prognostic implications of BRAF V600E in pediatric low-grade gliomas. *J Clin Oncol.* 2017;35(25):2934–41.
8. Kleinschmidt-DeMasters BK, Aisner DL, Birks DK, Foreman NK. Epithelioid GBMs show a high percentage of BRAF V600E mutation. *Am J Surg Pathol.* 2013;37(5):685–98.
9. Hyman DM, Puzanov I, Subbiah V et al. Vemurafenib in multiple nonmelanoma cancers with BRAF V600 mutations. *N Engl J Med.* 2015;373(8):726–36.
10. Turcan S, Rohle D, Goenka A et al. IDH1 mutation is sufficient to establish the glioma hypermethylator phenotype. *Nature.* 2012; 483(7390):479–83.
11. Eckel-Passow JE, Lachance DH, Molinaro AM et al. Glioma groups based on 1p19q, IDH, and TERT promoter mutations in tumours. *N Engl J Med.* 2015; 372(26):2499–508.
12. Van den Bent MJ, Brandes AA, Taphoorn MJ, et al. Adjuvant procarbazine, lomustine, and vincristine chemotherapy in newly diagnosed anaplastic oligodendroglioma: long-term follow-up of EORTC brain tumor group study 26951. *J Clin Oncol.* 2013; 31(3):344–50.
13. Cairncross G, Wang M, Shaw E et al. Phase III trial of chemoradiotherapy for anaplastic oligodendroglioma: Long-term results of RTOG 9402. *J Clin Oncol.* 2013; 31:337–43.
14. Hegi ME, Diserens AC, Gorlia T et al. MGMT gene silencing and benefit from temozolomide in glioblastoma. *N Engl J Med.* 2005; 352:997–1003.
15. Westphal M, Maire CL, Lamszus K. EGFR as a target for glioblastoma treatment: An unfulfilled promise. *CNS Drugs.* 2017; 31(9):723–35.
16. Sahm F, Schrimpf D, Stichel D et al. DNA methylation based classification and grading system for meningioma: a multicentre retrospective analysis. Lancet Oncol. 2017; 18(5):682–94.
17. Pfaff E, Al Damaty A, Balasubramanian GP et al. Brain stem biopsy in pediatric diffuse intrinsic pontine glioma in the era of precision medicine: the INFORM study experience. *Eur J Cancer.* 2019; 114:27–35.
18. Louveau A, Smirnov I, Keyes TJ et al. Structural and functional features of central nervous system lymphatic vessels. *Nature.* 2015; 523(7560):337–41.
19. Wen PY, Chang S, Van den Bent M et al. Response assessment in neuro oncology clinical trials. *J Clin Oncol.* 2017; 35(21):2439–49.
20. Law I, Albert NL, Arbizu J et al. Joint EANM/EANO/RANO guidelines/SNMMI procedure standards for imaging of gliomas using PET with radiolabelled amino acids and 18F-FDG. *Eur J Nucl Med Mol Imag.* 2019; 46(3):540–57.
21. Stummer W and Kamp M. The importance of surgical resection in malignant glioma. *Curr Opin Neurol.* 2009; 22:645–9.
22. Rossi M, Ambrogi F, Gay L et al. Is supratotal resection achievable in low-grade gliomas? Feasibility, putative factors, safety and functional outcome. *J Neurosurg.* 2019 May 17;132(6):1692–705.
23. Hart MG, Grant GR, Solyom EF, Grant R. Biopsy versus resection for high grade glioma. *Cochrane Database Syst. Rev.* 2019; 6:CD002034.
24. Ellison DW. Childhood medulloblastoma: Novel approaches to the classification of a heterogeneous disease. *Acta Neuropathol.* 2010; 120:305–16.
25. Leroy HA, Delmaire C, Le Rhun et al. High-field intraoperative MRI and glioma surgery: results after the first 100 consecutive patients. *Acta Neurochir (Wien).* 2019.
26. Stummer W, Pichlmeier U, Meinel T et al. Fluorescence-guided surgery with 5-aminolevulinic acid for resection of malignant glioma: a randomised controlled multicentre phase III trial. *Lancet Oncol.* 2006; 7:392–401.
27. Gerritsen JKW, Arends L, Klimek M et al. Impact of intraoperative stimulation mapping on high-grade glioma surgery outcome: a meta-analysis. *Acta Neurochir (Wien).* 2019; 16(1):99–107.
28. Westphal M, Hilt DC, Bortey E et al. A phase 3 trial of local chemotherapy with biodegradable carmustine (BCNU) wafers (Gliadel wafers) in patients with primary malignant glioma. *Neuro-Oncology.* 2003; 5:79–88.
29. Nieder C, Astner ST, Mehta MP et al. Improvement, clinical course, and quality of life after palliative radiotherapy for recurrent glioblastoma. *Am J Clin Oncol.* 2008; 31(3):300–5.
30. Shepherd SF, Laing RW, Cosgrove VP et al. Hypofractionated stereotactic radiotherapy in the management of recurrent glioma. *Int J Radiat Oncol Biol Phys.* 1997; 37(2):393–8.
31. Shanker M, Chua B, Bettington C, et al. Re-irradiation for recurrent high grade gliomas: a systematic review and analysis of treatment technique with respect to survival and risk of radionecrosis. *Neuro-Oncol. Pract.* 2018;npy019:1–12.
32. Sanghera P, Rampling R, Haylock H et al. The concepts, diagnosis and management of early imaging changes following therapy for glioblastomas. *Clin Oncol (Royal College of Radiologists).* 2012; 24:216–27.
33. Lawrence Y, Li A, Naqa I et al. Radiation dose-volume effects in the brain. *Int J Radiat Oncol Biol Phys.* 2010; 76 Supplement: S28–S35.
34. Mayo C, Martel M, Marks L et al. Radiation dose-volume effects of optic nerves and chiasm. *Int J Radiat Oncol Biol Phys.* 2010; 76 Supplement:S28–S35.
35. Belka C, Budach W, Kortmann RD, Bamberg M. Radiation induced CNS toxicity-molecular and cellular mechanisms. *Br J Cancer.* 2001; 85(9):1233–9.
36. Kirkpatrick JP, van der Kogel AJ, Schultheiss TE. Radiation dose-volume effects in the spinal cord. *Int J Radiat Oncol Biol Phys.* 2010; 76(3):S42–S49.
37. Vogelbaum MA, Brewer C, Barnett GH et al. First-in-human evaluation of the cleveland multiport catheter for convection-enhanced

delivery of topotecan in recurrent high-grade glioma: results of pilot trial 1. *J Neurosurg.* 2018 Apr 13;130(2):476–85.

38. Gilbert MR, Dignam JJ, Armstrong TS et al. A randomized trial of bevacizumab for newly diagnosed glioblastoma. *N Engl J Med.* 2014; 370(8):699–708.

39. Chinot OL, Wick W, Mason W et al. Bevacizumab plus radiotherapy-temozolomide for newly diagnosed glioblastoma. *N Engl J Med.* 2014; 370(8):709–22.

40. Paolillo M, Boselli C, Schinelli S. Glioblastoma under siege: An overview of current therapeutic strategies. *Brain Sci.* 2018 Jan;8(1):15.

41. Chinnaiyan P, Won M, Wen PY et al. A randomized phase II study of everolimus in combination with chemoradiation in newly diagnosed glioblastoma: results of NRG oncology RTOG 0913. *Neuro Oncol.* 2018; 20(5):666–673.

42. Rooney A, McNamara S, Mackinnon M et al. The frequency, clinical associations and longitudinal course of major depressive disorder in adults with cerebral glioma. *J Clin Oncol.* 2011; 29:4307–12.

43. Gnekow AK, Falkenstein F, von Hornstein S et al. Long-term follow-up of the multi-centre treatment study HIT-LGG-1996 for low-grade glioma in children and adolescents of the german speaking society of pediatric oncology and hematology. *Neuro Oncol.* 2012; 14(10):1265–84.

44. Jakola AS, Skjulsvik AJ, Myrmel KS et al. Surgical resection versus watchful waiting in low-grade gliomas. *Ann Oncol.* 2017; 28(8):1942–48.

45. Pignatti F, Van den Bent M, Curran D et al. Prognostic factors for survival in adult patients with cerebral low-grade glioma. *J Clin Oncol.* 2002; 20:2076–84.

46. Baumert BG, Hegi ME, van den Bent MJ et al. Temozolomide chemotherapy versus radiotherapy in high-risk low-grade glioma (EORTC 22033–26033): a randomised, open-label, phase 3 intergroup study. *Lancet Oncol.* 2016; 17(11):1521–32.

47. Karim A, Maat B, Hatlevoll R et al. A randomized trial on dose-response in radiation therapy of low grade cerebral glioma: European organization for research and treatment of cancer (EORTC) study 22844. *Int J Radiat Oncol Biol Phys.* 1996; 36:549–56.

48. Shaw E, Arusell R, Scheithauer B et al. A prospective randomized trial of low versus high dose radiation in adults with a supratentorial low grade glioma: Initial report of an NCCTG-RTOG-ECOG study. *J Clin Oncol.* 2002 May 1;20(9):2267–76.

49. Van den Bent M, Baumert B, Erridge SC et al. Interim results from the CATNON trial (EORTC study 26053–22054) of treatment with concurrent and adjuvant temozolomide for 1p/19q non co-deleted anaplastic glioma: a phase 3, randomized, open label intergroup study. *Lancet.* 2017; 390(10103).

50. Cancer Genome Atlas Research Network. Comprehensive genomic characterization defines human glioblastoma genes and core pathways. *Nature.* 2008; 455:1061–8.

51. Stupp R, Brada M, van den Bent M et al. High-grade glioma: ESMO clinical practice guidelines for diagnosis, treatment and follow-up. *Ann Oncol.* 2014; 25(suppl 3):iii93–101.

52. Sage W, Guilfoyle M, Luney C et al. Local alkylating chemotherapy applied immediately after 5-ALA guided resection of glioblastoma does not provide additional benefit. *J Neurooncol.* 2018; 136(2):273–280.

53. Walker MD, Green SB, Byar DP et al. Randomized comparisons of radiotherapy and nitrosoureas for the treatment of malignant glioma after surgery. *N Engl J Med.* 1980; 303:1323–9.

54. Niyazi M, Brada M, Chalmers AJ et al. ESTRO-ACROP guideline "target delineation of glioblastomas". *Radiother Oncol.* 2016; 118(1):35–42.

55. Stupp R, Hegi ME, Mason WP et al. Effects of radiotherapy with -concomitant and adjuvant temozolomide versus radiotherapy alone on survival in glioblastoma in a randomised phase III study: 5-year analysis of the EORTC-NCIC trial. *Lancet Oncol.* 2009; 10:459–66.

56. Perry JR, Laperriere N, O'Callaghan CJ et al. Short-course radiation plus temozolomide in elderly patients with glioblastoma. *N Engl J Med.* 2017; 376(11):1027–37.

57. Brada M, Stenning S, Gabe R et al. Temozolomide versus procarbazine, lomustine, and vincristine in recurrent high-grade glioma. *J Clin Oncol.* 2010; 28:4601–8.

58. Wick W, Weller M, van den Bent M et al. Bevacizumab and recurrent malignant gliomas: a European perspective. *J Clin Oncol.* 2010; 28:12e188–9.

59. Shaw EG, Wang M, Coons SW et al. Randomized trial of radiation therapy plus procarbazine, lomustine and vincristine chemotherapy for supratentorial adult low-grade glioma: initial results of RTOG 9802. *J Clin Oncol.* 2012; 30(25):3065–70.

60. Pajtler KW, Witt H, Sill M et al. Molecular classification of ependymal tumors across All CNS compartments, histopathological grades, and age groups. *Cancer Cell.* 2015; 27(5):728–43.

61. Pajtler KW, Mack SC, Ramaswamy V et al. The current consensus on the clinical management of intracranial ependymoma and its distinct molecular variants. *Acta Neuropathol.* 2017; 133(1): 5–12.

62. Lehman NL, Hattab EM, Mobley BC et al. Morphological and molecular features of astroblastoma, including BRAFV600E mutations, suggest an ontological relationship to other cortical-based gliomas of children and young adults. *Neuro Oncol.* 2017; 19(1):31–42.

63. Tonse R, Gupta T, Epari S et al. Impact of WHO 2016 update of brain tumor classification, molecular markers and clinical outcomes in pleomorphic xanthoastrocytoma. *J Neurooncol.* 2018; 136(2):343–50.

64. Shapey J, Danesh-Meyer HV, Kaye AH. Diagnosis and management of optic nerve glioma. *J Clin Neurosci.* 2011; 18(12):1585–91.

65. Pekmezci M, Villanueva-Meyer JE, Goode B et al. The genetic landscape of ganglioglioma. *Acta Neuropathol Commun.* 2018; 6(1):47.

66. Kaley T, Touat M, Subbiah V et al. BRAF inhibition in BRAF(V600)-mutant gliomas: Results from the VE-BASKET Study. *J Clin Oncol.* 2018:JCO2018789990.

67. Sievers P, Stichel D, Schrimpf D et al. FGFR1:TACC1 fusion is a frequent event in molecularly defined extraventricular neurocytoma. *Acta Neuropathol.* 2018; 136(2):293–302.

68. Sharma T, Schwalbe EC, Williamson D et al. Second-generation molecular subgrouping of medulloblastoma: an international meta-analysis of Group 3 and Group 4 subtypes. *Acta Neuropathol.* 2019.

69. Bi WL, Zhang M, Wu WW et al. Meningioma genomics: Diagnostic, prognostic and therapeutic applications. *Front Surg.* 2016; 3:40.

70. Smee R, Williams J, Kotevski D, Schneider M. radiotherapy as a means of treating meningiomas. *J Clin Neurosci.* 2019; 61:210–8.

71. Goldbrunner R, Minniti G, Preusser M et al. EANO guidelines for the diagnosis and treatment of meningiomas. *Lancet Oncol.* 2016; 17(9):e383–91.

72. Ferreri AJ, Reni M, Foppoli M et al. High-dose cytarabine plus high-dose methotrexate versus high-dose methotrexate alone in patients with primary CNS lymphoma: a randomised phase 2 trial. *Lancet.* 2009; 374(9700):1512–20.

73. Ferreri AJ, Cwynarski K, Pulczynski E et al. Chemoimmunotherapy with methotrexate, cytarabine, thiotepa, and rituximab (MATRix regimen) in patients with primary CNS lymphoma: results of the first randomisation of the International Extranodal Lymphoma Study Group-32 (IELSG32) phase 2 trial. *Lancet Haematol.* 2016; 3(5):e217–27.

74. Fox CP, Phillips EH, Smith J et al. Guidelines for the diagnosis and management of primary central nervous system diffuse large B-cell lymphoma. *Br J Haematol.* 2019; 184(3):348–63.

75. Houillier C, Taillandier L, Dureau S et al. Radiotherapy or autologous stem cell transplantation for primary CNS lymphoma in patients 60 years of age and younger: results of the intergroup ANOCEF-GOELAMS randomized phase II PRECIS study. *J Clin Oncol.* 2019; 37(10):823–33.

76. Kim J, Kim W, Cho J et al. A multimodal approach including craniospinal irradiation improves the treatment outcome of high-risk intracranial nongerminomatous germ cell tumors. *Int J Radiat Oncol Biol.* 2012; 84:625–31.

77. Goldman S, Bouffet E, Fisher PG et al. Phase II trial assessing the ability of neoadjuvant chemotherapy with or without second-look surgery to eliminate measurable disease for nongerminomatous germ cell tumors: A children's oncology group study. *J Clin Oncol.* 2015; 33(22):2464–71.

78. Murray MJ, Bartels U, Nishikawa R, Fangusaro J, Matsutani M, Nicholson JC. Consensus on the management of intracranial germ-cell tumours. *Lancet Oncol.* 2015; 16(9):e470–e778.

79. Walcott BP, Nahed BV, Mohyeldin A et al. Chordoma: Current concepts, management, and future directions. *Lancet Oncol.* 2012; 13:e69–76.

80. Stacchiotti S, Gronchi A, Fossati P et al. Best practices for the management of local-regional recurrent chordoma: a position paper by the chordoma global consensus group. *Ann Oncol.* 2017; 28(6):1230–42.

81. Liu J, Zheng M, Yang W et al. Impact of surgery and radiation therapy on spinal high-grade gliomas: a population-based study. *J Neurooncol.* 2018; 139(3):609–16.

82. Frisk G, Svensson T, Backlund LM et al. Incidence and time trends of brain metastases admissions among breast cancer patients in Sweden. *Br J Cancer.* 2012; 106:1850–3.

83. Sperduto PW, Berkey B, Gaspar LE et al. A new prognostic index and comparison to three other indices for patients with brain metastases: An analysis of 1,960 patients in the RTOG database. *Int J Radiat Oncol Biol Phys.* 2008; 70:510–14.

84. Mulvenna P, Nankivell M, Barton R et al. Dexamethasone and supportive care with or without whole brain radiotherapy in treating patients with non-small cell lung cancer with brain metastases unsuitable for resection or stereotactic radiotherapy (QUARTZ): results from a phase 3, non-inferiority, randomised trial. *Lancet.* 2016; 388(10055):2004–14.

85. Andrews DW, Scott CB, Sperduto PW et al. Whole brain radiation therapy with or without stereotactic radiosurgery boost for patients with one to three brain metastases: Phase III results of the RTOG 9508 randomised trial. *Lancet.* 2004; 363:1665–72.

86. Patchell RA, Tibbs PA, Walsh JW et al. A randomized trial of surgery in the treatment of single metastases to the brain. *N Engl J Med.* 1990; 322:494–500.

87. Kocher M, Soffietti R, Abacioglu U et al. Adjuvant whole-brain radiotherapy versus observation after radiosurgery or surgical resection of one to three cerebral metastases: Results of the EORTC 22952–26001 study. *J Clin Oncol.* 2011; 29:134–41.

88. Kayama T, Sato S, Sakurada K et al. Effects of surgery with salvage stereotactic radiosurgery versus surgery with whole-brain radiation therapy in patients with one to four brain metastases (JCOG0504): A phase III, noninferiority, randomized controlled trial. *J Clin Oncol.* 2018:JCO2018786186.

89. Slotman B, Faivre-Finn C, Kramer G et al. Prophylactic cranial irradiation in extensive small-cell lung cancer. *N Engl J Med.* 2007; 357:664–72.

2 ADULT OCULAR AND ORBITAL (OCULAR ADNEXA) TUMORS

P.N. Plowman, Rachel Lewis, and J.L. Hungerford

Tumors of the eye and of the ocular adnexa are much more common in adults than in children. Apart from choroidal nevi and benign papillomas of the eyelids, the most frequently encountered neoplasms are malignant. In contrast to those of children, many adult intra-ocular malignant neoplasms are metastatic, the treatment of which is considered in the context of the whole systemic relapse. For adult primary malignant intra-ocular tumors, the overall cure rates remain relatively low, although a trend towards earlier detection during routine eye testing has produced some improvement in outlook, as have more modern oncology therapies for established disease.

Unlike intra-ocular malignancies, the majority of adult adnexal neoplasms are primary tumors. This contrasts once again with the situation in children, where adnexal malignancies are commonly metastatic or related to a blood dyscrasia. Orbital malignant tumors may have relatively good cure rates in adults because they are only locally invasive. Death from such a neoplasm usually results from direct local extension rather than metastatic spread. The outlook is similarly good for most malignant tumors of the eyelids and conjunctiva, because they seem to have a lower propensity to regional and distant spread than their equivalents in other structures.

Benign tumors are common in the eye and its adnexa. The importance of these tumors is that many are associated with familial diseases (clinical genetics' opinion often needs consideration) and, because of their location, complex treatment may be required to preserve vision or to reduce cosmetic deficit.

Benign tumors of the eye

The more common benign intra-ocular tumors in adults are of melanocytic, smooth-muscle, or vascular origin.

Melanocytic tumors

Melanocytic tumors are overwhelmingly the most numerous. Nevi arise from uveal melanocytes in the iris, ciliary body, and choroid. There is no doubt that nevi may occasionally undergo malignant change and that most uveal tract malignant melanomas arise in this way. Choroidal nevi are extremely common, but the chance of malignant change has been estimated to be less than 1 in 500 during a 5-year period. It is impractical to propose regular follow-up for all innocent, flat nevi. Nevertheless, repeated examinations are advised for all iris nevi and for raised choroidal lesions, those developing orange lipofuscin pigment, those with an associated serous retinal detachment or visual field defect, and those with multiple nevi. Patients with ocular or oculodermal melanocytosis also have an increased risk of uveal melanoma and should undergo regular examination of the ocular fundi.

Smooth-muscle tumors

Smooth-muscle tumors are represented by leiomyomas, which are slow-growing, pale, and benign tumors. Leiomyomas are rare in the eye and have been described most frequently in the iris, with a few cases reported in the ciliary body. Re-evaluation of archival histological material suggests, however, that most so-called iris leiomyomas are really amelanotic benign melanocytic lesions. The only true ocular leiomyomas arise in the ciliary body, where they may grow quite large and are difficult to clinically distinguish from amelanotic melanomas. Ciliary-body leiomyomas are very circumscribed tumors that are easily excised from within the eye, the main indication for this procedure being exclusion of the alternative diagnosis of malignant melanoma.

Vascular tumors

Vascular tumors may occur in the retina but are more common in the choroid. Most retinal lesions are capillary hemangiomas, which may be solitary or multiple. New retinal hemangiomas may arise throughout life in the von Hippel–Lindau syndrome. They tend to grow and may ultimately lead to bilateral blindness from retinal detachment. Large capillary hemangiomas may respond to cryotherapy, but the best response rates are obtained by treating smaller lesions by cryotherapy or laser photocoagulation. For this reason, a policy of annual ocular assessment of von Hippel–Lindau patients from infancy is wise, with early treatment of all new tumors.

Cavernous hemangiomas are less common in the retina than tumors of the capillary type. The lesions are usually solitary, although the ocular tumor may be associated with skin or CNS vascular lesions as part of an inherited neuro-oculocutaneous syndrome, of which one bilateral case has been reported. The cavernous type of hemangioma rarely grows and is unlikely to lead to loss of vision unless it involves the macular area or unless it bleeds. Hemorrhage from one of these tumors may be treated by photocoagulation or cryotherapy.

Hemangiomas affecting the choroid are of cavernous type, though their histology and clinical behavior are different from those of cavernous hemangiomas occurring at other sites. They are of two types—circumscribed or diffuse. Most are circumscribed and first detected in adult life. Circumscribed choroidal hemangiomas are not associated with systemic abnormalities. A minority of hemangiomas are diffuse. Diffuse hemangiomas commonly present in children and young adults and are usually associated with vascular abnormalities of the skin and CNS, often as part of the Sturge–Weber syndrome. Choroidal hemangiomas grow slowly, if at all. Nevertheless, they may threaten vision by producing a localized or extensive serous retinal detachment. Serous exudation may be reduced by argon laser grid photocoagulation with retinal reattachment, but usually without destruction of the tumor. If detachment persists or recurs, sustained retinal reattachment and good tumor regression may be achieved by irradiating a circumscribed choroidal hemangioma to a dose of only 40 Gy to the apex of the lesion, using a radioactive scleral plaque.

Diffuse choroidal hemangiomas commonly produce extensive, blinding serous retinal detachment. These tumors are usually too extensive to respond to photocoagulation or to focal radiotherapy using a scleral plaque. Sustained retinal reattachment has been achieved in diffuse hemangioma by using fractionated external-beam radiotherapy to a dose of 20–40 Gy in 2–4 weeks, using a lens-sparing approach as introduced originally for retinoblastoma.[1] With more advanced radiotherapy techniques such as volumetric arc therapy (VMAT), the same dose distribution can be achieved.

Although usually there is no obvious hemangioma regression, the benefit of radiotherapy would appear to be both reduction in the leakage of serum by the tumor and vascular atrophy. Photodynamic therapy using a photosensitizing drug, verteporfin, in combination with focal laser application has been used to treat both circumscribed and diffuse-choroidal hemangiomas with encouraging short-term results.

Benign tumors of the eyelids, conjunctiva, and orbit

Benign tumors of the ocular adnexa are common and are of epithelial, vascular, neurogenic, melanocytic, or lacrimal-gland origin. Benign orbital tumors must be distinguished from idiopathic inflammatory pseudotumors.

Epithelial tumors

Epithelial tumors mainly comprise benign papillomas of the eyelid margin, which are extremely common and of viral origin. They are easily treated by shaving and light cautery to the base, but they tend to recur. Recurrent tumors may be managed by wedge excision. Seborrheic keratosis is particularly common in the elderly and may be treated by curettage. Cryotherapy may be performed for tumors of this type in pale-skinned individuals, but it should be avoided in those with darker coloring because it is likely to be followed by noticeable depigmentation.

Vascular tumors

Vascular tumors predominantly affect the orbit. In the adult, cavernous hemangioma is one of the most common primary orbital tumors. It usually presents in middle-aged women and is best managed by surgical resection via a lateral orbitotomy.

Peripheral nerve tumors

Peripheral nerve tumors are mostly neurofibromas. The majority of orbital neurofibromas in adults are solitary and not associated with neurofibromatosis. Recurrence after surgical excision is unusual. Schwannomas are much less common and are encapsulated tumors that rarely recur after surgical excision. Those arising in neurofibromatosis 1 may respond to the MEK inhibitor: selumetinib.

Melanocytic tumors

Melanocytic tumors are mainly nevocellular nevi, which are common in the skin of the eyelids and must be distinguished from pigmented basal-cell and squamous-cell lesions. Occasionally, a divided nevus is encountered that occupies the adjacent margins of both upper and lower eyelids and that has arisen from a single nevus by separation of the eyelids in embryonic life. Nevocellular nevi are best managed by infrequent observation. In oculodermal melanocytosis (nevus of Ota), there is widespread infiltration of the eyelid skin and of all ocular structures with plump melanocytes. The condition is most common in individuals of Asian and African extraction. Malignant change does not occur in the cutaneous element of nevus of Ota, but as well as being associated with an increased incidence of intra-ocular melanoma it may very occasionally be linked with the development of a primary orbital melanoma. Benign conjunctival nevi are frequently cystic. They are easily excised and, bearing in mind that malignant change can occur, this option should be considered as an alternative to long-term follow-up.

Lacrimal-gland tumors

These are usually of benign mixed-cell histology (e.g. pleomorphic adenoma) and are encapsulated. The whole affected lacrimal gland should be excised with the capsule intact via a lateral orbitotomy. Incisional biopsy is contraindicated because recurrence is common if the capsule is ruptured and there is a significant chance of malignant change in the recurrent tumor.

Primary malignant tumors of the eye in the adult

In contrast to those of children, the vast majority of adult intra-ocular malignancies arise in the uveal tract, and primary malignancies in the retina are very rare indeed.

Malignant tumors of the uveal tract

Malignant tumors of the uveal tract are predominantly malignant melanomas. Uveal melanoma is the most common of all primary intra-ocular tumors. The neoplasm is most commonly encountered in the choroid but also arises in the ciliary body and occasionally in the iris. This tumor was formerly managed by enucleation of the eye. The survival rate following enucleation has been shown to be dependent on the size of the tumor, histological cell type, tumor's position within the eye, presence or absence of extra-scleral extension, and age of the patient. Large melanomas, ciliary-body melanomas, and melanomas containing epithelioid cells or extending extra-sclerally have a relatively bad prognosis, particularly in the elderly. For large tumors, the overall mortality rate approaches 50%, and classically the mean interval reported from treatment to the development of metastases is 43 months. Metastases are rarely detectable at the time of diagnosis of the ocular primary.

The treatment of choice depends mainly on the location of the tumor within the eye and on its size.[2,3] The diagnosis of an intra-ocular tumor is usually based entirely on clinical criteria, with an accuracy of almost 98%, but fine-needle aspiration and cytology or formal biopsy through a scleral trap-door incision may be considered in cases of doubt that cannot be resolved by a period of observation with serial photographs and ultrasound measurements of tumor size, looking for evidence of growth.

Iris melanomas are generally relatively benign spindle-cell lesions, and overall mortality rates appear to be as low as 3%. Most iris tumors can be managed by observation alone, with treatment reserved for those that are documented to grow or that are large at presentation. In contrast to their counterparts in the iris, melanomas of the choroid, particularly those that develop in the ciliary body, are associated with particularly poor survival rates, of around 50% at 5 years for larger lesions.

Three main methods of conservative treatment are available: photocoagulation, radiation, and resection. Photocoagulation is applicable only to very small melanomas situated in the posterior choroid outside the macular arcades of vessels and not directly abutting the optic disc. Most of the reported experience has been obtained using xenon arc photocoagulation,[9] but in recent years argon and krypton lasers have been employed and the role of photosensitization with hematoporphyrin derivatives has been explored. Hyperthermia using diode laser-generated infrared radiation, the so-called transpupillary thermotherapy, has been employed with good short-term results. Photocoagulation and hyperthermia are not applicable to melanomas anteriorly located in the iris and ciliary body.

By contrast, local surgical resection is technically possible for some intra-ocular melanomas. Although easier to perform on small lesions arising anteriorly in the iris and ciliary body, the complication rate is higher than for tumors that develop posteriorly in the choroid and to which the method is most applicable.[4] The technique is limited to young, otherwise fit patients by the need for anesthesia, with profound hypotension a risk while cutting the highly vascular choroid. Tumors up to 15 mm in diameter may be excised, and overlying retinal detachment facilitates this operation. Local resection alone has a lower tumor control rate than plaque radiotherapy alone, so it is now advised that this operation should always be combined with adjuvant plaque therapy.[5]

Radiotherapy has been by far the most widely used treatment modality for the conservative therapy of intra-ocular melanomas and may be applicable to tumors in all locations within the uveal tract.[6] Melanoma is a radio-resistant neoplasm, whereas the lens of the eye and the choroid, retina, and optic nerve are relatively radiosensitive structures. A radiation-induced cataract can be safely removed, but radiation-induced chorioretinopathy and optic neuropathy are not amenable to treatment. The risk of these side effects increases at doses to the whole eye in excess of 50 Gy, whereas a tumor dose between 80 and 120 Gy is required to regress uveal melanoma.

The treatment methods employed have depended on the difficulty of confining this high dose to the vicinity of the ocular tumor and thereby of limiting the dose to the adjacent retina, choroid, and optic nerve. Until recently, it has only been possible to preserve the healthy structures of the eye by brachytherapy techniques, employing radioactive applicators temporarily sutured to the surface of the sclera over the base of the tumor within the eye. After initial successes with radon, the most widely used source was the cobalt-60 applicator, because the conveniently long half-life of this isotope allows the source to be re-used many times and because it is simple to reactivate. The γ-rays emitted by cobalt-60 are of high energy, and the external surface of the applicator cannot be effectively shielded. More recently, the low-energy β-ray-emitting ruthenium-106 and X-ray-emitting iodine-125 plaques used for RB treatments (Figure 2.1) have been employed to treat ocular melanomas up to 5 and 8 mm thick, respectively.[3]

These plaques can be shielded, which allows them to be used to treat anterior melanomas without damage to the eyelids and lacrimal apparatus, as well as making them safer to handle. A dose of 80–120 Gy is prescribed at the apex of the tumor at a dose rate of at least 0.4 Gy/h. Radiation-induced maculopathy and optic neuropathy limit the visual results of plaque therapy for tumors near the macula or optic disc. Because of the effects of the inverse square law, the dose received by the base of a neoplasm escalates substantially with increasing tumor thickness. Furthermore, the higher the dose at the base of the tumor, the larger the area of surrounding choroid and retina that receives a dose in excess of the 50 Gy above which there is a significant risk of ischemic damage to normal ocular structures (Figure 2.2). However, the intense dose to the tumor base may itself lead to infarction of the tumor, enhancing the tumoricidal effect.

Over the last two decades, it has become possible to avoid this important limitation of radioactive scleral plaques. The special properties of positively charged particulate external beam radiotherapy give this an advantageous dose distribution. Not only is the dose uniform from the base to apex of the tumor but the Bragg peak effect means that the entry dose is reduced and that the beam is extinguished behind the treated volume (Figure 2.3).

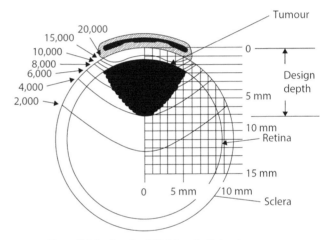

Dose distribution for CKA.3 (in cGy/6 days)

FIGURE 2.2 Dose distribution plot of 10-mm cobalt-60 applicator.

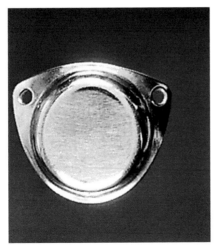 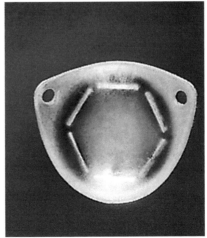

FIGURE 2.1 The iodine-125 ophthalmic applicator currently in use at St. Bartholomew's Hospital. Iodine-125 seeds are embedded in epoxy resin in a gold carrier.

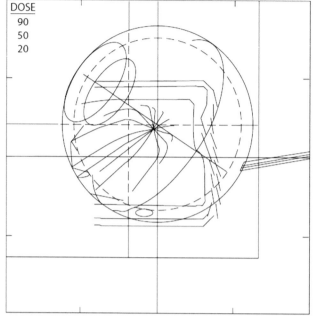

```
8411210            RIGHT EYE        8-SEP-84
PLANE WITHIN THE EYE
FIXATION LIGHT: POLAR 45 AZIMUTHAL 45 TWIST 0
EYE CENTER IS AT        0.50    0.40    0.00

DOSE
90
50
20

APERTURE IS: AP2
RANGE: 1.60        RANGE MODULATION: 1.60
PLANE POSITION PARALLEL TO BEAM X- -0.7 Y-0.0 Z-0.0
```

FIGURE 2.3 Computer-constructed plan for treatment by proton beam of an eye containing a malignant melanoma; 100%, 90%, and 50% isodose plots are shown and demonstrate the Bragg peak effect.

By employing protons or helium ions generated by a cyclotron or next-generation, linear accelerator-based, proton beam machines, these properties have allowed a high dose prescription of 60–70 Gy in 4 or 5 fractions to be delivered to ocular melanomas over 4–5 days, with the 50% isodose occurring within 2 mm of the tumor edge and with successful tumor regression. Survival rates have been comparable with those following enucleation.[8] Although charged particles can be used to treat melanomas that are too close to the optic disc to apply a radioactive scleral plaque or too thick for plaque brachytherapy, the surface-sparing advantages of the Bragg peak are progressively lost with increasing modulation of the beam to treat thicker and thicker tumors and tumors with anterior location. Consequently, eyelid damage limits the benefits of charged-particle therapy for larger and more anteriorly located melanomas. Moreover, the treatment of larger tumors may be followed by painful neovascular glaucoma, occasionally requiring enucleation.[8]

Gamma-knife stereotactic radiosurgery can also be used for the treatment of posterior uveal tract melanomas.[9] The treatment is delivered in one or two fractions, and this plainly contributes to the high rate of side effects, which are not dissimilar to those of charged-particle therapy. Nevertheless, with the new generation of proton beam machines becoming available, it is likely that proton therapy will dominate external-beam radiotherapy practice in the future.

When appropriately selected for radiotherapy, more than 90% of eyes can be retained.[10] The criterion of treatment success is shrinkage of the tumor or cessation of growth. Regression is slow and can continue episodically for 2 years or more. Melanomas less than 5-mm thickness will often regress to a flat scar, but larger tumors will usually have some residual thickness when regression ceases.

Enucleation is advised for large melanomas measuring more than 1.5 cm³ in volume. Ciliary-body melanomas occupying more than one-third of the circumference of the globe are too large to manage by resection or plaque therapy and are also best treated by enucleation. Circumscribed nodular extra-scleral extension may be managed by plaque therapy or by resection with a scleral graft, but extensive extra-scleral spread is better treated by removal of the eye. The presence of extra-scleral extension (Figure 2.4) reduces the survival rate and significantly increases the risk of orbital recurrence.[11,1] Orbital exenteration following enucleation for extra-scleral extension confers no survival advantage, and the risk of orbital recurrence can be substantially reduced by postoperative orbital radiotherapy.[12]

Prior to local therapy as outlined earlier, a baseline body scan (particularly with liver imaging in mind) is performed and subsequent post-treatment screening relies on serial liver function blood tests and/or imaging—more frequently in the early follow-up years.

It has long been recognized that cytogenetics can be prognostic in uveal melanoma, and loss of chromosome 3 (monosomy 3) is associated with poor prognosis. More recently, it has been realized that the biology of uveal melanoma differs from that of cutaneous melanoma. The vast majority (85–95%) of uveal melanoma is characterized by activating mutations in genes encoding the G-protein-alpha subunits *GNAQ* or *GNA11*, which lead to stimulation of the MAPK and phosphatidylinositol 3-kinase (PI3K)/ Akt pathways,[13–15] as well as the transcriptional co-activator Yes-associated protein 1 (YAP1) through the Trio-Rho/Rac signaling circuit. Additional mutations mutually exclusive to those in *GNAQ/11* have been identified in phospholipase C β4 (PLCB4) and the G-protein coupled receptor cysteinyl leukotriene receptor 2 (CYSLTR2), affirming the importance of the G-alpha signaling pathway in uveal melanoma.

Inactivating mutations in *BAP1*, a tumor suppressor gene located on chromosome 3p, are found in approximately 47% of primary uveal melanoma and 84% of metastatic uveal melanoma cases, consistent with the association between *BAP1* mutations

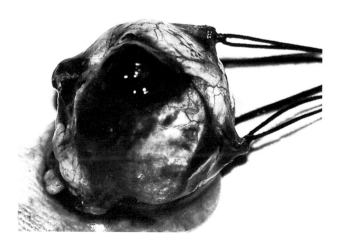

FIGURE 2.4 Enucleated eye, showing an encapsulated modular extra-scleral extension of malignant melanoma.

and poor prognosis.[16] Mutations in splicing factor 3B subunit 1 (*SF3B1*), involved in pre-messenger RNA splicing, while associated with more favorable prognostic features than *BAP1* mutations, are also found in cases of delayed metastasis, with a median of 8.2 years.[16,17] *EIF1AX* encodes for eukaryotic translation initiation factor 1A. These mutations are mutually exclusive from *BAP1* and *SF3B1* and are associated with a longer disease-free survival and a more favorable prognosis.

Unlike dermatological melanoma, B-RAF is rarely to never the driving oncogene in this disease and B-RAF inhibitors have virtually no role in therapeutics in this disease.

For patients with ocular melanocytosis, (dysplastic) nevi surveillance is advised as there is an increased risk of malignancy.

For patients with systemic relapse, cure is never possible. Immunotherapy has a modest response, for example, ipilimumab (a monoclonal antibody that targets the cytotoxic T lymphocyte associated antigen-4 [CTLA-4] receptor) has been demonstrated to be active—often in conjunction with a PD1 inhibitor such as nivolumab. So far, there have been small studies that demonstrate stability of metastatic ocular melanoma—response rates of circa 17% and stability rates of circa 50% with progression-free survival of a mean of 26 months—such that this is the current first-line approach.[17]

Current chemotherapy regimens include the intravenous co-administration of carboplatin and paclitaxel, which we have found to be superior to dacarbazine or temozolomide, but still have an objective response rate of less than 20%. In frail patients, we still might advise the less toxic, oral temozolomide first but with careful monitoring and use of the combined intravenous regime at the time of obvious progression.

With such lack of success with current systemic therapies, the recent results in researching molecular signaling pathway observations in this condition have brought new interest into the possible "druggable" targets in these tumor-specific, genetically/molecularly driven pathways.

As has been outlined above, the vast majority (85–95%) of uveal melanomas are characterized by activating mutations in genes encoding the G-protein-alpha subunits *GNAQ* or *GNA11*, which lead to stimulation of the MAPK and phosphatidylinositol 3-kinase (PI3K)/Akt pathways. Unfortunately, the use of MAPK pathway inhibitors has so far not led to major responses—perhaps 10% response rates.[18]

The various signaling pathways that are potential therapeutic targets in uveal melanoma include the MAPK, protein kinase C (PKC), and phosphoinositide 3-kinase (PI3K)/Akt/mammalian target of rapamycin (mTOR) pathways. Once again, these have not yet had a major effect in terms of clinical efficacy.

Developing from the monosomy 3 observations has come the discovery that BRCA-1-associated protein 1 (BAP1)—located on chromosome 3p21.1—is mutated in 85% of metastatic uveal melanomas, particularly in the higher risk cases. The fact that histone deacetylase inhibitors reverse the biochemical effects of BAP-1 functional loss by reversing H2A histone hyperrubiquitination may provide a druggable avenue to explore in therapeutics.[19]

In summary, although the new genetic discoveries regarding what drives ocular melanoma growth are potentially exciting, most are not yet ready for the clinic.

Given that the majority of first relapses from ocular melanoma occur in the liver, and not infrequently metachronously, liver-directed therapies may be appropriate for selected patients—surgery, radiofrequency ablation, and stereotactic body radiotherapy are all focal therapies that may be considered.

Malignant tumors of the retina

These are exceedingly uncommon. Cytologically malignant adenocarcinomas of the retinal pigment epithelium have been reported, although these lesions rarely, if ever, metastasize. They are pigmented and are usually a chance finding when an eye is removed for what is thought to be a malignant melanoma. For this reason, there are no data related to whether or not they can be managed conservatively.

Retinoblastoma, so important in children, is very rare in adult life.

Ocular lymphoma

Primary ocular lymphoma is a completely different disease from orbital lymphoma. Ocular lymphoma is a high-grade, usually B-cell, lymphoma with a strong predisposition to occur synchronously or metachronously in the brain and both eyes. The brain involvement is as solid mass disease (exactly as primary cerebral lymphoma—the same disease) and not leptomeningeal disease. This is the primary "oculocerebral" lymphoma; it usually presents to the ophthalmologist with involvement of the retina and vitreous, and the symptoms and signs can easily be confused with those of a posterior uveitis or vitritis, often delaying the diagnosis; vitreous biopsy is needed for diagnosis As there is no lymphatic connection from one orbit to the other, the bilateral ocular predisposition is of interest.

It is worth noting the (typically) different clinical picture when systemic lymphoma involves the eye. Here, the choroid is mainly involved—the lesions appearing as solid or well-defined creamy yellow choroidal lesions with a clear vitreous. With disease progression, both presentations merge and a systemic workup is always required.

Staging of primary ocular lymphoma requires expert binocular ophthalmoscopy and high-tesla MR imaging of the brain as the incidence of brain disease is common and therapy is directed to both sites. Spinal and systemic disease at presentation is unusual. Indeed the disease is often considered as one, i.e. primary central nervous system lymphoma with ocular involvement (PCNSLO). A body [18]FDG PET scan is recommended, although it is most frequently negative.

Treatment requires CNS and ocular penetrating drugs. Chemotherapy with high-dose methotrexate (at 3.5g/m^2 per course) plus cytosine arabinoside has been the "standard of care" until recently when more intensive regimens, with these two drugs plus thiotepa and rituximab have been added in the "Matrix protocol"[20]—followed by high-dose therapy with autologous stem cell transplant—in an attempt to increase cure rates and obviate the need for radiotherapy.

The routine addition of ocular and brain radiotherapy (even when scanning shows complete remission after four courses of standard pre-Matrix or similar chemotherapy) remained a slightly controversial topic but appeared to add to long-term disease-free survival modestly in the pre-Matrix era—at the expense of neuropsychological sequelae in long-term survivors. (Note that the order of high-dose methotrexate before brain radiotherapy is less morbid to the normal brain than vice versa.) Recently, the use of thiotepa has again been questioned and lower dose brain prophylactic radiotherapy (24 Gy) may be returning into first-line regimes. There have been a few deaths in the autograft series and there is now a continuing controversy as to the optimal best regime.

Nowadays, we usually employ radiotherapy in those patients who are not fit enough to receive the intensive chemotherapy. The controversy is then which patients to treat the only apparently afflicted eye versus those for whom it is indicated to widen the fields in the knowledge of the high risk of bilaterality and brain involvement risk—albeit metachronously.

Where radiotherapy is indicated (and we might note that this is indicated as sole therapy for the unusual low grade ocular lymphoma—as well as in elderly and frail patients), then for the patient who has presented with monocular disease, the eye receives 40–44 Gy conventionally fractionated.

If indicated (see above), it is advised to give prophylactic brain and contralateral eye radiotherapy at this time (30–34 Gy, conventionally fractionated).

Alternatives to systemic chemotherapy and radiotherapy include local chemotherapy into the eye—again for frail and elderly patients who are too unfit for high-dose systemic therapy: in unilateral cases, intravitreal methotrexate has been used in the dosage of 400 µg twice weekly for 4 weeks, followed by once weekly for 4 weeks, followed by once monthly for 12 months. It is used as a primary therapy as an alternative to radiotherapy or for cases of relapse. The risks associated are conjunctival injection and keratopathy. Sometimes these can be very severe which warrants the use of alternatives. Clinical remission is achieved after mean of 6.4 +/– 3.4 injection. Intravitreal rituximab, which is a chimeric anti-CD20 monoclonal antibody, can be used in the dosage of 1 mg/0.1 ml in cases which are unresponsive or cannot tolerate methotrexate.

The long-term prognosis of this rare lymphoma remains very guarded, with not more than 50% cure rates, notwithstanding aggressive chemoradiotherapy protocols such as those mentioned above.

Secondary deposits

Secondary deposits are usually seen in the uveal tract and only rarely seen in the retina, although choroidal metastases often present with a serous retinal detachment. The most common source of a choroidal metastasis is breast cancer. The ocular secondaries rarely present before the breast primary, and the deposits are commonly multiple and bilateral. The second most common source is lung cancer. An ocular deposit is, more often than not, detected before the lung primary and is usually solitary and unilateral. The treatment of ocular metastases is palliative and mainly by external-beam radiotherapy, although solitary metastases may be treated by plaque brachytherapy. Prior to radiotherapy for choroidal metastases, it is advisable to perform an MRI of the brain, as brain metastases frequently accompany ocular metastases and should be treated at the same radiotherapy session if present. It is legitimate to postpone irradiation for a short period and to watch for evidence of regression if the patient is to start chemotherapy, unless there is extensive retinal detachment, but our experience is that chemotherapy does not durably control these metastases and that radiotherapy maintains its important role in therapy. In the current era of genomically targeted therapy in oncology, we have seen responses of ocular metastases to tyrosine kinase inhibitors (TKI) (Figure 2.5), some of which are known to be active for brain metastases, but the ocular penetration of these drugs is less clear.

Photodynamic therapy may be employed to treat small, solitary choroidal metastases, metastases not controlled by radiotherapy, and rare new lesions arising in the previously irradiated choroid.

Primary malignant tumors of the eyelids, conjunctiva, and orbit/ocular adnexa

Like their benign counterparts, primary malignancies of the ocular adnexa are of epithelial, vascular, neurogenic, melanocytic, or lacrimal-gland origin.

Malignant epithelial tumors

These are relatively common. Basal-cell carcinoma is by far the most frequently encountered eyelid tumor, and the inner canthus is one of the most common sites for this neoplasm. The treatment of choice for eyelid basal-cell carcinomas depends on whether the tumor is of the nodular or the morpheic type and on its size, its location, and the presence or absence of infiltration of underlying periosteum and bone. Small lesions may be treated effectively by liquid nitrogen cryotherapy. Cryotherapy or surgical excision is to be preferred for small basal-cell carcinomas on the upper eyelid, as radiotherapy may lead to keratinization of the eyelid margin and thereby to ocular discomfort from corneal epithelial abrasion. Very high cure rates can be obtained from surgical resection provided that complete excision is confirmed by frozen section at the time of surgery, especially for morphea-type tumors. Extensive inner canthal lesions may be treated either by excision

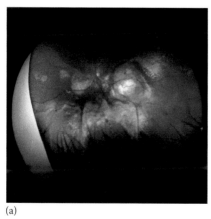 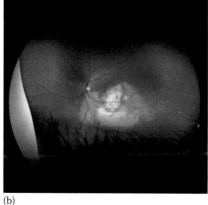

(a)   (b)

FIGURE 2.5 Ophthalmoscopic pictures of (a) before and (b) three months after therapy of an EGFR (exon 19 mutant) lung cancer with the orally administered TKI (tyrosine kinase inhibitory): osimertinib. Excellent response is demonstrated. (From Keshwani et al., 2020. With permission.)

or by a radiotherapy regime which is fractionated to reduce late effects (e.g. lacrimal duct stenosis, ectropion), although it is difficult to avoid epiphora with either approach. Radiotherapy is particularly suitable for tumors that have recurred after excision and for those tethered to the periosteum; once again, a fully fractionated regime is advised. We utilize an orthovoltage technique with an "internal" eye shield (i.e. contact lens of lead with a smoothed internal wall) placed (after local anesthetic desensitization of the cornea) between the lids to protect the eye from the radiation beam. Occasionally, orbital exenteration will be required for persistent or very extensive tumors.

Adenocarcinoma is the second most common primary eyelid malignancy, and most examples are sebaceous carcinomas. The eyelid is copiously supplied with glandular structures and is a site of predilection for this neoplasm, which may also arise in sebaceous glands in the caruncle or eyebrow. The tumor tends to be multifocal, and pagetoid spread from the lid on to the bulbar conjunctiva is characteristic. Diagnosis is difficult and often delayed because the tumor is mistaken for a simple meibomian cyst or for chronic conjunctivitis or blepharitis. Persistent or recurrent meibomian cysts and chronic, indeterminate "infections" of the conjunctiva and eyelid should therefore be subjected to biopsy. After melanoma, it has the highest mortality rate of all eyelid cancers and is best managed by wide excision. Where the orbit is invaded, orbital exenteration is recommended, and although radiotherapy may be considered when an advanced sebaceous carcinoma involves the only good eye, this neoplasm is not very radiosensitive.

Invasive squamous carcinoma is rare in the eyelid, often arising in an area of actinic keratosis. It may also arise in the conjunctiva, either de novo or in an area of pre-existing intra-epithelial squamous carcinoma. Surgical excision of eyelid lesions is to be preferred, and block dissection may be added in the rare instances in which regional lymph-node spread occurs. Tethered lymph glands may be better treated by carefully fractionated external-beam radiotherapy with ocular protection effected by a lead contact lens fitted behind the lids (after prior local anesthetic drops) each day before therapy. Metastasis from an eyelid primary is uncommon and death very rare.

The mortality rate is similarly low for conjunctival primary epithelial tumors. Most are intra-epithelial carcinoma-in-situ lesions that show a low propensity to develop into invasive carcinomas. The majority of these lesions are classified as "conjunctival (or corneal) intra-epithelial neoplasia" (CIN) by ophthalmologists. They have indistinct margins and may be multifocal. Consequently, they show a strong tendency to recur after simple excision. The risk of recurrence may be reduced by adjuvant cryotherapy, although very persistent lesions are best managed by radiotherapy, particularly if there is any histopathological evidence of an invasive element. Radiotherapy for bulbar conjunctival lesions is best administered using a strontium-90 β-ray source (and double-sided plaques are used for disease "creeping" onto the palpebral conjunctiva). Topical mitomycin C is effective in the treatment of CIN that has recurred after surgery and for the primary treatment of some extensive, and therefore irresectable, in-situ lesions. Mitomycin C therapy alone is not recommended for thick tumors or for invasive conjunctival carcinoma. Topical 5-fluorouracil has been found effective for squamous-cell carcinomas of the conjunctiva. Isolated case reports and small series have described the use of alfa 2b interferon in epithelial conjunctival tumors. Thick in-situ lesions should first be debulked and mitomycin C used in an adjuvant setting. Invasive tumors require wide excision. The long-term benefits of topical agents for epithelial tumors are yet to be defined.[21–23]

Malignant vascular tumors

Malignant vascular tumors may occur in the orbit but are uncommon. Hemangiopericytoma (solitary fibrous tumor) is a slow-growing, partially encapsulated tumor. If the capsule is not breached during surgical removal, a total cure is usually effected. Post-operative radiotherapy may be indicated. Local recurrence should be managed by orbital exenteration, and more distant relapse as for soft tissue sarcoma.

Malignant hemangioendothelioma is much less common. It is not encapsulated, and local recurrence is likely after attempted surgical excision unless a wide margin of normal tissue is excised. Recurrence should be managed by orbital exenteration. There is a high mortality rate from distant spread. Proton beam therapy may in the future widen the indications for radiotherapy in this population of patients.

Malignant neurogenic tumors

Malignant neurogenic tumors of neural crest origin may arise de novo or may develop in a pre-existing benign tumor, particularly in association with neurofibromatosis. Malignant schwannoma is an infiltrative tumor that tends to grow along neural channels and to present with pain. Local surgical excision is frequently followed by recurrence, and orbital exenteration may be required. Persistent local recurrence may be managed by radiotherapy. Death may occur from direct intra-cranial extension or from distant metastases.

Meningioma

Most of the meningiomas seen in the orbit represent direct orbital invasion by an intra-cranial tumor—usually from the sphenoid ridge but very occasionally a primary orbital meningioma may arise in the optic nerve sheath. Primary meningiomas of the orbit may be excised via a lateral orbitotomy, and the local recurrence rate after this operation is much less than that following the removal of an intra-cranial meningioma. Recurrent or subtotally resected Grade 2 menigiomata may be an indication for post-operative radiotherapy (versus close MR surveillance).

Optic nerve meningioma is a difficult condition to treat if the vision is to be preserved. However, we have good follow-up data on several scores of patients demonstrating durable stability of the growth pattern after conventionally fractionated radiotherapy to 45 Gy in 25 daily fractions—even including some patients with improvement in vision. It is obviously important that good-quality MRI assists in the radiotherapy planning—particularly as to whether the meningioma has spread back through the optic canal—so mandating coverage of the intra-cranial component in the radiation fields.

Malignant melanocytic tumors

Malignant melanocytic tumors are mostly melanomas. Their management is largely surgical. Malignant melanoma of the eyelid skin is extremely rare and is best managed by wide surgical excision. Malignant melanoma is more common in the conjunctiva (Figure 2.6), but nevertheless it is still rare. The majority of conjunctival melanomas arise in a pre-existing conjunctival lesion. Approximately 18% of tumors arise in a pre-existing nevus and 57% in primary acquired melanosis (PAM). PAM was formerly termed pre-cancerous melanosis and may be a manifestation of the atypical mole syndrome. Atypical melanocytes spread to involve much of the conjunctiva and on to the cornea and eyelid.[24–26] Ultimately, melanoma develops in most cases of PAM in which atypia are found, as indicated by biopsy

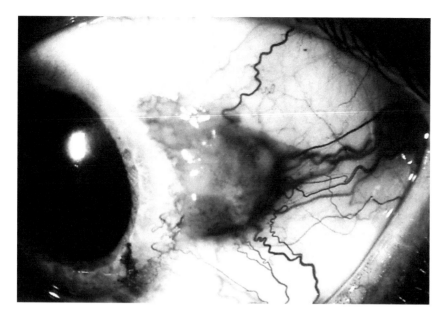

FIGURE 2.6   Conjunctival malignant melanoma arising in primary acquired melanosis.

or impression cytology,[27] and in most cases multifocal tumors develop sequentially.

Patients with PAM should have regular re-evaluations, looking for signs of a developing invasive melanoma. Cryotherapy is recommended to try to delay or prevent the onset of malignant change in PAM.[28] This treatment should be directed towards areas of acquired conjunctival pigmentation. Unfortunately, the success of this approach is limited by the facts that most patients with PAM do not present until the first melanoma has developed and that in some instances the melanosis is not pigmented and is therefore invisible. Eyelid skin melanomas are also associated with PAM,[29] and the conjunctival involvement may not be apparent or may be unsuspected at the time the lid tumor is diagnosed.

Survival rates are excellent following surgical excision of solitary bulbar conjunctival tumors not associated with PAM. The local recurrence rate is low after simple excision of melanomas that do not involve the corneo-scleral limbus and after en bloc lamellar corneo-scleral dissection of those that do. Recurrence after incomplete excision may be reduced by adjuvant cryotherapy or by β-ray radiotherapy. The effectiveness of adjunctive treatments with topical cytotoxics such as mitomycin C and 5-fluorouracil in reducing relapse after surgical excision of conjunctival melanoma or as a primary treatment is not fully evaluated. The value of these drugs in preventing the evolution of conjunctival melanomas from PAM is also not yet known. It is more difficult to eradicate a melanoma arising in the palpebral conjunctiva, partly because adjunctive treatments are more difficult to apply in this location. Accordingly, survival rates are poorer for such tumors. Additionally, melanomas arising in this location are more often than not associated with PAM, and other interrelated prognostic factors apply.

Tumors arising in unfavorable locations have 2.2 times the mortality of epibulbar melanomas. Unfavorable locations include the palpebral conjunctiva, the conjunctival fornices and plica, caruncle, and lid margin. Histology is relevant, and mixed-cell tumors have three times the mortality of spindle-cell lesions. Access to lymphatics may be the underlying reason why some locations are less prognostically favorable than others, and

lymphatic invasion carries a fourfold increase in mortality rate. Multifocal and thick tumors attract a worse prognosis than solitary, thin ones. The various risk factors conspire to make conjunctival melanoma arising in PAM a much more serious disease than melanoma arising de novo or in a nevus.

Because of their poor outlook, melanomas arising in the eyelid, conjunctival fornix, and, particularly, caruncle have all been traditionally managed by orbital exenteration. The role of exenteration was compared retrospectively in two groups of patients, one of which underwent the operation as the primary treatment of their disease and the other first underwent conservative treatment, with exenteration being reserved for palliative treatment.[30] The second group of patients was not seen to be disadvantaged by prior conservative surgery in terms of survival. The key to survival appeared to be the thickness of the largest tumor rather than the treatment method, with overall melanoma-related mortality ranging between nil in tumors with a maximum thickness of 1 mm and 50% in those in excess of 2-mm thickness. A particularly poor outcome was noted for caruncular melanoma, with six out of seven patients dying despite primary exenteration. These results had suggested that, where possible, a conservative approach should be tried first.

However, the activity of immunotherapy and the higher chance of a genomically targetable gene mutation in these extra-ocular melanomas argue that new analyses be made of the optimal therapy for this type of melanoma in the modern era.

The role for adjuvant therapy (e.g. immunotherapy) is not proven for these melanomas but needs to be considered in the modern era, as does genomically targeted therapy (especially where the BRAF gene seems to be the "driver." The likelihood for BRAF mutation as the driver for these extra-ocular melanomas is higher than for the uveal cases, and this should always be assessed as BRAF inhibitors (plus MEK inhibitors—to block the most common escape mutation in this situation)—will have important implications for therapy—in short, the appropriate therapy for skin melanoma cases should be considered.

Orbital recurrence is seen in large, neglected tumors and nasal recurrence in inner canthal lesions, probably because of implantation of tumor cells shed down the nasal passages. At

St. Bartholomew's Hospital, patients exenterated for large mela-nomas now receive adjunctive orbital radiotherapy, and those undergoing exenteration for inner canthal melanomas receive radiotherapy post-operatively to the ipsilateral nasal passages, in the hope of eliminating local recurrence. However, once again, in the modern era, the use of systemic immunotherapy and genomi-cally targeted therapy in lieu of or in addition to radiotherapy all needs consideration.

Malignant lacrimal-gland and duct tumors

The most common malignant tumor of the lacrimal gland is adenoid cystic carcinoma. This tumor is not encapsulated and is locally invasive. There is a high mortality rate, with death usually resulting from direct intra-cranial extension. The tumor grows rapidly, and the history of painful proptosis is short. The pain results from the infiltration of neural channels. Radical resection may be performed if adenoid cystic carcinoma does not extend to the orbital apex and appears to be confined within the periosteum. Radiotherapy should be considered post-operatively, and we usu-ally use volumetric arc therapy to treat the whole orbit to a dose of 50–55 Gy in 6 weeks. This is high-dose orbital radiotherapy, and there is ocular morbidity (dry eye, cataractogenesis, and some risk to the retina and of bulbar phthisis).

In the management of advanced disease or relapse, some ade-nocarcinomas of the lacrimal gland (rather like salivary gland carcinomas) may express androgen receptors and respond to androgen receptor inhibitors such as bicalutamide.[31] Again, like salivary gland carcinomas, some lacrimal gland cancers may be "driven" by an amplified HER-2 gene mutation and this should be checked as HER-2 directed therapy would then be appropri-ate.[32] It will be interesting to see if (like salivary gland carcino-mas) occasional lacrimal gland carcinomas are "driven by" NTRK fusion mutants (for which there are now potent small molecular inhibitors).

Chemotherapy response rates in advanced disease are suf-ficiently poor that adjuvant chemotherapy cannot be recom-mended. However, in the relapse situation, we would recommend a platinum-based doublet of chemotherapy agents—often with a taxane but also we have noted some partial responses with peme-trexed as the second agent.

Malignant lymphomas of the orbit

The orbit is one of the more common sites of extranodal origin of lymphoma, and orbital lymphoma is a disease that must be dis-tinguished from the rare ocular lymphoma (see above). Almost all orbital lymphomas are of B-cell origin; Hodgkin disease rarely affects the orbit.

Primary conjunctival lymphomas are now recognized as mucosa-associated lymphoid tissue (MALT) tumors—marginal-zone lymphoma (MZL)—and these comprise 44% of all orbital cases. Chronic antigenic stimulation (e.g. chlamydial infection or the autoimmune thyroid eye disease) may predispose to the development of these lymphomas. The recent discovery of the regression of conjunctival MALT lymphoma following treatment of the chlamydial infection with doxycycline[33] is a fascinating observation as it is entirely analogous to the discovery of gas-tric MALT lymphoma responding to anti-helicobacter therapy. Clearly, this needs to be further researched. Our group has dem-onstrated an association between orbital lymphoma and thyroid eye disease[34]—an autoimmune disease that, not surprisingly (and as for Hashimoto's disease, Sjogren's syndrome, etc.), predisposes to the formation of lymphoma after a period of time (>7 years).

Other histologies found are lymphoplasmacytic/lymphoplas-macytoid lymphoma (LPL) (24%), follicle center cell lymphoma (FCL) (12%), diffuse large cell lymphoma (12%), and rare types (e.g. mantle cell lymphoma) and, of course, orbital deposits from systemic lymphoma occur.[35–37]

The risk of development of extra-orbital disease and lymphoma-related death has been assessed in a recent UK analysis of almost 200 patients presenting to Moorfields Eye Hospital, London, and St. Bartholomew's Hospital from the 1980s, with a long follow-up. In this historic series, the risk of relapse by 5 years in patients pre-senting with localized disease is related to pathology, being 47% for MZL, 48% for LPL, 64% for FCL, 81% for DCL, and 95% for other histologies, with 5-year lymphoma-related mortality rates of 12%, 19%, 22%, 48%, and 53% respectively.[35–37] These data are of interest only as so far as to demonstrate the relative growth potential of the various types of lymphoma—the current cohort of low-grade and stage-1E orbital lymphoma is associated with a 95% chance of disease-free survival at 5 years.

Orbital lymphomas may be bilateral at presentation (16% in our analysis of 326 cases of primary orbital lymphoma), which is surprising given the absence of lymphatic connections between the two orbits but unsurprising when one considers the etiologi-cal factors contributing to the development of MALT lymphoma. Interestingly, in our series bilaterality at presentation doubled the risk of extra-orbital disease/relapse. Is it just doubling the chance because there are two orbits from which to spread? We are unsure.

Our analysis also examined other predicting clinical features for late relapse and death, the incidence of these two events being sequentially greater for patients with predominantly deep orbital presentations (and painful optic neuropathy was significantly prognostic as it marks for large orbital masses) and lacrimal-gland and eyelid (i.e. subcutaneous eyelid mass) presentations. These clinical features also marked for a greater likelihood of discov-ering systemic disease at presentation, as compared to a patient with a lengthy history of a unilateral conjunctival (MALT) lym-phoma mass.[35–37]

Diagnosis of orbital lymphoma is made by orbital scanning (preferably MRI) followed by biopsy for histology. Staging fol-lows—the authors do not perform bone marrow testing routinely on (otherwise) stage-1E or conjunctival MALT lymphomas as the positive rate is so low.

Where the disease is localized to the conjunctiva (no disease behind the equator of the globe on good-quality MRI of the orbit), the optimal treatment has changed over the last 10 years. The current algorithm for treatment of conjunctival marginal-zone lymphoma (no disease behind the conjunctival sac) entails a 6- to 8-week course of the antibiotic doxycycline—this is based on some observational data that chronic chlamydial infection of the conjunctiva can stimulate lymphocytes to neoplasia. If doxycy-cline does not effect regression, then we employ the single agent: rituximab (a monoclonal antibody aimed at the CD20 determi-nant of this B-cell lymphoma). This carries none of the risks of cytotoxic chemotherapy and may be enough to put these early and indolent lymphomas into remission. Our experience with 6 3-weekly rituximab infusions is that we see frequent remissions, although only some are durable. If the foregoing has not put the patient into remission, then the next step is radiotherapy. When radiotherapy is used, our current approach is with an anterior orthovoltage (250–300 KV) portal covering the conjunctival sac and with midline ocular shielding; this last is achieved with a plastic contact lens with a centrally mounted lead cylinder, which is placed carefully between the lids before each radiation frac-tion (after anesthetizing the conjunctiva with local anesthetic eye

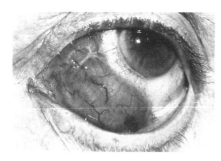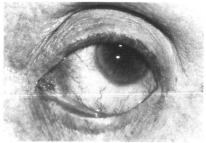

FIGURE 2.7 Subconjunctival deposit of lymphoma (left) before and (right) after treatment by fractionated radiotherapy.

drops) such that the cornea (and behind it the lens) is shielded from the primary beam. Our research demonstrated that an orthovoltage beam was superior to an electron beam, where there was more scatter inwards under the lead shield.

Where the disease is behind the equator of the globe on MR or not solely conjunctival, such a technique (utilized to prevent cataractogenesis) is inappropriate and volumetric arc therapy or a wedged pair of megavoltage portals is used to treat the entire orbit, mindful of the possible need to use bolus anteriorly where the disease comes very superficially anteriorly. The standard radiotherapy prescription is 30 Gy in 15 fractions over 21 days, although a higher dose—to 35 Gy—may be appropriate for the minority of bigger tumor masses.

For localized high-grade B-cell lymphomas, four cycles of rituximab with cyclophosphamide, Adriamycin, vincristine, and prednisolone (CHOP) – R-CHOP precedes radiotherapy to the orbit. Such chemotherapy is clearly appropriate for high-grade extra-orbital disease, whereas simpler chemotherapy is recommended or nowadays "Smart" drug therapy may be indicated.

Secondary deposits

Secondary deposits are uncommon in the ocular adnexa in adults, although they may occasionally be seen in the orbit. Breast carcinoma is the most common primary source. They are treated by radiotherapy (except the possible response to systemic options—including the TKIs instanced above for intra-ocular metastasis) may allow a very short period of observation on systemic therapy—but with careful monitoring of vision.

Radiotherapy is the therapy of choice with doses in the range of 40 Gy in 4 weeks or shorter fractionated courses, such as 30 Gy in 10 fractions, being delivered (Figure 2.7).

See boxes on Diagnosis and Treatment.

DIAGNOSIS

1) Most common benign adult intra-ocular tumors are melanocytic, smooth-muscle, or vascular in origin.
2) Benign tumors of the ocular adnexae are epithelial, vascular, neurogenic, melanocytic, or of lacrimal gland origin (e.g. pleomorphic adenoma).
3) Conjunctival lymphoma is often localized to the conjunctival sac and possibly driven by chronic chlamydial local infection. This may be why there is a bilateral predisposition.
4) Orbital lymphomas are commonly low-grade extra-nodal marginal-zone lymphoma (non-Hodgkin lymphoma), stage 1AE, and are easily curable.

5) Intra-ocular lymphoma is frequently high-grade B-cell lymphoma and often part of oculo-cerebral lymphoma.
6) Ocular melanoma differs from skin melanoma, rarely having BRAF mutation, and may have a lower response to immunotherapy. Monosomy of chromosome 3 confers a worse prognosis, and mutations in the BAP1 gene increase the metastatic potential of the tumor.
7) Lacrimal gland carcinoma, like salivary gland carcinoma, may express androgen receptors and be driven by Her-2 gene mutation.

TREATMENT

1) Diffuse choroidal hemangioma can be treated with photodynamic therapy or fractionated external beam radiotherapy.
2) Conjunctival lymphoma can be cured in 95% of patients with superficial kilovoltage radiotherapy using a lens-sparing technique. Some tumors respond to doxycycline antibiotic therapy alone.
3) High-grade intra-ocular lymphoma requires high-dose chemotherapy which penetrates the central nervous system. Stem cell transplant may obviate the need for whole-brain/ocular radiotherapy with its associated long-term sequalae.
4) Ocular melanoma can be treated with plaque brachytherapy or stereotactic radiotherapy with the intent of organ preservation. Otherwise enucleation or exenteration with or without post-operative radiotherapy can be employed with curative intent.
5) Metastatic ocular melanoma has a poor response rate to chemotherapy, and there is usually no target for BRAF inhibitors. Immunotherapy (CTLA-4 and PDL-1 targeted agents) does have some activity in these tumors.

References

1. Plowman PN, Harnett AN. Radiotherapy in benign orbital disease, I. Complicated ocular and orbital angiomas. *Br J Ophthalmol.* 1986; 72:286–8.
2. Hungerford JL. Uveal melanoma. *Eur J Cancer.* 1993; 29:1365–8.
3. Hungerford JL. Surgical treatment of ocular melanoma. *Melanoma Res.* 1993; 3:305–12.
4. Foulds WS. Current options in the management of choroidal melanoma. *Trans Ophthalmol Soc UK.* 1983; 103:28–34.

5. Damato BE, Paul J, Foulds WS. Risk factors for residual and recurrent melanoma after trans-scleral local resection. *Br J Ophthalmol.* 1996; 80:102–8.

6. Hungerford JL. Current trends in the treatment of ocular melanoma by radiotherapy. *Clin Exp Ophthalmol.* 2003; 31:8–13.

7. Seddon JM, Gragoudas ES, Egan KM et al. Relative survival rates after alternative therapies for uveal, melanoma. *Ophthalmology.* 1990; 97:769–77.

8. Foss AJ, Whelahan I, Hungerford JL et al. Predictive factors for the development of rubeosis following proton beam radiotherapy for uveal melanoma. *Br J Ophthalmol.* 1997; 81:748–54.

9. Zehetmayer M, Menapace R, Kitz K, Ertl A. Stereotatic radiosurgery for uveal melanoma. In: Kogelnik HD (ed.) *Progress in Radiooncology.* Bologna, Italy: Monduzzi, 1995. pp. 451–4.

10. Stallard HB. Radiotherapy for malignant melanoma of the choroid. *Br J Ophthalmol.* 1966; 50:147–55.

11. Starr HJ, Zimmerman LE. Extrascleral extension and orbital recurrence of malignant melanoma of the choroid and ciliary body. *Int Ophthalmol Clin.* 1962; 2:369–84.

12. Hykin PG, McCartney ACE, Plowman PN, Hungerford JL. Postenucleation orbital radiotherapy for the treatment of malignant melanoma of the choroid with extrascleral extension. *Br J Ophthalmol.* 1990; 74:36–9.

13. Chua V, Lapadula D, Randolph C et al. Dysregulated GPCR signalling and therapeutic options in uveal melanoma. *Mol Cancer Res.* 2017; 15(5): 501–6.

14. Moore AR, Ceruado E, Chen Y. Recurrent activating mutations of G-protein coupled receptor CYSLTR2 in uveal melanoma. *Nature Gen.* 2016; 48(6): 675–580.

15. Gupta MP, Lane AM, De Angelis NM et al. Clinical characterisitcs of uveal melanoma in patients with germline BAP1 mutations. *JAMA (Ophthalmol).* 2015; 133(8): 881–7.

16. Szalai E, Jiang Y, van Poppelen NM et al. Association of uveal melanoma metastatic rate with stochastic mutation rate and type of mutation. *JAMA (Ophthalmol).* 2018; 136(10):1115–20.

17. Pelster M, Gruschkus SK, Bassett R et al. Phase 2 study of ipilumumab and nivolumab in metastatic uveal melanoma. *Proc Am Soc Clin Oncol.* 2019 Abstract 9522.

18. Croce M, Ferrini S, Gangeri R. Targeted therapy of uveal melanoma: Recent failures and perspectives. *Cancers (Basel).* 2019; 11(6):846–55.

19. Landreville S, Agapova O, Matatali KA. Histone deacetylase inhibitors induce growth arrest in uveak melanoma. *Clin Cancer Res.* 2011; 18(2):408–16.

20. Schorb E, Fox C, Kasendra B et al. Induction chemo-immunotherapy with MATRIX regimen in patient with newly diagnosed PCNSL—A mutlicenter retrospective analysis. *Blood.* 2017; 130:376.

21. Wilson MW, Hungerford JL, George SM, Madreperla SA. Topical mitomycin C for the treatment of conjunctival and corneal epithelial dysplasia and neoplasia. *Am J Ophthalmol.* 1997; 124:303–11.

22. Midena E, Angeli CD, Valenti M et al. Treatment of conjunctival squamous cell carcinoma with topical 5-fluorouracil. *Br J Ophthalmol.* 2000; 84:268–72.

23. Kim JW, Abranson DH. Topical options for conjunctival neoplasms. *Clin Ophthalmol.* 2008; 2:503–15

24. Bataille V, Boyle J, Hungerford JL, Newton JA. Three cases of primary acquired melanosis of the conjunctiva as a manifestation of the atypical mole syndrome. *Br J Dermatol.* 1993; 128:86–90.

25. Paridaens ADA, Kirkness CM, Garner A, Hungerford JL. Recurrent malignant melanoma of the corneal stroma: A case of "black cornea." *Br J Ophthalmol.* 1992; 76:444–6.

26. Robertson DM, Hungerford JL, McCartney ACE. Pigmentation of the eyelid margin accompanying conjunctival melanoma. *Am J Ophthalmol.* 1989; 108:435–9.

27. Paridaens ADA, McCartney ACE, Curling OM et al. Impression cytology of conjunctival melanosis and melanoma. *Br J Ophthalmol.* 1992; 76:198–201.

28. Jakobiec FA, Rini FJ, Fraunfelder FT, Brownstein S. Cryotherapy for conjunctival primary acquired melanosis and malignant melanoma. *Ophthalmology.* 1988; 95:1058–70.

29. Hicks C, Liu C, Hiranandani M et al. Conjunctival melanoma after excision of a lentigo maligna melanoma in the ipsilateral eyelid skin. *Br J Ophthalmol.* 1994; 78:317–18.

30. Paridaens ADA, McCartney ACE, Minassian DC, Hungerford JL. Orbital exenteration in 95 cases of conjunctival malignant melanoma. *Br J Ophthalmol.* 1994; 78:520–8.

31. Park AH, Ho-Seok S, Cho KJ. Androgen receptor positive ductal adenocarcinoma of the naso lacrimal duct: A case report. *Am J Ophthalmol Case rep.* 2017; 5:33–37.

32. Arihara Y, Murase K, Kato J et al. Trastuzumab based combination chemotherapy in patients with human epidermal growth factor receptor—2 positive metastatic carcinoma ex-pleomorphic carcinoma. *Case Rep Oncol.* 2018; 11(3):835–41.

33. Ferreri AJM, Ponzini M, Guidoboni M et al. Regression of ocular adnexal lymphoma after chlamydia psittaci-eradicating antibiotic therapy. *J Clin Oncol.* 2005; 23:5067–73.

34. Nutting CM, Desai SS, Norton A, Rose GE, Plowman PN. Graves' ophthalmopathy predisposes to orbital lymphoma. *Eye.* 2006; 20:645–8.

35. Hardman-Lea S, Kerr-Muir M, Wotherspoon AC et al. Mucosal-associated lymphoid tissue lymphoma of the conjunctiva. *Arch Ophthalmol.* 1994; 112:1207–12.

36. Jenkins C, Rose GE, Bunce C et al. Histological features of ocular adnexal lymphoma (REAL) classification and their association with patient morbidity and survival. *Br J Opohthalmol.* 2000; 84:907–13.

37. Jenkins C, Rose GE, Bunce C et al. Clinical features associated with survival of patients with lymphoma of the ocular adnexa. *Eye.* 2003; 17:809–20.

38. Keshwani K, Roelofs L, Hay G et al. Treating choroidal metastases and improving vision with osimertinib in EGFR T790M mutated lung adenocarcinoma: A case report and review of literature. *Ocular Oncology and Pathology.* 2010. In press.

3 HEAD AND NECK CANCER

Lorcan O'Toole and Nicholas D. Stafford

Introduction

A multidisciplinary approach is essential in the management of head and neck cancers (HNC). Decision-making involves careful appraisal of available treatment options, and it is the patient who is the key decision-maker, once they have been properly informed of the risks and advantages of these options.

The multidisciplinary team (MDT) and clinic are based at specialist cancer centers which frequently adopt a hub and spoke model with outreach clinics attended by core MDT members.

A reasonable objective of the Specialist Centre (as practiced in the United Kingdom) is to see patients referred with suspected HNC within two weeks, obtain a diagnosis within 31 days, and commence definitive treatment within 31 days of diagnosis.

Comprehensive guidelines have been published for the management of HNC, such as the 2016 UK National Multidisciplinary guidelines and the regularly updated online US guidelines from the NCCN.[1,2]

Incidence

Worldwide, nearly 650,000 people develop HNC annually, accounting for approximately 5% of cancers overall. The ratio of males to females is 3:1. In the United Kingdom, the incidence of HNC increased by 31% between 1993–1995 and 2013–2015.

HNC is related to social deprivation and age. When the most deprived are compared with the most affluent incidence is doubled (European age standardization rate 21.7 vs. 10.3). The highest incidence rates are in older people; in the United Kingdom more than a fifth of new cases of HNC are diagnosed in patients 75 years and older.

Outcome

The outcomes for patients with HNC depend on the stage of disease at diagnosis, the anatomical subsite affected, age, gender, and the treatment administered. The EUROCARE 5 study[3] published in 2015 analyzed European cancer registries for the outcomes of HNC patients diagnosed between 1999 and 2007. Results demonstrate the poorest outcomes, in terms of 5-year relative survival (RS), to be 25% for hypopharynx compared to 59% for larynx cancers. The 5-year RS for localized hypopharynx cancer was 42% compared to 74% for larynx. However, 54% of patients were diagnosed with locally advanced or metastatic disease at presentation. Outcomes were significantly better for younger patients and for females.

Etiology

First-degree relatives of patients with HNC have a 3.5 times higher risk of developing the disease than the general population suggesting a genetic-based susceptibility. Environmental factors are particularly important in the etiology of HNC (Table 3.1). The two most important carcinogens are alcohol and tobacco functioning as co-carcinogens, the effect of both smoking and drinking is approximately 2.5 times greater than simply adding the risk from each.

Many other occupational and environmental toxins associated with HNC include hardwood dust, asbestos, pesticides, betel nut chewing, mouthwashes, and formaldehyde.

Viruses

Five viruses have been associated with HNC: human papilloma virus (HPV), herpes simplex virus (HSV), Epstein–Barr virus (EBV) (see "Nasopharynx" section later in this chapter), hepatitis C virus (HCV), and human immunodeficiency virus (HIV).

HPV is associated with tumors of the oral cavity, oropharynx, and larynx. Type 16 is the most prevalent, particularly in oropharyngeal tumors, and accounts for approximately 70% of cases in North America and Europe. Patients with HPV-related HNC are less likely to smoke or drink, are younger and more likely to have indulged in high-risk sexual behavior (oral sex with multiple partners). Survival is better in patients with HPV-positive tumors.

HSV type 1 is associated with HNC of the oral cavity. HCV antibodies are present in a significantly higher proportion of HPV-positive HNC compared to controls. There is a two- to threefold increase in HNC in patients with HIV positivity.

Problem of second primary tumors

The incidence of second primary tumors after initial treatment of an HNC is approximately 5% per year. A second primary, rather than simply a recurrence of the original tumor is defined by the following criteria:

- The new tumor must be separated from the site of the original tumor by at least 2 cm of normal epithelium, or it must be more than 3 years since the eradication of the original tumor.
- If the second tumor is in the lung, it should be solitary and, if less than 3 years from the time of diagnosis of the original tumor, the histological appearance should be different.

The second primary is synchronous if diagnosed within 6 months of the first or metachronous if greater than 6 months.

Overall, 10–30% of patients will develop a second malignancy. The majority of these second tumors occurs in the head and neck, lung, or esophagus and are associated with smoking and alcohol exposure. Only 10% of such patients survive for 5 years.

Assessment of patients

A full clinical history and general physical examination are essential both in relation to the HNC, presence of comorbidities, and the possibility of a second primary tumor.

The site of origin of the primary HNC, its size, appearance, and the involvement of adjacent structures should all be formally recorded. Standardized diagrams are helpful.

TABLE 3.1 Environmental Factors Potentially Implicated in the Cause of Head and Neck Cancer

Environmental Factor	Cancer Location
Alcohol	Oral cavity
	Pharynx
	Esophagus
	Larynx
Tobacco	Oral cavity
	Pharynx
	Esophagus
	Larynx
Betel nut/pan masala (a complex mixture of areca nut, tobacco, lime, cardamom, etc.)	Oral cavity
Thorium dioxide	Paranasal sinuses
HPV	Oropharynx
	Oral cavity
	Larynx
EBV	Nasopharyngeal carcinoma
Chromium dust/fumes	Nasal cavity and sinuses
Leather working	Nasal cavity and sinuses
Nickel dust/fumes	Nasal cavity and sinuses
Wood dust (e.g. beech)	Nasal cavity and sinuses
Iron deficiency	Post-cricoid carcinoma
Salt fish	Nasopharynx
HIV infection	Oral cavity
	Oropharynx

Outpatient fiber-optic endoscopy is performed but most patients will require formal assessment under anesthesia. Tissue diagnosis by biopsy of the primary is mandatory. Ultrasound-guided fine-needle aspiration cytology can be performed if there is doubt about whether enlarged nodes are reactive or involved by tumor. A negative result does not definitively exclude nodal involvement and occasionally a further core biopsy is required.

The following investigations should be considered in all patients:

- Full blood count.
- Liver function tests, urea, and electrolytes.
- Cross-sectional imaging appropriate to the primary tumor: Information is required particularly concerning the direct extension of tumor into bone, the extent of nodal disease, and the involvement of adjacent neurovascular structures. CT is particularly useful in evaluating the invasion of the laryngeal cartilage or spread into the pre-epiglottic or paraglottic spaces. MRI scanning is particularly useful for assessing oral cavity and oropharyngeal tumors and in the assessment of patients with amalgam-filled teeth.
- PET-CT scanning can provide further detail about the extent of primary and nodal involvement and the presence of metastases or synchronous second primaries.

General principles of surgery

Surgery can be associated with significant long-term morbidity and should, therefore, only be undertaken in those patients who are fit enough to withstand its effects and who are aware of the likely functional outcome. Apart from diversions of the airway or digestive tract, aimed at relieving symptoms, there is little role for palliative surgery. Surgery should only be undertaken when there is a realistic chance of curing the patient.

Patients undergoing major oral cavity or oropharyngeal tumor resections are usually given a temporary tracheostomy to safeguard the airway. Similarly, in patients undergoing major resections in whom the likelihood of an early return to normal swallowing is small, a gastrostomy will safeguard the airway from overspill and allow good and safe nutritional support during the early post-operative period. Having decided on major surgery, the following issues need to be considered:

- The extent of the excision that will be required to remove the tumor. Standard works talk of allowing a 2-cm rim of macroscopically normal tissue around the tumor. However, such a margin is not always feasible in the head and neck, and recourse to frozen-section analysis of excision margins is often necessary at the time of surgery. Positive histological margins are associated with a poorer prognosis.
- Reliance on frozen section for histological diagnosis of the primary tumor may be unwise. Although frozen-section analysis is reliable for squamous-cell carcinoma, it is notoriously unreliable for salivary gland malignancies. Whenever possible, a definitive histological diagnosis should be obtained prior to excisional surgery.
- Management of nodal disease. Certain primary tumor sites in the head and neck are associated with a high incidence of metastatic nodal disease, which may be too early to be clinically palpable or evident on scanning. Such sites include the nasopharynx, oropharynx, oral cavity, supraglottis, and hypopharynx. It is therefore logical to consider a prophylactic ipsilateral neck dissection when undertaking excision of a primary tumor at one of these sites. In the absence of palpable disease, a selective neck dissection is undertaken, sending off any suspicious-looking nodes for frozen-section analysis. A fully modified radical neck dissection for clinical N_0 disease is only justified if intra-operative frozen section proves positive.
- Reconstruction of the defect. Primary closure of a defect is often not feasible. If a comfortable primary closure cannot be achieved, consideration must be given to the use of transposed tissue.

The types of flaps or grafts available and the situations in which they are most commonly applied can be summarized as follows:

Free skin grafts:
- Split skin grafts can be used on a well-vascularized bed, for example, post-hemiglossectomy or post-buccal mucosa excision.

Local mucosal or skin flaps:
- Random: these flaps do not have a defined vessel supplying them. They are therefore relatively small.
- Axial: these flaps have a named blood supply. They can be cutaneous, e.g. the nasolabial flap. Local axial flaps should be used with care in instances where the surgical field has previously been irradiated.
- Distant axial flaps. These are distant in that the base of the flap is not immediately adjacent to the area of excision. They can be:
  - Cutaneous: e.g. the delto-pectoral flap.

– Myocutaneous: The two most popular myocutaneous flaps are the pectoralis major and the latissimus dorsi flaps. They can be used for "lining" or "cover".

- Osseomyocutaneous flaps: these are a variation of myocutaenous flaps and incorporate a portion of rib to provide reconstruction of the jaw.
- Free flaps. These are portions of tissue that carry an identifiable arterial supply and venous drainage, allowing their transfer and inset into the surgical defect with anastomosis of the vessels to appropriate vessels in the neck. The functional results following free-flap reconstructions may be excellent, but there are no randomized studies to prove their superiority over more traditional methods of reconstruction. Examples include:
  – The radial forearm flap which can be harvested with an attached, vascularized segment of radial bone and the groin flap (antero-lateral thigh flap).
  – The free fibular flap.
  – The rectus abdominis flap: Which can also be harvested with overlying skin. This provides a bulky flap, for example, for defects after glossectomy.
- A segment of jejunum can be harvested along with its vascular arcade and can be inset as an intact tube to provide a neopharynx.
- Pedicled viscera. Following a pharyngolaryngo-esophagectomy (e.g. for a post-cricoid or cervical esophageal carcinoma), the best way to reconstruct the upper digestive tract may be to mobilize and transpose the stomach into the neck.

Following total laryngectomy, the essence of speech restoration is to create a small fistula between the posterior wall of the trachea and the cervical esophagus. This allows air through a valve lying in the fistula into the pharynx.

Potential complications of head and neck surgery

These include:

- Fistula formation: the development of an oro-cutaneous or pharyngo-cutaneous salivary fistula can occur after any major excision involving resection of digestive tract mucosa via the neck. It is more commonly seen in patients who have previously undergone radiotherapy. A persistent fistula may indicate an early tumor recurrence.
- A chylous fistula is most likely to occur following a modified radical neck dissection. It usually settles spontaneously.
- Aspiration: after any major resection of the oral cavity or oropharynx, a reconstructive flap will need to be employed. This flap will be anesthetic and immobile and, not surprisingly, swallowing will suffer as a consequence. Depending on factors such as the site of the flap, the patient's age, and previous surgery/radiotherapy, the patient usually learns to compensate. However, in a minority long-term aspiration becomes a serious problem.
- Wound breakdown: this is rarely significant unless there is an associated fistula.
- Frozen shoulder: this is often seen following conventional radical neck dissection, in which the accessory nerve is divided. Post-operative physiotherapy may help.

General principles of radiotherapy

External-beam radiotherapy

Radiotherapy (RT) is an essential modality for cure, palliation, and adjuvant treatment of HNC.

When disease control rates can be similar, RT is often preferable to surgery because of its organ-sparing effect and better functional outcomes.

However, RT is still associated with high levels of both acute and chronic toxicities, which mandate careful consideration and discussion between the patient and the multidisciplinary team in formulating a management plan.

The current technique for RT delivery in most centers is intensity-modulated radiotherapy (IMRT).

IMRT has the advantage of enabling highly conformal dose distributions and better normal organ sparing. Several retrospective studies and prospective randomized trials[4] have been published demonstrating a reduction in radiation-induced late toxicity, particularly xerostomia, and better quality of life for patients following IMRT.

The first stage of IMRT is a treatment planning session. Patient immobilization is achieved using a thermoplastic mask which is crucial to the reproducibility of the planned daily treatment. A planning CT is performed with the patient in the mask. CT localization can be supplemented by image fusion with MRI or positron emission tomography (PET)-CT for better accuracy in tumor delineation.

The principals involved in HNC radiotherapy are no different from those that apply elsewhere in the body. The gross tumor volume (GTV) comprises the primary tumor and cervical node metastases, if present. The high-dose clinical target volume (CTV) is an isotropic expansion of the GTV by up to 10 mm to include a tissue volume that contains the GTV and possible microscopic subclinical extension. In addition to the high-dose CTV there may be an intermediate-dose CTV comprising a further expansion around the primary or involved nodal volumes. A low-dose CTV is drawn to include the remainder of the nodal levels not already included in high or intermediate dose but thought to be at risk of harboring subclinical metastases.

Consensus guidelines have been published to assist the oncologist with the CTV expansion around the primary tumor,[5] nodal CTV delineation,[6] and CTV delineation in post-operative radiotherapy.[7]

A detailed discussion on principles of target volume and organ-at-risk (OAR) delineation and dose constraints for head and neck tumors is covered in other works.[8,9]

A final expansion of CTV to planning target volume (PTV) allows for day-to-day variations in patient position on treatment.

The RT planner using the treatment planning system selects the most appropriate way to deliver radiation maximizing conformity and homogeneity of dose across the PTV while minimizing doses to normal tissues and OARs.

IMRT uses a simultaneous integrated boost technique concurrently delivering a different dose of radiotherapy per fraction per day to the different CTV volumes. While other regimens are in use, the most common radical RT dose is 70 Gy in 35 fractions over 7 weeks. Treatment is delivered by linear accelerators (LINACs) using 6-MV photons.

Modern LINACs have on-board cone-beam CT technology which allows for image-guided RT (IGRT). This imaging confirms accurate patient positioning and is used to adjust for day-to-day variations in patient positioning. Image-guided adaptive RT (IGART) is an evolution of IGRT where the changes in tumor size and position and that of OARs such as salivary glands can be monitored throughout treatment. If changes are deemed significant the RT plan can be adapted to ensure accuracy of tumor dose and OAR sparing.

Head and neck brachytherapy

The use of flexible radioactive sources (such as ^{192}Ir wire) as interstitial implants enables a high dose of radiation to be precisely localized. This technique can occasionally be indicated in the treatment of early or locally recurrent carcinomas of the lip, oral cavity, oropharynx, and nasopharynx. Implantation can also be used in the treatment of lymph nodes. Implants can be used as a means of boosting the external RT dose to the tumor, or to treat recurrence. The European Society for Radiotherapy and Oncology has published guidelines for the use of brachytherapy in the treatment of HNC.[10]

Heavy charged particles

Heavy charged particle treatment, in particular proton beam treatment, is increasingly being used in the treatment of head and neck cancers. Initially used for tumors in areas such as the brain stem where a quick and predictable falloff between the high dose volume and the OAR is critical, proton treatment is being investigated for a broader range of applications in areas such as the oropharynx and oral cavity.

Complications of radiotherapy

Acute RT reactions

Mucosal and skin reactions are the main acute toxicity problems. In a standard course of radical RT, mucosal reactions become apparent from about week 2 and skin reactions a little later. Skin reactions tend to settle within 2 weeks after RT, but mucosal reactions can take up to 8 weeks on average. The reaction begins with erythema and edema followed by a patchy exudate becoming confluent. Ulceration may occur in severe cases. During RT, a decrease in the rate of flow of saliva occurs within 10–14 days of the start of treatment. The effects of radiation on salivary function are at their maximum 4–6 weeks after the start of treatment. The serous acini are more sensitive to radiation than the mucinous acini, which means that the saliva changes and becomes thick and sticky. These thickened mucus secretions can be difficult for the patient to expectorate and lead to additional problems with nausea, taste disturbance, and decreased oral intake. Chemotherapy or anti-EGFR (epidermal growth factor receptor) treatment with radiotherapy shortens time to onset, exacerbates the severity, and prolongs the duration of mucositis and dermatitis.

Patients should be seen and examined at least once a week during treatment and reassured as to the expected sequence of events. Advice is best given as a set of written instructions, which are carefully explained to patients at the start of treatment and reinforced during weekly review. The major points are summarized in Box 3.1 and are outlined below.

BOX 3.1   INSTRUCTIONS FOR PATIENTS' SELF-CARE DURING RADIOTHERAPY TO THE HEAD AND NECK

SKIN CARE
- Avoid aftershave or astringent cosmetics.
- Wash gently, pat the skin dry, and avoid wet shaving.
- Avoid collars or other clothes that chafe the treated area.
- Try not to scratch the skin.

MUCOSAL CARE
- Stop smoking.
- Do not drink alcohol.
- Avoid hot or spicy foods.
- Use regular mouthwashes.
- Carry out careful dental hygiene.
- Chew sugar-free gum.
- Drink plenty of clear fluids.

DIET AND NUTRITION
- Follow a bland high-protein diet.
- Use dietary supplements.
- Take supplementary vitamins.
- Put food through blender if necessary.

CARE OF THE VOICE
- Rest the voice as much as possible.
- Do not try to force the voice.
- Speak slowly and quietly.
- Avoid dry or smoky atmospheres.
- Avoid excessive coughing.

Basic oral care

Careful supervision of oral hygiene is important, with prompt identification and management of any secondary infection such as oral candidiasis. Simple measures can reduce the duration and severity of the acute mucosal reaction, prominent among which are to stop smoking and avoid alcohol.

Frequent oral rinsing with bland solutions such as normal saline with sodium bicarbonate (1 L water with 1/2 teaspoon baking soda and 1/2 teaspoon salt) is helpful, and use of a soft toothbrush minimizes mucosal trauma. Other mouthwashes with local analgesics, coating agents, or oral rinses such as Difflam, Gelclair, Caphosol, and Mucilage are frequently employed.

Adequate analgesia is extremely important in the management of mucositis. Treatment follows the World Health Organization (WHO) ladder from paracetamol through to morphine. Liquid or soluble preparations are preferred.

Maintenance of adequate hydration and nutrition

All patients are routinely provided with dietetic support.

A prophylactic gastrostomy (RIG or PEG) should be considered to allow the maintenance of adequate and safe nutritional, fluid and medicinal intake during and after RT following detailed discussion on the pros and cons of this approach with the patient. Good oral intake is always preferable and should be maintained as long as possible by diet modification with soft and semi-liquid food along with oral nutritional supplements and generous analgesia. Even in the presence of tube feeding, maintaining oral fluid intake reduces the symptoms of excessive mucus production.

A reasonable approach is as follows:

1. A gastrostomy should be routinely considered for all patients receiving radical chemoradiotherapy to both sides of the neck.

2. A gastrostomy should be considered for patients having radical RT with large volumes encompassing all or a substantial part of the upper aerodigestive tract mucosa.
3. Other patients can be managed expectantly, and nasogastric tube feeding employed to maintain adequate and safe oral nutrition and hydration as required during RT.

Radiation dermatitis

Management is based on symptom control. It is important to instruct patients to gently clean and dry the skin in the radiation field before each irradiation session. In mild cases, topical moisturizers are used (e.g. aqueous creams) but not immediately prior to RT. In more severe cases, other topical treatments such as hydrogel (e.g. Intrasite Gel), hydrophilic dressings, topical steroids (e.g. hydrocortisone 1% cream), and silver sulfadiazine 1% cream can be considered.

Speech and safe swallow

Particularly when the larynx is within the treated area, speech therapy support is important in preventing unnecessary mucosal trauma and monitoring for silent aspiration.

Late effects of radiation

The late toxicities from RT can be seen as a continuation of acute toxicities many months after completion of treatment and the development of new toxicities months or years later. Many of these toxicities can be permanent. The structures at risk for late effects of radiotherapy to the head and neck are listed in Table 3.2.

Salivary glands

The incidence and severity of the effects of RT on the salivary glands depend on the mean dose of RT received.

RT plans aim to keep the mean parotid gland dose to <24 Gy particularly on the contralateral side. Shielding even a proportion of one parotid gland may preserve reasonable salivary flow in the longer term. In cases where this is not possible, salivary gland damage can lead to chronic xerostomia and can be associated with severe symptoms of dry mouth and rapidly progressive dental caries.

These symptoms can be ameliorated by the use of artificial saliva preparations and increased oral fluid intake. There is some evidence that pharmacological interventions such as pilocarpine

may benefit a proportion of patients but at the risk of additional side effects.

The return of salivary function is slow; it can take several years and is almost invariably incomplete.

Disturbances of taste

RT can also produce disturbances in taste, which occur early in the course of treatment and persist for many months. Failure to appreciate the texture and real taste of food is common and can exacerbate existing swallowing problems.

Dental

All patients undergoing RT to the head and neck require a restorative dentist's assessment and subsequent recommendations, which are aided by detailed information from the oncologist regarding proposed RT volumes and doses. Pre-treatment dental clearance is recommended only in cases of very bad dental caries. With a conservative approach, the majority of patients can keep their teeth and the risk of osteoradionecrosis (ORN) is minimized.

Radionecrosis

Soft tissue, cartilage, or bone necrosis are uncommon late complications of RT. Trivial trauma can occasionally produce significant necrosis of the pharyngeal mucosa. Laryngeal cartilage necrosis can cause chronic problems in relation to swallowing function. ORN is most commonly seen in relation to the mandible and is often precipitated by post-RT dental extraction. Treatment is usually with surgical debridement and antibiotics, but occasionally formal resection is required. If dental extractions are required post-RT, hyperbaric oxygen therapy has proved to be very helpful in reducing the incidence of ORN.

Muscles and soft tissue

Severe fibrosis of the muscles and tissues around the mandible can produce trismus. This may be severe and can affect both eating and speaking. Regular jaw-opening exercises, using rubber wedges of gradually increasing thickness, can prevent or ameliorate trismus. Such treatment must be started early.

Lymphoedema can commonly be seen after RT affecting mucosa internally or in the soft tissues of the neck. Symptoms are usually mild, but more severe cases will benefit from the input of a lymphoedema specialist.

Endocrine deficiency

When the thyroid gland is within the RT field, up to 50–60% of patients may develop biochemical hypothyroidism, which manifests as a raised thyroid-stimulating hormone level. Only about a third of these patients will develop clinical hypothyroidism. Risks of developing hypothyroidism are increased if there has been previous surgery to the neck.

Spinal cord damage

Lhermitte's sign is a transitory complication of RT to the cord, but its occurrence does not imply any increased risk of subsequent myelopathy. It typically occurs 3–15 months following the completion of treatment and is self-limiting.

The potentially fatal complication of RT induced myelopathy is exceptionally rare (<1%) when the maximum cord dose is kept below 55 Gy.

TABLE 3.2 Structures in the Head and Neck That Are Vulnerable to the Adverse Late Effects of Radiotherapy

Tissue	Total Dose at 2 Gy pf	Total Dose at 2.75 Gy pf	Sequel
Lens	6	5.5	Cataract
Retina	52	46	Loss of vision
Optic nerve	56	50	Loss of vision
Anterior eye	70	61	Dry eye
VIIIn	65	57	Hearing loss
Cranial nerves	65	57	CN palsy
Temporal lobe	55	48	Epilepsy dementia
Brainstem	54	48	Dysarthria, nystagmus, disturbed consciousness
Spinal cord	50	45	Myelopathy
Temporal bone	64	56	Osteonecrosis

Note: The doses given indicate a level at which approximately 5% of patients might be expected to experience the complication.
Abbreviations: CN, cranial nerve; pf, per fraction.

Neurotoxicity

Peripheral nerves are traditionally regarded as being relatively radioresistant; however it may be prudent to impose a dose constraint on the brachial plexus when high doses of RT are given to the mid and lower neck.

Tinnitus and sensorineural hearing loss

There is a dose–response relationship for the severity of the direct effects of RT on the cochlea. Tinnitus and high-frequency hearing loss after irradiation are increasingly seen with doses above 45 Gy and are exacerbated by concomitant cisplatin use. Post-RT middle ear effusion can cause similar symptoms but is self-limiting.

Optic structures

These structures are rarely within the RT field but have varying sensitivities to RT damage. The lens is most sensitive and a single fraction of 5 Gy is sufficient to produce cataract; however this can be easily be treated surgically.

The lacrimal apparatus and cornea can also be affected by high-dose radiation therapy (>70 Gy). Severe damage will cause a painful dry eye and sometimes enucleation is required.

High RT dose to the retina may cause exudative retinopathy, leading to impaired vision. Steroids and laser coagulation may buy some time but vision may ultimately be lost.

The tolerance to radiation of the optic nerve is higher than that of the retina, but if damage does occur, blindness is inevitable, and there is no effective treatment.

Second malignancy

While previous RT to the head and neck is associated with a small decrease in the risk of second primary HNC locally it may also be associated with a small increase of other in-field malignancies such as thyroid cancers and sarcomas up to 15 years after exposure.

General principles of combined treatment in head and neck carcinoma

In stage I and II disease, either surgery or definitive radiotherapy provides good local control, acceptable toxicity, and satisfactory functional outcome. For locally advanced disease (stage III and IV), a combined-treatment approach should be considered at MDT. Surgery followed by post-operative RT or chemoradiotherapy (CRT) frequently offers the highest chance of achieving cure, particularly in oral cavity cancers. CRT remains the gold standard in non-resectable disease including most locally advanced oropharyngeal tumors. It is also preferred in resectable patients when the anticipated functional outcome after surgery would be poor, e.g. organ-preserving CRT for locally advanced laryngeal cancers. However, the decision to omit surgery and offer organ-sparing CRT should always be taken at MDT, and informed patient preference is paramount to the final decision.

Post-operative radiotherapy and chemotherapy

The option of post-operative adjuvant RT/CRT should be considered at MDT in all cases. It is recommended for the following adverse prognostic features: (1) histologically positive (<1 mm), (2) close resection margins (<5 mm), (3) N2–3 disease, (4) T3–T4 primary, (5) perineural or vascular invasion, (6) positive surgical margin (where re-excision is not advised), (7) extracapsular nodal extension. Adjuvant CRT increases local control rates and

improves survival in groups 1, 6, and 7. Consideration of adjuvant RT alone is recommended in the presence of one or more of the remaining adverse prognostic features. CRT is given with cisplatin routinely and a RT dose of 60 Gy in 30 fractions. In cases where none of the adverse prognostic features are demonstrated, radiotherapy can safely be omitted.

Chemoradiotherapy

Concurrent CRT remains standard care for locally advanced disease where non-surgical treatment is indicated. The benefit of CRT over RT was summarized by the MACH-NC Collaborative Group meta-analysis as improving loco-regional control rates and giving a 6.5% increase in overall survival.[11] CRT also improves the rate of organ preservation.[12] The benefit of adding chemotherapy decreases with the patient's age and remains marginal over 70 years of age. Single-agent cisplatin is the most widely used option.

Induction chemotherapy (IC) followed by CRT is not proven to be more effective than CRT alone. Randomized controlled trials[13–15] have examined this strategy using a variety of regimens in both IC and CRT arms but, unfortunately, the results are inconsistent.

Radiotherapy combined with targeted therapies

CRT, although effective, causes significant toxicity.

Cetuximab, a monoclonal antibody inhibitor of EGFR is effective concurrent with RT in HNC. EGFR is a member of the family of receptor tyrosine kinases that convert extracellular signals to intracellular responses including increased cell proliferation, motility, adhesion, and invasion as well as induction of angiogenesis and inhibition of apoptosis.

RT with concurrent cetuximab compared to RT alone has shown a significant improvement in loco-regional control overall and disease-free survivals[16] with no difference in acute grade 3/4 in-field toxicities or quality of life.

Two phase III trials DeEscalate[17] and RTOG1016[18] have compared cisplatin-based CRT to cetuximab plus RT in good-prognosis (HPV p16+) oropharyngeal cancers and definitively found cisplatin CRT to be superior.

Cetuximab, however, does provide a valid alternative in cases where patients are unfit to receive platinum-based treatment.

Trials investigating the role of other targeted biological agents in conjunction with RT are underway. Checkpoint inhibitors which inhibit the programmed cell death receptor 1 (PD1) such as nivolumab and pembrolizumab are prominent in this research, which will almost certainly result in the introduction of these novel therapies to clinical practice. There is also interest in hypoxic sensitizers such as nimorazole, particularly in more elderly and infirm patients.

Palliative radiotherapy

Palliative RT is considered in cases of incurable head and neck cancer. The aim is to achieve symptom control and improvement of quality of life. Toxicity is minimized as lower RT doses are used compared to radical RT. The most frequent indication for palliative RT is to improve pain caused by local spread of cancer or distant bone metastases. Symptoms of tumor-related bleeding, dysphagia, and skin ulceration can sometimes benefit from palliative RT. Simple RT techniques are typically used with one direct or two fields. Total doses of 8 Gy in 1 fraction, 20 Gy in 5 fractions, and 30 Gy in 10 fractions are the most commonly used alternatives.

Palliative systemic therapy

Cytotoxic chemotherapy, EGFR inhibition, and checkpoint inhibitors may benefit patients with locally recurrent or metastatic disease in conjunction with best supportive care.

Because palliative chemotherapy carries significant risk of side effects, it is usually offered to patients with a good performance status and minimal co-morbidities. Cisplatin/5-fluorouracil is the most accepted palliative regimen. Methotrexate is used in some centers as a less toxic alternative with better compliance in administration. However, while median survival is similar response rates are higher with the doublet.

When cetuximab is added to cisplatin/5-fluorouracil chemotherapy, an improvement in response rate, progression-free and overall survival is seen as described in the landmark EXTREME trial.[19]

Immunotherapy with checkpoint inhibition has more recently become standard of care in palliative treatment of HNC patients. Nivolumab, given on progression of disease within 6 months of platinum-based treatment, is superior to conventional second-line chemotherapy (taxane or methotrexate) with less toxicity.[20] Pembrolizumab plus chemotherapy has shown improved overall survival compared to cetuximab chemotherapy in the first-line setting.[21]

Oligometastatic disease and re-irradiation

In selected cases of localized recurrence, re-irradiation can be considered. This treatment is feasible and provides durable locoregional control in some patients, particularly if preceded by surgery. Delivering a second course of RT to the same area in the head and neck is more challenging because of the side effects of prior therapy and concerns about the risks of high cumulative RT doses to normal structures. The irradiated volume should be restricted to the tumor with a limited margin without elective nodal irradiation. Advanced RT techniques like IMRT, stereotactic body radio surgery (SBRT), or proton therapy are recommended to minimize the dose near critical normal structures. Equivalent doses of 50–66 Gy in 25–33 fractions are commonly used. Chemotherapy or cetuximab may be used concurrently to achieve better results. The American College of Radiology has published guidelines for the use of re-irradiation in head and neck cancer.[22]

In cases of oligometastatic disease, particularly in the lung, consideration can be given to surgical resection or SBRT.

Rehabilitation

Rehabilitation after treatment of HNC is multidisciplinary. It is now standard practice to allocate a "key worker" to every new patient presented to the MDT. This person has the responsibility of referring them to other appropriate team members as and when necessary.

The main issues in the rehabilitation of head and neck cancer patients are summarized in Box 3.2.

BOX 3.2   SUMMARY OF ISSUES OF CONCERN IN THE REHABILITATION OF PATIENTS WITH HNC

PREVENTION OF SECOND PRIMARY TUMORS

- Change in smoking and drinking habits
- Chemoprevention
- Regular ENT assessment

PHYSIOTHERAPY

- After radical neck dissection or other major surgery

SPEECH THERAPY

- After laryngectomy
- Care of the voice during and after radiotherapy
- Swallowing and mastication problems (video-fluoroscopy)

PROSTHETICS/PROSTHODONTICS

- After major head and neck surgery

DENTAL CARE

- After radiotherapy (xerostomia and caries)

PSYCHOLOGICAL SUPPORT

- Accepting and dealing with diagnosis
- Specific issues related to perceived damage from treatment
- Relationships and sexuality
- Problems with body image

SOCIAL SUPPORT

- Financial and social worries
- Loss of earnings
- Homelessness
- Alcoholism

Palliative care

Overall, 50% of patients with HNC die from uncontrolled locoregional disease. Isolation, pain, cachexia, and fear can all combine to produce a miserable existence for these patients, which are challenging for palliative care specialists to control.

All patients in the palliative phase of their disease should be discussed in the MDT.

Staging

The prognosis of patients with HNC is related to the extent and spread of the tumor, the fitness, age, and comorbidities of the patient, and to treatment given. Traditional clinical staging systems concentrate primarily on those factors related to the tumor. The tumor, node metastases classification (TNM) is most commonly employed. The Union for International Cancer Control (UICC) TNM system for cancer has undergone several revisions, most recently the 8th in 2017.[23]

The primary tumor (T) is staged T1 to T4 based on location, size, and infiltration of surrounding tissues (Box 3.3).

Nodal disease is termed N1 to N3 based on size, location, and number of involved nodes (Box 3.4). Additional categories are used to describe when the tumor or lymph nodes cannot be assessed; TX or NX, where there is no evidence of primary tumor or nodal metastases or when only carcinoma in situ is seen; T0 or N0. Tumor and lymph nodes can be staged on clinical or pathological grounds; for the sake of clarity the clinical versions are used here. There are some important variations between anatomical tumor subsites which are discussed in the relevant sections below. Distant metastases are deemed present, M1, or absent, M0.

BOX 3.3   GENERIC T STAGING OF PRIMARY TUMOR, BASED ON UICC (2017; REF 23)

- *T1*: Tumor 2 cm or less
- *T2*: Tumor more than 2 cm but not more than 4 cm
- *T3*: Tumor more than 4 cm or with specified local extension
- *T4a*: More locally advanced tumor but possibly still resectable, invading bone, cartilage, skin, etc.
- *T4b*: Very locally advanced and likely unresectable with clear margins, encasing carotid artery, invading skull base, etc.

BOX 3.4   GENERIC N STAGING OF NODAL DISEASE, BASED ON UICC (2017; REF 23)

- *N1*: Metastasis in a single ipsilateral lymph node, 3 cm or less
- *N2a*: Metastasis in a single ipsilateral lymph node more than 3 cm but not more than 6 cm
- *N2b*: Metastasis in multiple ipsilateral lymph nodes, none more than 6 cm
- *N2c*: Metastasis in bilateral or contralateral lymph nodes, none more than 6 cm
- *N3a*: Metastasis in lymph node more than 6 cm
- *N3b*: Metastasis in a single or multiple lymph nodes with clinical extranodal extension

---

There are seven common anatomical levels used to describe neck nodes in HNC:

- *Level I*: Sub mental and submandibular triangle—bounded by bellies of digastric, mandible, and hyoid.
- *Level II*: upper jugular nodes—from skull base to hyoid.
- *Level III*: middle jugular nodes—from hyoid to cricoid.
- *Level IV*: lower jugular nodes—from cricoid to clavicle.
- *Level V*: posterior triangle nodes—between anterior border of trapezius, posterior border of sternocleidomastoid and clavicle.
- *Level VI*: anterior central nodes—from hyoid to suprasternal notch and bounded on each side by the carotid sheath.
- *Level VII*: nodes in the superior mediastinum inferior to the suprasternal notch.

TNM categories are organized into five groups designated stages based on prognosis (Table 3.3). Staging of HNC is uniform across most anatomical subsites but with important variations for HPV-positive oropharyngeal cancer, nasopharyngeal cancer, and unknown primary cervical nodes.

Squamous cell carcinoma of unknown primary presenting as a cervical lymph node

The UK guidelines (2016) make the following recommendations:

TABLE 3.3   UICC Stage Grouping for Head and Neck Cancer: Excepting Oropharynx HPV-Positive and Nasopharynx

Stage Group	T	N	M
0	Tis	N0	M0
I	T1	N0	M0
II	T2	N0	M0
III	T3	N0	M0
	T1	N1	M0
	T2	N1	M0
	T3	N1	M0
IVA	T4a	N0, N1	M0
	T1, T2, T3, T4a	N2	M0
IVB	Any	N3	M0
	T4b	Any	M0
IVC	Any	Any	M1

Note: Stage groupings, based on TNM, for cancer of the head and neck.
Source: Wittekind et al., 2017, with permission.

All patients presenting with confirmed cervical lymph node metastatic squamous cell carcinoma and no apparent primary site should undergo:

1. Positron emission tomography-computed tomography whole-body scan.
2. Panendoscopy and directed biopsies.
3. Bilateral tonsillectomy.
4. Tongue base mucosectomy can be offered if facilities and expertise exist.

While many HNC present as a neck node, following the diagnostic workup above only 1–3% will remain of true unknown primary site. Subsequent guidelines recommend:

5. Concomitant chemotherapy with radiation should be considered in patients with an unknown primary.
6. Concomitant chemotherapy with radiation should be offered to suitable patients in the post-operative setting, where indicated.
7. Neo-adjuvant chemotherapy can be used in gross "unresectable" disease.
8. Patients should be followed up at least every 2 months in the first 2 years and every 3 to 6 months in the subsequent years.
9. Patients should be followed up to a minimum of 5 years with a prolonged follow up for selected patients.
10. Positron emission tomography–computed tomography scan at 3 to 4 months after treatment is a useful follow-up strategy for patients treated by chemoradiation therapy.

Management is with curative intent but has not been clearly defined by the results of randomized controlled trials and falls broadly into two categories:

1. *Management of the neck.*
   Prognosis depends on the extent of neck involvement at presentation with survival for the N1 neck being approximately twice that of the N3 neck at 5 years.
   Single modality treatment either surgery or CRT is appropriate for the N1 neck without ECS (extracapsular extension).

For higher stage disease, neck dissection may be followed by RT or CRT (Close/positive margins, ECS) or CRT alone may be given particularly if there is HPV-related disease. RT to the bilateral neck should be considered for stage >/= N2.

2. *Management of possible primary sites.*

The traditional approach to treatment when the primary site cannot be defined has been to use extended-field radiotherapy, with a treatment volume that includes not only the neck nodes bilaterally but also the potential sites for the primary tumor. These would include the nasopharynx, piriform fossa, and whole of the larynx. The largest published experience of this strategy was from a Danish group citing outcomes over 20 years' follow up of 352 patients.[24] Most of these patients were treated with primary radiotherapy to the bilateral neck and possible primary sites. Those receiving the more comprehensive treatment had non-significantly better outcomes including overall survival, and the subsequent emergence rate of the primary site was 20% overall. A more recent publication of the outcomes of 52 patients, half of whom had neck dissection and were treated with comprehensive IMRT, reported only a 2% primary emergence rate and 88% overall survival rate at 5 years.[25]

Oral cavity

The oral cavity consists of the lips, oral tongue, floor of mouth, buccal mucosa, alveolus, retromolar trigone, and hard palate. Globally incidence varies considerably but in the UK oral cavity primaries make up about 28% of all HNC with an incidence of 5 per 100,000 of population per year.

While the nodal staging of these cancers follows the generic scheme (Box 3.4), T staging of oral cavity tumors is characterized by the emphasis on depth of tumor invasion (at <5 mm, 5–10 mm, or >10 mm) in addition to tumor dimension.[23]

Smoking and alcohol are the principal risk factors but betel nut use (in Asia), HPV infection, and UV exposure are also important.

Surgical treatment remains the preferred management option of both early and locally advanced cancers. RT or CRT is mainly employed as adjuvant therapy for locally advanced cancers with the field including the surgical tumor bed and both sides of the neck due to the high risk of nodal metastasis.

Lip

Lip cancer constitutes about 15% of all oral cancers. The biggest risk factor is exposure to UV light.

Over 90% are squamous, and over 90% are on the lower lip. Nodal involvement is rare at presentation (<5%) with poor differentiation and greater tumor thickness being the main risk factors. Upper lip cancers tend to have a much worse prognosis.

- Surgery is the primary treatment. Larger lesions may require a local advancement or transposition flap repair.
- There is no indication for routine treatment of local lymph nodes.
- Early lesions are equally well-treated with RT or surgery. Adjuvant RT/CRT improves local control when indicated.
- Five-year survival ranges from 80% for T1/2 tumors to 50% for T3/4 tumors.

Oral tongue

Approximately 40% of all oral cavity cancers arise in the mobile anterior 2/3 of the tongue.

Palpable lymphadenopathy is evident in 30–40% of patients at presentation and a further 30% have occult disease. Tumor thickness >4 mm is predictive of a 20% risk of nodal involvement.

Elective ipsilateral neck dissection should be offered in all surgical cases as it has been shown to improve overall and disease-free survival. Sentinel lymph node biopsy is increasingly being used in place of up front neck dissection.

Simple surgical excision with an adequate margin is effective for small lesions. A standard hemiglossectomy is appropriate for larger lesions not extending across the mid-line. Those crossing the mid-line require more extensive surgery usually with a mandibulotomy for access.

Primary RT/CRT is rarely indicated for oral tongue cancer, but adjuvant treatment is recommended for advanced cancers with the usual high-risk indicators. The high morbidity of adjuvant RT/CRT at this site means observation may be a valid approach for patients with lower risk indicators such as vascular/neural invasion.

Overall 5-year survival is 70% for stage I/II and 40% for stage III/IV.

Floor of mouth

These tumors comprise 15% of all oral cavity cancers. The risk of lymph node spread is high with more than half of patients harboring occult metastases at presentation.

Management is very similar to that of cancers of the anterior tongue. Presentation is often relatively late with tumor adherent to or eroding the mandible. In such cases, a marginal or a segmental mandibulectomy may be required.

A neck dissection, either radical, modified, or supraomohyoid, should be performed in continuity with the primary lesion.

Adjuvant RT/CRT is recommended for stage III/IV disease.

Overall 5-year survival is 90% for stage I/II and 50% for stage III/IV.

Buccal mucosa

These tumors comprise 15% of all oral cavity cancers.

Tumors may arise in a pre-existing area of submucous fibrosis and rarely present at T1 stage. Locoregional recurrence is higher than for other oral cavity sites.

Small tumors may be successfully treated by either surgery or radiotherapy; large tumors will require a combination of the two.

Overall 5-year survival is 75% for stage I/II and 50% for stage III/IV.

Alveolus, hard palate, and retromolar trigone

These tumors comprise 15% of all oral cavity cancers. Local recurrence rates are high. Lymph node involvement is seen in >20% of T2–T4 tumors.

Alveolar and retromolar trigone tumors can frequently be treated with marginal mandibulectomy, but segmental mandibulectomy is required for more advanced disease.

In cancers of the hard palate, the majority of cases demonstrate bone involvement, necessitating resection of palatal bone with reconstruction using a dental plate with or without an obturator.

Radical radiotherapy is associated with a significant risk of osteoradionecrosis, but adjuvant RT/CRT is given for the usual indications.

Overall, 5-year survival is approximately 70% for stage I/II disease and <50% for stage III/IV.

Oropharynx

The oropharynx comprises the base of tongue (posterior 1/3), vallecula, tonsils, soft palate, and posterior pharyngeal wall. Oropharyngeal cancers (OPC) have been increasing dramatically in incidence worldwide since the late 1990's. Most recent figures for the UK demonstrate an incidence of 5 per 100,000 persons per year in 2010–2012 or 25% of all HNC. Evidence demonstrates HPV (particularly genotype 16) as an independent risk factor now accounting for up to 70% of cases. Between 60% and 75% of patients have palpable cervical nodes at presentation, and the majority (around 70%) have T3 or T4 primaries.

The T staging for OPC deviates from the generic format in assigning a single T4 category for HPV-associated cancers. The N staging for HPV-positive OPC does not make a distinction for extranodal extension and attaches significance only to unilateral vs. contralateral/bilateral and to nodes greater or less than 6 cm.[23]

HPV-positive OPC has a significantly better prognosis than OPC caused by smoking, and this is reflected in a separate staging classification for HPV-positive patients (Table 3.4). Note the presence of T4 or N3 disease is classified as stage III.

Patients frequently present with neck node metastases with or without symptoms at the primary site. OPC can cause pain, a unilateral sore throat, referred otalgia, and/or dysphagia. Mucosal ulceration is common. Currently, management protocols for OPC do not distinguish between HPV status although it is an area of intense scientific interest and the subject of a number of clinical trials.

Base of tongue and soft palate

These are considered midline structures. Early stage I and II tumors can be treated with radical RT/CRT to both the primary tumor and bilateral neck nodes or with trans oral laser resection and neck dissection with adjuvant RT/CRT as indicated. RT/CRT is generally favored for the soft palate because of the greater likelihood of functional impairment with surgery. More advanced stage disease is managed with concurrent chemoradiotherapy due to frequent post-operative problems with speech and swallowing in this group.

Tonsil

RT/CRT or trans oral resection and neck dissection with adjuvant RT/CRT as indicated, are valid options for stage I/II tonsil primaries. Well-lateralized tumors of the tonsil have a low risk of

contralateral node involvement, and treatment is usually delivered to the primary site and ipsilateral neck lymph nodes. RT/CRT to the contralateral neck is usually indicated when the primary crosses the midline or when there are multiple ipsilateral nodes. Stage III/IV disease is usually treated with RT/CRT for organ preservation with surgery reserved for recurrent disease.

Posterior Wall

Posterior wall OPC is rare. These cancers are often advanced at the time of presentation, and prevertebral muscle involvement renders many inoperable. If the patient is fit for treatment, chemoradiotherapy is the preferred option for most cases.

Prognosis of OPC

Excellent survival has been demonstrated for HPV-positive OPC particularly in non-smokers. Even with N1/2 lymph node involvement, this group has a 3-year survival of about 90%. An intermediate 3-year survival of 70% is seen in patients who are HPV-positive with a >10 pack-year smoking history. The worst 3-year survival, of 46%, is seen in HPV-negative smokers (excluding those with T1/2 N0 disease) and HPV-negative nonsmokers with T4 disease.

Hypopharynx

Carcinoma of the hypopharynx is rare, accounting for approximately 5% of all HNC in the UK.

Only 15% of these tumors present at stage I/II with up to 70% having nodal metastases and 20% distant metastatic spread at diagnosis. Submucosal extension is common, and occasionally satellite lesions are seen.

Etiology is smoking, alcohol, and environmental pollution. Initial symptoms can be vague including dysphagia, odynophagia, and hoarseness followed by dyspnea, otalgia, and neck masses.

The main subsites are the pyriform sinus, posterior pharyngeal wall, and posterior cricoid space. Tumors arising on the lateral pharyngeal surface of the aryepiglottic folds are more appropriately considered with tumors of the supraglottic larynx.

The T staging and N staging of hypopharyngeal tumors follow the generic scheme but attach additional significance to fixation of the hemilarynx.[23]

Pyriform fossa

Approximately 70% of all hypopharyngeal tumors arise in the pyriform fossa. Approximately 5% are T1 tumors. Even small primary tumors may be associated with advanced neck disease and prophylactic treatment of the neck is therefore indicated in all N0 patients.

The majority of pyriform fossa cancers are treated with surgery followed by post-operative CRT, although single-modality treatment with surgery or RT alone can be effective in early-stage disease. In a minority of more advanced cases with good performance status, an organ-sparing treatment can be considered with induction chemotherapy followed by RT or up-front CRT. Patients with extensive cartilage or vocal cord infiltration are unsuitable for this approach.

Surgery for advanced disease usually entails pharyngo-laryngectomy and block dissection of the ipsilateral or bilateral neck. A permanent tracheostomy is inevitable. Reconstruction of the neo-pharynx may be required using either a skin flap (myocutaneous or free graft) or a visceral reconstruction (stomach). More advanced surgical techniques such as transoral robotic surgery

TABLE 3.4   **UICC Stage Grouping for Head and Neck Cancer: Oropharynx HPV-Positive**

Stage Group	T	N	M
0	Tis	N0	M0
I	T1, T2	N0, N1	M0
II	T1, T2	N2	M0
	T3	N0, N1, N2	M0
III	T1, T2, T3	N3	M0
	T4	Any N	
IV	Any T	Any N	M1

Note: Stage groupings, based on TNM, for cancer of the head and neck.
Source: Wittekind et al., 2017, with permission.

are increasingly being considered for advanced hypopharyngeal cancers.[26]

Post-cricoid

These rare tumors can be associated with a pre-existing post-cricoid web or Plummer–Vinson syndrome. They are similar in behavior to tumors of the upper third of the esophagus. Surgically, the best curative option is a total pharyngo-laryngo-esophagectomy and stomach transposition.

Posterior pharyngeal wall

See comments on posterior oropharyngeal wall tumors.

Prognosis of hypopharyngeal cancers

Five-year survival for early-stage tumors is approximately 50%. For more advanced tumors, this falls to below 30%. Overall, there is a discrepancy between disease-specific survival (52%) and overall survival (33%) which reflects the importance of intercurrent deaths and new primaries (often lung) in this group of patients.

Larynx

Approximately 20% of all HNC arises from the larynx with a male predominance. The main etiological factors are smoking and alcohol. The larynx is composed of three subsites, glottic, supraglottic, and subglottic. Most cancers occur in the glottis (70%) and tend to present early with hoarseness. There are three glottic subsites: Cord, anterior commissure, and posterior commissure. Nodal involvement at presentation is rare (<5%), reflecting the poor lymphatic supply to the vocal cords.

Supraglottic (25%) and subglottic (<5%) tend to present with more advanced disease. The supraglottis has a rich lymphatic plexus draining to the subdigastric and mid-cervical nodes while the subglottis drains to the lower cervical, paratracheal, and mediastinal nodes. Approximately half of supraglottic tumors arise from the lower supraglottis and half from the epilarynx, i.e. the suprahyoid supraglottis, the aryepiglottic fold, and the arytenoid. Approximately 50% of patients with epilaryngeal tumors are stage T4, and almost half have palpable nodes at presentation, compared with only 25% of patients with tumors of the lower supraglottis. Tumors of the epilarynx tend to behave more like pharyngeal tumors.

While the N staging of laryngeal cancers follows the usual pattern, the T staging is quite different, assigning importance to number of anatomic subsites involved, presence of vocal cord fixation, and cartilage involvement rather than the tumor dimensions.[23]

The presence of cord fixation as one of the defining features of a T3 tumor can arise through a variety of mechanisms: sheer tumor bulk, stenting the cord, cricoarytenoid joint involvement, disruption of the recurrent laryngeal nerve by tumor, or direct infiltration of the intrinsic muscles of the larynx. Cord mobility is better assessed on indirect or fiber-optic laryngoscopy rather than in the anesthetized, paralyzed patient. CT scanning is mandatory in staging laryngeal tumors to define the extent of cartilage invasion, evidence of local spread beyond the larynx, and nodal disease. Clinical staging of laryngeal tumors will frequently be escalated on imaging.

The patient who presents with stridor due to a laryngeal tumor usually has advanced disease, but careful assessment should take place if possible. To avoid tracheostomy, endoscopic debulking may be possible to secure the airway. Emergency laryngectomy

is rarely indicated and requires confirmation of tumor histology either beforehand or by frozen section at the time of surgery.

Management of laryngeal tumors

For carcinoma in situ of the vocal cord, simply stripping the cord can provide both material for diagnosis and, in the short-term at least, effective treatment. Endoscopic laser excision is now the best definitive treatment for in situ carcinoma of the larynx.

For early-stage glottic tumors (T1/T2) endoscopic laser excision offers local control rates as good as those obtained with RT. The criteria for suitability for laser excision include lack of involvement of the anterior commissure, fitness for anesthesia, and lack of paraglottic space or arytenoid involvement (as judged by CT). RT should remain the primary treatment of choice when laser excision is likely to result in significant deterioration in voice quality. Early-stage supraglottic and subglottic carcinomas can be treated with laser excision, robotic surgery, or RT, but elective treatment of the neck is required due to the higher risk of lymph node involvement.

The choice of treatment for locally advanced laryngeal carcinoma lies between surgery and organ-sparing CRT with salvage laryngectomy. For T3 and early T4 primaries, organ-sparing conservative treatment remains the preferred option. Rates of salvage laryngectomy are significantly lower for T3 vs. T4 disease (29% vs. 56%). The remaining T4 laryngeal cancers are treated with total laryngectomy as tumors showing cartilage invasion are much less likely to be cured by RT. Radical neck dissection is combined with laryngectomy in the presence of cervical lymphadenopathy. Postoperative RT/CRT is usually required after surgery.

Laryngectomy is also employed for patients whose tumors persist or recur after primary radiotherapy and in whom laser resection or robotic surgery is not indicated.

Laryngectomy after radiotherapy

The most common indication for this is residual or recurrent tumor. This may be clinically obvious, be suggested by serial CT scanning, or present as intractable "perichondritis." Diagnosis of tumor in relation to the latter may only be possible by careful examination of the laryngectomy specimen. Chronic pain, dysphonic voice, and airway compromise (which in itself sometimes necessitates a tracheostomy) will often lead the patient to request surgery even in the absence of overt tumor recurrence. Another indication is a larynx that is scarred and incompetent, usually several years post-RT. The symptoms usually precipitating the decision to proceed with surgery are chronic stridor, pain, and/or intractable aspiration.

Previous RT undoubtedly increases the complication rate for laryngectomy.

Prognosis of laryngeal cancers

Overall 5-year survival is around 90% for T1 tumors and 80% for T2 tumors. For T3 and T4 tumors this falls to 50–60%. As in other HNC sites disease-specific survival is 10–15% higher, reflecting the high rate of intercurrent deaths and second malignancies in these patients.

Nasopharynx

Nasopharyngeal carcinoma (NPC) is a rare cancer in the UK, accounting for just 2% of all HNC; however the incidence is 20–30 times higher in some Eastern countries. It is three times more common in men. Three main factors are important for the development NPC: genetic susceptibility, EBV infection, and dietary factors such as salted fish containing high nitrosamine levels.

The WHO histologic classification of NPC is the most widely used system:

- *Type I*: keratinizing squamous: 25% UK NPC is not related to EBV and behaves more like a typical HNC.
- *Type II + III*: non-keratinizing carcinoma differentiated (12%) and undifferentiated (63%): EBV associated.
- *Type IV*: Basaloid squamous: Very rare, associated with aggressive course and poor prognosis.

The staging for NPC is distinct from that for other head and neck cancers in that comparatively more advanced disease has a lower T and N staging. In terms of T stage, the extent of primary tumor infiltration of surrounding structures is assessed rather its dimensions. The appearance of involved lymph nodes below the cricoid cartilage and nodal masses greater than 6 cm are associated with higher N stage.[23]

The nasopharynx is difficult to assess clinically. CT scanning and MRI are essential to obtain accurate anatomical information about the primary and its spread. Most tumors originate in the fossa of Rosenmuller, and the earliest radiological sign is blunting of the angle at the Eustachian cushion. CT scanning has highlighted the importance of spread into the parapharyngeal space which cannot be assessed clinically. Around 30% of patients with clinically negative necks will have occult nodal involvement on imaging, which will also demonstrate involvement of the skull base in approximately 35% of cancers.

About 75% of patients have palpable neck nodes at presentation, and a neck mass is the presenting symptom in 40–50% of patients. The remaining patients usually present with nasal symptoms (obstruction and epistaxis) or with otological symptoms (deafness and tinnitus). Headache, often severe, central, and unresponsive to standard analgesics, usually indicates a locally advanced tumor. Between 20% and 25% of patients have cranial nerve palsies at presentation.

Management of NPC

RT/CRT is the primary radical treatment for NPC. Stage I and node negative stage II disease can be treated by RT alone. CRT with 3-weekly cisplatin is considered to be the standard regime. Induction chemotherapy has shown a benefit in disease-free survival but not overall survival on meta-analysis; however toxicity is substantial and may impair effective delivery of definitive CRT. A more recent RCT (randomized control trial) of induction cisplatin and gemcitabine chemotherapy plus CRT vs. CRT alone in 480 patients with locoregionally advanced NPC, has shown an absolute improvement in overall survival at 3 years of 5%.[27]

RT is targeted to the primary tumor and affected lymph nodes. IMRT is the gold standard although proton treatment may be advantageous in terms of reduced toxicity particularly with extensive involvement of the base of skull. The adjacent anatomical compartments considered at risk of microscopic spread from the tumor and the bilateral neck nodes (levels lb through V, and retropharyngeal nodes) are also irradiated to prophylactic dose. Even in N0 disease, elective bilateral nodal irradiation is recommended due to the high incidence of occult neck metastasis.

Management of recurrence

Approximately half of patients with locoregional recurrence will be found to have synchronous distant metastases and can be

TABLE 3.5   UICC Stage Grouping for Head and Neck Cancer: Nasopharynx

Stage Group	T	N	M
Stage 0	Tis	N0	M0
Stage I	T1	N0	M0
Stage II	T1	N1	M0
	T2	N0, N1	M0
Stage III	T1, T2	N2	M0
	T3	N0, N1, N2	M0
Stage IVA	T4	N0, N1, N2	M0
	Any T	N3	M0
Stage IVB	Any T	Any N	M1

Note: Stage groupings, based on TNM, for cancer of the head and neck.
Source: Wittekind et al., 2017, with permission.

offered palliative treatments. Salvage therapy offers the hope of long-term survival in selected patients with solely locoregional recurrence. For patients with nodal recurrence surgery is the treatment of choice. Patients with local recurrence can be treated by nasopharyngectomy or re-irradiation. If RT is chosen, highly selective treatment may be delivered by SRS, brachytherapy, or proton beam as they are potentially less toxic modalities than standard IMRT.

Prognosis of NPC

Overall survival by stage in Western countries will be inferior to that of Eastern countries due to the proportionally higher incidence of non-EBV associated disease. Staging of NPC differs from other sites and is shown in Table 3.5. Data from America suggest a 65–70% 5-year survival for stages I and II and a 40–60% 5-year survival for stages III and IV. Combined 5-year survival in England across all stages is 50%.

Tumors of the nasal cavity and paranasal sinuses

Tumors of the nose and paranasal sinuses are characterized by histological and anatomical heterogeneity and comprise approximately 4% of all HNC. Half occur in the nasal cavity and half in the sinuses. The T staging for the nasal cavity/ethmoid sinus and the maxillary sinus differs from the generic model in that tumor dimensions are not recorded, giving precedence to the extent of subsite involvement and boney invasion.[23] The nasal cavity subsites are the septum, the floor of the nasal cavity, the side walls of the nasal cavity, and the nasal vestibule (skin-covered area just inside the nostril). The majority of sinus cancers are seen in the maxillary and ethmoid regions; tumors of the sphenoid and frontal sinuses are very rare.

The etiology of this group of cancers are tobacco smoke, occupational exposure (e.g. hardwood dust), air pollution, and possibly HPV virus infection.

In contrast to other HNC sites there is a broad variety of histological variation. Overall squamous cell carcinoma comprises 50% and adenocarcinoma 20% while the remainder are accounted for by miscellaneous histologies including adenoid cystic, mucoepidermoid, melanoma, and sarcoma.

Nasal cavity tumors tend to present with obstruction (70%) and bleeding (40%). Sinus tumors initially have vague symptoms and the majority present with symptoms of local invasion such as pain, unilateral nasal obstruction, bleeding, and discharge.

Nasal cavity

Nodal involvement at presentation is uncommon (10% and 15%), so elective treatment of the neck is usually not indicated. Cancers of the nasal vestibule tend to present earlier than other nasal cavity subsites and behave more like skin cancers

Many tumors involve bone or cartilage, and primary surgery is therefore the preferred treatment. A lateral rhinotomy provides excellent access to tumors arising from the lateral nasal wall or septum. Endoscopic resection can be considered in some cases.

Adjuvant RT/CRT is indicated in most cases where the tumor is staged T2 or above. RT/CRT can be considered as a definitive treatment in inoperable patients or those who refuse surgery. The proximity of critical structures such as the ocular apparatus and brainstem can make delivery of the necessary RT dose difficult and lead either to compromises in irradiated volumes or significant risk of long-term toxicities. In the future the more widespread use of proton therapy may help ameliorate this problem.

Paranasal sinuses

Approximately 70–90% of tumors are T3 or T4 at presentation. Lymph node involvement at presentation or during 5-year follow-up is uncommon (<15%).

Surgical treatment remains the preferred option. For maxillary sinus tumors a radical maxillectomy is usually the minimum required. Orbital invasion may necessitate orbital exenteration. Tumors of the ethmoid sinus frequently involve the orbit, and the ipsilateral eye may have to be sacrificed. Extension superiorly into the anterior cranial fossa may necessitate craniofacial surgery. Sphenoid and frontal sinus tumors tend to present late, and surgery has little to offer due to the close anatomical proximity of crucial neurovascular structures.

RT is mainly employed as post-operative adjuvant therapy for such advanced cases. In some cases, neoadjuvant or adjuvant CRT is considered, extrapolating from results at other HNC sites. As in the nasal cavity the complexity of the target volume and close proximity of other vital structures lead either to compromises or increased risks. The field will often include the ipsilateral orbit and/or the adjacent skull base. Neck lymph nodes are included in the presence of cervical lymphadenopathy. In some centers, elective radiotherapy to the ipsilateral submandibular and upper cervical nodes is recommended in negative neck for T3/T4 tumors.

Prognosis of nasal cavity and paranasal sinus tumors

For nasal cavity tumors, overall and disease-free survival are similar at about 60% to 80% at 5 years but vary with histological type. Local recurrence is the predominant cause of treatment failure, and isolated nodal relapse is uncommon (<20%). Distant metastases are seen in <20% overall but are more common in certain histological subtypes such as adenoid cystic. The prognosis of nasal vestibule tumors is better overall and mirrors that of skin cancers by stage.

For the paranasal sinuses, maxillary tumors tend to do better. Overall 5-year survival varies according to T stage, from 60% for early tumors to less than 40% for T4 tumors. Failure of local control accounts for more than 80% of all failures. Only about 5–10% of patients relapse in the regional nodes. About 5% of patients develop distant metastases, and less than 5% develop second primaries

Inverting papilloma (Ringertz tumor)

This is not an HNC but a locally aggressive benign tumor usually found in the nasal cavity with a high risk of post-treatment recurrence if subperiosteal resection is not undertaken. Endoscopic surgery is increasingly being used. However approximately 5% will be found to have undergone malignant change with foci of squamous cell carcinoma seen on histological inspection post-resection.

The presence of malignant change in the excised specimen is an indication for consideration of postoperative RT.

Rare and unusual tumors of the head and neck

External auditory canal

The incidence in the United Kingdom at this site is less than 1/1,000,000 per annum. The majority of malignant tumors are squamous carcinomas.

Tumors of the medial bony canal may spread to the middle ear, so it may be difficult to differentiate them from middle ear carcinomas. CT and MRI are required to accurately delineate the extent of local infiltration. Lymph node metastases are rare (<5%).

A lateral petrosectomy (removing bone and soft tissues lateral to a sagittal plane running through the middle ear cleft) and post-operative RT or CRT, in more advanced stages, is the treatment of choice. Five-year survival is excellent if clear margins are obtained but falls to approximately 60% when the tumor cannot be completely removed surgically.

Middle ear

These tumors also have an incidence in the United Kingdom of less than 1/1,000,000 per annum. They cause severe otalgia and can produce palsies of one or more of the last six cranial nerves (a facial nerve palsy being the most common). Nodal spread is uncommon. Only about 20% of patients have T1 tumors at presentation.

These tumors are best managed by a combination of surgery and post-operative RT/CRT to the tumor bed, pre- and post-auricular lymph nodes. The clinically negative neck does not require dissection.

About 30% of patients present with disease that is too far advanced to permit radical therapy, in which case palliative RT may be an option.

Surgery and RT for carcinoma of the middle ear will produce a 5-year survival rate of around 40-60%. Failure to control local disease is the usual cause of treatment failure.

Paragangliomas

Paragangliomas are slow-growing neuroendocrine tumors arising from extra adrenal autonomic paraganglia. Overall incidence is low (2/100,000 per annum), and females outnumber males by approximately 3 to 1.

About 10% of head and neck paragangliomas will display malignant behavior and 5% will secrete catecholamines. Only 5–10% of paragangliomas metastasize, primarily to local lymph nodes. Around 20% of patients will have multiple tumors. This is particularly true of familial cases. The symptoms and clinical findings depend on the site of origin.

The simplest classification of paragangliomas is by site:

- Middle ear = glomus tympanicum
- Jugular bulb ± middle ear = glomus jugulare
- Parapharyngeal = glomus vagale
- Carotid bifurcation = carotid body tumor/chemodectoma

The choice of treatment lies between surgical resection and RT. The former is the treatment of choice in fit, operable patients. Older patients, or those in whom surgical resection would produce unacceptable morbidity, are best treated with RT. Stereotactic body radiotherapy (SBRT) is increasingly being used for jugular and skull base paragangliomas. Five-year survival for malignant paragangliomas is approximately 80% for regionally confined and only 10% for those with distant metastases.

Olfactory neuroblastoma

These tumors arise from the olfactory epithelium in the roof of the nasal cavity with an incidence of only one case per 5 million population per year.

Patients usually present with anosmia, nasal obstruction, nasal discharge, or epistaxis. The Kadish system has been used for clinical staging:

- A: confined to the nasal cavity
- B: involvement of the paranasal sinuses
- C: spread beyond the nasal cavity or paranasal sinuses

Treatment is primarily surgical, with craniofacial resection being the standard procedure. Post-operative RT should be given to patients with high-grade tumors, or those in whom excision is incomplete. Inoperable tumors, or tumors in patients who are unfit for surgery, can be treated with radical RT. Because of the complexity of the target volume and close vicinity of multiple organs at risk, proton treatment is increasingly being considered both for adjuvant and radical cases.

Combined surgery and RT lead to a 5-year survival of 65%.

Late recurrence, beyond 10 years, is typical of this tumor. Distant metastases occur in up to 20% of patients. There is limited experience with chemotherapy in metastatic disease, but cisplatin-based regimens may be considered in patients of good performance status.

Mucosal melanomas

Less than 10% of melanomas occurring in the head and neck arise from mucosa. The nose, paranasal sinuses, and oral cavity are the commonest sites, 20% are multifocal, and lymphatic spread is seen in approximately 10–20%.

Surgery offers the best chance of long-term local control although the anatomical location means clear margins are frequently difficult to obtain. Post-operative RT should be considered where there is doubt about the adequacy of the surgical margins; although a survival benefit has not been shown, local recurrence risk is reduced. For patients whose tumors are inoperable, RT alone can provide effective palliation. Adjuvant immunotherapy can be considered as an option because of its effectiveness in cutaneous melanoma, but clinical trial evidence is currently lacking.

Most patients will develop metastatic disease, usually in the lung. Imatinib may offer significant therapeutic benefit in metastatic disease harboring the KIT mutation. Overall, 5-year survival is less than 25%.

Key learning points

- Successful management of HNC requires a multiprofessional, multidisciplinary approach with the individual patient placed firmly at the center of the decision-making process.
- Although the majority of head and neck cancers are squamous carcinomas, these tumors are remarkably heterogeneous, both biologically and clinically. There are no universal rules for managing head and neck cancer.
- Systemic therapies (cytotoxic, biological, and immunomodulatory) have a limited but increasingly important role to play in the treatment of HNC. At least some of this benefit is related to their local radio-sensitizing effects when given concurrently with radiotherapy.
- Technical developments in surgery and radiotherapy continue to decrease the toxicity and long-term morbidity associated with the treatment of HNC.

References

1. Paleri V, Roland N. Introduction to the United Kingdom national multidisciplinary guidelines for head and neck cancer. *J Laryngol Otol.* 2016; 130(S2): S3–4.
2. https://www.nccn.org/professionals/physician_gls/default.aspx.
3. Gatta G, Botta L, Sánchez MJ et al. Prognoses and improvement for head and neck cancers diagnosed in Europe in early 2000s: The EUROCARE-5 population-based study. *Eur J Cancer.* 2015; 51:2130–2143.
4. Nutting CM, Morden JP, Harrington KJ et al. Parotid-sparing intensity modulated versus conventional radiotherapy in head and neck cancer (PARSPORT): A phase 3 multicentre randomised controlled trial. *Lancet Oncol.* 2011; 12:127–36.
5. Grégoire V, Evans M, Le QT et al. Delineation of the primary tumour clinical target volumes (CTV-P) in laryngeal, hypopharyngeal, oropharyngeal and oral cavity squamous cell carcinoma: AIRO, CACA, DAHANCA, EORTC, GEORCC, GORTEC, HKNPCSG, HNCIG, IAG-KHT, LPRHHT, NCIC CTG, NCRI, NRG Oncology, PHNS, SBRT, SOMERA, SRO, SSHNO, TROG consensus guidelines. *Radiother Oncol.* 2018; 126(1):3–24.
6. Gregoire V, Levendag P, Ang KK et al. CT-based delineation of lymph node levels and related CTVs in the node-negative neck: DAHANCA, EORTC, GORTEC, NCIC, RTOG consensus guidelines. *Radiother Oncol.* 2003; 69:227–36.
7. Gregoire V, Eisbruch A, Hamoir M et al. Proposal for the delineation of the nodal CTV in the node-positive and the post-operative neck. *Radiother Oncol.* 2006; 79:15–20.
8. Chao KC, Apisarnthanarax S, Ozyigit G, editors. *Practical Essentials of Intensity Modulated Radiation Therapy.* 3rd ed. Philadelphia, PA: Lippincott Williams & Wilkins, 2014.
9. Lee TF, Fang FM. Quantitative analysis of normal tissue effects in the clinic (QUANTEC). *Int J Radiat Oncol Biol Phys.* 2010; 76(3Suppl):S3–9.
10. Kovács G, Martinez-Monge R, Budrukkar A et al. GEC-ESTRO ACROP recommendations for head & neck brachytherapy in squamous cell carcinomas: 1st update—Improvement by cross sectional imaging-based treatment planning and stepping source technology. *Radiother Oncol.* 2017; 122(2): 248–54.
11. Pignon JP, le Maître A, Maillard E et al. Meta-analysis of chemotherapy in head and neck cancer (MACH-NC): An update on 93 randomised trials and 17,346 patients. *Radiother Oncol.* 2009; 92:4–14.
12. Forastiere AA, Goepfert H, Maor M et al. Concurrent chemotherapy and radiotherapy for organ preservation in advanced laryngeal cancer. *N Engl J Med.* 2003; 349:2091–8.
13. Haddad R, O'Neill A, Rabinowits et al. Induction chemotherapy followed by concurrent chemoradiotherapy (sequential chemoradiotherapy) versus concurrent chemoradiotherapy alone in locally

advanced head and neck cancer (PARADIGM): a randomised phase 3 trial. *Lancet Oncol.* 2013; 14(3):257.

14. Cohen EE, Karrison TG, Kocherginsky M et al. Phase III randomized trial of induction chemotherapy in patients with N2 or N3 locally advanced head and neck cancer. *J Clin Oncol.* 2014; 32(25):2735.

15. Ghi MG, Paccagnella A, Ferrari D et al. Induction TPF followed by concomitant treatment versus concomitant treatment alone in locally advanced head and neck cancer. A phase II–III trial. *Ann Oncol.* 2017; 28(9):2206.

16. Bonner JA, Harari PM, Cohen RB et al. Radiotherapy plus cetuximab for locoregionally advanced head and neck cancer: 5-Year survival data from a phase 3 randomized trial, and relation between cetuximab-induced rash and survival. *Lancet Oncol.* 2010; 11:21–8.

17. Mehanna H, Robinson M, Hartley A et al. Radiotherapy plus cisplatin or cetuximab in low-risk human papillomavirus-positive oropharyngeal cancer (De-ESCALaTE HPV): an open-label randomised controlled phase 3 trial. *Lancet.* 2019; 393(10166):51.

18. Gillison ML, Trotti AM, Harris J et al. Radiotherapy plus cetuximab or cisplatin in human papillomavirus-positive oropharyngeal cancer (NRG Oncology RTOG 1016): a randomised, multicentre, non-inferiority trial. *Lancet.* 2019; 393(10166):40.

19. Vermorken JB, Mesia R, Rivera F et al. Platinum-based chemotherapy plus cetuximab in head and neck cancer. *N Engl J Med.* 2008; 359:1116–27.

20. Harrington KJ, Ferris RL, Blumenschein G Jr et al. Nivolumab versus standard, single-agent therapy of investigator's choice in recurrent or metastatic squamous cell carcinoma of the head and neck (CheckMate 141): health-related quality-of-life results from a randomised, phase 3 trial. *Lancet Oncol.* 2017; 18(8):1104.

21. Cohen EEW, Soulières D, Le Tourneau C et al. Pembrolizumab versus methotrexate, docetaxel, or cetuximab for recurrent or metastatic head-and-neck squamous cell carcinoma (KEYNOTE-040): a randomised, open-label, phase 3 study. *Lancet.* 2019; 393(10167):156.

22. McDonald M, Lawson J, Garg MK et al. ACR appropriateness criteria retreatment of recurrent head and neck cancer after prior definitive radiation: Expert panel on radiation oncology-head and neck cancer. *Int J Radiat Oncol Biol Phys.* 2011; 80:1292–98.

23. Wittekind C, Brierley JD, Gospodarowicz MK. *TNM Classification of Malignant Tumours.* 8th ed. Oxford: Wiley Blackwell, 2017.

24. Grau C, Johansen LV, Jakobsen J et al. Cervical lymph node metastases from unknown primary tumours. Results from a national survey by the Danish Society for Head and Neck Oncology. *Radiother Oncol.* 2000; 55(2):121.

25. Frank SJ, Rosenthal DI, Petsuksiri J et al. Intensity-modulated radiotherapy for cervical node squamous cell carcinoma metastases from unknown head and-neck primary site: M. D. Anderson cancer center outcomes and patterns of failure. *Int J Radiat Oncol Biol Phys.* 2010; 78: 1005–10.

26. Dziegielewski PT, Kang SY, Ozer E. Transoral robotic surgery (TORS) for laryngeal and hypopharyngeal cancers. *J Surg Oncol.* 2015; 112(7):702.

27. Zhang Y, Chen L, Hu GQ, et al. Gemcitabine and cisplatin induction chemotherapy in nasopharyngeal carcinoma. *NEJM.* 2019; 381(12):1124.

4 THYROID

Kate Newbold and Clive Harmer

Introduction

The thyroid follicular cell can give rise to a wide variety of neoplasms, ranging from incidental papillary microcarcinoma, which has no effect on life expectancy despite minimal treatment, to lethal anaplastic cancer, which is invariably fatal despite aggressive treatment. The majority of cases occur in young adults, but thyroid cancer can affect any age group. The age-standardized incidence in the United Kingdom has increased by around two-and-a-half times over the last 30 years from only 900 cases per year being diagnosed between 1990 and 1994 (1.7 per 100,000) to 3500 between 2014 and 2016 (5.7 per 100,000).[1] This figure is predicted to rise by 74% in the UK between 2014 and 2035, to 11 cases per 100,000 people by 2035.

Mortality rates remain low and have decreased in the UK by 47% since the 1970s.[1] Most patients are cured; therefore, morbidity caused by treatment should not exceed that caused by the disease. With increasing incidence of small and indolent thyroid cancers, care should be taken not to expose patients to treatments inconsistent with their prognosis. Management of thyroid cancer demands multidisciplinary care, including consultation with the pathologist, surgeon, oncologist, endocrinologist, and nuclear physician.

Epidemiology

Thyroid cancer is the most common endocrine malignancy, but it remains rare, accounting for only 1% of all cancers in the United Kingdom.[1] Incidence rates vary widely: the highest in North America of 15.1 per 100,000 in women can be compared with the lowest rates in central Africa, where rates in women are 1.2 per 100,000. U.K. rates remain lower than the European average. These geographical differences are probably caused by environmental and dietary factors such as iodine intake rather than by race or heredity.[2] The incidence has been increasing, partly reflecting past use of radiotherapy for benign childhood conditions and long-term survival in patients treated with radiotherapy and partly due to increased detection with ultrasonography and incidental findings following scans such as positron emission tomography (PET)/computed tomography (CT) and carotid Doppler ultrasounds carried out for other purposes. The incidence is strongly related to both age and sex. Thyroid cancer is rare in children, with incidence increasing steadily with age. Age-specific incidence rates rise from around age 10–14 slowly in males and more rapidly in females, with the highest rates between 50 and 54 years for females and between 85 and 89 years for males.[1] The ratio between men and women is 1:2.7, that is, 3.2 per 100,000 in men and 8.1 per 100,000 in women in the United Kingdom.[1]

Etiology

Radiation exposure increases the incidence of well-differentiated thyroid cancer. Individual radiation exposure is increasing mainly due to the medical use of ionizing radiation in diagnostic imaging. It is reported that radiation exposure has doubled in the United States from 1980 to 2006.[3] Age at exposure is inversely related to the risk. American studies from the 1950s showed that between 32% and almost 100% of children with thyroid cancer had received prior irradiation for a variety of conditions including enlarged thymus, tonsils, adenoids, or acne. In Belarus, the most affected country after Chernobyl, the incidence increased to 13.5 per 100,000 children in 2000 compared with the usual incidence of less than 1 per 100,000. The majority of cases occurred in children under the age of 10 years at the time of the accident, with at least two-thirds younger than 5.[4] In a cohort of childhood cancer survivors, 7.5% of all secondary malignancies were thyroid cancers.[5] Judicious use of diagnostic imaging is therefore advised in children. In fact, the American Thyroid Association has issued guidance for thyroid shielding during diagnostic dental x-rays for both children and adults.[6] A second type of radiation exposure to the thyroid is from radioisotopes that concentrate in the gland. A meta-analysis reported that the relative risk of developing a thyroid cancer following treatment for thyrotoxicosis with radioiodine was 1.99 (95% confidence interval [CI]: 0.92–1.33) and a dose effect was observed at doses greater than 1 Gy.[7] The latent period is at least 3–5 years, with most cases occurring between 20 and 40 years after exposure.

Thyroid tumors can be produced in animals by iodine deficiency or drugs. A common factor in these experimental conditions is prolonged stimulation by the thyroid-stimulating hormone (TSH). A sequence of reversible hyperplasia followed by irreversible hyperplasia and in some cases, by the subsequent development of follicular carcinoma has been noted.[8] Evidence of primary TSH-related induction of thyroid tumors in humans is not convincing. However, papillary carcinoma is more common in iodine-rich areas such as islands, whereas a number of case-controlled studies have strongly suggested that low dietary iodine content is responsible for the increased rates of follicular and anaplastic cancer in areas of endemic goitre.[9] Because of the strong female predominance, the influence of sex-hormone status has been investigated. A pooled analysis of case-control studies also confirmed a weak association of menstrual and reproductive factors with thyroid cancer risk.[10] The biological basis of these epidemiological observations could be that estrogen acts as a growth promoter on thyrocytes. Some experimental evidence suggests that thyrocytes express estrogen receptors, and estrogens may stimulate thyrocyte growth in cell-culture systems. It has also been shown that tamoxifen inhibits the growth of papillary cancer cells both *in vitro* and *in vivo*.

Differentiated thyroid cancer (DTC), specifically papillary thyroid carcinoma (PTC) and follicular thyroid carcinoma (FTC), comprises 95% of all thyroid malignancies, of which about 5% are familial. These may be associated with syndromes that are composed of predominately non-thyroidal tumors, including Cowden's disease (PTEN-hamartoma tumor syndrome), Pendred syndrome, Werner syndrome, Carney complex type 1, and familial adenomatous polyposis/Gardner's syndrome. Other conditions with less established links to the development of DTC include ataxia-telangiectasia syndrome, McCune Albright syndrome, and Peutz–Jeghers syndrome. There remain some families with preponderance to DTC with no established genotype–phenotype correlation such as PTC with multinodular goiter or PTC with renal cell carcinoma.[11]

Pathogenesis

Although thyroid follicular cells can give rise to both benign and malignant tumors, the evidence to support an adenoma to carcinoma multi-step pathogenesis is not universally accepted. Malignant transformation is due to the activation of proto-oncogenes or the inactivation of tumor suppressor genes in combination with environmental factors. Defects to the tyrosine kinase receptor genes are commonly found in thyroid cancer. The interaction of these receptors with growth factors leads to the activation of the mitogen-activated protein kinase (MAPK) pathway through RAS and BRAF proteins, resulting in uncontrolled cell division. A pan-cancer study using The Cancer Genome Atlas (TCGA) showed that PTC is a tumor with one of the lowest tumor mutational burdens, usually with only a single driver gene alteration.[12] This provides some explanation of the indolent nature of thyroid cancer compared with other solid tumors. The fact that the development of thyroid cancer occurs following single gene alterations suggests that these could be potential therapeutic targets to provide effective disease control.[13]

PTC usually shows single mutations: BRAF 40–45%, RET/PTC rearrangements 10–20%, and RAS point mutations 10–20%. Prognosis is generally very good in these tumors. However tumors with multiple gene mutations, e.g. BRAF V600E together with TERT promoter or TP53, PIK3CA, AKT1, have an adverse prognosis. The coexistence of BRAF V600E and TERT promoter mutations correlates with lymph node metastasis, multifocality, distant metastasis, tumor recurrence, extrathyroidal extension, and disease specific mortality.[14] This pattern of mutations is seen in those differentiated thyroid cancers that transform to poorly differentiated or anaplastic thyroid cancer.

Follicular variant PTC (fvPTC) has a genotype similar to FTC with RAS mutations, BRAF K601E mutations, and PAX8/PPARG rearrangements. A subgroup of fvPTC has recently been reclassified as non-invasive follicular thyroid neoplasm with papillary like nuclei (NIFTP). These tumors show an absence of BRAF V600E, the presence of RAS mutations, and PAX8/PPARG translocations and are now not considered malignant tumors.

FTC differs from PTC with mutations seen in NRAS, HRAS, and KRAS genes in 40–50%, PAX8/PPARG rearrangements in up to 35%, and PTEN and PIK3CA in 5–10%. Hurtle cell variant shows a much lower frequency of RAS and PAX8/PPARG and absence of PTEN and PIK3CA. BRAF V600E mutations are very rare in FTC.

Pathology and natural history

Thyroid tumors can originate from the follicular epithelium, from parafollicular or C cells, or from non-epithelial stromal elements. The World Health Organization (WHO) classifies malignant epithelial thyroid tumors as papillary carcinoma, follicular carcinoma, medullary carcinoma, and undifferentiated (anaplastic) carcinoma.[15] The American Joint Committee on Cancer (AJCC) tumor, nodes, metastases (TNM) eighth edition classification is recommended to assist in making management decisions and for the uniformity of case-series reporting.

Papillary carcinoma

Papillary carcinoma is the most common type, comprising 80% of all thyroid malignancies. These tumors are almost three times as common in women as in men, with a peak incidence in the third and fourth decades. The histological hallmarks are branching papillae arranged on a fibrovascular stalk. Tumor cells are cuboidal with a homogeneous cytoplasm and characteristic hypochromatic nuclei with absent nucleoli (Orphan Annie eyes) and may contain laminated calcified psammoma bodies (Figure 4.1a). Features of papillary cancer include an infiltrating pattern of growth, multi-focality (up to 75% of cases), and spread to the regional lymph nodes. Obvious cervical adenopathy is seen in 50% of patients at presentation but reported in as many as 90% of those who undergo elective node dissection. Hematogenous metastases are less common and mainly involve the lungs; lung involvement at diagnosis occurs in 5–10% of cases in adults but may be in up to 25% of children. Certain variants of papillary cancer, such as tall cell, columnar, and diffuse sclerosing variants, have been shown to be more aggressive. Follicular variant of papillary thyroid carcinoma (FV-PTC) is a common variant of PTC; the long-term outcome remains excellent and similar to that of classical PTC.[16]

Follicular carcinoma

Follicular carcinoma accounts for 5–20% of thyroid tumors and is also three times more common in females than in males, but it tends to present in midlife. It lacks the diagnostic features of papillary cancer. It may be extremely difficult to diagnose when well differentiated, as the appearance is similar to that of both normal thyroid and benign follicular adenoma. The presence of capsular or vascular invasion is often the only feature to denote malignancy (Figure 4.1b). Depending on the degree of invasiveness, it may be described as minimally or widely invasive. This distinction defines the less favorable prognosis associated with the latter. Lymph node metastases are less common than in papillary tumors, but hematogenous spread to bones and lungs is present in 14% of patients at diagnosis.

Hürthle-cell carcinoma was previously considered a variant of follicular cancer and is composed of cells that exhibit oncocytic changes (Figure 4.1c). However, it is now recognized as a distinct pathological entity because of its different oncogenic expression. The majority of Hürthle-cell tumors are benign, but malignancy is documented in local recurrence and distant metastases. Histopathological studies have shown that either capsular or vascular invasion is a reliable criterion of malignancy. Although they are usually well differentiated and produce thyroglobulin, these tumors rarely take up iodine. This is a contributory factor to their poorer prognosis than other follicular carcinomas.[17]

Insular carcinoma is a form of poorly differentiated tumor arising from follicular cells with behavior intermediate between differentiated and undifferentiated carcinoma, characterized by a nested growth pattern and prominent vascularity. It invades both lymphatics and veins, resulting in nodal and distant metastases with poor prognosis.[18]

Microcarcinoma

Microcarcinoma is defined by the WHO to be a tumor 1 cm or less in maximum dimension. Incidence ranges from 0.5% to 14%; however, this is strongly dependent on the accuracy and extent of pathological review.[19] Microcarcinomas make up 30% of all DTC and are largely responsible for the increase in incidence of DTC over the last decade.[20] In patients undergoing surgery for benign thyroid disease, particularly Hashimoto's, rates of incidental microcarcinoma have been reported to be 2–49.9%.[21–23] Rates of detection at autopsy are around 8%.[24] Metastases to regional lymph nodes are not uncommon, with rates between 12% and 50%,[25–32] but distant metastases are extremely unusual, rarely causing significant morbidity or mortality (0–0.9%).[26,33,34]

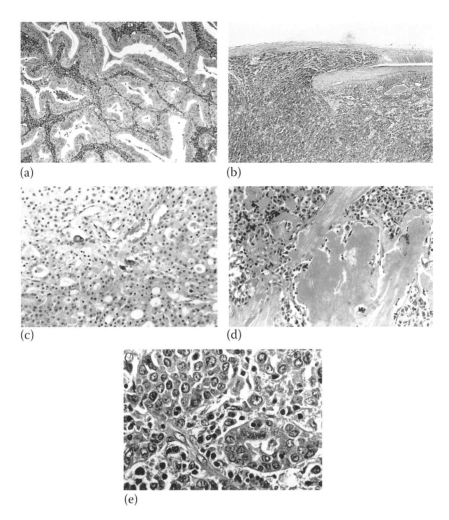

FIGURE 4.1   (a) Papillary cancer, tall cell variant; (b) follicular cancer, showing capsular invasion; (c) Hürthle-cell carcinoma; (d) medullary carcinoma with amyloid stroma; (e) non-Hodgkin lymphoma of mucosa-associated lymphoid tissue type.

Anaplastic carcinoma

Anaplastic thyroid cancer is one of the most aggressive of all malignancies and one of the most lethal. There are 70–90 new cases annually in the United Kingdom, accounting for 3% to 4% of all thyroid cancers.[35] The incidence has been reported to be decreasing due to more accurate diagnosis, more aggressive management of DTC, and increased dietary iodine. It is most common in the elderly, with 75% of the patients being over 60 years old. Most series quote a ratio of men to women of 1:3. It may be associated with a long history of goiter; a significant number of cases are probably associated with a pre-existing DTC.[36]

These tumors also arise from the follicular cell. However, the natural history, clinical presentation, and outcome reflect their undifferentiated biology with rapid growth and invasive characteristics. Histological variants include small cell, giant cell, and spindle cell, although these subtypes have no known prognostic significance.

Patients present with a rapidly enlarging collar of tumor and confluent lymphadenopathy often invading the trachea, larynx, or esophagus, resulting in stridor, hoarseness, or dysphagia. The majority die within 6 months of the first symptom from aggressive loco-regional disease. All anaplastic thyroid cancers are TNM Stage IV. A small proportion (2–6%) may be diagnosed as

an incidental finding in a thyroidectomy specimen. At diagnosis, 25–50% of patients have pulmonary metastases, and at death, this figure approaches 100%.

Medullary carcinoma

Medullary carcinoma of the thyroid (MTC) accounts for 7% of all thyroid tumors but 14% of all thyroid cancer mortality. Sporadic MTC accounts for 70–80% of cases, with the remainder being familial. Hereditary MTC can occur alone—familial medullary thyroid carcinoma (FMTC)[37]—or as the thyroid manifestation of multiple endocrine neoplasia (MEN) type II syndromes (MEN IIa and MEN IIb), as shown in Table 4.1. These are autosomal

TABLE 4.1   MTC Syndromes

Phenotype	Frequency (%)	Presentation
Sporadic MTC	80	MTC
MEN IIa	9	MTC, pheochromocytoma, hyperparathyroidism
MEN IIb	3	MTC, pheochromocytoma, neuromas (see Figure 4.2), Marfanoid habitus
FMTC	8	MTC

dominant disorders caused by germline mutations in the RET proto-oncogene, located on the long arm of chromosome 10, band q11.2, which codes for a tyrosine kinase receptor.

Medullary carcinoma arises from the parafollicular or "C" cells, which are of neural crest origin and secrete calcitonin as well as other peptides: carcinoembryonic antigen (CEA), adrenocorticotrophic hormone, serotonin, bradykinin, prostaglandin, and vasoactive intestinal peptide. Immunohistochemical staining for calcitonin granules is the most accurate method to establish the diagnosis (Figure 4.1d). Fewer than 20% of sporadic tumors are bilateral, but in the familial syndromes, medullary cancer is usually bilateral and multi-centric. At presentation, involvement of cervical or mediastinal lymph nodes is seen in 11–75% of patients and distant metastases (to lung, bone, and liver) in 12%.

Lymphoma of the thyroid

Lymphoma of the thyroid is rare, representing 2% of thyroid malignancies and 2% of extra-nodal lymphomas. Chronic autoimmune stimulation, as in Hashimoto's thyroiditis, is a predisposing factor. There is a strong female predominance, and the median age at diagnosis is in the seventh decade, similar to that of anaplastic cancer, from which it must be distinguished (Figure 4.1e). An analysis of the U.S. National Cancer Database published in 2019 identified 3466 patients between 2004 and 2015. The median all-cause survival was 11.6 years (CI: 11.1 to 12.1 years). The majority were diffuse large B cell lymphoma (DLBCL, 59.5%), with marginal zone lymphoma (18.3%) and follicular and Burkitt lymphoma (8% and 1.9%, respectively) making up the rest.[38] Mucosa-associated lymphoid tissue (MALT) is a form of marginal zone lymphoma and is characterized by a low grade of malignancy, slow growth rate, and a tendency for late relapse or second lymphomas in other MALT sites.[37]

Patients present with a rapidly enlarging, painless neck mass; one-third of the patients experience compressive symptoms. Symptoms also include fever, night sweats, and weight loss, but these are rare.[39]

Rare tumors

There exists a subset of rare thyroid tumors that exhibit aggressive behavior and have a poor prognosis. These include thymus-like tumors; mucoepidermoid carcinoma; mixed medullary follicular cancers; teratomas; and sarcomas, including angiosarcoma and liposarcoma.[40] The thyroid is also commonly affected by metastases originating from other primary tumor sites.[41]

Diagnostic evaluation

Palpable thyroid nodules are present in 4–7% of all adults; age, gender, history of exposure to ionizing radiation, and method by which the nodules are detected all significantly influence the findings of different retrospective studies. In most series, a 5–15% risk of cancer in all thyroid nodules for the total population is reported.[42] Investigations should be directed towards selecting those with an increased risk of malignancy. However, no single clinical feature, physical finding, or laboratory test is pathognomonic for the detection of thyroid cancer, except for the serum calcitonin level in medullary carcinoma and fine-needle aspiration cytology (FNAC). With significant advances in the understanding of the molecular mechanisms of thyroid cancer, there has been much interest in diagnostic molecular markers such as RET-PTC, RAS, and BRAF V600E mutations; galectin 3; and gene expression markers, mRNA and microRNA. It is likely that

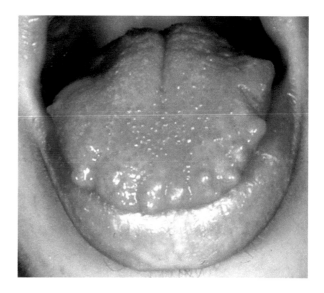

FIGURE 4.2 Patient with multiple endocrine neoplasia IIb demonstrating neuromas of the tongue. Neuromas may also involve the buccal mucosa, eyelid, conjunctiva, and glans penis.

a combination of molecular and cytological testing will increasingly become part of the routine diagnostic workup.[11] Exposure to ionizing radiation, extremes of age, a family history of thyroid cancer or MEN syndromes (Figure 4.2), and other inherited disorders such as Gardner's syndrome and Cowden's disease increase the suspicion of cancer. Although not specific for malignancy, a history of rapid growth, pain, hoarseness, or airway obstruction is of concern. On examination of the neck, attention should be paid to the size, consistency, mobility, and number of nodules as well as to the presence of enlarged lymph nodes. The risk of malignancy is greater in a solitary nodule (5–15%) than in multiple nodules; a dominant nodule or a nodule that changes size in a multinodular goiter requires further investigation. Cervical adenopathy is the most consistent feature of malignancy with a thyroid mass, but it lacks specificity.

Ultrasonography is an essential adjunct to clinical examination for assessment of nodule size, detection of multiple nodules, and assisting in FNAC. A hyperechoic nodule with well-defined margins is more likely to be benign. In contrast, a nodule that appears hypoechoic with irregular margins, microcalcification, and increased blood flow should raise suspicion. Despite these features, ultrasound cannot reliably distinguish benign from malignant lesions, and FNAC is still required.

The most important investigation for evaluating thyroid nodules remains FNAC; diagnostic accuracy ranges from 70% to 95%, depending on the skills of the operator and the reporting cytopathologist. The report should be defined as inadequate (Thy1), benign (Thy2), follicular (Thy3a and Thy3f), suspicious (Thy4), or malignant (Thy5).[43] Inadequate samples should be followed by repeat FNAC under ultrasound guidance. The malignant potential of follicular neoplasms cannot be determined cytologically; therefore, surgical excision in the form of thyroid lobectomy is advised. Molecular testing may be helpful but is not yet in routine use in the United Kingdom. FNAC is adequate to diagnose anaplastic cancer, but histopathology is required to distinguish the subtypes of primary thyroid lymphoma by immunohistochemistry and ascertain MALT status.

Radionuclide imaging with iodine (^{131}I) or sodium pertechnetate (^{99m}Tc) is of limited value in the initial evaluation of thyroid nodules since the advent of FNAC. Cold nodules are more likely to be malignant, but warm and hot nodules can also be malignant.

Following thyroidectomy and radioiodine ablation of remnant thyroid tissue, diagnostic whole-body ^{131}I scanning is highly specific; focuses of uptake correspond to thyroid cancer metastases. Less well-differentiated tumors may concentrate so little ^{131}I that the diagnostic scan will prove false negative. Locating these tumors may be helpful in planning alternative treatment, including surgical resection. Fluorodeoxyglucose (FDG) positron emission tomography co-registered with computed tomography (18FDG-PET/CT) may be useful, and the sensitivity of the investigation can be increased by preparing the patient with recombinant human TSH (rhTSH).[44] Imaging modalities for the investigation of rising calcitonin in MTC include indium-111 (^{111}In) octreotide, gallium-68 dotatate PET/CT, fluorine 18 DOPA (dihydroxyphenylalanine)-PET/CT, fluorine 18FDG-PET/CT, and [123]I *meta*-iodobenzylguanidine (mIBG).[45]

CT or magnetic resonance imaging (MRI) can define tumor extension to structures such as trachea or vessels and nodal involvement in the neck or mediastinum. Imaging of the chest may reveal micronodular disease in the lungs not shown on chest x-ray. MRI is preferred to avoid the use of iodinated contrast, which reduces uptake of subsequent radioiodine therapy.

Tumor, nodes, metastases

All patients must have their diagnosis confirmed histologically and their TNM stage recorded. The clinical classification is essential to select and evaluate therapy and provides data to estimate prognosis.

Management of differentiated thyroid cancer

DTC is one of the most controversial malignancies in terms of treatment. Almost every stage of management decision making involves debate: the extent of initial surgery, need for lymph node dissection, role of radioactive iodine ablation, value of dosimetry in radioiodine therapy, degree of TSH suppression, and role of adjuvant external-beam radiotherapy (EBRT). The reasons for these ongoing controversies are that DTC is rare and its behavior is indolent. Due to a lack of prospective studies, the potential for relapse may be either underestimated, resulting in patients receiving inadequate treatment, or overstated, so that patients are over-treated.

Certain factors have been linked to the behavior of DTC and are used to determine prognosis. In most studies, age is found to be the most important predictor of outcome; a significant increase in mortality is seen over the age of 40 years (Figure 4.3). Males tend to fare worse than females. Tumor size, extension, and grade are also related to the risks of recurrence and survival (Figure 4.4). Patients with papillary cancer fare better than those with well-differentiated follicular carcinoma. Less well-differentiated follicular tumors show a significantly higher relapse rate and shorter survival. Some series have reported that the ratio of positive to negative lymph nodes following resection is predictive of recurrent disease, whereas others rely on the absolute number of positive nodes and the presence of extra-nodal extension.[46,47] The results of multivariate analysis for 1390 patients with DTC treated at the Royal Marsden Hospital, London, United Kingdom, between 1929 and 1999 are shown in Table 4.2.[48]

Based on these prognostic factors, several scoring systems have been developed to help in assessing individual patient risk of dying from cancer and planning treatment (AGES, AMES, GAMES, and MACIS). None of these systems is perfect, but all succeed in identifying high-risk and low-risk patients.[49,50] Prognosis in the low-risk group is excellent, with cancer-specific mortality lower than 1% at 30 years.[51] The recurrence and survival rates are strikingly different in the high-risk group. A post-ablation assessment at 9–12 months with stimulated serum thyroglobulin (Tg) and neck ultrasound scan (USS) allows potential modification of the initial static risk estimate based on response to ablation. This dynamic risk stratification using a combination of clinicopathological factors plus treatment response criteria allows a more individualized approach to treatment, follow-up, and prognostication.[52] Such a selective approach may spare many patients the

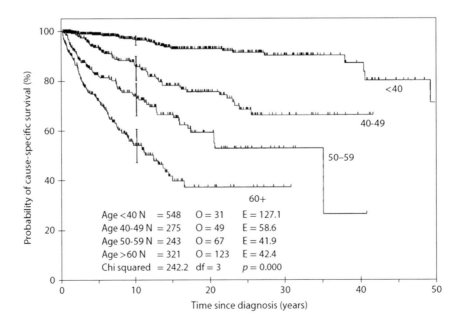

FIGURE 4.3 Differentiated thyroid cancer: Royal Marsden Hospital experience 1929–1999 (1390 patients). Cause-specific survival according to age.

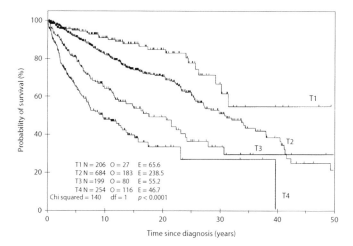

FIGURE 4.4 Differentiated thyroid cancer: Royal Marsden Hospital experience 1929–1999 (1390 patients). Survival according to tumor stage.

TABLE 4.2 Prognostic Factors for Survival, Local Recurrence, and Distant Recurrence for 1390 Patients with Differentiated Thyroid Cancer Treated at the Royal Marsden Hospital between 1929 and 1999

	HR (95% CI)		
Factor	Survival	Local recurrence	Distant recurrence
Age (years)			
≤40	1.0	1.0	1.0
40–49	2.5 (2.3–2.7)	1.4 (1.3–1.6)	1.8 (1.6–2.1)
50–59	6.2 (5.6–6.8)	2.1 (1.9–2.3)	3.3 (2.9–3.7)
≥60	15.3 (13.9–16.8)	2.9 (2.7–3.2)	6.0 (5.3–6.8)
	$p < 0.001$	$p < 0.001$	$p < 0.001$
T stage			
T1	1.0	1.0	1.0
T2	1.9 (1.7–2.1)	1.7 (1.5–1.9)	1.8 (1.6–2.1)
T3	3.5 (3.1–3.9)	2.8 (2.5–3.2)	3.4 (2.9–3.9)
T4	6.5 (5.8–7.2)	4.8 (4.2–5.4)	6.2 (5.4–7.2)
T4	6.5 (5.8–7.2)	4.8 (4.2–5.4)	6.2 (5.4–7.2)
	$p < 0.001$	$p < 0.001$	$p < 0.001$
M stage			
M0	1.0	1.0	1.0
M1	6.9 (5.4–8.7)	0.92 (0.51–1.6)	3.9 (2.6–6.0)
	$p < 0.001$	NS	$p < 0.001$
Surgery			
NT/TT	1.0	1.0	1.0
ST/HT/L	1.89 (1.49–2.4)	1.8 (1.38–2.36)	1.87 (1.3–2.5)
B/E	4.66 (3.56–6.1)	3.48 (2.49–4.85)	3.72 (2.5–5.5)
	$p < 0.001$	$p < 0.001$	$p < 0.001$
Iodine ablation			
No	1.0	1.0	1.0
Yes	0.67 (0.55–0.82)	0.39 (0.31–0.50)	0.4 (0.3–0.58)
	$p < 0.001$	$p < 0.001$	$p < 0.001$
Grade			
I	1.0	1.0	1.0
II	2.6 (2.3–2.9)	2.0 (1.7–2.3)	2.6 (2.1–3.1)
III	6.6 (5.9–7.5)	3.8 (3.3–4.5)	6.7 (5.6–8.0)
	$p < 0.001$	$p < 0.001$	$p < 0.001$

Note: This table shows Cox proportional hazards regression model for multivariate analysis.

Abbreviations: B, biopsy; E, enucleation; HT, hemi-thyroidectomy; L, lobectomy; NS, not significant; NT, near-total thyroidectomy; ST, subtotal thyroidectomy; TT, total thyroidectomy.

morbidity of unnecessarily aggressive treatment and follow-up without compromising outcome.

Surgical treatment

Surgery remains the initial and potentially curative treatment for DTC. However, there is no universal agreement as to the extent of surgical procedure required. The minimum requirement is complete excision of all macroscopic disease, which usually demands ipsilateral lobectomy and isthmusectomy.[53] Most studies have shown a significant reduction in local recurrence rates following total (or near-total) thyroidectomy, with some also reporting improved overall survival (OS).[54,55]

Other advantages in favor of total thyroidectomy are that post-operative follow-up using Tg is facilitated, as well as subsequent ^{131}I therapy if this becomes necessary. The main argument against radical surgery, that is, morbidity, is less important now that experienced surgeons are reporting reduced complication rates. Vocal-cord paralysis occurs in only 1–3% and permanent hypocalcemia in 1–6% in most specialist centers following total or near-total thyroidectomy.

The conclusion of a meta-analysis of 2318 patients was that there was no difference in recurrence or long-term complication rates between patients undergoing total thyroidectomy and those undergoing total thyroidectomy + prophylactic central compartment neck dissection.[56]

The surgical management of lateral neck lymph node metastases is also controversial. If clinically apparent nodal disease is present, most surgeons recommend a modified neck dissection preserving the sternomastoid, spinal accessory nerve, and internal jugular vein. Simple node excision, previously known as "berry picking," is not recommended. If nodes are clinically involved, we favor a selective node dissection of levels II, III, IV, and VI; thyroid cancer rarely spreads to submandibular or posterior cervical lymph nodes (levels I and V).

Endocrine treatment

TSH is the main regulator of thyroid function, differentiation, and proliferation. Binding of TSH to its receptor on thyroid cells primarily activates a cyclic adenosine monophosphate cascade, leading to thyroid hormone synthesis and release as well as to the expression of thyroid-specific genes, including those encoding Tg and thyroperoxidase. DTC retains some degree of thyroid-specific gene expression and function similar to normal thyroid cells; therefore, it is responsive to stimulation by TSH. In thyroid cancer cell lines, TSH has been shown to stimulate vascular endothelial growth factor (VEGF) secretion and angiogenesis. Thus, TSH may promote growth in some thyroid cancers.[57]

The beneficial effect of TSH suppression has not been assessed in prospective studies. However, available data suggest that thyroxine reduces the risk of recurrence, tumor progression, and death from thyroid cancer.[56] It is generally accepted that a TSH level below 0.1 mU/L is desirable, but there is no evidence that undetectable TSH levels offer any advantage over low but detectable levels. The benefits of long-term TSH suppression in patients with a low risk of recurrence are not confirmed, and therefore, a risk-stratified level and duration of TSH suppression should be adopted to minimize the skeletal and cardiac morbidity of TSH suppression, as recommended by both American and European thyroid associations[59,60] (Figure 4.5).

Radioactive iodine ablation of residual thyroid tissue

The value of post-operative ^{131}I to ablate residual normal thyroid is still debated. Arguments in favor of remnant ablation are that it permits subsequent identification by a whole-body scan of any residual or metastatic carcinoma and increases the sensitivity of Tg measurement for follow-up. Most importantly, several retrospective studies have documented that it decreases tumor recurrence and death.[55,61] However, the beneficial effect of ^{131}I ablation can be seen mainly in patients who are at high risk of recurrence, such as those with larger tumors, extrathyroid extension, and involved lymph nodes, as well as those with residual disease.[62] In low-risk patient groups, and especially in those with microcarcinoma, prognosis is so favorable after surgery alone that little further improvement is possible with ^{131}I ablation.[63]

The optimal activity of ^{131}I required to achieve successful ablation has been a subject of much debate, with doses ranging between 1.1 and 3.7 GBq. The advantages of administering the smallest effective dose of ^{131}I are patient convenience and lower cost as well as a reduced risk of treatment-related complications from lower whole-body radiation exposure. In 2012, two prospective randomized controlled trials compared 1.1 GBq with 3.7 GBq; success of ablation was the common primary endpoint.[64,65] Both reported non-inferiority of the lower activity with a lower rate of adverse events. All patients had undergone total thyroidectomy with an R0 resection. Most were staged T1 N0 or T2 N0, and therefore, 1.1 GBq has become the recommended activity for these patients. In one of the trials,[64] 23% of the patients had T3 tumors and 16% had N1 disease, but for both of these subgroups, no difference was observed in ablation success rate between 1.1 and 3.7 GBq. In these subgroups, the final choice of activity

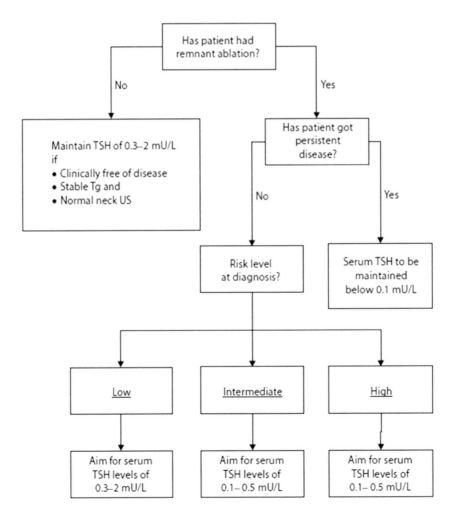

FIGURE 4.5   Risk-stratified thyroid-stimulating hormone suppression.

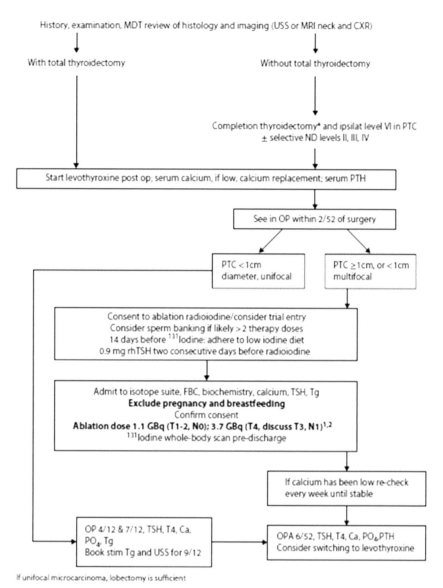

History, examination, MDT review of histology and imaging (USS or MRI neck and CXR)

With total thyroidectomy | Without total thyroidectomy

Completion thyroidectomy* and ipsilat level VI in PTC ± selective ND levels II, III, IV

Start levothyroxine post op; serum calcium, if low, calcium replacement; serum PTH

See in OP within 2/52 of surgery

PTC <1cm diameter, unifocal | PTC ≥1cm, or <1cm multifocal

Consent to ablation radioiodine/consider trial entry
Consider sperm banking if likely >2 therapy doses
14 days before ^{131}Iodine: adhere to low iodine diet
0.9 mg rhTSH two consecutive days before radioiodine

Admit to isotope suite, FBC, biochemistry, calcium, TSH, Tg
Exclude pregnancy and breastfeeding
Confirm consent
Ablation dose 1.1 GBq (T1-2, N0); 3.7 GBq (T4, discuss T3, N1)[1,2]
^{131}Iodine whole-body scan pre-discharge

If calcium has been low re-check every week until stable

OP 4/12 & 7/12, TSH, T4, Ca, PO$_4$, Tg
Book stim Tg and USS for 9/12

OPA 6/52, TSH, T4, Ca, PO$_4$,PTH
Consider switching to levothyroxine

If unifocal microcarcinoma, lobectomy is sufficient

FIGURE 4.6 Management of differentiated thyroid carcinoma. Ca, calcium; CXR, chest x-ray; FBC, full blood count; MDT, multidisciplinary team; ND, neck dissection; OP, outpatients; PO$_4$, phosphate; PTC, papillary thyroid carcinoma; PTH, parathyroid hormone; rhTSH, recombinant human thyroid-stimulating hormone; stim Tg, stimulated thyroglobulin; Tg, thyroglobulin. (Data from Mallick et al., 2012.)

should be decided on an individual case basis, taking all prognostic factors into consideration. Patients with higher stages of disease should continue to receive 3.7 GBq (Figure 4.6).

To optimize iodine uptake by both residual normal thyroid and cancer, TSH stimulation is necessary prior to ablation. This rise in TSH can be achieved by withdrawing the patient from his or her thyroid hormone replacement, but this results in hypothyroidism and morbidity. A TSH rise can also be achieved by the administration of rhTSH as an intramuscular injection, which permits the patient to remain euthyroid. The uncertainty over whether ablation rates differ between patients who are given rhTSH and those prepared with standard withdrawal has been resolved by the previously discussed randomized trials.[64,65] Both studies reported ablation success rate to be as good after rhTSH as after thyroid hormone withdrawal (THW) for patients with low to intermediate risk who received either 1.1 or 3.7 GBq. Use of rhTSH is associated with better quality of life[66] and has been

shown to be of benefit to patients and society[67,68]; most importantly, it reduces radiation exposure to normal tissues compared with THW by preserving normal renal function and hence, excretion of the radioiodine.[69,70] After ablation, ^{131}I whole-body scans are obtained (Figure 4.7). Single-photon emission computed tomography (SPECT)/CT scanning improves the localization of iodine uptake and should be used where possible. Historically, ablation success was determined by a diagnostic scan performed at 6–12 months. This is no longer universally practiced except in patients with anti-Tg antibodies, when serum Tg becomes invalid. The current recommended criterion for successful ablation is an undetectable serum Tg (<1 µg/L) following rhTSH stimulation in association with a negative neck ultrasound at 9–12 months.[59] Provided that these criteria are met and there are no adverse features, no further treatment is required. If the results prove abnormal, further imaging and treatment are required. If therapeutic radioiodine is indicated, this should be repeated at 6- to

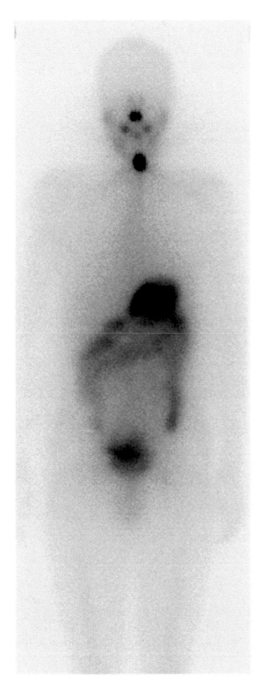

FIGURE 4.7 Post-ablation Iodine 131 whole-body scan.

12-month intervals until uptake disappears and the Tg becomes undetectable (Figure 4.8).

Follow-up

Annual follow-up comprising clinical examination and estimation of free T4, TSH, and Tg is essential to ensure normal thyroid function with appropriate TSH suppression and to detect recurrent tumor. Early discovery of recurrence is of paramount prognostic significance for both cure and survival.[71] Local or regional relapse develops in 5–20% of patients with DTC. Most relapses occur during the early years of follow-up, but they may be detected even after 40 years; follow-up should therefore be lifelong.

Recurrence in the thyroid bed or cervical lymph nodes may be discovered by palpation. Ultrasonography or MRI delineates disease extent. Serum Tg is usually elevated, although it may be undetectable in 20% of patients on thyroxine who have isolated lymph node metastasis.[72]

Surgery is the treatment for loco-regional recurrence; complete resection should be attempted. Even if disease cannot be completely removed, surgical debulking facilitates the subsequent use of radioiodine. If surgical removal would result in unacceptable morbidity or has to be incomplete, both radioiodine treatment and EBRT should be used to control local disease.[73,74] The outcome for patients with loco-regional recurrence is closely related to its site, initial prognostic factors, and response to treatment.

Treatment of metastatic disease

Distant metastases develop in 5–23% of patients with DTC, mainly in lung and bone and less frequently in liver and brain. Both univariate and multivariate analyses have highlighted the adverse prognostic effect on survival of older age at the time of discovery of metastases.[71,75] Treatment comprises repeated doses of radioiodine. Activities ranging from 3.7 to 11.1 GBq at 3- to 9-month intervals have been employed; many centers use a dose of 5.5 GBq at 6-month intervals (Figure 4.9). There is no maximum limit to the cumulative ^{131}I dose that can be given to patients with persistent disease, provided that individual doses do not exceed 2 Gy total-body exposure, progressive improvement can be documented, and each pre-treatment blood count confirms the absence of bone-marrow damage.

A whole-body scan after iodine administration provides scintigraphic assessment of disease. Diagnostic scanning using a tracer dose of iodine is not necessary prior to therapy and may have an adverse effect, because tumor stunning by the diagnostic dose may reduce the uptake of therapeutic [131]I.[76,77] A significant proportion of patients with residual tumor, as evidenced by an elevated Tg, demonstrate a negative diagnostic scan, but uptake can be documented in the post-therapy scan.[78,79]

The real benefit of iodine treatment has been questioned; however, at least one large study clearly demonstrated its independent prognostic benefit on survival. Younger patients with limited-volume disease, mainly in the lungs, who achieve a complete response to radioiodine treatment have been consistently shown to have the best prognosis, with a 15-year survival of 89%.[71] In contrast, older patients and those with large metastases or bone involvement are less likely to respond.[80] Although distant metastases, particularly in the lung, may remain stable for years, there is evidence that early treatment may affect outcome. Microscopic foci are more radiosensitive; complete response was reported in 82% of patients with uptake in lung metastases not seen on chest radiography but in only 15% of those with visible micronodules or macronodules.[81] Bone lesions demonstrate a low response rate to radioiodine; surgical excision, when possible, or EBRT should be added.[82,83] Advanced radiotherapy delivery techniques such as stereotactic body radiation therapy (SBRT) may be used. Surgical resection with curative intent for patients with a solitary deposit not concentrating iodine and those with bulky disease resistant to iodine has achieved a 5-year post-metastasectomy survival of 46%.[84]

Sometimes, metastases persist despite the administration of substantial ^{131}I therapy doses. This may be the consequence of rapid turnover of radioiodine in tumor. The effective half-life in metastases responding to therapy has been shown to be more

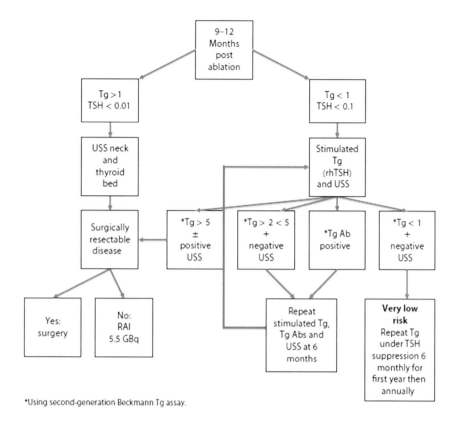

FIGURE 4.8 Post-ablation follow-up of differentiated thyroid carcinoma. GBq, gigabecquerels; RAI, radioiodine; rhTSH, recombinant human thyroid-stimulating hormone; Tg, thyroglobulin; USS, ultrasound scan thyroid bed and neck.

than twice as long as in those not responding: 5.5 days compared with 2.5 days.[85] In a retrospective review of 400 patients, FDG-PET positivity was a strong adverse predictor of survival on multivariate analysis (in addition to age), suggesting that these patients should be treated more aggressively.[86]

Various interventions have been attempted to try to increase iodine avidity (e.g. retinoic acid derivatives) or to increase retention (e.g. lithium) but have shown disappointing results.[87–90] Selective MAPK pathway antagonists have been shown to increase the expression of the sodium iodide symporter (NIS) and uptake of iodine in mouse models. Treatment with selumetinib, an MEK inhibitor, has demonstrated improved radioiodine avidity in a small study,[91] but Phase 3 data are required, and entry into clinical trials is encouraged.

Dosimetry of ^{131}I therapy

Historically, the use of radioiodine has been empirical. Fixed activities of 1.1–3.7 GBq for remnant ablation and 3.7–7.5 GBq for therapy are still administered based on experience and likely side effects. However, measurement of the absorbed dose (in gray) has several advantages. One is that patients are not overtreated, and overall radiation exposure is kept as low as possible. Second, it is the only way to determine whether further ^{131}I therapy will be effective, so that alternative treatment can be considered in unsuccessful cases. But the most important reason for basing iodine therapy on lesion dosimetry is that optimizing the administered dose gives the highest probability that the lesion will be eradicated. Because information suggests that a stunning effect occurs with incomplete or inadequate therapy and it may be permanent, the most effective strategy is to attempt

to eradicate a tumor with either a single ^{131}I administration or as few treatments as possible. Preliminary analysis of 25 dosimetry studies in patients with metastatic lesions showed a wide variation in radiation absorbed dose (5–621 Gy) from a fixed administered ^{131}I activity of 5.5 GBq.[92] There was evidence of a dose–response relationship explaining the spectrum of clinical response (Figure 4.10). This huge variation in absorbed dose highlights the technical difficulty in dosimetric measurements. Calculations are based on two major assumptions: one is that radioactivity is uniformly distributed throughout the tumor, and the second is that washout of ^{131}I is governed by a single exponential function. If either of these assumptions is inaccurate, errors will be introduced into the dosimetry estimates. In addition, errors on each parameter (percentage uptake, target activity, half-life, and mass) will contribute to a combined error of absorbed dose.[93] Therefore, quantitative imaging-based dosimetry with ^{131}I SPECT/CT or [124]I PET/CT assessment remains within the research setting, and there is currently insufficient evidence to recommend its routine use.[94,95]

Complications of radioiodine treatment

Radioiodine therapy is well tolerated, with only a few patients experiencing mild nausea within the first 24 hours post administration. Radiation thyroiditis may occur in the first week following ablation, characterized by pain, swelling, and local tenderness in the neck. Acute sialadenitis affecting the parotid or submandibular glands occasionally occurs within 48 hours of administration and may last a few days. A liberal fluid intake is encouraged to minimize this effect. Sialadenitis may persist into a chronic phase, with episodes recurring over years; about 70%

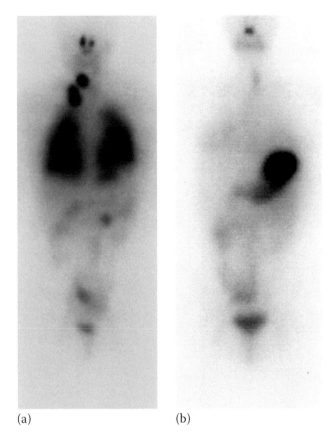

(a)   (b)

FIGURE 4.9 (a) Whole-body scan following an ablation dose of 3 GBq ^{131}I demonstrating diffuse lung metastases plus uptake in the right side of the neck. (b) Following repeated ^{131}I therapy, the last post-therapy whole-body scan demonstrates complete eradication of tumor.

may show a significant decrease in salivary function, which can result in xerostomia, and this appears to be dose related.[96]

Most patients demonstrate a transient slight reduction in platelet and white cell counts after ^{131}I therapy, which is of no clinical importance. These effects reach a nadir at 4–6 weeks after therapy,

with recovery in the majority by 6 months. Myelodysplasia leading to aplastic anemia is rare and likely to occur only in patients with extensive bone metastases who have received a high cumulative whole-body dose in excess of 2 Gy per treatment.[97] Acute radiation pneumonitis and chronic pulmonary fibrosis have been reported in patients with diffuse functioning lung metastases following single therapeutic activities exceeding 9 GBq. A 6- to 12-month interval between iodine doses may reduce the risk of this complication. If serial lung function tests indicate early damage, future doses can be fractionated.

Because DTC occurs in women of childbearing age and young men, the possibility that iodine treatment may affect fertility has created concern. A temporary increase in follicular stimulating hormone (FSH) levels has been noted following ^{131}I treatment in both male and female patients, indicating temporary gonadal dysfunction. A positive correlation between FSH levels and the cumulative activity of iodine has also been reported.[98] Regarding female patients, no significant difference was observed in fertility rates, birth rates, or prematurity among women treated with radioiodine and those not treated.[99,100] Among 406 patients under the age of 40 years, temporary amenorrhea and minor menstrual irregularities were seen in 20%; 427 normal children were born to 276 women, and only one patient was unable to conceive.[101] If pregnancy is deferred for 6 months after radioiodine, there is no risk to the fetus; contraception should be discussed. Fertility is not impaired, although there is a reported small increased risk of miscarriage if pregnancy occurs within 1 year of ablation.[102] In males, a 4-month period of avoidance of fathering a child is recommended, and therefore, contraception should also be discussed with male patients. If more than two therapy doses are anticipated, consideration should be given to sperm banking.

The carcinogenic hazard of ^{131}I in the treatment of DTC has been the subject of several reports. Lifetime incidence of second cancers is low, affecting around 0.5% of patients.[103–107] Only one of three cohort studies showed an increased but non-significant risk of leukemia (relative risk about 2). The risk of leukemia increases with a high cumulative dose (>18.5 GBq) and the use of additional EBRT. Patients who have a high cumulative dose of radioactive iodine may also be more likely to develop second solid malignancies (in e.g. the bladder, colorectal, breast, and salivary glands).[103,107] The total cumulative activity should therefore be kept as low as possible.

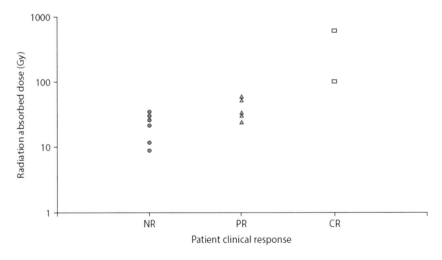

FIGURE 4.10 Dose–response relationship in radioiodine therapy for patients with metastatic thyroid cancer. CR, complete response; NR, no response; PR, partial response.

External-beam radiotherapy and systemic therapies

The role of EBRT in the management of DTC remains controversial because many reports are presented with no distinction between adjuvant (post-operative) EBRT and treatment of macroscopic residual disease. There are no prospective randomized controlled trials. Radiotherapy does not prevent simultaneous administration of radioiodine, although ^{131}I should be given first, as its uptake may be diminished after radiotherapy; if there is good uptake by the tumor, EBRT may become unnecessary. EBRT to the neck has significant acute and late morbidity, and the indication should be very carefully considered.

Farahati et al.[108] suggest that adjuvant EBRT should be restricted to patients older than 40 years with locally advanced tumors (pT_4) that are non-iodine avid. Treatment improved local control in those aged over 40 years with invasive papillary cancer and lymph node involvement from 22% to 90% at 10 years ($p = 0.01$). Tsang et al.[109] reported on 207 patients (155 papillary and 52 follicular) with post-operative residual microscopic disease. In papillary carcinoma, those irradiated had a 10-year cause-specific survival of 100% and a local relapse-free rate of 93%, with a cause-specific survival of 95% ($p = 0.038$) and a local relapse-free rate of 78% ($p = 0.01$). Radiotherapy did not significantly affect cause-specific survival or local relapse-free rate in follicular tumors.

The presence of gross inoperable macroscopic disease is another indication for EBRT. In our retrospective study, complete regression was achieved in 37.5% and partial regression in 25%.[110] Similarly, Chow et al.[111] reported an improvement in local control from 24% to 56% at 10 years ($p < 0.001$). Irradiation is also effective for advanced and recurrent inoperable Hürthle-cell carcinoma, claiming a relatively more important role because this tumor takes up iodine less frequently.[18]

Despite the small study size, the 5-year local recurrence rates from Birmingham, United Kingdom, indicate a possible dose response.[112] These were 63% following a dose of less than 50 Gy but only 15% and 18% for doses of 50–54 Gy and more than 54 Gy, respectively. Most patients had either macroscopic or microscopic residual disease.

Our policy is to use EBRT infrequently, because high dose is required and side effects are unavoidable. Intensity-modulated radiotherapy should be the technique of choice, as it permits optimal target dose delivery while minimizing toxicity (Figure 4.11). The aim is to deliver 60 Gy in 30 daily fractions to the post-operative bed over 6 weeks using 4–6 MV photons.[113] A brisk cutaneous erythema is invariable, with radiation esophagitis requiring liquid analgesia, liberal hydration, and adequate dietary intake. Symptoms resolve within 2 weeks after completion of treatment; laryngitis and dysphonia also resolve completely. Late effects include dysphagia, which may develop months or years later, caused by stricture or motility changes as a result of muscle or nerve damage.

Palliative radiotherapy is indicated for fungating nodes, bleeding, stridor, dysphagia, and superior vena caval obstruction due to progressive inoperable disease. Bone metastases causing pain, vertebral involvement threatening the spinal cord, long bone involvement if there is a potential for fracture, and brain metastases should also be treated, although surgical intervention should be considered. Tumor in lung or mediastinum can be treated if unresectable. Stereotactic radiotherapy, where available, should be considered for well-defined lesions, enabling delivery of higher doses and minimizing irradiation of surrounding normal tissue.

Chemotherapy in DTC has been superseded by targeted therapies. It can, however, be considered in patients with good performance status who have symptomatic, radioiodine-refractory, locally advanced, or metastatic disease when targeted therapies are unavailable or have proved unsuccessful. The agents used are doxorubicin and cisplatin, but durable responses are uncommon.

Efficacy has been demonstrated in Phase 2 studies for several targeted agents, including axitinib, motesanib, sorafenib, pazopanib, Lenvatinib, and thalidomide. Sorafenib, a multikinase inhibitor targeting VEGF receptors, platelet-derived growth

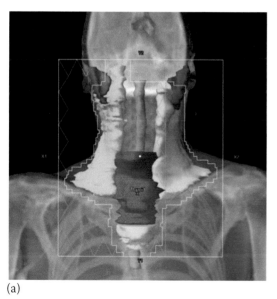

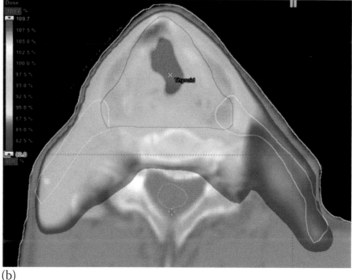

(a) (b)

FIGURE 4.11 Intensity-modulated radiotherapy (IMRT) for post-operative irradiation of thyroid bed and neck. (a) IMRT provides variable dose delivery to target while maintaining tolerance to organs at risk: 65 Gy to thyroid bed (red), 60 Gy to dissected neck (green), 54 Gy to elective nodal regions (cyan), spinal cord (pale pink), and parotid glands (magenta). (b) Color wash of dose levels demonstrates the ability to conform different dose levels to target while sparing organs at risk, for example, spinal cord using IMRT.

factor receptors, BRAF, RET, and c-KIT, was the first agent to show benefit in terms of progression-free survival (PFS) in this setting in a Phase 3 randomized controlled trial. The DECISION trial enrolled 417 patients with locally advanced or metastatic radioactive iodine-refractory DTC. Patients had progression within the prior 14 months as defined by the Response Evaluation Criteria in Solid Tumors. Those who had undergone previous treatment with targeted therapy or chemotherapy were excluded. Patients were randomly assigned to 400 mg of sorafenib orally twice daily or to placebo. If the disease progressed, patients on placebo were allowed to cross over to treatment. The majority of patients in both groups had distant metastases. The study met its primary endpoint of PFS, 10.8 versus 5.8 months in the placebo arm, with a statistically significant hazards regression (HR) of 0.587, $p < 0.0001$. Median OS had not been reached, and it is noteworthy that this secondary endpoint will be affected by the large proportion of patients in the placebo arm (71%) who crossed over to treatment. No complete response was seen in the study. Partial response (PR) was seen in 12.2% of patients in the sorafenib arm and 0.5% in the placebo arm. The median duration of PR was 10.2 months. Sorafenib reduced target lesion size in 73% of patients compared with 27% in the placebo arm, and this reduction in tumor volume was often sufficient to alleviate symptoms. The most frequent adverse events were hand and foot skin reactions, diarrhea, alopecia, rash, fatigue, and hypertension. Dose modification due to side effects was more common with sorafenib (77.8%) than placebo (30.1%), and 18.8% of patients discontinued sorafenib due to adverse events compared with 3.8% of patients receiving placebo.[114] Lenvatinib was the second kinase inhibitor to show a PFS benefit over placebo in iodine-refractory thyroid cancer.[115] Lenvatinib has activity against VEGFR1-3, FGFR1-4, PDGFR α, RET, and KIT. The SELECT study was a Phase 3, randomized, double blind, placebo controlled, multicenter trial that recruited 392 patients from 21 countries. Patients required a diagnosis of metastatic or locally advanced DTC with evidence of radioiodine resistance and radiological progressive disease within the last 13 months. One line of prior multikinase inhibitor use was allowed. Patients were randomized to receive lenvatinib at 24 mg per day taken continuously versus placebo. At the time of progression, cross over to the lenvatinib arm was allowed; 95.6% of eligible patients opted for this. The primary end point of PFS reached statistical significance with a median of 18.3 months for lenvatinib versus 3.6 months for placebo (HR 0.21; 99% CI 0.14–0.31; $p < 0.001$). Response rates were seen in 64% of patients taking lenvatinib versus 1.5% of those on placebo. The secondary endpoint of OS did not reach significance (HR 0.73; 95% CI 0.50–1.07; $p = 0.10$).[115]

As with sorafenib, patients taking lenvatinib experienced many of the side effects common to this class of drugs; 75.9% within the lenvatinib group and 9.9% of the placebo group experienced Grade 3 or more toxicity. The most common side effects were hypertension, diarrhea, fatigue, weight loss, decreased appetite, and rash. Six (2.3%) deaths in the lenvatinib group were felt to be treatment related. These included three deaths not otherwise specified, one pulmonary embolism, one deterioration of general health, and one hemorrhagic stroke. Of the lenvatinib group, 67.8% required a dose reduction, and 14.2% stopped treatment due to adverse events, most commonly due to hypertension and fatigue.[115] A subsequent analysis[116] showed that most adverse events occurred early and were responsive to dose reductions.

Trials addressing the superiority of one systemic therapy over another have not yet been performed. The optimal timing for the initiation of these therapies remains to be determined, as does the optimal duration of use and agent selection. All have side effects, some of which require drug interruptions, dose reductions, or discontinuation of therapy. It is important when considering the initiation of such therapies to take into account the balance between potential benefit, quality of life, toxicity, and cost. Treatment should be started only when both progressive disease and troublesome symptoms occur.

Management of anaplastic carcinoma

Patients with anaplastic carcinoma present with rapidly progressive local and regional nodal disease. Prognosis is dismal, with a median survival of only 6 months from the original symptom. Local growth results in upper airway and esophageal obstruction. Maximal surgical debulking should be attempted, leaving residual tumor for treatment by radiation and/or chemotherapy.[117] Unfortunately, initial surgery is rarely possible, and anaplastic cancer is the least radiosensitive of all thyroid tumors. Doses lower than 50 Gy given in conventional fractionation are associated with a very low probability of local control. A total of 50–60 Gy administered over 5–6 weeks achieved local response in fewer than 45% of patients, but 75% still died from local disease progression.[118]

In an attempt to improve local control, alternative approaches have been investigated, including accelerated radiotherapy and chemotherapy. Clinical and some laboratory data on the proliferation rate suggest that the tumor-doubling time is less than 5 days, making accelerated radiotherapy attractive. In our series of 17 patients treated twice daily, 5 days a week, to a dose of 60.8 Gy in 32 fractions over 20–24 days, significant response was achieved in 59% (including three patients with a complete clinical response). Unfortunately, there was a corresponding increase in treatment toxicity that was unacceptable; Grade 3–4 esophagitis occurred in more than 90% of patients and persisted for several weeks. Survival remained poor, with almost all patients dying within 6 months of treatment.[119]

Better response rates are reported with combined chemotherapy and radiotherapy, particularly if the latter is a hyperfractionated schedule.[120] Doxorubicin is the most effective agent, and low doses in combination with radiation appear to have a synergistic effect. In a study from Sweden, 22 patients were treated with hyperfractionated accelerated radiotherapy (46 Gy in 29 fractions, each of 1.6 Gy, twice daily) concurrently with 20 mg of doxorubicin weekly ≥3, followed by debulking surgery. Despite the patients' advanced ages (over 60 years) and locally extensive disease, such aggressive treatment was feasible. Local control was achieved in 77%, and in those undergoing surgery, none demonstrated local failure; 9% of patients survived for more than 2 years.[121] Control of local disease is important both for palliation and if there is to be any chance of prolonging survival. But because almost all patients who achieve local control still die from metastatic disease, an effective systemic treatment is needed. No response was observed in distant metastases in either the Swedish study[121] or the French study[120] employing doxorubicin (60 mg/m²) plus cisplatin (90 mg/m²) and radiation.

Fosbretabulin, a vascular disrupting agent, selectively targets tumor neovasculature, leading to a reduction in tumor blood flow and central necrosis. A Phase 2 study (FACT trial) randomized carboplatin and paclitaxel with and without fosbretabulin. This was the first drug regimen to suggest improved survival from a median of 4.0 to 5.2 months (HR 0.72). It was shown that 1-year survival more than doubled with fosbretabulin (25.5% vs. 8.7%).[122] However, accrual for this study did not reach the target, and therefore, these results are not statistically significant. Dabrafenib, a B-Raf enzyme inhibitor (150 mg twice daily), together with trametinib, a MEK inhibitor (2 mg daily), was studied in a prospective, non-randomized clinical trial in patients with anaplastic thyroid carcinoma (ATC) expressing the *BRAF V600E* mutation.[123] Data on 23 evaluable patients showed an overall response rate of 61% (95% CI: 39%, 80%). A complete or partial response was seen in 57% of patients; 64% of the patients had a response duration of at least 6 months, and the median OS was 80% at 1 year. There will have been some selection bias in this study, as patients who did not have an Eastern Cooperative Oncology Group performance status of 0–1 and patients who were unable to swallow pills were excluded; both factors are unfortunately common in patients presenting with ATC.[123] This does provide some encouragement for treatment response in this subset of patients with good performance status. Ongoing studies are also investigating the role of this drug combination in the neoadjuvant setting to enable surgical resection in good responders.[124] Treatment with single agent B-Raf inhibition has not been so promising, one study reporting just two responses in seven patients with *BRAF* mutated ATC.[125]

Targeted therapies in combination with immunotherapy are an avenue of current research, and data are awaited.

Management of medullary thyroid cancer

Total thyroidectomy with routine dissection of lymph nodes in the central compartment of the neck and lateral cervical nodes, if involved, is the optimal surgical treatment. Total thyroidectomy is indicated, because in more than 90% of familial and about 20% of sporadic cases, disease is multi-centric and bilateral. The incidence of local recurrence is lower in patients treated by radical surgery.[126] Cervical lymph node involvement at presentation ranges from 15% to 75%. A modified neck dissection with preservation of the sternomastoid muscle, spinal accessory nerve, and internal jugular vein is indicated if metastatic nodes are found during sampling.[127] Bilateral neck dissection has been recommended,[128] because adequacy of the initial operation is a prerequisite for cure, although with improved radiological staging, surgical resection of clinically involved nodal regions only is increasingly preferred to reduce morbidity.[129] Excision of mediastinal lymph nodes, if involved, should be attempted. Ideally, calcitonin will fall to an undetectable level post-operatively. Measurement of serum calcitonin and CEA levels should be repeated at annual follow-up, together with clinical evaluation. Lifelong thyroxine is prescribed at physiological dose; there is no advantage in TSH suppression.

Unfortunately, elevated calcitonin levels often persist following surgery. The most common sites of residual disease are nodes in the neck and mediastinum; distant metastases may involve the liver, lungs, or skeleton. Non-invasive imaging for detecting occult disease includes USS, contrast-enhanced CT with dual-phase sequences through the liver, indium-111 (^{111}In) octreotide, gallium-68 dotatate PET/CT, ^{18}F-DOPA PET/CT, ^{18}F-FDG-PET/CT, and ^{123}I-mIBG.[45]

Residual MTC is usually progressive, as reflected by a rise in calcitonin levels over time. This progressive increase can continue from the first post-operative measurement but may not appear until after a long latent period. In a series from the Mayo Clinic, only 11 of 31 patients with raised calcitonin but negative imaging developed overt recurrent disease when followed for a mean period of 12 years. Re-operation for clinically documented local recurrence did not result in normalization in calcitonin levels. However, OS values at 5 and 10 years were 90% and 86%, respectively.[130] Analysis of calcitonin-doubling times in 65 patients with

abnormal calcitonin levels after total thyroidectomy and bilateral lymph node dissection by the French Neuro-Endocrine Tumour Group revealed that all 41 with a doubling time of more than 2 years were alive at the end of the study (3–30 years). On univariate analysis, TNM stage and doubling time were significant predictors of survival, but only the latter was significant on multivariate analysis ($p = 0.002$).[131]

The role of post-operative radiotherapy is controversial due to a lack of prospective studies; retrospective series comparing surgery alone with surgery plus radiotherapy are subject to selection bias. Favorable responses in terms of tumor reduction and local control have been reported.[132] At the Institut Gustave-Roussy, Villejuif, France, survival of 68 patients treated with surgery alone was similar to that of 59 patients who received post-operative radiotherapy. However, in patients with involved lymph nodes, 5-year survival improved significantly with post-operative radiotherapy, from 36% to 81%.[133]

In summary, EBRT should be considered only after optimal surgery is performed and if there is significant risk of local recurrence. This may be where there is macroscopic residual disease or microscopic residual disease on the background of large-volume disease. EBRT should not be used to consolidate inadequate surgery.[128] Palliative radiotherapy can play a valuable role in unresectable disease and to improve pain control of bone metastases. SBRT may be useful for small well-defined tumors, permitting delivery of higher doses.

Patients with metastatic MTC may survive for years with minimal symptoms and apart from medication to control diarrhea, may not require other treatment. Chemotherapy is now rarely used. Doxorubicin produces symptomatic response in fewer than 30% of cases; most are partial and of short duration. The same response rate is obtained when doxorubicin is used in combination with other drugs. The selective uptake of ^{131}I-mIBG and ^{111}In-octreotide by 30–50% of medullary cancers generated interest in their potential use, but treatment is relatively ineffective.[134] Treatment with unlabeled somatostatin analogues may help to control severe diarrhea from metastatic disease.

Targeted therapies are the modality of choice for inoperable progressive and symptomatic disease. Vandetanib and cabozantinib (both tyrosine kinase inhibitors) showed PFS advantage over placebo in prospective randomized controlled trials of 11 months and 7 months, respectively.[135,136] Of note, there has not yet been any OS advantage. Ongoing clinical trials are addressing the question of sequencing of these drugs (Figure 4.12).

There are preliminary data for RET-specific inhibitors in patients with RET-altered tumors. Two agents are currently under investigation with response rates of 56%[137] and 63%[138] in medullary thyroid cancers previously treated with cabozanitinib or vandetanib. Phase 3 trials of these drugs are planned.

The clinical course of MTC varies widely. In our series, OS was 72% at 5 years, 56% at 10 years, 40% at 15 years, and 30% at 20 years.[139] Outcomes from a cohort of 66 patients with germline RET mutations showed OS at 10 years of 94%; 38% had loco-regional recurrence within 10 years of initial treatment, and 27% had distant metastases at 10 years. Predictors of distant recurrence were tumor size, lymph node involvement, and pre- and post-operative CEA, but interestingly, not calcitonin. Patients with tumors bearing the M918T mutation (typically seen in MEN IIb) had a significantly higher rate of distant relapse than those with other mutations, with a 10-year distant recurrence-free survival of 0%, compared with 83% in all other patients ($p < 0.001$); however, 10-year OS rates were similar in spite of this (100% vs. 92%; $p = 0.49$).[140] These outcome data relate to populations treated, in the majority, before the advent

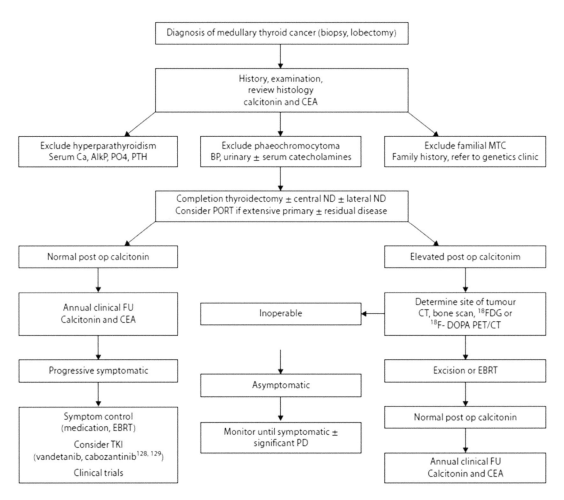

FIGURE 4.12   Management of medullary thyroid cancer. FU, follow-up; ND, neck dissection; PORT, post-operative radiotherapy; TKI, tyrosine kinase inhibitor.

of targeted therapies, and the impact of these agents on survival is awaited.

Management of familial medullary thyroid cancer (MEN IIa and IIb)

The RET proto-oncogene is a 21-exon gene on chromosome 10q 11-2 that encodes for a tyrosine kinase transmembrane receptor. The goal of screening for MEN II is to identify gene carriers early in an attempt to modify the outcome of the disease. The two manifestations that are life-threatening are MTC and pheochromocytoma. There is compelling evidence for both that early intervention will improve outcome.[141]

Genetic testing should be performed soon after birth. Family members found not to be gene carriers by RET mutation analysis do not require further genetic or biochemical testing, and no tests need to be performed on their descendants. Adults who are gene carriers are at high risk of developing MTC; total thyroidectomy with central lymph node dissection should be performed after exclusion of pheochromocytoma. For the management of children found to be gene carriers, serum calcitonin monitoring and the timing of prophylactic thyroidectomy depend on the RET mutation, which reflects the degree of risk of developing MTC.[129] In MEN IIb, total thyroidectomy should be performed as soon as possible, even for patients under 2 years of age.[129] Surgery is well tolerated, and the risks of recurrent

laryngeal nerve damage or hypoparathyroidism are no greater than in older children.[141] In MEN IIa, total thyroidectomy can be delayed until the child is older, but it is usually recommended before the age of 10 years.

Annual measurement of urinary catecholamines and metanephrines on a 24-hour specimen provides outpatient screening to detect pheochromocytoma. Elevated epinephrine or an elevated epinephrine to norepinephrine ratio is the most commonly observed pattern. Basal or exercise-stimulated plasma catecholamines provide an alternative method of screening. MRI is used to confirm pheochromocytoma. In most cases, abnormalities involve both adrenals, and bilateral adrenalectomy is recommended.[142] The procedure is well tolerated but must be preceded by α-blockade and then β-blockade for 7–10 days.

Measurement of serum calcium should be performed annually in MEN IIa gene carriers to screen for hyperparathyroidism. Once hypercalcemia is documented, serum intact parathyroid hormone should be measured to confirm the diagnosis. The majority of patients with hyperparathyroidism have diffuse but unequal multi-glandular hyperplasia, with only a small proportion (10–15%) having a single adenoma. There is controversy regarding total parathyroidectomy with immediate autotransplantation versus subtotal parathyroidectomy.

The value of genetic screening is beyond doubt. However, it is important that family members are counselled regarding the impact of a positive genetic test.

Management of thyroid lymphoma

Most patients with primary thyroid lymphoma present with a rapidly enlarging mass plus confluent cervical/mediastinal lymphadenopathy (stage II$_E$), but in about one-third of the patients, tumor is confined to the thyroid gland (I$_E$). Hematology; biochemistry; FDG-PET/CT scan; and bone-marrow aspirate plus trephine are required for staging. These patients are often elderly and may require urgent therapy to relieve airway obstruction, making full staging impracticable until later. Thyroid lymphomas as a whole were shown to have an overall all-cause median survival of 11.6 years (mean 9.0 years) with a 75% 5-year and 59% 10-year survival in the retrospective analysis of 3466 patients within the National Cancer Database in the United States.[143]

Treatment is based on the pathological sub-type as with nodal lymphomas. Surgery to debulk the tumor is neither feasible nor necessary. The combination of radiotherapy preceded by immuno-chemotherapy (R-CHOP: rituximab, cyclophosphamide, doxorubicin, vincristine, and prednisolone) is standard practice for DLBCL[144] and results in 5-year survival rates of 65–90%.[145]

The more indolent MALT lymphoma is treated with radiotherapy as a single-modality treatment with excellent outcomes. A complete response rate of almost 100%, a relapse rate of around 30%, a salvage rate of more than 50%, and an overall cause-specific survival of almost 90% at 5 and 10 years has been reported.[146] Primary Hodgkin's disease of the thyroid is very rare and treated in a similar fashion to extra-nodal Hodgkin's at any other site.

All cases of thyroid lymphoma should be referred to the local lymphoma multidisciplinary team for either transfer of management or joint care.

Future prospects

Individualization of treatment is the aim of all oncological management, and thyroid cancer is no exception. A better understanding of baseline clinical factors; histopathological staging; and increasingly, molecular pathology is likely to play a larger part in initial management decision making. Risk stratification based on these factors should be dynamic, allowing the drift of individuals between risk categories based on response to treatment. This will enable a tailored approach to adjuvant therapies, intensity of follow-up, and degree of TSH suppression.

A prospective randomized multicenter trial, IoN[147] (Iodine or Not), is comparing total thyroidectomy, TSH suppression, and low-dose radioactive iodine ablation with total thyroidectomy and TSH suppression only in low-risk patients with DTC. This builds on the results from the earlier U.K. study[64] addressing the question of benefit of radioiodine ablation in patients with low risk of recurrence.

The fundamental problem for recurrent or metastatic iodine-negative disease is decreased expression of the NIS. In these patients, options for treatment are limited. There has been interest in the interplay between activation of the MAPK pathway and downregulation of NIS expression: a Phase 2 study of the tyrosine kinase inhibitor selumetinib in combination with radioiodine reported an increase in iodine avidity with consequent improvement in clinical outcome.[91] This may be a new chapter in the re-differentiation story, and Phase 3 data are awaited.

Targeted therapies have shown promise for all subtypes of thyroid cancer, and further development of agents increasingly specific in their pathway blockade will hopefully improve efficacy and reduce drug-induced morbidity. Combinations of kinase inhibitors, possibly together with immunotherapy, may also provide further progress in the management of advanced disease.

The Butterfly Thyroid Cancer Trust (www.butterfly.org.uk) is a patient-led organization that provides information and support. The Association for Multiple Endocrine Neoplasia Disorders is a similar patient-led organization (www.amend.org.uk). The British Thyroid Foundation Cancer Group has also published a patient information leaflet for patients (www.btf-thyroid.org).

Key learning points

- The incidence of thyroid cancer has increased significantly over the past decades. However, mortality rates have fallen, possibly reflecting earlier diagnosis and improved treatment.
- Fine-needle aspiration cytology represents the gold-standard investigation for evaluating thyroid nodules.
- Age is the single most important independent predictor of recurrence and survival in DTC. Tumor size, grade, extension, and presence of metastases also predict outcome.
- Surgery remains the initial and potentially curative treatment for DTC and medullary carcinoma.
- Remnant ^{131}I ablation post thyroidectomy reduces the risk of loco-regional recurrence and cause-specific mortality in DTC, particularly in patients with adverse prognostic features.
- Radioiodine therapy is the mainstay of treatment for metastatic DTC: a significant proportion of patients can be cured, and durable palliation can be achieved in others.
- Targeted therapies provide a therapeutic option in locally advanced and metastatic disease.

References

1. Cancer Research UK. Thyroid Cancer Statistics. http://www.cancerresearchuk.org/cancer-info/cancerstats/types/thyroid/uk-thyroid-cancer-statistics. Accessed September 2019.
2. Waterhouse JA. Epidemiology of thyroid cancer. In: Preece PE, Rosen RD, Maran AGD (eds.), *Head and Neck Oncology for the General Surgeon*. London, UK: WB Saunders, 1991, pp. 1–10.
3. Mettler FA. Jr, Bhargavan M, Thomadsen BR et al. Nuclear medicine exposure in the United States, 2005–2007: Preliminary results. *Semin Nucl Med*. 2008; 38:384–91.
4. Becker DV, Robbins J, Beebe GW et al. Childhood thyroid cancer following the Chernobyl accident: A status report. Endocrinol Metab Clin North Am. 1996; 25(1):197–211.
5. Black P, Straaten A, Gutjahr P. Secondary thyroid carcinoma after treatment for childhood cancer. *Med Pediatr Oncol*. 1998; 31(2):91–5.
6. American Thyroid Association. American Thyroid Association (ATA) Issues Policy Statement on Minimizing Radiation Exposure from Medical, Dental Diagnostics. http://www.thyroid.org/american-thyroid-association-ata-issues-policy-statement-on-minimizing-radiation-exposure-from-medical-dental-diagnostics/. Accessed September 2014.
7. Hieu TT, Russell AW, Cuneo R et al. Cancer risk after medical exposure to radioactive iodine in benign thyroid diseases: A meta-analysis. *Endocr-Relat Cancer*. 2012; 19(5):645–55.
8. Schaller RT Jr, Stevenson JK. Development of carcinoma of the thyroid in iodine-deficient mice. *Cancer*. 1966; 19(8):1063–80.
9. Franceschi S, Levi F, Negri E et al. Diet and thyroid cancer: A pooled analysis of four European case-control studies. *Int J Cancer*. 1991; 48(3):395–8.

10. Negri E, Dal Maso L, Ron E et al. A pooled analysis of case-control studies of thyroid cancer. II. Menstrual and reproductive factors. *Cancer Cause Control.* 1999; 10(2):143–55.

11. Son EJ, Nosé V. Familial follicular cell-derived thyroid carcinoma. Front Endocrinol (Lausanne). 2012; 3:61.

12. TCGA, *Cell* 159, 676–690, October 23, 2014.

13. Song and Park. *Endocr Metab.* 2019; 34:1–10.

14. Huang et al. *Diagn Pathol.* 2019; 14:74.

15. Hedinger C, Williams E, Sobin L. *World Health Organization: Histological Typing of Thyroid Tumours.* Berlin, Germany: Springer-Verlag, 1988, pp. 9–11.

16. Yu X, Schneider D, Leverson G et al. Follicular variant of papillary thyroid carcinoma is a unique clinical entity: A population-based study of 10,740 cases. *Thyroid.* 2013; 23(10):1263–8.

17. Bowen J, Haq M, Rhys-Evans P, Harmer C. Hürthle cell carcinoma: Prognostic factors affecting survival. *Clin Oncol.* 2004; 16(7):S29.

18. Kazaure HS, Roman SA, Sosa JA. Insular thyroid cancer: A population-level analysis of patient characteristics and predictors of survival. *Cancer.* 2012; 118(13):3260–7.

19. Neuhold N, Schultheis A, Hermann M et al. Incidental papillary microcarcinoma of the thyroid—further evidence of a very low malignant potential: A retrospective clinicopathological study with up to 30 years of follow-up. *Ann Surg Oncol.* 2011; 18(12):3430–6.

20. Hughes DT, Haymart MR, Miller BS, et al. The most commonly occurring papillary thyroid cancer in the United States is now a microcarcinoma in a patient older than 45 years. *Thyroid.* 2011; 21:231–6.

21. deMatos PS, Ferreira AP, Ward LS. Prevalence of papillary microcarcinoma of the thyroid in Brazilian autopsy and surgical series. *Endocr Pathol.* 2006; 17(2):165–73.

22. Pakdaman MN, Rochon L, Gologan O, et al. Incidence and histopathological behavior of papillary microcarcinomas: Study of 429 cases. *Otolaryngol Head Neck Surg.* 2008; 139(5):718–22.

23. Bradly DP, Reddy V, Prinz RA, et.al. Incidental papillary carcinoma in patients treated surgically for benign thyroid diseases. *Surgery.* 2009; 146(6):1099–104.

24. Ramos AM, Sales Ade O, Barbalho de Mello LE et al. Absence of peritumoral fibrosis or inflammatory infiltrate may be related to clinical progression of papillary thyroid microcarcinoma. *Int J Surg Pathol.* 2009; 17(6):432–7.

25. Cheema Y, Olson S, Elson D et al. What is the biology and optimal treatment for papillary microcarcinoma of the thyroid? *J Surg Res.* 2006; 134(2):160–2.

26. Corapcioglu D, Sak SD, Delibasi T et al. Papillary microcarcinomas of the thyroid gland and immunohistochemical analysis of expression of p53 protein in papillary microcarcinomas. *J Transl Med.* 2006; 4:28.

27. Lee J, Rhee Y, Lee S et al. Frequent, aggressive behaviors of thyroid microcarcinomas in Korean patients. *Endocr J.* 2006; 53(5):627–32.

28. Lim DJ, Baek KH, Lee YS et al. Clinical, histopathological, and molecular characteristics of papillary thyroid microcarcinoma. *Thyroid.* 2007; 17(9):883–8.

29. Gülben K, Berberogˇlu U, Celen O et al. Incidental papillary microcarcinoma of the thyroid—factors affecting lymph node metastasis. *Langenbecks Arch Surg.* 2008; 393(1):25–9.

30. So YK, Son YI, Hong SD et al. Subclinical lymph node metastasis in papillary thyroid microcarcinoma: A study of 551 resections. *Surgery.* 2010; 148(3):526–31.

31. Park YJ, Kim YA, Lee YJ et al. Papillary microcarcinoma in comparison with larger papillary thyroid carcinoma in BRAF (V600E) mutation, clinicopathological features, and immunohistochemical findings. *Head Neck.* 2010; 32(1):38–45.

32. Lim YC, Choi EC, Yoon YH, Kim EH, Koo BS. Central lymph node metastases in unilateral papillary thyroid microcarcinoma. *Br J Surg.* 2009; 96(3):253–7.

33. Wada N, Duh QY, Sugino K et al. Lymph node metastasis from 259 papillary thyroid microcarcinomas: Frequency, pattern of occurrence and recurrence, and optimal strategy for neck dissection. *Ann Surg.* 2003; 237(3):399–407.

34. Hay ID, Hutchinson ME, Gonzalez-Losada T et al. Papillary thyroid microcarcinoma: A study of 900 cases observed in a 60-year period. *Surgery.* 2008; 144:980–7.

35. South East Knowledge and Intelligence—Cancer. http://www.ociu.nhs.uk/. Accessed September 2014.

36. Rosai J, Carcangiu M, DeLellis R. Tumours of the thyroid gland. In: *Atlas of Tumour Pathology.* Washington, DC: Armed Forces Institute of Pathology, 1992.

37. Hyer SL, Newbold K, Harmer C. Familial medullary thyroid cancer: Clinical aspects and prognosis. *Eur J Surg Oncol.* 2005; 31(4):415–9.

38. Vardell Noble V, Ermann DA, Griffin EK, et al. Primary thyroid lymphoma: An analysis of the national cancer database. *Cureus.* 2019; 11(2): e4088.

39. Harrington KJ, Michalaki VJ, Vini L et al. Management of non-Hodgkin's lymphoma of the thyroid: The Royal Marsden Hospital experience. *Br J Radiol.* 2005; 78(929):405–10.

40. Mitra A, Fisher C, Rhys-Evans P et al. Liposarcoma of the thyroid. *Sarcoma.* 2004; 8:91–6.

41. Wood K, Vini L, Harmer C. Metastases to the thyroid gland: The Royal Marsden experience. *Eur J Surg Oncol.* 2004; 30(6):583–8.

42. Mazzaferri EL. Thyroid cancer in thyroid nodules: Finding a needle in the haystack. *Am J Med.* 1992; 93(4):359–62.

43. The Royal College of Pathologists. *Pathology: The Science Behind the Cure.* http://www.rcpath.org/Resources/RCPath/Migrated%20Resources/Documents/G/g089guidanceonthereportingofthyroidcytologyfinal.pdf. Accessed September 2014.

44. Leboulleux S, Schroeder PR, Busaidy NL et al. Assessment of the incremental value of recombinant thyrotropin stimulation before 2-[18F]-Fluoro-2-deoxy-D-glucose positron emission tomography/computed tomography imaging to localize residual differentiated thyroid cancer. *J Clin Endocrinol Metab.* 2009; 94(4):1310–6.

45. Treglia G, Castaldi P, Villani MF et al. Comparison of 18F-DOPA, 18F-FDG and 68 Ga-somatostat in analogue PET/CT in patients with recurrent medullary thyroid carcinoma. *Eur J Nucl Med Mol Imaging.* 2012; 39(4):569–80.

46. Schneider DF, Mazeh H, Chen H et al. Lymph node ratio predicts recurrence in papillary thyroid cancer. *Oncologist.* 2013; 18(2):157–62.

47. Randolph GW, Duh QY, Heller KS et al. American Thyroid Association Surgical Affairs Committee's Taskforce on Thyroid Cancer Nodal Surgery. The prognostic significance of nodal metastases from papillary thyroid carcinoma can be stratified based on the size and number of metastatic lymph nodes, as well as the presence of extranodal extension. *Thyroid.* 2012; 22(11):1144–52.

48. Vini L, A'Hern R, Fisher C et al. Differentiated thyroid cancer: The Royal Marsden experience. *Br J Cancer.* 1999; 8(Suppl. 2):112.

49. Cady B, Rossi R. An expanded view of risk-group definition in differentiated thyroid carcinoma. *Surgery.* 1988; 104(6):947–53.

50. Loree TR. Therapeutic implications of prognostic factors in differentiated carcinoma of the thyroid gland. *Semin Surg Oncol.* 1995; 11(3):246–55.

51. Hay ID, Grant CS, van Heerden JA et al. Papillary thyroid microcarcinoma: A study of 535 cases observed in a 50-year period. *Surgery.* 1992; 112(6):1139–46.

52. Tuttle RM, Tala H, Shah J et al. Estimating risk of recurrence in differentiated thyroid cancer after total thyroidectomy and radioactive iodine remnant ablation: Using response to therapy variables to modify the initial risk estimates predicted by the new American Thyroid Association staging system. *Thyroid.* 2010; 20(12):1341–9.

53. Rhys-Evans P, See A, Harmer C. Cancer of the thyroid gland. In: Rhys-Evans P, Montgomery P, Gullane P (eds.), *Principles and Practice of Head and Neck Oncology.* London, UK: Martin Dunitz, 2003, pp. 405–30.

54. Hay ID, Grant CS, Taylor WF et al. Ipsilateral lobectomy versus bilateral lobar resection in papillary thyroid carcinoma: A retrospective analysis of surgical outcome using a novel prognostic scoring system. *Surgery.* 1987; 102(6):1088–95.

55. Mazzaferri EL, Jhiang SM. Long-term impact of initial surgical and medical therapy on papillary and follicular thyroid cancer. *Am J Med.* 1994; 97(5):418–28.

56. Wang T, Cheung K, Farrokhyar F et al. A meta-analysis of the effect of prophylactic central compartment neck dissection on locoregional recurrence rates in patients with papillary thyroid cancer. *Ann Surg Oncol.* 2013; 20(11):3477–83.

57. Soh EY, Sobhi SA, Wong MG et al. Thyroid-stimulating hormone promotes the secretion of vascular endothelial growth factor in thyroid cancer cell lines. *Surgery.* 1996; 120(6):944–7.

58. Mazzaferri EL. Papillary thyroid carcinoma: Factors influencing prognosis and current therapy. *Semin Oncol.* 1987; 14(3):315–32.

59. American Thyroid Association (ATA) Guidelines Task force on Thyroid Nodules and Differentiated Thyroid Cancer, Cooper DS, Doherty GM, Haugen BR et al. Revised American Thyroid Association management guidelines for patients with thyroid nodules and differentiated thyroid cancer. *Thyroid.* 2009; 19(11):1167–214.

60. Pacini F, Schlumberger M, Dralle H et al. European Thyroid Cancer Taskforce. European consensus for the management of patients with differentiated thyroid carcinoma of the follicular epithelium. *Eur J Endocrinol.* 2006; 154:787–803.

61. Vini L, Harmer C. Radioiodine treatment for differentiated thyroid cancer. *Clin Oncol (R Coll Radiol).* 2000; 12(6):365–72.

62. Taylor T, Specker B, Robbins J et al. Outcome after treatment of high-risk papillary and non-Hürthle-cell follicular thyroid carcinoma. *Ann Intern Med.* 1998; 129(8):622–7.

63. Nixon IJ, Ganly I, Patel SG et al. The results of selective use of radioactive iodine on survival and on recurrence in the management of papillary thyroid cancer, based on Memorial Sloan-Kettering Cancer Center risk group stratification. *Thyroid.* 2013; 23(6):683–94.

64. Mallick U, Harmer C, Yap B et al. Ablation with low-dose radio iodine and thyrotropin alpha in thyroid cancer. *N Engl J Med.* 2012; 366(18):1674–85.

65. Schlumberger M, Catargi B, Borget I et al. Thyroïde refractaires network for the essai stimulation ablation equivalence trial. Strategies of radioiodine ablation in patients with low-risk thyroid cancer. *N Engl J Med.* 2012; 366(18):1663–73.

66. Lee J, Yun MJ, Nam KH et al. Quality of life and effectiveness comparisons of thyroxine withdrawal, triiodothyronine withdrawal, and recombinant thyroid-stimulating hormone administration for low-dose radioiodine remnant ablation of differentiated thyroid carcinoma. *Thyroid.* 2010; 20(2):173–9.

67. Borget I, Corone C, Nocaudie M et al. Sick leave for follow-up control in thyroid cancer patients: Comparison between stimulation with thyrogen and thyroid hormone withdrawal. *Eur J Endocrinol.* 2007; 156(5):531–8.

68. Mernagh P, Suebwongpat A, Silverberg J et al. Cost-effectiveness of using recombinant human thyroid-stimulating hormone before radioiodine ablation for thyroid cancer: The Canadian perspective. *Value Health.* 2010; 13(2):180–7.

69. Ma C, Xie J, Liu W et al. Recombinant human thyrotropin (rhTSH) aided radioiodine treatment for residual or metastatic differentiated thyroid cancer. *Cochrane Database Syst Rev.* 2010; (11):CD008302.

70. Reiners C, Lassmann M, Luster M. Recombinant human thyrotropin: Safety and quality of life evaluation. *J Endocrinol Invest.* 2012; 35(Suppl. 6):30–5.

71. Schlumberger M, Challeton C, de Vathaire F et al. Radioactive iodine treatment and external radiotherapy for lung and bone metastases from thyroid carcinoma. *J Nucl Med.* 1996; 37(4):598–605.

72. Schlumberger M, Baudin E. Serum thyroglobulin determination in the follow-up of patients with differentiated thyroid carcinoma. *Eur J Endocrinol.* 1998; 138(3):249–52.

73. O'Connell ME, A'Hern RP, Harmer CL. Results of external beam radiotherapy in differentiated thyroid carcinoma: A retrospective study from the Royal Marsden Hospital. *Eur J Cancer.* 1994; 30A(6):733–9.

74. Haq M, Harmer C. Non-surgical management of thyroid cancer. In: Mazzaferri E, Harmer C, Mallick U, Kendall-Taylor P (eds.), *Practical Management of Thyroid Cancer.* London, UK: Springer-Verlag, 2006, pp. 171–91.

75. Haq M, Harmer C. Differentiated thyroid carcinoma with distant metastases at presentation: Prognostic factors and outcome. *Clin Endocrinol.* 2005; 63(1):87–93.

76. Park HM, Perkins OW, Edmondson JW et al. Influence of diagnostic radioiodines on the uptake of ablative dose of iodine-131. *Thyroid.* 1994; 4(1):49–54.

77. Siddiqi A, Foley RR, Britton KE et al. The role of 123I-diagnostic imaging in the follow-up of patients with differentiated thyroid carcinoma as compared to 131I-scanning: Avoidance of negative therapeutic uptake due to stunning. *Clin Endocrinol.* 2001; 55(4):515–21.

78. Fatourechi V, Hay ID, Mullan BP et al. Are post-therapy radioiodine scans informative and do they influence subsequent therapy of patients with differentiated thyroid cancer? *Thyroid.* 2000; 10(7):573–7.

79. Pineda JD, Lee T, Ain K et al. Iodine-131 therapy for thyroid cancer patients with elevated thyroglobulin and negative diagnostic scan. *J Clin Endocrinol Metab.* 1995; 80(5):1488–92.

80. Haq M, McCready R, Harmer C. Treatment of advanced differentiated thyroid carcinoma with high activity radioiodine therapy. *Nucl Med Commun.* 2004; 25(8):799–805.

81. Maxon HR, Thomas SR, Samaratunga RC. Dosimetric considerations in the radioiodine treatment of macrometastases and micrometastases from differentiated thyroid cancer. *Thyroid.* 1997; 7(2):183–7.

82. Marcocci C, Pacini F, Elisei R et al. Clinical and biologic behavior of bone metastases from differentiated thyroid carcinoma. *Surgery.* 1989; 106(6):960–6.

83. Niederle B, Roka R, Schemper M et al. Surgical treatment of distant metastases in differentiated thyroid cancer: Indication and results. *Surgery.* 1986; 100(6):1088–97.

84. Vini L, Harmer C, Goldstraw P. The role of metastasectomy in differentiated thyroid cancer. *Eur J Surg Oncol.* 1998; 24:348.

85. Maxon HR, Thomas SR, Hertzberg VS et al. Relation between effective radiation dose and outcome of radioiodine therapy for thyroid cancer. *N Engl J Med.* 1983; 309(16):937–41.

86. Robbins RJ, Wan Q, Grewal RK et al. Real-time prognosis for metastatic thyroid carcinoma based on FDG-PET scanning. *J Clin Endocrinol Metab.* 2006; 91(2):498–505.

87. Koong SS, Reynolds JC, Movius EG et al. Lithium as a potential adjuvant to 131I therapy of metastatic, well differentiated thyroid carcinoma. *J Clin Endocrinol Metab.* 1999; 84(3):912–6.

88. Handkiewicz-Junak D, Roskosz J, Hasse-Lazar K et al. 13-cis-Retinoic acid re-differentiation therapy and recombinant human thyrotropin-aided radioiodine treatment of non-functional metastatic thyroid cancer: A single-center, 53-patient phase 2 study. *Thyroid Res.* 2009; 2(1):8.

89. Oh SW, Moon SH, Parkdo J et al. Combined therapy with 131I and retinoic acid in Korean patients with radioiodine-refractory papillary thyroid cancer. *Eur J Nucl Med Mol Imaging.* 2011; 38(10):1798–805.

90. Short SC, Suovuori A, Cook G et al. A phase II study using retinoids as redifferentiation agents to increase iodine uptake in metastatic thyroid cancer. *ClinOncol (RCollRadiol).* 2004; 16(8):569–74.

91. Ho AL, Grewal RK, Leboeuf R et al. Selumetinib-enhanced radio iodine uptake in advanced thyroid cancer. *N Engl J Med.* 2013; 368(7):623–32.

92. Vini L, Chittenden S, Pratt B et al. In vivo dosimetry of radioiodine in patients with metastatic differentiated thyroid cancer. *J Nucl Med.* 1998; 25:904.

93. Flower MA, McCready VR. Radionuclide therapy dose calculations: What accuracy can be achieved? *Eur J Nucl Med.* 1997; 24(12):1462–4.

94. Lassmann M, Hänscheid H, Verburg FA et al. The use of dosimetry in the treatment of differentiated thyroid cancer. *Q J Nucl Med Mol Imaging.* 2011; 55(2):107–15.

95. Lassmann M, Hänscheid H, Chiesa C et al. EANM Dosimetry Committee series on standard operational procedures for pretherapeutic dosimetry I: Blood and bone marrow dosimetry in differentiated thyroid cancer therapy. *Eur J Nucl Med Mol Imaging.* 2008; 35(7):1405–12.

96. Hyer S, Kong A, Pratt B et al. Salivary gland toxicity after radioiodine therapy for thyroid cancer. *Clin Oncol.* 2007; 19(1):83–6.
97. Benua R, Cicale NR, Sonenberg M et al. The relation of radioiodine dosimetry to results and complications in the treatment of metastatic thyroid cancer. *Am J Roentgenol Radium Ther Nucl Med.* 1962; 87:171–82.
98. Pacini F, Gasperi M, Fugazzola L et al. Testicular function in patients with differentiated thyroid carcinoma treated with radioiodine. *J Nucl Med.* 1994; 35(9):1418–22.
99. Dottorini ME, Lomuscio G, Mazzucchelli L et al. Assessment of female fertility and carcinogenesis after iodine-131 therapy for differentiated thyroid carcinoma. *J Nucl Med.* 1995; 36(1):21–7.
100. Schlumberger M, de Vathaire F, Ceccarelli C et al. Exposure to radioactive iodine-131 for scintigraphy or therapy does not preclude pregnancy in thyroid cancer patients. *J Nucl Med.* 1996; 37(4):606–12.
101. Vini L, Hyer S, Al Saadi A et al. Prognosis for fertility and ovarian function after treatment with radioiodine for thyroid cancer. *Postgrad Med J.* 2002; 78(916):92–3.
102. Bal C, Kumar A, Tripathi M et al. High-dose radioiodine treatment for differentiated thyroid carcinoma is not associated with change in female fertility or any genetic risk to the offspring. *Int J Radiat Oncol Biol Phys.* 2005; 63:449–55.
103. Rubino C, de Vathaire F, Dottorini ME et al. Second primary malignancies in thyroid cancer patients. *Br J Cancer.* 2003; 89(9):1638–44.
104. Sawka AM, Thephamongkhol K, Brouwers M et al. A systematic review and meta-analysis of the effectiveness of radioactive iodine remnant ablation for well-differentiated thyroid cancer. *J Clin Endocrinol Metab.* 2004; 89:3668–76.
105. de Vathaire F, Schlumberger M, Delisle MJ et al. Leukaemia and cancers following iodine-131 administration for thyroid cancer. *Br J Cancer.* 1997; 75:734–9.
106. Sandeep TC, Strachan MW, Reynolds RM et al. Second primary cancers in thyroid cancer patients: A multinational record linkage study. *J Clin Endocrinol Metab.* 2006; 91:1819–25.
107. Schroeder T, Kuendgen A, Kayser S et al. Therapy-related myeloid neoplasms following treatment with radioiodine. *Haematologica* 2012; 97(2):206–12.
108. Farahati J, Reiners C, Stuschke M et al. Differentiated thyroid cancer. Impact of adjuvant external radiotherapy in patients with perithyroidal tumor infiltration (stage pT4). *Cancer.* 1996; 77(1):172–80.
109. Tsang RW, Brierley JD, Simpson WJ et al. The effects of surgery, radioiodine, and external radiation therapy on the clinical outcome of patients with differentiated thyroid carcinoma. *Cancer.* 1998; 82(2):375–88.
110. O'Connell ME, A'Hern RP, Harmer CL. Results of external beam radiotherapy in differentiated thyroid carcinoma: A retrospective study from the Royal Marsden Hospital. *Eur J Cancer.* 1994; 30A(6):733–9.
111. Chow SM, Law SC, Mendenhall WM et al. Papillary thyroid carcinoma: Prognostic factors and the role of radioiodine and external radiotherapy. *Int J Radiat Oncol Biol Phys.* 2002; 52(3):784–95.
112. Ford D, Giridharan S, McConkey C et al. External beam radiotherapy in the management of differentiated thyroid cancer. *Clin Oncol (R Coll Radiol).* 2003; 15(6):337–41.
113. Nutting CM, Convery DJ, Cosgrove VP et al. Improvements in target coverage and reduced spinal cord irradiation using intensity-modulated radiotherapy (IMRT) in patients with carcinoma of the thyroid gland. *Radiother Oncol.* 2001; 60(2):173–80.
114. Brose MS, Nutting CM, Jarzab B et al. Sorafenib in radioactive iodine-refractory, locally advanced or metastatic differentiated thyroid cancer: a randomised, double-blind, phase 3 trial. *Lancet.* 2014; 384(9940):319–28.
115. Schlumberger M, Tahara M, Wirth LJ et al. Lenvatinib versus placebo in radioiodine-refractory thyroid cancer. *N Engl J Med.* 2015; 372(7):621–30.
116. Haddad RI, Schlumberger M, Wirth LJ et al. Incidence and timing of common adverse events in Lenvatinib-treated patients from the SELECT trial and their association with survival outcomes. *Endocrine.* 2017.
117. McIver B, Hay ID, Giuffrida DF et al. Anaplastic thyroid carcinoma: A 50-year experience at a single institution. *Surgery.* 2001; 130(6):1028–34.
118. Levendag PC, De Porre PM, van Putten WL. Anaplastic carcinoma of the thyroid gland treated by radiation therapy. *Int J Radiat Oncol Biol Phys.* 1993; 26(1):125–8.
119. Mitchell G, Huddart R, Harmer C. Phase II evaluation of high dose accelerated radiotherapy for anaplastic thyroid carcinoma. *Radiother Oncol.* 1999; 50(1):33–8.
120. Schlumberger M, Parmentier C, Delisle MJ et al. Combination therapy for anaplastic giant cell thyroid carcinoma. *Cancer.* 1991; 67(3):564–6.
121. Tennvall J, Lundell G, Wahlberg P et al. Anaplastic thyroid carcinoma: Three protocols combining doxorubicin, hyperfractionated radiotherapy and surgery. *Br J Cancer.* 2002; 86(12):1848–53.
122. Sosa JA, Balkissoon J, Lu SP et al. Thyroidectomy followed by fosbretabulin (CA4P) combination regimen appears to suggest improvement in patient survival in anaplastic thyroid cancer. *Surgery.* 2012; 152(6):1078–87.
123. Subbiah V, Kreitman RJ, Wainberg ZA et al. Dabrafenib and trametinib treatment in patients with locally advanced or metastatic BRAF V600-mutant anaplastic thyroid cancer. *J Clin Oncol.* 2018; 36(1):7–13.
124. Cabanillas ME, Ferrarotto R, Garden AS et al, Neoadjuvant BRAF- and immune-directed therapy for anaplastic thyroid carcinoma. *Thyroid.* 2018; 28(7):945–51.
125. Hyman DM, Puzanov I, Subbiah V et al. Vemurafenib in multiple nonmelanoma cancers with BRAF V600 mutations. *N Engl J Med.* 2015; 373(8):726–36.
126. Modigliani E, Franc B, Niccoli-sire P. Diagnosis and treatment of medullary thyroid cancer. *Baillieres Best Pract Res Clin Endocrinol Metab.* 2000; 14(4):631–49.
127. Dralle H, Scheumann GF, Proye C et al. The value of lymph node dissection in hereditary medullary thyroid carcinoma: A retrospective, European, multicentre study. *J Intern Med.* 1995; 238(4):357–61.
128. Scollo C, Baudin E, Travagli JP et al. Rationale for central and bilateral lymph node dissection in sporadic and hereditary medullary thyroid cancer. *J Clin Endocrinol Metab.* 2003; 88(5):2070–5.
129. American Thyroid Association Guidelines Task Force, Kloos RT, Eng C, Evans DB et al. Medullary thyroid cancer: Management guidelines of the American Thyroid Association. *Thyroid.* 2009; 19(6):565–612.
130. van Heerden JA, Grant CS, Gharib H et al. Long-term course of patients with persistent hypercalcitoninemia after apparent curative primary surgery for medullary thyroid carcinoma. *Ann Surg.* 1990; 212(4):395–400.
131. Barbet J, Campion L, Kraeber-Bodere F et al. Prognostic impact of serum calcitonin and carcinoembryonic antigen doubling-times in patients with medullary thyroid carcinoma. *J Clin Endocrinol Metab.* 2005; 90(11):6077–84.
132. Fife KM, Bower M, Harmer CL. Medullary thyroid cancer: The role of radiotherapy in local control. *Eur J Surg Oncol.* 1996; 22(6):588–91.
133. Schlumberger M, Gardet P, de Vathaire F. External radiotherapy and chemotherapy in MTC patients. In: Calmettes C, Guliana J (eds.), *Medullary Thyroid Carcinoma.* Paris, France: Inserm/John Libbey, 1991, pp. 213–20.
134. Kaltsas G, Rockall A, Papadogias D et al. Recent advances in radiological and radionuclide imaging and therapy of neuroendocrine tumours. *Eur J Endocrinol.* 2004; 151(1):15–27.
135. Wells SA Jr, Robinson BG, Gagel RF et al. Vandetanib in patients with locally advanced or metastatic medullary thyroid cancer: A randomized, double-blind phase III trial. *J Clin Oncol.* 2012; 30(2):134–41.
136. Elisei R, Schlumberger MJ, Müller SP et al. Cabozantinib in progressive medullary thyroid cancer. *J Clin Oncol.* 2013; 31(29):3639–46.
137. Wirth L, Sherman E, Drilon A et al. Registrational results of LOXO-292 in patients with RET-altered thyroid cancers *Ann Oncol.* 2019; 30(suppl_5):v851–v934.

138. Subbiah V, Gainor JF, Rahal R et al. Precision targeted therapy with BLU-667 for RET-driven cancers. *Cancer Discov.* 2018; 8(7):836–49.

139. Hyer SL, Vini L, A'Hern R et al. Medullary thyroid cancer: Multivariate analysis of prognostic factors influencing survival. *Eur J Surg Oncol.* 2000; 26(7):686–90.

140. Spanheimer PM, Ganly I, Chou J et al. Long-term oncologic outcomes after curative resection of familial medullary thyroid carcinoma. *Ann Surg Oncol.* 2019; 26(13):4423–4429

141. Wells SA Jr, Chi DD, Toshima K et al. Predictive DNA testing and prophylactic thyroidectomy in patients at risk for multiple endocrine neoplasia type 2A. *Ann Surg.* 1994; 220(3):237–47.

142. Heshmati HM, Gharib H, van Heerden JA et al. Advances and controversies in the diagnosis and management of medullary thyroid carcinoma. *Am J Med.* 1997; 103(1):60–9.

143. Vardell Noble V, Ermann DA, Griffin EK et al. Primary thyroid lymphoma: An analysis of the national cancer database. *Cureus.* 2019; 11(2):e4088.

144. Yahalom J, Illidge T, Specht L et al. Modern radiation therapy for extranodal lymphomas: Field and dose guidelines from the International Lymphoma Radiation Oncology Group. *Int J Radiat Oncol Biol Phys.* 2015; 92(1):11–31.

145. Stein SA, Wartofsky L. Primary thyroid lymphoma: A clinical review. *J Clin Endocrinol Metab.* 2013; 98(8):3131–8.

146. Laing RW, Hoskin P, Hudson BV et al. The significance of MALT histology in thyroid lymphoma: A review of patients from the BNLI and Royal Marsden Hospital. *Clin Oncol (R Coll Radiol).* 1994; 6(5):300–4.

147. Is Ablative Radio-iodine Necessary for Low Risk Differentiated Thyroid Cancer Patients? UK Clinical Trials Gateway. IoN (CRUK). http://www.ukctg.nihr.ac.uk/trialdetails/NCT01398085. Accessed September 2014.

Useful websites

https://oncologypro.esmo.org/guidelines/Endocrine-Cancers/Thyroid-cancer

www.cancer.gov/cancertopics/types/thyroid

http://seer.cancer.gov/statfacts/html/thyro.html

www.ncin.org.uk/cancer_type_and_topic_specific_work/cancer_type_specific_work/head_and_neck_cancers/head_and_neck_cancer_hub/

www.cancer.net/cancer-types/thyroid-cancer

www.cancerresearchuk.org/cancer-help/type/thyroid-cancer/

www.british-thyroid-association.org

www.british-thyroid-association.org/Guidelines/

www.thyroidcanceralliance.org

www.amend.org.uk

5 ENDOCRINE AND NEUROENDOCRINE TUMORS

Natasha Shrikrishnapalasuriyar, P.N. Plowman, Márta Korbonits, and Ashley B. Grossman

Introduction

In 1966, Pearse first described the cytochemical and ultrastructural properties that were shared by several apparently disparate cell series in the body—initially adrenomedullary chromaffin cells, enterochromaffin cells, the corticotroph, the melanotroph, the pancreatic islet B cell, and the thyroid C cell. Pearse later proposed the generic name APUD for these cells from the initial letters of their common cytochemical characteristics, which include *Amine Precursor Uptake and Decarboxylase* activity within the cells.[1] Since then, the list of APUD cells has expanded enormously. The structural and chemical similarity of APUD cells to neurons suggested a neural crest origin. Indeed, APUD cells of the adrenal medulla and carotid body are of principally neuroectodermal lineage, and the ultrastructural similarity is true for all APUD cells, although we now know that many such cells develop *in situ*. Pearse considered these cells as "neuroendocrine" programmed cells derived from determined precursors arising in the embryonic epiblast, or in one of its principal early descendants. They are best conceived as constituting a diffuse neuroendocrine system (DNES), which may be regarded as a third division of the nervous system, the products of which suppress, amplify, or modulate the activities of the other two divisions.[2]

The DNES may be divided into central and peripheral divisions: The first contains the cells of the hypothalamo–pituitary axis and the pineal gland, whereas the cells of the second division are primarily located in the gastrointestinal tract, lung, and pancreas, where they comprise the gastro-entero-pancreatic (GEP), bronchial, and thymic endocrine cells. Generally, tumors arising from the second group are included under the broad rubric "neuroendocrine tumors" (NETs). More recent concepts have tended to decrease the emphasis on a truly discrete and distinct neuroendocrine "network" and also on their presumed embryological commonality. In particular, in the gut most neuroendocrine cells may differentiate *in situ* from precursors common to other cell types.

This chapter deals with many NETs, although pineal tumors and medullary carcinoma of the thyroid are covered in more detail in their respective chapters. The management of pituitary tumors is discussed first, followed by some of the more important neoplastic conditions in other organs. Adrenomedullary and related tumors are then discussed, plus the embryologically unrelated adrenocortical cancer, and finally NETs.

Pituitary tumors

Tumors of the pituitary gland represent around 10% to 15% of all intracranial tumors.[3] This figure is usually based on mass lesions of the pituitary, which present with visual field defects or local destructive or compressive changes, and it is now realized that small, hormonally active pituitary tumors are considerably less rare. Indeed, "microadenomas" of the pituitary can be found in nearly a quarter of autopsy specimens. These tumors can be functioning or non-functioning depending on their size. Small tumors present due to their consequent endocrinopathy, most commonly reproductive or sexual dysfunction. In comparison, large tumors present with mass effects causing visual disturbance, headache, or hypopituitarism. Pituitary tumors are considered benign tumors; however, some are difficult to manage due to recurrence despite current treatment modalities, and for this reason it has recently been suggested that all should be considered as pituitary neuroendocrine tumors (PitNETs). In this section, we will cover the classification of pituitary tumors and their treatment, and focus on prolactinomas—the most common pituitary tumor.

Classification

In 2017, the World Health Organisation (WHO) changed the classification of pituitary adenomas.[4,5] The new classification describes pituitary adenomas according to their adenohypophyseal lineage and transcription factors, and their clinical and prognostic factors. There are three main pathways of adenohypophyseal cell differentiation and their consequent transcription factors. Corticotrophs are determined by the T-box transcription factor (T-Pit), while somatotrophs, lactotrophs, and thyrotroph are characterized by pituitary transcription factor-1 (Pit1).[4,5] Gonadotrophs involve Steroidogenic Factor 1 (SF-1). The original distinction between "typical" and "atypical" tumors has been removed, and it is now suggested that the Ki-67 proliferation index alone be used to indicate the degree of aggressiveness. Immunostaining for p53 should not be routine but can be used in some circumstances, as can (rarely) electron microscopy. Thus, all such tumors are considered to have the propensity of an aggressive course, but metastases specifically define a pituitary carcinoma.

Table 5.1 represents the anterior pituitary hormones with their secreting cells and their consequent endocrinopathies. Classification can also be shown by their staining properties, although the original acidophilic and basophilic staining is no longer routinely recommended and has been replaced by immunostaining for their respective pituitary hormones (or their subunits), and in some cases with transcription factors.[6] Pituitary tumors can be differentiated with regard to their size: Microadenomas (<1 cm) and macroadenomas (>1 cm). Secretory tumors of the neurohypophysis have not been described.

Presentation

Secretory tumors usually present in terms of their clinical syndrome, and thus acromegaly or gigantism with GH-secreting tumors, Cushing's disease with ACTH-secreting tumors, and amenorrhea/galactorrhea in women and sexual dysfunction in men with prolactinomas. Non-functioning tumors more usually present with space-occupying features such as visual loss, including the classical (but nevertheless uncommon) bitemporal hemianopia, and headache; diplopia due to impingement on the 3rd, 4th, and 6th cranial nerves is infrequent except in cases of pituitary apoplexy. Hypopituitarism can be present with any large tumor, and may also be a presenting feature. It should also be emphasized that recent advances have indicated that almost all so-called non-functioning pituitary adenomas are in fact silent or "whispering" gonadotroph tumors.[7]

TABLE 5.1 Anterior Pituitary Hormones and Associated Endocrinopathies

Adenoma Cell Origin	Hormone	Syndrome
Somatotroph	Growth hormone	Acromegaly/gigantism
Lactotroph	Prolactin	Prolactinoma
Thyrotroph	TSH	Hyperthyroidism
Gonadotrophs	LH/FSH	Hypogonadism, very rarely hypergonadism
Corticotrophs	ACTH	Cushing's disease

Treatment

The clinical behavior of a pituitary tumor can be variable, with some behaving in a quiescent manner, growing slowly over time, others enlarging rapidly. Indications for early transsphenoidal surgery are visual loss due to pressure on the optic chiasm, nerves, or tracts, or a secretory syndrome. Most surgery nowadays is transsphenoidal and generally endoscopic, and should be performed by an experienced surgeon. However, at least 30% of patients with non-functioning adenomas will show tumor regrowth 0.4–3.7 years after surgery, with an increased risk of tumor progression in the presence of residual tumor.[8] It is particularly important in the management of pituitary disorders that the objectives of treatment are clarified. In the case of pituitary tumors, the principal problems are due to the local mass effects of the lesion, especially visual impairment, headache, partial or complete hypopituitarism, and the distant (target tissue) effects of any hormonal hypersecretion. Treatment thus needs to be directed towards reversing the neurological impairment and avoiding its recurrence, replacing any endocrine deficits, and normalizing the levels of any elevated hormones. The disruption of the patient's lifestyle should be minimized; this implies careful consideration of the necessity for long-term medication, with its possible side-effects, and the frequency of outpatient visits and inpatient reassessments. It is difficult to optimize all these objectives simultaneously, as it is usually the case that the more radical therapy with the highest probability of tumor sterilization will be most likely to induce long-term endocrine sequelae. Furthermore, individual patients may differ in their requirements for the normalization of their endocrine status and their desire to avoid medication. Not all neuroendocrine changes defined by subtle alterations during complex test procedures necessitate therapeutic intervention. It is evident, therefore, that a range of treatment options can often be made available, and a therapeutic plan optimized according to the needs and wishes of the individual patient.

Prolactinomas

Prolactin-secreting pituitary adenomas (prolactinomas) are the most common functional pituitary tumor and account for 40% of all pituitary adenomas.[9] Microprolactinomas, measuring less than 1 cm, are contained in the pituitary fossa, whereas macroprolactinomas are larger than 1 cm and may cause local compression and displacement of adjacent structures due to their expansion beyond the pituitary fossa.

Macroprolactinomas

Clinical symptoms are the consequence of direct effects of hyperprolactinemia, or of tumor expansion due to local compression either of the anterior pituitary (hormonal deficits) or of adjacent structures. Usually, serum prolactin levels are markedly increased in prolactinomas and correlate with tumor size, but mild hyperprolactinemia can be present in patients with hypothalamic or pituitary lesions of other etiology due to compression of the hypophyseal blood vessels and consequent loss of the dopaminergic inhibitory tone. In general, there is a rough correlation between tumor size and prolactin level: With macroprolactinomas levels are rarely less than 2000 mU/L, which is 4–5 times the upper limit of the normal value (<450 mIU/l; c.20 ng/L). Prolactin release is predominantly regulated by the inhibitory action of hypothalamic dopamine, and any disruption of the portal vasculature causing a decrease in dopamine delivery to the lactotrophs would also result in an increase in prolactin levels. Thus, non-functioning or other non-prolactin secreting pituitary tumors may present with hyperprolactinemia as well, although very rarely above 2000 mU/L.[10]

Diagnostic imaging techniques such as computed tomography (CT) and, particularly, magnetic resonance imaging (MRI) with or without gadolinium, allow the visualization of a pituitary adenoma and whether there is extra-sellar extension, and the exclusion of a possible hypothalamic lesion.

Direct effects of prolactin cause amenorrhea or oligomenorrhoea in women, occasionally with galactorrhea, with consequent evidence of estrogen deficiency. Prolactin causes a decrease in libido and erectile function in men, but this is compounded by partial or severe testosterone deficiency. It should be noted as well that very high levels of serum prolactin (usually >250,000 mU/L) can "saturate" the assay and lead to artefactual low levels being measured, the so-called "hook-effect."

Treatment of macroprolactinomas involves dopamine agonists in the first instance, principally cabergoline. Dopamine agonists should be initiated with the aim of lowering prolactin levels, decreasing tumor size, and causing a restoration of gonadal function.[9] Cabergoline is the primary choice for patients due to its higher efficacy in normalizing prolactin levels and causing tumor shrinkage. In a systematic review, cabergoline achieved a 62% reduction in tumor size and 67% reduction in resolution of abnormal visual fields.[11] It is administered once or twice a week at a dose of 0.5 mg, but a total weekly dose of up to 3 to 4 mg may occasionally be required in patients. Bromocriptine is an alternative treatment, but studies have shown that patient compliance with cabergoline is greater due to fewer side-effects, and bromocriptine needs to be taken at least once daily. Side-effects include nausea and dizziness, but these usually reduce over time, and it should be advised to take this medication with food. There have been reports that high doses of cabergoline, as used in Parkinson's disease, may cause cardiac valvular problems, but if this occurs in patients with prolactinomas it is likely to be very rare; nevertheless, some authorities advise regular echocardiographic assessment. More importantly, "impulse control disorders" may present with pathological gambling, hypersexuality, or other psychopathological problems, and needs to be specifically queried in all patients on long-term dopamine agonists.[12]

The usual surgical treatment of prolactinomas is transsphenoidal surgery. Around 10% of patients may require surgery if they do not respond to dopamine agonists or if visual field deficits do not improve over 4–6 weeks. Other indications for surgery include apoplexy, with macroprolactinomas, or intolerance or resistance to dopaminergic agonists. Morbidity is low in experienced hands, with a rate of less than 1% to 2% for major complications (cerebrospinal fluid [CSF] rhinorrhea and meningitis, ischemic stroke, or intracranial hemorrhage and visual loss), and of approximately 5% for minor complications; surgically induced diabetes insipidus is usually transient. Transsphenoidal surgery for macroprolactinomas is rarely curative, as small residual tumoral rests remain.

In a large series, transsphenoidal surgery induced remission in 56% of patients with macroprolactinomas (normalization of post-operative prolactin levels), with a recurrence rate of 13% (including microadenomas and macroadenomas) at 10 years.[13] The addition of post-operative standard external-beam radiotherapy to this regimen decreased the risk of recurrence from 50% to 3% or less at 10 years, but is not routinely recommended.[14]

Malignant prolactinomas are defined as those demonstrating metastatic spread. It should be stated that these are extremely rare, 0.1–0.2% of all pituitary tumors, and when seen the prognosis is poor.[15] Treatment for malignant prolactinomas is difficult and survival is often less than 1 year.[9] Conventional chemotherapy agents rarely show positive effects on malignant prolactinomas, but studies have shown that temozolomide, an oral alkylating agent, can be highly effective, at least in the short term.[16]

In summary, dopamine agonist therapy has transformed the management of macroprolactinomas, and surgery has been limited to patients demonstrating residual chiasmal compression after attempted tumor shrinkage or in those patients showing intolerance or resistance. Such surgery is rarely curative and may occasionally have to be complemented by radiotherapy. There remains uncertainty concerning the optimal long-term therapy; some centers advise tumor control with dopamine agonist therapy alone, whereas others suggest that definitive treatment with radiotherapy will lead to gradual sterilization of the tumor, with a low medium-term risk of hypopituitarism. However, the evidence in favor of radiation-induced cerebrovascular disease, and the (slight risk of) induction of second tumors, has led to a decrease in enthusiasm for radiotherapy in this situation. With either approach, long-term close surveillance is necessary. It should be emphasized that radiotherapy, radiosurgery, or proton bean therapy should only be managed by those with modern collimated equipment and experience in treating these tumors. A small proportion of patients may eventually be weaned off dopamine agonists with persisting normalization of serum prolactin levels.

Microprolactinomas

Microprolactinomas have a prevalence of up to 10% in adults, as revealed by some autopsy series, although hyperprolactinemia is produced by these tumors in only 0.1% of female patients.[17] The prevalence in men is much lower (0.005%), presumably due to their different hormonal milieu. There is, however, no evidence that estrogen-containing oral contraceptives are oncogenic. It was formerly thought that there was "functional" or "idiopathic" hyperprolactinemia (up to 4000–6000 mIU/L),[18] but it is likely that all such patients actually harbor microprolactinomas, increasingly detectable with modern MRI. However, it is important to exclude primary hypothyroidism, and a number of drugs, which may increase prolactin (anti-emetics such as metoclopramide, most classical anti-psychotics, and possibly some of the newer anti-psychotics and anti-depressants). High-resolution MRI scans reveal abnormalities of the pituitary fossa in the majority of these patients. In this context, most women with serum prolactin levels persistently above 1000 mIU/L are likely to have microprolactinomas. Most clinical centers would recommend primary therapy with cabergoline as treatment for secondary amenorrhea in such patients; resistance to this drug is rare, and there is little cross-intolerance between different agonists. Occasionally after treatment with a dopamine agonist, serum prolactin may return to a level much lower than previously, such that therapy may be discontinued; this tends to occur particularly following a pregnancy. Very rarely, there is progression from a microadenoma

to a macroadenoma, with a gradual increase in tumor size and prolactin level and the onset of local compressive symptoms. In such a case, the treatment should be adapted to that appropriate for a macroprolactinoma, but it should be emphasized that this is extremely rare.

Treatment involves cabergoline, starting with 0.25 mg once a week and increasing over 2–3 weeks to 0.5 mg once or twice a week. Resistance due to intolerable side-effects may occasionally be responsive to an alternative dopamine agonist such as bromocriptine or quinagolide, but this is a rare occurrence. Most data on safety in inducing conception have been obtained with bromocriptine, with more than 20 years' evidence of a lack of teratogenicity or problems in pregnancy. To date, cabergoline and quinagolide appear to be equally safe, but the relative long-term experience is more limited. However, many would not switch from cabergoline to bromocriptine for the induction of conception.

In an Italian study with 2–5 years of follow-up,[19] withdrawal of long-term cabergoline used as primary therapy resulted in recurrent hyperprolactinemia at rates of 31% and 36% in patients with microprolactinomas and macroprolactinomas, respectively (although levels remained lower than those before treatment), but in the absence of tumor re-growth. The estimated rate of recurrence at 5 years was higher if a residual tumor was visible on MRI at the time of cabergoline withdrawal. These results suggest that it is safe to interrupt long-term cabergoline treatment under careful monitoring during follow-up, as there probably exists a persistent anti-tumoral effect of cabergoline that is additive to the natural evolution of some microprolactinomas.

If a patient's symptoms are minimal, it may be prudent in some cases to avoid treatment altogether. The natural history of microprolactinomas is generally benign, and many patients only require reassurance. There are, however, three conditions in which treatment may be initiated. First, hyperprolactinemia may cause subtle changes in sexual function and libido so every patient should at least be offered a trial of a dopamine agonist to assess their clinical response. Second, hyperprolactinemia is associated with estrogen deficiency and long-term osteoporosis, and therefore should necessarily be treated when it causes either complete amenorrhea or low circulating estradiol levels.[20] Finally, all patients should be followed up long-term to monitor the possible progression to a macroprolactinoma. An alternative approach is to simply treat the patient with some form of estrogen replacement therapy to induce regular withdrawal bleeds and minimize the risk of osteoporosis. The risk of tumor growth is minimal, but does require monitoring.[21]

Microprolactinomas appear to be extremely uncommon in men. It has been suggested that this is because the principal clinical symptom of poor libido or erectile failure is not brought early to medical attention and the patients are only seen if they progress to a macroprolactinoma some 10 years later. Whatever the case, the treatment of a male microprolactinoma follows the same guidelines as in the female.

Finally, a number of patients with apparent hyperprolactinemia and a relative absence of symptoms may have macroprolactinemia, where biochemical assays show a spuriously elevated level due to prolactin's association with an immunoglobulin. This can be established by various techniques, but it is a vital test in all patients with hyperprolactinemia in whom the clinical and hormonal correlates are discordant. As noted above, one additional caveat is that in some prolactin assays the presence of very high prolactin levels will saturate the assay antibody and may show a spuriously low or even normal level of prolactin—the "hook effect." This would confound the interpretation of very large prolactinomas, which would be misdiagnosed as non-functioning adenomas and thus treated surgically. Most laboratories are aware of this and will dilute out samples in which this may be a confounder, and in any case modern assays are usually robust up to 1,000,000 mIU/L.

In summary, microprolactinomas generally have a benign natural history, and therapy must take this into account. The mainstay of treatment is dopamine agonist therapy, supplemented where necessary by transsphenoidal surgery. Radiotherapy should only be considered where the tumor gives evidence of high growth characteristics such as local invasiveness or very high serum prolactin levels, or there is resistance to dopamine agonist therapy and surgery is ineffective by itself. As with the therapy of macroprolactinomas, there may be a risk of cardiac valvular defects with long-term high-dose use, and impulse control disorders may be missed unless critically considered.

Pituitary tumors during pregnancy

The management of prolactinomas during pregnancy can be challenging for endocrinologists. During pregnancy, the pituitary gland increases in size due to increase in serum estrogens, which can increase tumor size and cause mass effects. The risk of tumor enlargement occurs in 3% in microadenomas and 32% in macroadenomas.[22] An MRI should be carried out prior to conception to document tumor size and therefore serve as a baseline if there is evidence of tumor expansion. There are few data to be found on the teratogenicity of these agents, and therefore it is advisable to discontinue dopamine agonists when confirmed pregnant, with the exception of women with invasive macroprolactinomas, although there is equally no evidence of harmful effects.[9,22] Women taking bromocriptine during early pregnancy did not show any higher incidence of miscarriages or congenital malformations than the general population. The same results have been found with cabergoline showing no significant difference in the occurrence of premature delivery or neonatal malformations. Patients with large macroadenomas causing mass effects should continue with bromocriptine and can undergo transsphenoidal surgery in the second trimester if vision is compromised or the tumor continues to advance.[22] Clinical observation is used to monitor prolactinomas during pregnancy, and one should not rely on prolactin levels. Any new signs of mass effect or tumor size increase on MRI indicate that bromocriptine should be restarted.

Non-functioning adenomas ("functionless" tumors)

A significant proportion (30–40%) of large pituitary tumors are apparently functionless, as they are not associated with a hypersecretory syndrome, although a number may be capable of secreting a hormonal product in very low quantities, and the great majority—if not all—exhibit positive immunostaining for glycoprotein hormones, mainly gonadotrophins or their subunits. In 10% of these tumors pro-opiomelanocortin-derived products can be detected, and about 2% immunostain for GH. These tumors represent the so-called silent corticotroph adenomas, gonadotrophinomas, or somatotrophinomas. Indeed, most tumors are on the spectrum of secretory characteristics, with very few being truly "null cell tumors."[23] These tumors usually present due to mass effects consequent on their size and with visual defects and headache, but partial or complete hypopituitarism is often present on dynamic testing.

The principal treatment for functionless tumors is surgical.[24] Surgery is used to decompress the visual pathways, and nowadays this is almost always transsphenoidal in all but the most massive tumors.[25] As functionless pituitary tumors sometimes express dopamine and/or somatostatin receptors, early work suggested that pre-treatment with bromocriptine or somatostatin derivatives might cause tumor shrinkage, similar to that seen with prolactinomas. However, prospective studies of patients carefully followed up for prolonged periods previously suggested that any shrinkage that does occur is relatively minor or, even if more important, is observed in a small number of patients and does not generally obviate the need for surgery.[26–29] It is conceivable that the slight but definite evidence of a decrease in apparent tumor size is due to a diminution in size of the normal lactotrophs or somatotrophs, and that once this occurs the inevitable tumor progression is seen. However, more recent studies with cabergoline have demonstrated true tumor shrinkage in patients treated with cabergoline with residual tumor following transsphenoidal surgery. Newer somatostatin analogues with selectivity for somatostatin receptor subtypes more characteristic of the non-functioning tumors, or mixed dopamine-somatostatin ligands, may prove to be more useful.

If the surgeon believes that they have achieved complete clearance, and if the tumor shows no obvious evidence of invasiveness, many centers would follow this with serial MRI scans (the first at 3–6 months) to assess recurrence. However, a number of surveys in the 1990s demonstrated significant recurrence rates, even in those tumors thought to have been removed completely, of the order of 50% at 10 years.[30,31] More recently, Laws et al.[13] reported better results, with 16% recurrence at 10 years (but only 6% requiring re-operation) and 83% of patients being alive and without evidence of disease. Post-operative improvement of visual deficits occurred in 87% and normalization of hormone secretion in 27% of patients. Our current policy is to re-image the tumor annually for 5 years post-operatively, and then at intervals thereafter; radiotherapy is reserved for patients showing tumor re-growth or for those with invasive or aggressive characteristics radiologically or pathologically, or both. Following radiotherapy, the rate of recurrence has been much less than 5% at 10 years. We have not seen clear evidence of second tumors or neurocognitive defects using our current prescription, although a second-tumor rate, particularly meningioma, of up to 3% at 10 years, has been reported. The radiotherapy is generally administered fractionated as an external beam via 3–5 portals over 5 weeks, but with discrete targets a single dose of focused radiation—radiosurgery—can be used as long as the tumor is clear of the optic apparatus. However, if tumors recur in the absence of radiotherapy, it is likely that further recurrence will be seen even after a second or even third operation.

There remain the group of patients whose serum prolactin varies between 1,000 and 6,000 mU/L, who may have either a prolactin-secreting tumor or a functionless tumor causing stalk compression-induced hyperprolactinemia. Both categories respond to cabergoline with a normalization of serum prolactin, but only the former is likely to show tumor regression. A short trial of cabergoline may be appropriate to test the response of the tumor, but this must be monitored extremely carefully by serial visual-field testing and MRI scanning, as recourse to surgery is important in non-responders.

Silent corticotroph tumors and gonadotrophin-secreting and thyroid-stimulating hormone (TSH)-secreting tumors should be treated as functionless tumors. Some silent corticotroph tumors may progress to clinical Cushing's disease and should be treated particularly vigorously. TSH-secreting tumors present with clinical and biochemical thyrotoxicosis with inappropriately non-suppressed TSH levels; they are usually macroadenomas, and are generally sensitive to somatostatin analogues, which may be given as a therapeutic trial; gonadotrophinomas may occasionally respond to gonadotrophin-releasing hormone (GnRH) antagonists (and, infrequently, to GnRH agonists), but most often require surgery.[32]

In summary, the primary approach to the functionless tumor is surgical, transsphenoidal in the great majority, followed by a policy of regular imaging and close monitoring, with radiotherapy being reserved for aggressive or recurrent tumors.

Acromegaly

Acromegaly is a rare condition, with an annual incidence of about 3–5 cases per million.[33] Its prevalence in the United Kingdom is approximately 85 per million population, although this may be a significant underestimate. There is a high mortality from acromegaly if left untreated, approximately twice the normal standardized mortality rate. Acromegaly is due to an excess of growth hormone (GH) most commonly due to a GH-secreting pituitary tumor or can be due to hypothalamic or neuroendocrine tumors which secrete GH-releasing hormone. Acromegaly can occur alongside other endocrine tumors and be part of multiple syndromes including MEN1, Carney complex, McCune–Albright, and SDHx-related pituitary adenomas. It can also present as familial isolated pituitary adenoma (FIPA).

Clinically, the features of acromegaly depend on the levels of serum IGF-1 and GH, and are contingent upon the duration of the delay in diagnosis. Typical features develop over many years and include visual disturbance due to mass effects, joint discomfort, mandibular prognathism and overbite, infertility, or menstrual irregularities; changes in hand and foot size are seen, and excessive sweating is very common. Acromegaly is associated with conditions such as type 2 diabetes, hypertension, and obstructive sleep apnea. There is a higher prevalence of colorectal neoplasms in patients with acromegaly. GH-producing tumors slowly grow and patients present usually over the age of 50 years. A common clinical manifestation is joint pain which affects around 70% at the time of diagnosis.[34] In younger patients the diagnosis may be less obvious, while onset before epiphyseal fusion leads to gigantism.

Transsphenoidal surgery is the treatment of choice for intrasellar microadenomas, non-invasive macroadenomas, and tumors causing mass effect. Normalization and biochemical control of IGF-1 and induction of a safe level of GH (<1 ng/L) occurs in about 80% of patients with microadenomas and 40–50% of those with macroadenomas following surgery in expert hands.

Medical treatment is recommended for patients who decline surgery, are unfit, or despite surgery have active disease. First-line medical treatment is the use of somatostatin receptor ligands (SRL), with cabergoline and GH receptor antagonists held in reserve for treatment failure. SRLs are effective in controlling GH/IGF-1 hypersecretion and reduce tumor size, but are completely effective in hormonal control in only around 30% of patients. Octreotide LAR and Lanreotide Autogel are the SRLs in general use, activating the somatostatin receptor subtype 2, while second generation somatostatin analogues include pasireotide, which acts on the subtype 5 receptor (amongst others) and may be considered in cases of resistance to octreotide or lanreotide. However, nearly 70% of patients develop impaired glycemic control with pasireotide, which needs to be taken into consideration, especially in patients with pre-existing diabetes.[35] The dopamine agonist cabergoline can be used in conjunction with first-line somatostatin analogues in patients who have mildly elevated IGF-1 at baseline, but is of limited efficacy.

Pegvisomant, a GH receptor antagonist, is used in patients who have persistently elevated IGF-1 levels despite maximal medical therapy or who are unable to take pasireotide. It is almost always effective when given at a sufficient dose, and is administered via a daily, weekly, or twice-weekly subcutaneous injection.[35]

Radiotherapy is reserved for patients unresponsive to current medical therapy or with invasive and/or progressive tumors. External beam fractionated radiotherapy is given in the first instance, which can be supplemented by focused radiosurgery for small residual lesions. Serum GH and IGF1 levels fall slowly over time, with the most rapid fall seen over the first 2 years.

Cushing's disease

Cushing's disease is defined as the symptoms and signs of excess glucocorticoids secondary to a pituitary tumor. In general, Cushing's syndrome is most commonly seen in patients being administered pharmacological doses of corticosteroids, but once this has been excluded exogenous sources need to be sought. Patients show a redistribution of fat stores centrally, catabolic effects such as myopathy, thin skin, easy bruising and osteoporosis, and metabolic changes including diabetes, hypertension, and occasionally hypokalemia. The diagnosis is made on the demonstration of abnormal cortisol secretion, classically in terms of an elevated urinary free cortisol. However, more sensitive techniques such as a failure to suppress cortisol secretion to dexamethasone, either overnight or in more prolonged testing, or an absence of the normal circadian rhythmicity confirmed with late-night serum or salivary cortisol, are usually employed. Once such excess glucocorticoid changes are confirmed, measurement of plasma ACTH will differentiate between ACTH-independent causes (adrenal adenoma or carcinoma, very rarely bilateral micronodular or macronodular hyperplasia) and those which are ACTH-dependent: Most ACTH-dependent cases are due to a pituitary tumor, but ectopic causes need to be considered.[36]

As the pituitary tumors in Cushing's disease are usually small, with a mean diameter of 6 mm, they may not be easily visible even on MRI scanning. Bilateral petrosal sinus sampling for ACTH will confirm the diagnosis of Cushing's disease as opposed to an ectopic source.

Treatment will usually comprise transsphenoidal surgery, which in the best hands will show an immediate cure rate of 80–90%; post-operatively, the patients with be adrenally insufficient, and will require steroid cover until their own pituitary–adrenal axis recovers. Some 15–20% will eventually recur, and then consideration will need to be given to bilateral adrenalectomy or some form of radiotherapy. In patients with mild disease, cabergoline or long-acting pasireotide may be trialed, but neither are uniformly effective and the latter can cause significant hyperglycemia. Adrenostatic medical therapy with metyrapone, ketoconazole, and/or the glucocorticoid-receptor blocker mifepristone are useful for urgent control of hypercortisolemia, and in emergency situations parenteral etomidate has a role.

Familial isolated pituitary adenomas (FIPA)

FIPA is an autosomal dominant condition characterized by the presence of pituitary adenomas in two or more members of a family without associated clinical or genetic abnormalities of other syndromic disease (such as MEN1, Carney complex or pheochromocytomas/paragangliomas).[37] Around 4% to 5% of the cases were suggested to occur in a familial setting, either isolated or as part of an endocrine tumor syndrome,[38] but current data suggest a higher proportion of familial cases and the recent establishment of familial isolated pituitary adenoma as a separate clinical entity is expected to increase this prevalence.[39]

Though the genetic abnormalities that lead to pituitary tumorigenesis are diverse and incompletely described to date, mutations in a variety of genes are known causes of pituitary adenomas or blastomas, either isolated or "as part of a syndrome." The inherited conditions that, to date, are known to predispose to pituitary adenomas include multiple endocrine neoplasia type 1 (MEN1), multiple endocrine neoplasia type 4 (MEN4), Carney complex, and MAX and mutations in *DICER1*[40] and succinate-dehydrogenase (*SDH*) genes.[41] In families with FIPA, some 20% show a mutation in the AIP gene, and such germline mutations are also seen in around 4% of patients with sporadic adenomas. In gigantism, the proportion showing AIP mutations rises to over 30%.

As noted earlier, AIP accounts for some 20% of FIPA families, especially where GH-secreting tumors, and some prolactinomas, predominate. Very rarely, duplication of an orphan receptor may cause very early (<4 years) gigantism, X-linked acrogigantism (XLAG).

Multiple endocrine neoplasia 1 (MEN1)

In 1954, Wermer[42] reported the first clinical description of a family with an association of pituitary tumors, hypercalcemia, and pancreatic adenomas. Multiple endocrine neoplasia 1 (MEN1) is a syndrome characterized by the development of tumors mainly in endocrine but also non-endocrine organs (Table 5.2).[43]

The three main components of the syndrome are hyperparathyroidism, entero-pancreatic endocrine tumors, and pituitary adenomas. In addition, endocrine components of the syndrome include thymic and bronchial carcinoids, adrenal cortex non-functioning tumors, and, very rarely, pheochromocytomas. Skin lesions include lipomas, facial angiofibromas and collagenomas.

The diagnosis of MEN1 can be established by three ways shown in Figure 5.1.

The prevalence of MEN1 detected from post-mortem studies is estimated to be 0.25%, although in general the population prevalence is in the region of 1:40,000. It is seen in up to 18% of young patients with primary hyperparathyroidism, 16–38% in patients with gastrinomas, but less than 3% in patients with pituitary tumors.[43] The observation of loss of heterozygosity (LOH) of chromosome 11q13 in tumors from MEN1 patients led to the mapping, in 1988 and later cloning, in 1997, of the *MEN1* gene. This gene spans 7.2 kb of genomic sequence, contains an 1,830-bp coding region with 10 exons (the first is not translated) and encodes a 610 amino-acid protein, menin.[44] *MEN1* mutations are detected in 90–95% of MEN1 patients. *MEN1* is considered a tumor suppressor gene because heterozygous inactivating mutations predispose to neoplasia and the majority of MEN1-related

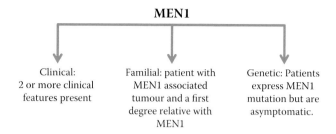

FIGURE 5.1 Diagnosis of MEN1.

tumors show LOH at 11q13.[45–47] MEN1 has an autosomal dominant pattern of inheritance but can occur sporadically as a new mutation. Penetrance is variable and age- and organ-specific, but the hyperparathyroidism usually presents by the fifth decade.[48] It should be emphasized that there is little genotype–phenotype correlation in MEN1.

Primary hyperparathyroidism (PHPT) is the most common endocrinopathy (90%) of MEN1 with hypercalcemia presenting by the age of 50 years. PHPT can remain asymptomatic for a long period of time, and it can manifest as reduced bone mass by the age of 35 years. Patients detected to have a MEN1 mutation should be screened annually for the development of primary hyperparathyroidism. Almost all patients have parathyroid hyperplasia, so the most recommended treatment is 3½ gland parathyroidectomy, with concurrent removal of the thymus. A subtotal parathyroidectomy causes a 20–60% chance of reoccurrence of hypercalcemia within 10 years, but such recurrence is usually mild and can be treated with the calcium-receptor agonist cinacalcet, if necessary.

Pituitary tumors occur in about 30–40% of MEN1, presenting as oligomenorrhea/amenorrhea in women and sexual dysfunction in men. Prolactinomas predominate (62%), but NFPAs (15%), somatotrophinomas (9%) and corticotropinomas (4%), and rarely thyrotropinomas, are also seen.[49,50] A pituitary adenoma is the first manifestation of MEN1 in around 17% of patients (ranging from 10% to 25%). Pituitary adenomas in the context of MEN1 arise at a younger age (mean 35 years) than in patients with sporadic pituitary adenomas.[49] The earliest age of presentation that has been reported is 5 years.[51] From 10% to 39% of tumors secrete more than one hormone, usually PRL/GH.[49,52] The majority of these tumors are macroadenomas (76–85%), and around half of them are invasive.[53] About 4% of patients present multiple adenomas. Whether such tumors are more aggressive than their sporadic counterparts has been the subject of debate, but in our experience they are not usually problematic. Pancreatic tumors are discussed in more detail later in this chapter.

Multiple endocrine neoplasia 4 (MEN4)

A new MEN syndrome was described initially in rats (MENX) in 2000 by Franklin et al.; the human homologue is referred to as[54] MEN4, and is caused by the germline mutation in cyclin-dependent kinase inhibitor (CDKN1B) coding for the tumor suppressor gene p27. The most common phenotypic features of patients with MEN4 are parathyroid and pituitary adenomas. The first case of MEN4 was detected in 2006 in a three-generation family with the father who had acromegaly, a brother who had severe hypertension who died at age 39 years, and a female (proband) who had a somatotrophinoma causing acromegaly. The clinical manifestations of MEN4 have similarities to MEN1. PHPT caused by

TABLE 5.2 Manifestations of MEN1

Manifestation	%
Primary hyperparathyroidism	95
Enteropancreatic tumors	30–70
Pituitary adenomas	20–25
Gastrinomas	40
Insulinomas	10
Gastric neuroendocrine tumors	10

parathyroid neoplasia affects approximately 80% of MEN4; however, it presents at a later age (mean age 56 years) than in MEN1 and with a female predominance. MEN4 appears to be extremely rare.

Pituitary tumors: Growth areas

Transsphenoidal surgery is remarkably successful for the removal and often cure of the majority of pituitary tumors. However, while medical therapy is also available for prolactin-, GH-, ACTH-, and TSH-secreting tumors, with varying degrees of success, apparently non-functioning tumors are largely unresponsive to medical therapy. Current research suggests such medical approaches will become available for all types of pituitary tumor in the future, allowing for effective and well-tolerated alternatives to surgery.

Medullary thyroid carcinoma

Medullary thyroid carcinoma (MTC) is a rare thyroid cancer accounting for 3% of all thyroid cancers in adults and 10% in children.[55] Seventy five percent of MTC occurs sporadically while the remaining 25% are part of a familial syndrome.[56] Familial MTC can be subdivided into MEN2 (MEN-2A), MEN3 (MEN-2B), and familial medullary thyroid carcinoma (FMTC) without an MEN syndrome. MEN2 presents with pheochromocytomas (around 50%) and tumors of the parathyroid gland, whereas MEN 3 present with MTC, pheochromocytomas, and neuromas of the gastro-intestinal tract and/or mouth, but no parathyroid tumors. These have an autosomal dominant pattern of inheritance and occur due to mutations in the *RET* proto-oncogene, a tyrosine kinase receptor, located at chromosome 10q11-2. Somatic *RET* mutations have also been detected in some sporadic MTCs. The distinction between a hereditary syndrome and a sporadic manifestation is important, as the clinical presentation, prognosis, and therapeutic approach differ. In general, there is a strong genotype–phenotype correlation, with 85% of patients with MEN2 showing a codon 634 mutation[57] and MEN3 generally a mutation in the intracellular domain at codon 918.

Clinically, MTC can either be indolent and remain unchanged for many years or progress aggressively and then be associated with a high mortality. MTC arise from the parafollicular C cells of the thyroid gland, which secrete a specific peptide called calcitonin. This peptide is used as a diagnostic marker in MTC,[55] and in some cases CEA is also a useful marker. Mortality in MEN3 is from MTC and intestinal ganglioneuromatosis rather than pheochromocytoma, due to the improved detection and management of pheochromocytoma. MTC in the setting of MEN3 is the most aggressive, with invasive carcinoma and lymph-node metastases often present in the first years of life.[58] MTC as part of MEN2 is the next most aggressive, with hyperplasia or invasive carcinoma with lymph-node metastases detected slightly later but still in the first decade.[59] MTC in the setting of FMTC is less aggressive, classically occurring in the second or even third decades of life. As pheochromocytomas in the context of MEN have a peak incidence in the fourth to fifth decade of life, some of these MTCs are misclassified as FMTC. MTC can occur in infancy whereas MTC is less aggressive in MEN2.

Prevention or cure of MTC is by surgery.[60] Surgery should be ideally performed before malignant progression. In circumstances in which screening has been carried out in adults with an elevated baseline calcitonin, surgery consists of total thyroidectomy with central lymph node dissection. Lateral neck dissection is performed when the primary tumor is greater than 1 cm or when there is evidence of nodal disease on preoperative neck ultrasound.

If the calcitonin levels are elevated after thyroid surgery, consideration of repeat surgery is necessary. If there is no evidence of distant metastases and if local disease is found in the neck and/or mediastinum, then repeat surgery should be considered. The role of adjunctive external beam radiotherapy remains unclear.

In MEN2B (MEN3), MTC occurs early and aggressively and therefore thyroidectomy should be carried out at a young age. The age at which a prophylactic thyroidectomy occurs depends on the position of the *RET* gene codon. For mutations that occur on codons 883, 918, or 922, thyroidectomy should occur before 6 months of age due to the aggressiveness of these carriers.[61] The average life expectancy if a thyroidectomy does not occur is approximately 21 years of age. For the common 634 mutation in MEN2A, thyroidectomy by the age of 5 years is recommended. For other mutations, specific guidelines for that mutation should be followed.

Symptomatic relief for patients with MEN consists of somatostatin analogues for the diarrhea and/or flushing, and antimotility agents. However, as noted below, the therapy of recurrent and metastatic medullary thyroid cancer has changed.

RET is a transmembrane receptor protein-tyrosine kinase that is required for the development of the nervous system/neural crest and several other tissues. The mechanism of activation of RET by its glial-cell derived neurotrophic factor (GDNF) ligands requires additional GDNF family receptor-α (GFRα) co-receptors (GFRα1/2/3/4). RET point mutations have been reported in multiple endocrine neoplasia (MEN2A, MEN2B) and medullary thyroid carcinoma. RET fusion proteins have been reported in papillary thyroid and non-small cell lung adenocarcinomas. There has been much recent interest and clinical benefit from the use of the RET inhibitors in the therapy of metastatic medullary thyroid cancer. Vandetanib and cabozantinib have been licensed and are of proven efficacy; recently, a more potent agent, *Blue-667*, has become available and looks more promising still. This last drug has activity in the brain (of more importance in the RET-driven lung cancers than medullary carcinoma of thyroid). Side-effects such as hypertension, ECG changes, and blood test abnormalities are usually minor but close monitoring is required—as for all cancer patients on tyrosine kinase inhibitors.

Radionuclide therapy with ^{131}I-MIBG or ^{177}Lu-dotatate radionuclide therapy has a place in those patients with tracer scan positive disease and carries the advantage of relatively few side-effects. Repetitive therapy is delivered at 3–6-month intervals—usually four administrations at our institutions (the "tail-end" scan after each therapy dose predicting the usefulness of subsequent therapy doses). However, it seems that tracer uptake for either analogue is uncommon.

Conventional chemotherapy has limited efficacy in patients with MTC. Immunotherapy has no established role in the therapy of this disease at present.

Medullary thyroid carcinoma: Growth areas

Current agents such as tyrosine kinase inhibitors (TKIs) are moderately effective but suffer from significant side-effect profiles. A series of other related TKIs are under development and trial, and appear to be considerably more effective and less burdened by serious adverse events. It is likely that assessment of specific somatic mutation status using whole-exome screening will allow for the customized use of such agents in the near future.

Pheochromocytomas and paragangliomas

Pheochromocytomas originate from the chromaffin cells of the sympathetic chain and account for 0.1–0.6% of cases of secondary hypertension.[62] Ninety percent originate from the adrenal medulla, and about 10% originate from sympathetic and parasympathetic ganglia, known as extra-adrenal pheochromocytomas or better as paragangliomas. Pheochromocytomas commonly secrete norepinephrine (noradrenaline) and epinephrine (adrenaline); however, in some cases they predominantly secrete dopamine, especially when more malignant or from head-and-neck paragangliomas.

Previously, only 10% of cases were identified as an inherited origin; however, recently some 30% of such tumors have been shown to be of a germline mutation in at least 20 genes.[63] Germline mutations in different genes have been found to cause familial pheochromocytomas. Succinate dehydrogenase (SDH) mutations are frequent cause of familial pheochromocytomas. SDH mutations occur on different subunits B, D, C, A, and AF2 (Table 5.3),[64] with SDHB mutations showing a particularly aggressive course and a high incidence of malignancy. Hereditary pheochromocytomas are frequently found in MEN2 and syndromes (50%) with an autosomal dominant pattern with mutations in the *RET* proto-oncogene, as noted earlier: These are almost always benign, and frequently bilateral.

About 15–20% of patients with Von Hippel–Lindau (VHL) disease develop pheochromocytomas.[63,65] VHL is due to a mutation in VHL tumor suppressor gene located on chromosome 3p25-26. This multisystem disorder causes hemangioblastomas in the spinal cord and brain alongside tumors in other organs such as kidneys, pancreas, and adrenal glands. The syndrome demonstrates marked phenotypic variability and accounts for approximately a third of patients with CNS hemangioblastoma and 50% of patients with apparently isolated familial pheochromocytoma.[65] VHL patients are at a high risk of developing adrenal tumors and, therefore, glucocorticoid and mineralocorticoid replacement are mandatory if bilateral surgery is performed. However, cortical-sparing laparoscopic surgery is being increasingly attempted

The other genes shown in Table 5.3 include TMEM127 and MAX, while in many cases the germline syndromes predispose to paragangliomas rather than pheochromocytomas. Paragangliomas are more often prone to metastasis than pheochromocytomas, and are less often secretory. Approaching 20 germlines genes have been identified to date with these tumors.

The clinical manifestations of pheochromocytomas usually result from catecholamine secretion, which may occur at rest or be precipitated by physical activity, emotion, certain drugs such as hydrocortisone, and tyramine-rich food. Hypertension, either paroxysmal or sustained (in 50% of patients) is the most common manifestation, found in about 90% of patients. Episodes of hypotension, either postural or alternating with hypertension, can also occur. Headache is common in about 80–90% of cases and truncal sweating can be seen in 60–70%. The triad of headache, sweating, and palpitations is suggestive of a diagnosis of pheochromocytoma, the major differential diagnosis being anxiety or panic attacks.[62]

Biochemical diagnosis is based on increased catecholamine metabolites. Plasma or urinary fractionated metanephrines (normetanephrine and metanephrine) are highly sensitive and form the basis for specific screening tests that detect secretory pheochromocytomas and paragangliomas: Plasma 3-methoxytyramine, a metabolite of dopamine, is used as a potential marker of malignancy.[66]

Conventional CT and MRI scanning make an important contribution to localizing small adrenal, extra-adrenal, or metastatic lesions; however, despite these scans having a high sensitivity (95%), specificity remains around 75–80%. MRI is most useful for patients with skull base and neck paragangliomas, post-operative surgical clips, and allergy to CT contrast, and is also best for screening and in children to minimize radiation exposure.

Classically, ^{123}I-MIBG scintigraphy was considered to provide approaching 100% detection for adrenal pheochromocytomas, but may be negative for small lesions or those with extensive necrosis. However, its sensitivity is low for paragangliomas (56% to 75%), and most recently the presence of somatostatin receptors revealed by ^{68}Ga-dotatate PET scanning may offer the best functional imaging for both pheochromocytomas and paragangliomas, with ^{18}F-FDOPA PET scanning also having a place. ^{18}F-fluorodeoxyglucose can also be used in patients with

TABLE 5.3   **Hereditary Syndromes Associated with Pheochromocytomas and Paragangliomas**

Hereditary Syndromes Associated with Pheochromocytomas and Paragangliomas	Localization	Clinical Features
Von Hippel–Lindau (VHL) Pheochromocytomas in about 10–20%. 5% are malignant	3p25.5	Benign, adrenal often bilateral pheochromocytomas Retinal angiomas, renal cell carcinoma
Multiple endocrine neoplasia (MEN) MEN 2 and MEN 3	10q11.2	Adrenal bilateral pheochromocytomas (MEN2 medullary thyroid carcinoma, hyperparathyroidism) MEN2B Marphanoid signs
SDHB	1p36.1-p35	Malignant, solitary sympathetic paraganglioma
SDHD	11q23	Benign (usually), head and neck paraganglioma, maternal imprinting
SDHC	1q23.3	Mostly head and neck paraganglioma
SDHA	5p15	Abdominal paragangliomas, rarely pheochromocytomas
SDHAF2	11q12.2	Head and neck paragangliomas Maternal imprinting
Neurofibromatosis type 1 (pheochromocytomas in < 5%)	17q11.2	Adrenal pheochromocytomas Café au lait spots Mucosal and cutaneous neurofibromas Inguinal or axillary freckles Iris hamartomas (Lisch nodules)
TMEM27	2q11.2	Benign, adrenal bilateral pheochromocytomas but more paragangliomas
MAX	14q23.3	Adrenal Bilateral often malignant pheochromocytomas

metastatic disease and is preferred over ^{123}I-MIBG scintigraphy unless ^{131}I-MIBG therapy is being considered.[62]

The mainstay of treatment for pheochromocytomas requires surgical resection, following a minimum of 7–10 days' blockade with either oral phenoxybenzamine, where available, or doxazosin in effective doses to normalize blood pressure. Any β-adrenoceptor blockade should be reserved for complementing α-adrenoceptor blockade after this has been shown to be effective: A target blood pressure at rest is 130/80 mmHg, with some advising the necessity for a postural drop, although in our experience this is not always necessary. Improved preoperative medical preparation and modern anesthesia and surgical techniques have resulted in a low perioperative mortality of less than 1% in major centers.[67]

Radiation therapy has not been proved to be effective but may help in controlling symptomatic bone disease. Chemotherapy using a combination of cyclophosphamide, vincristine, and dacarbazine has shown a high response rate and symptomatic improvement, but no clear effect on long-term survival.[68] Monotherapy with temozolomide, especially with SDHx-mutated tumors, has shown some good responses.

Targeted radiotherapy with ^{131}I-MIBG is used to slow tumor progression. This relatively straightforward radionuclide therapy is used at 3–6 monthly intervals—the justification of the next administration being predicted by the uptake of the preceding dose (best assessed by the "tail-end" scan after that dose and, of course, the patient's improvement or not, serial catecholamine levels, and imaging), and we usually give up to six doses in responders. More recently, radionuclide therapy (PRRT) with ^{177}Lu-dotatate is becoming a new and arguably better (in terms of dose delivery to cancer) radiopharmaceutical therapy.[69] Sunitinib and cabozantinib can also be tried. Assessment of response follows the same guidelines as for MIBG.

Pheochromocytomas and paragangliomas: Growth areas

It is likely that more germline and somatic mutations will be identified, and thus allow for the personalized use of targeted agents. Cell line, animal, and early clinical studies also indicate that combination therapy with targeted agents against parallel signaling pathways will be more effective than currently used agents, and indeed combinatorial regimens of re-purposed drugs with minimal side-effects and low cost may prove effective treatments for malignant tumors. It is also likely that newer targeted radionuclides, possibly loaded with alpha-particle emitters, will be in more widespread use.

Adrenocortical cancer (ACC)

Adrenal tumors are found in around 2–10% of the population, and those with hormone-producing and biochemically active tumors can lead to severe morbidity and mortality.[70] Surgery remains the mainstay of treatment and metastatic disease remains rare. Current endocrine guidelines emphasize that a non-functioning lesion <4 cm with a Hounsfield unit <10 does not need any further follow-up imaging, whereas intermediate lesions need further assessment with FDG PET/CT to help with the diagnosis.[70]

In the presence of an adrenal mass lesion, the two concerns are secretory capacity and malignancy. It is usually straightforward to exclude primary hyperaldosteronism and a pheochromocytoma, so the critical point is to assess the possibility of adrenal malignancy, either primary or secondary. Adrenocortical cancer

(ACC) is rare and accounts for 0.5–2% cases of incidentally discovered mass lesions per year.[71] ACC presents as a bimodal distribution, with the first peak being in children at the age of 5 and the second peak in the fourth and fifth decades of life with a slightly greater prevalence in women. It can occur sporadically or as part of hereditary syndrome such as MEN1 (very rarely) or the Li–Fraumeni syndrome, p53 germline mutations being seen in up to 50% of children with ACC (Table 5.4).[72] The incidence of ACC is increasing due to greater detection of adrenal incidentalomas in the general population. In patients presenting clinically, around half present with signs of steroid hormone excess (Cushing's syndrome, virilization in women, or a feminizing tumor in men, very rarely with aldosterone secretion), the remainder with abdominal mass effects.

Hypercortisolism is the most common presenting hormone excess which causes symptoms of diabetes mellitus, muscles weakness, atrophy, and osteoporosis. Adult ACC can be associated with virilization alone or a mixed syndrome of virilization and Cushing's syndrome. Excessive release of androgens causes hirsutism and virilization, which is a common presentation in children. Hypokalemia and hypertension may occur due to the saturation of the renal enzyme 11-HSD2 which leads to activation of the mineralocorticoid receptor by high levels of glucocorticoids.[73]

The exact genetics related to ACC development in these hereditary conditions is unknown. It has been thought that the Wnt/β-catenin pathway and IGF-2 over expression has been linked as well as the germline *TP53* mutations and dysregulation of the Gap 2/mitosis transition and the IGF-1 receptor (IGF1R) signaling. The overexpression of IGF-2 is one of the most important mechanisms of adrenocortical tumorigenesis. IGF-2 is found on 11p15 and encodes a growth factor that is expressed through the paternal allele. The maternal allele is silenced.[73]

Survival depends on the stage at presentation, with an overall 5-year survival of 82% for stage 1 extending to 13% for stage IV. Tumors greater than 6 cm have a 25% chance of being malignant compared to 2% of tumors less than 4 cm. The Weiss score was created in 1984 for evaluating ACC based on nine histopathological criteria and has been used widely. A score of three histopathological features is suggestive of malignancy. In addition, the Ki-67 labeling index has been used with a cut off of 10% suggesting malignant potential.

The mainstay of treatment is surgery with a complete margin-negative resection. When a high level of suspicion of ACC exists, open surgical oncological resection is recommended as lymph removal may improve diagnostic accuracy and therapeutic outcome. Laparoscopic adrenalectomy can be considered for tumors with a size up to 6 cm without any evidence of local invasion, but biopsy is contraindicated when there is suspicion of malignancy as there is a risk of seeding. For residual or inoperable tumors, the mainstay of therapy is the adrenolytic drug mitotane; its mode of action is unclear but it directly suppresses the adrenal cortex

TABLE 5.4　Hereditary Syndromes and ACC

Syndrome	Prevalence in ACC Patients	Gene Mutation
Li–Fraumeni syndrome	50–80% of children (founder effect in Brazilian cohort) 3% of adults	TP53 mutation
Lynch syndrome	3% of adults	MSH2, MSH6, MSH1
MEN1	Rare in adults	MENIN
FAP	<1%	APC

and modifies the peripheral metabolism of steroids. Mitotane is administered orally in increasing doses to a maintenance daily dose establishing a "therapeutic level" of 14–20g/L. Levels above this cause nausea, fatigue, and severe neurological disturbance, as mitotane is stored in lipid-rich tissues including the myelin sheath. Lower levels appear to be less effective therapeutically. It should also be noted that patients will often require hydrocortisone replacement once any evidence of Cushing's syndrome is treated, and that *serum* cortisol estimations are highly unreliable in this situation. Chemotherapy with etoposide, platinum, and doxorubicin is standard first-line therapy; the usefulness of second-line chemotherapy is questionable. Immunotherapy has not been markedly successful in therapy so far.[72]

It is important to realize that metastatic malignancy is commonly seen in the adrenal, and in most cases the primary lesion is obvious and there is little diagnostic difficulty. It is rare for adrenal function to be altered except in bilateral disease—usually from lung cancer. Occasionally, biopsy of such a lesion will confirm the source, and with oligo-metastatic disease surgery may be indicated.

Adrenocortical tumors: Growth areas

The outlook for adrenocortical carcinoma remains grim, and it is not expected that there will be any major improvement in chemotherapy regimens. There is extensive research on the molecular genetics of such tumors, and it seems likely that only through a thorough understanding of the deranged pathways will effective targeted agents be developed. Unfortunately, there is little likelihood of such new agents appearing in the immediate future.

Neuroendocrine tumors

Neuroendocrine tumors (NETs) can arise from many sites, but the majority are within the gastro-entero pancreatic axis and have been subdivided into foregut, midgut, and hindgut NETs. Classically, all were termed "carcinoids," as it was realized that they demonstrated some carcinoma-like features, but nowadays it is generally agreed to use the term NET as a more general descriptor (although in the lung the term carcinoid is currently retained). Midgut NETs histologically are argentaffin positive and immunostain for serotonin.[74] The 2010 WHO classification introduced a grading system based on mitotic count and Ki-67 proliferation index. Gastro-enteropancreatic NETs are classified as NET grade 1, NET grade 2, and neuroendocrine carcinoma (NET grade 3).[75] More recently, at least for the pancreas, grade 3 tumors have been sub-divided into grade 3 NETs (well-differentiated, Ki-67 usually < 55%) and grade 3 neuroendocrine carcinomas (NECs, poorly differentiated, Ki-67 > 55%).

NETs are diverse due to their difference in clinical presentation, behavior, and prognosis.[76] Previously known as islet cell tumors, pancreatic neuroendocrine tumors (pNETs) have an incidence of around 0.43 per 100,000/year.[77] The majority of these tumors are silent or non-functioning in terms of secretion, but due to the improvements in diagnostic techniques and symptoms we are now detecting these tumors earlier. Non-functioning pNETs can present with mass effects or hemorrhage, but increasingly are being detected as part of a genetic syndrome program or are incidentally found on CT or MR scanning. Pancreatic NETs are not infrequently found in conjunction with patients who have MEN1; other examples of genetic syndromes include Von Hippel–Lindau, MEN4, tuberosis sclerosis, and neurofibromatosis type 1(NF1). Zollinger–Elllison syndrome—gastrinomas—and insulinomas are especially seen in patients with MEN1.

Multiple genes are involved in the development of NET, which have been associated with different abnormalities including point mutations, gene deletions, DNA methylation, chromosomal loss, and gain. Foregut NETs show frequent deletions and mutations of the MEN1 gene whereas midgut NETs show loss of chromosome 18, 11q, and 16q, while hindgut NETs express transforming growth factor alpha and the epidermal growth factor receptor.[74] NETs can develop in the lungs where the most frequent cause is due to the loss of chromosome 3p and p53 mutation, and chromosomal loss of 5q21 is associated with aggressive tumors. Pancreatic NETs have never sat comfortably with other foregut-derived NET, showing different genomics and behavior. Pancreatic NETs from MEN1 patients show a loss of chromosome 11, and around 30% of these tumors may show a loss of chromosomes at 3, 6, 8, 10, 18, 21.[74]

While many pNETs have no clear functional syndrome, some present with symptoms and signs related to their hormonal oversecretion (see Table 5.5). In other cases, when the tumor is large, the patient may present with symptoms of jaundice, weight loss, and abdominal/back pain, and thus can mimic the presentation of pancreatic adenocarcinoma. In these cases, it is especially important that the histopathologist is clearly aware of the differential diagnosis. Table 5.5 shows the prevalence of different types of pancreatic neuroendocrine tumors and their clinical manifestations.[77]

"Carcinoid tumors"

Midgut carcinoid tumors are small intestinal NETs derived from serotonin-producing enterochromaffin cells, and have an incidence of approximately 0.67–0.81 per 100,000/year. NETs arising from the midgut may present incidentally, or with bowel obstruction. Tumor growth may be slow and without clinical features until it metastasizes to the liver, in which case secretory products may leak into the circulation and cause a carcinoid syndrome in one-third of cases. The principal product, 5HT or serotonin, is associated with watery diarrhea and flushing, and occasionally bronchospasm, although other neuroactive agents may be involved. The 5HT is also pro-fibrotic and may cause a desmoplastic response in the gut, or valvular cardiac defects—carcinoid heart disease. In such cases the valvular abnormalities are usually right-sided tricuspid and pulmonary incompetence, although if there is a patent foramen ovale there may occasionally be left-sided defects. The carcinoid syndrome is essentially diagnosed on the basis of 24-hour urinary 5HIAA excretion, although many foods can also elevate 5HIAA, and newer plasma assays are becoming available.

TABLE 5.5 **Pancreatic Neuroendocrine Tumors and Their Clinical Manifestations**

NET	Clinical Manifestation	%
Pancreatic islet cell tumors		
Gastinomas	Zollinger–Ellison syndrome	16–30
Insulinomas	Whipple triad (hypoglycemic symptoms, documented hypoglycemia, and resolution with glucose)	35–40
Vipomas	Watery diarrhea and hypokalemia	<10
Glucagonomas	Migratory necrolytic erythema, glucose intolerance, diarrhea	<10
Somatostatinomas	Gall bladder disease, diabetes, steatorrhea	<10

Colorectal NETs

The incidence of colorectal NETs is on the rise and is approximately 0.2–0.86 per 100,000/year. These have an aggressive nature and have often spread at the time of diagnosis. The mainstay of treatment is a colectomy with retention of lymph nodes. Tumor sizes <2 cm can often be managed endoscopically.

Lung neuroendocrine tumors

These are rare neoplasms which can be subdivided into subtypes: Typical carcinoid, atypical carcinoid, large cell neuroendocrine lung carcinoma, small cell lung carcinoma (SCLC). Patients often present with cough, hemoptysis, wheezing, and respiratory infections, but many are now being diagnosed incidentally. Not infrequently they are associated with ectopic ACTH secretion, and very occasionally a carcinoid syndrome. The WHO classifies these subtypes according to their mitotic index and the presence of necrosis. Surgical resection remains the mainstay of treatment for lung NETs. Complete anatomic resection with systemic nodal dissection is the best choice.[78] If incomplete or recurrent, treatment options are as for other NETs (see below). Thymic NETs can be especially aggressive, and in 25% of cases are associated with ectopic ACTH, and in 25% with MEN1.

A formal staging system has been provided by the European Neuroendocrine Tumor Society (ENETS), as noted earlier, and this should be used in conjunction with the TNM system.

Treatment

This is a complex area, and for detailed discussion the European Neuroendocrine Tumor Society (ENETS) has produced a set of guidelines which are readily available (www.ENETS.org). Therefore, only a brief outline will be given here.

All patients should be staged by the TNM system, and histopathology obtained to grade the tumor. Chromogranin A is a rather non-specific and not highly sensitive blood test, but is useful for patient follow-up. The newer *NETest* is under development and may prove helpful in the future. In addition to routine cross-sectional imaging with CT/MR, it is advised that functional radionuclide imaging with ^{111}In-octreotide or preferably with ^{68}Ga-dotatate PET scanning, with CT or MR co-registration, should be routinely performed at baseline, and thereafter at intervals.

The only curable option is surgery, but this should also be considered even in the presence of metastatic disease. General guidelines advice for a midgut primary (the typical low Ki-67 index tumor) is for it to be surgically removed whenever possible, and other metastases, particularly liver metastases, to be surgically removed (or ablated by other focal techniques) if the tumor bulk can be reduced by at least 70%. In the face of residual tumor, octreotide LAR or Lanreotide Autogel, usually at doses of 30 mg or 120 mg per month respectively, have been shown to retard tumor progression in the PROMID and CLARINET trials. These agents are also highly successful at inhibiting endocrine hypersecretion from pNET or in the carcinoid syndrome. For localized lesions in the liver, some form of hepatic embolization, with or without chemo-embolization, can be useful, or radiofrequency ablation or related technique can be used for small isolated hepatic metastases. However, their effects on overall survival have not been clearly demonstrated.

For grade 2 tumors, standard chemotherapy regimens include temozolomide or capecitabine with lomustine (an oral chemotherapy regime that is derived from the original Mayo Clinic: 5-fluorouracil and streptozotocin regime). Many centers are now using the combination of temozolomide and capecitabine. Grade 3 carcinomas usually are treated with a platinum-containing agent and etoposide.

Following the major international NETTER-1 trial, patients with progressive disease showing uptake on the ^{68}Ga-dotatate PET scan are well treated with beta-emitting radionuclides including ^{177}Lu-dotatate, generally given as intravenous infusions of specific activity around 7000 MBq (with an amino-acid infusion) on 4 occasions separated by 6–8 weekly intervals. ^{90}Y-octreotate has also been used but is more nephrotoxic.

The tyrosine inhibitor (TKI) inhibitor sunitinib has been shown to produce some increase in progression-free survival in pNET and latterly pazopanib may the preferred TKI as it has activity again VEGF and FGFR positive tumors. TKI therapy should be considered for all progressive low-to-intermediate grade tumors.

mTOR is a serine-threonine protein kinase and is part of the pI3Kinase/AKT/mTOR extracellular pathway, signaling growth and cell division. This path is frequently upregulated in NET. Everolimus is a potent inhibitor of the downstream mechanistic part of this pathway (in which PTEN also is part). Everolimus has activity against advanced GI tract and pancreatic NETs. Whether mTOR versus TKI should be used first against advancing NET may be best determined by next-generation sequencing of the individual NET, and particularly the PTEN/AKT/PI3K/mTOR status.

Overall, our recommendation for systemic therapy for advanced/metastatic NET for low to intermediate grade (1–2) NET would be for radioisotope therapy in the first instance, where possible. For relapse through this, then smart drug therapy (mTOR inhibition or TKI) can be tried, with chemotherapy as the last line of therapy but especially for higher-grade tumors. For high grade (3), chemotherapy is first-line therapy. With the increasing spectrum of smart drugs available for (less than grade 3) NET, genomic analyses may become the key determinant for first-line therapy.

Lastly, we call attention to the embryological origin of the site of GI NET being a determinant of behavior, and note that the recent observations that midgut colon cancer differs in many ways (genomically and behaviorally) from hindgut colon cancer suggest that this embryological distinction in origin is not confined to NET.

Immunotherapy has little place in the treatment of these tumors except for grade 3 tumors unresponsive to chemotherapy. It is imperative that due to the relative rarity of these tumors, and the complexity of the treatments available, all patients are discussed at a center of excellence by an experienced multidisciplinary team.[78,79]

Neuroendocrine tumors: Growth areas

There has been considerable research into the molecular alterations in NETs, with some positive data on somatic mutations in pNETs, and epigenetic changes in midgut tumors. Current research is concentrating on developing new targeted agents personalized to the specific changes in any given patient, while clinically the optimal sequencing of therapies is a major topic of active exploration.

Key learning points

- Pituitary tumors can be secretory or non-secretory.
- Non-secretory pituitary tumors present with space-occupying effects including headache, visual loss, and hypopituitarism.
- In most cases the initial treatment of choice is transsphenoidal surgery, except for prolactinomas when the dopamine agonist cabergoline is highly effective.

- A number of germline syndromes are associated with pituitary tumors and should be actively sought.
- Medullary thyroid carcinoma may be part of a genetic syndrome; even when metastatic it may be indolent and active surveillance only required: New TKIs are available for progressive disease.
- Pheochromocytomas and paragangliomas require assessment with metanephrines, and are very often part of a germline syndrome requiring family studies. When metastatic, novel radionuclide therapy is in active use including new radiolabeled targeted agents.
- Small benign adrenocortical tumors are common and often require little investigation or follow-up. Conversely, adrenocortical carcinoma is often a rapidly lethal disease; mitotane is currently the mainstay of therapy.
- Neuroendocrine tumors are becoming increasingly common, and require active therapy with surgery, somatostatin analogues, targeted agents, and radionuclide therapy. They should be assessed and initially treated in "centers of excellence" with dedicated multidisciplinary teams.

References

1. Pearse AG. Common cytochemical and ultrastructural characteristics of cells producing polypeptide hormones (the APUD series) and their relevance to thyroid and ultimobranchial C cells and calcitonin. *Proc R Soc Lond B Biol Sci.* 1968; 170(1018):71–80.
2. Pearse AG, Takor T. Embryology of the diffuse neuroendocrine system and its relationship to the common peptides. *Fed Proc.* 1979; 38(9):2288–94.
3. Lines KE, Stevenson M, Thakker RV. Animal models of pituitary neoplasia. *Mol Cell Endocrinol.* 2016; 421:68–81.
4. Inoshita N, Nishioka H. The 2017 WHO classification of pituitary adenoma: overview and comments. *Brain Tumor Pathol.* 2018; 35(2):51–6.
5. Nishioka H, Inoshita N. The 2017 WHO classification of pituitary tumors. *No Shinkei Geka.* 2019; 47(6):597–606.
6. Syro LV, Rotondo F, Ramirez A et al. Progress in the diagnosis and classification of pituitary adenomas. *Front Endocrinol (Lausanne).* 2015; 6:97.
7. Drummond J, Roncaroli F, Grossman AB, Korbonits M. Clinical and pathological aspects of silent pituitary adenomas. *J Clin Endocrinol Metab.* 2019; 104(7):2473–89.
8. Raverot G, Burman P, McCormack A et al. European society of endocrinology clinical practice guidelines for the management of aggressive pituitary tumours and carcinomas. *Eur J Endocrinol.* 2018; 178(1):G1–G24.
9. Melmed S, Casanueva FF, Hoffman AR et al. Diagnosis and treatment of hyperprolactinemia: an Endocrine Society clinical practice guideline. *J Clin Endocrinol Metab.* 2011; 96(2):273–88.
10. Korevaar T, Wass JA, Grossman AB, Karavitaki N. Disconnection hyperprolactinaemia in nonadenomatous sellar/paraparasellar lesions practically never exceeds 2000 mU/l. *Clin Endocrinol (Oxf).* 2012; 76(4):602–3.
11. Wang AT, Mullan RJ, Lane MA et al. Treatment of hyperprolactinemia: a systematic review and meta-analysis. *Syst Rev.* 2012; 1:33.
12. Noronha S, Stokes V, Karavitaki N, Grossman A. Treating prolactinomas with dopamine agonists: always worth the gamble? *Endocrine.* 2016; 51(2):205–10.
13. Laws ER, Jane JA. Neurosurgical approach to treating pituitary adenomas. *Growth Horm IGF Res.* 2005; 15 Suppl A:S36–41.
14. Brada M, Rajan B, Traish D et al. The long-term efficacy of conservative surgery and radiotherapy in the control of pituitary adenomas. *Clin Endocrinol (Oxf).* 1993; 38(6):571–8.
15. Moscote-Salazar LR, Satyarthee GD, Calderon-Miranda WG et al. Prolactin secreting pituitary carcinoma with extracranial spread

presenting with pathological fracture of femur. *J Neurosci Rural Pract.* 2018; 9(1):170–3.
16. Dworakowska D, Grossman AB. Aggressive and malignant pituitary tumours: state-of-the-art. *Endocr Relat Cancer.* 2018; 25(11):R559–R75.
17. Miyai K, Ichihara K, Kondo K, Mori S. Asymptomatic hyperprolactinaemia and prolactinoma in the general population—mass screening by paired assays of serum prolactin. *Clin Endocrinol (Oxf).* 1986; 25(5):549–54.
18. Prescott RW, Johnston DG, Taylor PK et al. The inability of dynamic tests of prolactin and TSH secretion to differentiate between tumorous and non-tumorous hyperprolactinemia. *J Endocrinol Invest.* 1985; 8(1):49–54.
19. Colao A, Di Sarno A, Cappabianca P et al. Withdrawal of long-term cabergoline therapy for tumoral and nontumoral hyperprolactinemia. *N Engl J Med.* 2003; 349(21):2023–33.
20. Koppelman MC, Kurtz DW, Morrish KA et al. Vertebral body bone mineral content in hyperprolactinemic women. *J Clin Endocrinol Metab.* 1984; 59(6):1050–3.
21. Corenblum B, Donovan L. The safety of physiological estrogen plus progestin replacement therapy and with oral contraceptive therapy in women with pathological hyperprolactinemia. *Fertil Steril.* 1993; 59(3):671–3.
22. Almalki MH, Alzahrani S, Alshahrani F et al. Managing prolactinomas during pregnancy. *Front Endocrinol (Lausanne).* 2015; 6:85.
23. Mercado M, Melgar V, Salame L, Cuenca D. Clinically non-functioning pituitary adenomas: Pathogenic, diagnostic and therapeutic aspects. *Endocrinol Diabetes Nutr.* 2017; 64(7):384–95.
24. Kreutzer J, Fahlbusch R. Diagnosis and treatment of pituitary tumors. *Curr Opin Neurol.* 2004; 17(6):693–703.
25. Harris PE, Afshar F, Coates P et al. The effects of transsphenoidal surgery on endocrine function and visual fields in patients with functionless pituitary tumours. *Q J Med.* 1989; 71(265):417–27.
26. Bevan JS, Webster J, Burke CW, Scanlon MF. Dopamine agonists and pituitary tumor shrinkage. *Endocr Rev.* 1992; 13(2):220–40.
27. Grossman A, Ross R, Charlesworth M et al. The effect of dopamine agonist therapy on large functionless pituitary tumours. *Clin Endocrinol (Oxf).* 1985; 22(5):679–86.
28. Lohmann T, Trantakis C, Biesold M et al. Minor tumour shrinkage in nonfunctioning pituitary adenomas by long-term treatment with the dopamine agonist cabergoline. *Pituitary.* 2001; 4(3):173–8.
29. Pivonello R, Matrone C, Filippella M et al. Dopamine receptor expression and function in clinically nonfunctioning pituitary tumors: comparison with the effectiveness of cabergoline treatment. *J Clin Endocrinol Metab.* 2004; 89(4):1674–83.
30. Gittoes NJ, Bates AS, Tse W et al. Radiotherapy for non-function pituitary tumours. *Clin Endocrinol (Oxf).* 1998; 48(3):331–7.
31. Turner HE, Stratton IM, Byrne JV, Adams CB, Wass JA. Audit of selected patients with nonfunctioning pituitary adenomas treated without irradiation—a follow-up study. *Clin Endocrinol (Oxf).* 1999; 51(3):281–4.
32. Tampourlou M, Ntali G, Ahmed S et al. Outcome of nonfunctioning pituitary adenomas that regrow after primary treatment: A study from two large UK centers. *J Clin Endocrinol Metab.* 2017; 102(6):1889–97.
33. Vasilev V, Daly A, Zacharieva S, Beckers A. Management of acromegaly. *F1000 Med Rep.* 2010; 2:54.
34. Lugo G, Pena L, Cordido F. Clinical manifestations and diagnosis of acromegaly. *Int J Endocrinol.* 2012; 2012:540398.
35. Melmed S, Bronstein MD, Chanson P et al. A consensus statement on acromegaly therapeutic outcomes. *Nat Rev Endocrinol.* 2018; 14(9):552–61.
36. Sharma ST, Nieman LK, Feelders RA. Cushing's syndrome: epidemiology and developments in disease management. *Clin Epidemiol.* 2015; 7:281–93.
37. Beckers A, Aaltonen LA, Daly AF, Karhu A. Familial isolated pituitary adenomas (FIPA) and the pituitary adenoma predisposition due to mutations in the aryl hydrocarbon receptor interacting protein (AIP) gene. *Endocr Rev.* 2013; 34(2):239–77.

38. Melmed S. Acromegaly pathogenesis and treatment. *J Clin Invest.* 2009; 119(11):3189–202.

39. Couldwell WT, Cannon-Albright L. A heritable predisposition to pituitary tumors. *Pituitary.* 2010; 13(2):130–7.

40. de Kock L, Sabbaghian N, Plourde F et al. Pituitary blastoma: a pathognomonic feature of germ-line DICER1 mutations. *Acta Neuropathol.* 2014; 128(1):111–22.

41. Xekouki P, Pacak K, Almeida M et al. Succinate dehydrogenase (SDH) D subunit (SDHD) inactivation in a growth-hormone-producing pituitary tumor: a new association for SDH? *J Clin Endocrinol Metab.* 2012; 97(3):E357–66.

42. Wermer P. Genetic aspects of adenomatosis of endocrine glands. *Am J Med.* 1954; 16(3):363–71.

43. Thakker RV. Multiple endocrine neoplasia type 1 (MEN1) and type 4 (MEN4). *Mol Cell Endocrinol.* 2014; 386(1–2):2–15.

44. Lemos MC, Thakker RV. Multiple endocrine neoplasia type 1 (MEN1): analysis of 1336 mutations reported in the first decade following identification of the gene. *Hum Mutat.* 2008; 29(1):22–32.

45. Bertolino P, Tong WM, Galendo D, Wang ZQ, Zhang CX. Heterozygous Men1 mutant mice develop a range of endocrine tumors mimicking multiple endocrine neoplasia type 1. *Mol Endocrinol.* 2003; 17(9):1880–92.

46. Crabtree JS, Scacheri PC, Ward JM et al. A mouse model of multiple endocrine neoplasia, type 1, develops multiple endocrine tumors. *Proc Natl Acad Sci U S A.* 2001; 98(3):1118–23.

47. Pannett AA, Thakker RV. Somatic mutations in MEN type 1 tumors, consistent with the Knudson "two-hit" hypothesis. *J Clin Endocrinol Metab.* 2001; 86(9):4371–4.

48. Brandi ML, Gagel RF, Angeli A et al. Guidelines for diagnosis and therapy of MEN type 1 and type 2. *J Clin Endocrinol Metab.* 2001; 86(12):5658–71.

49. Vergès B, Boureille F, Goudet P et al. Pituitary disease in MEN type 1 (MEN1): data from the France-Belgium MEN1 multicenter study. *J Clin Endocrinol Metab.* 2002; 87(2):457–65.

50. Benito M, Asa SL, Livolsi VA, West VA, Snyder PJ. Gonadotroph tumor associated with multiple endocrine neoplasia type 1. *J Clin Endocrinol Metab.* 2005; 90(1):570–4.

51. Farrell WE, Azevedo MF, Batista DL et al. Unique gene expression profile associated with an early-onset multiple endocrine neoplasia (MEN1)-associated pituitary adenoma. *J Clin Endocrinol Metab.* 2011; 96(11):E1905–14.

52. Trouillas J, Labat-Moleur F, Sturm N et al. Pituitary tumors and hyperplasia in multiple endocrine neoplasia type 1 syndrome (MEN1): a case-control study in a series of 77 patients versus 2509 non-MEN1 patients. *Am J Surg Pathol.* 2008; 32(4):534–43.

53. Goudet P, Bonithon-Kopp C, Murat A et al. Gender-related differences in MEN1 lesion occurrence and diagnosis: a cohort study of 734 cases from the Groupe d'etude des Tumeurs Endocrines. *Eur J Endocrinol.* 2011; 165(1):97–105.

54. Pellegata NS, Quintanilla-Martinez L, Siggelkow H et al. Germline mutations in p27Kip1 cause a multiple endocrine neoplasia syndrome in rats and humans. *Proc Natl Acad Sci U S A.* 2006; 103(42):15558–63.

55. Roy M, Chen H, Sippel RS. Current understanding and management of medullary thyroid cancer. *Oncologist.* 2013; 18(10):1093–100.

56. Choi YS, Kwon HJ, Kim BK et al. A case of medullary thyroid carcinoma with de novo V804M RET germline mutation. *J Korean Med Sci.* 2013; 28(1):156–9.

57. Raue F, Frank-Raue K. Genotype-phenotype relationship in multiple endocrine neoplasia type 2. Implications for clinical management. *Hormones (Athens).* 2009; 8(1):23–8.

58. Lundgren CI, Delbridg L, Learoyd D, Robinson B. Surgical approach to medullary thyroid cancer. *Arq Bras Endocrinol Metabol.* 2007; 51(5):818–24.

59. Modigliani E, Cohen R, Campos JM et al. Prognostic factors for survival and for biochemical cure in medullary thyroid carcinoma: results in 899 patients. The GETC Study Group. Groupe d'étude des tumeurs à calcitonine. *Clin Endocrinol (Oxf).* 1998; 48(3):265–73.

60. Fleming JB, Lee JE, Bouvet M et al. Surgical strategy for the treatment of medullary thyroid carcinoma. *Ann Surg.* 1999; 230(5):697–707.

61. Jarzab B, Szpak-Ulczok S, Wloch J, Czarniecka A, Krajewska J. Timing and criteria for prophylactic thyroidectomy in asymptomatic RET carriers—the role of Ct serum level. *Thyroid Res.* 2013; 6 Suppl 1:S9.

62. Lenders JW, Duh QY, Eisenhofer G et al. Pheochromocytoma and paraganglioma: an endocrine society clinical practice guideline. *J Clin Endocrinol Metab.* 2014; 99(6):1915–42.

63. Jafri M, Maher ER. The genetics of phaeochromocytoma: using clinical features to guide genetic testing. *Eur J Endocrinol.* 2012; 166(2):151–8.

64. Karasek D, Shah U, Frysak Z, Stratakis C, Pacak K. An update on the genetics of pheochromocytoma. *J Hum Hypertens.* 2013; 27(3):141–7.

65. Jalbani IK, Nazim SM, Abbas F. Pheochromocytoma associated with von Hippel-Lindau disease in a Pakistani family. *Urol Ann.* 2015; 7(1):120–3.

66. van Berkel A, Lenders JW, Timmers HJ. Diagnosis of endocrine disease: biochemical diagnosis of phaeochromocytoma and paraganglioma. *Eur J Endocrinol.* 2014; 170(3):R109–19.

67. Lenders JWM, Eisenhofer G. Update on modern management of pheochromocytoma and paraganglioma. *Endocrinol Metab (Seoul).* 2017; 32(2):152–61.

68. Otoukesh S, Cooper CJ, Lou W et al. Combination chemotherapy regimen in a patient with metastatic malignant pheochromocytoma and neurofibromatosis type 1. *Am J Case Rep.* 2014; 15:123–7.

69. Mak IYF, Hayes AR, Khoo B, Grossman A. Peptide receptor radionuclide therapy as a novel treatment for metastatic and invasive phaeochromocytoma and paraganglioma. *Neuroendocrinology.* 2019; 109(4):287–98.

70. Crona J, Beuschlein F, Pacak K, Skogseid B. Advances in adrenal tumors 2018. *Endocr Relat Cancer.* 2018; 25(7):R405–R20.

71. Aghamohammadzadeh N, Faraji A, Bozorgi F, Faraji I, Moghadaszadeh M. Primary hyperaldostronisim as initial presentation of adrenal cortical carcinoma with liver metastasis: a case report. *Int J Hematol Oncol Stem Cell Res.* 2013; 7(2):38–42.

72. Else T, Kim AC, Sabolch A et al. Adrenocortical carcinoma. *Endocr Rev.* 2014; 35(2):282–326.

73. Almeida MQ, Bezerra-Neto JE, Mendonça BB, Latronico AC, Fragoso MCBV. Primary malignant tumors of the adrenal glands. *Clinics (Sao Paulo).* 2018; 73(suppl 1):e756s.

74. Leotlela PD, Jauch A, Holtgreve-Grez H, Thakker RV. Genetics of neuroendocrine and carcinoid tumours. *Endocr Relat Cancer.* 2003; 10(4):437–50.

75. Kim JY, Hong SM, Ro JY. Recent updates on grading and classification of neuroendocrine tumors. *Ann Diagn Pathol.* 2017; 29:11–6.

76. Gao L, Natov NS, Daly KP et al. An update on the management of pancreatic neuroendocrine tumors. *Anticancer Drugs.* 2018; 29(7):597–612.

77. McKenna LR, Edil BH. Update on pancreatic neuroendocrine tumors. *Gland Surg.* 2014; 3(4):258–75.

78. Tsoli M, Chatzellis E, Koumarianou A, Kolomodi D, Kaltsas G. Current best practice in the management of neuroendocrine tumors. *Ther Adv Endocrinol Metab.* 2019; 10:2042018818804698.

79. Kunz PL, Reidy-Lagunes D, Anthony LB et al. Consensus guidelines for the management and treatment of neuroendocrine tumors. *Pancreas.* 2013; 42(4):557–77.

6 BREAST CANCER

Amy Case, Gwenllian Edwards, and Catherine Pembroke

Epidemiology

Globally, breast cancer is the most frequently diagnosed cancer among women, with an estimated 1.67 million new cancer cases diagnosed in 2012.[1,2] In less developed countries, it is the leading cause of cancer death in women, whilst in developed regions it is now second after lung cancer. The incidence rates are highest in western and northern Europe, Australia/New Zealand, and North America and lowest in Asia and Middle Africa.[3] These worldwide differences have been attributed to changes in body weight, fat intake, early age at menarche, reproductive patterns such as fewer pregnancies and later age at first birth, late age at menopause, use of oral contraceptives, hormone replacement therapy, alcohol consumption, and lack of physical activity. The impact of environmental and cultural changes has been highlighted by studies of migration patterns to the United States, with rising incidences of breast cancer amongst subsequent generations.[4] The age-specific incidence rates rise steadily between the ages of 35 and 70 years, and then more sharply over 70 years, with over 25% of diagnoses made in the over-75 group. The highest incidence is seen in females aged between 85 and 89 years.[5]

Women in the United Kingdom have a one in seven lifetime risk of developing breast cancer.[6] In 2016 approximately 55,200 new cases of breast cancer were diagnosed in the United Kingdom (54,500 [>99%] cases were in females and 360 [<1%] in males), with 11,563 deaths. Since the 1970s, the mortality rate from breast cancer in the United Kingdom for all age groups has decreased by 38%. The reduction is attributed to the national mammographic screening program and access to more effective treatments. The 5-year survival for breast cancer in the UK varies from 99% in stage I, to 15% 5-year survival for stage IV disease.[7]

Molecular genetics

Human cancers can either be inherited via the germline of a carrier or otherwise occur sporadically due to exposure to a variety of widely differing mutagens. The prevailing theory of carcinogenesis is that of Boveri's somatic mutations[8] which postulates that cancer derives from a single somatic cell which has accumulated successive DNA mutations. These mutations are thought to occur in genes that govern the pathways for cell growth, proliferation, and adhesion such as the MAPK, RB/E2F, P13K/AKT/mTOR, and TP53 pathways.[9]

Alterations in genes that are in involved in normal growth and proliferation can lead to overexpression or enhanced function of that gene's protein product. These alterations are often responsible for the development of sporadic cancers, which account for the majority of breast cancers. Genes that are activated and overexpressed in 20–30% of breast cancers include the oncogenes HER2, *Bcl-2*, *Cyclin D1* and *c-Myc*, *RAS*, *ER*, and *RAS*. Genes inactivated somatically in varying proportions of breast cancers include the *CHK2*, *Rb*, *TP53*, and *NM23* tumor suppressor genes.[10] Human epidermal growth factor receptor 2 (HER2) overexpression is reported in approximately a third of patients and is generally associated with a more aggressive phenotype.

Interestingly it is virtually never seen in lobular breast cancers.[11] Estrogen receptor (ER) expression is noted in approximately 80% of breast cancers.

Germline mutations in the tumor suppressor genes BRCA1 and BRCA2 account for about 2% and 1%, respectively, of breast cancer incidence and are the most common cause of both hereditary breast and ovarian cancers. Affected individuals are born heterozygous for the gene defect resulting in mutation carriers having the loss of one of their wildtype alleles, and random loss of the other wildtype allele through loss of heterozygosity or other somatic mutation leads to breast cancer.[12] A meta-analysis of 10 studies has reported that the mean cumulative risks of breast cancer by age 70 years for BRCA1 and BRCA2 mutation carriers were 57% and 49%, respectively, and ovarian cancer risks were 40% for BRCA1 and 18% for BRCA2 mutation carriers, respectively.[13] The molecular basis of the cellular effect in both syndromes is a defect in DNA repair by homologous recombination, rendering the genome prone to mutation, a state referred to as genomic instability.[14] Less commonly, Li–Fraumeni, ataxia telangiectasia, Cowden, and Lynch (also known as hereditary non-polyposis colorectal cancer) are other hereditary syndromes that demonstrate an increased susceptibility to breast and/or ovarian cancer.

Continued efforts to elucidate the molecular nature of breast cancer are now providing targets for effective therapies to be developed against specific cellular pathways which are known to be aberrant in breast cancers. Some of these agents have significantly changed the landscape of breast cancer treatment over the past decade and will hopefully continue to improve expected survival from the disease.

Pathology

Pathogenesis and molecular classification

The breast is a modified sweat gland with 15–20 duct systems converging on the nipple. Stereomicroscopy of whole-breast sections supports the origin of most breast carcinomas from the terminal duct lobular unit. Recognizable precursor lesions of invasive carcinoma include DCIS.[15] The intraduct components of invasive tumors share the same grade as the invasive disease and have a very similar genetic profile. Similarly, the grade of pure DCIS is usually correlated with the grade of an invasive recurrence. Local recurrences after breast conservation treatment of invasive disease are usually the same grade as the primary lesion. All these features suggest a highly stable genotype that is determined at an early stage in breast cancer development. Genotyping of precursor lesions and invasive cancers is advancing rapidly, and characteristic patterns of DNA losses and gains are associated with different histological types of disease and different grades of malignancy. In some instances, these are already characterized at the level of the gene, for example, loss of the adhesion molecule E-cadherin on the long arm of chromosome 16 in lobular carcinoma.[16]

Future classifications of breast cancer are likely to include gene expression profiles. For example, five subgroups identified on the basis of differing expression profiles have been reported to have different prognoses.[17] The prognosis of the basal-like and HER2-positive clusters is significantly worse than that of the predominantly ER-positive luminal categories. HER2 status is currently confirmed by fluorescent in situ hybridization (counting gene copy number) and, as for ER positivity, gene expression status can increasingly be established using immunohistochemical analyses of specific proteins (Figure 6.1). Thus, the basal-like tumors can be identified by positive staining for cytokeratins 5 and 14 as well as by ER-negative, progesterone receptor (PR)-negative, and HER2-negative status. Such tumors are often deficient in BRCA1 protein and may be more sensitive to DNA cross-linking agents such as platinum compounds. With the recent surge in utilization of immune-directed therapies in many cancers the expression of programmed cell death ligand 1 (PDL1) is now beginning to be studied. PDL1 has been found to be upregulated in as many as 20% of tumor samples and again is most typically associated with basal breast cancers.[18] Expression and protein profiling are currently a very active research area. Given this level of diversity, to allow a personalized approach to management and accurate prognostication, it is vital that pathological evaluation of all breast cancers include immunohistochemistry (IHC) for ER (using a standardized methodology such as Allred or H-score), PR, and HER2. Where IHC gives a borderline result for HER2 (+3 being positive and +2 ambiguous), gene amplification via in situ hybridization should be undertaken to further define HER2 status.[19]

Traditional histological classification

Most breast malignancies arise from epithelial elements and are adenocarcinomas. Based on the growth pattern and cytologic features of the lesions, in situ carcinomas of the breast are either ductal (also known as intraductal carcinoma) or lobular. Invasive breast carcinomas consist of several histological subtypes; invasive ductal carcinoma accounts for 75%, invasive lobular carcinoma accounts for 8–10%, and medullary carcinoma accounts for 1–2% of all invasive breast cancers.[20] Tubular, mucinous, and papillary carcinomas are three other subtypes of invasive breast cancer, which have a better prognosis than other subtypes and together account for 5% of invasive cancers.

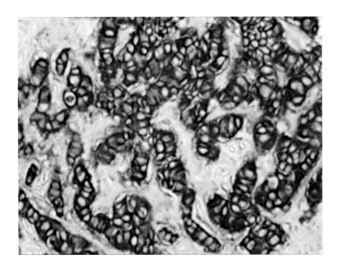

FIGURE 6.1 Breast cancer tissue showing strong membrane staining with anti-human epidermal growth factor receptor 2 antibody (3+).

Duct carcinoma in situ

DCIS comprises a heterogeneous group of lesions characterized by proliferation of malignant cells within the mammary ductal system, with no evidence of invasion into the surrounding stroma. Most patients more commonly present with screen-detected microcalcification with no breast-related symptoms or signs on physical examination. Less common presentations include mass, nipple discharge, or other soft tissue change. DCIS is nearly always unilateral, in contrast to lobular carcinoma in situ (LCIS). The Van Nuys Prognostic Index classifies DCIS according to the risk of local recurrence after breast-preserving surgery is proposed.[21] This index distinguishes high-nuclear- and non-high-nuclear-grade lesions, the latter being subdivided according to the presence or absence of comedo-type necrosis.

Lobular carcinoma in situ

LCIS, a non-invasive lesion arising from the lobules and terminal ducts of the breast, is not identified by mammography or by clinical examination but detected as an incidental finding on breast biopsies performed for other reasons. It is predominantly found in premenopausal women and is typically multicentric in the breast and often (35%) bilateral. LCIS has long been regarded as an indicator of elevated cancer risk rather than as a pre-malignant condition in its own right, but new data challenge this model. It is associated with an approximately 30% lifetime risk of developing invasive carcinoma, usually ductal and usually (>60%) in the ipsilateral breast.

Clinical presentation and investigation

The presentation of breast cancer may vary from a simple palpable mass, to nipple inversion, blood-stained nipple discharge, skin tethering, peau d'orange, or axillary adenopathy. A thorough personal history including menopausal status and family history is vital, and clinical assessment should include bilateral breast and locoregional nodal examinations. All patients should undergo a triple assessment consisting of bilateral mammography, ultrasound, and a core needle biopsy.

Bilateral mammography is undertaken in all women over the age of 40 (with a concerning breast symptom) and in those between 35 and 40 with a clinical score of or above 3 (BIRADS), followed by ultrasound and core needle biopsy. Digital breast tomosynthesis (further detailed in the screening section) is established as an integral assessment tool with many centers offering DBT as the mammographic standard in symptomatic breast imaging. Mammographic abnormalities that are not visible on ultrasound undergo stereotactic biopsy. Stereotactic biopsy may also be undertaken using tomosynthesis. Clinically concerning findings that are occult on imaging undergo clinical biopsy. The axilla is assessed with ultrasound in all cases and any suspicious nodes are biopsied. Magnetic resonance imaging (MRI) of the breasts is reserved for those with occult disease on conventional imaging, lobular cancer, multi-focal disease, or prior to neo-adjuvant therapy. Radiological marker clip insertion should be considered in small or very subtle abnormalities.

Typical mammographic features of screen-detected cancer include spiculate densities, clusters of fine calcifications (Figure 6.2), retraction or thickening of the overlying skin or nipple, and enlarged axillary nodes. The investigation of a screen-detected impalpable abnormality requires core biopsy guided by targeted ultrasound, or stereotactic biopsy using mammography.

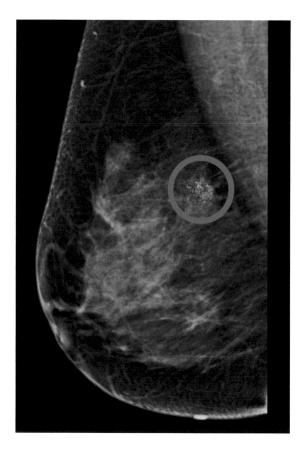

FIGURE 6.2 Microgram illustrating microcalcification.

If negative, this is followed by wire-guided excision biopsy (<10 g) to establish a histological diagnosis, and assess biomarker status (estrogen receptor ER, progesterone receptor PR, and HER2). Specimen radiography, following wide local excision, is important to confirm that the radiological abnormality has been removed in its entirety.

If the core biopsy confirms malignancy (ductal carcinoma in situ [DCIS] can be difficult to distinguish from invasive cancer on core biopsy), the extent of abnormalities on mammography will influence the type and extent of primary surgery, and the surgical management of the axilla. Palpable DCIS is treated in a similar fashion to invasive malignancy; if there is strong suspicion of invasive malignancy, vacuum biopsy may be undertaken to gain more tissue, thus more histological information and accurate preoperative diagnosis.

Subsequent staging depends on clinical stage and risk. For the majority of early-stage disease, simple investigations, such as hematology and biochemistry tests, should suffice. Further radiological staging is considered according to symptomology, or in those with locally advanced disease, i.e. clinically positive axilla >4 nodes, ≥5cm primary tumor, or aggressive biology (for example, inflammatory breast cancer, which has a high risk of de novo secondary disease).[22] When indicated staging includes a computed tomography (CT) scan of the chest and/or abdomen and/or pelvis. Isotope bones scans are not routinely undertaken in most institutions unless there are symptoms not explained by CT. When skeletal metastases are present, bone scintigraphy is indicated to assess extent of disease, particularly in the appendicular skeleton, and plain radiography may be required to assess risk of pathological fracture. MRI may be helpful in differentiating between benign and metastatic bone disease, to assess for

cord or neural compromise, or where there is strong suspicion of skeletal or neurological (including meningeal) disease which is not established with usual modalities. There is currently no role for routine 18F-FDG PET/CT in the assessment of locoregional disease although it can be useful in characterizing distant disease when standard imaging is indeterminate[23] (Table 6.1).

Staging

Clinical and pathologic staging is routinely used to obtain baseline prognostic information, to compare results from clinical trials and across institutions, and for choosing optimum local and systemic treatment options. The tumor node metastasis (TNM) staging system for breast cancer is commonly followed but periodic revisions of TNM staging are essential due to advances in imaging techniques and treatments that impact survival. The *AJCC Cancer Staging Manual (eighth edition)* was published in 2017, and made important changes, including the addition of biomarkers such as ER, PR, and HER2 status into prognostic staging.[24] New to the eighth edition is the "Prognostic Stage Group," which incorporates these biomarkers, and histological grade, to create a more accurate predictors of outcome. Though not mandatory for staging, genomic profiling using Oncotype Dx® score has also been incorporated in staging for the first time. An example of prognostic staging using this information is given in Tables 6.2 and 6.3.[24,25]

Screening

Mammography remains the main imaging modality for the screening of breast cancer. In the UK, two-view (medio-lateral and cranio-caudal) digital mammography is currently offered every 3 years to all women between the ages of 50 and 70 years. In 2012, an independent panel reviewed the evidence of the benefits and harms of breast screening in the context of the UK breast-screening programs.[26] The report concluded that screening reduces breast cancer mortality but at the cost of over-diagnosis. The review estimates that while screening prevents about 1,300 breast cancer deaths per year, for every one breast cancer death prevented, about 3 over-diagnosed cases are identified and treated. That said, the report also suggests that of the 307,000 women aged 50–52 years who are invited to begin screening every year, just over 1% would have an over-diagnosed cancer in the next 20 years. On balance, given the estimated 20% reduction in breast cancer mortality in women invited to screening, the panel concluded that the UK breast-screening programs confer significant benefit and should continue, but clear communication of these harms and benefits to women is vital. Similar conclusions regarding the overall net benefit of screening were reached by the International Agency for Research on Cancer in 2014.[27]

There is controversy and currently no consensus about screening in the 40-49-year age group. The UK Age trial looked at the effect of screening from the age of 40 on breast cancer mortality rates. The trial compared annual mammography between the ages of 40 and 48 years, to entering the screening program at 50 and having 3 yearly mammograms. After a median of 17 years of follow-up, the study found a significant reduction in breast cancer mortality in the group who were screened between 40 and 48, but this was only seen for the first 10 years after intervention, and the overall breast cancer incidence was similar between both groups.[28] A 2009 meta-analyses of 8 trials, including UK Age and the NBSS-1 Canadian trial, reported a relative risk reduction of

TABLE 6.1   TNM Classification of Breast Cancer

T	Primary Tumor
Tis	Carcinoma in situ
	Tis (DCIS) Ductal carcinoma in situ
	Tis (LCIS)* Lobular carcinoma in situ
	Tis (Paget) Paget disease of the nipple not associated with invasive tumor or DCIS in the underlying breast
T1	Tumor ≤2 cm in greatest dimension
	T1mi Microinvasion ≤0.1 cm in greatest dimension
	T1a >0.1 cm but ≤0.5 cm in greatest dimension
	T1b >0.5 cm but ≤1 cm in greatest dimension
	T1c >1 cm but ≤2 cm in greatest dimension
T2	Tumor >2 cm but ≤5 cm in greatest dimension
T3	Tumor >5 cm in greatest dimension
T4	Tumor of any size with direct extension to skin (ulceration or macroscopic nodules) and/or chest wall (includes ribs, intercostal muscles, serratus anterior muscle, but not pectoral muscle adherence or invasion)
T4a	Extension to chest wall
T4b	Ulceration and/or ipsilateral satellite nodules and/or edema (including peau d'orange), not meeting the criteria for inflammatory carcinoma
T4c	Both 4a and 4b above
T4d	Inflammatory carcinoma
N	Regional lymph nodes

Clinical (cN):

N1	Metastasis to movable ipsilateral level I, II axillary node(s)
N2	Metastasis in fixed ipsilateral level I, II axillary node(s) *or* in clinically detected* ipsilateral internal mammary lymph node(s) in the *absence* of clinically evident axillary lymph node metastasis
N2a	Metastasis in axillary lymph node(s) fixed to one another or to other structures
N2b	Metastasis in clinically detected** internal mammary lymph node(s) in the absence of clinically evident axillary lymph node metastasis
N3	Metastasis in ipsilateral infraclavicular (level III) lymph node(s) with or without level I and II lymph node involvement; or in clinically detected** ipsilateral internal mammary lymph node(s) in the *presence* of clinically evident axillary lymph node metastasis; or metastasis in ipsilateral supraclavicular lymph node(s) with or without axillary or internal mammary lymph node involvement
	N3a Metastasis in infraclavicular lymph node(s)
	N3b Metastasis in internal mammary and axillary lymph nodes
	N3c Metastasis in supraclavicular lymph node(s)

Pathological (pN):

Based on axillary lymph node dissection, +/− sentinel node biopsy (SNB); if based solely on SNB, the suffix (sn) is added, e.g. pN(sn). Note internal mammary nodes are not routinely sampled at SNB or ANC

Isolated tumor cells (≤0.2mm or <200 cells in a single histological section) are not designated as positive nodes

The suffix (i+) denotes identification of malignant cells by immunohistochemistry, e.g. pN0(i+)

The suffix (mol+) denotes positive molecular findings by reverse transcriptase polymerase chain reaction (RT-PCR), e.g. pN0(mol+)

M	Distant metastasis

cM0(i+) No clinical or radiographic evidence, but molecularly or microscopically detected tumor cells in blood (CTCs), bone marrow or other non-regional nodal tissue no larger than 0.2 mm

M1	Distant metastasis detected by clinical and radiographic means and/or histologically proven metastases larger than 0.2 mm (pM)

Source: Adapted from AJCC 8th ed., 2017.

Notes: The ptn pathological classification requires the examination of a resected primary carcinoma with no gross tumor at the margins of resection. In addition, X in each category (e.g., TX) indicates the stage cannot be assessed; 0 (e.g., T0) indicates there is no evidence for the stage.

*   Lobular carcinoma in situ is now classed as a benign entity and as such has been removed from the TNM staging in the 8th edition.

**   "Clinically detected" is defined as detected by imaging studies (excluding lymphoscintigraphy), clinical examination, or highly suspicious fine-needle aspiration cytology (FNAC).

15% in favor of screening in those aged between 39 and 49 years.[29] The AgeX trial is a cluster-randomized trial investigating age extension of the UK breast screening program from 50–70 to 47–73 years. It aims to recruit 6 million women and run over 17 years, and its first results are expected in the mid-2020s.[30]

Digital mammography is more accurate for pre- and perimenopausal women presenting with dense, glandular breasts and has now replaced screen-film mammography in most Western countries.[31] Digital breast tomosynthesis (DBT) is a three-dimensional technique during which a series of low-dose images are acquired from an X-ray tube moving in an arc over the breast. The TOMMY trial[32] compared DBT in conjunction with digital mammography to 2D mammography alone, and found an improvement in specificity but only marginal increases in sensitivity. Similarly to 2D mammography, there is the potential for dense, glandular breasts to reduce the detection accuracy of DBT and an additional MRI is often suggested.[33] Although DBT has been widely adopted, long-term data regarding its impact on clinical outcomes are awaited.

TABLE 6.2 **Anatomical Stage Grouping**

Stage Group	T	N	M
Stage 0	Tis	N0	M0
Stage IA	T1*	N0	M0
Stage 1B	T0,1	N1mi	M0
Stage IIA	T0	N1	M0
	T1*	N1	M0
	T2	N0	M0
Stage IIB	T2	N1	M0
	T3	N0	M0
Stage IIIA	T1	N2	M0
	T2	N2	M0
	T3	N1, N2	M0
Stage IIIB	T4	N0, N1, N2	M0
Stage IIIC	Any T	N3	M0
Stage IV	Any T	Any N	M1

Source: Adapted from AJCC 8th ed., 2017.
* T1 includes T1mi.

Identification of high-risk groups

Family history identifies a minority of patients at increased lifetime risk of breast cancer due to a mixture of shared environmental and genetic factors. Definitions vary, but the average lifetime risk of 8% in the United Kingdom is increased to 12–25% if the family has just one or two first-degree relatives diagnosed with breast cancer before the age of 50 years, or two first-degree or second-degree relatives on the same side of the family with breast

or ovarian cancer (these scenarios apply to 4% of the female population in the United Kingdom). Women with three or more first-degree or second-degree relatives with breast or ovarian cancer on the same side of the family, a history of bilateral tumors, male breast cancer, or sarcoma or women aged less than 40 years at diagnosis have a 25–50% lifetime risk of breast cancer (applies to 1% of the female population). Nevertheless, this leaves 95% of the female population with a lifetime risk of less than 12%.

Women at intermediate or high risk according to the aforementioned factors are offered referral to a specialist risk service, comprising clinical genetics, breast oncology, and counsellors.[34] Women with an increased risk of breast cancer should be "breast aware" and follow advice regarding self-examination provided to all women. Intermediate risk women aged from 40 to 49 should attend annual clinical breast examination and digital mammography.

Women who inherit proven *BRCA1* or *BRCA2* mutations have a 60–80% lifetime risk of breast cancer and a significant risk of ovarian cancer.[35,36] Several studies have demonstrated that, for high-risk patients, MRI is more sensitive at detecting early cancers and therefore is now the standard of care for many.[37–40] As such, annual MRI (in addition to mammography) should be offered from the age of 30 years to those with high risk or known BRCA1/2 mutation, and may be considered from the age of 20 for those with a TP53 mutation. European guidance suggests enhanced screening begins at 10 years younger than the youngest familial case.[41] In addition, women with *BRCA 1* mutations, in view of their elevated risk of ovarian cancer, are often referred for annual pelvic ultrasounds. Women at high risk (>25%) of breast cancer may wish to consider further measures, including bilateral prophylactic mastectomies and reconstruction (and

TABLE 6.3 **Recommended Adjuvant Therapy by Intrinsic Subtype**

Intrinsic Subtype	Biomarker Status	Recommended Therapy	Comments
Luminal A-like	ER + (strongly) HER2 − Ki67 low (or low grade) PR +	ET alone in the majority of cases	Chemotherapy should be avoided in stage I/II disease, especially when there is a low genetic score. Consider chemotherapy if grade 3 or high tumor burden.
Luminal B-like (HER2-negative)	ER + (variable degree of expression) HER2 − Ki 67 high (or high grade) PR low	ET + chemotherapy	Population of highest uncertainty. Prognostic features such as LN status should be considered, along with patient co-morbidities and preferences. In LN-negative disease, genetic recurrence score can be helpful. In LN-positive disease, chemotherapy should be considered given the current uncertainty about the efficacy of genetic scoring in this group.
Luminal B-like (HER2-positive)	ER + HER2 + Any Ki67 Any PR	ET + chemotherapy + anti-HER2 therapy	No data to support omission of chemotherapy in this group. In small, LN-negative disease (pT1pN0) could consider single-agent paclitaxel with anti-HER2. Dual anti-HER2 therapy (trastuzumab + pertuzumab) is indicated in LN-positive disease Data awaited regarding adjuvant neratinib.
HER2-positive	HER + ER − PR −	Chemotherapy + dual anti-HER2 therapy	In pT1a/b adjuvant trastuzumab alone can be considered.
Triple-negative	ER − PR − HER2 −	Chemotherapy	Can consider omitting chemotherapy in very small disease (pT1a). Neoadjuvant rather than adjuvant therapy is suggested in stage II/III disease. BRCA1/2 positive—consider alkylating agent (no consensus about platinum in adjuvant setting). Potential to avoid chemotherapy in certain histological subtypes (secretory, juvenile apocrine, adenoid cystic).

Sources: Adapted from ESMO, 2015; St. Gallen, 2017; NICE Guidance, 2018.
Abbreviations: ER = estrogen receptor, HER2 = human epidermal growth factor 2 receptor, PR = progesterone receptor, Ki67 is a proliferation marker, ET = endocrine therapy, LN = lymph node.

oophorectomy in the case of *BRCA1* mutation carriers). These interventions are taken only after careful consideration, including psychological counseling.[42]

Breast cancer prevention therapy

A systematic review of 7 randomized controlled trials of tamoxifen or raloxifene in women without pre-existing breast cancer concluded that tamoxifen and raloxifene reduce the incidence of invasive breast cancer by 7 to 9 cases in 1,000 women over 5 years compared with placebo.[43] Although the trials were not powered for mortality, breast cancer–specific and all-cause mortality rates were not statistically significantly reduced by either medication. Extended follow-up of the IBIS I study of tamoxifen has demonstrated a long period of protection, with a breast cancer identified in 7% in the tamoxifen group versus 9.8% in the placebo group with a median follow-up of 16 years.[44]

Data for the use of aromatase inhibitors (AI) for the prevention of breast cancer come from two main trials. The National Cancer Institute of Canada (NCIC) MAP.3 trial suggested that the steroidal AI, exemestane is an effective agent, reducing risk by 53%.[45] The IBIS II trial of the non-steroidal AI anastrozole versus placebo in high-risk postmenopausal women revealed that anastrozole also reduced the risk of all breast cancer by 53%.[46] Long-term follow-up for both of these agents is required to ascertain whether this risk reduction is durable.

Most guidance recommends that tamoxifen is discussed with those in the high-risk population, and anastrozole or exemestane in the postmenopausal group. The decision to use tamoxifen should take into consideration the adverse effects including endometrial cancer, thromboembolic events and cataracts, and the risk of osteoporosis considered with an AI. [47]

Surgery for early breast cancer

Surgery remains the primary curative treatment for the majority of patients with DCIS or invasive breast cancer. Historically, radical mastectomy formed the basis of surgical breast cancer management until the late twentieth century when breast-conserving techniques were introduced. Breast cancer screening, introduced in the United Kingdom in 1988, has subsequently detected an increased number of early breast cancers, of which a significant proportion will receive breast-conserving surgery (BCS). Axillary surgery has also revolutionized in recent years with the use of sentinel node sampling to assess axillary node involvement, thus preventing patients from undergoing unnecessary axillary clearance, which can be associated with debilitating sequelae.

Primary surgery

The two main surgical options in breast cancer management are BCS in conjunction with adjuvant radiotherapy and mastectomy. Randomized trials have supported equivalent survival between the two methods when BCS is combined with radiotherapy in early-stage disease.[48] The main advantage of BCS over mastectomy is a more cosmetically acceptable breast post-surgically. It is best clinical practice to offer the patient choice between the two methods if appropriate. Absolute contraindications to BCS and radiotherapy include multicentric disease, large tumor to breast size (although neoadjuvant chemotherapy may be considered), diffuse microcalcifications on imaging, or previous radiotherapy affecting the breast. Special clinical consideration should be given to patients who are pregnant (as radiotherapy is contraindicated), although BCS could potentially be performed in the third trimester and radiotherapy postnatally. Patients with connective tissue disorders may not be suitable for radiotherapy as long-term radiation complications may be exacerbated in this group.[49]

Wide local excision is the most common BCS procedure and entails complete excision of the tumor down to the pectoral muscle, ensuring an adequate surrounding margin of normal breast tissue. Titanium clips are placed at the base of the tumorectomy before parenchymal reconstitution of the excision defect, to aid adjuvant radiotherapy planning.[50] For impalpable tumors, preoperative wire localization can guide surgical location of the tumor. Adequate radial excision margins are imperative for local tumor control. A 5- to 10-mm margin of normal breast tissue provides histologically acceptable results in the majority of patients.[51] Although there is no consensus on what is considered a close margin, less than 2 mm is usually considered unacceptable.[52] In cases where this is not achieved, patients should be consulted regarding re-excision or mastectomy if appropriate. The rate of local recurrence following BCS may be increased if patients are young, have involved lymph nodes, or have ER-negative tumors and in the absence of adjuvant radiotherapy.[53] Oncoplastic breast surgery (OBS) is a developing field that blends surgical oncology techniques with reconstructive/plastic surgery, attempting to provide clinically adequate tumor excision with preservation of breast shape and appearance. This may be of benefit, for example, in patients with large tumors where breast contour would inevitably be deformed post-excision with standard BCS techniques. To date, long-term outcomes have been reported as being equivocal between standard BCS and OBS, although no prospective studies have been reported.[54]

For patients who are advised or who opt to have a mastectomy, the UK National Institute for Clinical Excellence (NICE) recommends that all patients should be offered breast reconstruction.[55] However, audits have shown in England between 2008 and 2009 that only 31% of patients who had a mastectomy had subsequent reconstruction, suggesting more robust discussion is required with the patient during surgical consultation.[56] Reconstruction may be performed at the time of surgery (immediate reconstruction) or as a subsequent procedure (delayed reconstruction) (Figure 6.3). Varying techniques are used to achieve reconstruction of the breast mound. One involves the insertion of an implant under the pectoralis major, which may be of fixed volume or an adjustable tissue expander that requires injections of saline in incremental amounts over time to increase mound size.[50] Reconstruction may also involve using the patient's own tissue (autologous reconstruction). A "pedicle flap" involves the rotation of a flap consisting of skin, fat, and muscle from the patient's back or abdomen up to the breast area while a section remains intact, thus maintaining its own blood supply.[41] A "free flap" involves complete excision of a similar flap, usually from the patient's abdomen, buttock, or thigh. This flap is then attached to the mastectomy site with microvascular techniques being employed to anastamose the original blood supply to the recipient vessels[56] (Figure 6.4). The Michigan Breast Reconstruction Outcomes Study demonstrated that 2 years after reconstruction patients who underwent an autologous reconstruction were in general more satisfied with the aesthetics of their reconstruction compared to those who received implants/tissue expanders.[57] Patients who undergo breast reconstruction may proceed to have chest wall radiotherapy if required, although some retrospective studies report increased rates of late adverse effects including fat and flap necrosis, induration, and infection.[58]

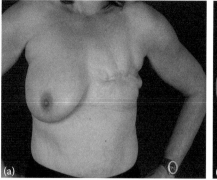
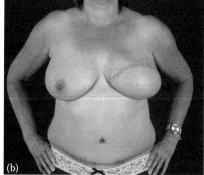

FIGURE 6.3 Left delayed reconstruction.

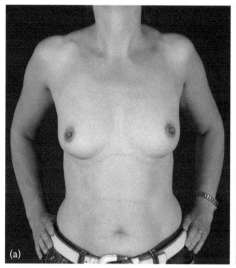
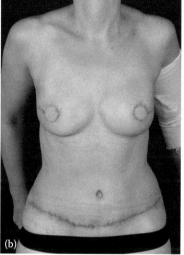

FIGURE 6.4 Bilateral immediate deep inferior epigastric artery flap.

Axillary surgery

Axillary staging is imperative in patients undergoing surgery for invasive breast cancer or extensive DCIS, for prognostication and consideration of additional surgical, cytotoxic, and radiotherapy treatment. As clinical axillary assessment is unreliable, all patients should undergo preoperative axillary ultrasound assessment, with fine-needle aspiration or core biopsy of any suspicious nodes. Historically, surgical assessment of the axilla entailed axillary lymph node dissection (ALND). This technique entails the removal of all tissue below the axillary vein within the boundaries of the axilla, sparing the long thoracic nerve. In current practice, this procedure is reserved for patients who have positive lymph nodes diagnosed preoperatively. This procedure often carries significant morbidity, primarily lymphoedema of the ipsilateral arm, stiffening or "freezing" of the shoulder, and damage to the intercostobrachial nerve. The most common surgical method of assessing axillary involvement is sentinel lymph node biopsy (SLNB). SLNB considers breast lymphatic drainage as a chain of lymph nodes. If the first lymph node in the chain is not affected with metastatic disease, the remainder of the chain should also be cancer-free and no further treatment to the axilla is required. SLNB involves the injection of a radiolabeled colloid into the breast preoperatively with Patent Blue V dye injected in the same region during initial breast surgery. A Geiger counter then locates the sentinel node. The ALMANAC trial supported SLNB as a safe and effective alternative to ALND in nodal staging for early breast cancer, with reduced arm morbidity and increased quality of life.[59]

In recent years, research has focused on de-escalating axillary treatment, with the aim of reducing the co-morbidity of ALND for those with modest lymphatic involvement. Micrometastatic disease (0.2–2mm) is prognostically equivalent to node negative disease, and no further treatment is required. This was confirmed by the IBCSG 23-01 study, in which patients with one or more SLN micrometastases were randomized to ALND or no axillary treatment, and found no difference in disease-free survival at 10 years.[60]

When clinically occult macrometastatic disease is discovered at SLNB, there is evidence that suggests ALND can be avoided in the case of limited disease. The ACOSOG-Z0011 trial reported non-inferiority between ALND versus omission of ALND after 10 years of follow-up in a population of patients with T1–T2 disease and 1–2 SLN containing macrometastases following BCS followed by adjuvant tangential breast radiotherapy.[61] This trial, however, was subject to criticism for closing to recruitment early, including many patients with micometastatic disease only, and using high tangent

WBRT (thereby treating axillary levels 1 and 2). The currently recruiting POSNOC trial is randomizing patients with clinically node negative disease and 1–2 SLN macrometastases to either adjuvant systemic therapy alone, or adjuvant therapy in addition to ALND or axillary radiotherapy, with a primary end point of axillary recurrence at 5 years. Its results will provide more clarity in this setting. As described later, the AMAROS trial studied those with T1–2 primary breast cancer, clinically node negative, positive SLNB, and randomized them to ALND or axillary radiotherapy, and found comparable 5-year axillary recurrence rates between groups (0.43 versus 1.19% respectively).[62] Practice has now shifted to reserve ALND for those with extensive axillary involvement.[19]

In the neoadjuvant setting, post- as opposed to pre-chemotherapy SLNB is favored. Patients with clinically node-positive disease prior to NACT should have the macrometastatic nodes clipped. Dual mapping of a minimum of four lymph nodes, including the clipped node, should be performed to minimize false negative rates. Management of these patients was outlined in a consensus document in 2019, which is summarized in Figure 6.5.[63] Patients with residual macrometastatic nodal disease should receive an ALND as there is little evidence to suggest axillary radiotherapy is a suitable alternative. Trials such as the ATENC study and NSABP B-51/Radiation Therapy Oncology Group 1304 study will explore this clinical question.

Adjuvant therapy

The primary aim of adjuvant treatment is to improve local control and increase overall survival (OS). The post-operative surgical specimens provide the vital pathological information needed by a breast multidisciplinary team (MDT) to stage the cancer and identify key prognostic and predictive indices to aid in adjuvant treatment decision-making. It is equally important that the MDT considers age, co-morbidities, and performance status of the patient when making such decisions.

Prognostic and predictive indices

Conventional pathological features of invasive carcinomas correlating with prognosis include:

- ER/PR/HER2 status and proliferation markers
- Number of involved lymph nodes
- Histological subtype
- Tumor size
- Grade
- Lympho-vascular invasion
- Status of surgical margins (in breast-conserving surgery)

Pathological node status is the single most powerful prognostic indicator, node-positive patients having, on average, a 10-year

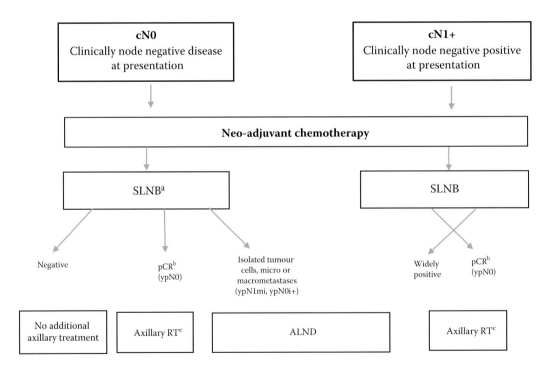

a Inc N0 disease, SLNB may be carried out before or after neoadjuvant chemotherapy with comparable identification and false positive rates, though standard practice is post chemotherapy SLNB

b In the subgroup where there is pathological evidence of disease response (such as fibrosis) in nodes previously thought to be negative clinically, there is no trial data with regards to management so they should be managed as pCR in previously node positive group

c There is no firm evidence regarding axillary radiotherapy following pCR at SNB following NACT. Further evidence is awaited before this approach becomes standard practice.

FIGURE 6.5   Axillary management following adjuvant chemotherapy. (From Gandhi et al., 2019.)

survival of 40% compared with 80% for node-negative women after locoregional therapy alone. A variety of predictive scoring systems are available to predict the likelihood of recurrence. These are compiled from multivariate analyses which generate algorithms based on pathological tumor size, grade, and node status, and separate patients into prognostic groups. The best known until recently was the Nottingham Prognostic Index (NPI): NI = 0.2 × – Pathological tumor size (centimeters) + Node stage/level (1–3) + Grade (1–3).[64] This has now been superseded by online prognostication and treatment benefit tools. In the United Kingdom, PREDICT has been designed to help clinicians and patients estimate the benefits of hormone therapy, chemotherapy, and anti-HER2 therapy on breast cancer survival following surgery. The model was derived from cancer registry information on 5,694 women treated in East Anglia, England, during 1999–2003, and breast cancer mortality models for ER-positive and ER-negative tumors were constructed using Cox proportional hazards, adjusted for known prognostic factors and mode of detection (symptomatic versus screen detected). The model has been validated in two data sets from the West Midlands Cancer Intelligence Unit and British Columbia. This model has been updated to include prognostic effect of HER2 and Ki-67 status.[65] The tool divides women into three categories: Low-risk, intermediate-, and high-risk, relating to a 3%, 3–5%, and >5% absolute 10-year survival benefit from chemotherapy respectively. It should be noted that PREDICT is less accurate for women <30 years with ER-positive disease, for those older than 70, is not validated in men, and may under-represent some ethnic groups.

Even using these prognostic models, decisions around adjuvant chemotherapy are complex and traditionally have been made on the assumption that clinically undetectable microscopic disease is present. In addition, there is a wide interpatient variation in response to chemotherapy, and at present we risk treating patients with inherently chemo-insensitive disease with a potentially toxic treatment that will offer them little benefit. It is hoped that genetic profiling will help to distinguish patients who are higher risk and stand to benefit from chemotherapy, from low-risk patients, and will help to predict response to chemotherapy, thus potentially sparing some patients unnecessary, costly, and potentially harmful treatment.

Gene expression profiling has been used to identify and develop molecular signatures, which complement pathological staging and augment prognostic stratification of patients to aid in this decision-making process. There are now several validated gene expression profiles available, including the Oncotype DX Breast Recurrence Score (known as Oncotype DX), EndoPredict, MammaPrint, and Prosigna. At present, there are no data directly comparing PREDICT with tumor profiling, and it should also be noted that clinical trials have each tested a single technology and the competing assays have not been compared directly to one another to date. Current UK guidance recommends that tumor profiling tests can be considered in women with early disease that is hormone receptor–positive (ER, PR, or both), HER2-negative, and lymph node–negative (including micrometastases), if they are intermediate-risk using PREDICT or NPI, and if the information provided by profiling would help them make a decision about chemotherapy.[66]

The Oncotype DX score quantifies expression of 21 genes (16 cancer-related and 5 reference) from a sample of breast cancer tissue to quantify the 10-year risk of distant recurrence, and provides a recurrence score of 0–100. It has arguably one of the more widely used assays, and was first validated in 2004, in a retrospective analysis of 668 samples collected from the National Surgical Adjuvant Breast and Bowel Project (NSABP) B-14 trial.

This study validated the Oncotype Dx recurrence score to quantify the likelihood of distant recurrence in patients with node-negative, ER-positive breast cancer who had been treated with tamoxifen.[67] The recurrence score was also predictive of response to tamoxifen, with further analysis confirming the association between the recurrence score and the risk of locoregional and distant recurrence.[68]

The TAILOR X trial was a non-inferiority study of 6,711 women, with hormone receptor–positive, HER2-negative, node-negative disease, who were randomly allocated to either endocrine therapy alone or chemotherapy plus endocrine therapy.[69] Those aged over 50 with a recurrence score of <26 showed no survival benefit with adjuvant chemotherapy. Women aged <50 years with a recurrence score of 16–25 did demonstrate some survival benefits with chemotherapy. ASCO now recommends that women with hormone-receptor positive, node negative disease with an Oncotype DX score of <26 aged over 50 have little benefit from chemotherapy, and this group can be offered endocrine therapy alone. Chemotherapy should only be offered in those with scores of 16–25 who are <50 years, and to all with a score of >26.[70]

The benefit of genomic profiling in the node-positive setting is less clear. The OPTIMA trial is a non-inferiority study that is comparing management guided by the Prosigna genomic test to standard management (i.e. chemotherapy) in the high-risk population.[71] The trial is actively recruiting, the results of which are awaited. The RxPONDER trial is evaluating the benefit for the Oncotype Dx test in those patients with 1–3 nodes positive, the results of which are expected in 2022.[72]

Adjuvant systemic therapy

Adjuvant chemotherapies have contributed significantly to the reduction in breast cancer mortality. Information gained from clinico-pathological assessment, and where appropriate, gene expression profiling, should be combined with individual patient factors such as fitness, co-morbidities, and preferences, to create an adjuvant treatment plan that is tailored to the patient and the biology of their disease. The molecular phenotype will govern the type of adjuvant therapy offered, as summarized in Table 6.3.

The following regimens are used in practice, though the most frequent contain an anthracycline and/or taxane:

- Anthracycline and/or taxane, for example fluorouracil, epirubicin, cyclophosphamide (FEC), or FEC-T (3 cycles of the former followed by 3 cycles of docetaxel or 12 weeks of paclitaxel).
- Cyclophosphamide, methotrexate, fluorouracil (CMF).
- AC (doxorubicin and cyclophosphamide).
- Non-anthracycline based chemotherapy, such as TC (docetaxel, cyclophosphamide) or weekly paclitaxel, can be considered in selected patients for whom cardiotoxicity is a greater risk.
- Dose-dense scheduling (i.e. 2-weekly rather than 3-weekly) can be considered for highly proliferative disease.

Current UK practice suggests the inclusion of both anthracyclines and taxanes when proposing adjuvant chemotherapy for breast cancer.[73] The 2011 Early Breast Cancer Trialists' Collaborative Group (EBCTCG) meta-analysis assessed both anthracycline-based regimens and CMF. It concluded that both regimens were effective in reducing recurrence, breast cancer–associated mortality, and overall mortality compared to no chemotherapy.[74] Greater reductions in recurrence and survival were seen when comparing ER-negative with ER-positive disease.

When comparing CMF with anthracycline-based regimens, outcomes are similar; however, there is a benefit where a higher cumulative dose of anthracycline is used. The following year, EBCTCG looked at the addition of taxanes to adjuvant regimens. The addition of a taxane led to a 2.8% improvement in breast cancer–specific survival correlating with a reduction in breast cancer mortality by a third and 3.2% improvement in OS.[75] In contrast, the UK TACT trial explored the use of taxanes in a large cohort of patients and found no additional survival benefit for a sequential anthracycline–taxane regimen (FEC-docetaxel) over FEC alone, but there was an expected increase in grade 3 and 4 toxicities.[76] This conflicting picture is further marred by the lack of information about biological subtypes of the cancers treated in an era before routine determination of HER2 status. Weekly paclitaxel is generally better tolerated than 3-weekly 75 mg/m^2 docetaxel but is more time- and resource-intensive for both hospital and patient.

Dose-dense scheduling has been validated to reduce disease recurrence and reduce 10-year mortality rate by 3%. This can be achieved by reducing 3-weekly schedules to 2-weekly intervals, and can be considered in highly proliferative tumors.[77]

Treatment duration ranges from 4 to 8 cycles (12–24 weeks) depending on regime and recurrence risk. Support with granulocyte colony-stimulating factor (G-CSF should be considered with dose-dense schedules).[41] Data looking specifically at the elderly population are lacking; however, there should be no upper age-limit of when to offer adjuvant chemotherapy. Decisions should be made following thorough assessment of the patient's physical fitness and detailed discussion of the risks and benefits.

ER-positive, HER2-negative disease

Most cases of luminal A (ER/PR-positive/HER2-negative) cancer will not require chemotherapy, unless there is a high burden of nodal disease rendering it high risk of relapse. Luminal B (ER-positive, PR/HER2-negative) cancers can be considered for chemotherapy unless they are characterized as low-risk following pathological staging or genetic profiling. In the premenopausal setting, the beneficial effect of chemotherapy is likely to be partly due to treatment-induced ovarian suppression.

HER2-positive disease

In 2005, two US studies of adjuvant chemotherapy combined with the HER2-targeting monoclonal antibody trastuzumab (Herceptin) were published, which started a revolution in the adjuvant treatment of HER2-positive early breast cancer. The first interim analysis demonstrated that the addition of trastuzumab therapy was associated with a 33% reduction in the risk of death,[78] and the effect remained similar when combined with the European HERA[79] and BCIRG 006[80] trial results in the 2012 Cochrane review.[81] There is clear substantial evidence to recommend the use of trastuzumab in HER2-positive disease in both node-positive and node-negative disease where the primary tumor is more than 1 cm. Unfortunately, there is little evidence to guide the treatment of smaller tumors, although many clinicians feel that it should be advocated, as HER2 positivity confers a poorer prognosis regardless of tumor size. The duration of treatment remains debatable but 12 months of therapy remains the standard of care as there was no additional benefit seen in the 2-year arm of HERA. More recently, the PERSEPHONE trial compared 6 versus 12 months of adjuvant trastuzumab and reported non-inferiority at 6 months with fewer adverse side effects. This may open the door to similar future studies and ultimately

de-escalation of treatment duration in some low-risk groups.[82] The trials clearly demonstrated that trastuzumab is associated with increased cardiac toxicity, and these concerns have been addressed by the publication of many guidelines including the National Cancer Research Institute (NCRI) recommendations for cardiac monitoring, which use a user-friendly traffic light system to guide the clinician.[83] With close adherence to such guidelines, cardiac toxicity has become a very manageable toxicity.

Trastuzumab is thought to work synergistically with chemotherapy, and therefore the adjuvant trials have been in combinations with either anthracycline, anthracycline–taxane,[74,78] or docetaxel–carboplatin. It has become standard practice to give concurrent trastuzumab and taxane, whereas concurrent anthracycline–trastuzumab cycles present concerns for combined cardiac toxicity and have generally been avoided. For those with lower risk pathological staging (pT1a/bN0) single-agent paclitaxel in combination with trastuzumab is often considered to avoid the anthracycline-associated toxicity.[84,85]

In more recent years, dual anti-HER2 targeted therapy, with both adjuvant trastuzumab and pertuzumab, has become the new standard of care for HER2-positive patients in the node-positive setting. Pertuzumab is a monoclonal antibody with a complementary mechanism of action to that of trastuzumab. It inhibits HER2 heterodimerization with other HER family receptors, thus inducing cell-mediated cytotoxicity. The APHINITY trial was a prospective randomized controlled trial (RCT) of 4,805 HER2-positive patients randomized to receive either placebo or pertuzumab for 1 year in addition to the standard of care (chemotherapy and trastuzumab).[86] The addition of pertuzumab was found to be associated with a significantly higher invasive-disease free survival of 7.1% versus 8.7% in the placebo group, with the biggest effect seen in those with lymph-node involvement or hormone receptor–negative disease. The evidence for the impact on overall survival is awaiting maturity.

Trials are emerging regarding the role of neratinib, an irreversible HER1, HER2, and HER4 tyrosine kinase inhibitor in ER-positive, HER2-positive breast cancer. The ExteNET trial randomized patients to either 1 year of neratinib or placebo, commencing on the completion chemotherapy and 1 year of adjuvant trastuzumab.[87] At 5 years of follow-up, patients in the neratinib group had significantly fewer invasive disease-free survival events than those in the placebo group (116 versus 163 events; stratified hazard ratio 0.73), and the invasive disease-free survival was 90.2% in the neratinib group, and 87.7% in the placebo group. Further investigation regarding the possible role of neratinib in the adjuvant setting is awaited.

Further agents have been investigated in the adjuvant setting, but to date neither lapatinib (ALTTO trial)[88] or bevacizumab (BETH study)[89] have shown any benefit to disease-free survival.

Hormone receptor–negative, HER2-negative disease (triple-negative breast cancer, TNBC)

In the absence of any targetable hormone or HER2 receptors, chemotherapy is the only adjuvant systemic therapy available to those with TNBC. Chemotherapy should be considered for all TNBC patients but could potentially be avoided to those with pT1a (≤5 mm) following a discussion of the risks and benefits with the patient.[90]

The combination of anthracycline and taxane plus or minus a platinum agent should remain the foundation of chemotherapy regimens for TNBC.[91] The evidence for offering a platinum-based chemotherapy remains uncertain but it has been found to

TABLE 6.4   **Endocrine Therapy for ER-Positive Invasive Breast Cancer**

	Premenopausal	Postmenopausal	Men
Endocrine therapy	Tamoxifen [a] + Consider ovarian suppression [b]	Aromatase inhibitor (AI)—steroidal or non-steroidal *or* Tamoxifen (if low risk, AI not tolerated or AI contra-indicated)	Tamoxifen
Duration	≥5 years Consider extended therapy up to 10 years	Extended therapy with an AI for ≥5 years can be offered to women who have been taking tamoxifen for 2–5 years[c]	Sparsity of data for male population

[a] If tamoxifen contra-indicated, GnRH agonist + AI should be considered.

[b] If risk of recurrence high enough to consider chemotherapy, then ovarian suppression should be discussed, especially if menses return within 2 years of chemotherapy. There are also emerging data regarding role of the aromatase inhibitor, exemestane + ovarian suppression in premenopausal group (SOFT-TEXT).

[c] Patients becoming postmenopausal while on tamoxifen should then switch to an AI for 5 years.

be effective in managing TNBC, especially those with BRCA1/2 mutations.

Many TNBC patients, given the less favorable biology of their disease, will receive chemotherapy in the neo-adjuvant setting (fully described below). TNBC patients with residual invasive disease at the time of surgery following neoadjuvant chemotherapy have a higher risk of relapse. The CREATE X trial assigned patients with HER2-negative residual invasive disease following standard neoadjuvant chemotherapy to receive post-surgical adjuvant treatment with capecitabine or placebo, and reported a higher rate of overall survival of 89.2% versus 83.6% at 5 years respectively. Subset analysis of patients with TNBC revealed that the rate of disease-free survival was 69.8% in the capecitabine group, compared to 56.1% in the control group. In the ER-positive group, this difference was much less pronounced. The role of adjuvant capecitabine remains a topic of debate, and has not universally become standard practice. Other agents being appraised in the post-neoadjuvant chemotherapy setting include PARP inhibitors, CDK 4/6 inhibitors, and ado-trastuzumab emtansine, for all of which published data are anticipated. The C-TRAK trial is currently evaluating the benefit of measuring circulating DNA as a guide to instigate immunotherapy and prevent recurrence; recruitment is ongoing.[92]

Chemotherapy timing

In addition to easing patient anxiety, early commencement of adjuvant chemotherapy has a beneficial effect on clinical outcome. A retrospective review investigating the impact of time between surgery and chemotherapy and survival demonstrated 5-year survival of 89% versus 78% when comparing those who started chemotherapy between weeks 8 and 12 and those who started between weeks 12 and 24 post-surgery, with relapse survival rates of 82% and 69% respectively.[93] Endocrine treatment is usually started sequentially following chemotherapy treatment.

Adjuvant endocrine therapy

The EBCTCG meta-analyses, most recently updated in 2011, continue to provide clear evidence that adjuvant endocrine therapies significantly reduce disease recurrence and mortality in women with ER-positive early breast cancer. For women with ER-positive early breast cancer, adjuvant endocrine therapies have accordingly become the standard of care and have relatively low toxicity.

For women with ER-positive early breast cancer, adjuvant endocrine therapy is well-established as a cost-effective and relatively low-toxicity treatment that significantly reduces disease recurrence and mortality. Tamoxifen is a non-steroidal anti-estrogen, which acts by preventing estrogen binding at one of the

activating sites of the estrogen receptor and can be used in both pre- and postmenopausal women. Tamoxifen binds selectively to one of two activating domains on the estrogen receptor (AF-2). This means that some estrogenic activity remains in tissues. Thus choice of endocrine therapy depends on menopausal status and is summarized in Table 6.4.

Adjuvant tamoxifen

The 2011 EBCTCG systematic overview confirmed that in women with ER-positive disease 5 years of adjuvant tamoxifen reduce the annual breast cancer death rate by about a third throughout the first 15 years of follow-up (relative risk [RR]: 0.71 in years 0–4, 0.66 in years 5–9, and 0.68 in years 10–14).[94] These RR reductions appear to be independent of the use of chemotherapy and of patient age, nodal status, or PR status. In ER-weak disease, trials confirm that tamoxifen has no significant impact on recurrence or breast cancer mortality.[95]

Recently, the benefits, and possible adverse effects, of longer duration tamoxifen have been tested in the "adjuvant Tamoxifen Treatment offer more (aTTom)" and "Adjuvant Tamoxifen Longer against Shorter (ATLAS)" trials. Both these trials have reported that for women with ER-positive disease continuing tamoxifen for 10 years' total duration results in further reductions in both recurrence and mortality, particularly after year 10. These results, taken together with the results from previous trials, suggest that 10 years of tamoxifen treatment overall can reduce breast cancer mortality by about half during the second decade after diagnosis.[96,97] The risks and potential implications of additional years of endocrine therapy should be discussed with patients including the impact of ongoing menopausal symptoms, increased risk of thromboembolism, bone density loss, and teratogenic risk. The cumulative risk of endometrial cancer in the ALTAS study in years 5–14 was 3.1% in the group who took tamoxifen for 10 years, versus 1.6% in the 5-year group (mortality 0.4 versus 0.2%).

Adjuvant aromatase inhibitors

Aromatase inhibitors (AI), such as anastrozole, letrozole, and exemestane, block the peripheral conversion of androstenedione to estrogen via the inhibition of the aromatase enzyme and are ineffective before menopause. In postmenopausal women, the third-generation AIs suppress circulating estrogen levels by approximately 98%.[98,99]

A series of adjuvant trials with AIs including over 30,000 women have been completed and have established the place of AIs in the management of postmenopausal women with breast cancer. AIs have been explored (1) as replacement for tamoxifen,[100] (2) following 2–3 years of tamoxifen,[101] (3) following 5 years of tamoxifen,[102] and (4) as an extended therapy over 10 years. Updated results from the Arimidex or Tamoxifen Alone or in Combination (ATAC) trial,[103] Breast International Group (BIG) 1-98 Femara-Tamoxifen trial,[104] and Intergroup Exemestane Study[105] all showed a small but statistically significant improvement in relapse-free survival (and in some cases OS) for the AIs over tamoxifen when administered in the first 5 years. The MA17 trial (testing letrozole 2.5 mg daily after 5 years of tamoxifen) also reported a significantly superior DFS in favor of letrozole (and a significant OS benefit), with the consequence that this option has become standard of care for high-risk patients who have completed 5 years of adjuvant tamoxifen therapy.[102] To date, there is limited evidence of the value of extending AI therapy to 10 years. Although extended treatment reduces the rate of disease recurrence and contra-lateral breast cancer, the absolute effect is modest, and the MA.17R trial found no difference in overall survival with the additional treatment.[106] In terms of choice of agent, a recent study has reported equivalent efficacy between anastrozole and letrozole.[107]

Aromatase inhibitors are beneficial in terms of reduced risk of endometrial cancer and venous thromboembolism compared to tamoxifen. However, more recently it has become clear that the side-effect profile of AIs is also a problem for some patients (slightly increased odds of developing cardiovascular disease, bone health issues, and arthralgia) such that some authors have suggested that the optimum approach involves a switch from tamoxifen to an AI to reduce this toxicity and provide the best balance between efficacy and toxicity.[108]

Adjuvant ovarian suppression

The 2005 overview by EBCTCG evaluated almost 8,000 women below the age of 50 years with ER-positive or ER-unknown disease randomized into trials of ovarian ablation/suppression (OAS) (approximately half had chemotherapy as well).[109] In patients less than 50 years old randomized to ovarian ablation versus no other systemic treatment for ER-positive or ER-unknown disease, suppression of ovarian function achieved a 30% reduction in the annual odds of breast cancer mortality. In young women who wish to preserve fertility, the use of gonadotrophin-releasing hormone (GnRH) agonists is a reasonable, safe, and reversible alternative to surgery or radiotherapy ablation. Although, in practice, the generally accepted standard endocrine therapy is tamoxifen, OAS appears to be equally effective, and the two modalities have not been directly compared in randomized trials.

Combined adjuvant endocrine therapies

The rationale for combining endocrine therapies in younger women, who are less likely to develop permanent amenorrhea as the result of adjuvant chemotherapy, is that these women may be at higher risk of relapse compared to older, premenopausal patients with chemotherapy-induced amenorrhea.

In premenopausal women aged <35 years with high-risk ER-positive cancer, ovarian function suppression (OFS) in combination with an AI should be considered. The 2018 combined analysis of the SOFT-TEXT[110] trials reported absolute improvements in 8-year DFS of 4% in those receiving OFS plus tamoxifen/exemestane compared to tamoxifen alone. The benefit appeared greater for those that received OFS plus AI (exemestane) with a DFS of 7% compared to tamoxifen alone. Those who were <35 years of age were found to have a rate of freedom from distant recurrence at 8 years of 82.4%, 77.5%, and 73.8% in those that received OFS plus exemestane, OFS plus tamoxifen, and tamoxifen alone respectively. Overall survival data are awaiting maturity.

In contrast, in postmenopausal women adjuvant concurrent tamoxifen and anastrozole has no advantage over tamoxifen alone and is inferior to anastrozole alone,[103] the explanation for the inferiority of combined treatment being that tamoxifen acts as an estrogen agonist in the estrogen-depleted environment induced by the AI.

Adjuvant bisphosphonates

It has become standard practice to offer adjuvant bisphosphonates to postmenopausal women with node-positive or node-negative high-risk breast cancer.[111,112] Optimal choice of bisphosphonate and dosing strategy is unclear, but as there are most data for zoledronic acid or sodium clodronate, these are favored by both UK NICE and ASCO guidelines. Zoledronic acid is administered 6-monthly for 3–5 years, and clodronate given daily for 2–3 years.

Bisphosphonates impair osteoclast maturation and development, and inhibit osteoclastic bone resorption and reduce the rate of bone turnover. It is also postulated that high osteoclast activity could be associated with excess production of growth factors, which could aid the survival of micrometastases. Bisphosphonates also affect T-cell function, thus altering the tumor microenvironment. The Early Breast Cancer Trialists' Collaborative Group (EBCTCG) meta-analyses of adjuvant bisphosphonates in early breast cancer concluded that their addition reduced breast cancer recurrence in the bone and improved breast cancer survival.[113] In all women, the absolute 10-year risk was reduced by 1.4% for distant recurrence, 1.1% for bone recurrence, and 1.7% for breast cancer mortality. Greater benefit was demonstrated in postmenopausal women, with the absolute reduction in breast cancer mortality of 3.3%, 3.4% for distant recurrence, 2.2% for bone recurrence, and 2.3% for all-cause mortality. Although some deem this as modest, such reductions are comparable with those seen with the addition of taxane chemotherapy. It should be noted that associated side effects include renal impairment, osteonecrosis of the jaw, and hypocalcemia. Women should be counselled regarding the risk of osteonecrosis of the jaw (0–0.7%),[114] and adequate dental checks should be carried out prior to commencement of treatment and at intervals thereafter. Data are awaited regarding the use of denosumab in this setting.

Radiotherapy

It has long been established that BCS followed by whole-breast radiotherapy is a safe alternative to mastectomy (Figure 6.6). A meta-analysis from the EBCTCG showed that radiotherapy after BCS in pN0 disease (n = 7,287) reduced the 10-year risk of locoregional or distant first recurrence from 31.0% to 15.6% and reduced the 15-year risk of breast cancer death from 20.5% to 17.2%. Similar benefits were seen in pN+ disease (n = 1,050), where radiotherapy reduced the 10-year recurrence risk from 63.7% to 42.5% and the 15-year risk of breast cancer death from 51.3% to 42.8%.[115]

Radiotherapy scheduling

Conventionally fractionated whole-breast radiotherapy (WBRT) offers 1.8 to 2 Gy daily fractions over 5 weeks to a total dose of 45–50 Gy. Great efforts have been made to investigate hypofractionated regimens (40–42.5 Gy in 15–16 fractions) in an attempt to reduce strain on resources within radiotherapy departments

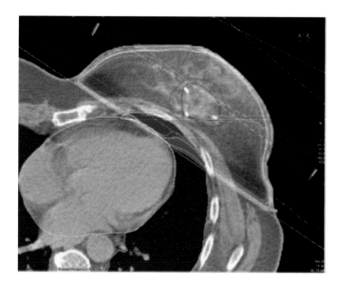

FIGURE 6.6 A typical breast radiotherapy plan using tangential wedged fields.

and improve patient experience. A recent meta-analysis confirmed no differences in breast cancer specific survival, 10-year mortality, cosmesis, or late radiation toxicity when conventional WBRT was compared to hypofractionated schedules. The 10-year follow-up from the large (n = 2,236) UK START A and START B trials demonstrated that hypofraction is safe and effective irrespective of age, grade, and nodal status.[116] The American Society of Radiation Oncology (ASTRO) now recommends hypofractionated WBRT (40–42.5 Gy in 15–16 fractions) as the new standard for WBRT.[117] The concept of extreme WBRT hypofractionation has been further investigated by the UK FAST-Forward and FAST-Forward lymphatics trials. These trials aim to prove non-inferiority when extreme WBRT hypofractionation schedules (27 Gy in 5 fractions, 26 Gy in 5 fractions) are compared to the UK 40 Gy in 15 fractions standard.[118] Both trials are closed to recruitment.

Omitting radiotherapy

In highly selected, low-risk subsets it may be reasonable to discuss the omission of WBRT following BCS. Elderly patients (aged >65 years) with ER-positive HER-negative small (<3 cm) tumors receiving a minimum of 5 years of adjuvant hormone treatment appear to have modest benefits in local control following WBRT with no survival advantage. The CALGB 9343 trial demonstrated small gains in 10-year local control (98% versus 90%) with no significant differences in survival, in those who received 5 years of adjuvant tamoxifen with or without WBRT respectively.[119] The PRIME 2 trial reported higher but small absolute rates of 5-year ipsilateral breast tumor recurrences (IBTR) (1.3% and 4.1%) with no differences in regional recurrence, distant metastases, contralateral cancers, and overall survival when adjuvant WBRT was omitted.[117] Rates of local relapse appear to occur in linear fashion over time and therefore follow-up for at least 10 years is required to salvage any IBTR that occur. If omission of radiotherapy is considered, compliance with endocrine therapy must be stressed as a critical component of treatment as anticipated relapse risk would be considerably higher. The PRIMETIME phase 3 trial is actively recruiting and investigating the selective avoidance of radiotherapy for low-risk subsets identified by immunohistochemical profiling.[120]

Tumor bed boost

A radiotherapy boost to the tumor bed following WBRT intends to optimize local control by reducing recurrence rates. The European Organization for Research and Treatment of Cancer (EORTC) recruited 5,318 women with stage 1/2 early breast cancer and randomized them to receive conventional WBRT (50 Gy in 25 fractions) with or without a boost of 16 Gy in 8 fractions delivered by electrons, photons, or iridium.[191] A median follow-up of 17.2 years demonstrated first-failure local breast recurrence rates of 9% versus 13% and salvage mastectomy rates of 79% versus 75% in favor of those who received a boost, yet no overall survival benefit was seen. The absolute benefit was greatest in young women under 40 years with local recurrences of 36% versus 24.4% reported. A later subgroup analysis was performed which demonstrated age (≤50 years), high-grade tumors, and DCIS correlated with later relapses, and in patients with all 3 features, a boost reduced 20-year local relapse from 38% to 9% (hazard ratio [HR] = 0.21, p = 0.002). When discussing the benefits of a boost with patients it is important to discuss that long-term cosmesis is less favorable as severe fibrosis occurred in 5.2% of women who received a boost and 1.8% of those who did not.[121,122] Much of the evidence has been to offer sequential treatment; however the concept of offering a simultaneous integrated boost has been addressed by the UK IMPORT HIGH and the US trials, the results of which are awaited.[123]

Partial breast irradiation

Greater understanding of the short- and long-term toxicities associated with WBRT suggests we should be investigating ways to minimize normal tissue exposure whilst maintaining the same level of tumor control. The rationale for offering partial breast irradiation (PBI) followed the observation that the majority of ipsilateral breast tumor recurrences (IBTR) occur in close proximity to the tumor bed.[124] Advances in radiotherapy techniques allow for accurate localization of surgical titanium clips, enabling more precise matching of radiotherapy target volumes.

The IMPORT LOW trial demonstrated in a low-risk subgroup of women (predominantly ≥50 years, ≤3 cm, node negative. Grade 1/2, ER-positive and HER2-negative) 40 Gy in 15 fractions PBI was non-inferior to WBRT in terms of 5-year local recurrence rates (0.5% versus 1.1% respectively). Patients reported less acute and long-term cosmetic effects following PBI with improvement in overall breast appearances (p = 0.007) and breast hardness (p = 0.002).[125] The UK Royal College of Radiologists 2016 Consensus statement has now suggested that PBI should be considered for patients meeting the above criteria.[126]

Accelerated partial breast irradiation

The concept of accelerated partial breast irradiation (ABPI) for early-stage, low-risk disease suggests that targeting the area at most risk of recurrence whilst sparing the normal adjacent tissues (heart, lung, and ipsilateral breast) allows for further hypofractionation of dose and shorter treatment time.

I) *Interstitial brachytherapy*

Interstitial brachytherapy was the first APBI technique introduced with the most mature follow-up data. It involves the geometric positioning of about 10 to 20 catheters in tissue surrounding the lumpectomy at the time of surgery or shortly after. Homogenous dose is delivered to the tumor bed with a defined margin (typically 1–2 cm) using high-dose-rate radioactive sources temporarily after-loaded. The Groupe Européen de Curiethérapie of the European Society for Radiotherapy and Oncology (GEC-ESTRO) demonstrated equivalent 5-year IBTRs when WBRT was compared to APBI with significantly fewer late skin effects in those who received the latter.

II) *Intraoperative radiation therapy*

Intraoperative radiotherapy (IORT), given peri- or post-operatively, offers a single dose of 20–21 Gy via low-energy kilovoltage (kV) X-rays or electrons. IORT does have the important advantage in that radiation is administered in a single fraction, decreasing utilization of radiation treatment units and improving patient experience. However, IORT is a resource-intensive therapy requiring specialized training and costly machines with the potential to shift the burden of treatment onto surgical waiting lists. With trial evidence awaiting maturity and concerns regarding delivery of radiation without pathological confirmation of margin or lymph node status, this is not yet regarded as standard practice.

Two large phase III prospective trials compared IORT with electrons (ELIOT) or kV (TARGIT) with WBRT.[127,128] They both reported acceptable cosmetic rates with equivalent survivals in both arms but higher rates of IBTR in the IORT groups. The ELIOT trial demonstrated 5-year IBTR of 4.4% versus 0.4% in the IORT and WBRT respectively, although those in low-risk subgroups had better outcomes.[127] The TARGIT trial has insufficient follow-up (median 2 years and 5 months), but did show encouraging 5-year IBTR rates of 3.3% versus 1.3% in the IORT and WBRT respectively.[128]

III) *External beam accelerated partial breast irradiation*

Recent technological advances in image guidance and intensity-modulated radiotherapy (IMRT) have allowed for accurate localization and delivery of PBI. Evidence to prove efficacy and acceptable toxicity as well as the optimal dose and fractionation remains to be determined.

A prospective study randomized 520 women aged $\geq$40 years with tumors measuring <2.5 cm to receive WBRT (50 Gy in 25 fractions) or ABPI (30 Gy in 5 daily fractions). They reported at 5 years comparable survival and local recurrences but significantly improved early and late cosmetic outcomes in those who received ABPI (p = 0.045). The NSABP-B39/RTOG 0413 trial and Canadian OPAR trials who also investigate WBRT versus ABPI are closed and awaiting publication.[129]

Concern has been raised regarding the optimal dose and timing of ABPI following the RAPID trial which randomized women to received WBRT (42.5–50 Gy in 16–25 fractions) with ABPI (38.5 Gy in 10 fractions twice daily). They reported on significantly worse grade 1–2 cosmesis at 3 years in those who received ABPI (29% versus 16.5%) with telangiectasia and breast induration significantly worse in the experimental arm. The authors suggest that a 6-hour treatment time interval was not sufficient to allow for normal tissue repair.[130]

Post-mastectomy radiotherapy

It is recommended that patients with higher risks of local recurrence (T3–4, $\geq$4 positive lymph nodes, and excision margin <1 mm) should be offered post-mastectomy radiotherapy (PMRT). The recent EBCTCG meta-analysis investigated outcomes following PMRT in node-negative, node-positive (1–3), and $\geq$4 lymph node-positive. The meta-analysis showed no benefit to PMRT in the node-negative setting. They did, however, demonstrate significant improvements in both local recurrences (10-year gain 10.6%) and breast cancer mortality (20-year gain 8.1%) in those with 1–3 node-positive lymph nodes.[131] It is now recommended that PMRT should be offered to all node-positive patients.

Axillary radiotherapy

For patients presenting with T1/2 tumors (i.e. <5 cm) and positive macrometastatic ($\geq$2 mm) sentinel lymph nodes following BCS or mastectomy, axillary radiotherapy would be an acceptable alternative to axillary lymph node dissection (ALND). Axillary radiotherapy (typically levels 1–3) has the obvious advantage of sparing the patient from a second surgery but is also associated with lower rates of lymphedema (5-year 11% versus 23%). The AMAROS trial, conducted by the EORTC, randomized 4,806 patients with unifocal disease meeting the above criteria to ALND or axillary radiotherapy. They reported equivalent and low rate of axillary recurrences with no significant differences in disease-free and overall survivals at 5 and 10 years.[62]

Regional nodal irradiation

Regional nodal radiotherapy (RNI) typically refers to the supra- and infraclavicular plus/minus internal mammary lymph node regions, and should be considered in patients deemed at higher risk of locoregional relapse. There is consensus that RNI should be offered to those with $\geq$4 macrometastatic axillary lymph nodes but controversy remains for those with 1–3 nodes involved. This follows the MA20 and EORTC trials which both demonstrated reduced recurrence rates associated with RNI.[132,133] The MA20 trial randomized 1,800 women (90% with any node-positive disease, 85% of whom with 1–3 lymph node) to received RNI+WBI or WBI alone. They demonstrated improvements in 10-year disease-free survival (77 versus 82% HR0.76) but not overall survival.[132] The similarly designed EORTC trial randomized 4,000 women (43% of whom had 1–3 nodes positive) to receive RNI (including medial supraclavicular fossa and internal mammary) or not following WBI. With a median follow-up of 10.9 months, the arms that received RNI demonstrated significantly improved breast cancer mortality rates (12.5% versus 14.4%; HR0.82) with a trend towards OS (82.3% versus 80.7% HR 0.87) and improved DFS (72% versus 69%).[133] It is important to note that RNI was associated with higher degrees of toxicity (pneumonitis and lymphedema) and therefore should be reserved for those in whom the absolute benefit is expected to be greater than the associated risk.

The UK Royal College of Radiologists 2016 Consensus Statement suggests that internal mammary irradiation (IMNI) should be offered in T4 and/or $\geq$4 axillary lymph node macrometastases or any node-positive with central or medial disease. This statement follows a Danish prospective population-based cohort study of 3,090 patients who treated right-sided early-stage node-positive breast cancer patients with IMNI and left-sided not and demonstrated 3.7% 8-year survival benefit. The difference, however, was more pronounced in those with central/medial disease and or $\geq$4 positive lymph nodes with 8-year survivals of 72.2% versus 64.8% with or without IMNI respectively.[134]

Radiotherapy following neoadjuvant chemotherapy

There is no clear consensus on the most appropriate adjuvant radiotherapy techniques required following neoadjuvant chemotherapy (NACT). With some older data suggesting that NACT can be associated with higher rates of local recurrence,[135] there is a reluctance to down-grade radiotherapy based on pathological response or molecular subgroup. In the absence of prospective data to guide our approach, it is recommended to offer post-operative WBRT following BCS regardless of response to treatment. For post-mastectomy patients, chest wall radiotherapy is reserved for those with positive residual nodal disease or stage III disease regardless of response. In patients who present with stage III cancer or who have residual node-positive disease following NACT, it is recommended to offer regional nodal radiation. This recommendation follows evidence to suggest greater than 10% risk of locoregional recurrence in those with persistently positive nodes following NACT.[136]

Radiotherapy for ductal carcinoma in situ

Radiotherapy for DCIS following BCS significantly reduces the odds of in-breast recurrence (both invasive and non-invasive), but it does not appear to affect odds of distant recurrence or mortality. The decision to offer WBRT following BCS for DCIS should be discussed with the patient, and made on a balance of risks versus benefits. The Van Nuys Prognostic Index suggests a management strategy based on a score representing low, intermediate, and high risks of recurrence.[137] It is recommended that those scoring ≥7 should be offered adjuvant WBRT following BCS.

A meta-analysis in 2009 demonstrated the IBTR benefit of radiotherapy (hazard ratio [HR], 0.49) following BCS. All subgroups analyzed (margin status, age, and grade) benefited from the addition of radiotherapy which translated into a number needed to treat of nine women to prevent one IBTR.[138] In patients having low-risk disease (small, low grade, and large margin >10 mm), there is the potential to omit the radiotherapy, although there is a lack of randomized prospective data.

Radiotherapy toxicities

Whole-breast radiotherapy can be associated with some short- and long-term toxicities. The acute side effects typically involve the treated area (skin and muscle) as well as fatigue. The incidence of acute skin dermatitis can be reduced by using modern techniques such as IMRT and a careful skin care routine.[139]

As survival rates improve we become increasingly aware of the importance of long-term side effects associated with WBRT. Women may notice cosmetic differences with changes in breast appearance, color, shape, and size. Offering a tumor bed boost is associated with a greater degree of fibrosis and poorer cosmetic outcomes. Other important long-term sequelae are lymphedema, cardiac risk, pneumonitis, brachial plexopathies, rib fractures, and second malignancies.

Lymphoedema can be a disabling condition of the arm caused by disruption of the lymphatic system either by surgery, disease, or radiotherapy. Axillary radiotherapy is generally reserved for those with a positive sentinel node or those with remaining macroscopic disease. The AMAROS study suggested 11% 5-year lymphedema rates following axillary radiotherapy with the estimated risk significantly higher when given following axillary surgery.[62] The association with cardiac risk and WBRT was well-described by a population-based case-control study who demonstrated the rates of major coronary events increased linearly with the mean cardiac dose received. They reported an increase of 7.4% over a patient's cardiac risk per gray mean cardiac dose received. The increase started within the first 5 years after radiotherapy and continued into the third decade after radiotherapy.[140] It is important to remember that this study used historical data and older radiotherapy techniques, prior to the use of IMRT and deep inspiratory breath hold scans. Nevertheless it is important to

measure the mean cardiac dose to ensure it is within acceptable tolerance levels and to discuss the anticipated risks, particularly in those at most risk of cardiac disease. Radiation pneumonitis can present with cough, dyspnea, and a low-grade fever and is typically self-limiting requiring a short course of steroids. The risk of developing pneumonitis is related to the volume and dose of lung irradiated so it is important to measure ipsilateral lung dose and respect tolerance limits carefully. Brachial plexopathy did occur with older radiotherapy techniques where matching of nodal fields was frequently done poorly, resulting in significant overlap and overdosing of the plexus. At its most severe this would result in permanent loss of ipsilateral arm function and pain which is now thankfully rare given the newer techniques. Other potential toxicities, although very rare, include rib fractures, pericarditis, and secondary malignancies. There are data to suggest that there is an increase in relative risk of developing secondary malignancies such as lung and esophageal cancer; the absolute risk remains small but should be considered when weighing up the risks and benefits of offering WBRT.[141]

Locally advanced disease

Neoadjuvant chemotherapy

Alternating the sequence of treatments via the use of neoadjuvant chemotherapy is usually considered in patients who have large, locally advanced, or inflammatory breast cancer. Initiating chemotherapy prior to surgery may downstage tumors, initially considered to be inoperable, or may allow the consideration of BCS rather than mastectomy for tumors too large to consider this approach at presentation. It is also postulated to be more effective at managing micrometastatic disease than in the adjuvant setting. Where chemotherapy is initiated in the neoadjuvant setting, present guidance advises that all chemotherapy should be administered pre-operatively (rather than further chemotherapy being given in the post-operative setting).[19] In summary, a neoadjuvant approach may be considered in the following circumstances:

- Tumor >2 cm, with biology that would necessitate chemotherapy
- Locally advanced or large tumor where mastectomy would otherwise be required
- Stage II or III HER2+ or TNBC, particularly where response may de-escalate surgical approach

Prior to neoadjuvant chemotherapy, tumor burden should be accurately assessed with MRI or ultrasound, and histological assessment including ER/PR and HER2 status must be available. All patients undergoing neoadjuvant endocrine or chemotherapy, where there is an intention for breast conservation, should have a radiological marker clip inserted and be reassessed during and at the end of neoadjuvant treatment.

Historically it has been difficult to compare the efficacy of neoadjuvant and adjuvant chemotherapy due to differences in most trials in the approach to breast-conserving surgery after tumor shrinkage. A 2018 meta-analysis of ten trials conducted by the EBCTCG aimed to minimize these confounding factors and compare data. They compared the same chemotherapy in the pre- and post-operative setting and reported a 15-year local recurrence rate of 21.4% versus 15.9% respectively with no significant differences in distant recurrence rate or breast cancer mortality. It should be noted that the results were from an era before anti-HER2 therapy, and there were differences between studies with regards to adjuvant radiotherapy and axillary managements.[142]

Regarding optimal chemotherapy regimen choice, multiple studies, including the NSABP B27 trial, have supported the addition of a taxane to an anthracycline-containing regimen, with improvements in both clinical response and pCR, although with no difference in OS or DFS.[143] The NeoSphere study was practice-changing for those with HER2-positive disease, in which dual anti-HER2 therapy with pertuzumab and trastuzumab in combination with docetaxel was found to result in a 45.8% pCR rate compared to 29% with trastuzumab and docetaxel alone. A subgroup analysis of those with ER-negative tumors found an even higher pCR of 63.2%.[144] These results were supported by the 5-year analysis in 2016, and suggested an association with pCR and longer progression-free survival (PFS) (85% at 5 years' pCR versus 76% without pCR).[145] As such, neoadjuvant chemotherapy with dual anti-HER2 therapy has become standard practice for HER2-positive patients requiring neo-adjuvant treatment in the UK.[146]

The addition of a platinum in addition to anthracycline-containing regimens has been found to be beneficial for those with TNBC in the neoadjuvant setting, with pCR rates as high as 60% when carboplatin was added to a regime containing taxane, anthracycline, and cyclophosphamide.[147–149] Further data are awaited with regards to possible additional efficacy in the BRCA1/2 mutated groups.

In the case of residual disease following neoadjuvant chemotherapy (i.e. no pCR), the risk of recurrence is higher, and clinical trials are evaluating post-neoadjuvant therapy with a variety of agents in this setting (as described earlier).

Neoadjuvant endocrine therapy

For postmenopausal women with ER-positive breast cancer, neoadjuvant endocrine treatment has been proposed as an appropriate approach after its established efficacy in the adjuvant setting and the increasing recognition that chemotherapy may be less effective in ER-positive HER2-negative disease. In the past, neoadjuvant endocrine therapy was only given to older and frail patients with ER-positive breast cancer. However, recent studies of this therapy in fit postmenopausal women showed that improved surgical outcomes and clinical response with upfront endocrine therapy were not age-related.[87] This area of research was ignited by the use of AIs rather than tamoxifen in this group of women. For example, the letrozole P024 trial randomized 337 postmenopausal women with ER-positive and/or PR-positive primary untreated breast cancer to once-daily letrozole (2.5 mg) or tamoxifen (20 mg) for 4 months prior to surgery.[88] At baseline, none of the patients were considered to be a candidate for BCS. The overall objective response rate (ORR) (clinical palpation) was statistically significantly superior in the letrozole group, 55% versus 36%. Secondary end points of ultrasound response (35% versus 25%), mammographic response (34% versus 16%), and BCS (45% versus 35%) all favored the AI. Regression analysis demonstrated that patients receiving letrozole were more than twice as likely to achieve a clinical response as patients receiving tamoxifen (odds ratio [OR], 2.23). These findings have been confirmed in several further studies, and current research centers on the use of predictive markers of benefit in this setting (e.g. Ki67, molecular signatures) and using this approach as a test bed for new signal-pathway inhibitors. In the United Kingdom, the Perioperative Endocrine Therapy for Individualizing Care (POETIC) trial has successfully completed

randomizing over 4,000 ER-positive early breast cancer patients to 2 weeks of pre-surgical treatment with a non-steroidal AI or no pre-surgical treatment. This study is the largest of its kind and provides a unique opportunity for in-depth analysis of the determinants of tumor response and resistance to estrogen deprivation, as well as testing the role of pre-surgical therapy for improved biomarker-based (surrogate) estimates of prognosis. It is currently in the follow-up phase and results are eagerly awaited.

Locoregional recurrence

Breast cancer can recur locoregionally in the treated breast, the chest wall (Figure 6.7), and the axilla. It affects a small percentage of patients overall, more commonly with a more advanced stage at presentation or if adjuvant treatments were not given. It may be the first symptom of secondary breast cancer relapse; but in the absence of any distant disease, aggressive management with the aim of cure is appropriate. This would include surgery if operable, radiotherapy if involving an untreated area, and further adjuvant hormone therapy if the disease is hormone receptor–positive. The risk of later secondary relapse is high, and the CALOR[150] pre-publication results suggest a significant benefit for adjuvant chemotherapy following surgical resection of recurrent disease, which is hormone receptor–negative.

Secondary breast cancer

Secondary breast cancers are often defined as synchronous, i.e. presenting with metastatic disease at initial diagnosis, or metachronous, i.e. distant disease following previous radical treatment. Although the natural history is quite heterogeneous, it is almost always incurable. The proportion of those treated for early breast cancer who later develop secondary disease may be as high as 20–30%, with 6–10% of women presenting with synchronous disease.[151] Treatment is increasingly based on a better understanding of the underlying biology of the different molecular subgroups, although good multidisciplinary care allowing tailored monitoring of disease, control of symptoms, and support to maintain quality of life is crucial. Median overall survival for all secondary breast cancer patients is now exceeding 2 years,[3] although this does range significantly depending on molecular

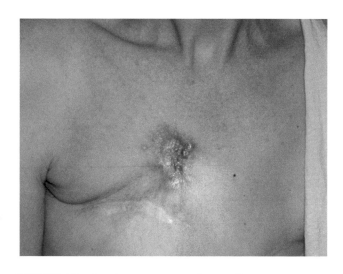

FIGURE 6.7 Local recurrence on chest wall.

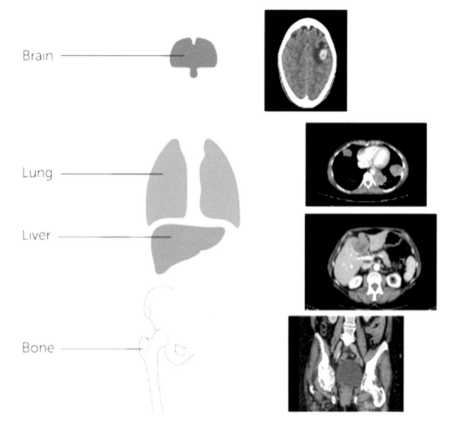

FIGURE 6.8 Typical metastatic sites and computed tomography appearance. (Courtesy of the patient information website of Cancer Research UK, London, UK, http://www.cancerresearchuk.org/cancerhelp.)

subgroups. An observational cohort study of French patients with metastatic breast cancer found the overall survival (OS) of the whole cohort to be 37.22 months. OS was 42.12 months in the hormone receptor (ER)–positive/HER2-negative cohort and 44.9 months in the ER-positive/HER2-positive cohort. Survival was much shorter in the triple-negative cohort, with an OS of 14.52 months.[152]

As treatment choices in the metastatic setting depend on immunohistochemical profiling, it is important that accessible metastatic sites are biopsied as changes can occur between primary and secondary disease. Data suggest that the discordance in receptor status can be as much as 30% for ER (most commonly positive to negative) and 5% (negative to positive) for HER2[153] resulting in significant alterations in subsequent treatments.

Although the patterns of secondary relapse between patients cover a very wide spectrum (Figure 6.8), some common patterns are discernible:

- The skeleton is very commonly involved and can be the only site of disease.
- Liver, lung, and cerebral metastases tend to be multiple.
- Multiple adjacent nodal sites of involvement are common.
- Pleural involvement is usually ipsilateral to the involved breast.
- Involvement of the serosal peritoneum and other abdominopelvic sites is typical of lobular cancer metastasis.

Table 6.5 lists the key disease- and patient-related factors in treatment decision-making for secondary breast cancer.[154]

TABLE 6.5 Factors to Consider When Making Treatment Decisions in Secondary Breast Cancer

Disease-Related Factors	Patient-Related Factors
Disease-free interval	Patient preferences
Previous therapies and response	Biological age
Biological factors (HR, HER2)	Menopausal status
Tumor burden (number and site of metastases)	Co-morbidities and performance status
Need for rapid disease/symptom control	Socio-economic and psychological factors
	Available therapies in the patient's country

Source: Cardoso et al., 2012. With permission.

Hormonal and targeted therapy in the metastatic setting

Patients with ER-positive metastatic breast cancer often show excellent response rates to endocrine therapy alone (response rate 32–38%),[154] or to endocrine therapies in combination with other targeted agents. With the exception of patients presenting with a high burden of visceral metastases in either impending or established crisis, endocrine treatment alone or in combination with a cyclin D kinase (CDK) 4/6 inhibitor for postmenopausal patients is often the first line treatment of choice. The choice of endocrine agent depends on the menopausal status of the patient, prior treatment history, and HER2 status.

Hormone receptor–positive, HER2-negative breast cancer in postmenopausal women

For postmenopausal women with ER-positive/HER2-negative metastatic breast cancer, the first-line options include aromatase inhibitors (AIs), tamoxifen, or AIs in combination with CDK4/6 inhibitors. AIs are the preferred first-line endocrine agents as they have shown a survival advantage compared to tamoxifen. A meta-analysis of 23 randomized trials (n = 8,504 patients) comparing the efficacy of AIs as the first-line treatment for postmenopausal women with advanced breast cancer has shown that treatment with an AI resulted in an improvement in OS compared to tamoxifen (HR, 0.89) and other endocrine therapies (HR, 0.87).[155] Data regarding the choice of AIs suggest that AIs are comparable in efficacy, with exemestane and anastrozole treatment resulting in a similar ORR (15% in both groups) and OS (31 and 33 months, respectively).[156] Tamoxifen should be considered as first line in patients with osteoporosis and increased fracture risk and also in patients who do not tolerate AIs due to toxicities.

Seminal trials on the use of CDK4/6 inhibitors in combination with endocrine therapy are changing the landscape of treatment for hormone receptor–positive, HER2-negative advanced breast cancers. Both the PALOMA and MONALEESA trials have studied the addition of CDK4/6 inhibitors to AIs in the first-line metastatic setting and have shown significant improvements in PFS of 10.3 months and 9.3 months respectively when compared to AIs alone.[157,158] This will be discussed in more detail later in this chapter.

The options in the second line include:

- Steroidal AI (exemestane) use after a non-steroidal AI (letrozole/anastrozole) and vice versa
- Tamoxifen or fulvestrant alone or in combination with abemaciclib or ribociclib
- Endocrine therapy plus the mammalian target of rapamycin (mTOR) inhibitor everolimus

It appears as though there is little difference in efficacy between the AIs in the second-line setting.[159] A systematic review of nine studies to evaluate the use of steroidal AIs (exemestane) in the second-line setting after treatment failure with non-steroidal AI (anastrozole or letrozole) has reported a clinical benefit rate for exemestane use that ranged from 12% to 55% and an overall response rate that ranged from 2% to 26%.[160] Fulvestrant is the only endocrine therapy that works by downregulating estrogen receptors, whereas AIs' mechanism of action is to deplete estrogen. Previous studies comparing fulvestrant and AIs failed to show any significant differences in their ORR or OS.[161,162] It appears, however, that the effect of fulvestrant is dose-dependent as these previous studies administered a dose of 250 mg monthly (which is lower than that used in clinical practice). More recently the FALCON trial did demonstrate an improved PFS with fulvestrant prescribed at 500 mg monthly compared with anastrozole (HR, 0.8, 95% CI 0.637 to 0.999).[163] Fulvestrant has also been studied in combination with the CDK4/6 inhibitor abemaciclib within the MONARCH 2 trial in patients who have progressed on endocrine therapy. It has shown an improved PFS of 16.4 months versus 9.3 months when compared to endocrine therapy alone.[164]

Resistance (de novo or acquired) to endocrine therapies in hormone receptor–positive breast cancer eventually results in relapse, and one of the emerging mechanisms of resistance is aberrant activation of the mTOR intracellular signaling pathway, which can be explored as a potential target to overcome this resistance. The BOLERO-2 trial, combining exemestane with everolimus, improved PFS in patients with hormone receptor–positive advanced breast cancer previously treated with non-steroidal AIs.[165] The 724 women were randomly assigned to exemestane (25 mg daily) plus placebo or exemestane plus everolimus (10 mg daily) treatment. An ORR (9.5% versus 0.4%) and a PFS (median, 6.9 versus 2.8 months; HR for mortality, 0.43, 95%CI, 0.35 to 0.54) were observed relative to those in the placebo-controlled group. Everolimus was, however, associated with grade 3/4 side effects, including stomatitis, 8%; dyspnea, 4%; elevated liver enzymes, 3%; and pneumonitis, 3%. The trial concluded that everolimus combined with an AI is an option in patients with hormone receptor–positive advanced breast cancer previously treated with non-steroidal AIs. However, the risks of significant toxicities must be taken into account.

Following progression on two or more lines of endocrine therapy in the postmenopausal setting, the choice of later lines of treatment is very much dependent on patient choice, wellbeing, disease burden, and rate of progression. For patients who chose, or are only suitable for endocrine monotherapy, tamoxifen could be considered but it must be recognized that the expected response rates are low. In a combined analysis of two randomized trials the ORR of tamoxifen following the AI anastrozole was shown to be 10% with a clinical response rate, defined as ORR plus 6 months of stable disease, of 49%.[166] Another alternative option includes the use of progestin. Studies have reported response rates of around 25% and median duration of response of 15 months for progestational agents (megestrol acetate and medroxyprogesterone acetate) in metastatic breast cancer, but these were mainly studied in patients who progressed on tamoxifen, and no data are available for its activity after the use of an AI.[167]

PIK3CA mutations have been found in over 40% of estrogen receptor-positive breast cancers.[168] PIK3CA encodes the alpha catalytic subunit of PI3K which is a component of phosphoinositide 3-kinase/protein kinase B/mechanistic target of rapamycin (PI3K/AKT/mTOR) signaling pathway, a pathway with a central role in cell growth, survival, and angiogenesis. Mutations in PIK3CA have been identified as a potential mechanism for endocrine resistance in estrogen receptor-positive breast cancers. Alpelisib is a PI3K inhibitor which has recently been studied in combination with fulvestrant in patients with advanced hormone receptor–positive breast cancers who have received prior treatment with an AI either in the adjuvant or advanced setting. This phase III, randomized study of 572 patients revealed that patients with an identified PIK3CA mutation had a PFS of 11.0 months in the alpelisib plus fulvestrant group compared with 5.7 months in the fulvestrant plus placebo group (HR for progression or death, 0.65; 95%CI, 0.50 to 0.85; p < 0.001). In the cohort without a PIK3CA mutation the hazard ratio was 0.85 (95%CI, 0.58 to 1.25).[169] No trial data yet exist on whether the combined use of PIK3CA inhibitors with CDK4/6 inhibitors and AIs would have a synergistic anti-tumor effect.

Premenopausal women

The options for ER-positive/HER2-negative metastatic breast cancer patients who are premenopausal include tamoxifen, ovarian suppression or ablation, or AI plus ovarian suppression. Ovarian ablation involves a bilateral surgical oophorectomy, whereas ovarian suppression is achieved with a GnRH analogue. In premenopausal women, meta-analysis of four studies has shown that the activity of tamoxifen is similar to ovarian ablation with no significant differences in the risk of disease progression (OR, 0.86) or the risk of death (OR, 0.94).[170] In another meta-analysis that compared a GnRH agonist plus tamoxifen to a GnRH agonist alone, the PFS (HR, 0.70) and OS (HR, 0.78) were significantly improved with the combined therapy.[171] A trial of premenopausal women who were treated with letrozole plus goserelin (for ovarian suppression) suggests that the administration of a GnRH agonist plus an AI may be effective in premenopausal women, with similar time to progression among premenopausal and postmenopausal women (9.5 versus 9 months, respectively).[172] It is therefore unclear at present whether combined treatment is superior to ovarian suppression alone or not, and treatment decisions are often made on individual case-by-case basis.

Ovarian suppression or ablation can be used in order to permit premenopausal women to embark on analogous treatment strategies as those pursued by their postmenopausal counterparts. Adopting the approach of ovarian suppression combined with AI in premenopausal women therefore allows access to the CDK4/6 inhibitors which are associated with significant improvements in PFS compared to endocrine treatment alone. None of the first-line CDK4/6 studies looked at the activity of these agents in premenopausal women in the absence of ovarian suppression; however a subgroup analysis of premenopausal women receiving ovarian suppression within the PALOMA-3 trial showed that they derived a similar benefit from CDK4/6 inhibitor plus AI combination as the overall study population.[157]

Targeted therapy in the metastatic setting

BOLERO-2 was the first of many studies to explore the potential of combining new therapeutic targets with endocrine therapy to overcome endocrine resistance. Since then, many trials have continued to focus on the combination of targeted agents and AIs. The most promising of these trials have focused on targeting the CDK4/6 pathway which has been found to be overactive in breast cancers. Consistent benefits are being observed with CDK4/6 inhibitors in combination with AIs or fulvestrant in both the front-line and subsequent-line setting which are now changing the paradigm of treatment in advanced breast cancers.

PALOMA-2, a phase III double-blind, randomized study of 666 postmenopausal women with hormone receptor–positive, HER2-negative advanced breast cancer comparing palbociclib and letrozole against letrozole alone revealed a median PFS of 24.8 months versus 14.5 months (HR for disease progression or death, 0.58, 95%CI, 0.46 to 0.72, p < 0.001) and an objective response rate (ORR; 42% versus 35%).[157] Similarly the phase III MONALEESA–2 study compared the use of the CDK4/6 inhibitor ribociclib used in addition to letrozole with letrozole alone in the first-line setting. Median PFS was found to be 25.3 months versus 16.0 months (HR, 0.586, 95% CI, 0.457 to 0.704) in favor of combined therapy.[158] Abemaciclib, another CDK4/6 inhibitor, is now FDA-approved in combination with an AI for postmenopausal women in the first-line metastatic setting following results of the MONARCH 3 trial. PFS was significantly increased in the abemaciclib arm (HR 0.54; 95% CI, 0.42 to 0.72, p < 0.000021) as median PFS was not reached, compared to 14.7 months in the AI plus placebo arm.[173] The most notable toxicities seen with these agents across all studies appear to be neutropenia, leukopenia, and elevated liver enzymes.

The use of CDK4/6 inhibitors in combination with endocrine therapy has also been assessed in the "subsequent line" setting. MONALEESA 3 compared ribociclib plus fulvestrant versus fulvestrant alone and included patients who were either treatment-naïve or had progressed after one line of endocrine therapy in the advanced setting. It revealed a consistent favorable treatment effect in both the treatment-naïve and previously treated groups with (HR 0.557; 95%CI, 0.415 to 0.812) and (HR 0.565; 95%CI, 0.428 to 0.744)

respectively.[173] A further two trials looking at the CDK4/6 inhibitors palbociclib and abemaciclib in combination with fulvestrant have also reported similarly positive impacts on PFS. Both trials included patients who had progressed whilst on, or within 12 months of discontinuing adjuvant endocrine therapy, or who had progressed whilst receiving first-line endocrine therapy in the advanced setting. PALOMA 3 which combined palbociclib with fulvestrant reported a median PFS of 9.5 months (95% CI 9.2–11.0) in the fulvestrant plus palbociclib group and 4.6 months (3.5–5.6) in the fulvestrant plus placebo group (hazard ratio 0.46, 95% CI 0.36–0.59, p < 0.0001).[174] MONARCH 2, a global, multicenter, phase III study of 669 women comparing the abemaciclib and fulvestrant combination with fulvestrant alone in patients who had received prior endocrine therapy showed a median PFS of 16.4 months versus 9.3 months (HR 0.553; 95%CI, 0.449–0.681, p < 0.001).[164]

HER2-directed therapy in the metastatic setting

HER2 is overexpressed in approximately 20% of breast cancers. The use of agents targeted against the HER2 receptor have significantly improved the prognosis of patients who have HER2-positive breast cancers, and therefore are recommended for use in the first-line setting.

Targeted agents currently available for the treatment of HER2-positive breast cancers include the monoclonal antibodies trastuzumab and pertuzumab; a small-molecule tyrosine kinase inhibitor, lapatinib; and an antibody–cytotoxic drug conjugate of trastuzumab and a microtubule inhibitor DM1 named ado-trastuzumab-emtansine (Kadcyla).

HER2-directed therapy should be the primary component of therapy in patients with HER2-positive disease irrespective of their hormone receptor status. In patients with hormone receptor–positive disease, endocrine therapy can be combined with HER2-directed therapy plus chemotherapy in the first line, or is more typically used sequentially following completion of chemotherapy cycles. In most cases, it is usual for HER2 therapy to be given in conjunction with chemotherapy. Endocrine monotherapy is not recommended for hormone receptor–positive and HER2-positive disease. The TANDEM study randomly assigned 207 postmenopausal patients to treatment with the combination of anastrozole plus trastuzumab or anastrozole alone.[175] Anastrozole plus trastuzumab therapy showed a significant improvement in PFS (median, 5 months versus 2 months) but no significant improvement in OS (28.5 months versus 23.9 months) compared to single-agent anastrozole. HER2-directed therapy in combination with an AI is therefore certainly an option for patients who are unsuitable for treatment with chemotherapy.

Data derived from the phase III CLEOPATRA trial strongly support the use of a triple-agent regimen with trastuzumab, pertuzumab, and taxane chemotherapy combined. This study included patients who had received HER2-directed therapy in the adjuvant setting as well as those who were naïve to directed therapy. The 808 women were all treated with trastuzumab and docetaxel, and were also randomly assigned to receive additional treatment with either pertuzumab or placebo. The addition of pertuzumab resulted in an overall response rate (ORR) 80% versus 69%, with an improved median PFS of 19 versus 12 months (HR 0.62, 95% CI, 0.51 to 0.75) and OS (median, 56.5 versus 40.8 months; HR 0.68; 95%CI, 0.56 to 0.84).[175] The trial used up to six cycles of docetaxel, and HER2-directed therapy or placebo was continued until disease progression or unacceptable toxicities were encountered. For

TABLE 6.6　Chemotherapy for Secondary Breast Cancer

	Regimens	Common Schedule	Route
Single agents			
Anthracycline	Epirubicin, Doxorubicin	3-weekly or weekly	IV bolus
Taxane	Docetaxel Paclitaxel Nab-paclitaxel	3-weekly Weekly 3-weekly or weekly	IV infusion
Fluoropyrimidine	Capectiabine	Days 1–14 every 3 weeks	Oral
Vinca alkaloid	Vinorelbine	Days 1, 8 every 3 weeks	Oral or IV bolus
Novel	Eribulin	Days 1, 8 every 3 weeks	IV bolus
Combinations			
	FEC: 5-FU, epirubicin, cyclophospahmide	3-weekly	IV bolus
	Gemcitabine, paclitaxel	Days 1, 8 every 3 weeks	IV infusion
	Docetaxel, capecitabine	3-weekly	IV infusion and oral

patients who have previously received HER2-directed therapy in the adjuvant setting it is recommended that first-line treatment in the metastatic setting should be with trastuzumab, taxane, and pertuzumab provided that there has been six months or more of a treatment-free interval since completion of adjuvant therapy, and that the patient remains clinically suitable for triple therapy. The chemotherapy partner used in CLEOPATRA and many other first-line trials is docetaxel, though other taxanes, vinorelbine,[176] and capecitabine[177] are all effective (Table 6.6).

Should there be less than a 6-month treatment-free interval after completion of HER2-directed therapy in the adjuvant setting or progression after first-line treatment in the advanced setting it is reasonable to consider the use of ado-trastuzumab-emtansine (Kadcyla) as a second-line therapy. Its role was evaluated in the phase III MARIANNE study; 1095 patients who had not previously received treatment in the advanced setting were randomly assigned to one of three treatment arms which included trastuzumab plus taxane, Kadcyla plus placebo, and pertuzumab plus Kadcyla. Kadcyla showed non-inferiority, but not superiority to the other two arms in the first line setting.[178] It has also shown significant activity in patients pre-treated with HER2-targeting therapy within the EMILIA and TH3RESA studies and as such is now commonly used in the second-line setting. Both studies found significant improvements in PFS within the Kadcyla arms with hazard ratios of 0.65 and 0.52 respectively.[179,180]

Lapatinib is a small-molecule tyrosine kinase inhibitor directed against the HER2 and EGFR pathways. Its clinical effectiveness has been studied in combination with capecitabine in patients who have progressed on trastuzumab. Initial results of a phase III trial of 399 women who received either lapatinib and capecitabine in combination or capecitabine alone did reveal an improved time to progression and a trend towards improved OS; however there was no statistically significant difference in median OS (67.7 weeks for lapatinib plus capecitabine versus 66.6 weeks for capecitabine monotherapy [HR 0.78; 95% CI 0.55 to 1.12, $p = 0.177$]).[180] In the UK, NICE guidance does not recommend the combination of lapatinib and capecitabine.

Chemotherapy

Despite the lack of direct evidence from clinical trials for improvements in OS compared to best supportive care, it is widely recognized that advanced breast cancer can be very sensitive to cytotoxic chemotherapy, and some regimens have been shown to have superior survival over comparator therapy.[180]

Single-agent therapies are generally recommended due to lower toxicity, though combination therapies are associated with higher response rates and are useful if a rapid response is required. Table 6.6 shows established agents and combinations. Anthracyclines, taxanes, and capecitabine are particularly effective (with few trials comparing treatments or sequences/strategies), and many patients will be fit for multiple lines of therapy, so the real art is making the best choice with the individual at each stage. Where there is evidence of clinical benefit, courses of 18–24 weeks are standard, though treatment to progression is feasible for some agents, particularly capecitabine. There is no high-level evidence that the latter improves overall outcome.

Eribulin, a non-taxane microtubule dynamics inhibitor, is now an option for patients who have progressed after at least two previous lines of chemotherapy, which include an anthracycline or a taxane, and capecitabine. It was studied within the EMBRACE trial ($n = 762$), comparing its impact on OS with treatment of the physician's choice. A significant and clinically meaningful improvement in OS, 13.1 versus 10.6 months, was shown, which challenged the notion that an improved OS with additional lines of therapy is an unrealistic expectation in patients with heavily pre-treated disease.[181]

Metastatic triple-negative breast cancer

Tumors with poor or no hormone sensitivity, nor HER2 receptor overexpression, carry a relatively poor prognosis, with a median survival of approximately 12–15 months in the metastatic setting.[182] Further sub-classifications based on molecular biology show promise for discovery of targeting intracellular pathways, but current treatment is based on cytotoxic chemotherapy. Responses can be profound but not usually sustained, and there are by nature no treatments available to allow maintenance of response.

Recent developments have, however, been made with the use of immunotherapy in patients whose tumors express the programmed cell death ligand (PDL-1) at a level of greater than 1%. IMpassion 130 compared the use of nab-paclitaxel chemotherapy either with the immunotherapy atezolizumab or a placebo. Overall, there was only a modest improvement in PFS from 7.2 months to 5.5 months (HR, 0.8; 95%CI, 0.69 to 0.92) and no statistically significant improvement in the OS. However, in a subset analysis of patients with PDL-1 positive tumors improved PFS and OS were observed; OS (21.3 months versus 15.5 months; HR 0.62, 95%CI 0.45–0.86).[183] Further studies are underway to determine the benefit of immunotherapies in this setting either used alone or in combination with other systemic therapies or radiation.

BRCA1-deficient tumors have an RNA expression profile and basal cytokeratin expression phenotype similar to triple-negative tumors of the basal-like group and are thought to be particularly sensitive to the DNA adducts induced by platinum due to BRCA-dependent DNA repair defects. Consequently, platinum agents are widely used in triple-negative disease as a whole and are being studied. The UK TNT trial compared docetaxel with carboplatin first line, but failed to demonstrate a statistically significant OS benefit in all-comers. A benefit in PFS was seen in the BRCA1/2 mutant population however.[184]

Inhibitors of poly ADP-ribose polymerase (PARP inhibitors) such as olaparib and talazoparib have certainly shown clinical benefits within the BRCA1/2 mutant population[185,186] and continue to hold promise as treatments for the wider group of triple-negative cancers, but in early trials their benefits seem to be limited to BRCA-deficient cancers. Talazoparib was studied within the phase III EMRACA trial, comparing the PARP inhibitor against single-agent capecitabine, vinorelbine, eribulin, or gemcitabine in the metastatic setting. An improved PFS relative to chemotherapy (8.6 months versus 5.6 months, HR 0.64, 95%CI 0.41–0.71) was concluded in addition to reported improvements in quality of life as well as improved tolerance of the drug in the talazoparib arm.[186]

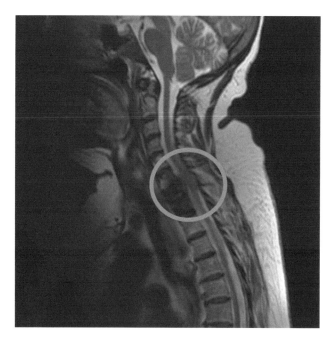

FIGURE 6.9 Magnetic resonance image showing spinal cord compression.

Complications of metastatic breast cancer

Bone metastases

Bone is the most common site of metastases, and approximately 70% of patients dying from metastatic breast cancer have evidence of bone metastases at post-mortem analysis.[187] Skeletal complications from bony metastases also referred to as skeletal-related events (SREs) are responsible for major morbidity and include hypercalcemia, pathologic fracture, spinal cord compression (Figure 6.9), and the need for radiotherapy treatment or surgery to bone. Bone metastases are the common cause of cancer-related pain affecting the patient's quality of life, but bone pain is not included in the definition of SREs and is instead measured as a separate outcome in clinical trials. Management options for bone metastases include systemic therapies (chemotherapy, endocrine therapy, and targeted therapies), local therapies (radiotherapy and surgery), and bone-targeting agents (osteoclast inhibition) that reduce SREs such as denosumab and bisphosphonates.

Bisphosphonates interfere with tumor-mediated lysis by inhibiting osteoclast recruitment and function. In women with breast cancer who have clinically evident bony metastases, data from clinical trials and meta-analysis have established that the use of bisphosphonates (oral or intravenous) reduces the frequency of SREs by approximately one-third compared with no bisphosphonate therapy or placebo.[188–191] A Cochrane review to assess the effect of bisphosphonates and other bone agents on SREs has concluded that bisphosphonates reduced the SRE risk in patients with bony metastatic disease by 14% compared with placebo or no bisphosphonates.[192] Treatment with bisphosphonates also resulted in delays in median time to SREs and improvement in bone pain and global quality of life. However, bisphosphonate treatment did not appear to affect survival in women with breast cancer bony metastases. The optimal timing of the initiation of bisphosphonate therapy and the duration of treatment are uncertain. International practice guideline groups have not expressed

a preference on which bone-directed agent should be chosen, though in the case of bisphosphonates there is a general trend to use zoledronic acid intravenous infusion on a monthly basis. The UK NCRI phase III trial (ZICE) comparing intravenous zoledronic acid treatment with oral ibandronate in metastatic breast cancer patients with bone metastases has concluded that oral ibandronate is inferior to zoledronic acid in terms of the SRE rate, but both were similar in delaying time to first SRE.[193] Toxicities of bisphosphonates include renal toxicity and osteonecrosis of the jaw (ONJ). ONJ can cause significant morbidity and distress to a cancer patient and, therefore, every effort should be made to avoid it. Dental surveillance and good oral care are essential in its prevention.

Denosumab is a monoclonal antibody-targeting receptor activator of nuclear factor κB ligand (RANKL), a key component in the pathway for osteoclast formation and activation. Osteoclast inhibition can also be achieved by targeting RANKL with denosumab, which has shown efficacy in the treatment of postmenopausal osteoporosis and in patients with breast cancer who are at risk for cancer therapy-induced bone loss. In patients with bone metastases from breast cancer, denosumab has demonstrated efficacy in delaying the time to first SRE compared with zoledronic acid.[194] In the above-mentioned Cochrane review denosumab reduced the risk of developing SREs compared with bisphosphonates by 22%.[192] In the United Kingdom, NICE has recommended the use of denosumab as an option for preventing SREs in breast cancer patients with bony metastases.[195] The lack of renal monitoring requirement and the convenience of subcutaneous injection with denosumab make it a potential treatment option for breast cancer patients with bony metastases.

Radiotherapy is a very effective treatment for breast cancer patients with painful skeletal metastases. Patients have at least a 65% chance of worthwhile pain relief, with complete response in about 20%, as judged by self-assessment questionnaires. No clear evidence for a dose response has emerged for the short-term relief of bone pain. The long-term effectiveness of a single fraction of 8 Gy compared to multi-fraction schedules has been established using patient self-assessments for 12 months in 761 patients with uncomplicated metastatic bone pain, more than half with breast cancer.[196]

Pathological fracture of a long bone is a complication that should be prevented as often as possible by periodic review of femoral radiographs in patients with known skeletal disease. It is difficult to predict pathological fracture, but erosion of more than half the cortical thickness is an indication for an orthopedic opinion concerning prophylactic surgical fixation or pinning. There is no randomized evidence related to the contribution of post-surgical radiotherapy, or the optimal dose, but 20 Gy in 5 fractions is commonly prescribed.

Other significant complications of metastatic disease include spinal cord compression, hypercalcemia, pleural effusions, and brain and meningeal metastasis. The management of these complications requires a good multidisciplinary approach involving an oncologist, surgeons, and palliative care teams.

Oligometastatic breast cancer

Patients presenting with oligometastatic breast cancers may benefit from stereotactic radiotherapy (SABR). The phase II SABR-COMET ($n = 99$) trial compared SABR with standard of care treatments in patients with oligometastatic cancers (visceral as well as bony metastatic disease).[197] It revealed promising results with an improved median OS (41 months versus 28 months; hazard ratio 0.57, 95% CI 0.30–1.10; $p = 0.090$) in the SABR group, though a further phase III trial is required to show conclusive OS benefits. A further study in which 48 women with breast cancer oligometastatic disease received SABR to their radiologically apparent sites of disease concluded that of those treated, benefits were more profound in the bone-only cohort. Five- and 10-year OS were reported as 83% and 75% respectively after SABR to bony disease, suggesting that patients presenting with bone-only oligometastatic breast cancer could expect to survive longer than 10 years.[198]

Acknowledgments

We would like to thank Dr Aisling Butler (Consultant Radiologist at Velindre Cancer Centre) for her contribution and expertise. We thank Thomas Rackley, Sharath Gangadhara, Elin Evans, Simon Waters, and Peter Barrett-Lee, the authors of the previous edition, whose chapter we have adapted and modified. We also thank Miss Dai Nguyen (Consultant Plastic Surgeon at Morriston Hospital, Swansea, Wales) for providing the high-quality breast reconstruction photos.

References

1. Ferlay J, Soerjomataram I, Dikshit R et al. Cancer incidence and mortality worldwide: Sources, methods and major patterns in GLOBOCAN 2012. Int J Cancer. 2015; 136(5):E359–86. doi:10.1002/ijc.29210

2. Bray F, Ferlay J, Soerjomataram I. Global cancer statistics 2018: GLOBOCAN estimates of incidence and mortality worldwide for 36 cancers in 185 countries. CA Cancer J Clin. 2018; 68(6):394–424.

3. Jemal A, Bray F, Center MM, Ferlay J et al. Global cancer statistics. [Erratum appears in CA Cancer J Clin. 2011; 61(2):134]. CA Cancer J Clin. 2011.

4. Parkin DM, Bray F, Ferlay J et al. Global cancer statistics, 2002. CA Cancer J Clin. 2005; 55(2):74–108. doi:10.3322/canjclin.55.2.74

5. UK CR. No title. https://www.cancerresearchuk.org/health-profe ssional/cancer-statistics/statistics-by-cancer-type/breast-cancer #heading-Zero. Accessed August 8, 2019.

6. UK CR. No title. https://www.cancerresearchuk.org/health-profe ssional/cancer-statistics/statistics-by-cancer-type/breast-cancer/ risk-factors#ref1. Accessed August 8, 2019.

7. UK CR. Breast cancer survival by stage at diagnosis. https://ww w.cancerresearchuk.org/health-professional/cancer-statistics/stat istics-by-cancer-type/breast-cancer/survival#heading-Three.

8. Sonnenschein C, Soto AM. Theories of carcinogenesis: An emerging perspective. Semin Cancer Biol. 2008; 18(5): 372–377). Academic Press. doi:10.1016/j.semcancer.2008.03.012

9. Hanahan D, Weinberg RA. Hallmarks of cancer: The next generation. Cell. 2011; 144(5):646–74. doi:10.1016/j.cell.2011.02.013

10. CHEK2-Breast Cancer Consortium. Low-penetrance susceptibility to breast cancer due to CHEK2* 1100delC in noncarriers of BRCA1 or BRCA2 mutations. Nature Genetics. 2002; 31(1):55.

11. Slamon DJ, Leyland-Jones B, Shak S et al. Use of chemotherapy plus a monoclonal antibody against her2 for metastatic breast cancer that overexpresses HER2. N Engl J Med. 2001; 344(11):783–92. doi:10.1056/NEJM200103153441101

12. O'Donovan PJ, Livingston DM. BRCA1 and BRCA2: Breast/ovarian cancer susceptibility gene products and participants in DNA double-strand break repair. Carcinogenesis. 2010; 31(6):961–7.

13. Chen S, Parmigiani G. Meta-analysis of BRCA1 and BRCA2 penetrance. J Clin Oncol. 2007; 25(11):1329. doi:10.1200/JCO.2006.09.1066

14. Venkitaraman AR. Cancer susceptibility and the functions of BRCA1 and BRCA2. Cell. 2002;108(2):171–82. doi:10.1016/S0092-8674(02)00615-3

15. Lakhani SR. In-situ lobular neoplasia: Time for an awakening. Lancet. 2003; 361(9352):96. doi:10.1016/S0140-6736(03)12240-4

16. Simpson PT, Reis-Filho JS, Gale T, Lakhani SR. Molecular evolution of breast cancer. J Pathol. 2005; 205(2):248–54. doi:10.1002/path.1691

17. Sørlie T, Perou CM, Tibshirani R et al. Gene expression patterns of breast carcinomas distinguish tumor subclasses with clinical implications. Proc Natl Acad Sci U S A. 2001; 98(19):10869–74doi:10.1073/pnas.191367098

18. Sabatier R, Finetti P, Mamessier E et al. Prognostic and predictive value of PDL1 expression in breast cancer. Oncotarget. 2015; 6(7):5449. doi:10.18632/oncotarget.3216

19. Cardoso F, Kyriakides S, Ohno S et al. Early breast cancer: ESMO clinical practice guidelines for diagnosis, treatment and follow-up. Ann Oncol. 2019; 30(8):1194–220.

20. Li CI, Uribe DJ, Daling JR. Clinical characteristics of different histologic types of breast cancer. Br J Cancer. 2005; 93(9):1046–52. doi:10.1038/sj.bjc.6602787

21. Silverstein MJ. The University of Southern California/Van Nuys prognostic index for ductal carcinoma in situ of the breast. Am J Surg. 2003 2003; 186(4):337–43. doi:10.1016/S0002-9610(03)00265-4

22. Copson E, Shaaban A, Maishman T et al. The presentation, management and outcome of inflammatory breast cancer cases in the UK: Data from a multi-centre retrospective review. Breast. 2018; 42:133–41.

23. Lim HS, Yoon W, Chung TW et al. FDG PET/CT for the detection and evaluation of breast diseases: Usefulness and limitations. RadioGraphics. 2007; 27(suppl_1):S197–213. doi:10.1148/rg.27si075507

24. Hortobagyi GN, Connolly JL, D'Orsi CJ et al. AJCC Cancer Staging Manual. 8th Edition. 2017. doi:10.1007/978-3-319-40618-3_48

25. Giuliano AE, Edge SB, Hortobagyi GN. Eighth edition of the AJCC cancer staging manual: breast cancer. Ann Surg Oncol. 2018; 25(7):1783–85.

26. Marmot MG, Altman DG, Cameron DA et al. The benefits and harms of breast cancer screening: An independent review. Br J Cancer. 2013; 108(11):2205–40.

27. Lauby-Secretan B, Scoccianti C, Loomis D et al. Breast-cancer screening—Viewpoint of the IARC working group. N Engl J Med. 2015; 372(24):2353–8. doi:10.1056/nejmsr1504363. https://www.rcr.ac.uk/system/files/publication/field_publication_files/bfco2016_breast-consensus-guidelines.pdf

28. Moss SM, Wale C, Smith R et al. Effect of mammographic screening from age 40 years on breast cancer mortality in the UK Age

trial at 17 years' follow-up: A randomised controlled trial. *Lancet Oncol.* 2015; 16(9):1123–32. doi:10.1016/S1470-2045(15)00128-X

29. Tyne K, Nygren P. Screening for breast cancer: Systematic evidence review Update for the U.S. Preventive services task force. *Science (80-).* 2009; 151(10):727–W242. doi:10.1059/0003-4819-151-10-200911170-00009.Screening

30. ClinicalTrials.gov. Bethesda (MD): National Library of Medicine (US). 2000 Feb 29. Identifier NCT01081288, Extending the National Health Service (NHS) Breast Screening Age Range (AgeX); 2010 Mar 5 [cited 2019 Aug 12]. Available from: https://clinicaltrials.gov/ct2/show/NCT01081288.

31. Pisano ED, Hendrick RE, Yaffe MJ et al. Diagnostic accuracy of digital versus film mammography: Exploratory analysis of selected population subgroups in DMIST. *Radiology.* 2008; 246(2):376–83. doi:10.1148/radiol.2461070200

32. Gilbert FJ, Tucker L, Gillan MGC et al. The TOMMY trial: A comparison of TOMosynthesis with digital mammography in the UK NHS breast screening programme—A multicentre retrospective reading study comparing the diagnostic performance of digital breast tomosynthesis and digital mammography with digital mammography alone. *Health Technol Assess (Rockv).* 2015; 19(4):1–166. doi:10.3310/hta19040

33. Vourtsis A, Berg WA. Breast density implications and supplemental screening. *Eur Radiol.* 2019; 29(4):1762–77.

34. Vasen HFA, Haites NE, Evans DGR et al. Current policies for surveillance and management in women at risk of breast and ovarian cancer: A survey among 16 European Family Cancer Clinics. *Eur J Cancer.* 1998; 34(12):1922–6. doi:10.1016/S0959-8049(98)00288-3

35. Ford D, Easton DF, Stratton M et al. Genetic heterogeneity and penetrance analysis of the BRCA1 and BRCA2 genes in breast cancer families. *Am J Hum Genet.* 1998; 62(3):676–89.

36. Beral V, Bull D, Doll R et al. Familial breast cancer: Collaborative reanalysis of individual data from 52 epidemiological studies including 58 209 women with breast cancer and 101 986 women without the disease. *Lancet.* 2001; 358(9291):1389–99. doi:10.1016/S0140-6736(01)06524-2

37. Phi XA, Houssami N, Hooning MJ et al. Accuracy of screening women at familial risk of breast cancer without a known gene mutation: Individual patient data meta-analysis. *Eur J Cancer.* 2017; 85(May):31–8. doi:10.1016/j.ejca.2017.07.055

38. Leach MO. Screening with magnetic resonance imaging and mammography of a UK population at high familial risk of breast cancer: A prospective multicentre cohort study (MARIBS). *Lancet.* 2005; 365(9473):1769–78. doi:10.1016/S0140-6736(05)66481-1

39. Warner E, Messersmith H, Causer P et al. Systematic review: Using magnetic resonance imaging to screen women at high risk for breast cancer. *Ann Intern Med.* 2008; 148(9):671–9. doi:10.7326/0003-4819-148-9-200805060-00007

40. Saadatmand S, Geuzinge HA, Rutgers EJT et al. MRI versus mammography for breast cancer screening in women with familial risk (FaMRIsc): a multicentre, randomised, controlled trial. *Lancet.* 2019; 20(8):1136–47. doi:10.1016/S1470-2045(19)30275-X

41. Senkus E, Kyriakides S, Ohno S et al. Primary breast cancer: ESMO clinical practice guidelines for diagnosis, treatment and follow-up. *Ann Oncol Off J Eur Soc Med Oncol.* 2015; 26 Suppl 5(Supplement 5):v8–30. doi:10.1093/annonc/mdv298

42. Hopwood P. Genetic risk counselling for breast cancer families. *Eur J Cancer.* 1998; 34:1477–79.

43. Nelson HD, Smith MEB, Griffin JC, Fu R. Use of medications to reduce risk for primary breast cancer: A systematic review for the U.S. preventive services task force. *Ann Intern Med.* 2013; 158(8):604–14. doi:10.7326/0003-4819-158-8-201304160-00005

44. Cuzick J, Sestak I, Cawthorn S et al. Tamoxifen for prevention of breast cancer: Extended long-term follow-up of the IBIS-I breast cancer prevention trial. *Lancet Oncol.* 2015; 16(1):67–75. doi:10.1016/S1470-2045(14)71171-4

45. Goss PE, Ingle JN, Alés-Martínez JE et al. Exemestane for breast-cancer prevention in postmenopausal women. *N Engl J Med.* 2011; 364:2381–91.

46. Cuzick J, Sestak I, Forbes JF et al. Anastrozole for prevention of breast cancer in high-risk postmenopausal women

(IBIS-II): An international, double-blind, randomised placebo-controlled trial. *Lancet.* 2014; 383(9922):1041–48. doi:10.1016/S0140-6736(13)62292-8

47. Thorat MA, Cuzick J. Europe PMC funders group preventing invasive breast cancer using endocrine therapy. 2018; 34(Suppl 1):1–17. doi:10.1016/j.breast.2017.06.027.Preventing

48. Mastectomy or lumpectomy? The choice of operation for clinical stages I and II breast cancer. The Steering Committee on Clinical Practice Guidelines for the Care and Treatment of Breast Cancer. Canadian Association of Radiation Oncologists. *CMAJ.* 1998; 158(3):S15–S21.

49. Wo J, Taghian A. Radiotherapy in setting of collagen vascular disease. *Int J Radiat Oncol Biol Phys.* 2007; 69(5):1347–53. doi:10.1016/j.ijrobp.2007.07.2357

50. Berry MG, Gomez KF. Surgical techniques in breast cancer: An overview. *Surg (United Kingdom).* 2013; 31(1):32–6. doi:10.1016/j.mpsur.2012.10.013

51. Kearney TJ, Morrow M. Effect of reexcision on the success of breast-conserving surgery. *Ann Surg Oncol.* 1995 Jul 1;2(4):303-7. doi:10.1007/BF02307061

52. Law TT, Kwong A. Surgical margins in breast conservation therapy: How much should we excise? *South Med J.* 2009; 102(12):1234–7. doi:10.1097/SMJ.0b013e3181bfd420

53. Miles RC, Gullerud RE, Lohse CM et al. Local recurrence after breast-conserving surgery: Multivariable analysis of risk factors and the impact of young age. *Ann Surg Oncol.* 201; 19(4):1153–9. doi:10.1245/s10434-011-2084-6

54. Fitoussi AD, Berry MG, Famà F et al. Oncoplastic breast surgery for cancer: Analysis of 540 consecutive cases. *Plast Reconstr Surg.* 2010; 125(2):454–62. doi:10.1097/PRS.0b013e3181c82d3e

55. Yarnold J. Early and locally advanced breast cancer: Diagnosis and treatment national institute for health and clinical excellence guideline 2009. *Clin Oncol.* 2009; 21(3):159–60.doi:10.1016/j.clon.2008.12.008

56. Jeevan R, Cromwell D, Browne J et al. National mastectomy and breast reconstruction audit. *NHS Inf* Cent. 2011.

57. Alderman AK, Kuhn LE, Lowery JC, Wilkins EG. Does patient satisfaction with breast reconstruction change over time? Two-year results of the Michigan breast reconstruction outcomes study. *J Am Coll Surg.* 2007; 204(1):7–12. doi:10.1016/j.jamcollsurg.2006.09.022

58. Afolabi OO, Lalonde DH, Williams JG. Breast reconstruction and radiation therapy: A Canadian perspective. *Can J Plast Surg.* 2012; 20(1):43–6. doi:10.1177/229255031202000106

59. Mansel RE, Fallowfield L, Kissin M et al. Randomized multicenter trial of sentinel node biopsy versus standard axillary treatment in operable breast cancer: The ALMANAC trial. *J Natl Cancer Inst.* 2006; 98(9):599–609. doi:10.1093/jnci/djj158

60. Galimberti V, Cole BF, Viale G et al. Axillary dissection versus no axillary dissection in patients with breast cancer and sentinel-node micrometastases (IBCSG 23–01): 10-year follow-up of a randomised, controlled, phase 3 trial. *Lancet.* 2018; 19(October):1385–93. doi:10.1016/S1470-2045(18)30380-2

61. Giuliano AE, Ballman KV, McCall L et al. Effect of axillary dissection vs. no axillary dissection on 10-year overall survival among women with invasive breast cancer and sentinel node metastasis: The ACOSOG Z0011 (Alliance) randomized clinical trial. *JAMA—J Am Med Assoc.* 2017; 318(10):918–26. doi:10.1001/jama.2017.11470

62. Donker M, van Tienhoven G, Straver ME et al. Radiotherapy or surgery of the axilla after a positive sentinel node in breast cancer (EORTC 10981–22023 AMAROS): A randomised, multicentre, open-label, phase 3 non-inferiority trial. *Lancet Oncol.* 2014; 15(12):1303–10. doi:10.1016/S1470-2045(14)70460-7

63. Gandhi A, Coles C, Makris A et al. Axillary surgery following neoadjuvant chemotherapy—Multidisciplinary guidance from the Association of Breast Surgery, Faculty of Clinical Oncology of the Royal College of Radiologists, UK Breast Cancer Group, National Coordinating Committee for Breast. *Clin Oncol.* 2019; 31(9):664–8. doi:10.1016/j.clon.2019.05.021

64. Todd JH, Dowle C, Williams MR et al. Confirmation of a prognostic index in primary breast cancer. *Br J Cancer.* 1987; 56(4):489–92. doi:10.1038/bjc.1987.230

65. PREDICT. https://breast.predict.nhs.uk/.
66. National Institute for Health and Care Excellence N. Tumour profiling tests to guide adjuvant chemotherapy decisions in early breast. December 2018. https://www.nice.org.uk/guidance/dg34/resources/tumour-profiling-tests-to-guide-adjuvant-chemotherapy-decisions-in-early-breast-cancer-pdf-1053750722245.
67. Paik S, Shak S, Tang G et al. A multigene assay to predict recurrence of tamoxifen-treated, node-negative breast cancer. *N Engl J Med.* 2004; 351:2817–26.
68. Mamounas EP, Tang G, Fisher B et al. Association between the 21-gene recurrence score assay and risk of locoregional recurrence in node-negative, estrogen receptor-positive breast cancer: Results from NSABP B-14 and NSABP B-20. *J Clin Oncol.* 2010; 28(10):1677. doi:10.1200/JCO.2009.23.7610
69. Sparano JA, Gray RJ, Makower DF et al. Adjuvant chemotherapy guided by a 21-gene expression assay in breast cancer. *N Engl J Med.* 2018; 379(2):111–21. doi:10.1056/NEJMoa1804710
70. Andre F, Ismaila N, Henry NL et al. Use of biomarkers to guide decisions on adjuvant systemic therapy for women with early-stage invasive breast cancer: ASCO clinical practice guideline update—Integration of results from TAILORx. *J Clin Oncol.* 2019; 37(22):1956–64. doi:10.1200/jco.19.00945
71. Stein RC, Dunn JA, Bartlett JMS et al. OPTIMA prelim: A randomised feasibility study of personalised care in the treatment of women with early breast cancer. *Health Technol Assess (Rockv).* 2016; 20(10):201. doi:10.3310/hta20100
72. Tamoxifen citrate, letrozole, anastrozole, or exemestane with or without chemotherapy in treating patients with invasive RxPONDER breast cancer. https://clinicaltrials.gov/ct2/show/NCT01272037.
73. National Institue for Health and Care Excellence (NICE). Early and locally advanced breast cancer: diagnosis and management. [NG101] Published July 2018.
74. Palmieri C, Jones A. The 2011 EBCTCG polychemotherapy overview. *Lancet.* 2012; 379(9814):390–92. doi:10.1016/S0140-6736(11)61823-0
75. Albain K, Anderson S, Arriagada R et al. Comparisons between different polychemotherapy regimens for early breast cancer: Meta-analyses of long-term outcome among 100 000 women in 123 randomised trials. *Lancet.* 2012; 379(9814):432–44. doi:10.1016/S0140-6736(11)61625-5
76. Ellis P, Barrett-Lee P, Johnson L et al. Sequential docetaxel as adjuvant chemotherapy for early breast cancer (TACT): an open-label, phase III, randomised controlled trial. *Lancet.* 2009; 373(9676):1681–92. doi:10.1016/S0140-6736(09)60740-6
77. Gray R, Bradley R, Braybrooke J et al. Abstract GS1-01: Increasing the dose density of adjuvant chemotherapy by shortening intervals between courses or by sequential drug administration significantly reduces both disease recurrence and breast cancer mortality: An EBCTCG meta-analysis of 21,000 women in 16 randomized trials. In *Cancer Research* 2018; 78:4. Amer Assoc Cancer Research. doi:10.1158/1538-7445.sabcs17-gs1-01
78. Romond EH, Perez EA, Bryant J et al. Trastuzumab plus adjuvant chemotherapy for operable HER2-positive breast cancer. *New England Journal of Medicine.* 2005; 353(16):1673–84.
79. Goldhirsch A, Gelber RD, Piccart-Gebhart MJ et al. 2 years versus 1 year of adjuvant trastuzumab for HER2-positive breast cancer (HERA): an open-label, randomised controlled trial. *The Lancet.* 2013; 382(9897):1021–28. doi:10.1016/S0140-6736(13)61094-6.
80. Slamon D, Eiermann W, Robert N et al. Adjuvant trastuzumab in HER2 positive breast cancer. *NEJM.* 2011; 365(14):1273–83.
81. Moja L, Tagliabue L, Balduzzi S et al. Trastuzumab containing regimens for early breast cancer Cochrane database of systematic reviews. 2012; (4). doi:10.1002/14651858.CD006243.pub2.www.cochranelibrary.com
82. Earl HM, Hiller L, Vallier A et al. 6 versus 12 months of adjuvant trastuzumab for HER2-positive early breast cancer (PERSEPHONE): 4-year disease-free survival results of a randomised phase 3 non-inferiority trial. *The Lancet.* 2019 Jun 29;393(10191):2599-612. doi:10.1016/S0140-6736(19)30650-6.
83. Jones AL, Barlow M, Barrett-Lee PJ et al. Management of cardiac health in trastuzumab-treated patients with breast cancer: updated United Kingdom National Cancer Research Institute recommendations for monitoring. *Br J Cancer.* 2009; 100(5):684–92. doi:10.1038/sj.bjc.6604909
84. Tolaney SM, Barry W, Dang CT. Adjuvant paclitaxel and trastuzumab for node-negative, HER2-positive breast cancer. *N Engl J Med.* 2015; 372:134–41. doi:10.1056/NEJMoa1406281
85. Joerger M, Thürlimann B, Huober J. Small HER2-positive, node-negative breast cancer: who should receive systemic adjuvant treatment? *Annals of Oncology.* 2011; 22(1):17–23. doi:10.1093/annonc/mdq304
86. von Minckwitz G, Procter M, de Azambuja E et al. Adjuvant pertuzumab and trastuzumab in early HER2-positive breast cancer. *N Engl J Med.* 2017; 377(2):122–31. doi:10.1056/nejmoa1703643
87. Martin M, Holmes FA, Ejlertsen B et al. Neratinib after trastuzumab-based adjuvant therapy in HER2-positive breast cancer (ExteNET): 5-year analysis of a randomised, double-blind, placebo-controlled, phase 3 trial. *The Lancet Oncology.* 2017; 18(12):1688–700. doi:10.1016/S1470-2045(17)30717-9
88. Piccart-Gebhart M, Holmes E, Azambuja E De et al. Adjuvant lapatinib and trastuzumab for early human epidermal growth factor receptor 2—positive breast cancer: Results from the randomized phase III adjuvant Lapatinib and/or Trastuzumab treatment optimization trial. *J Clin Oncol.* 2019; 34(10):1034–42. doi:10.1200/JCO.2015.62.1797
89. Slamon D, Swain S, Buyse M. Abstract S1–03: Primary results from BETH, a phase 3 controlled study of adjuvant chemotherapy and trastuzumab ± bevacizumab in patients with HER2-positive, node-positive or high risk node-negative breast cancer. Abstracts: Thirty-Sixth Annual CTRC-AACR San Antonio Breast Cancer Symposium. https://cancerres.aacrjournals.org/content/73/24_Supplement/S1-03#. Published 2013. Accessed September 20, 2008.
90. Curigliano G, Burstein HJ, Winer EP et al. De-escalating and escalating treatments for early-stage breast cancer: The St. Gallen International Expert Consensus conference on the primary therapy of early breast cancer 2017. *Ann Oncol.* 2017; 28(8):1700–12. doi:10.1093/annonc/mdx308
91. Blum JL, Flynn PJ, Yothers G et al. Anthracyclines in early breast Cancer: The ABC trials—USOR 06–090, NSABP B-46-I/USOR 07132, and NSABP B-49 (NRG Oncology). *J Clin Oncol.* 2017; 35(23):2647–55. doi:10.1200/JCO.2016.71.4147
92. ClinicalTrials.gov [Internet]. Bethesda (MD): National Library of Medicine (US). 2000 Feb 29. Identifier NCT03145961, A trial using ctDNA blood tests to detect cancer cells after standard treatment to trigger additional treatment in early stage triple negative breast cancer patients (c-TRAK-TN); 2017 May 9 [cited 2019 Sep 20]; [10 pages]. Available from: https://clinicaltrials.gov/ct2/show/NCT03145961.
93. Lohrisch C, Paltiel C, Gelmon K et al. Impact on survival of time from definitive surgery to initiation of adjuvant chemotherapy for early-stage breast cancer. *J Clin Oncol.* 2006; 24(30):4888–94. doi:10.1200/JCO.2005.01.6089
94. Abe O, Abe R, Enomoto K et al. Relevance of breast cancer hormone receptors and other factors to the efficacy of adjuvant tamoxifen: Patient-level meta-analysis of randomised trials. *Lancet.* 2011; 378(9793):771–84. doi:10.1016/S0140-6736(11)60993-8
95. Abe O, Abe R, Enomoto K et al. Tamoxifen for early breast cancer: An overview of the randomised trials. *Lancet.* 1998; 351(9114):1451–67. doi:10.1016/S0140-6736(97)11423-4
96. Gray RG, Rea D, Handley K et al. aTTom: Long-term effects of continuing adjuvant tamoxifen to 10 years versus stopping at 5 years in 6,953 women with early breast cancer. *J Clin Oncol.* 2013; 31(18S):5. doi:10.1200/jco.2013.31.18_suppl.5
97. Davies C, Pan H, Godwin J et al. Long-term effects of continuing adjuvant tamoxifen to 10 years versus stopping at 5 years after diagnosis of oestrogen receptor-positive breast cancer: ATLAS, a randomised trial. *Lancet.* 2013; 381(9869):805–16. doi:10.1016/S0140-6736(12)61963-1

98. Demers LM. Effects of fadrozole (CGS 16949A) and Letrozole (CGS 20267) on the inhibition of aromatase activity in breast cancer patients. *Breast Cancer Res Treat.* 1994; 30(1):95–102. doi:10.1007/BF00682744

99. Geisler J, King N, Anker G et al. In vivo inhibition of aromatization by exemestane, a novel irreversible aromatase inhibitor, in postmenopausal breast cancer patients. *Clin Cancer Res.* 1998; 4(9):2089–93.

100. Cianfrocca ME, Gradishar WJ. Results of the ATAC (arimidex, tamoxifen, alone or in combination) trial after completion of 5 years' adjuvant treatment for breast cancer. *Breast Dis.* 2006; 17(2):188. doi:10.1016/S1043-321X(06)80466-2

101. Coombes RC, Hall E, Gibson LJ et al. A randomized trial of exemestane after two to three years of tamoxifen therapy in postmenopausal women with primary breast cancer. *N Engl J Med.* 2004; 350(11):1081–92. doi:10.1056/NEJMoa040331

102. Goss PE, Ingle JN, Martino S et al. Randomized trial of letrozole following tamoxifen as extended adjuvant therapy in receptor-positive breast cancer: Updated findings from NCIC CTG MA.17. *J Natl Cancer Inst.* 2005; 97(17):1262–71. doi:10.1093/jnci/dji250

103. Cuzick J, Sestak I, Baum M et al. Effect of anastrozole and tamoxifen as adjuvant treatment for early-stage breast cancer: 10-year analysis of the ATAC trial. *Lancet Oncol.* 2010; 11(12):1135–41. doi:10.1016/S1470-2045(10)70257-6

104. Coates AS, Keshaviah A, Thürlimann B et al. Five years of letrozole compared with tamoxifen as initial adjuvant therapy for postmenopausal women with endocrine-responsive early breast cancer: Update of study BIG 1–98. *J Clin Oncol.* 2007; 25(5):486–92. doi:10.1200/JCO.2006.08.8617

105. Bliss JM, Kilburn LS, Coleman RE et al. Disease-related outcomes with long-term follow-up: An updated analysis of the intergroup exemestane study. *J Clin Oncol.* 2012; 30(7):709–17. doi:10.1200/JCO.2010.33.7899

106. Goss PE, Ingle JN, Pritchard KI et al. Extending aromatase-inhibitor adjuvant therapy to 10 years. *N Engl J Med.* 2016; 375(3):209–19. doi:10.1056/NEJMoa1604700

107. Smith I, Yardley D, Burris H et al. Comparative efficacy and safety of adjuvant letrozole versus anastrozole in postmenopausal patients with hormone receptor-positive, node-positive early breast cancer: Final results of the randomized phase III femara versus anastrozole clinical evaluation. *J Clin Oncol.* 2017; 35(10):1041–48. doi:10.1200/JCO.2016.69.2871

108. Amir E, Seruga B, Niraula S et al. Toxicity of adjuvant endocrine therapy in postmenopausal breast cancer patients: A systematic review and meta-analysis. *J Natl Cancer Inst.* 2011; 103(17):1299–309. doi:10.1093/jnci/djr242

109. Clarke M, Collins R, Davies C et al. Ovarian ablation in early breast cancer: Overview of the randomised trials. *The Lancet.* 1996; 348(9036):1189–96. doi:10.1016/S0140-6736(96)05023-4

110. Francis PA, Pagani O, Fleming GF et al. Tailoring adjuvant endocrine therapy for premenopausal breast cancer. *N Eng J Med.* 2018; 379(2):122–37.

111. NICE Advice. Early breast cancer (preventing recurrence and improving survival): *adjuvant Bisphosphonates.* 2017:1–44. nice.org.uk/guidance/es15.

112. Dhesy-Thind S, Fletcher GG, Blanchette PS et al. Use of adjuvant bisphosphonates and other bone-modifying agents in breast cancer: A Cancer Care Ontario and American Society of Clinical Oncology clinical practice guideline. *J Clin Oncol.* 2017; 35(18):2062–81. doi:10.1200/JCO.2016.70.7257

113. Coleman R, Gray R, Powles T et al. Adjuvant bisphosphonate treatment in early breast cancer: Meta-analyses of individual patient data from randomised trials. *Lancet.* 2015; 386(10001):1353–61. doi:10.1016/S0140-6736(15)60908-4

114. O'Carrigan B, Wong MH, Willson ML, Stockler MR, Pavlakis N, Goodwin A. Bisphosphonates and other bone agents for breast cancer. Cochrane database of systematic reviews. 2017(10). doi:10.1002/14651858.CD003474.pub3.www.cochranelibrary.com

115. Early Breast Cancer Trialists' Collaboration Group. Effect of radiotherapy after breast-conserving surgery on 10-year recurrence and 15-year breast cancer death: Meta-analysis of individual patient data for 10 801 women in 17 randomised trials. *Lancet.* 2011; 378(9804):1707–16. doi:10.1016/S0140-6736(11)61629-2

116. Haviland JS, Owen JR, Dewar JA et al. The UK Standardisation of Breast Radiotherapy (START) trials of radiotherapy hypofractionation for treatment of early breast cancer: 10-year follow-up results of two randomised controlled trials. *Lancet Oncol.* 2013; 14(11):1086–1094. doi:10.1016/S1470-2045(13)70386-3

117. Kunkler IH, Williams LJ, Jack WJL et al. Breast-conserving surgery with or without irradiation in women aged 65 years or older with early breast cancer (PRIME II): a randomised controlled trial. *Lancet Oncol.* 2015; 16(3):266–73. doi:10.1016/S1470-2045(14)71221-5

118. Tsang Y, Venables K, Yarnold J. Quality assurance analysis of participating centres' protocol compliance to a UK multicentre hypofractionated breast (FAST) trial. *Br J Radiol.* 2012; 85(September):647–53. doi:10.1259/bjr/32249628

119. Hughes KS, Schnaper LA, Bellon JR et al. Lumpectomy plus tamoxifen with or without irradiation in women age 70 years or older with early breast cancer: Long-term follow-up of CALGB 9343. 2013; 31(19). doi:10.1200/JCO.2012.45.2615

120. Kirwan CC. It's PRIMETIME. Postoperative avoidance of radiotherapy: Biomarker selection of women at very low risk of local recurrence. *Clin Oncol (R Coll Radiol).* 2016; 28(9):594–6. doi:10.1016/j.clon.2016.06.007

121. Bartelink H, Maingon P, Poortmans P et al. Whole-breast irradiation with or without a boost for patients treated with breast-conserving surgery for early breast cancer: 20-year follow-up of a randomised phase 3 trial. *Lancet Oncol.* 2015; 16(1):47–56. doi:10.1016/S1470-2045(14)71156-8

122. Jones HA, Antonini N, Hart AAM et al. Impact of pathological characteristics on local relapse after breast-conserving therapy: A subgroup analysis of the EORTC boost versus no boost trial. *J Clin Oncol.* 2019; 27(30):4939–47. doi:10.1200/JCO.2008.21.5764

123. Donovan EM, Ciurlionis L, Fairfoul J et al. Planning with intensity-modulated radiotherapy and tomotherapy to modulate dose across breast to reflect recurrence risk (IMPORT High trial). *Int J Rad Oncol Biol Phys.* 2011; 79(4):1064–72. doi:10.1016/j.ijrobp.2009.12.052

124. Mannino M, Yarnold JR. Local relapse rates are falling after breast conserving surgery and systemic therapy for early breast cancer: Can radiotherapy ever be safely withheld? *Radiother Oncol.* 2009; 90(1):14–22. doi:10.1016/j.radonc.2008.05.002

125. Coles CE, Griffin CL, Kirby AM et al. Partial-breast radiotherapy after breast conservation surgery for patients with early breast cancer (UK IMPORT LOW trial): 5-year results from a multicentre, randomised, controlled, phase 3, non-inferiority trial. *Lancet.* 2017; 390(10099):1048–60. doi:10.1016/S0140-6736(17)31145-5

126. Royal College of Radiologists (RCR). Postoperative radiotherapy for breast cancer: UK consensus statements. November 2016.

127. Veronesi U, Orecchia R, Maisonneuve P et al. Intraoperative radiotherapy versus external radiotherapy for early breast cancer (ELIOT): a randomised controlled equivalence trial. *Lancet Oncol.* 2013; 14(13):1269–77. doi:10.1016/S1470-2045(13)70497-2

128. Vaidya JS, Wenz F, Bulsara M et al. Risk-adapted targeted intraoperative radiotherapy versus whole-breast radiotherapy for breast cancer: 5-year results for local control and overall survival from the TARGIT-A randomised trial. 2014; 383:603–13. doi:10.1016/S0140-6736(13)61950-9

129. Leonard KL, Hepel JT, Hiatt JR et al. The effect of dose-volume parameters and interfraction interval on cosmetic outcome and toxicity after 3-dimensional conformal accelerated partial breast irradiation. *Radiat Oncol Biol.* 2013; 85(3):623–9. doi:10.1016/j.ijrobp.2012.06.052

130. Olivotto IA, Whelan TJ, Parpia S et al. Interim cosmetic and toxicity results from RAPID: A randomized trial of accelerated partial breast irradiation using three-dimensional conformal external beam radiation therapy. *J Clin Oncol.* 2013; 31(32):4038–45. doi:10.1200/JCO.2013.50.5511

131. McGale P, Taylor C, Correa C et al. (Early Breast Cancer Trialists' Collaborative Group). Effect of radiotherapy after mastectomy and

axillary surgery on 10-year recurrence and 20-year breast cancer mortality: meta-analysis of individual patient data for 8135 women in 22 randomised trials. *Lancet*. 2014; 383(9935):2127–35. doi:10.1016/S0140-6736(14)60488-8

132. Whelan TJ, Olivotto IA, Parulekar WR et al. Regional nodal irradiation in early-stage breast cancer. *NEJM*. 2015; 373(4ne):307–16. doi:10.1056/NEJMoa1415340

133. Poortmans PM, Collette S, Kirkove C et al. Internal mammary and medial supraclavicular irradiation in breast cancer. *NEJM*. 2015; 373(4):317–27. doi:10.1056/NEJMoa1415369

134. Thorsen LBJ, Thomsen MS, Berg M et al. CT-planned internal mammary node radiotherapy in the DBCG-IMN study: Benefit versus potentially harmful effects. *Acta Oncol*. 2014; 53(8):1027–34. doi:10.3109/0284186X.2014.925579

135. Asselain B, Barlow W, Bartlett J et al. (Early Breast Cancer Trialists' Collaborative Group E). Articles long-term outcomes for neoadjuvant versus adjuvant chemotherapy in early breast cancer: meta-analysis of individual patient data from ten randomised trials. *Lancet Oncol*. 2018; 19(1):27–39. doi:10.1016/S1470-2045(17)30777-5

136. Mamounas EP, Anderson SJ, Dignam JJ et al. Predictors of locoregional recurrence after neoadjuvant chemotherapy: Results from combined analysis of national surgical adjuvant breast and bowel project B-18 and B-27. *J Clin Oncol*. 2012; 30(32):3960–6. doi:10.1200/JCO.2011.40.8369

137. Poller DN, Barth A, Slamon DJ et al. Prognostic classification of breast ductal carcinoma in situ. *Lancet*. 1995; 345(8958):1154–7.

138. Goodwin A, Parker S, Ghersi D, Wilcken N. Post-operative radiotherapy for ductal carcinoma in situ of the breast—A systematic review of the randomised trials. *Breast*. 2009; 18(3):143–9.

139. Shah C, Wobb J, Grills I et al. Use of intensity modulated radiation therapy to reduce acute and chronic toxicities of breast cancer patients treated with traditional and accelerated whole breast irradiation. *PRRO*. 2012; 2(4):e45–e51. doi:10.1016/j.prro.2012.01.008

140. Darby SC, Ewertz M, McGale P et al. Risk of ischemic heart disease in women after radiotherapy for breast cancer. *NEJM*. 2013; 368(11):987–98. doi:10.1056/NEJMoa1209825

141. Taylor C, Correa C, Duane FK et al. Estimating the risks of breast cancer radiotherapy: Evidence from modern radiation doses to the lungs and heart and from previous randomized trials. *J Clin Oncol*. 2019; 35(15). doi:10.1200/JCO.2016.72.0722

142. Asselain B, Barlow W, Bartlett J et al. Long-term outcomes for neoadjuvant versus adjuvant chemotherapy in early breast cancer: meta-analysis of individual patient data from ten randomised trials. *Lancet Oncol*. 2018; 19(1):27–39. doi:10.1016/S1470-2045(17)30777-5

143. Rastogi P, Anderson SJ, Bear HD et al. Preoperative chemotherapy: Updates of national surgical adjuvant breast and bowel project protocols B-18 and B-27. *J Clin Oncol*. 2008; 26(5):778–85. doi:10.1200/JCO.2007.15.0235

144. Gianni L, Pienkowski T, Im YH et al. Efficacy and safety of neoadjuvant pertuzumab and trastuzumab in women with locally advanced, inflammatory, or early HER2-positive breast cancer (NeoSphere): A randomised multicentre, open-label, phase 2 trial. *Lancet Oncol*. 2012; 13(1):25–32. doi:10.1016/S1470-2045(11)70336-9

145. Gianni L, Pienkowski T, Im YH et al. 5-year analysis of neoadjuvant pertuzumab and trastuzumab in patients with locally advanced, inflammatory, or early-stage HER2-positive breast cancer (NeoSphere): a multicentre, open-label, phase 2 randomised trial. *Lancet Oncol*. 2016; 17(6):791–800. doi:10.1016/S1470-2045(16)00163-7

146. National Institute for Health and Care Excellence N. Pertuzumab for adjuvant treatment of early stage breast cancer. Technology appraisal guidance [TA424]. Published December 2016 https://www.nice.org.uk/guidance/ta424.

147. Sikov WM, Berry DA, Perou CM et al. Impact of the addition of carboplatin and/or bevacizumab to neoadjuvant once-per-week paclitaxel followed by dose-dense doxorubicin and cyclophosphamide on pathologic complete response rates in stage II to III triple-negative breast cancer: CALGB 40603 (Alliance). *J Clin Oncol*. 2015; 33(1):13–21. doi:10.1200/JCO.2014.57.0572

148. Loibl S, O'Shaughnessy J, Untch M et al. Addition of the PARP inhibitor veliparib plus carboplatin or carboplatin alone to standard neoadjuvant chemotherapy in triple-negative breast cancer (BrighTNess): a randomised, phase 3 trial. *Lancet Oncol*. 2018; 19(4):497–509. doi:10.1016/S1470-2045(18)30111-6

149. Von Minckwitz G, Schneeweiss A, Loibl S et al. Neoadjuvant carboplatin in patients with triple-negative and HER2-positive early breast cancer (GeparSixto; GBG 66): A randomised phase 2 trial. *Lancet Oncol*. 2014; 15(7):747–56. doi:10.1016/S1470-2045(14)70160-3

150. Aebi S, Gelber S, Anderson SJ et al. Chemotherapy for isolated locoregional recurrence of breast cancer (CALOR): a randomised trial. *Lancet* 2014; 15(2): 156–63. doi:10.1016/S1470-2045(13)70589-8

151. Secondary Breast Cancer Taskforce. Breast Cancer Care. Improving the care of people with metastatic breast cancer final report. 2008.

152. Gobbini E, Ezzalfani M, Bachelot T et al. Time trends of overall survival among metastatic breast cancer patients in the real-life ESME cohort. *Eur J Cancer*. 2018; 96:17–24. doi:10.1016/j.ejca.2018.03.015

153. Zotano G, Marti E, Chaco I et al. Prospective evaluation of the conversion rate in the receptor status between primary breast cancer and metastasis: results from the GEICAM 2009-03 ConvertHER study. *Breast Cancer Res Treat*. 2014; 143:507–15. doi:10.1007/s10549-013-2825-2

154. Cardoso F, Fallowfield L, Costa A et al. ESMO Guidelines Working Group. Locally recurrent or metastatic breast cancer: ESMO Clinical Practice Guidelines for diagnosis, treatment and follow-up. *Ann Oncol*. 2011; 22(6):vi25–vi30. doi:10.1093/annonc/mdr372

155. Mauri D, Pavlidis N, Polyzos NP, Ioannidis JPA. Survival with aromatase inhibitors and inactivators versus standard hormonal therapy in advanced breast cancer: Meta-analysis. *JNCI* 2006; 98(18):1285–91. doi:10.1093/jnci/djj357

156. Campos SM, Guastalla JP, Subar M. A comparative study of exemestane versus anastrozole in patients with postmenopausal breast cancer with visceral metastases. *Clin Breast Cancer*. 2009; 9(1):39–44.

157. Finn RS, Martin M, Rugo HS et al. Palbociclib and letrozole in advanced breast cancer. *NEJM*. 2016; 375(20):1925–36. doi:10.1056/NEJMoa1607303

158. Hortobagyi GN, Stemmer SM, Burris HA et al. Updated results from MONALEESA-2, a phase III trial of first-line ribociclib plus letrozole versus placebo plus letrozole in hormone receptor-positive, HER2-negative advanced breast cancer. *Annals of Oncology*, 29(7), 2018, pp.1541-1547. doi:10.1093/annonc/mdy155

159. Rose C, Vtoraya O, Pluzanska A et al. An open randomised trial of second-line endocrine therapy in advanced breast cancer: comparison of the aromatase inhibitors letrozole and anastrozole. *Eur J Cancer*. 2003; 39:2318–27. doi:10.1016/S0959-8049(03)00630-0

160. Beresford M, Tumur I, Chakrabarti J et al. A qualitative systematic review of the evidence base for non-cross-resistance between steroidal and non-steroidal aromatase inhibitors in metastatic breast cancer. *Clin Oncol*. 2011; 23(3):209–15. doi:10.1016/j.clon.2010.11.005

161. Howell A, Pippen J, Elledge RM et al. Fulvestrant versus anastrozole for the treatment of advanced breast carcinoma: A prospectively planned combined survival analysis of two multicenter trials. *Cancer*. 2005; 104(2):236–39. doi:10.1002/cncr.21163

162. Chia S, Gradishar W, Mauriac L et al. Double-blind, randomized placebo controlled trial of fulvestrant compared with exemestane after prior nonsteroidal aromatase inhibitor therapy in postmenopausal women with hormone receptor—Positive, advanced breast cancer: Results from EFECT. *J Clin Oncol*. 2019; 26(10). doi:10.1200/JCO.2007.13.5822

163. Robertson JFR, Bondarenko IM, Trishkina E et al. Fulvestrant 500 mg versus anastrozole 1 mg for hormone receptor-positive advanced breast cancer (FALCON): an international, randomised, double-blind, phase 3 trial. *Lancet*. 2016; 388(10063):2997–3005. doi:10.1016/S0140-6736(16)32389-3

164. Sledge GW, Toi M, Neven P et al. MONARCH 2: Abemaciclib in combination with fulvestrant in women with HR+/

HER2—Advanced breast cancer who had progressed while receiving endocrine therapy. *J Clin Oncol.* 2019; 35(25). doi:10.1200/JCO.2017.73.7585

165. Pritchard KI, Lebrun F, Beck JT et al. Everolimus in postmenopausal hormone- receptor–positive advanced breast cancer. *NEJM.* 2012; 366:520–9.

166. Thürlimann B, Robertson JF, Nabholtz JM et al. Efficacy of tamoxifen following anastrozole ("Arimidex") compared with anastrozole following tamoxifen as first-line treatment for advanced breast cancer in postmenopausal women. *Eur J Cancer.* 2003; 39:2310–17. doi:10.1016/S0959-8049(03)00602-6

167. Willemse PH, Van Der Ploeg E, Sleijfer DT et al. A randomized comparison of megestrol acetate (MA) and medroxyprogesterone acetate (MPA) in patients with advanced breast cancer. *Eur J Cancer Clin Oncol.* 1990; 26(3):337–43.

168. The Cancer Genome Atlas Network. Comprehensive molecular portraits of human breast tumours. *Nature.* 2012; 490:61–70. doi:10.1038/nature11412

169. Andre F, Ciruelos E, Rubovszky G et al. Alpelisib for PIK3CA-mutated, hormone receptor-positive advanced breast cancer. *NEJM.* 2019; 380:1929–40.

170. Crump M, Sawka CA, DeBoer G. An individual patient-based meta-analysis of tamoxifen versus ovarian ablation as first line endocrine therapy for premenopausal women with metastatic breast cancer. *Breast Cancer Res Treat.* 1997; 44(3):201–10.

171. Klijn BJGM, Blamey RW, Boccardo F et al. Hormone (LHRH) agonist versus LHRH agonist alone in premenopausal advanced breast cancer: A meta-analysis of four randomized trials. *J Clin Oncol.* 2019; 19(2):343–53.

172. Park I, Ro J, Lee K et al. Phase II parallel group study showing comparable efficacy between premenopausal metastatic breast cancer patients treated with letrozole plus goserelin and postmenopausal patients treated with letrozole alone as first-line hormone therapy. *J Clin Oncol.* 2010; 28(16):2705–11.

173. Goetz MP, Toi M, Campone M et al. MONARCH 3: Abemaciclib as initial therapy for advanced breast cancer. *J Clin Oncol.* 2017; 35(32):3638–46.

174. Cristofanilli M, Turner NC, Bondarenko I et al. Fulvestrant plus palbociclib versus fulvestrant plus placebo for treatment of hormone-receptor-positive, HER2-negative metastatic breast cancer that progressed on previous endocrine therapy (PALOMA-3): final analysis of the multicentre, double-blind. *Lancet Oncol.* 2016; 17(4):425–39. doi:10.1016/S1470-2045(15)00613-0

175. Kaufman B, Mackey JR, Clemens MR et al. Trastuzumab plus anastrozole versus anastrozole alone for the treatment of postmenopausal women with human epidermal growth factor receptor 2-positive, hormone receptor-positive metastatic breast cancer: Results from the randomized phase III TAnDEM study. *J Clin Oncol.* 2009; 27(33):5529–37.

176. Andersson M, Lidbrink E, Bjerre K et al. Phase III randomized study comparing docetaxel plus trastuzumab with vinorelbine plus trastuzumab as first-line therapy of metastatic or locally advanced human epidermal growth factor receptor 2-positive breast cancer: The HERNATA study. *J Clin Oncol.* 2011; 29(3):264–71.

177. von Minckwitz G, Schwedler K, Schmidt M et al. Trastuzumab beyond progression: Overall survival analysis of the GBG 26/BIG 3–05 phase III study in HER2-positive breast cancer. *Eur J Cancer.* 2011; 47(15):2273–81.

178. Perez E, Barrios C, Eiermann W et al. Trastuzumab emtansine with or without pertuzumab versus trastuzumab plus taxane for human epidermal growth factor receptor 2-positive, advanced breast cancer: Primary results from the phase III MARIANNE study. *J Clin Oncol.* 2017; 35(2):141–8.

179. Verma S, Miles D, Gianni L et al. Trastuzumab emtansine for HER2-positive advanced breast cancer. *NEJM.* 2012; 367(19):1783–91.

180. Krop IE, Kim SB, González-Martín A et al. Trastuzumab emtansine versus treatment of physician's choice for pretreated HER2-positive advanced breast cancer (TH3RESA): a randomised, open-label, phase 3 trial. *Lancet Oncol.* 2014; 15(7):689–99.

181. Cortes J, O'Shaughnessy J, Loesch D et al. Eribulin monotherapy versus treatment of physician's choice in patients with metastatic breast cancer (EMBRACE): A phase 3 open-label randomised study. *Lancet.* 2011; 377(9769):914–23.

182. Kassam F, Enright K, Dent R et al. Survival outcomes for patients with metastatic triple-negative breast cancer: Implications for clinical practice and trial design. *Clin Breast Cancer.* 2009; 9(1): 29–33.

183. Schmid P, Adams S, Rugo H et al. Atezolizumab and nab-paclitaxel in advanced triple-negative breast cancer. *NEJM.* 2018; 379(22):2108–21.

184. Tutt A, Tovey H, Cheang MC et al. Carboplatin in BRCA1/2-mutated and triple-negative breast cancer BRCAness subgroups: the TNT trial. *Nat Med.* 2018; 24(5):628–37.

185. Robson M, Im S, Senkus E et al. Olaparib for metastatic breast cancer in patients with a germline BRCA mutation. *NEJM.* 2017; 377(6):523–33.

186. Litton J, Rugo H, Hurvitz S et al. Talazoparib in patients with advanced breast cancer and a germline BRCA mutation. *NEJM.* 2018; 379(8):753–63.

187. Coleman R. Clinical features of metastatic bone disease and risk of skeletal morbidity. *Clin Cancer Res.* 2006; 12(20 pt 2):6243s–6249s.

188. Ross J, Saunders Y, Edmonds P et al. Systematic review of role of bisphosphonates on skeletal morbidity in metastatic cancer. *BMJ.* 2003; 327(7413):469.

189. Pavlakis N, Schmidt R, Stockler M. Bisphosphonates for breast cancer. *Cochrane Database Syst Rev.* 2005; 20(3):CD003474.

190. Machado M, Crus L, Tannus G, Fonseca M. Efficacy of clodronate, pamidronate, and zoledronate in reducing morbidity and mortality in cancer patients with bone metastasis: A meta-analysis of randomized clinical trials. *Clin Ther.* 2009; 31(5):962–79.

191. Hillner B, Ingle J, Chlebowski R et al. American Society of Clinical Oncology 2003 update on the role of bisphosphonates and bone health issues in women with breast cancer. *J Clin Oncol.* 2003; 21(21):4042–57.

192. O'Carrigan B, Wong M, Wilson M et al. Bisphosphonates and other bone agents for breast cancer. *Cochrane Database Syst Rev.* 2017; 10:CD003474.

193. Barrett-Lee PP, Casbard A, Abraham J et al. Abstract PD07-09: Zoledronate versus ibandronate comparative evaluation oral ibandronic acid versus intravenous zoledronic acid in treatment of bone metastases from breast cancer: a randomised, open label, non-inferiority phase 3 trial. *Lancet Oncol.* 2014; 15(1):114–22. doi:10.1016/S1470-2045(13)70539-4

194. Stopeck A, Lipton A, Body J et al. Denosumab compared with zoledronic acid for the treatment of bone metastases in patients with advanced breast cancer: A randomized, double-blind study. *J Clin Oncol.* 2010; 28((35)):5132–39.

195. Ford J, Cummins E, Sharma P et al. Systematic review of the clinical effectiveness and cost-effectiveness, and economic evaluation, of denosumab for the treatment of bone metastases from solid tumours. *Health Technol Assess (Rockv).* 2013; 17(29):1–386.

196. Yarnold JR, on behalf of the Bone Pain Trial Working Party. 8 Gy single fraction radiotherapy for the treatment of metastatic skeletal pain: randomised comparison with a multifraction schedule over 12 months of patient follow-up. *Radiother Oncol.* 1999; 52(2):111–21.

197. Palma D, Olson R, Harrow S et al. Stereotactic ablative radiotherapy versus standard of care palliative treatment in patients with oligometastatic cancers (SABR-COMET): a randomised, phase 2, open-label trial. *Lancet.* 2019; 393(10185):2051–58.

198. Milano M, Katz A, Zhang H et al. Oligometastatic breast cancer treated with hypofractionated stereotactic radiotherapy: Some patients

Useful websites

www.predict.nhs.uk/
Predict is an online tool that can be used by patients and clinicians to aid in adjuvant treatment decisions based on histological features of the breast cancer.
www.adjuvantonline.com/index.jsp

The purpose of Adjuvant! is to help health professionals and patients with early cancer discuss the risks and benefits of getting additional therapy (adjuvant therapy: usually chemotherapy, hormone therapy, or both) after surgery.

www.pinkribbonfoundation.org.uk/

The Pink Ribbon Foundation is an impartial and committed organization responsible for bringing together individuals, charities, and organizations to fight breast cancer.

www.cancer.gov/cancertopics/types/cancersbodylocation/breast

www.esmo.org/Guidelines-Practice/Clinical-Practice-Guidelines/Breast-Cancer

http://seer.cancer.gov/statfacts/html/breast.html

www.ncin.org.uk/cancer_type_and_topic_specific_work/cancer_type_specific_work/breast_cancer/

www.lifemath.net/cancer/breastcancer/outcome/index.php

Web-based prognosis calculator.

http://pathways.nice.org.uk/pathways/early-and-locally-advanced-breast-cancer?fno=1

http://pathways.nice.org.uk/pathways/advanced-breast-cancer?fno=1

www.cancerresearchuk.org/cancer-help/type/breast-cancer/

www.cancer.net/cancer-types/breast-cancer

www.breastcancercare.org.uk

UK support and information for women with breast cancer. Breast Cancer Care runs four centers, three in England and one in Scotland, that offer talks and courses and peer support across the regions. There is a free helpline and free "moving forward" post-treatment courses run with the NHS.

www.thehaven.org.uk

Free emotional, nutritional, and physical support for women with breast cancer in the United Kingdom. The Haven operates centers in London, Hereford, and Leeds that give breast cancer patients a free, personalized program of therapy from yoga to acupuncture to cookery workshops. Patients outside these areas can still access classes online.

www.breastcancergenetics.co.uk

Helpline and support for women with breast cancer in the family. Provides personal stories from women who have opted for preventative mastectomy.

www.willow.org

Phone, web, and group help for women with breast cancer. Breast Cancer Support. Canada offers a free phone line staffed by volunteers with personal experience of the disease. There is an online community and information on everything you need to know.

www.cbcsf.ca

Cash for breast cancer patients. Women undergoing treatment for breast cancer and facing financial difficulties can apply to the Canadian Breast Cancer Support Fund for help.

http://beyondtheshock.com

Video files and stories about breast cancer and surviving it. Newly diagnosed women can watch educational videos about cancer, ask questions about the disease, and view video stories from survivors.

www.bcna.org.au/

Get support for your breast cancer. Breast Cancer Network Australia gives women face-to-face group support or online networking. You can also read personal stories and leaf through the local services directory.

www.bcaus.org.au

This Australian Breast Cancer Forum does what it says on the tin.

7 LUNG CANCER

Michael Flynn and Nadia Yousaf

Epidemiology and etiology

Lung cancer remains the most common cancer worldwide after non-melanocytic skin cancer and is now the third most common cancer in the United Kingdom.[1] Over half of patients are diagnosed at a late stage,[2] with up to 40% presenting via emergency services.[3] Across all stages of lung cancer, survival is still poor, although recently there is a trend towards improvements, with 37% of patients surviving 1 year.

There is significant geographical variation in incidence, which often closely mirrors rates of smoking. Using the UK as an example, incidence rates in the north of England and Scotland reflect regional variations in smoking prevalence of up to 25%. The incidence of lung cancer increases with age; it is extremely rare under the age of 40, with the majority of cases occurring in the 70 and over age group. The incidence of lung cancer in men in the UK has been falling and has almost halved since the 1970s; conversely, in women, it has increased by almost 70% over the same time span. This is probably due to the change in smoking trends over the years. For women, lung cancer has overtaken breast cancer as the commonest cause of cancer death.

Of note, approximately 10% of lung cancer occurs in never-smokers. Statistics show that this proportion is higher for women (20%) and Asian populations (50%). The reasons for this are unclear, but it may be due to different environmental factors including exposure to radon, asbestos, passive smoking, and other pollutants. Asbestos exposure contributes to the largest number of deaths, and silica, diesel oil, mineral oils, arsenic, dioxin, benzopyrene, and radon exposure accounts for the majority of the remaining cases. Therefore, occupations at risk include miners, workers in construction and manufacturing, farmers, and painters.

The health risks of indirect (passive) smoking are difficult to quantify, but the incidence of lung cancer and ischemic heart disease is increased. It is estimated that a non-smoker living in a smoking household is exposed to the equivalent of 1% of the cigarettes actively smoked. In this non-smoking population, the risk of developing lung cancer is increased by 24%. The knowledge that lung cancer occurs in never-smokers and other epidemiological data have underpinned several large studies of heritable risk alleles and revealed significant heterogeneity in genetic susceptibility.

Histopathological classification

Traditionally, lung cancers have been subdivided based on histological appearances under a light microscope. The two most common epithelial subtypes, neuroendocrine tumors and non-small-cell lung cancer (NSCLC), are incorporated within the 2015 World Health Organization (WHO) classification.[4]

Neuroendocrine tumors

These consist of high-grade neuroendocrine tumors (HG NET) such as small-cell lung cancer (SCLC) and large cell neuroendocrine or more indolent carcinoid tumors. HG NET are usually associated with a history of heavy smoking and are typically found in the major bronchi. These tumors are frequently observed to secrete antidiuretic hormone, calcitonin, and adrenocorticotrophic hormone in either an autocrine or a paracrine manner. Macroscopically, tumors are friable with a pinky cut surface. Microscopically, SCLCs are characterized by the presence of small cells with large pleomorphic nuclei and scanty cytoplasm. The majority of SCLCs express thyroid transcription factor-1 (TTF-1) as well as neuroendocrine markers such as chromogranin, synaptophysin, and CD56. At the molecular level, G to T transversion mutations, which are characteristic of smoking, are common. SCLC tumors show a high density of somatic DNA aberrations, and allelic loss of tumor suppressor genes is commonest, with *p53* and *Rb* being universally affected.[5]

Non-small-cell lung cancer

The 2015 WHO classification encourages diagnostic precision, made possible with the greater availability of immunohistochemistry and molecular techniques, and is at the forefront of the international effort to reduce NSCLC not-otherwise-specified diagnosis rates. There are now several driver mutations that have been identified in NSCLC, and those in adenocarcinoma and squamous cell carcinoma are specifically depicted in Table 7.1. Some of the commonest molecular techniques used to identify these are summarized in Table 7.2. The table shows the applications of each technique for the different types of aberrations that may be encountered in lung cancer. Targeted exome sequencing on tissue or blood is being increasingly utilized to sequence a focused panel of genes as costs and turnaround times have reduced. Polymerase chain reaction (PCR) technology can also be used to target more specific areas of the genome, identifying single gene mutations and their RNA counterparts in tissue or in circulating tumor cells in blood. Fluorescent in-situ hybridization (FISH) makes use of microscopy to identify fusion and amplification products of fluorescently labeled genes, and although it has been transformational for identifying common fusion/amplifications such as anaplastic lymphoma kinase (ALK), it is also labor-intensive. Immunohistochemistry can be a very cheap, widely performed assay, which can be highly sensitive and specific for identifying protein products of fusions/amplifications such as ALK.

Squamous cell carcinoma (SCC) now accounts for up to 30% of patients diagnosed with NSCLC in Western countries, occurring usually in men and typically related to smoking. Historically, these tumors were stereotypically found proximally in the major bronchi, but increasing numbers are now found more peripherally. Macroscopically, these tumors appear as firm lesions with a pale-grey, gritty surface and can be cavitating. Microscopically, the hallmarks of squamous differentiation are apparent, with prominent intercellular bridges and keratinization. Immunohistochemical staining with antibodies against cytokeratin 5, 6, p40, and p63 increases confidence in the diagnosis. Molecularly, SCC has been shown to demonstrate recurrent mutations in 11 genes, including mutation of TP53 in almost all sampled cases. Significantly altered pathways included NFE2L2

TABLE 7.1   Commonest Molecular Aberrations Found in Lung Adenocarcinomas and Squamous Cell Carcinomas

Adenocarcinoma
KRAS (25.5%)
Wild-type (20.8%)
EGFR (16.1%)
NF-1 (8.1%)
BRAF (6.9%)
MET exon 14 (4.2%)
ALK (3.9%)
NRG1 (3.2%)
DDR2 (2.9%)
RIT1 (2.2%)
HER2 (1.9%)
ROS1 (1.7%)
NTRK1 (1.7%)
RET (0.7%)
Squamous cell carcinoma
Other or wild-type (55%)
FGFR (20%)
PIK3CA (12%)
PTEN loss (10%)
DDR2 (3%)

and KEAP1 in 34%, squamous differentiation genes in 44%, phosphatidylinositol-3-OH kinase pathway genes in 47%, and CDKN2A and RB1 in 72% of tumors.[6] None of these commonest mutations in SCC are currently targetable.

Adenocarcinomas account for the majority of NSCLC diagnoses. Macroscopically, they form irregular round masses, whose cut surfaces often have a myxoid appearance. Microscopically, varying patterns of glandular differentiation are seen. TTF-1 is positive in 75%–100% of lung adenocarcinomas and can help differentiate a primary lung adenocarcinoma from a metastasis. Molecularly, adenocarcinomas have been more specifically characterized.[7] Adenocarcinomas in never-smokers are more likely to have a single oncogenic driver. There is a 75% chance of a targetable oncogenic driver being identified in these patients, with the commonest genetic aberrations including those in epidermal growth factor receptor (EGFR), ALK, ROS1, RET, and NTRK1. KRAS, another common mutation found in adenocarcinomas, is showing early evidence of being targetable.

PD-L1 expression and tumor mutational burden (TMB)

PD-1 is a negative co-stimulatory receptor, expressed mainly on activated T cells and to varying degrees in tumor tissues, which downregulates excessive immune responses by binding to its ligands, PD-L1 and PD-L2.[8] It is already well established that PD-L1 positivity predicts response to immunotherapy and is correlated with both progression-free survival (PFS) and overall survival (OS) in those treated with immune-checkpoint inhibitors.[9] However, variability in the significance of these correlations and the cutoff level at which they are observed across clinical trials suggests the picture is more nuanced. Reasons for this include the variable sensitivity of each of the assays used to quantify PD-L1 expression and the lack of specificity of the cell types on which it is being quantified. However, a recent publication of work within the pivotal academic and industrial collaboration BLUEPRINT, which assessed the feasibility of harmonizing the clinical use of five independently developed commercial PD-L1 immuno-histochemistry assays, has provided evidence for interchangeability in the sensitivity of at least three assays, although there remains great variability in the best way in which to assess their applicability.[10]

The TMB is defined as the total number of nonsynonymous mutations per coding area of a tumor genome. The utility of TMB as a prognostic biomarker is becoming increasingly evident across tumor types. Higher TMB has been shown to predict a favorable outcome from PD-1/PD-L1 blockade across diverse tumors, including NSCLC.[11] Specifically, a high density of neoepitopes stemming from either somatic driver or passenger mutations may permit more ready immune detection after immune-checkpoint inhibition, leading to destruction of cells bearing these mutation-associated neoantigens.[12] However, there are challenges in the definition of thresholds of higher TMBs and variability in whether TMB is expressed as the total number of mutations per exome, or mutations per megabase differ between studies, which makes inter-study interpretation of its utility as a predictive biomarker difficult to ascertain.

Prevention and screening

Primary prevention

Anti-smoking public health policies have resulted in significant changes to UK law in recent years, resulting in a ban on tobacco advertising alongside a ban on smoking within enclosed public places. There is evidence that the overall decline in smoking in the United Kingdom has been influenced by such strategies.

Screening

The majority of patients with lung cancer present with advanced disease, for which curative treatments are not possible. However, a number of large studies definitively show that screening both results in significant stage shift and reduces lung cancer mortality.

The American National Lung Cancer Screening study was a large randomized trial involving more than 50,000 participants.[13] High-risk individuals were randomized between annual

TABLE 7.2   Assays Used to Identify Specific Mutations, Gene Rearrangements, or Amplifications at the DNA, RNA, and Protein Level

Category	Mutation	Gene rearrangement	Amplification
DNA	Direct sequencing	FISH	FISH
	PCR-based methods	NGS	qPCR
	NGS		NGS
RNA		RT-PCR (fusion transcript)	Real-time PCR (mRNA overexpression)
Protein	IHC (mutation-specific antibody)	IHC (protein expression)	IHC (protein overexpression)

Abbreviations: FISH: fluorescent in-situ hybridization; IHC: immunohistochemistry; NGS: next generation sequencing; qPCR: quantitative polymerase chain reaction; RT-PCR: reverse transcriptase polymerase chain reaction.

low-dose computed tomography (LDCT) and chest X-ray (CXR). A higher proportion of Stage I cancers were identified in the LDCT arm than in the CXR arm (54% vs. 36%), which translated to a significant 20% mortality benefit. NELSON, the equivalent European based study recruiting in Belgium and the Netherlands and the second largest screening program internationally, was also recently reported. Significant stage shift was noted; that is, approximately 70% of patients were Stage I/II in the screening arm, while 70% of patients in the observation arm were Stage III/IV.[14] In addition, there was a 26% reduction in mortality.

Diagnosis and staging

Clinical features

The vast majority of patients with lung cancer present with symptomatic disease, with approximately 40% being diagnosed after an emergency presentation. Symptoms can be non-specific, especially in patients with pre-existing comorbidities such as chronic obstructive pulmonary disease. Recurrent chest infections in a smoker must be taken seriously and prompt further investigation, as this is the most common presenting finding. The development of a new cough or hemoptysis or change in character of an existing cough is also common, as is weight loss. Chest or shoulder pain can also occur and is often a feature of local invasion. New onset or progressive dyspnea can be due to extrinsic or intrinsic airway obstruction, lymphangitis, pulmonary emboli, or pleural/pericardial effusions. Cancer involving the recurrent laryngeal nerve may present with dysphonia. Fever may be due to obstructive pneumonia or less frequently due to metastases. The median interval between symptom onset and diagnosis is about 4 months. This delay occurs because symptoms are often of gradual onset and against a background of chronic obstructive airways disease in smokers. HG NET has a high mitotic rate and metastasizes early. Symptoms from HG NET occur earlier and are more varied than those from NSCLC, including paraneoplastic syndromes, some preceding the diagnosis by many months.

Extrathoracic metastases

Common sites of metastases include the liver, bone, adrenal glands, and brain. Liver metastases are seen in more than 35% of patients at autopsy, and characteristic symptoms are pain and a feeling of fullness. Bone lesions occur in about 25% of patients. These are usually lytic and occur most commonly in the spine, pelvis, and femur. Brain metastases are particularly common in SCLC and adenocarcinoma, seen in up to 44% of patients at autopsy. They can present with focal neurological deficits, with features of raised intracranial pressure such as headaches and vomiting, with impaired mental function, or with personality changes. The incidence of adrenal metastasis may be as high as 30%, although patients often remain asymptomatic.

Diagnosis

Some asymptomatic patients will have abnormalities identified incidentally on CXR or computed tomography. Patients presenting with suggestive symptoms or an abnormal CXR should have a contrast-enhanced computed tomography (CECT) scan of the chest and abdomen; appearances may allow differentiation between benign and malignant processes within the lung and also permit staging. The CECT scan should be performed before a diagnostic procedure, thus providing information on the position of the tumor and the presence of metastases, allowing clinicians

to determine the most appropriate method of obtaining a tissue diagnosis. Diagnosis can be confirmed by mediastinoscopy or endobronchial ultrasound (EBUS) of affected mediastinal nodes, especially if this will change clinical management. If present, metastatic disease is the preferable biopsy site to stage and attain a diagnosis concurrently.

Staging

Precise staging is important to give patients and carers accurate prognostic information, decide on the most effective treatment, and allow comparison between different treatments and institutes. The international standard for lung cancer staging is TNM, with subgroup-amalgamated disease stage groups. The original TNM system adopted by the Union for International Cancer Control (UICC) was updated in 2018 (UICC version 8), underpinned by data from the International Association for the Study of Lung Cancer (IASLC) staging bank of approximately 100,000 lung cancers, and has yielded some important changes from the seventh edition (Table 7.3).

CECT staging is limited by poor sensitivity and specificity, particularly in relation to size-congruent lymph node metastasis or liver metastasis. ^{18}F-fluorodeoxyglucose positron emission tomography (FDG-PET) scans are of additional benefit in assessing distant metastatic disease in patients who are being considered for radical treatment. However, in patients with enlarged mediastinal nodes on CECT, a high false-positive rate of greater than 15% is observed, even using combined imaging. Mediastinal nodes should be pathologically verified by transbronchial needle aspiration, EBUS, or mediastinoscopy, if clinically relevant, in those with features of N2 or N3 involvement on CECT or FDG-PET. Asymptomatic brain metastasis may be present, and brain imaging is recommended for patients undergoing radical therapy.

SCLC was previously divided into limited and extensive stages using the Veteran's Affairs system. About 30% of patients have limited disease, which is defined as disease confined to one hemithorax with regional metastases, including hilar, ipsilateral, and

TABLE 7.3 Differences between TNM 7 and 8 Staging Systems

T/N/M	TNM 7	TNM 8
T	–	Tis
	–	Tmi
	–	Tss
	T1a ($\leq$2)	T1a ($\leq$1)
	T1b	T1b (1–2)
		T1c (2–3)
	T2a (>3–5)	T2a (>3–$\leq$4)
	T2b (>5–7)	T2b (>4–$\leq$5)
	T3 (>7)	T4
	T3—atelectasis or pneumonitis involving whole lung	T2—atelectasis or pneumonitis irrespective of involving lobe or whole lung
	T3—tumor involving main bronchus (<2 cm distance to carina)	T2—tumor involving main bronchus (irrespective of distance to carina)
	T3—invasion of diaphragm	T4—invasion of diaphragm
N	No change	No change
M	M1b—distant metastasis	M1b—single extrathoracic metastasis
		M1c—multiple extrathoracic metastasis

contralateral mediastinal and supraclavicular nodes, and ipsilateral pleural effusions (whether or not the cytology is positive). Extensive-stage disease was defined as disease beyond this, including distant lymph node, brain, liver, bone, bone marrow, and intra-abdominal soft-tissue metastases. UICC version 8 staging continues to incorporate a TNM classification for SCLC, reflective of NSCLC and validated on several thousand SCLC cases.

Management of non-small-cell lung cancer

Stage I/II

Although there is little evidence from randomized controlled studies evaluating the benefits of surgery, many observational studies show a survival advantage. Surgical resection remains the prime modality of curative treatment for NSCLC. Resectability depends on tumor location and stage and on the patient's ability to tolerate the procedure. Due to lifestyle factors, patients with lung cancer often have other comorbidities such as airways disease or ischemic heart disease. Therefore, British Thoracic Society guidelines define fitness for surgery, with particular reference to age, pulmonary function, cardiovascular fitness, nutrition, weight loss, and performance status (PS). Patients with Stage I and II tumors should be offered resection if preoperative assessment suggests that such a procedure would be safe. Optimal surgery for Stage I and II disease involves lobectomy, systematic lymph node dissection, and pleural lavage. In patients with poor pulmonary function, more limited resections can be considered and include segmentectomy and wedge resection. A systematic review including 13 observational studies comparing segmentectomy and lobectomy has shown 5-year survival rates of 62% and 80%, respectively, with increased loco-regional recurrence in those undergoing limited resection.[15] Minimally invasive video-assisted thoracic surgery is being increasingly used for lung resection. Meta-analyses of randomized and non-randomized trials have shown similar outcomes compared with open lobectomy but importantly, shorter hospital stays and fewer complications.[15]

In patients with a central tumor, more extensive surgery such as a pneumonectomy may be appropriate but requires good pulmonary reserve. In patients with compromised lung function, sleeve resection can be considered, although there is a higher risk of loco-regional recurrence, with post-operative complication rates being similar.[15]

Mortality rates following pneumonectomy are 6%–8%, whereas after lobectomy, the rate is only 3%. Morbidity is high, with about 20% of patients having minor complications and 10% suffering from major problems such as emboli and pulmonary insufficiency. Studies examining quality of life (QoL) post resection have shown that preoperative levels are not achieved until at least 6 months after surgery.

Treatment failure results from local relapse in about a third of patients and from metastatic spread in the remainder, with fewer than 10% of patients developing brain metastases. The majority of local relapses occur within the first 2 years following surgery, providing an argument for close follow-up during this period. In addition to recurrent disease, a proportion of patients develop a second primary lung cancer. Resection of new primary lung cancers should be performed if possible, even in the circumstance of synchronous lung cancer, although survival is poor (~25%) even for low-stage disease.

Although a systematic review of trials comparing stereotactic body radiotherapy (SBRT) with lobectomy for Stage I disease has demonstrated inferior recurrence rates for SBRT,[16] for patients unfit for surgery, this is a reasonable treatment option. SBRT delivers higher doses per fraction and fewer fractions than conventional radiotherapy (RT). Conventional fractionation RT is reserved for patients with tumors that are not amenable to surgery or SBRT. Treatment schedules vary, but most studies have used the biological equivalent of 60 Gy in 30 fractions of 2 Gy. The use of hyperfractionated schedules has been investigated. A randomized controlled trial comparing continuous hyperfractionated accelerated radiotherapy (54 Gy in 1.5 Gy fractions three times a day over 12 days) with conventional radiotherapy (60 Gy in 2 Gy fractions daily for 6 weeks) demonstrated a 22% reduction in the risk of death.[17] However, this regimen has been poorly taken up due to practical problems with delivery. There is no long-term data on alternative ablative techniques such as radiofrequency or microwave ablation, and therefore, these are not currently recommended.

Adjuvant cisplatin doublet chemotherapy is usually offered to patients with greater than Stage IIb lung cancer and a good PS due to a demonstrated absolute survival benefit of 5% at 5 years[18] in Stage II disease.

Stage III

Stage III disease is a heterogeneous group, ranging from patients with large tumors and no lymph node involvement to those with involvement of fixed, bulky contralateral mediastinal nodes (N3). The current standard of care for these patients is concomitant chemoradiation followed by 1 year of durvalumab. When given after chemoradiation, durvalumab confers a 10% OS benefit at 2 years,[19] with longer-term data pending. The role of durvalumab following sequential chemoradiation is not yet known, but in patients with a poor PS, this treatment strategy may be adopted to reduce the risk of esophagitis and myelosuppression at the expense of disease control.

The role of surgery in the management of Stage III disease is limited. Randomized studies conducted in the pre-durvalumab era have not demonstrated a survival benefit from induction chemotherapy followed by surgery versus chemoradiation.[20]

Post-operative radiotherapy for those patients undergoing surgery

In an attempt to reduce the risk of local recurrence following surgery, several studies have investigated post-operative radiotherapy. Patients with involved positive post-operative margins or N2 disease may benefit from consolidation radiotherapy to reduce the risk of local recurrence; for all other patients, post-operative radiotherapy has been shown to be detrimental.[15] The results of the LungART study, which compared post-operative conformal radiotherapy with no post-operative radiotherapy in patients who had completely resected NSCLC and N2 mediastinal disease, are awaited.

Advanced Stage III/IV

For the last three decades, first-line systemic therapy for most patients with advanced or metastatic NSCLC has consisted of platinum-doublet chemotherapy. Modest improvements in outcomes were made 15 years ago with the introduction of pemetrexed chemotherapy and more controversially, with the addition of the antiangiogenic agent bevacizumab for patients with non-squamous NSCLC,[21,22] but the potential for durable benefit has been difficult to realize.

However, more recently, there have been significant paradigm shifts, and several factors have become important in choosing the correct treatment. Improvements in molecular subtyping of NSCLC, with the upfront identification of oncogenic drivers and PD-L1 status, and in the availability of newer therapies, including immunotherapies, have resulted in the widespread adoption of a dichotomy of therapeutic approaches in advanced disease. This division into "oncogenic-driven" lung cancer, in which an identified oncogenic mutation has been identified and can be targeted (Figure 7.1), and "immunogenic" lung cancer, in which PD-L1 expression informs whether single agent immunotherapy or immunotherapy/chemotherapy ± antiangiogenic combination is the treatment recommendation (Figure 7.2), has widespread application. Specific considerations on deciding on appropriate systemic therapy are covered in the following subsections.

Absence/presence of driver mutations

Several targeted therapies have been developed to address molecular addiction in the subset of tumors harboring actionable aberrations, including inhibitors of EGFR, ALK, and ROS proto-oncogene 1 receptor tyrosine kinase (ROS1). Cancers with these mutations should be treated with targeted therapies upfront, and improvements in survival vs. chemotherapy have been shown. In addition, these tumors show low response rates to immune-checkpoint inhibition (ICPI).

Other driver mutations, including B-Raf (BRAF), rearranged during transfection (RET), human epidermal growth factor receptor 2 (HER2), and neurotrophic tropomyosin receptor

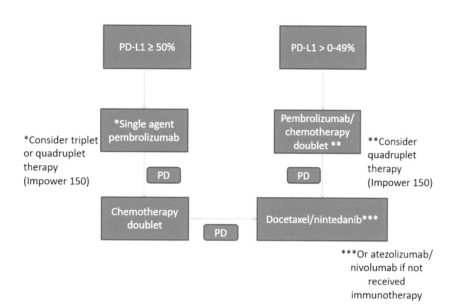

FIGURE 7.1   Treatment algorithm for non-oncogene-addicted NSCLC.

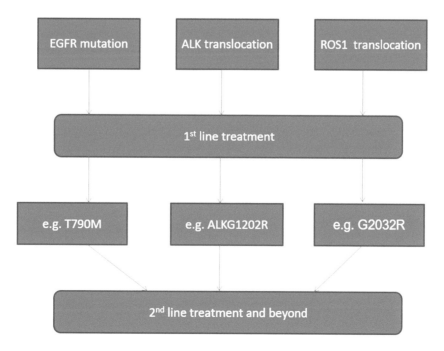

FIGURE 7.2   Oncogene-addicted NSCLC.

kinase (NTRK), and MET can be targeted, but usually in the second-line setting, as superiority to chemotherapy has not been established.

However, the ultimate emergence of resistance remains a clinical problem and necessitates repeat molecular analysis of the tumor at the point of progression to elucidate the resistance mechanism and to inform further lines of therapy (Figure 7.1).

Helpfully, as the technology for identification of mutations including ctDNA has evolved, the need to routinely obtain repeat invasive tumor biopsies has declined, permitting a window into the patient's current mutational burden, especially when biopsies are difficult to obtain. One of the major limitations of ctDNA technology currently is, however, its inability to pick up small-cell transformation.

PD-L1; >50% and <50%

Many pivotal trials have demonstrated the superiority of immunotherapy with or without chemotherapy (Tables 7.4 and 7.5), but important questions remain. There is a lack of evidence as to what strategy to adopt after the cessation of immunotherapy due to progression or toxicity or after the prescribed 2 years of treatment. Similarly, some populations have historically been excluded from immunotherapy clinical trials due to, for example, autoimmune disease, viral hepatitis, or HIV. There is now data to support the relative safety of ICPI in hepatocellular carcinoma,[23] HIV,[24] and autoimmunity,[25] and ongoing trials are looking at each of these patient subpopulations.

TABLE 7.4   Pivotal First-Line Immunotherapy Phase III Studies

Trial	Stratifier	Treatment	mPFS (months)	mOS (months)	Treatment-related AEs, grade 3–5 (%)
KEYNOTE-024	PD-L1 TPS ≥50%	Pembrolizumab	10.3	30.0	31
		Platinum + pemetrexed/gemcitabine/paclitaxel	6.0	14.2	53
Checkmate 026	PD-L1 ≥5%	Nivolumab	4.2	14.4	18
		Platinum + pemetrexed/gemcitabine/paclitaxel	5.9	13.2	52
KEYNOTE-042	PD-L1 TPS ≥1%	Pembrolizumab	5.4	16.7	18
		Platinum + pemetrexed/paclitaxel	6.5	12.1	41
IMpower150	Non-squamous	Atezolizumab + bevacizumab + platinum + paclitaxel	8.3	19.2	59
		Bevacizumab + platinum + paclitaxel	6.8	14.7	50
KEYNOTE-407	Squamous	Pembrolizumab + platinum + paclitaxel	6.4	15.9	70
		Placebo + platinum + paclitaxel	4.8	11.3	68
Checkmate 227	PD-L1 negative	Nivolumab + platinum/pemetrexed or gemcitabine	5.6	NR	54
		Platinum/pemetrexed or gemcitabine	4.7	NR	38
Checkmate 227	Tumor mutational burden ≥10 mutations/Mb	Nivolumab + platinum/pemetrexed or gemcitabine	7.2	23.0	32
		Platinum/pemetrexed or gemcitabine	5.5	16.7	37
KEYNOTE-189	Non-squamous	Pembrolizumab + platinum/pemetrexed	8.8	NR	57
		Placebo + platinum/pemetrexed	4.9	11.3	65
MYSTIC	PD-L1 ≥25%	Durvalumab	4.7	16.3	15
		Platinum/pemetrexed or gemcitabine or paclitaxel	5.4	12.9	35
	PD-L1 ≥25%	Durvalumab + tremilimumab	3.9	11.9	24
		Platinum/pemetrexed or gemcitabine or paclitaxel	5.4	12.9	35
	TMB ≥15 mut/Mb	Durvalumab + tremilimumab		16.5	24
		Platinum/pemetrexed or gemcitabine or paclitaxel		10.5	35

Abbreviations: AEs: adverse events; mOS: median overall survival; mPFS: median progression-free survival.

TABLE 7.5   Pivotal Phase III Immunotherapy Studies after First-Line Treatment

Trial	Stratifier	Treatment	mPFS (mo)	mOS (mo)	Treatment-related AEs, grade 3–5 (%)
Checkmate 017	Squamous	Nivolumab	3.5	9.2	7
		Docetaxel	2.8	6.0	55
Checkmate 057	Non-squamous	Nivolumab	2.3	12.2	10
		Docetaxel	4.2	9.4	54
KEYNOTE 10	PD-L1 ≥1%	Pembrolizumab 10[a]	4.0	12.7	16
		Pembrolizumab 2[a]	3.9	10.4	13
		Docetaxel	4.0	8.5	35
OAK	–	Atezolizumab	2.8	13.8	15
		Docetaxel	4.1	9.6	43

Note   [a]mg/kg

Squamous versus non-squamous histopathology

Many of the molecular driver mutations that can be targeted currently are found predominantly in adenocarcinomas, but this may change as drugs targeting specific SCC mutations are trialed. There are differences in the responses to immunotherapy across the subtypes, which may influence decision making. Also, some chemotherapy regimens, including pemetrexed, are preferred in non-squamous subtypes.

Number of sites of metastatic disease

Significant improvements in the identification of patients with oligometastatic disease (usually defined as those with fewer than five metastatic sites of disease) in the diagnostic pathway, largely by the widespread adoption of positron emission tomography/ computed tomography (PET-CT) together with refinements in minimally invasive surgical technique and improvements in systemic treatment options, have resulted in the more aggressive treatment of this subgroup of patients. This treatment usually involves radical treatment to both primary and metastatic site(s). There are prospective data to support the OS benefit of this approach.[26] However, much of the data collected in this and other trials was prior to the widespread adoption of immunotherapy, and so follow-on studies are required comparing ablative approaches with the continuation of modern systemic therapy regimens alone.

First-line systemic chemotherapy strategies

It would be useful to briefly highlight the current first-line, maintenance, and second-line treatment chemotherapeutic options, specifically for those patients in whom immunotherapy may not be a therapeutic option.

First-line platinum-doublet regimens showed a significant increase in objective response rates and a 5% absolute benefit in OS at 1 year in patients with a PS of 0 to 1. Cisplatin-containing regimens may confer a slight advantage in OS over carboplatin-containing regimens, especially in adenocarcinoma, but with more nausea and fatigue reported.[27] The optimal duration of treatment is unclear despite a number of randomized clinical trials having been set up to answer this question. Current standards are four to six cycles of platinum-doublet chemotherapy. For patients with non-squamous histology, treatment with platinum-pemetrexed (a multitargeted antifolate agent) should be considered. Other standard regimens used contain platinum in combination with third-generation agents such as gemcitabine, vinorelbine, paclitaxel, and docetaxel. Direct comparisons of the different combinations of these third-generation agents plus platinum have generally shown no obvious superiority.[28] Importantly, outcomes for patients with squamous histology were inferior with pemetrexed. The addition of targeted therapy with bevacizumab, a humanized monoclonal antibody that blocks the binding of all vascular endothelial growth factor A isoforms to the receptor, has been investigated, and conflicting results have been demonstrated, with a small OS benefit of this drug compared with carboplatin/paclitaxel in the ECOG 4599 Phase III study,[22] whereas the Phase III AVAiL trial[21] failed to confirm an OS benefit for bevacizumab in combination with gemcitabine–cisplatin compared with chemotherapy alone, and therefore, the addition of bevacizumab has not been universally adopted.

Both switch maintenance with a single non-cross-reactant agent and continuation maintenance of a single non-platinum agent following non-progression of four to six cycles of platinum-doublet chemotherapy have been investigated as strategies to prolong PFS and OS, with a maintenance pemetrexed approach widely adopted.[29,30] The strategy remains controversial, as the OS benefit is small, many patients in the control arms did not receive second-line therapy, and QoL due to toxicity may be of concern.

Second-line systemic chemotherapy regimens

Evidence for second-line chemotherapeutic options remains scant due to the historically poorer prognosis of those patients with advanced lung cancer. However, in selected adenocarcinoma patients without a targetable mutation, treatment with docetaxel and nintedanib has been shown to improve OS by approximately 2 months compared with docetaxel alone (12.6 vs. 10.3).[31]

Immunotherapeutics

In this landscape of stagnation of improvements in the treatment of advanced disease, there has been the relatively recent approval of monoclonal antibodies targeting programmed death 1 (PD-1) or its ligand programmed death ligand 1 (PD-L1). PD-1 blockade is postulated to work in the activation of T cells, i.e. to restore the immune function of exhausted T cells following extended or high levels of antigen exposure, as occurs, for example, in advanced lung cancer. This approach has significantly improved the treatment and outlook for patients with advanced NSCLC, particularly in patients without a targetable oncogene. The initial proof of principle that anti–PD-(L)1 antibodies could effectively harness the antitumor activity of T cells was demonstrated in patients with previously treated advanced NSCLC. Since then, these treatments have quickly moved to the first-line setting both as monotherapy and in combination with chemotherapy. Within less than a decade, immunotherapy has transformed from being largely dismissed to a near universal component of treatment of patients with advanced disease. Figure 7.1 provides a therapeutic algorithm in non-oncogene-addicted, or immunogenic, NSCLC.

First-line, PD-L1 ≥50%

The pivotal KEYNOTE-024 Phase III randomized study evaluated the administration of pembrolizumab 200 mg every 3 weeks versus platinum-based chemotherapy in treatment-naïve, advanced, ≥50% PD-L1 NSCLC, permitting crossover on progression. Median PFS was 10.3 months with pembrolizumab versus 6.0 months with chemotherapy, and the hazard ratio for disease progression or death was 0.50 (p < 0.001).[32] KEYNOTE-024 met its primary endpoint and, with significant improvement in OS, OS rates, and duration of response, has established a new standard of single agent pembrolizumab in those patients with PD-L1 expression >50%, though some clinicians may continue to advocate triplet regimens in patients with a greater burden of disease.[33] The IMpower150 trial, which did not specifically stratify patients according to PD-L1 status, showed significant improvements in progression-free and overall survival with atezolizumab plus bevacizumab, carboplatin and paclitaxel versus bevacizumab, and carboplatin and paclitaxel in chemotherapy-naïve patients with non-squamous NSCLC.[34] Of note, a subgroup analysis of IMpower150 showed that for those with EGFR mutations previously treated with targeted therapies, there was also a small OS benefit derived from the quadruplet regimen.[35] Clinician choice as to whether to opt for a quadruplet regimen may be linked to factors such as patient PS or contraindications to vascular endothelial growth factor (VEGFR)-targeted treatment. There are as yet no head-to-head comparisons of triplet versus quadruplet regimens.

First-line, PD-L1 0–49%

The subset analysis of those patients with PD-L1 expression between 1% and 49% enrolled within the similarly designed KEYNOTE-042 (PD-L1 >1%) showed that pembrolizumab outperformed standard doublet chemotherapy.[33] Because of the utilization of a subset analysis together with no chemotherapy combination comparator arm, health regulators are reluctant to license pembrolizumab monotherapy in the intermediate expressing subgroup. A couple of larger Phase III studies testing the combination of immunotherapy with chemotherapy in both advanced non-squamous (KEYNOTE-189) and squamous (KEYNOTE-407) carcinomas have made this approach standard of care in those patients with 0–49%PD-L1 expression (Figure 7.1). As earlier, the quadruplet regimen of atezolizumab, bevacizumab, and carboplatin plus paclitaxel may be favored in selected patients for reasons discussed previously, remembering that currently there are no trials comparing triplet with quadruplet regimens.

Second-line, PD-L1 >1%

Four Phase III studies (Table 7.4) in previously treated NSCLC had similar designs evaluating PD-(L)1 inhibitors versus standard of care (docetaxel) as second-line therapy among patients with advanced NSCLC and reached a similar conclusion that PD-(L)1 inhibitors improved OS.[33]

Encouragingly, long-term follow-up of the Phase I nivolumab study in patients with NSCLC shows a 5-year OS survival of 16%. This suggests that especially in those patients who may have more "immunogenic"-driven cancers, there is a hope of longer-term benefit.[36] However, there remains only a minority of patients who achieve this durable benefit from immunotherapy. Important questions remain about how treatment should be selected and managed for individual patients. Treatment approaches moving forward are likely to explore new biomarkers and combination approaches, but the challenges of selecting the patient who is likely to be able to tolerate the additional toxicity that such combination approaches may induce will be paramount in decision making.

Immune-related adverse events and their management

Increasing use of immune-checkpoint inhibitors has exposed a discrete group of immune-related adverse events (irAEs). Many of these are driven by the same immunologic mechanisms responsible for the drugs' therapeutic effects, namely blockade of inhibitory mechanisms that suppress the immune system and protect body tissues from an acute or chronic immune response.[37] Skin, gut, endocrine, lung, and musculoskeletal adverse events are relatively common, whereas cardiovascular, hematologic, renal, and neurologic adverse events occur much less frequently. Although the majority of irAEs are mild to moderate in severity, serious and occasionally life-threatening events are reported, with treatment-related deaths occurring in up to 2% of patients. irAEs typically have a delayed onset and prolonged duration compared with adverse events from chemotherapy, and effective management depends on early recognition and prompt intervention with immunomodulatory strategies.

Molecularly directed treatment of lung cancer

Significant advances have been made over the past 15 years in the identification of molecular changes that lead to the development of NSCLC. The term "driver" mutation was coined to describe a transforming somatic aberration. Such abnormalities usually constitutionally activate signaling pathways crucial for cell proliferation and survival and result in uninhibited tumor growth. This results in over-reliance or "addiction," usually by activation of receptor tyrosine kinases (RTKs). Around 50% of adenocarcinomas are underpinned by a druggable ("actionable") somatic aberration. A much smaller number have been identified in SCC. Such aberrations are usually mutually exclusive and can be therapeutically targeted to modify the natural history of the disease. Figure 7.2 depicts an algorithm for the treatment of oncogene-addicted lung cancer.

Since the groundbreaking work in the early 2000s that linked specific mutations in the tyrosine kinase domain of the EGFR gene to exceptional responses to EGFR tyrosine kinase inhibitors, personalized therapeutic approaches have dramatically changed the management of advanced NSCLC. This initial discovery inspired subsequent efforts to identify other actionable subsets, ultimately leading to approval of drugs targeting unique molecular drivers, including ALK, ROS1, and BRAF. With sequential use of increasingly potent targeted therapies, patients with NSCLC now live up to 3–4 years compared with 1 year for those without targetable mutations. However, despite these remarkable gains, targeted therapies rarely produce cures, and nearly all patients with NSCLC will eventually succumb to their disease. The insights gained in the development of resistance have inspired a new wave of therapeutic approaches that seek to bypass resistance mechanisms through early introduction of the most potent therapies and investigation of combination strategies.[38]

EGFR mutations and EGFR-targeted therapies

EGFR is a member of the human epidermal growth factor receptor 2 (HER2) family of transmembrane receptors and is overexpressed in the majority of lung cancers. EGFR-activating mutations are observed in approximately 15% to 20% of patients with non-small-cell lung cancer.

In 2004, three separate studies identified activating mutations in the tyrosine kinase domain (exons 18–21) of EGFR. Two common mutations (in-frame micro-deletions in exon 19 and the exon 21 L858R missense mutation) account for nearly 90% of all mutations observed. These mutations are associated with a marked response to the tyrosine kinase inhibitors (TKIs) erlotinib and gefitinib with an improved PFS from approximately 5 months with chemotherapy to 11 months. The remaining less frequent mutations include G719X (4%), L861X (1%), and S768I (1%) mutations, and exon 20 insertions (2%–9%) are associated with sensitivity, partial sensitivity, or primary EGFR TKI therapy resistance. EGFR mutation prevalence varies contingent on population, being more common in Southeast Asian patients, never-smokers, and women and having a prevalence of less than 15% in adenocarcinomas in European populations. These mutations occur almost exclusively in tumors that are TTF-1 positive. EGFR mutation seems prognostic compared with wild-type tumors with retrospective molecular analysis of the BR.21 trial of erlotinib versus placebo, demonstrating a superior OS for patients on placebo with EGFR mutations compared with wild-type patients.[39]

In those with an EGFR mutation, first-line treatment with an EGFR TKI drug (erlotinib, gefitinib or afatinib, dacomitinib, or osimertinib) has been shown to improve PFS and OS compared with chemotherapy, as has the addition of VEGFR2 inhibitor to erlotinib, which significantly improved PFS. Of relevance, the earlier first-generation TKIs have poorer central nervous system

(CNS) penetration.[40] OS data from these trials are confounded by subsequent treatment with EGFR TKI. Trials reporting QoL have demonstrated a marked benefit for EGFR TKI therapy. Unfortunately, resistance to treatment eventually develops. Mechanisms of resistance have been widely studied and usually involve T790M allele over-representation (resulting in a reduced gefitinib/erlotinib affinity) in approximately 50% of patients. Other mechanisms, such as MET or HER2 amplification or transformation to SCLC, have also been described. The cause for resistance in up to 15% of patients remains unknown.

The compound osimertinib is a third-generation TKI, which was granted Food and Drug Administration (FDA) approval in March 2017 based on targeting EGFR T790M resistance. The compound has received additional FDA and European Medicines Agency (EMA) approval as first-line therapy with improvement in PFS by suppressing the activating mutation and preventing the rise of the dominant resistance clone. Repeat tissue and plasma analyses on therapy have revealed insights into multiple mechanisms of resistance, including novel second site EGFR mutations, activated bypass pathways such as MET amplification, HER2 amplification, RAS mutations, BRAF mutations, PIK3CA mutations, and novel fusion events.[38] Strategies to understand and predict patterns of mutagenesis are still just beginning, and technologies to understand synthetically lethal dependencies and track cancer evolution through therapy are being explored. The expansion of combination therapies is aimed at targeting minimal residual disease and bypass pathways early based on projected resistance. Table 7.6 highlights differences in mechanisms of resistance to first- and second-generation EGFR inhibitors vs. osimertinib. In addition to standard chemotherapy, patients who become resistant to osimertinib now have the options of atezolizumab, bevacizumab, or carboplatin plus paclitaxel after a subgroup analysis of IMpower 150[35] demonstrated a small OS advantage in patients with EGFR-sensitizing mutations.

ALK translocations and inhibitors

ALK is a member of the insulin receptor superfamily of RTKs and is normally expressed only in the CNS in healthy adults, playing a role in neuronal cell differentiation. The ligand for ALK is not currently known, but binding leads to receptor dimerization and subsequent activation of a number of proliferative and pro-survival pathways such as mitogen-activated protein kinase (MAPK), PI3K, and JAK-STAT. Somatic ALK fusions with EML4 in NSCLC were first described in 2007. Subsequently, other ALK fusion partners have been reported. The fusion protein has an activated ALK, leading to ligand-independent dimerization and constitutive activation. ALK fusion proteins have been identified in approximately 2%–7% of adenocarcinomas, predominantly of

signet ring subtype. Clinically, these patients tend to be younger, are never-smokers, present with advanced disease, and have a high incidence of brain metastases.

In 2011, the FDA approved the first-generation ALK TKI crizotinib for treatment of chemotherapy-resistant ALK-rearranged NSCLC. Subsequent Phase III studies demonstrated that crizotinib was superior to chemotherapy in TKI-naïve patients across all lines of therapy. Despite durable responses, a majority of patients relapse within a year of initiating crizotinib. In the largest series to date evaluating molecular mediators of crizotinib resistance, acquired mutations in the ALK tyrosine kinase domain were detected in 20% of crizotinib-resistant clinical specimens, and ALK amplification was identified in 8% of resistant tumors.[41] In addition to these on-target mechanisms, off-target mechanisms (e.g., activation of EGFR and other bypass signaling pathways, epithelial-to-mesenchymal transformation, and SCLC transformation) have been described.

More potent and selective second-generation ALK TKIs (ceritinib, alectinib, and brigatinib) have been subsequently developed and approved for the treatment of crizotinib-refractory ALK-rearranged NSCLC. Second-generation ALK TKIs induce responses in approximately 50% of patients who have progressed on crizotinib and result in disease stabilization for the majority of remaining patients, confirming that ALK-rearranged NSCLCs that relapse on crizotinib remain addicted to ALK signaling. Interestingly, the structural differences of the second-generation ALK TKIs lead to distinct resistance profiles.[41] As a result, approximately 50% of tumors progressing on a second-generation ALK TKI will harbor an ALK resistance mutation, but the spectrum of resistance mutations differs for each TKI; the most common mutation encountered, ALKG1202R, is highly refractory and confers resistance to multiple second-generation TKIs. A recent Phase III trial comparing alectinib with crizotinib in the first-line setting demonstrated a markedly superior PFS with alectinib (34.8 months vs. 10.9 months), leading to approval of alectinib as first-line treatment. The highly potent and selective third-generation ALK TKI lorlatinib, a drug designed to overcome the ALK mutations implicated in first- and second-generation TKI resistance, continues to be developed within clinical trials. Lorlatinib is thought to have the potential to overcome all clinically observed single ALK resistance mutations, including the G1202R mutation.[38]

Other targetable molecular aberrations

ROS1 is another member of the insulin receptor superfamily of RTK with marked sequence homology to ALK. ROS1 is not expressed in the normal lung. Furthermore, the function of wild-type ROS1 is poorly understood, and the ligand is unknown. Several ROS1 fusion partners, the most frequent of which is CD74, have recently been identified in 1% to 2% of patients with NSCLC.[38] These lead to constitutive activation of RTKs and subsequent phosphorylation of MAPK, PI3K, and JAK-STAT. ROS1 fusions occur in a similar clinical population as ALK fusions. Crizotinib, a multitargeted TKI that potently targets ROS1, is the only currently approved therapy for treatment of ROS1-rearranged NSCLC. Approval was based on an expansion cohort of the PROFILE 1001 Phase I study, in which crizotinib induced an overall response rate of 72% with a PFS of 19.2 months. Despite impressive responses, most patients will relapse within 2 years, and in the largest cohort of crizotinib-resistant ROS1-rearranged NSCLC cases, most of the tumors harbored ROS1 mutations (i.e., on-target resistance). The most frequently observed resistance

TABLE 7.6   Commonest Mutations after Treatment with First-/Second-Generation TKIs and Third-Generation TKIs in EGFR-Mutant NSCLC

First- and Second-Generation	Third-Generation
T790M (60%)	T790M loss (30%)
Unknown (20%)	Unknown (30%)
HER2 amplification (10%)	MET amplification (15%)
MET amplification (3%)	PIK3CA (7%)
Small-cell transformation (4%)	KRAS (3%)
	HER2 amplification (2%)
	Small-cell transformation (5%)

mutation was the solvent front G2032R, which is analogous to ALKG1202R. The multitargeted TKI cabozantinib has preclinical activity against the solvent front mutations that have been identified in crizotinib resistance, including G2032R and D2033N. Lorlatinib is also a potent inhibitor of ROS1.

HER2 is a member of the c-ErbB family and is overexpressed in about 20% of NSCLCs. HER2 does not have a known ligand but is activated by dimerizing with other family members. Mutations in the HER2 tyrosine kinase domain are observed in about 2% of NSCLCs; they are more common in females, adenocarcinomas, and never-smokers.[38] They usually comprise in-frame insertions in exon 20 codons 774–781, resulting in increased adenosine triphosphate binding affinity, consequent phosphorylation of HER2/ EGFR3, and subsequent activation of the MAPK pathway. Retrospective analyses suggest that drugs such as trastuzumab or afatinib may be useful in this group of patients.

The Raf family (A-RAF, B-RAF, and C-RAF) of threonine kinases are implicated in a number of tumors, most commonly in melanoma. Three different loci for activating missense *BRAF* mutations (exons 11, 15, and V6000E) have been identified in around 5% of lung adenocarcinomas resulting in the activation of the MAPK pathway.[38] V600E accounts for around 60% of *BRAF* mutations and occurs mainly in adenocarcinomas with micropapillary features. It does not appear to be related to smoking status, but it is associated with an aggressive phenotype and a poor OS. *BRAF* TKIs (vemurafenib or dabrafenib) are active against V600E. Other *BRAF* missense mutations in exons 11 and 15 have been identified in adenocarcinomas and more rarely in SCCs. These lead to *BRAF* activation, possibly via conformal changes to the G loop or through loss of AKT inhibition due to conformal changes at the AKT phosphorylation site.

The small G protein RAS is a family of membrane-associated threonine kinases (N-Ras, H-Ras, and K-Ras), and when activated by growth factors, cytokines, and hormones, it leads to activation of the MAPK pathway via downstream activation of MEK. A somatic point mutation in *KRAS* was first identified in patients with adenocarcinoma almost 30 years ago, and subsequently, it was noted that these mutations occur in up to a quarter of NSCLCs, most commonly in codons 12 and 13, and less frequently in codon 61. *KRAS* mutations have been seen more frequently in women and in smokers. These point mutations result in impaired GTPase activity, leading to constitutive ligand-independent activation of *KRAS*. Over the years, the impact of *KRAS* mutations on survival has been investigated in a number of studies with mixed results. More recently, a large meta-analysis was conducted of 53 heterogeneous (both early- and advanced-disease) studies involving over 5000 patients, which was published between 1999 and 2003 and demonstrated that *KRAS* mutations were associated with a poor prognosis (hazard ratio, 1.4; 95% confidence interval, 1.18–1.65).[42] Despite this, some controversy remains; a prospective analysis of *KRAS* status and prognosis in 480 patients undergoing post-operative adjuvant radiotherapy or chemoradiotherapy did not identify *KRAS* mutations as being independently prognostic. Direct inhibition of mutant *KRAS* has proved clinically difficult; however, the discovery of an allosteric pocket of KRAS has led to the development of an allosteric G12C-mutant-specific inhibitor, which stabilizes KRAS in an inactive form and is moving into clinical development. For example, the KRAS inhibitor AMG 510 gave a response rate of 20% in heavily pretreated solid tumors (NCT03600883).

RET-rearrangements are seen in 1% to 2% of NSCLCs. The most frequent fusion partner is KIF5B (72%).[43] Although no drugs have been approved for RET-rearranged NSCLCs, several multitargeted RET inhibitors (cabozantinib, lenvatinib, and vandetanib) have been approved for medullary thyroid cancer, which commonly harbors activating RET point mutations. BLU-667 and LOXO-292 are newer compounds, which have demonstrated impressive activity and tolerability in early-phase studies of RET-rearrangement-positive NSCLC.

Various mutations in the PIK3A pathway or MET have also been identified but are not mutually exclusive. The role of these as driver mutations is uncertain, but they may be involved in resistance treatments. MET exon 14–skipping somatic mutations in splice sites of exon 14 promote RNA splicing–based skipping of MET exon 14, which increases MET stability by allowing the protein to escape from ubiquitin-mediated degradation. Genetic alterations leading to MET exon 14 skipping occur in approximately 2–3% of NSCLC and are particularly enriched in tumors with adenosquamous or sarcomatoid histology.[44] MET skipping alterations predict sensitivity to MET-directed drugs. For example, 10 (66%) of the first 15 patients treated with crizotinib in an expansion cohort of the PROFILE 1001 study achieved a response to therapy.

Management of small-cell lung cancer

SCLCs and large cell neuroendocrine tumors are both high-grade carcinomas of neuroendocrine origin. Both share similar gene expression profiles and have an aggressive clinical course, often presenting at an advanced stage with distant metastatic disease. Although they are initially very sensitive to both chemotherapy and radiotherapy, cure is rarely achieved, as rapid treatment-resistant relapse is common. Although progress has been made in understanding the molecular abnormalities that underpin these high-grade neuroendocrine malignancies, advances in clinical practice have not been forthcoming despite many trials, and prognosis has not changed significantly over the years. Without treatment, the median survival from diagnosis of SCLC is 6 weeks for patients with extensive disease and 12 weeks for limited disease.

Limited-stage

Thoracic radiotherapy and chemotherapy

Approximately a third of patients diagnosed with SCLC will have limited disease (T1-4 N1-3 M0) at diagnosis. Two meta-analyses comparing chemotherapy with chemotherapy plus radiotherapy have clearly demonstrated improved local tumor control (24% vs. 47%) and a significant survival advantage with bi-modality treatment (an absolute benefit of 5.4% at 3 years).

Four cycles of platinum-based combination regimens are standard of care due to increased response rates and improved OS; the most frequently used is cisplatin/carboplatin plus etoposide. Chemotherapy given as soon as possible after diagnosis is associated with improvement in QoL even where the treatment is palliative. Supportive treatment with granulocyte colony-stimulating factor reduces the depth and duration of neutropenia during standard chemotherapy for SCLC, leading to fewer infections and a higher proportion of patients receiving the planned dose on time.

A landmark trial in 1999 comparing concurrent cisplatin and etoposide with either 45 Gy radiotherapy given hyperfractionated (twice daily) or once daily demonstrated a 4 month improvement in median survival (23 vs. 19 months) and a 10% absolute improvement in survival at 5 years (26% vs. 16%) but with more frequent grade 3 esophagitis. Although this resulted in the acceptance of twice-daily concurrent chemotherapy as standard in parts of the United States and Europe, it has not been widely adopted in the United Kingdom. More recent studies have prospectively demonstrated that doses of 70 Gy delivered once daily over 7 weeks concurrently with chemotherapy are safe for patients with limited SCLC and a good PS,[45] but further randomized trials are required to demonstrate the superiority of higher doses of once-daily radiotherapy to the current standard of care.

Extensive-stage

For patients presenting with extensive-stage SCLC, first-line treatment with platinum-etoposide doublet chemotherapy had been the standard of care. However, recently, it has been demonstrated that atezolizumab added to the etoposide doublet demonstrated superior PFS and OS compared with chemotherapy alone.[46]

Chemotherapy following relapse

Despite dramatic responses to first-line therapy, the majority of SCLC patients relapse with chemo-resistant disease. In general, patients who develop disease progression more than 3 months from the completion of first-line therapy obtain the best results with second-line chemotherapy. Although second responses can be obtained by re-introducing the first-line regimen, particularly in patients with remissions of more than 6 months, the use of drugs that have not previously been used results in improved responses. O'Brien et al. randomized 141 patients with relapsed SCLC to receive oral topotecan or best supportive care (BSC) and demonstrated that topotecan extended survival (OS, 26 vs. 14 weeks) and improved QoL.[47] Intravenous topotecan has shown similar efficacy to cyclophosphamide, doxorubicin, and vincristine chemotherapy with a median survival of approximately 25 weeks. Recently, the combination of nivolumab and ipilimumab and nivolumab alone were shown to demonstrate antitumor activity in the relapsed setting with durable responses and manageable safety profiles in previously treated patients with SCLC.[48]

Prophylactic cranial irradiation

Up to 50% of SCLC patients achieving remission develop brain metastases within 2 years. A meta-analysis of 987 patients in seven randomized controlled trials comparing prophylactic cranial irradiation (PCI) with no PCI in patients with complete response following induction chemotherapy and limited-stage SCLC reported that survival was significantly increased in the patients receiving PCI, with a 16% reduction in risk of death and a 5.4% increase in survival at 3 years.[49] The risk of brain metastases was reduced by 54%. There was no significant difference between doses of radiation received, although there was a trend towards better survival in patients receiving higher radiation doses.

Patients with extensive-stage SCLC are unlikely to have a complete response to chemotherapy. Nonetheless, a 6 week improvement in OS and a significant reduction in symptomatic brain metastasis were reported in the EORTC randomized trial of PCI in patients with at least a partial response to chemotherapy.[49] More recently, patients without brain metastases randomized to PCI or observation showed no significant difference in survival.[50] Periodic magnetic resonance imaging of the head rather than PCI is therefore recommended in this patient population.

Management of CNS metastatic disease

The role of whole brain radiotherapy (WBRT) in the management of brain metastasis was called into question in 2016 by the QUARTZ study. This was a pragmatic randomized Phase III non-inferiority study comparing WBRT with BSC in patients with brain metastasis unsuitable for surgical resection or stereotactic radiosurgery (SRS). The study was slow to recruit, with the majority of patients PS 2, and did not show any difference in survival, QoL, or dexamethasone use between the groups. Median OS was only 9 weeks in both arms. Therefore, patients with a poor PS are not treated with WBRT, but there is probably a role for WBRT in patients with a good PS, particularly in the immunotherapy era, when brain metastasis should be treated before starting such therapy due to the risk of increased brain edema.

A few other pivotal studies have investigated the specific role of systemic therapy in patients with multiple brain metastases. It has been demonstrated that pemetrexed-cisplatin is an effective and well-tolerated regimen as first-line therapy for NSCLC patients with brain metastases. The BRAIN study demonstrated encouraging efficacy of bevacizumab with first-line paclitaxel and carboplatin in patients with NSCLC and asymptomatic, untreated brain metastases.

More specific targeting of brain metastases, including with SRS and newer-generation TKIs with better brain penetration, have resulted in significant improvements in PFS and OS in specific patient subpopulations. The adoption of SRS in the management of oligometastases to the brain has expanded, with some pivotal studies summarized in Table 7.7. SRS is currently commissioned

TABLE 7.7   **Summary of Randomized Trials Involving SRS and WBRT**

Trial	Patient Inclusion	% Single Brain Tumors	Primary Endpoint	Local Control (1 Year %)	Distant Control (1 Year %)	mOS (Months) (1 Year Rate)	Functional Outcomes
WBRT + SRS	1–3 brain metastases, KPS ≥70, maximum diameter 4 cm	56	Overall survival	82	NR	6.5	No difference in mental status
WBRT (RTOG 9508)		56		71		4.9	More patients' KPS improved with WBRT and SRS (12%) vs. WBRT alone (4%), $p = 0.03$
SRS	1–4 metastases, KPS ≥70, maximum diameter 3 cm	49	Brain tumor recurrence	72.5	36.3	28.4%	No difference in MMSE or neurologic functional preservation
SRS + WBRT (JRSOG99-1)		48		88.7	58.5	38.5% (NS)	
SRS	1–3 metastases, WHO performance status ≤2, stable disease or asymptomatic synchronous primary tumor	68	Duration of functional independence based on a WHO >2	69 (2 year)	52 (2 year)	10.9	No difference in time to WHO >2 in patients who had WBRT (10.0 months) vs. observation (9.5 months)
WBRT+SRS (EORTC 22952-26001)		66		81	67	10.7 (NS)	

Abbreviations: KPS: Karnofsky Performance Score; MMSE: Mini-Mental State Examination.

for <10 cc of disease independent of the number of lesions. In addition, there is evidence that after resection of brain metastases, SRS is important. Specifically, SRS of the surgical cavity in patients who have had complete resection of one, two, or three brain metastases significantly lowers local recurrence compared with that noted for observation alone.[51] Thus, the use of SRS after brain metastasis resection could be an alternative to WBRT. As described earlier, in those patients with oncogene-addicted disease, newer-generation TKIs have better CNS penetration with resulting improved CNS response rates.

Symptom control, prognostication, and increasing role of palliative care early in the cancer pathway

As chemotherapy and radiotherapy provide clinical benefit with an improvement in symptoms in the majority of patients with lung cancer, specialist palliative care has traditionally been reserved for the terminal stages of disease. However, the importance of early specialist palliative care intervention has been demonstrated in a randomized controlled study. Patients with advanced lung cancer undergoing active treatment were randomized between early and late palliative care support.[52] A significant improvement in QoL, a reduction in depressive symptoms, and less aggressive end-of-life care were observed in patients randomized to early palliative care. Importantly and perhaps surprisingly, despite similar chemotherapy uptake in both study arms, a significant improvement in OS was observed in patients receiving early specialist palliative care (11.6 vs. 8.9 months).

Specific symptoms can be improved with interventions including external-beam radiotherapy and endobronchial debulking or stenting, which can improve breathlessness associated with endobronchial obstruction. Pleural effusions can be relieved by drainage of fluid and pleurodesis to prevent re-accumulation. Immediate relief from symptoms of superior vena cava obstruction (SVCO) can be achieved by radiological stent insertion. Both denosumab and bisphosphonates improve pain and skeletal events resulting from bone metastases.

Future directions and questions to be addressed

Management options in special populations: The elderly and PS ≥2 population

Older patients often have considerable co-morbidity, the biology of their tumors may be different, and the physiological changes of ageing need to be considered. The evidence for the treatment of this population comes from trials designed for older patients and those in which no upper age was set and in which a subset analysis was performed; in these latter trials, it could be argued that the patients were highly selected. Separately, patients with poorer PS are often excluded from clinical trials, so evidence of the safety and efficacy of newer agents within health economic constraints is extremely limited. As immunotherapy uptake has exploded, and these agents are generally considered better tolerated, the number of trials addressing their value in this subpopulation is expanding.

Beyond consolidation durvalumab

A discrepancy between FDA and EMA durvalumab licensing and PACIFIC trial inclusion criteria with regard to specific PD-L1 cutoff points has created some conflict as to what

the eligibility criteria are in different countries. In the United Kingdom, a PD-L1 expression of >1% is required prior to Cancer Drugs Fund approval. It is still not clear whether PD-L1 expression is a relevant biomarker in Stage III disease.

In addition, just as neoadjuvant chemotherapy continues to divide health authority recommendations, the question must surely be raised as to whether giving upfront immunotherapy to selected patients prior to surgery may improve outcomes. There are arguments for a hypothesis that a neoadjuvant over an adjuvant immunotherapy approach may result in superior outcomes, including that the presence of the tumor may become a source of infiltrating immune cells and neoantigens. Neoadjuvant studies also permit the monitoring of molecular changes in sequential tumor samples. Trials addressing this question include the use of both pembrolizumab and nivolumab. One Phase II study is recruiting patients with NSCLC Stage II/III given two cycles of pembrolizumab (NCT03197467). In a similarly designed study, patients with untreated Stage I–IIIA NSCLC underwent neoadjuvant therapy with two cycles of nivolumab (NCT03732664). Results for both studies are pending.

Other important questions that remain include whether immunotherapy should be given together with radiotherapy and chemotherapy concomitantly or sequentially, and which is the optimal chemotherapy regimen to be given alongside it. Due to the significant improvements in OS observed in the PACIFIC trial, an important question is whether surgery will start to play a more niched role in the management of N2 disease.

Upfront treatment with newer-generation TKIs vs. sequential treatment

The third-generation EGFR inhibitor osimertinib, which was initially developed for T790M-mediated resistance, has now been approved for upfront use for EGFR-mutant NSCLCs. The longer PFS compared with first-generation EGFR inhibitors is probably the result of suppression of potential resistance by T790M clones, increased CNS penetration, and increased selectivity for the activating mutant over wild-type EGFR, allowing improved drug dosing while minimizing toxicity. Similarly, for ALK-rearranged NSCLC, alectinib has now supplanted the first-generation ALK inhibitor crizotinib as first-line treatment. Alectinib more potently suppresses ALK kinase activity and can overcome most crizotinib-resistant mutations. A recent retrospective analysis of a cohort of patients that received sequential treatment of crizotinib followed by alectinib reported a time to second progression of 22.6 months, which is considerably shorter than the PFS of 34.8 months of first-line alectinib in the ALEX study. Perhaps, upfront use of the most dynamic ALK inhibitor, lorlatinib, will be propelled into first-line use. Importantly, separately from the question of whether retrospective versus real-time head-to-head and first- versus third-generation studies would be required for licensing, regulators such as the National Institute for Health and Care Excellence will need to carefully peruse the evidence for the most cost-effective approach on a population level.

Immunotherapy in advanced disease: How to elevate the tail on the survival curve; beyond PD-L1 and TMB biomarkers

Long-term follow-up in the Phase I nivolumab study in patients with NSCLC shows a 5-year OS survival of 16%. The future focus in order to raise the tail on this survival curve must surely be not only duration of treatment and combination approaches but also how best to select patients for specific treatments. Other biomarkers of interest that are being developed over and above PD-L1 and TMB include infiltrating and circulating immune cell gene expression signatures, T cell repertoires, and specific bacterial colonization signatures within gut microbiome studies.

Tumor development is associated with the generation of an immunosuppressive tumor milieu, and therefore, consideration of the influence of multiple cell types, extracellular matrix, and metabolic mediators becomes important. Each of these components potentially represents a hurdle to T cells and their antitumor immune responses, which may also specifically be influenced by immunotherapy. Strategies to influence the tumor microenvironment are expanding and include the use of metabolic mediators such as epacadostat. In addition, adoptive T cell therapies are becoming increasingly relevant in clinical practice. Chimeric antigen receptors (CARs) are engineered antigen receptor proteins consisting of an antigen-binding region and T cell receptor (TCR) signaling domains. With this technology, T cells are genetically modified to express CARs, expanded ex vivo, and adoptively transferred to patients, acting to redirect T cells' effector functions upon binding to antigens on tumor cells. There are a number of trials being developed in lung cancer with these technologies.

The future clinical utility of immuno-oncology will probably be a more personalized treatment package taking into account the immune landscape, the immunogenicity of the tumor (TMB), and PD-L1. Mainstreaming of these tests into routine clinical practice will likely be significantly accelerated by the expansion of artificial intelligence into healthcare technology.

Key learning points

- Lung cancer remains the most common cancer worldwide after non-melanocytic skin cancer.
- Due to recently introduced lung cancer screening programs in the United States and Europe, there has been a significant improvement in the percentage of lung cancers diagnosed at earlier stages.
- The 2015 WHO classification of lung cancer encourages enhanced diagnostic precision made possible by the greater availability of immunohistochemistry and molecular techniques.
- The original TNM system adopted by the UICC was updated in 2018 (UICC version 8) and has yielded some important changes from the seventh edition.
- In Stage III disease, the practice-changing PACIFIC study showed a significant PFS and OS benefit when consolidation durvalumab, a PD-L1 inhibitor, was given post concomitant chemoradiotherapy.
- Improvements in molecular subtyping of NSCLC, with the upfront identification of oncogenic drivers and PD-L1 status, and in the availability of newer therapies including immunotherapies have resulted in the widespread adoption of a dichotomy of therapeutic approaches in advanced disease.
- In extensive-stage SCLC, the addition of atezolizumab to the carboplatin-etoposide doublet demonstrated superior PFS and OS compared with chemotherapy alone.

References

1. Lung cancer statistics [Internet]. Cancer Research UK. 2015 [cited 2019 Apr 28]. Available from: https://www.cancerresearchuk.org/health-professional/cancer-statistics/statistics-by-cancer-type/lung-cancer

2. NLCA annual report 2018 [Internet]. RCP London. 2019 [cited 2019 Jun 1]. Available from: https://www.rcplondon.ac.uk/projects/outputs/nlca-annual-report-2018

3. Newsom-Davis T. The route to diagnosis: emergency presentation of lung cancer. Lung Cancer Manage. 2017; 6(2):67–73.

4. Travis WD, Brambilla E, Nicholson AG et al. The 2015 World Health Organization classification of lung tumors: Impact of genetic, clinical and radiologic advances since the 2004 classification. J Thorac Oncol. 2015; 10(9):1243–60.

5. George J, Lim JS, Jang SJ et al. Comprehensive genomic profiles of small-cell lung cancer. Nature. 2015; 524(7563):47–53.

6. Cancer Genome Atlas Research Network. Comprehensive genomic characterization of squamous cell lung cancers. Nature. 2012; 489(7417):519–25.

7. Cancer Genome Atlas Research Network. Comprehensive molecular profiling of lung adenocarcinoma. Nature. 2014; 511(7511):543–50.

8. Pardoll DM. The blockade of immune checkpoints in cancer immunotherapy. Nat Rev Cancer. 2012; 12(4):252–64.

9. Aguiar PN Jr, De Mello RA, Hall P et al. PD-L1 expression as a predictive biomarker in advanced non-small-cell lung cancer: updated survival data. Immunotherapy. 2017; 9(6):499–506.

10. Tsao MS, Kerr KM, Kockx M et al. PD-L1 Immunohistochemistry comparability study in real-life clinical samples: Results of blueprint phase 2 project. J Thorac Oncol. 2018; 13(9):1302–11.

11. Rizvi NA, Hellmann MD, Snyder A et al. Cancer immunology. Mutational landscape determines sensitivity to PD-1 blockade in non-small cell lung cancer. Science. 2015; 348(6230):124–8.

12. Anagnostou V, Smith KN, Forde PM et al. Evolution of neoantigen landscape during immune checkpoint blockade in non-small cell lung cancer. Cancer Discov. 2017; 7(3):264–76.

13. National Lung Screening Trial Research Team, Church TR, Black WC et al. Results of initial low-dose computed tomographic screening for lung cancer. N Engl J Med. 2013; 368(21):1980–91.

14. De Koning H, Van Der Aalst C, Ten Haaf K, Oudkerk M. PL02.05 effects of volume CT lung cancer screening: Mortality results of the NELSON randomised-controlled population based trial. J Thorac Oncol. 2018; 13(10):S185.

15. Lim E, Baldwin D, Beckles M et al. Guidelines on the radical management of patients with lung cancer. Thorax. 2010; 65 Suppl 3:iii1–27.

16. Wang S, Wang X, Zhou Q et al. Stereotactic ablative radiotherapy versus lobectomy for stage I non-small cell lung cancer: A systematic review. Thorac Cancer. 2018; 9(3):337–47.

17. Saunders M, Dische S, Barrett A et al. Continuous, hyperfractionated, accelerated radiotherapy (CHART) versus conventional radiotherapy in non-small cell lung cancer: mature data from the randomised multicentre trial. CHART Steering committee. Radiother Oncol. 1999; 52(2):137–48.

18. Pignon J-P, Tribodet H, Scagliotti GV et al. Lung adjuvant cisplatin evaluation: a pooled analysis by the LACE Collaborative Group. J Clin Oncol. 2008; 26(21):3552–9.

19. Antonia SJ, Villegas A, Daniel D et al. Overall survival with durvalumab after chemoradiotherapy in stage III NSCLC. N Engl J Med. 2018; 379(24):2342–50.

20. Jeremić B. Induction therapies plus surgery versus exclusive radiochemotherapy in stage IIIA/N2 non-small cell lung cancer (NSCLC). Am J Clin Oncol. 2018; 41(3):267–73.

21. Reck M, von Pawel J, Zatloukal P et al. Overall survival with cisplatin-gemcitabine and bevacizumab or placebo as first-line therapy for nonsquamous non-small-cell lung cancer: results from a randomised phase III trial (AVAiL). Ann Oncol. 2010; 21(9):1804–9.

22. Sandler A, Gray R, Perry MC et al. Paclitaxel-carboplatin alone or with bevacizumab for non-small-cell lung cancer. N Engl J Med. 2006; 355(24):2542–50.

23. Zhu AX, Finn RS, Cattan S et al. KEYNOTE-224: Pembrolizumab in patients with advanced hepatocellular carcinoma previously treated with sorafenib. J Clin Orthod. 2018; 36(4_suppl):209.

24. Gonzalez-Cao M, Martinez-Picado J, Karachaliou N et al. Cancer immunotherapy of patients with HIV infection. Clin Transl Oncol. 2019; 21(6):713–20.

25. Kehl KL, Yang S, Awad MM et al. Pre-existing autoimmune disease and the risk of immune-related adverse events among patients receiving checkpoint inhibitors for cancer. *Cancer Immunol Immunother.* 2019; 68(6):917–26.

26. Gong H-Y, Wang Y, Han G, Song Q-B. Radiotherapy for oligometastatic tumor improved the prognosis of patients with non-small cell lung cancer (NSCLC). *Thorac Cancer.* 2019; 10(5):1136–40.

27. Ardizzoni A, Boni L, Tiseo M et al. Cisplatin- versus carboplatin-based chemotherapy in first-line treatment of advanced non-small-cell lung cancer: an individual patient data meta-analysis. *J Natl Cancer Inst.* 2007; 99(11):847–57.

28. Schiller JH, Harrington D, Belani CP et al. Comparison of four chemotherapy regimens for advanced non-small-cell lung cancer. *N Engl J Med.* 2002; 346(2):92–8.

29. Ciuleanu T, Brodowicz T, Zielinski C et al. Maintenance pemetrexed plus best supportive care versus placebo plus best supportive care for non-small-cell lung cancer: a randomised, double-blind, phase 3 study. *Lancet.* 2009; 374(9699):1432–40.

30. Paz-Ares L, de Marinis F, Dediu M et al. Maintenance therapy with pemetrexed plus best supportive care versus placebo plus best supportive care after induction therapy with pemetrexed plus cisplatin for advanced non-squamous non-small-cell lung cancer (PARAMOUNT): a double-blind, phase 3, randomised controlled trial. *Lancet Oncol.* 2012; 13(3):247–55.

31. Reck M, Kaiser R, Mellemgaard A et al. Docetaxel plus nintedanib versus docetaxel plus placebo in patients with previously treated non-small-cell lung cancer (LUME-Lung 1): a phase 3, double-blind, randomised controlled trial. *Lancet Oncol.* 20140; 15(2):143–55.

32. Reck M, Rodríguez-Abreu D, Robinson AG et al. Pembrolizumab versus chemotherapy for PD-L1-positive non-small-cell lung cancer. *N Engl J Med.* 2016; 375(19):1823–33.

33. Peters S, Reck M, Smit EF et al. How to make the best use of immunotherapy as first-line treatment for advanced/metastatic non-small-cell lung cancer. *Ann Oncol.* 2019; 30(6):884–96.

34. Socinski MA, Jotte RM, Cappuzzo F et al. Atezolizumab for first-line treatment of metastatic nonsquamous NSCLC. *N Engl J Med.* 2018; 378(24):2288–301.

35. Reck M, Mok TSK, Nishio M et al. Atezolizumab plus bevacizumab and chemotherapy in non-small-cell lung cancer (IMpower150): key subgroup analyses of patients with EGFR mutations or baseline liver metastases in a randomised, open-label phase 3 trial. *Lancet Respir Med.* 2019; 7(5):387–401.

36. Five-year Survival Rate For Nivolumab-treated Advanced Lung Cancer Patients Much Higher Than Historical Rate [Internet]. [cited 2019 May 11]. Available from: https://www.aacr.org/News room/Pages/News-Release-Detail.aspx?ItemID=1031

37. Puzanov I, Diab A, Abdallah K et al. Managing toxicities associated with immune checkpoint inhibitors: consensus recommendations from the society for immunotherapy of cancer (SITC) toxicity management working group. *J Immunother Cancer.* 2017; 5(1):95.

38. Yoda S, Dagogo-Jack I, Hata AN. Targeting oncogenic drivers in lung cancer: Recent progress, current challenges and future opportunities. *Pharmacol Ther.* 2019; 193:20–30.

39. Tsao M-S, Sakurada A, Cutz J-C et al. Erlotinib in lung cancer—Molecular and clinical predictors of outcome. *N Engl J Med.* 2005; 353(2):133–44.

40. Mok TS, Wu Y-L, Ahn M-J t al. Osimertinib or platinum-pemetrexed in EGFR T790M-positive lung cancer. *N Engl J Med.* 2017; 376(7):629–40.

41. Gainor JF, Dardaei L, Yoda S et al. Molecular mechanisms of resistance to first- and second-generation ALK inhibitors in ALK-rearranged lung cancer. *Cancer Discov.* 2016; 6(10): 1118–33.

42. Riely GJ, Marks J, Pao W. KRAS mutations in non-small cell lung cancer. *Proc Am Thorac Soc.* 2009; 6(2):201–5.

43. Gautschi O, Milia J, Filleron T et al. Targeting RET in patients with RET-rearranged lung cancers: Results from the global, multicenter RET registry. *J Clin Oncol.* 2017; 35(13):1403–10.

44. Schrock AB, Frampton GM, Suh J et al. Characterization of 298 patients with lung cancer harboring MET exon 14 skipping alterations. *J Thorac Oncol.* 2016; 11(9):1493–502.

45. Bogart JA, Herndon JE 2nd, Lyss AP et al. 70 Gy thoracic radiotherapy is feasible concurrent with chemotherapy for limited-stage small-cell lung cancer: analysis of cancer and leukemia group B study 39808. *Int J Radiat Oncol Biol Phys.* 2004; 59(2):460–8.

46. Horn L, Mansfield AS, Szczęsna A et al. First-line atezolizumab plus chemotherapy in extensive-stage small-cell lung cancer. *N Engl J Med.* 2018; 379(23):2220–9.

47. O'Brien M, Eckardt J, Ramlau R. Recent advances with topotecan in the treatment of lung cancer. *Oncologist.* 2007; 12(10):1194–204.

48. Antonia SJ, López-Martin JA, Bendell J et al. Nivolumab alone and nivolumab plus ipilimumab in recurrent small-cell lung cancer (CheckMate 032): a multicentre, open-label, phase 1/2 trial. *Lancet Oncol.* 2016; 17(7):883–95.

49. Hann CL, Rudin CM. Management of small-cell lung cancer: incremental changes but hope for the future. *Oncology.* 2008; 22(13):1486–92.

50. Takahashi T, Yamanaka T, Seto T et al. Prophylactic cranial irradiation versus observation in patients with extensive-disease small-cell lung cancer: a multicentre, randomised, open-label, phase 3 trial. *Lancet Oncol.* 2017; 18(5):663–71.

51. Mahajan A, Ahmed S, McAleer MF et al. Post-operative stereotactic radiosurgery versus observation for completely resected brain metastases: a single-centre, randomised, controlled, phase 3 trial. *Lancet Oncol.* 2017; 18(8):1040–8.

52. Temel JS, Greer JA, Muzikansky A et al. Early palliative care for patients with metastatic non-small-cell lung cancer. *N Engl J Med.* 2010; 363(8):733–42.

8 ESOPHAGEAL CANCER

Jennifer Kahan, Carys Morgan, Kieran Foley, and Thomas Crosby

Introduction

Carcinoma of the esophagus is the seventh most common cancer in the world, with an incidence of over half a million cases per year; it accounts for approximately 5% of cancer-related deaths and was responsible for one in every 20 cancer deaths in 2018.[1] Seventy percent of cases occur in men, and there is a twofold to threefold difference in incidence and mortality between the sexes.

There are two main histological subtypes of esophageal cancer (squamous cell and adenocarcinoma) with differing risk factors. There has been a rapid increase in the incidence of adenocarcinoma (AC) of the distal esophagus and gastro-esophageal junction (GEJ) in affluent Western populations, whereas on a worldwide basis, squamous cell carcinoma (SCC) of the upper esophagus remains the more common type. There is marked geographic variation in the incidence of both forms of the disease, reflecting the different etiological factors.[2,3]

Survival from esophageal cancer remains poor in part due to a high proportion of cases (about 70%) presenting with advanced stage disease. The overall 5- and 10-year survival rates are only around 13% and 10%, respectively.[4] Treatment of esophageal cancer is therefore challenging, and although there have been significant advances in surgical and radiotherapy (RT) techniques over the past 20 years, alongside the use of multimodality therapy, we are yet to see significant improvements in outcomes. Clinical research remains vital in order to elucidate the most effective treatments while minimizing the significant toxicities associated with some treatment modalities.

Epidemiology and etiological factors

The two main histological subtypes of esophageal cancer are adenocarcinoma seen in the distal esophagus, GEJ, and gastric cardia and SCC of the thoracic and cervical esophagus. During the past 50 years, there has been a change in the incidence of the two common histological subtypes in western populations. In the 1960s, 90% of cases were squamous carcinomas; but the rapid rise in adenocarcinomas of the lower esophagus and gastric cardia has reversed this.

Squamous cell carcinoma

Squamous carcinomas usually develop in the upper and middle third of the esophagus and occur most commonly in southeastern and central Asia, including China and Iran, and southern and eastern Africa, with reducing frequency in most western countries.

Squamous esophageal cancer shows greater geographical variation in incidence than any other cancer. Differences are found both between local areas of the same region and between different ethnic groups within regions. This suggests that environmental factors play an important part in its etiology. In the western population, the two major risk factors of smoking and excess alcohol ingestion are synergistic in effect[5]; the reduction in cigarette smoking is likely to be a significant factor in the fall in incidence. A diet low in fruit and green vegetables is associated with an increased risk. It is important to note that many of the risk factors for squamous carcinoma of the esophagus are associated with a lower socio-economic status[6] and an increased lifetime risk of 10–15% of other cancers of the aero-digestive tract.

In some geographical areas, high rates of disease have clear causal relationships with a particular risk factor: for example, the association with betel nut chewing in the Indian subcontinent,[7–9] ingestion of hot drinks like Mate in some South American countries,[10,11] and dietary factors such as a diet high in nitrosamines in areas like China.[12] In other parts of the world, the etiology is much less clear. The high incidence in parts of eastern and southern Africa is not well explained, and the disease is seen occurring often at much younger ages with less of a gender bias. Malawi has the highest incidence worldwide.[1] The true reason for this pattern has not been elucidated, although a number of possibilities are postulated, including exposure to chemical carcinogens and exposure to inhaled biomass smoke.[13] Infective causes such as an association with the HIV epidemic in sub-Saharan Africa do not appear to fully explain this pattern, with incidence rates stable despite the rise of HIV infection. In a recent review, the potential risk factors are considered, and ongoing work is needed in this area.[14] Of note, there have been many studies and meta-analyses investigating the association of human papillomavirus (HPV) infection with esophageal SCC. Overall, it is likely that HPV infection is important in a subset of SCC of the esophagus, but the association is not as clear as that seen in cervical and oropharyngeal SCC. The prevalence of HPV infection in two large meta-analyses was 22–40%.[15]

Other known risk factors for esophageal SCC include structural abnormalities such as achalasia, which increases the risk up to 16-fold[16,17]; caustic strictures are also associated with SCC,[18] and Plummer–Vinson syndrome is a condition associated with esophageal web formation in the post cricoid region and with an increased risk of SCC.[19] Lastly, Tylosis palmaris (type A) is an autosomal dominant condition now known to be due to mutations in *RHBDF2* located on chromosome 17q25.1, and this condition leads to a very high lifetime risk of developing the disease (95% by the age of 70).[20]

Adenocarcinoma

The incidence of esophageal adenocarcinoma has increased in western Europe and North America around six-fold since 1975[3] and is highest in the United States and in Norway. There has been a similar increase in adenocarcinoma of the gastric cardia.

The major risk factors for adenocarcinoma are gastro-esophageal reflux disease (GERD),[21] obesity,[22,23] and Barrett's esophagus.[24] A Swedish case-controlled study suggested that people who had suffered from recurrent reflux 5 years earlier were nearly eight times more likely to develop adenocarcinoma of the esophagus than those who had not,[21] especially when symptoms were severe. This was regardless of whether Barrett's esophagus was also present.

Barrett's esophagus describes a process whereby an abnormal intestinal-type columnar epithelium replaces esophageal squamous epithelium damaged by refluxed gastric contents; this leads to an excess risk of developing an adenocarcinoma that may be 30–125 times the average for an age group. Gastro-esophageal reflux and Barrett's esophagus both occur with greatest frequency in white males.

Obesity is a strong risk factor, accounting for a threefold increase, but in contrast to SCC, cigarette smoking is associated with only a small increase in risk, and high alcohol consumption does not appear to influence the risk of developing the disease. The use of aspirin and other non-steroidal anti-inflammatories has been found to be protective, as has a diet high in fruit and vegetables.[25]

The most common site of esophageal adenocarcinoma is the GEJ. Adenocarcinomas are often associated with endoscopic evidence of Barrett's esophagus, where they may present as an ulcer or a mass, or there may be no endoscopic abnormality.[26] Early adenocarcinomas not associated with Barrett's esophagus usually arise from an ulcer, plaque, or nodule at the GEJ.[27]

See further Table 8.1.

Rarer histological subtypes

These include small-cell carcinomas, neuroendocrine tumors, gastrointestinal (GI) stromal tumors, melanomas, leiomyosarcomas, and adenoid cystic tumors. In general, the management of these cancers depends on the histological subtype rather than the tissue of origin.

Pathology

Apart from the clear histopathological differences between esophageal SCC and adenocarcinoma, two important pieces of work from The Cancer Genome Atlas project (TCGA) recently described the molecular and genomic features of esophageal and gastric cancer. In the case of esophageal cancer, a comprehensive molecular analysis of 164 esophageal cancer cases was carried out, and molecular subtypes were described.

Esophageal squamous carcinomas unsurprisingly were closer to squamous cancers seen in other organs such as head and neck or cervix. Three molecular subgroups of SCC were described, with frequent genomic amplifications of *CCND1* and *SOX2* and/or *TP63* seen.[28]

Junctional adenocarcinomas resembled the previously described chromosomally unstable variant (CIN) of gastric cancer, suggesting that this is one disease entity, although some

differences were identified, such as increased DNA hypermethylation in the esophageal adenocarcinomas. *ERBB2*, *VEGFA*, and *GATA4* and *GATA6* were also more commonly amplified.[29] The classification and understanding of the differences in pathophysiology may help in designing future studies and identifying new treatment approaches.

Barrett's esophagus is a premalignant condition associated with a 1% lifetime risk of developing esophageal adenocarcinoma. The squamous epithelium of the lower esophagus is damaged by reflux and replaced by a type of columnar epithelium resembling that seen in the stomach and intestine.

Barrett's esophagus may lead to the development of dysplasia, and tumors may arise in an associated ulcer or mass. The sequence from metaplasia through degrees of dysplasia to invasive adenocarcinoma is associated with genetic changes such as loss of *TP53* function, loss of heterozygosity of the *Rb* gene, overexpression of cyclins D1 and E, and inactivation of p16 and p27. Amplification of *MYC* and *K*- and *H-RAS* occurs late in the transition to adenocarcinoma. A high proportion of adenocarcinomas have foci of gastric- or intestinal-type lining in the immediate vicinity of the tumor and elsewhere in the esophagus.

Clinical presentation

Both adenocarcinomas and squamous cell carcinomas have similar clinical presentations.

Dysphagia due to obstruction of the esophagus by the tumor is the most common presenting symptom.[30] This is often progressive over some weeks to months, leading to alteration in diet and difficulty in managing solid foods. Often, at the time of diagnosis, the patient has made significant changes to their nutritional intake. This is often accompanied by weight loss, which may be exacerbated by the onset of tumor-related anorexia. Regurgitation of saliva, mucus, or food can also occur in patients with advanced disease.

A commonly used dysphagia grading system is helpful for assessment of progression of dysphagia and response to intervention, such as a stent.[31]

- Grade 1, patient has difficulty with some foods such as bread and meat.
- Grade 2, patient is able to eat a soft diet.
- Grade 3, patient only manages a liquid diet.
- Grade 4, complete dysphagia (including saliva).

TABLE 8.1 Risk Factors for Cancer of the Esophagus

Risk Factors	Squamous Cell	Adenocarcinomas
Social factors	Smoking	Obesity
	Excessive alcohol	Smoking
	Betel nut chewing	
	Lower socioeconomic status	
Dietary factors	Low fruit and green vegetables	
	High consumption of N-nitroso compounds	
	Ingestion of high-temperature drinks	
Associated conditions	Achalasia, associated with 16-fold increase in risk	Gastro-esophageal reflux
	Tylosis palmaris Type A may increase risk due to absence of tumor suppressor gene on 17q25.1	Barrett's esophagus
	Plummer–Vinson syndrome	
Associated infections	HPV	
	HIV	
Protective factors		Aspirin
		Diet high in fruit and vegetables

Patients may develop symptomatic lymphadenopathy, or widespread disease may be apparent on imaging. Lymphatic drainage follows the arterial supply, and thus, the upper third of the esophagus typically drains to the deep cervical lymph nodes, the middle third to posterior mediastinal lymph nodes, and the lower third to the left gastric and coeliac groups of lymph nodes. In addition to regional node spread, the rich submucosal plexus means that upper-third tumors can spread to coeliac nodes and lower-third to supraclavicular and deep cervical nodes in up to 30% of cases. This spread is classified as distant or M1 disease.

Distant metastases to the liver, bone, and lung are seen in nearly 30% of patients at diagnosis but are more common in gastroesophageal adenocarcinoma. In addition, bone marrow invasion can be detected in up to 40% of cases using immunohistochemical techniques.[32] Patients may present with symptoms of metastatic disease such as back pain, early satiety, upper abdominal fullness, or pain due to liver involvement or local infiltration.

Patients may describe pain, often a retrosternal discomfort, odynophagia, or a retrosternal burning sensation. Aspiration pneumonia is infrequent, and hoarseness may occur in locally advanced disease if the recurrent laryngeal nerve is invaded. Chronic GI blood loss from esophageal cancer is common, resulting in iron-deficiency anemia. However, patients seldom notice blood in regurgitated food. Frank hematemesis and melena are also uncommon.

Tracheo-bronchial fistula is a late complication of esophageal cancer. Fistulae are caused by direct invasion through the esophageal wall and into the main bronchi, presenting with intractable coughing or recurrent pneumonia, and in these cases, prognosis is usually very limited.

Diagnosis and staging

Diagnosis

Upper GI endoscopy is the initial investigation of choice in patients with dysphagia or aged 55 and over with weight loss and upper abdominal pain, reflux, or dyspepsia, and should be performed within 2 weeks of presentation (National Institute for Health and Clinical Excellence [NICE] 2017[33]). Early esophageal cancer may appear as a superficial plaque or ulceration and more advanced lesions as a stricture, an ulcerated mass, a circumferential mass or a large ulcer. Biopsy of the abnormal area provide the diagnosis in more than 90% of cases. Once carcinoma is histologically confirmed, the patient should be referred to an upper GI cancer multidisciplinary team (MDT) for appropriate treatment decisions and planning. MDT management has been associated with improved patient outcomes after cancer treatments.[34]

Staging

In common with many solid tumors, esophageal cancer is staged according to the Union of International Cancer Control (UICC) Tumour Node Metastasis (TNM) classification (see Table 8.2).[35]

Where possible, each patient is assigned a clinical stage (cTNM) for squamous cell carcinoma or for adenocarcinoma, which provides further prognostic information and guides management decisions (Table 8.3).

Staging modalities

Initially, patients with a confirmed diagnosis of esophageal cancer have a computed tomography (CT) examination of the thorax

TABLE 8.2   Definition of Primary Tumor/Regional Lymph Node/Distant Metastasis (TNM) Stages for Esophageal Cancers

stage	T	N	M
is	Carcinoma in situ	–	–
1	(Invasion of) lamina propria, muscularis mucosae, or submucosa	1–2 regional nodes	Distant
1a	Lamina propria or muscularis mucosae		
1b	Submucosa		
2	Muscularis propria	3–6 regional nodes	
3	Adventitia	7+ regional nodes	
4	Adjacent structures		
4a	Pleura, pericardium, azygos vein, diaphragm, or peritoneum		
4b	Adjacent structures (aorta, vertebral body, trachea)		

Source: Compiled from Sobin and Gospodarowicz, 2017.
Note: Additionally, Stage X indicates that a primary tumor cannot be assessed, and Stage 0 indicates no evidence of primary tumor.

TABLE 8.3A   Clinical Staging of SCC of the Esophagus

T	Tis	T1	T2	T3	T3	T1–3	T4	T1–4	T1–4
+N	N0	N0–1	N0–1	N0	N1	N2	N0–2	N3	N0–3
+M	M0	M0	M0	M0	M0	M0	M0	M0	M1
=cStage	0	I	II	II	III	III	IVA	IVA	IVB

Source: Data from Sobin and Gospodarowicz, 2017.

TABLE 8.3B   Clinical Staging of Adenocarcinomas of the Esophagus

T	Tis	T1	T1	T2	T2	T3–4a	T1–4a	T4b	T1–4	T1–4
+N	N0	N0	N1	N0	N1	N0–1	N2	N0–2	N3	N0–3
+M	M0	M0	M0	M0	M0	M0	M0	M0	M0	M1
=cStage	0	I	IIA	IIB	III	III	IVA	IVA	IVA	IVB

Source: Data from Sobin and Gospodarowicz, 2017.

and abdomen with intravenous (IV) contrast unless contraindications exist. The main purpose of this baseline staging CT is to assess for distant metastases, most commonly seen in the liver, lungs, peritoneum, or thoracic/abdominal lymph nodes.[36] Distant metastases currently preclude potentially curative treatment such as surgery or definitive chemoradiotherapy (dCRT). If the local disease is deemed un-resectable, then radical RT may still be considered.[37] Provided that the disease is potentially curable, patients are then referred for a positron emission tomography (PET) examination combined with CT (PET/CT).

Radioactive ^{18}F-fluorodeoxyglucose (^{18}F-FDG) is injected during PET/CT. The main advantage of PET/CT is the greater sensitivity for detecting distant metastases compared with contrast-enhanced CT (71% versus 52%, respectively).[38] PET/CT can change management decisions in up to 38% of patients.[33] Detecting distant metastatic disease is important, because patients can avoid undergoing major intervention when the chances of survival are poor. Quality of life must be considered, because surgical patients who die within 2 years of esophagectomy never fully regain their quality of life.[39]

Provided no distant metastases are detected, an endoscopic ultrasound (EUS) can be considered for locoregional staging. EUS is the superior imaging modality for T-staging, with studies describing accuracy of more than 80%.[40] Due to its superior contrast resolution, the individual layers of the esophageal wall are well visualized compared with CT and PET. EUS also benefits from temporal imaging, which is useful to assess adherence to adjacent structures, such as the descending aorta. EUS can detect small volumes of ascites and pericardial effusion, and if necessary, suspicious areas can be biopsied by fine-needle aspiration (FNA).[41] In about 30% of cases, the scope may not traverse a tumor-induced stenosis. In these cases, miniature EUS probes or a non-optical wire-guided echo endoscope may be helpful.[42]

However, N-staging of esophageal cancer is suboptimal. In general terms, all staging modalities tend to under-stage the number of involved lymph nodes.[43] In one meta-analysis, the sensitivity of CT, EUS, and PET/CT for the detection of lymph node metastases was 50%, 80%, and 57%, and the specificity was 83%, 70%, and 85%, respectively.[38] However, a recent radiological-pathological study revealed that a large proportion of lymph node metastases were classified as micro-metastases (82% measured less than 6 mm), which cannot be accurately detected on current imaging techniques.[43] Accurate N-staging remains a clinical challenge in esophageal cancer.

Less evidence exists for re-staging esophageal cancer after neoadjuvant treatment. The utility of PET response quantification has been investigated. The MUNICON-1 trial demonstrated that an SUV_{max} reduction of 35% after 2 weeks of neoadjuvant chemotherapy predicted response at the end of the 12-week cycle.[44] In addition, the trial showed that discontinuation of chemotherapy in metabolic non-responders did not affect their prognosis and prevented further exposure to potential side effects of treatment. Subsequently, the MUNICON-2 trial added RT to neoadjuvant chemotherapy in non-responders. The trial found that PET responders had improved 2-year overall survival compared to PET non-responders (71% vs. 42%), although this difference did not reach statistical significance ($p = 0.10$).[45]

In contrast, the value of EUS in re-staging esophageal cancer is doubtful. The accuracy of EUS post neoadjuvant therapy is poor (59% for both T-stage and N-stage) and does not accurately detect tumor down-staging even when a complete pathological response is achieved.[46] Accuracy is reasonable in patients with minimal tumor response but relatively poor in patients with a substantial local response, in whom fibrosis may be indistinguishable from residual tumor.[47]

Laparoscopy is an important final investigation for patients with apparently operable GEJ cancers, especially with disease extension below the diaphragm. Previously unrecognized peritoneal and liver metastases may be seen.

Treatment

Introduction

It is now clear that squamous cancers and adenocarcinomas should be considered separately and require differing approaches. For patients with adenocarcinomas (AC) that appear resectable and who are sufficiently fit, surgery remains the mainstay of therapy. Squamous cell carcinomas (SCC) are more often considered for definitive non-surgical management. Previous studies usually included both histological subtypes, leading to difficulty in determining optimum management within each cancer type. Additionally, the location of disease has an impact on treatment

options, patients with tumors of the upper third of the esophagus are usually offered non-surgical therapy in order to avoid the extensive surgery that would otherwise be required, while the treatment of Siewert type III junctional disease closely follows the management of gastric cancers.

We will consider the management of early disease, locally advanced disease, and advanced disease in turn, examining the evidence for a different management approach in SCC and AC.

All patients with esophageal cancer should be managed by an MDT to deliver the most appropriate treatment and support required. Co-morbidities, performance status, histological diagnosis, and stage of disease should be considered. Nutritional status should be addressed and dietetic support offered.

Barrett's esophagus

Barrett's esophagus is a precancerous condition characterized by abnormal replacement of the squamous epithelium of the lower esophagus by a columnar-type epithelium resembling that in the stomach and intestine. Barrett's esophagus may progress through a series of cellular changes of metaplasia, dysplasia, and neoplasia cumulating in esophageal AC. The intermediate stages of dysplasia can be graded into low-grade and high-grade dysplasia according to the degree of abnormal cellular architecture.

The true risk of progression from Barrett's esophagus to esophageal adenocarcinoma is difficult to accurately predict. In general, the higher the grade of dysplasia, the higher the risk of malignancy. Patients with no dysplasia but with intestinal metaplasia (abnormal epithelium but no evidence of dysplasia) would have the lowest risk.

The accurate classification of Barrett's esophagus is challenging; there may be sampling errors and inter-observer variation in biopsy interpretation leading to diagnostic misclassification.[48,49] Strategies to improve accurate classification include multiple biopsy sampling, diagnosis on at least two occasions, confirmation by two specialist histopathological experts, and confirmation by an independent pathologist with expertise in esophageal histopathology external to the original institution each time—all in the context of an MDT.

Screening and early detection

Currently, there are no simple, reliable, and cost-effective screening tests for esophageal cancer that have been adopted into clinical practice.

The evidence for endoscopic surveillance programs in patients with Barrett's esophagus is controversial. A large, population-based cohort study in Denmark surveilled over 11,000 patients diagnosed with Barrett's esophagus between 1992 and 2009. The overall incidence of AC was 2.9 cases per 1000 person-years, representing 7.6% of the total new cases of AC in the country. This equates to an annual risk of 0.12%, or one case of AC per 860 person-years. The authors concluded that routine surveillance of these patients is of doubtful value.[24] However, given that surveillance correlates with earlier cancer detection and consequently improved survival, the British Society of Gastroenterology (BSG) recommends surveillance in these patients. This is the standard of care in the United Kingdom.[50]

There is interest in developing alternative, less invasive methods for screening. The Barrett's Esophagus Screening Trial 2 (BEST2)[51] was a multicenter case-control study evaluating a non-endoscopic immunocytological device, called a Cytosponge®, for Barrett's esophagus screening. The trial aimed to reduce the need for endoscopic assessment in low-risk patients with Barrett's esophagus.

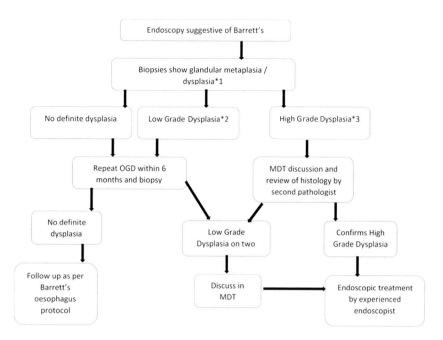

FIGURE 8.1 Management of Barrett's esophagus.

The specificity for diagnosing Barrett's esophagus was 92.4% with sensitivity of 79.9% (increasing to 87.2% in ≥3 cm lesions), and patients rated it favorably. The trial concluded that the Cytosponge-TFF3 test was safe and acceptable and had accuracy comparable to that of other screening tests.[51] Further development of such tools is likely, as they can pose a simple and inexpensive approach to diagnose Barrett's esophagus in patients with reflux symptoms who otherwise warrant endoscopy.

See further Figure 8.1.

Low-grade dysplasia

Low-grade dysplasia in the context of Barrett's esophagus can be treated with radiofrequency ablation or referral for endoscopic resection. This is provided patients are selected via an MDT experienced in managing Barrett's esophagus, and intervention should only be carried out by endoscopists experienced in treating Barrett's esophagus. Patients require long-term follow-up due to risk of recurrent disease.[48,49,50,52,53]

If the patient does not undergo endoscopic eradication therapy, surveillance endoscopy should be performed every 6 months for 1 year and then annually until there is reversion to non-dysplastic Barrett's.

There is as yet no adequate evidence on the efficacy and safety of endoscopic radiofrequency ablation for Barrett's esophagus without dysplasia; these cases should continue endoscopic follow-up.

Alternative methods to achieve eradication include photodynamic therapy, which can be considered for flat high-grade dysplasia. However, argon plasma coagulation, laser ablation, and multi-polar electrocoagulation are not recommended within NICE unless as part of a clinical trial.[49]

High-grade dysplasia

Endoscopic therapy can be considered as an alternative to esophagectomy for people with high-grade dysplasia and intramucosal cancer (T1a), taking into account individual patient preferences and general health. Endoscopic therapy is particularly suitable for patients who are considered unsuitable for surgery or who do not wish to undergo esophagectomy.[49] These techniques are discussed in detail later. In addition to endoscopic mucosal resection, ablative therapy should be considered, e.g. radiofrequency ablation, to completely remove residual flat dysplasia, taking into consideration the side-effect profiles[49] (Figure 8.1).

1) If no dysplasia is found on biopsy, a repeat biopsy is required after 6 months of maximal acid suppression. Two pathologists, ideally in different centers, should review any biopsies.
2) If low-grade dysplasia is identified at two separate endoscopies, options for treatment should be discussed at MDT.
3) High-grade dysplasia confirmed by two pathologists should be discussed at MDT and offered endoscopic therapy at an experienced center.

Early/locoregional disease (T1-2, N0, M0)

Early disease includes patients with a T1–T2 tumor and no evidence of nodal involvement or metastasis (N0, M0) on appropriate staging investigations. In patients who are fit, operative management is usually the treatment of choice.

The role of preoperative treatment in early, localized disease is uncertain. A randomized controlled trial (RCT) of 195 patients with early (Stage I and II) esophageal cancer showed that the addition of neoadjuvant CRT with cisplatin and fluorouracil did not improve R0 resection rates or survival and in fact, worsened postoperative mortality.[54] A retrospective multicenter European study showed that the addition of neoadjuvant therapy had no effect upon survival or recurrence, and no significant difference was observed between groups in terms of morbidity and mortality. Nodal disease was observed in 50% of patients at the time of surgery, with 20% of patients having pN2/N3 disease.[55] Based on current evidence, early disease (cT2N0) should be managed with surgery alone despite the high rate of nodal involvement.

Endoscopic treatment techniques

Endoscopic treatment options such as endoscopic mucosal resection (EMR) and endoscopic submucosal dissection (ESD) may be the preferred management of T1a disease. These were originally used in the management of premalignant disease such as high-grade dysplasia but are also well-tolerated and effective treatments for superficial early esophageal malignancy.[56] Circumferential EMR should be carefully considered, as there is a high incidence of stricture formation.

- EMR: Endoscopic mucosal resection
  - EMR is an endoscopic approach in which the neoplastic epithelium is excised, thus allowing a definitive histologic diagnosis.
  - Techniques may involve submucosal injection to separate mucosal and submucosal lesions from the muscularis propria and then suctioning to lift and cut the lesion.
  - There are various indications, including dysplastic Barrett's and early esophageal cancers (T1a) as well as large bowel lesions such as sessile colonic neoplasms.
- ESD: Endoscopic submucosal dissection
  - A specialist endoscopy technique that uses a modified needle knife (ESD-knife) to remove the lesion by dissecting through the submucosa, thus removing mucosal and submucosal tumors *en bloc* irrespective of the size of the lesion.
  - ESD has been found to improve *en bloc* curative resection and local recurrence rates compared with EMR but was more time-consuming and had higher rates of bleeding and perforation complications.[57,58] Indications include tumors of the upper GI tract, from the esophagus to the duodenum.
- Radiofrequency ablation
  - A bipolar electrode is used to ablate areas of dysplasia.
  - Highly effective in ablating Barrett's mucosa and associated dysplasia and in preventing progression of disease.
  - Does not have the same risks as photodynamic therapy and argon plasma coagulation, which are associated with esophageal stenosis and sub-squamous foci of Barrett's esophagus ("buried Barrett's").[49,50]

Endoscopic management is reserved for tumors that are small (<2 cm), non-ulcerating, well-differentiated, and involving less than 1/3 of the esophageal circumference. It is reported that endoscopic management has comparable cure rates to surgical resection for T1a adenocarcinomas in specialist centers.[59] Although the risk of lymph node metastases increases significantly when the submucosa is invaded, low-risk superficial T1b tumors may also be treated by endoscopic means.

In the squamous epithelium, only high-grade intraepithelial neoplasia or carcinomas of T1a affecting the mucosa without other risk factors (i.e. no lymphatic vessel invasion [L0], no venous invasion [V0], no ulceration G1/2, mucosa infiltration grade m1 or m2) are considered for endoscopic management. ESD would be a preferred treatment, as the likelihood of both *en bloc* resection and R0 resection is higher with ESD than with EMR.[58]

All endoscopically resected specimens should be reviewed by a specialist pathologist and discussed at an expert MDT meeting. If an R1 resection is confirmed, further alternative treatments (i.e. surgery or CRT) should be offered.

Surgical management

Surgery is the mainstay of treatment for most patients with esophageal adenocarcinoma who have technically resectable disease and are medically fit. It is also an option for patients with squamous carcinomas of the mid-distal esophagus. However, only 30–40% of patients will have surgically resectable disease at presentation. There are a number of surgical approaches for local disease, which vary between centers and surgeons.

Total esophagectomy

A total esophagectomy is required for locoregional AC, but the exact surgical method varies between centers and surgeons. International multicenter studies suggest that surgery should be provided in specialist high-volume treatment centers, which have lower morbidity rates and better infrastructure to deal with complications.[55,60]

Many surgeons, particularly in the United Kingdom, favor a two-stage radical transthoracic esophagectomy (Ivor Lewis approach). The stomach and coeliac nodes are mobilized via an abdominal incision, and the esophagus and mediastinal nodes via a right fifth interspace thoracotomy; the stomach and esophageal remnant are anastomosed. An alternative total thoracic, three-stage (McKeown) surgical approach can be adopted, when additional neck exploration and dissection are required.

Radical *en bloc* surgical resection and reconstruction involves thoracoabdominal resection that can include stomach, spleen, and removal of the posterior mediastinum. The stomach or colon is used to reconstruct the alimentary canal. This has greater complication rates, including necrosis or anastomotic leak, and necessitates a prolonged recovery.[61]

Both total and radical esophagectomy techniques have better survival outcomes than trans-hiatal esophagectomy. A trans-hiatal esophagectomy has less morbidity but higher rates of inadequate margins and local failure.[62] It is usually reserved for patients not fit enough to withstand more aggressive surgery. However, with the development of definitive non-surgical treatment options, surgery with a high failure rate may appear less favorable.

Pulmonary complications occur in more than half of patients after open esophagectomy; the development of minimally invasive and hybrid-minimally invasive esophagectomy aims to reduce surgical complications and improve recovery.

Two multicenter RCTs compared open transthoracic and minimally invasive transthoracic esophagectomy for resectable AC. They demonstrated reduced pulmonary complications and decreased perioperative morbidity, thus providing evidence for the short-term benefits of minimally invasive esophagectomy with decreased morbidity while preserving oncological effectiveness.[63] Laparoscopic gastric mobilization is now considered a standard procedure.[64]

There is uncertainty about the optimal surgical technique, although most specialist upper GI surgeons in the United Kingdom use a traditional or hybrid-minimally invasive assisted Ivor Lewis two-stage approach. If surgery is not possible due to feasibility, patient fitness, or patient preference, a definitive non-surgical treatment should be discussed. The combined treatment of CRT should be offered as a superior treatment over RT alone in those who are fit.

Minimizing operative risk

The combination of less invasive surgical techniques, better patient selection, extensive preoperative assessment, and enhanced postoperative care have led to a fall in postoperative complications.[63] Thirty-day mortality has reduced from 10.3% to 1.9% in the last few years in the United Kingdom.[65] However, 33% of patients suffered postoperative complications following esophagectomy. The majority (74%) of these complications were cardiopulmonary.

Risk factors for perioperative morbidity and mortality include poor cardiac and/or pulmonary function; advanced age; tumor stage; impaired general health, including diabetes mellitus and peripheral vascular disease; chronic use of steroids; and smoking.[66] Careful preoperative assessment includes optimization of risk factors and assessment of health reserves with techniques such as cardiopulmonary exercise (CPEX). CPEX is able to predict postoperative complications in other surgical specialties, and it is thought that the inability to deliver 800 ml min^{-1} m^{-2} oxygen and a lower anaerobic threshold (AT) correlate with increasing perioperative risks.[67]

Not only has patient selection improved, but the optimization of patients prior to surgery has also developed. This has been termed "prehabilitation." Following major surgical intervention, all patients experience an acute drop in physiological reserve/functional capacity followed by a recovery and rehabilitation phase. A low physiological reserve may increase the risk of perioperative complications and failure to complete full perioperative management. Therefore, the aim of prehabilitation is active preparation of patients to improve physiological reserve between surgical consultation and surgery, and it is based on physical management, nutritional care, and psychological preparation.[68] The PREHAB trial[69] aims to evaluate the efficacy of prehabilitation compared with conventional care in patients with gastroesophageal cancer with perioperative chemotherapy. While outcomes are awaited, all patients should receive dietician input and nutritional optimization with enteral or parenteral nutrition, as required.[70]

Enhanced Recovery After Surgery programs (ERAS/ERP) have resulted in improved short-term outcomes after surgery and have been widely integrated into surgico-oncological pathways. This has reduced length of stay and readmissions following surgery.

Locally advanced disease cT3-4 or cN1-3 M0

The vast majority of patients presenting with symptoms have locally advanced disease at the time of diagnosis. In locally advanced disease, surgery alone is not a recommended standard treatment. Surgery alone results in a failure to get clear resection margins (R0) in approximately 30% of T3 disease and 50% of T4 disease. There is clear evidence to support the use of preoperative and perioperative treatment to improve both R0 resection and survival in patients with operable locally advanced disease.

The use of definitive CRT (dCRT) should be offered to patients who are unfit for surgery and those who have disease that is not surgically resectable (e.g. T4 into aorta). Patients with locally advanced SCC should be offered definitive dCRT as an alternative to surgical management, as there are similar survival outcomes (see dCRT section).

Neoadjuvant/perioperative treatment
Pre/perioperative chemotherapy

The rationale behind neoadjuvant chemotherapy is to improve operability by tumor shrinkage and down-staging, which increases the likelihood of R0 resection, and simultaneously treating occult metastatic disease as early as possible. The disadvantage is that chemotherapy will delay surgery for non-responders

who will potentially progress and will also experience the side effects of neoadjuvant treatment without any benefit. This being said, neoadjuvant chemotherapy in both SCC and AC appears to achieve consistently good clinical response rates, ranging from 47% to 61%.[71]

There was initially uncertainty about the use of neoadjuvant treatment due to conflicting data from early studies. The U.S. Intergroup study[72] randomized patients to perioperative treatment with three cycles of cisplatin and 5-FU before and after surgery (if a response was seen) or surgery alone and found no significant survival difference (2-year survival of 35% versus 37%, p = NS). In contradiction to the Intergroup data, the U.K. MRC OE02 trial supported preoperative chemotherapy.[73] This study randomized 802 patients to two cycles of preoperative cisplatin and 5-FU or surgery alone and found a survival advantage at 2 years for patients who had preoperative therapy (43% versus 34%; p = 0.004). Both studies included both AC and SCC. This became standard of care in the United Kingdom and most European centers, but longer-term survival remained poor, with 5-year survival in this radically treated group of only 23%.

Subsequent meta-analysis also favored a small benefit to neoadjuvant chemotherapy with improvement in R0 resection and survival rates, although it was associated with some increased preoperative toxicity.[71,74–76]

There is much debate about the specific regimen that should be used pre/perioperatively in esophageal cancer. One approach is perioperative chemotherapy guided by the MAGIC[77] study, which was a gastric cancer study but also included resectable AC of the GEJ and the lower esophagus (25%). It demonstrated survival benefit with the use of a perioperative epirubicin, cisplatin, and continuous infusion 5-fluorouracil [5-FU] (ECF) chemotherapy regimen compared with surgery alone. In the intention-to-treat (ITT) analysis, patients who received perioperative chemotherapy had a 5-year survival of 36%, compared with 23% in patients treated with surgery alone. Progression-free survival (PFS) was also improved by perioperative chemotherapy.

The proportion of patients completing the postoperative chemotherapy in these studies was low, so interest arose in delivering more chemotherapy upfront as a neoadjuvant treatment. The MRC OE05 study[78] assessed whether increasing the duration of neoadjuvant chemotherapy in esophageal AC further improved survival when compared with the current standard regimen. Patients were recruited to either standard preoperative chemotherapy (as per OE02) or to four cycles of preoperative epirubicin, cisplatin and capecitabine (ECX). No significant benefit with additional chemotherapy was seen.

The MRC MAGIC-B/ST03[79] trial investigated the role of bevacizumab in combination with perioperative chemotherapy and also included those with junctional AC of the esophagus. This study found that the addition of bevacizumab in the unselected population did not improve overall survival (OS), and there were increased wound healing complications, including a higher anastomotic leak rate seen with bevacizumab in the junctional group.[79]

More recently, the FLOT-4 study was a practice-changing study of perioperative chemotherapy.[80] It randomized 716 patients with ≥T2 and/or clinically N+ gastroesophageal AC to receive either 5-FU 2600 mg/m^2 (24-hour infusion), leucoverin 200 mg/m^2, oxaliplatin 85 mg/m^2, docetaxel 50 mg/m^2 (FLOT) every 2 weeks, 4 cycles before and after surgery, or ECF/ECX 3 cycles before and after surgery. This demonstrated superior R0 resection rate, PFS, and OS with perioperative FLOT. Median OS of 50 months compared with 35 months with ECF/ECX was seen, and the 3-year OS rate was 57% versus 48%. FLOT also improved PFS, with a median PFS of 30 months compared with 18 months. There was more Grade 3 and 4 neutropenia in the FLOT arm, but it was otherwise reasonably well-tolerated, and this is now considered a regimen of choice.

Neoadjuvant chemoradiotherapy

An alternative approach to neoadjuvant/perioperative chemotherapy is the use of neoadjuvant CRT (nCRT).

In 2009, a Phase III trial reported outcomes of nCRT in GEJ tumors. It suggested postoperative mortality rates increased from 3.8% to 10% with the addition of CRT, despite an improved 3-year OS (27.7 vs. 47.4%).[81] This discouraged the widespread uptake of nCRT in Europe due to concerns regarding increased postoperative risk, although within North America, a preference for treating with nCRT remained.[76,82]

With ongoing advances in RT techniques and the widespread uptake of nCRT in other tumor sites, renewed interest in nCRT has led to increased research in this area.

A large Dutch RCT (CROSS Trial)[83] compared nCRT + surgery with surgery alone in 368 patients with locally advanced esophageal cancers T1N1 or T2–T3 N0. AC accounted for 75% of patients, SCC for 23%, and large cell undifferentiated cancers for 2%. The CRT arm received weekly carboplatin (AUC2) and paclitaxel for 5 weeks with concurrent RT (41.4 Gy in 23# 5 days a week) followed by surgery. Complete resection was found in 92% of the CRT group versus 69% in surgery alone ($p < 0.0001$), and a pathological complete response was achieved in 29% of patients receiving CRT. Reassuringly, the postoperative complications were similar in both arms, and in-hospital mortality was 4% for both groups. Median OS was statistically significant in the CRT group 49.4 months versus 24 months when patients received surgery alone.

NeoSCOPE was a U.K. trial examining oxaliplatin-capecitabine (OxCap) versus carboplatin-paclitaxel (CarPac) based nCRT with RT to a dose of 45 Gy in 25 fractions over 5 weeks. Both arms received induction OxCap chemotherapy (2×3 week cycles of oxaliplatin 130 mg/m^2 day 1, capecitabine 625 mg/m^2 bd days 1–21). Pathological complete response was seen in 29.3% and 11.1% CarPacRT and OxcapRT arms, respectively. Corresponding R0 resection rates were 80.5% and 72.2%, respectively. It concluded that while both regimens were well tolerated, only CarPacRT warranted further evaluation.

The exact optimal neoadjuvant or perioperative schedule treatment is still a controversial area for a number of reasons. Some earlier trials included patients with AC and SCC without adequate randomization to account for histological differences. There is no direct comparison of chemotherapy + surgery versus CRT + surgery, although currently, there are two studies in Europe comparing perioperative chemotherapy with neoadjuvant CRT in esophageal and junctional adenocarcinoma. The NeoAEGIS study[84] is currently recruiting patients and randomizing between perioperative chemotherapy (ECX or FLOT) and the CROSS regime, and the German trial ESOPEC[85] study has completed recruitment.

Definitive chemoradiotherapy (dCRT)

This is an option for patients with disease that is locally advanced and inoperable (T4b disease) in whom the disease can be encompassed in a radiation field. dCRT is also an option for those considered unfit for surgery. Patients with SCC should be offered dCRT as an alternative to surgical management, as similar survival outcomes are demonstrated.[70]

RT alone can be used for patients unfit for chemotherapy, although this is less effective as a single modality.[86,87]

RTOG 85-01 from the Radiation Therapy Oncology Group (RTOG) was the first study to show the benefit of combination therapy over RT alone. Patients were recruited between 1985 and 1990 and randomized between CRT and RT alone. The study included patients with both AC and SCC (although 90% were SCC) and T1–3 N0–1 M0 disease. In the CRT group ($n = 134$), patients received 50 Gy in 25 fractions over 5 weeks, plus four cycles of intravenous cisplatin and infusional fluorouracil. The RT alone group ($n = 62$) received 64 Gy in 32 fractions over 6.4 weeks. The trial stopped early, as interim analysis found significant benefit in the combined CRT group.[86] The long-term survival data at 5 years showed that the CRT group had OS of 26% (95% confidence interval 15–37%) compared with 0% following RT alone. A significantly better median survival (14 vs. 9.3 months) was also reported.[88] The comparative surgical survival rate at the time was 5–10% at 5 years.

The RT techniques of the time would now be considered outdated, but this trial led the way for the use of definitive CRT as a standard of care in the non-surgical management of locally advanced esophageal cancer. This approach was confirmed in a subsequent metanalysis.[89]

Within RTOG 85-01, there was a high locoregional failure rate (46% of patients in the CRT group had recurrence or persistence of disease in the esophagus at 12 months). A subsequent trial, INT 0123, compared escalated doses of RT in an aim to reduce local failure. Again, this included both AC and SCC and included concurrent chemotherapy with cisplatin and 5-FU (as in RTOG 85-01), but patients were randomized between 50.4 Gy and an escalated RT dose of 64.8 Gy (1.8 Gy per fraction, five fractions per week).[90]

Higher RT dose was not associated with a higher median survival (13 vs. 18 months) or lower incidence of locoregional persistent or recurrent disease (56% vs. 52%) in this study. In addition, the high-dose RT arm was also associated with significantly more toxicity and a higher rate of toxic deaths (9% vs. 2%). However, this study was carried out in the era before conformal three-dimensional RT and used techniques that are now outdated, which may in part explain the results. Locoregional recurrence remains high following dCRT, so dose escalation is now an area of interest once more with modern RT techniques and staging protocols.

The SCOPE 1 trial[91] was the first United Kingdom–based multicenter trial involving radiotherapy of the esophagus. It tested the addition of cetuximab to definitive CRT and included a comprehensive RT trials quality assurance (RTQA) program and detailed RT protocol. The trial reported that the use of cetuximab was associated with greater toxicity, lower doses of dCRT, and worse survival. Despite this, the overall disease control and OS in the standard dCRT arm were superior to any previous published multicenter studies, which was felt to be attributable to the standardization of high-quality RT with robust RTQA assessment. This study was pivotal in standardizing esophageal RT planning in the United Kingdom through its use of a trials quality assurance program, but it did not recommend cetuximab in combination with standard dCRT.[91]

The current U.K. dCRT trial, SCOPE 2, is assessing dose escalation in the era of modern radiation techniques, and in this study, volumetric modulated arc therapy (VMAT) is mandated with four-dimensional (4-D) CT planning and robust on-treatment verification, alongside a detailed RT protocol and QA program.[92]

There is interest in reducing toxicity and improving efficacy of chemotherapy used in dCRT, and alternatives to cisplatin-5FU have been explored.

A French intergroup study (PRODGE 5/ACCORD17) performed a Phase II/III study comparing the chemotherapy schedule folinic acid, 5-fluorouracil and oxaliplatin (FOLFOX4) with the standard RTOG regimen. In this study, 267 patients were randomized and six cycles of FOLFOX4 were used, three prior to RT and three concurrently with RT. Similar results were observed between treatment groups regarding clinical complete response rate (44% vs. 43%), PFS, and OS (median survival 20.2 vs. 17.5 months, survival rate at 3 years 19.9% vs. 26.9%, hazard ratio (HR) = 0.94, p = 0.70). Relative dose intensity of 5-FU and platinum was comparable in both treatment groups, as was the percentage of patients with premature stop of chemotherapy and overall toxicity. However, fewer toxic deaths occurred in the FOLFOX4 group compared with dCRT with cisplatin and 5-FU (1% vs. 6%).[93]

The neoadjuvant CROSS trial regimen used a weekly carboplatin-paclitaxel regime with neoadjuvant CRT. This was a well-tolerated regime and gained high acceptance in Europe, raising interest in investigating taxane-based chemotherapy with dCRT.

Definitive chemoradiotherapy regimens

The standard definitive treatment regimen involves four courses of platinum based chemotherapy (cisplatin or carboplatin if necessary) with a fluoropyrimidine combined with an RT dose of 50.4 Gy in 1.8 Gy fractions or 50 Gy in 25 fractions (2 Gy per fraction). An alternative regime involves six cycles of oxaliplatin/5-FU/folinic acid (FOLFOX).

The length of disease that is "encompassable" by a radiation field is a balance between achieving dose constraints to organs at risk and the chance of achieving clinical benefit over systemic therapy alone. The usual "accepted" maximum field length is 17–20 cm.

- Radiotherapy
  - Standard dose 50–54 Gy in 1.8–2 Gy fractions
- Concurrent chemotherapy
  - Standard regimen: four cycles platinum/fluoropyrimidine
  - Alternatives include FOLFOX and interest in weekly carboplatin/paclitaxel as per CROSS trial in definitive setting

dCRT in SCC

There are clear data that AC and SCC are different, with differing response to RT, and this led to specific trials to identify the optimum management of SCC.

Two Phase III studies have compared dCRT with a surgical approach (neoadjuvant CRT and surgery) in mainly squamous carcinomas. Stahl et al.[90] randomized 172 patients with locally advanced SCC of the esophagus to either induction chemotherapy followed by chemoradiotherapy (40 Gy) + surgery (arm A) or the same induction chemotherapy followed by chemoradiotherapy (at least 65 Gy) without surgery (arm B). Local PFS was better in the surgery group (2-year PFS, 64.3% versus 40.7%), but treatment-related mortality significantly increased in the surgery group compared with the CRT group (12.8% vs. 3.5%, respectively). This resulted in an equivalent OS between the two treatment groups. Stahl et al. concluded that the addition of surgery to CRT improves local tumor control but does not increase survival of patients with locally advanced esophageal SCC.

A further French study[54] also showed equivalent outcomes in SCC treated with dCRT compared with nCRT+ surgery. This study recruited 444 patients of SCC type. Survival times were comparable; early death was higher with surgery, as was local tumor control. A meta-analysis included six studies comparing definitive CRT with surgery in mainly SCC. Three of the studies were primary surgery alone with no preoperative treatment. It showed no difference in OS but a trend to more cancer-related deaths in the definitive (chemo-)radiation arms, predominantly due to a higher risk of locoregional progression, and more treatment-related deaths after surgery.[94]

These studies have led to the conclusion that dCRT is a valid option for locally advanced SCC of the esophagus and should be offered to patients alongside the surgical option. However, due to the higher local recurrence rate, patients fit for surgical salvage require appropriate and timely follow-up, including regular endoscopy with biopsies and CT imaging as standard.

> Definitive treatment options for locally advanced esophageal SCC include either, neoadjuvant CRT + surgery *or* dCRT + close surveillance (and salvage surgery if required).[56]

dCRT in AC

At present, there is less evidence for equivalence in AC, and indications for CRT include patients unfit for surgery or who choose non-surgical management and those with locally advanced inoperable disease. This would include T4b disease (involving aorta, trachea, heart, or great vessels) although not T4a (crura, pleura, or pericardium).

Summary of recommendations

Adenocarcinoma of the esophagus

Even accepting the limitations of current data, there appears to be a clear advantage to neoadjuvant treatment in locally advanced disease, and European Society for Medical Oncology (ESMO)[56] guidelines conclude that perioperative chemotherapy for a duration of 8–9 weeks in the preoperative phase (as well as 8–9 weeks in the postoperative phase if feasible) or preoperative CRT (41.4–50.5 Gy) should be considered standard in locally advanced AC of the esophagus and GEJ. The recent data on perioperative FLOT has now made this regime a standard of care for esophago-gastric junctional tumors.

Recommendation for management of adenocarcinomas:

- Direct comparison of nCRT and CRT is lacking, but trials are ongoing.
- Perioperative chemotherapy with FLOT or ECF is a current standard of care.
- Or nCRT 41.4–50.4 Gy in 1.8–2.0 Gy with weekly carboplatin-paclitaxel as per CROSS trial can be considered.
- In the event of complete clinical response, patients should still proceed to surgery.

Squamous cell cancers (SCC) of the esophagus

As mentioned earlier, the Intergroup, OE02, and CROSS studies included SCC. The proportion of patients with SCC in the CROSS trial was 23%. It compared nCRT + surgery with surgery alone and found a doubling of the median OS in the ITT analysis.

Trials comparing dCRT and CRT + surgery in SCC suggest equivalent OS[54,90] although noting that the non-operative strategy was associated with higher local tumor recurrence rates. Therefore, it is reasonable to offer nCRT and surgery or definitive CRT with close surveillance in these patients.[56] Consider salvage surgery for local tumor persistence or progression[95] in those who are fit enough. Both treatment options are recommended as definitive management options for locally advanced SCC of the esophagus. There are no randomized trials comparing nCRT + surgery versus definitive CRT and salvage surgery on demand.

Recommendations in the treatment of SCC:

- Surgery alone is not recommended in >T1b.
- Neoadjuvant chemotherapy and CRT in locally advanced disease
  - Increases R0 resection
  - Improves local control
  - Improves OS survival.
- CROSS indicated that CRT has superior outcomes to surgery alone.
- dCRT and CRT + surgery have equivalent OS outcomes.
- Definitive management options therefore include either nCRT + surgery or definitive CRT with close surveillance and consider salvage surgery for local tumor.

Postoperative adjuvant therapy

Adjuvant treatment following surgery is not usually the optimum treatment approach. Most evidence supports neoadjuvant or perioperative treatment (Table 8.4). In practical terms, postoperative treatment can be poorly tolerated following major surgery, with delays in commencing treatment and non-completion of treatment regimens, and RT fields are harder to define. A significant number of cases, however, are upstaged following pathological review, and in this situation, the options and evidence for adjuvant treatment are lacking, with varied practice and no clear consensus.

There is little evidence for adjuvant therapy for squamous carcinoma of the esophagus, although a single Japanese study compared adjuvant cisplatin and 5-FU with surgery alone, and the 5-year disease-free survival rate (the primary endpoint) was significantly better with chemotherapy (55% versus 45%), but OS was not significantly different (61% versus 52%).[96]

There are no randomized trials exploring the benefit of adjuvant chemotherapy (vs. surgery alone) in patients with esophageal or junctional AC, although a benefit has been suggested by a few non-randomized studies[97] and a large retrospective analysis.[98] There are studies of differing adjuvant chemotherapy regimens.

There are a number of adjuvant chemoradiotherapy gastric cancer studies. Some of these have included junctional AC. The U.S. Intergroup 0116 study[99] changed practice in the United States. Patients (n = 556) with resected T1–T4, N0, or N1 gastric or GEJ adenocarcinoma (20% of cases in this study) were randomly assigned to observation alone or adjuvant chemoradiotherapy. A regime of 45 Gy sandwiched between three cycles of Mayo Clinic schedule 5-FU was used. Three-year DFS and OS rates (50% versus 41%) were significantly better with combined-modality therapy in this study. Patients with GEJ tumors appeared to derive the same benefit. However, only 64% of all patients completed the planned treatment, and this trial has been criticized for inadequate surgical quality assurance, with a high proportion of D0 lymphadenectomies, leading to the suggestion that CRT made up for poor surgical technique. This approach became a standard for treatment of gastric cancer in the United States.

CALGB 80101 was also a mainly gastric study, which compared the Intergroup 0116 protocol with the addition of postoperative ECF before and after the concurrent RT. This study included completely resected T3 or node positive gastric or GEJ tumors (percentage unreported). Five-year OS was not significantly better with the addition of multi-agent chemotherapy[100] (44% in both groups) in this study.

In Europe, the Dutch CRITICS[101] trial enrolled some patients with proximal gastric and junctional tumors and compared perioperative chemotherapy with preoperative chemotherapy and adjuvant CRT. There was no significant difference in survival seen with multimodality treatment post-operatively in this group. Fewer than 50% completed the planned treatment, underlining the rationale for neoadjuvant treatment if possible.[101]

Available data has not conclusively resolved the issue of whether there is any benefit to adjuvant treatment in patients who have not received preoperative treatment, and an optimal regime has not been defined. Current ESMO guidelines suggest that adjuvant chemotherapy with or without radiotherapy is reasonable.

TABLE 8.4   Summary of Major Trials Investigating Neoadjuvant/Perioperative Treatment

Study	Tumor	Chemotherapy Regime	Outcome
US intergroup[72]	AC, SCC	3× cycles cis/5-FU vs. surgery alone peri-operatively (before and after surgery)	No difference in 2-year OS 35% versus 37%, p = NS
UK OE02[73]	AC, SCC	2× cycles cis/5-FU vs. surgery alone	Improved 2-year OS 43% versus 34%; p = 0.004
Dutch CROSS[83]	AC 75%, SCC 25%	CRT: 5 weeks of weekly carboplatin AUC 2 and paclitaxel concurrent RT (41.4 Gy in 23# 5 days a week) vs. no CRT	Median OS improved in CRT group 49.4 months versus surgery alone 24 months; p = 0.003
OE05[78]	AC	2× cycles cis/5-FU (as per OE02) vs. 4× ECX (epirubicin, cisplatin, and capecitabine)	Median survival was not improved by chemotherapy escalation: OS 23.4 months CF versus 26.1 months ECX
MAGIC[77]	AC, mainly gastric, 11% junctional tumors, 14% lower esophageal adenocarcinoma	3× ECX epirubicin, cisplatin, infusional 5-FU vs. surgery alone peri-operatively	5-year OS improved with neoadjuvant chemotherapy: 36%, versus 23% in surgery alone
FLOT[80]	Gastroesophageal AC >T2 and/or clinically N+	4 cycles FLOT (docetaxel, oxaliplatin, LV, 5-FU (24-hour infusion) every 2 weeks) vs. ECF peri-operatively	PFS of 30 months compared with 18 months Median OS of 50 months versus 35 months with ECF 3-year OS rate 57% versus 48%

Salvage surgery after definitive chemoradiotherapy

Local recurrence occurs within the first year in 10–30% of patients treated with dCRT.[36] For patients who would be considered suitable for salvage surgery, it is reasonable to offer regular radiological follow-up to identify early recurrence. Optimal surveillance strategies are an ongoing area of research, but current review may include 6-monthly imaging/esophago-gastro-duodenoscopy for 3 years and thereafter annually for up to 5 years. Salvage surgery may be considered depending on extent of disease and patient factors such as performance status and fitness for major surgery. Suitable patients should be discussed within an MDT. Patients will require repeat staging investigations including CT-PET and EUS prior to a decision regarding feasibility of surgery. Survival benefit is limited but has been shown in a large multicenter study suggesting that salvage surgery after dCRT can offer acceptable short- and long-term outcomes in selected patients at experienced centers.[95] Persistent cancer after dCRT seems to be more biologically aggressive, with poorer survival compared with recurrent cancer. The OS at 3 years was 40.9% in the resistant disease group and 56.2% in the recurrent disease group ($p = 0.046$). DFS again was lower in the resistant group (36.6% vs. 51.6%; $p = 0.095$), and such surgery is associated with an increased in-hospital mortality rate and increased morbidity. Informed discussion with patients of the potential high risks and poor outcomes is an integral part of the decision-making process for salvage surgery.

Management of the cervical esophagus

The cervical esophagus is 6–8 cm long and extends from the cricopharyngeus to the thoracic inlet, where it is contiguous with the thoracic esophagus. Carcinoma of the cervical esophagus, usually SCC, is relatively uncommon, accounting for fewer than 5% of all esophageal cancers.[102,103] Locally advanced disease is often present at diagnosis. In one report, tracheal invasion and vocal cord paralysis were evident in 35% and 24% of patients, respectively.[104]

Treatment choices include surgery, RT, and combined-modality treatment. Where surgical resection is required, a radical approach involving pharyngo-laryngo-esophagectomy and reconstruction is necessary. This includes removal of the thyroid gland usually involves a radical neck dissection.[105] Thus, the management of cervical esophageal cancers is more closely related to that of SCC of the head and neck than of malignancies of the more distal portions of the esophagus. This is major surgery and can be justified only for cases that have undergone the most careful selection and where suitable surgical and supportive care expertise is available.

CRT is generally preferred over surgery for disease in the cervical esophagus. Long-term outcomes appear similar between surgical and non-surgical management, and non-surgical management avoids extensive surgery with laryngectomy. In one series of 32 patients treated with CRT and salvage surgery, the 10-year survival rate was 27%, and 15 of the 32 patients successfully preserved their larynx.[106] Other studies have reported cases of potentially resectable cervical esophageal carcinomas treated initially with CRT or surgery and found no difference in 5-year OS, although almost a third of CRT patients required salvage surgery. They recommend that CRT is offered as a first-line treatment for larynx-preserving treatment.[107]

Complications of radiotherapy

Radiation esophagitis

Radiation esophagitis is common and develops in the second and third weeks of treatment. It is often perceived by patients as a sensation of obstruction, can vary in severity, and may require analgesia and a modification to the diet. A bismuth-chelating agent such as sucralfate may improve mucosal protection, but some patients prefer simple aspirin and hydrocortisone mucilage or its equivalent given orally. Radiation-induced esophagitis is exacerbated by concurrent chemotherapy, and robust nutritional and fluid support is often required to speed recovery in radically treated patients. All patients should have regular nutritional assessment and dietetic support before, during, and after treatment. Patients with significant dysphagia prior to treatment or those with significant weight loss or long radiation fields should be considered for prophylactic enteral feeding tube placement. A recent analysis of nutritional status and intervention within the SCOPE trial showed that pre-treatment assessment and correction of malnutrition can improve survival outcomes in patients treated with dCRT.[108]

Radiation pneumonitis

This may produce a dry cough even some months after treatment has been completed. It may be precipitated by intercurrent infection and may recur with subsequent infections. A hazy shadowing, corresponding to the boundaries of the radiation treatment fields, is sometimes seen on plain X-ray imaging. It may respond to soluble prednisolone (15 mg twice a day) and gradual tapering of the dose once symptoms have been controlled. Appropriate gastric protection is required when steroids are used.

Fistula formation

Broncho-esophageal fistulas may occur as a result of tumor that has invaded the tracheo-bronchial tree. Tumors thought to be invading in this way should only be irradiated with great caution, usually only after bronchoscopic assessment and if necessary, the placement of a covered stent. The incidence of fistula formation during CRT was 6% in one series[88] and accounted for one-half of all tracheo-esophageal fistulas in association with esophageal cancer. A fistula, when present, gives rise to explosive coughing and choking following a sip of water or any other fluid. For patients with persistent fistulas, symptomatic management may include covered airway and esophageal stents. In a similar manner, breakdown of tumor may occur where it is infiltrating large blood vessels, with disastrous results and catastrophic hemorrhage, which may be preceded by one or more minor episodes of hemoptysis. This is a rare phenomenon (despite the not uncommon finding of T4b disease) and needs to be weighed up with the risk of direct tumor invasion if not treated.

Late complications

The late complications of radical RT include mediastinal fibrosis and post-radiation stricture. The latter is managed by recurrent dilatations, although this poses a risk of perforation, and caution is always advised. It is important to consider frequent endoscopic dilatation for benign fibrotic strictures during the first 6 months post RT to prevent the development of late chronic stricturing. The prevalence of malignant and non-malignant post-RT strictures was roughly equal in one series.[89] The majority of patients with benign strictures were successfully dilated and had a 12-month survival rate of 88% compared with 19% for those with malignant strictures. Radiation damage to the spinal cord may occur where tolerance is exceeded, usually due to adverse patient geometry. This is very rare with modern planning and dosimetry. Palliative patients treated with opposed portals may occasionally experience transient radiation myelopathy with sensations such as electric shocks in the arms or legs following neck flexion (Lhermitte's sign). These symptoms are generally self-limiting without specific treatment.[95]

Advanced/metastatic disease

Palliation

Many patients will have advanced inoperable disease at diagnosis or are in poor physical condition, and definitive primary treatment is simply not appropriate. Some patients will receive radical treatment but will have resistant or recurrent disease (which may be local recurrence or distant metastatic spread). There are a number of treatments available for relief of symptoms, including endoscopic procedures, RT, and systemic therapies. The aim should be to prolong and maximize quality of life.

Management of dysphagia

Endoscopic stenting (self-expanding metal stents [SEMS]) can be used for relief of dysphagia secondary to luminal obstruction and are a quick and straightforward way of relieving malignant obstruction. This is an appropriate option up front for patients with dysphagia who are unlikely to proceed to other palliative therapies and may be offered prior to palliative chemotherapy where dysphagia is severe. There are complications, including discomfort, stent migration, perforation or malposition of the stent, and tumor overgrowth leading to further obstruction. In distal esophageal tumors, acid reflux can be problematic following stent placement. Stent placement therefore should be considered for Grade 3 or 4 dysphagia. Endoscopic dilatation will have limited efficacy in malignant obstruction, and relief of dysphagia is usually short lived.

Alternative treatment options include single dose intraluminal brachytherapy (even after previous external beam RT), which may help significantly with dysphagia.[109]

Palliative external beam radiotherapy can be offered to patients with symptomatic primary esophageal tumors in the context of metastatic or inoperable disease. Palliative dose and fractionation options are varied depending on patient fitness and extent of disease. It should be borne in mind that radiotherapy does not work immediately, and following treatment, it can take up to 6 weeks to see a benefit; therefore, severe symptoms or complete dysphagia are better managed with insertion of an esophageal stent if feasible. The addition of RT following insertion of an esophageal stent has recently been investigated in a randomized trial.[110] Results are awaited.

Palliative RT doses include:

30 Gy in 10 fractions treating daily for 2 weeks
20 Gy in five fractions treating daily for 1 week
8 Gy in a single fraction (used to gain hemostasis)
Higher-dose palliation: 40 Gy in 15 fractions over 3 weeks

Higher-dose palliative RT is sometimes appropriate to improve local symptoms, particularly in symptomatic disease of the upper third of the esophagus, where esophageal stenting is not an option. Dysphagia can be difficult to manage, and local invasion can lead to distressing symptoms. RT may also be used following palliative chemotherapy, particularly in patients with locally advanced disease. Further studies are needed to evaluate this approach, as additional benefit in terms of effect on survival or dysphagia-free survival is not clear.[111]

An international study of 220 patients assessed the benefit of palliative CRT compared with palliative RT alone for dysphagia. The addition of chemotherapy to palliative RT showed a non-significant improvement in dysphagia but at a cost of increased toxicity. This study suggested that a short course of RT alone can be considered a safe and well-tolerated treatment for malignant dysphagia in the palliative setting.[70]

It is essential to manage pain and nutrition in advanced disease. Occasionally, feeding options through a gastrostomy or jejunostomy can be provided to ensure adequate nutritional status when an esophageal stent is not possible. A careful deliberation of the holistic management of patients with poor prognosis is required prior to instigating enteral nutrition as part of supportive care. It is important to also ensure that patients receive social and psychological support by identifying and addressing the needs of the patients as well as their carers.[49,70]

Palliative chemotherapy

When choosing palliative systemic chemotherapy for patients with incurable esophageal or junctional cancers, the primary aim should be to improve or maintain quality of life. Improvements in outcome with more intensive chemotherapy regimens, such as docetaxel, cisplatin, and 5-FU, have been shown to be offset by significantly more toxicity.[64] Poor performance status, age <60, and metastatic disease were independent predictors of poor survival.[112]

In metastatic gastroesophageal AC, chemotherapy has been shown to be effective in improving symptoms and OS. Patients with good performance status can be offered combination chemotherapy. The use of a platinum-fluoropyrimidine doublet is regarded as standard of care for HER2-negative disease. HER2 (human epidermal growth factor receptor 2) testing should be offered to all patients with metastatic/advanced AC of the esophagus, and patients with HER2+ve disease should be treated with a trastuzumab-containing regimen (in combination with cisplatin and capecitabine or 5-FU).[56,70]

Research has established equivalence of the oral fluoropyrimidine, capecitabine, to 5-FU. A meta-analysis of the results of the REAL-2 and ML17032 trials demonstrated that capecitabine is non-inferior to 5-FU for OS and PFS in advanced esophagogastric cancer. Patients treated with capecitabine combinations were significantly more likely to have an objective response to treatment and superior OS. The REAL2 trial in addition compared oxaliplatin with cisplatin containing regimes and found that they were at least equivalent with respect to OS although with a different toxicity profile; hence, in the United Kingdom, oxaliplatin and capecitabine is most often used first line, as it is given as an outpatient regimen with less hydration required.

Currently, the only biologically targeted therapy in routine use in esophagogastric cancer is trastuzumab following the results of the Trastuzumab in Gastric Cancers (ToGA)[113] trial. The ToGA study was a large randomized controlled trial comparing trastuzumab with chemotherapy or chemotherapy alone. OS was improved to 13.8 months compared with 11.1 months with the addition of trastuzumab. The difference was most marked in those with tumors with the highest level of HER2 overexpression, where median OS was 16 months. The addition of alternative HER2 targeted treatments in first- and second-line settings (including TDM1,[114] pertuzumab,[115] and lapatanib[116]) has not been shown to be beneficial in studies to date.

Maintenance therapy following completion of first-line chemotherapy is currently the subject of a U.K. clinical trial. The PLATFORM study[117] is a multicenter trial with an adaptive design allowing new novel treatments to be added and ineffective ones to be discontinued as the study progresses. Currently, maintenance treatment is not recommended in HER2-negative disease.

Treatment of advanced disease in the elderly can be challenging, as patients are often frailer with more comorbidity, and the balance of risks and benefits of systemic anti-cancer therapy needs to be considered. A recently presented study (the GO2 study) found that frail and elderly patients with advanced gastroesophageal cancer may be safely and successfully treated with dose-reduced chemotherapy. In this Phase III trial, low doses of oxaliplatin/capecitabine performed similarly to intermediate and high doses of the regimen, with improved quality of life. The lowest dose offered was non-inferior in terms of PFS with less toxicity.[118] This may help decision making in this setting, where previous studies have excluded frailer patients.

Second-line chemotherapy is proven to prolong survival compared with best supportive care (BSC) in gastroesophageal AC.[119] Patients who had relapsed within 6 months of platinum-fluoropyrimidine chemotherapy with a good performance status were randomized to docetaxel or BSC in the COUGAR trial. OS improved to 5.5 months from 3.6 months, and docetaxel is recommended as an option for second-line treatment. An alternative is weekly paclitaxel.[120]

Biological agents

Genomic landscaping and detailed biological descriptions of esophago-gastric cancer are needed to aid the development of treatment options and treatment targeting. The complex and diverse biology of esophago-gastric cancer has meant that most studies using a non-selective approach to treatments have failed to show any benefit.

Biologically targeted drugs such as those targeting epidermal growth factor receptor (EGFR) overexpression have been evaluated in a number of studies. The EXPAND trial evaluated cetuximab + capecitabine or cisplatin for patients with locally advanced or metastatic AC of the GEJ or stomach. No benefit was seen in the unselected population.[121] Panitumumab in addition to chemotherapy was not beneficial in the REAL3 study.[122] The EGFR inhibitor gefitinib was not effective as a second-line treatment in esophageal cancer in unselected patients and did not improve OS. These studies have clearly demonstrated the need for identification of predictive biomarkers and the importance of translational work within ongoing studies.

Pathways of neoangiogenesis have also been considered as potential targets. Bevacizumab, a vascular endothelial growth factor A (VEGF-A) inhibitor, was evaluated in the AVAGAST study and did not lead to an improvement in OS in combination with chemotherapy.[123] Ramucirumab is a monoclonal antibody that binds VEGF2 receptors, and although it has a license for treatment of advanced gastric/GEJ tumors, it is not funded within the United Kingdom as monotherapy or in conjunction with chemotherapy. A large multicenter trial showed only a 2.66-month greater median OS with ramucirumab plus paclitaxel compared with placebo plus paclitaxel.[124] Although this is a small benefit, paclitaxel in combination with ramucirumab is an option for second-line therapy. The REGARD trial assessed ramucirumab as a single agent after platinum and fluoropyrimidine therapy, and improvements in median OS did reach significance (5.2 months for the ramucirumab arm vs. 3.8 months in the placebo arm).[125]

Additional biological targets undergoing investigation include c-MET, a transmembrane tyrosine kinase receptor associated with poorer survival when overexpressed, and the mTOR and PI3kinase pathway.

Immunotherapy

There are a number of studies on immunotherapy agents in the advanced setting with some mixed results. The recent Phase III KEYNOTE-181 study evaluated the anti–programmed death 1 (PD-1) antibody pembrolizumab compared with paclitaxel in the second-line setting for both esophageal AC and SCC. Those with

SCC appeared to benefit more from pembrolizumab than from paclitaxel. However, the survival benefits did not meet statistical significance.[126]

In the second-line setting for AC, the KEYNOTE-061 study compared pembrolizumab with paclitaxel, and in this study, the PD-1 inhibitor did not significantly improve OS compared with chemotherapy.[127] The Food and Drug Administration has therefore approved pembrolizumab for patients with advanced esophageal SCC that has progressed despite two or more lines of standard treatment in patients with a combined PD-L1 score of 10 or greater.

The use of first-line pembrolizumab in the KEYNOTE-062 trial was recently presented (ASCO 2019) and showed that for patients with (PD-L1)-positive, HER2-negative advanced gastric or junctional AC, first-line therapy with pembrolizumab resulted in non-inferior OS compared with standard chemotherapy. Additionally, treatment with pembrolizumab led to an improvement in OS among patients with tumors that had high levels of PD-L1 expression. In those with a PD-L1 expression >10, the median OS was 17.4 months with pembrolizumab and 10.8 months for those receiving chemotherapy. Two-year OS was 39% vs. 22% for standard chemotherapy. Because of the study design, this subgroup was not analyzed for statistical significance, but the data are encouraging.[128]

The anti-PD-1 monoclonal antibody nivolumab is licensed for treatment of chemo-refractory gastro-esophageal cancer in Japan, based on the results of the ATTRACTION-02 trial, which compared nivolumab with placebo after at least two lines of chemotherapy in three Asian countries. Patients treated with nivolumab had a significantly improved median OS (4.14 months with placebo to 5.32 months with nivolumab), and survival at 1 and 2 years more than doubled for patients who were treated with nivolumab (26.6% versus 10.9%). In non-Asian patients. the CheckMate 032 trial was a non-randomized Phase I/II trial of nivolumab monotherapy and combination nivolumab + ipilimumab (anti-CTLA4) in PD-L1-unselected gastro-esophageal cancer patients. Responses were observed in PD-L1-positive and negative tumors, and median OS for nivolumab-treated patients regardless of biomarker status was 6.2 months. Phase II data suggest a potential benefit in SCC, and further studies are needed in this area to elucidate which patients benefit and to assess future biomarkers. There are ongoing studies of combined immunotherapy and other immunotherapy agents in this setting.

Recommendations for management of metastatic esophageal carcinoma

First-line chemotherapy

- Request HER2 analysis if AC
- Offer entry to clinical trials where available
- HER2-positive AC:
  - Cisplatin and capecitabine or 5-FU in combination with trastuzumab for 4–6 cycles followed by maintenance trastuzumab until progression
- HER2-negative AC or SCC:
  - Doublet treatment: 5-FU or capecitabine in combination with cisplatin or oxaliplatin

Second-line palliative chemotherapy

- Docetaxel or weekly paclitaxel
- Weekly paclitaxel with ramucirumab (in AC)

Supportive measures

- Palliative care involvement and support
- Nutritional support and supplementary feeding
- Consider stent or palliative radiotherapy for malignant obstruction with dysphagia

Future improvements

While there have been improvements in treatment and outcomes for patients with esophageal cancer, these have been at a slower pace than seen in other cancer types, leading to this disease sometimes being labeled as "a cancer of unmet need."

Patients tend to present with advanced disease, in which objective responses are not commonly greater than 50%, survival is less than 12 months, and a significant proportion die within 3 months of starting palliative cytotoxic therapy, which has significant toxicities. Unfortunately, even the majority of those selected for potentially curative therapy do not have long-term disease control. There is therefore a need to focus not just on more effective treatments but also on reducing the use of ineffective treatment and selecting the right treatment for the right person.

Major improvements will come from prevention and early detection of the disease. Incidence can be reduced through public health measures to tackle known etiological factors, for example smoking cessation, reducing alcohol intake, changing methods of food processing and cooking, and developing national obesity strategies. Earlier detection will likely see the need for development of simple, low-cost, accessible, and acceptable triage tests using new technologies such as the Cytosponge or breath testing assays.

It is hoped that a better understanding of the genomic landscape of esophageal cancer will reveal driver mutations and actionable targets in the near future. The pace of these developments will depend on how well the clinical, science, and translational communities can work together to collect data, generate hypotheses, and test these in high-quality clinical studies.

The surgical community will focus on patient selection, the further role of minimal access approaches, and programs to reduce variation in surgical technical quality.

RT development will need to enhance precise delivery of treatments, incorporating imaging techniques (online imaging, 4-D planning) to allow for movement, and use new technologies such as proton beam therapies. Such new technologies may allow safe dose escalation, and current studies will determine whether these are more effective and associated with manageable toxicities. It is possible that dose escalation could be selected based on disease molecular profiles.

Systemic therapies will look to biological biomarkers to guide therapy but also to select those who are not likely to benefit, so that relatively ineffective treatment can be avoided. The role of immunotherapy will be thoroughly explored over the next decade, and how these agents work together with other cytotoxic and targeted agents and alongside localized treatments will be investigated. It will be important to incorporate the whole "multi-omic" platform as well as diagnostic and patient phenotypic information into a multi-parametric decision tool to select the right patient for the right treatment.

In addition, patients will need to be assessed using appropriate physiological and holistic needs assessments and supported through information provision. This will enable patients to be empowered to make the right decisions for themselves. Health optimization programs will be necessary to ensure that patients are prepared as well as possible mentally, psychologically, and physically to navigate their way through these complex treatment pathways.

With these approaches and the support of the clinical and scientific community, we are hopeful that significant improvements in the outcomes and experience of patients with esophageal cancer will be possible.

Key learning points

- SCC and AC of the esophagus/GEJ should be considered differing disease entities, and different management principles apply.
- Early T1a/b disease can be considered for endoscopic or surgical management in centralized, experienced centers, after discussion at specialist MDT.
- Locally advanced disease is managed with multimodality therapy, which may involve perioperative chemotherapy or nCRT and surgery. There is uncertainty regarding the optimal treatment. dCRT can be considered as a primary treatment option for SCC of the esophagus and for patients with AC who are unfit for surgery or with inoperable locally advanced disease.
- For squamous carcinomas, the addition of surgery to chemoradiotherapy improves local tumor control but does not increase survival of patients with locally advanced esophageal SCC.
- Involvement in clinical trials and RTQA has standardized esophageal radiotherapy planning in the United Kingdom, improving clinical outcomes, and with modern RT techniques (4-D planning/VMAT), dose escalation is being investigated.
- Platinum-fluoropyrimidine doublet chemotherapy remains the standard of care for metastatic disease with the addition of trastuzumab in AC with overexpression of HER2. Trials using biological therapies in unselected patients have not shown significant improvements in outcomes, and immunotherapies are being explored with mixed results to date.

References

1. Bray F, Ferlay J, Soerjomataram I, Siegel RL, Torre LA, Jemal A. Global cancer statistics 2018: GLOBOCAN estimates of incidence and mortality worldwide for 36 cancers in 185 countries. *CA: A Cancer Journal for Clinicians.* 2018; 68(6):394–424. doi:10.3322/caac.21492

2. Arnold M, Laversanne M, Brown LM, Devesa SS, Bray F. Predicting the future burden of esophageal cancer by histological subtype: International trends in incidence up to 2030. *Am J Gastroenterol.* 2017; 112(8):1247–1255. doi:10.1038/ajg.2017.155

3. Blot WJ, McLaughlin JK. The changing epidemiology of esophageal cancer. *Semin Oncol.* 1999; 26(5):2–8.

4. Cancer Research UK. Oesophagal cancer statistics. Accessed August 18, 2020. Available from: https://www.cancerresearchuk.org/health-professional/cancer-statistics/statistics-by-cancer-type/oesophageal-cancer

5. Pandeya N, Olsen CM, Whiteman DC. Sex differences in the proportion of esophageal squamous cell carcinoma cases attributable to tobacco smoking and alcohol consumption. *Cancer Epidemiol.* 2013; 37(5):579–584. doi:10.1016/j.canep.2013.05.011

6. Gammon MD, Schoenberg JB, Ahsan H et al. Tobacco, alcohol, and socioeconomic status and adenocarcinomas of the esophagus and gastric cardia. *J Natl Cancer Inst.* 1997; 3;89(17):1277–1284. doi:10.1093/jnci/89.17.1277

7. Phukan RK, Ali MS, Chetia CK, Mahanta J. Betel nut and tobacco chewing; potential risk factors of cancer of oesophagus in Assam, India. *Br J Cancer.* 2001; 85(5):661–667. doi:10.1054/bjoc.2001.1920

8. Wu MT, Lee YC, Chen CJ et al. Risk of betel chewing for oesophageal cancer in Taiwan. *Br J Cancer.* 2001; 85(5):658–660. doi:10.1054/bjoc.2001.1927

9. Akhtar S, Sheikh AA, Qureshi HU. Chewing areca nut, betel quid, oral snuff, cigarette smoking and the risk of oesophageal squamous-cell carcinoma in South Asians: A multicentre case-control study. *Eur J Cancer.* 2012; 48(5):655–661. doi:10.1016/j.ejca.2011.06.008

10. Victora CG, Muñoz N, Day NE et al. Hot beverages and oesophageal cancer in southern brazil: A case-control study. *Int J Cancer.* 1987; 39(6):710–716. doi:10.1002/ijc.2910390610

11. Okaru AO, Rullmann A, Farah A et al. Comparative oesophageal cancer risk assessment of hot beverage consumption (coffee, mate and tea): The margin of exposure of PAH vs. very hot temperatures. *BMC Cancer.* 2018. doi:10.1186/s12885-018-4060-z

12. Siddiqi M, Tricker AR, Preussmann R. The occurrence of preformed N-nitroso compounds in food samples from a high risk area of esophageal cancer in Kashmir, India. *Cancer Lett.* 1988. doi:10.1016/0304-3835(88)90038-9

13. Okello S, Akello SJ, Dwomoh E et al. Biomass fuel as a risk factor for esophageal squamous cell carcinoma: A systematic review and meta-analysis. *Environ Heal A Glob Access Sci Source.* 2019. doi:10.1186/s12940-019-0496-0

14. McCormack VA, Menya D, Munishi MO et al. Informing etiologic research priorities for squamous cell esophageal cancer in Africa: A review of setting-specific exposures to known and putative risk factors. *Int J Cancer.* 2017. doi:10.1002/ijc.30292

15. Hardefeldt HA, Cox MR, Eslick GD. Association between human papillomavirus (HPV) and oesophageal squamous cell carcinoma: A meta-Analysis. *Epidemiol Infect.* 2014. doi:10.1017/S0950268814000016

16. Leeuwenburgh I, Scholten P, Alderliesten J et al. Long-term esophageal cancer risk in patients with primary achalasia: A prospective study. *Am J Gastroenterol.* 2010. doi:10.1038/ajg.2010.263

17. Brücher BLDM, Stein HJ, Bartels H, Feussner H, Siewert JR. Achalasia and esophageal cancer: Incidence, prevalence, and prognosis. *World J Surg.* 2001. doi:10.1007/s00268-001-0026-3

18. Appelqvist P, Salmo M. Lye corrosion carcinoma of the esophagus. A review of 63 cases. *Cancer.* 1980. doi:10.1002/1097-0142(19800515)45:10<2655::AID-CNCR2820451028>3.0.CO;2-P

19. Aday U, Gündeş E, Ali Çetin D, Çiyiltepe H, Başak K, Duman M. Long-term evolution of squamous-cell cancer in Plummer-Vinson syndrome. *Prz Gastroenterol.* 2017; 12(3):226–228. doi:10.5114/pg.2017.70477

20. Iwaya T, Maesawa C, Ogasawara S, Tamura G. Tylosis esophageal cancer locus on chromosome 17q25.1 is commonly deleted in sporadic human esophageal cancer. *Gastroenterology.* 1998. doi:10.1016/S0016-5085(98)70426-3

21. Lagergren J, Bergström R, Lindgren A, Nyrén O. Symptomatic gastroesophageal reflux as a risk factor for esophageal adenocarcinoma. *N Engl J Med.* 1999; 340(11):825–31. doi:10.1056/NEJM199903183401101

22. Kubo A, Corley DA. Body mass index and adenocarcinomas of the esophagus or gastric cardia: A systematic review and meta-analysis. *Cancer Epidemiol Biomarkers Prev.* 2006. doi:10.1158/1055-9965.EPI-05-0860

23. Lagergren J, Bergström R, Nyrén O. Association between body mass and adenocarcinoma of the esophagus and gastric cardia. *Ann Intern Med.* 1999. doi:10.7326/0003-4819-130-11-199906010-00003

24. Hvid-Jensen F, Pedersen L, Drewes AM, Srøensen HT, Funch-Jensen P. Incidence of adenocarcinoma among patients with Barrett's esophagus. *N Engl J Med.* 2011. doi:10.1056/NEJMoa1103042

25. van den Brandt PA, Goldbohm RA, van 't Veer P et al. A large-scale prospective cohort study on diet and cancer in The Netherlands. *J Clin Epidemiol* 1990; 43:285–295.

26. Paraf F, Flejou JF, Pignon JP et al. Surgical pathology of adenocarcinoma arising in Barrett's esophagus. *Am J Surg Pathol.* 1995; 19:183–91.

27. Johansson J, Johnsson F, Walther B et al. Adenocarcinoma in the distal esophagus with and without Barrett's esophagus. Differences in symptoms and survival rates. *Arch Surg.* 1996; 131:708–13.

28. Kim J, Park YS, Bowlby R et al. Integrated genomic characterization of oesophageal carcinoma. *Nature.* 2017; 541(7636):169–74. doi:10.1038/nature20805

29. Bass AJ, Thorsson V, Shmulevich I et al. Comprehensive molecular characterization of gastric adenocarcinoma. *Nature* 2014. doi:10.1038/nature13480

30. Schlansky B, Dimarino AJ, Loren D, Infantolino A, Kowalski T, Cohen S. A survey of oesophageal cancer: Pathology, stage and clinical presentation. *Aliment Pharmacol Ther.* 2006; 23(5):587–93. doi:10.1111/j.1365-2036.2006.02782.x

31. Mellow MH, Pinkas H. Endoscopic laser therapy for malignancies affecting the esophagus and gastroesophageal junction: analysis of technical and functional efficacy. *Arch Intern Med.* 1985. doi:10.1001/archinte.1985.00360080117017

32. Thorban S, Roder JD, Nekarda H et al. Immunocytochemical detection of disseminated tumor cells in the bone marrow of patients with esophageal carcinoma. *J Natl Cancer Inst.* 1996; 88:1222–7.

33. National Institute of Clinical Excellence. Suspected cancer: recognition and referral NICE guideline [NG12]. Published date: June 23, 2015 Last updated: July 26, 2017. https://www.nice.org.uk/guidance/ng12

34. Stephens MR, Lewis WG, Brewster AE et al. Multidisciplinary team management is associated with improved outcomes after surgery for esophageal cancer. *Dis Esophagus.* 2006. doi:10.1111/j.1442-2050.2006.00559.x

35. Sobin LH, Gospodarowicz MK WC. UICC *TNM Classification of Malignant Tumours.* 8th ed. Oxford, UK: Wiley and Blackwell, 2017.

36. Allum WH, Blazeby JM, Griffin SM et al. Guidelines for the management of oesophageal and gastric cancer. *Gut.* 2011; 60(11):1449–72. doi:10.1136/gut.2010.228254

37. Crosby T, Hurt CN, Falk S et al. Chemoradiotherapy with or without cetuximab in patients with oesophageal cancer (SCOPE1): A multicentre, phase 2/3 randomised trial. *Lancet Oncol.* 2013; 14(7):627–37. doi:10.1016/S1470-2045(13)70136-0

38. van Vliet EPM, Heijenbrok-Kal MH, Hunink MGM, Kuipers EJ, Siersema PD. Staging investigations for oesophageal cancer: A meta-analysis. *Br J Cancer.* 2008; 98(3):547–57. doi:10.1038/sj.bjc.6604200

39. Blazeby JM, Farndon JR, Donovan J, Alderson D. A prospective longitudinal study examining the quality of life of patients with esophageal carcinoma. *Cancer.* 2000. doi:10.1002/(SICI)1097-0142(20000415)88:8<1781::AID-CNCR4>3.0.CO;2-G

40. Puli S-R, Reddy J-B, Bechtold M-L et al. Staging accuracy of esophageal cancer by endoscopic ultrasound: a meta-analysis and systematic review. *World J Gastroenterol.* 2008; 14(10):1479–90. doi:10.3748/wjg.14.1479

41. Vazquez-Sequeiros E, Norton ID, Clain JE et al. Impact of EUS-guided fine-needle aspiration on lymph node staging in patients with esophageal carcinoma. *Gastrointest Endosc.* 2001; 53(7):751–57. doi:10.1067/MGE.2001.112741

42. Morgan MA, Twine CP, Lewis WG et al. Prognostic significance of failure to cross esophageal tumors by endoluminal ultrasound. *Dis Esophagus.* 2008. doi:10.1111/j.1442-2050.2008.00809.x

43. Foley KG, Christian A, Fielding P, Lewis WG, Roberts SA. Accuracy of contemporary oesophageal cancer lymph node staging with radiological-pathological correlation. *Clin Radiol.* 2017. doi:10.1016/j.crad.2017.02.022

44. Javeri H, Xiao L, Rohren E et al. Influence of the baseline 18F-fluoro-2-deoxy-D-glucose positron emission tomography results on survival and pathologic response in patients with gastroesophageal cancer undergoing chemoradiation. *Cancer.* 2009.

45. Zum Büschenfelde CM, Herrmann K, Schuster T et al. 18 F-FDG PET-guided salvage neoadjuvant radiochemotherapy of adenocarcinoma of the esophagogastric junction: The MUNICON II trial. *J Nucl Med.* 2011. doi:10.2967/jnumed.110.085803

46. Bowrey DJ, Clark GWB, Roberts SA et al. Serial endoscopic ultrasound in the assessment of response to chemoradiotherapy for carcinoma of the esophagus. *J Gastrointest Surg.* 1999. doi:10.1016/S1091-255X(99)80098-5

47. Beseth BD, Bedford R, Isacoff WH, Holmes EC, Cameron RB. Endoscopic ultrasound does not accurately assess pathologic stage of esophageal cancer after neoadjuvant chemoradiotherapy. *Am Surg.* 2000.

48. Shaheen NJ, Falk GW, Iyer PG, Gerson LB. ACG clinical guideline: Diagnosis and management of Barrett's esophagus. *Am J Gastroenterol.* 2016. doi:10.1038/ajg.2015.322

49. NICE. *Barrett's Oesophagus: Ablative Therapy*, 2010. National Institute for Health and Care Excellence. https://www.nice.org.uk/guidance/cg106/resources/barretts-oesophagus-ablative-therapy-pdf-35109332329669.

50. Fitzgerald RC, Di Pietro M, Ragunath K et al. British Society of Gastroenterology guidelines on the diagnosis and management of Barrett's oesophagus. *Gut.* 2014. doi:10.1136/gutjnl-2013-305372

51. Ross-Innes CS, Debiram-Beecham I, O'Donovan M et al. Evaluation of a minimally invasive cell sampling device coupled with assessment of trefoil factor 3 expression for diagnosing Barrett's esophagus: A multi-center case–control study. *PLoS Med.* 2015. doi:10.1371/journal.pmed.1001780

52. di Pietro M, Fitzgerald RC. Revised British Society of Gastroenterology recommendation on the diagnosis and management of Barrett's oesophagus with low-grade dysplasia. *Gut.* 2018. doi:10.1136/gutjnl-2017-314135

53. American gastroenterological association medical position statement on the management of Barrett's esophagus. *Gastroenterology.* 2011. doi:10.1053/j.gastro.2011.01.030

54. Mariette C, Dahan L, Mornex F et al. Surgery alone versus chemoradiotherapy followed by surgery for stage I and II esophageal cancer: Final analysis of randomized controlled phase III trial FFCD 9901. *J Clin Oncol.* 2014. doi:10.1200/JCO.2013.53.6532

55. Markar SR, Gronnier C, Pasquer A et al. Role of neoadjuvant treatment in clinical T2N0M0 esophageal cancer: Results from a retrospective multi-center European study. *Eur J Cancer.* 2016. doi:10.1016/j.ejca.2015.11.024

56. Lordick F, Mariette C, Haustermans K, Obermannová R, Arnold D, on behalf of the ESMO Guidelines Committee clinicalguidelines@esmo org. Oesophageal cancer: ESMO clinical practice guidelines for diagnosis, treatment and follow-up. *Ann Oncol.* 2016. doi:10.1093/annonc/mdw329

57. Noordzij IC, Curvers WL, Schoon EJ. Endoscopic resection for early esophageal carcinoma. *J Thorac Dis.* 2019; 11(Suppl 5):S713–22. doi:10.21037/jtd.2019.03.19

58. Cao Y, Liao C, Tan A et al. Meta-analysis of endoscopic submucosal dissection versus endoscopic mucosal resection for tumors of the gastrointestinal tract. *Endoscopy.* 2009. doi:10.1055/s-0029-1215053

59. Pech O, Behrens A, May A et al. Long-term results and risk factor analysis for recurrence after curative endoscopic therapy in 349 patients with high-grade intraepithelial neoplasia and mucosal adenocarcinoma in Barrett's oesophagus. *Gut.* 2008. doi:10.1136/gut.2007.142539

60. Birkmeyer JD, Siewers AE, Finlayson EVA et al. Hospital volume and surgical mortality in the United States. *N Engl J Med.* 2002. doi:10.1056/NEJMsa012337

61. Collard JM, Otte JB, Fiasse R et al. Skeletonizing en bloc esophagectomy for cancer. *Ann Surg.* 2001. doi:10.1097/00000658-200107000-00005

62. Hulscher JBF, Van Sandick JW, De Boer AGEM et al. Extended transthoracic resection compared with limited transhiatal resection for adenocarcinoma of the esophagus. *N Engl J Med.* 2002. doi:10.1056/NEJMoa022343

63. Biere SSAY, Van Berge Henegouwen MI, Maas KW et al. Minimally invasive versus open oesophagectomy for patients with oesophageal cancer: A multicentre, open-label, randomised controlled trial. *Lancet.* 2012. doi:10.1016/S0140-6736(12)60516-9

64. Mariette C, Meunier B, Pezet D et al. Hybrid minimally invasive versus open oesophagectomy for patients with oesophageal cancer: A multicenter, open-label, randomized phase III controlled trial, the MIRO trial. *J Clin Oncol.* 2015. doi:10.1200/jco.2015.33.3_suppl.5

65. Maynard M, Chadwick G, Varagunam M et al. National oesophago-gastric cancer audit 2017. *R Coll Surg Engl.* 2017.

66. Durkin C, Schisler T, Lohser J. Current trends in anesthesia for esophagectomy. *Curr Opin Anaesthesiol.* 2017. doi:10.1097/ACO.0000000000000409

67. Howells P, Bieker M, Yeung J. Oesophageal cancer and the anaesthetist. *BJA Educ.* 2017. doi:10.1093/bjaed/mkw037

68. Tew GA, Ayyash R, Durrand J, Danjoux GR. Clinical guideline and recommendations on pre-operative exercise training in patients awaiting major non-cardiac surgery. *Anaesthesia.* 2018. doi:10.1111/anae.14177

69. Roy B Le, Pereira B, Bouteloup C et al. Effect of prehabilitation in gastro-oesophageal adenocarcinoma: Study protocol of a multicentric, randomised, control trial-the PREHAB study. *BMJ Open.* 2016. doi:10.1136/bmjopen-2016-012876

70. NICE guidelines. Oesophago-gastric cancer: assessment and management in adults. Published: January 24, 2018 http://www.nice.org.uk/guidance/ng83

71. Ronellenfitsch U, Schwarzbach M, Hofheinz R et al. Preoperative chemo(radio)therapy versus primary surgery for gastroesophageal adenocarcinoma: Systematic review with meta-analysis combining individual patient and aggregate data. *Eur J Cancer.* 2013. doi:10.1016/j.ejca.2013.05.029

72. Kelsen DP, Ginsberg R, Pajak TF et al. Chemotherapy followed by surgery compared with surgery alone for localized esophageal cancer. *N Engl J Med.* 1998. doi:10.1056/NEJM199812313392704

73. Girling DJ, Bancewicz J, Clark PI et al. Surgical resection with or without preoperative chemotherapy in oesophageal cancer: A randomised controlled trial. *Lancet.* 2002. doi:10.1016/S0140-6736(02)08651-8

74. Kranzfelder M, Schuster T, Geinitz H, Friess H, Büchler P. Meta-analysis of neoadjuvant treatment modalities and definitive non-surgical therapy for oesophageal squamous cell cancer. *Br J Surg.* 2011. doi:10.1002/bjs.7455

75. Allum WH, Stenning SP, Bancewicz J, Clark PI, Langley RE. Long-term results of a randomized trial of surgery with or without pre-operative chemotherapy in esophageal cancer. *J Clin Oncol.* 2009. doi:10.1200/JCO.2009.22.2083

76. Sjoquist KM, Burmeister BH, Smithers BM et al. Survival after neoadjuvant chemotherapy or chemoradiotherapy for resectable oesophageal carcinoma: An updated meta-analysis. *Lancet Oncol.* 2011. doi:10.1016/S1470-2045(11)70142-5

77. Chua YJ, Cunningham D. The UK NCRI MAGIC trial of perioperative chemotherapy in resectable gastric cancer: Implications for clinical practice. *Ann Surg Oncol.* 2007. doi:10.1245/s10434-007-9423-7

78. Alderson D, Cunningham D, Nankivell M et al. Neoadjuvant cisplatin and fluorouracil versus epirubicin, cisplatin, and capecitabine followed by resection in patients with oesophageal adenocarcinoma (UK MRC OE05): An open-label, randomised phase 3 trial. *Lancet Oncol.* 2017. doi:10.1016/S1470-2045(17)30447-3

79. Cunningham D, Stenning SP, Smyth EC et al. Peri-operative chemotherapy with or without bevacizumab in operable oesophagogastric adenocarcinoma (UK Medical Research Council ST03): Primary analysis results of a multicentre, open-label, randomised phase 2–3 trial. *Lancet Oncol.* 2017. doi:10.1016/S1470-2045(17)30043-8

80. Homann N, Pauligk C, Luley K et al. Pathological complete remission in patients with oesophagogastric cancer receiving preoperative 5-fluorouracil, oxaliplatin and docetaxel. *Int J Cancer.* 2012. doi:10.1002/ijc.26180

81. Stahl M, Walz MK, Stuschke M et al. Phase III comparison of preoperative chemotherapy compared with chemoradiotherapy in patients with locally advanced adenocarcinoma of the esophagogastric junction. *J Clin Oncol.* 2009. doi:10.1200/JCO.2008.17.0506

82. Walsh TN. Oesophageal cancer: Who needs neoadjuvant therapy? *Lancet Oncol.* 2011. doi:10.1016/S1470-2045(11)70158-9

83. Shapiro J, van Lanschot JJB, Hulshof MCCM et al. Neoadjuvant chemoradiotherapy plus surgery versus surgery alone for oesophageal or junctional cancer (CROSS): Long-term results of a randomised controlled trial. *Lancet Oncol.* 2015. doi:10.1016/S1470-2045(15)00040-6

84. Reynolds JV. Protocol Number: ICORG 10–14. Version number/ date: Version 8, 27th August 2015. List of amendments to date: Version 2, 4th July 2011; Version 3, 21st March 2012; Version 4, 22nd November 2013; Version 5, 19th November 2014; Version 6, 30th January 2015. 2015:1–154.

85. Hoeppner J, Lordick F, Brunner T et al. ESOPEC: Prospective randomized controlled multicenter phase III trial comparing perioperative chemotherapy (FLOT protocol) to neoadjuvant chemoradiation (CROSS protocol) in patients with adenocarcinoma of the esophagus (NCT02509286). *BMC Cancer.* 2016. doi:10.1186/s12885-016-2564-y

86. Herskovic A, Martz K, al-Sarraf M et al. Combined chemotherapy and radiotherapy compared with radiotherapy alone in patients with cancer of the esophagus. *N Engl J Med.* 1992. doi:10.1056/NEJM199206113262403

87. Brusselaers N, Mattsson F, Lagergren J. Hospital and surgeon volume in relation to long-term survival after oesophagectomy: Systematic review and meta-analysis. *Gut.* 2014. doi:10.1136/gutjnl-2013-306074

88. Cooper JS, Guo MD, Herskovic A et al. Chemoradiotherapy of locally advanced esophageal cancer: Long-term follow-up of a prospective randomized trial (RTOG 85–01). *J Am Med Assoc.* 1999. doi:10.1001/jama.281.17.1623

89. Wong RK, Malthaner R. Combined chemotherapy and radiotherapy (without surgery) compared with radiotherapy alone in localized carcinoma of the esophagus. *Cochrane Database Syst Rev.* 2010. doi:10.1002/14651858.cd002092.pub3

90. Stahl M, Stuschke M, Lehmann N et al. Chemoradiation with and without surgery in patients with locally advanced squamous cell carcinoma of the esophagus. *J Clin Oncol.* 2005. doi:10.1200/JCO.2005.00.034

91. Crosby T, Hurt C, Falk S et al. SCOPE 1: A phase II/III trial of chemoradiotherapy in esophageal cancer plus or minus cetuximab. *J Clin Oncol.* 2013. doi:10.1200/jco.2013.31.4_suppl.lba3

92. Crehange G, Bertaut A, Peiffert D et al. Exclusive chemoradiotherapy with or without dose escalation in locally advanced esophageal carcinoma: The CONCORDE study (PRODIGE 26). *J Clin Oncol.* 2017. doi:10.1200/jco.2017.35.15_suppl.4037

93. Conroy T, Galais MP, Raoul JL et al. Definitive chemoradiotherapy with FOLFOX versus fluorouracil and cisplatin in patients with oesophageal cancer (PRODIGE5/ACCORD17): Final results of a randomised, phase 2/3 trial. *Lancet Oncol.* 2014. doi:10.1016/S1470-2045(14)70028-2

94. Pöttgen C, Stuschke M. Radiotherapy versus surgery within multimodality protocols for esophageal cancer: A meta-analysis of the randomized trials. *Cancer Treat Rev.* 2012. doi:10.1016/j.ctrv.2011.10.005

95. Markar S, Gronnier C, Duhamel A et al. Salvage surgery after chemoradiotherapy in the management of esophageal cancer: Is it a viable therapeutic option? *J Clin Oncol.* 2015; 33(33):3866–3873.

96. Ando N, Iizuka T, Ide H et al. Surgery plus chemotherapy compared with surgery alone for localized squamous cell carcinoma of the thoracic esophagus: A Japan Clinical Oncology Group Study - JCOG9204. *J Clin Oncol.* 2003. doi:10.1200/JCO.2003.12.095

97. Armanios M, Xu R, Forastiere AA et al. Adjuvant chemotherapy for resected adenocarcinoma of the esophagus, gastro-esophageal junction, and cardia: Phase II trial (E8296) of the Eastern Cooperative Oncology Group. *J Clin Oncol.* 2004. doi:10.1200/JCO.2004.06.533

98. Speicher PJ, Englum BR, Ganapathi AM et al. Adjuvant chemotherapy is associated with improved survival after esophagectomy without induction therapy for node-positive adenocarcinoma. *J Thorac Oncol.* 2015. doi:10.1097/JTO.0000000000000384

99. Macdonald JS, Smalley SR, Benedetti J et al. Chemoradiotherapy after surgery compared with surgery alone for adenocarcinoma of the stomach or gastroesophageal junction. *N Engl J Med.* 2001; 345(10):725–30. doi:10.1056/NEJMoa010187

100. Fuchs CS, Enzinger PC, Meyerhardt J et al. Adjuvant chemodiotlherapy with epirubicin, cisplatin, and fluorouracil compared with adjuvant chemoradiotherapy with fluorouracil and leucovorin after curative resection of gastric cancer: Results from CALGB

101. Cats A, Jansen EPM, van Grieken NCT et al. Chemotherapy versus chemoradiotherapy after surgery and preoperative chemotherapy for resectable gastric cancer (CRITICS): an international, open-label, randomised phase 3 trial. *Lancet Oncol.* 2018; 19(5):616–28. doi:10.1016/S1470-2045(18)30132-3

102. Lei D, Pan X, Luan X et al. Surgical management of cervical esophageal carcinoma. *Zhonghua Er Bi Yan Hou Ke Za Zhi.* 2002.

103. Mendenhall WM, Sombeck MD, Parsons JT, Kasper ME, Stringer SP, Vogel SB. Management of cervical esophageal carcinoma. *Semin Radiat Oncol.* 1994. doi:10.1016/S1053-4296(05)80066-9

104. Collin CF, Spiro RH. Carcinoma of the cervical esophagus: Changing therapeutic trends. *Am J Surg.* 1984. doi:10.1016/0002-9610(84)90370-2

105. Triboulet JP, Mariette C, Chevalier D, Amrouni H. Surgical management of carcinoma of the hypopharynx and cervical esophagus: Analysis of 209 cases. *Arch Surg.* 2001. doi:10.1001/archsurg.136.10.1164

106. Bidoli P, Bajetta E, Stani SC et al. Ten-year survival with chemotherapy and radiotherapy in patients with squamous cell carcinoma of the esophagus. *Cancer.* 2002. doi:10.1002/cncr.10233

107. Takebayashi K, Tsubosa Y, Matsuda S et al. Comparison of curative surgery and definitive chemoradiotherapy as initial treatment for patients with cervical esophageal cancer. *Dis Esophagus.* 2017. doi:10.1111/dote.12502

108. Cox S, Powell C, Carter B et al. Role of nutritional status and intervention in oesophageal cancer treated with definitive chemoradiotherapy: Outcomes from SCOPE1. *Br J Cancer.* 2016; 115(2):172. doi:10.1038/bjc.2016.129

109. Homs MYV, Steyerberg EW, Eijkenboom WMH et al. Single-dose brachytherapy versus metal stent placement for the palliation of dysphagia from oesophageal cancer: Multicentre randomised trial. *Lancet.* 2004. doi:10.1016/S0140-6736(04)17272-3

110. Adamson D, Blazeby J, Nelson A et al. Palliative radiotherapy in addition to self-expanding metal stent for improving dysphagia and survival in advanced oesophageal cancer (ROCS: Radiotherapy after Oesophageal Cancer Stenting): Study protocol for a randomized controlled trial. *Trials.* 2014. doi:10.1186/1745-6215-15-402

111. Penniment MG, De Ieso PB, Harvey JA et al. Palliative chemoradiotherapy versus radiotherapy alone for dysphagia in advanced oesophageal cancer: a multicentre randomised controlled trial (TROG 03.01). *Lancet Gastroenterol Hepatol.* 2018. doi:10.1016/S2468-1253(17)30363-1

112. Okines AFC, Norman AR, McCloud P, Kang YK, Cunningham D. Meta-analysis of the REAL-2 and ML17032 trials: Evaluating capecitabine-based combination chemotherapy and infused 5-fluorouracil-based combination chemotherapy for the treatment of advanced oesophago-gastric cancer. *Ann Oncol.* 2009. doi:10.1093/annonc/mdp047

113. Bang YJ, Van Cutsem E, Feyereislova A et al. Trastuzumab in combination with chemotherapy versus chemotherapy alone for treatment of HER2-positive advanced gastric or gastro-oesophageal junction cancer (ToGA): A phase 3, open-label, randomised controlled trial. *Lancet.* 2010. doi:10.1016/S0140-6736(10)61121-X

114. Thuss-Patience PC, Shah MA, Ohtsu A et al. Trastuzumab emtansine versus taxane use for previously treated HER2-positive locally advanced or metastatic gastric or gastro-oesophageal junction adenocarcinoma (GATSBY): An international randomised, open-label, adaptive, phase 2/3 study. *Lancet Oncol.* 2017; 18(5):640–53. doi:10.1016/S1470-2045(17)30111-0

115. Tabernero J, Hoff PM, Shen L et al. Pertuzumab plus trastuzumab and chemotherapy for HER2-positive metastatic gastric or gastro-oesophageal junction cancer (JACOB): final analysis of a double-blind, randomised, placebo-controlled phase 3 study. *Lancet Oncol.* 2018; 19(10):1372–84. doi:10.1016/S1470-2045(18)30481-9

116. Hecht JR, Bang Y-J, Qin SK et al. Lapatinib in combination with capecitabine plus oxaliplatin in human epidermal growth factor receptor 2–positive advanced or metastatic gastric, esophageal, or gastroesophageal adenocarcinoma: TRIO-013/LOGiC—A

100. (continued) 80101 (Alliance). *J Clin Oncol.* 2017. doi:10.1200/JCO.2017.74.2130

randomized phase III trial. *J Clin Oncol.* 2015; 34(5):443–51. doi:10.1200/JCO.2015.62.6598

117. Cafferkey C, Chau I, Thistlethwaite F, Petty RD, Starling N, Watkins D, Rao S, Saffery C, Patel B, Peckitt C, Cunningham D. PLATFORM: Planning treatment of oesophago-gastric (OG) cancer—A randomised maintenance therapy trial. *J Clin Oncol.* 2016 34:4.

118. Hall PS, Swinson D, Waters JS et al. Optimizing chemotherapy for frail and elderly patients (pts) with advanced gastroesophageal cancer (aGOAC): The GO2 phase III trial. *J Clin Oncol.* 2019; 37(15_suppl):4006. doi:10.1200/JCO.2019.37.15_suppl.4006

119. Ford HER, Marshall A, Bridgewater JA et al. Docetaxel versus active symptom control for refractory oesophagogastric adenocarcinoma (COUGAR-02): An open-label, phase 3 randomised controlled trial. *Lancet Oncol.* 2014. doi:10.1016/S1470-2045(13)70549-7

120. Lee K-W, Maeng CH, Kim T-Y et al. A phase III study to compare the efficacy and safety of paclitaxel versus irinotecan in patients with metastatic or recurrent gastric cancer who failed in first-line therapy (KCSG ST10-01). *Oncologist.* 2019; 24(1):18–24. doi:10.1634/theoncologist.2018-0142

121. Lordick F, Kang Y-K, Chung H-C et al. Capecitabine and cisplatin with or without cetuximab for patients with previously untreated advanced gastric cancer (EXPAND): a randomised, open-label phase 3 trial. *Lancet Oncol.* 2013; 14(6):490–9. doi: 10.1016/S1470-2045(13)70102-5

122. Waddell T, Chau I, Cunningham D et al. Epirubicin, oxaliplatin, and capecitabine with or without panitumumab for patients with previously untreated advanced oesophagogastric cancer (REAL3): a randomised, open-label phase 3 trial. *Lancet Oncol.* 2013; 14(6):481–9. doi:10.1016/S1470-2045(13)70096-2

123. Ohtsu A, Shah MA, Van Cutsem E et al. Bevacizumab in combination with chemotherapy as first-line therapy in advanced gastric cancer: A randomized, double-blind, placebo-controlled phase III study. *J Clin Oncol.* 2011. doi:10.1200/JCO.2011.36.2236

124. Wilke H, Muro K, Van Cutsem E et al. Ramucirumab plus paclitaxel versus placebo plus paclitaxel in patients with previously treated advanced gastric or gastro-oesophageal junction adenocarcinoma (RAINBOW): A double-blind, randomised phase 3 trial. *Lancet Oncol.* 2014. doi:10.1016/S1470-2045(14)70420-6

125. Fuchs CS, Tomasek J, Yong CJ et al. Ramucirumab monotherapy for previously treated advanced gastric or gastro-oesophageal junction adenocarcinoma (REGARD): an international, randomised, multicentre, placebo-controlled, phase 3 trial. *Lancet.* 2014; 383(9911):31–9. doi:10.1016/S0140-6736(13)61719-5

126. Doi T, Bennouna J, Shen L et al. KEYNOTE-181: Phase 3, open-label study of second-line pembrolizumab vs. single-agent chemotherapy in patients with advanced/metastatic esophageal adenocarcinoma. *J Clin Oncol.* 2016. doi:10.1200/jco.2016.34.15_suppl.tps4140

127. Shitara K, Özgüroğlu M, Bang YJ et al. Pembrolizumab versus paclitaxel for previously treated, advanced gastric or gastro-oesophageal junction cancer (KEYNOTE-061): A randomised, open-label, controlled, phase 3 trial. *Lancet.* 2018. doi:10.1016/S0140-6736(18)31257-1

128. Tabernero J, Bang Y-J, Fuchs CS et al. KEYNOTE-062: Phase III study of pembrolizumab (MK-3475) alone or in combination with chemotherapy versus chemotherapy alone as first-line therapy for advanced gastric or gastroesophageal junction (GEJ) adenocarcinoma. *J Clin Oncol.* 2016. doi:10.1200/jco.2016.34.4_suppl.tps185

9 HEPATOCELLULAR CARCINOMA

Daniel H. Palmer and Philip J. Johnson

Introduction

Hepatocellular carcinoma (HCC) is the fifth commonest malignancy and the third commonest cause of cancer death. There is a wide geographic variation in HCC incidence. In particular, in sub-Saharan Africa and the Far East, it is a major public health problem, largely related to endemic chronic hepatitis B virus infection. Incidence and mortality are increasing in the West, reflecting an increasing burden of chronic liver disease. Although progress towards effective therapy has been slow, low-cost vaccines against the hepatitis B virus and anti-viral treatment are reducing the incidence of this malignancy. After considering briefly the etiological factors and the clinicopathological features of HCC, this chapter describes therapeutic options, grouped broadly into surgery, locoregional treatments, and systemic therapies.

Incidence

Hepatocellular carcinoma is the commonest primary liver malignancy and is one of the most common malignancies globally. The highest annual incidence rates, of up to 100 per 100,000, occur in parts of southern Africa and the Far East (Table 9.1).[1] Some estimates suggest that male Chinese carriers of the hepatitis B virus (HBV), who may comprise up to 15 per cent of males in certain populations, carry a lifetime risk of developing the tumor of over 20 per cent. HCC is much less common in northern Europe, the USA, and Australia, although incidence is increasing in direct proportion to the increasing burden of chronic liver disease. Previously this was driven, in part, by chronic hepatitis C virus (HCV) infection, although the introduction of direct-acting anti-viral drugs which can effectively cure the disease will likely reduce its impact on cancer incidence. However, alcohol and fatty liver disease related to obesity and type II diabetes are underpinning the ongoing increasing incidence.[2] In most series, between 10 per cent and 20 per cent of primary liver tumors are accounted for by biliary/gall bladder cancers (see Chapter 11) and about 1 per cent by primary hepatic sarcomas. Liver metastases are found at approximately 1 per cent of all autopsies, and the liver is involved in up to 40 per cent of adult patients with primary extra-hepatic malignancies who come to autopsy. Up to 75 per cent of primary tumors drained by the portal venous system will have spread to involve the liver before death occurs.[3] As such, the liver is the most common organ to be involved by malignancy.

Hepatocellular carcinoma

Etiology, risk factors, and prevention

Knowledge of risk factors for HCC development (Box 1) provides opportunities for interventional strategies that may reduce incidence and to identify high-risk populations who may be suitable for screening programs. The wide geographic variation in incidence indicates the importance of environmental factors. Globally, the most important of these are chronic infection with HBV and HCV and exposure to aflatoxin. In one study that followed 22,000 Chinese males, 15 per cent of whom were HBV carriers, for up to 9 years, the development of HCC was almost exclusively confined to the HBV group, with a relative risk approaching 100.[4] A HBV vaccination program began in Taiwan in the early 1980s, first inoculating neonates born to carrier mothers, and then extended to all neonates and children. The incidence, per 100,000 population, of HCC in children aged 6–9 years declined from 0.52 for those born between 1974 and 1984 to 0.13 for those born between 1984 and 1986.[5] Evidence also suggests that anti-viral therapy in patients with chronic hepatitis B may also decrease the incidence of subsequent HCC development.[6]

BOX 1   MAJOR RISK FACTORS FOR HEPATOCELLULAR CARCINOMA

Chronic liver disease (usually at the stage of cirrhosis)
Chronic viral hepatitis type B
Chronic hepatitis type C
Dietary exposure to aflatoxin
Increasing age
Male gender

The epidemiological evidence linking chronic HCV infection and HCC is similar to that for HBV.[7,8] Since HCV has no reverse transcriptase activity and, unlike HBV, does not integrate into the host genome, its oncogenic potential has generally been attributed to the chronic liver disease that chronic HCV infection may cause. However, there are data indicating that the HCV replicative lifecycle may engage potentially oncogenic pathways including the mitogenic MAP kinase pathway and angiogenic VEGF signaling, which may influence response to molecularly targeted therapies such as sorafenib (see below). The development of direct acting anti-viral agents (DAAs) has transformed the management of HCV, with most patients achieving sustained virological response, such that HCV-associated HCC is likely to decrease in coming years.[9]

Aflatoxin, formed by the fungus *Aspergillus flavus*, which grows on cereals stored under warm, damp conditions, is one of the most potent hepatic carcinogens, particularly in HBV-infected individuals. In several high-HCC-incidence areas of the world, a clear relationship between intake and the incidence of HCC has been established, both by conventional dietary assessment[10] and by the use of biomarkers.[11,12] As well as the obvious approach of improving grain storage to reduce aflatoxin exposure, the possibility of chemoprevention is an area of active research.[13,14]

Hepatocellular carcinoma usually arises in a cirrhotic liver, although the cirrhosis is not always symptomatic and, indeed, the development of HCC may be the first indication of the underlying chronic liver disease. Males with cirrhosis are at significantly higher risk of developing HCC than females, suggesting a potential role for sex hormones in HCC etiology.[15]

TABLE 9.1   Typical Age-Adjusted Incidence Rates per 100,000 of Population in Various Countries

	Country	Male	Female
Low-incidence areas	UK	1.6	0.8
	USA (white)	2	1
	Australia	1.1	0.5
	Germany	4	1.2
	Denmark	3.6	2.3
Intermediate-incidence areas	Italy	7.5	3.5
	Spain	7.5	4
	Romania	11.8	7.9
	Argentina	8	5
High-incidence areas	Japan	20	5
	Hong Kong	32	7
	Zimbabwe	65	25
	Senegal	25	9
	Taiwan	85	–

Many registries do not distinguish between hepatocellular carcinoma and other primary liver tumors

Anatomy of the liver

Recognition of the segmental anatomy of the liver has been important in allowing more refined operative techniques for surgical resection.[16] The portal vascular supply and the bile ducts define two functional hepatic lobes, the line of demarcation running from the gall bladder bed to the inferior vena cava. Each of these two lobes is split into four segments, none of which has any surface markings (Figure 9.1). The standard surgical resections are based on this description (Figure 9.2). The left, right, and middle hepatic veins drain the conventional "anatomical" left and right lobes, as defined by the falciform ligament, respectively. Whereas the normal liver parenchyma receives about 70 per cent of its blood supply from the portal vein, the dominant blood supply to liver tumors is from the hepatic artery. This forms the rationale for several therapeutic approaches, including hepatic artery occlusion and regional chemotherapy (see "Locoregional Therapies" section).

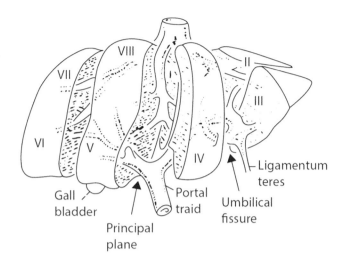

FIGURE 9.1   Segmental anatomy of the liver.

Symptoms and presentation

The most common mode of presentation for primary liver tumors is the triad of abdominal pain, weight loss, and hepatomegaly. In addition, patients may present with signs of hepatic decompensation, such as jaundice, ascites, encephalopathy, or variceal hemorrhage.[17] Rarely, presentation is with spontaneous rupture of the tumor with sudden onset of severe abdominal pain with shock, and paracentesis revealing bloodstained ascitic fluid.[18] Rarer presentations include hypoglycemia, hypercalcemia, and polycythemia. HCC is increasingly diagnosed pre-symptomatically by screening patients with cirrhosis using serial ultrasound examinations and/or estimations of alpha-fetoprotein (AFP).

Diagnosis

Dynamic triphasic computed tomography (CT) and contrast-enhanced magnetic resonance imaging (MRI) will classically show enhancement in the arterial phase with relative

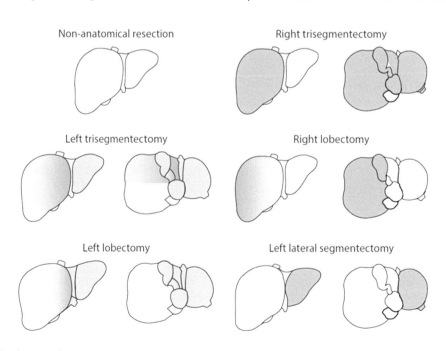

FIGURE 9.2   Standard surgical resections.

hypovascularity ("wash-out") in the early portal phase. In a patient with known cirrhosis and a mass greater than 2 cm in diameter, this radiological appearance is considered diagnostic of HCC without the need for histological confirmation according to both AASLD and EASL guidelines.[19] Cross-sectional imaging is also required to assess the extent of disease for treatment planning. In particular, size, number, and distribution of tumors can be established, as well as the presence of macrovascular (portal vein) invasion and extra-hepatic disease. Although contrast-enhanced CT and MRI are the best current imaging modalities, both techniques may miss up to 30 per cent of lesions (as detected in the explanted liver following liver transplantation), especially those smaller than 1 cm.[20]

The first serologic assay for the detection and clinical follow-up of HCC was alpha-fetoprotein (AFP). Serum AFP is elevated in 50–70 per cent of HCCs.[21] It is of value in the diagnosis of HCC in patients with cirrhosis and has been used as a screening tool in high-risk populations (see "Screening" section). However, levels up to 500 ng/mL can occur in benign liver diseases, especially chronic active hepatitis and fulminant hepatic failure. Nevertheless, a rising AFP is strongly suggestive of HCC. AFP is also useful in monitoring the effect of treatment and for the detection of disease recurrence or progression following treatment. It may also be of prognostic value with higher values associated with a worse prognosis (see "Staging and Prognosis"). The other commonly used assay is for des-gamma-carboxy prothrombin protein (DCP, or PIVKA-II). Levels of this protein are increased in up to 90 per cent of patients with HCC, but may also be elevated in patients with vitamin K deficiency, chronic active hepatitis, or metastatic carcinoma.[22]

Histology

For patients with a liver mass not fulfilling the imaging criteria (as defined above), the diagnosis of HCC must be made histologically. Fine-needle biopsy may be limited by sampling error/missing small lesions, and by difficulty in distinguishing well-differentiated HCC from dysplasia or from adenoma or even normal liver. Some groups believe that biopsy may risk tumor seeding along the needle track and recommend avoidance of the procedure in candidates for surgical resection or transplantation. The presence of bile in tumor cells is diagnostic of HCC. There are several histological subtypes. The most typical pattern is microtrabecular, which differs from normal liver by the absence of portal tracts or bile ducts. Other patterns include acinar, pseudoglandular, and scirrhous, but histological type is not of prognostic significance, with the exception of the fibrolamellar variant characterized by tumor cords with collagen strands. Fibrolamellar HCC typically occurs in younger patients (mean 26 years) without underlying chronic liver disease and AFP is not elevated.[25,26] In this setting, resection rates are higher and prognosis is better (median survival 5 years), although this may reflect the younger age, absence of cirrhosis, and low AFP, all of which are associated with a better prognosis, rather than being directly related to the histological subtype.[27]

Screening

In view of the limited therapeutic options for HCC once the lesion is greater than 4–5 cm in diameter and the fact that high-risk groups can be identified, screening is a logical approach, and there is some limited evidence that it does decrease disease-specific mortality.[23] Current guidelines suggest that those in a high-risk group undergo 6-monthly ultrasound examinations. Serial AFP estimation has also been used as a screening test, but current evidence suggests that it is insufficiently sensitive to be used as a screening tool.[19,24] The GALAD score (comprising **g**ender, **a**ge, **L**3 isoform of AFP, **A**FP, and **D**CP) has been developed as a statistical model to determine the risk of HCC in individuals with chronic liver disease, with significantly better performance than each biomarker individually, and may be elevated even before cancers are radiologically detectable, suggesting a potentially useful role in surveillance.[28] GALAD has been validated in a US study, performing better than ultrasound for early HCC detection.[29]

Natural history

Symptomatic HCC is usually rapidly fatal and untreated patients typically die within 12 months of the onset of symptoms. Geddes and Falkson[30] reported a mean duration of symptoms of 5 months before death in South African Bantu mineworkers; in China, the mean survival time from symptoms/diagnosis is less than 3 months. In the West, patients without underlying cirrhosis survive longer[16] (Figure 9.3) and survival up to 3 years may occur, particularly in patients who present without symptoms, vascular invasion, or extra-hepatic metastases.[31] The prognosis of patients with other primary liver tumors is equally poor. The only exceptions are the rare epithelioid hemangioendothelioma and the equally rare variant of HCC fibrolamellar carcinoma (see above). Both have a rather better prognosis, with a median survival of around 5 years. As local treatment becomes more effective, symptomatic lung, bone, and lymph-node metastases are more frequently detected.

Staging and prognosis

For most cancers, prognosis is predominantly related to tumor stage. However, most HCCs occur on a background of cirrhosis that independently contributes to prognosis.[32] For the majority of patients, the prognosis of HCC remains poor, with treatments other than surgery having little impact on survival. TNM staging for HCC ranges from I (a single tumor with no vascular invasion, no regional lymph node involvement, and no distant metastases) to IV (any extent of tumor, any regional lymph node involvement, and distant metastases); see ref. 36 for full details. Tumor size is a key prognostic factor, with survival approaching 3 years for tumors less than 3 cm but only 3 months for those larger than 8 cm.[33] Vascular invasion increases with tumor size, but is an

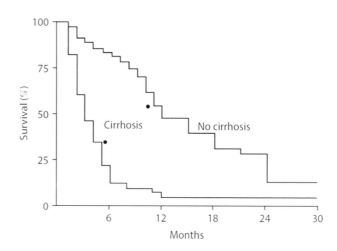

FIGURE 9.3   Cumulative survival curves for patients with hepatocellular carcinoma with and without cirrhosis. (Reproduced with permission from Melia et al., 1984.)

independent prognostic factor; even large tumors can have a good prognosis following surgical resection in the absence of vascular invasion.[34,35]

Following surgical resection, a key determinant of prognosis remains, as for other tumors, the TNM tumor stage.[36] Nevertheless, this can still be refined by the inclusion of other tumor-related and patient-related factors and may be further improved by emerging biological markers. Further, TNM can only be applied once a patient has been deemed resectable, which has already taken into account liver function and performance status, themselves markers of prognosis.

Underlying cirrhosis may limit prognosis independently of tumor-related factors, and the degree of liver dysfunction influences treatment options such as surgical resection, chemoembolization, and systemic therapies, which require sufficient hepatic reserve to be performed safely. Prognostic models for HCC are therefore complex and should take into account tumor stage, degree of liver impairment, patient fitness, and treatment efficacy. Systems omitting any of these are likely to be of limited value (e.g. the Child–Pugh score takes into account only the underlying liver function, and TNM only tumor-related factors). Attempts have been made to refine this system by incorporating more detailed tumor information and liver function (e.g. the Cancer of the Liver Italian Programme [CLIP] and Chinese University Prognostic Index [CUPI]), but these have not been widely applied (Table 9.2).[37,38] The Barcelona Clinic Liver Cancer (BCLC) algorithm has been widely adopted, particularly in the West, assigning patients with very early/early (0/A), intermediate (B), advanced (C), or terminal (D) stages according to tumor extent, liver function, and performance status, with associated guidelines for evidence-based treatment and prognosis for each stage.[39] Thus stage 0/A patients are suitable for curative-intent therapies (surgical resection/local ablative techniques/liver transplantation); stage B patients are suitable for other loco-regional therapies (typically transarterial chemoembolization, TACE); stage C patients are candidates for systemic anti-cancer therapy; and stage D for supportive care.

Treatment

Resection, transplantation, and local ablation may be considered potentially curative treatments, but none of these has been compared to an untreated group in large randomized controlled trials and evidence for benefit is based on comparison with historical controls. Thus, the best 5-year survival rate in untreated series is less than 20 per cent, whereas with transplantation, resection,

or ablations the comparable figures range from 40 per cent to 70 per cent.

Liver resection

Resectability of a tumor depends on its size, location, relation to blood vessels, and underlying liver function. In patients without cirrhosis, up to 75 per cent of the liver can be removed safely. However, resection in patients with cirrhosis is associated with significant morbidity and mortality, although this has fallen to less than 5 per cent with improvements in surgical technique, postoperative management, and anatomical resections combined with better patient selection. Nonetheless, only 10–20 per cent of patients are suitable for resection, although this may increase as screening programs detect tumors at an earlier stage. Survival is better for small (<5 cm), solitary tumors with negative resection margins and an absence of vascular invasion or lymph-node involvement, with 5-year survival rates up to 70 per cent.[40,41] Several techniques to increase the proportion of patients suitable for resection and to improve surgical outcomes have been utilized. These include neo-adjuvant techniques such as portal vein embolization and selective internal radiotherapy (SIRT), which aim to induce hypertrophy of the contralateral lobe to increase the size of the future liver remnant after resection and, with SIRT, also provide active treatment to the tumor which may result in downstaging prior to resection.

Liver transplantation

Liver transplantation has the potential to treat both tumor and underlying cirrhosis. A major limitation to transplantation is the supply of donor organs, and therefore accurate assessment of tumor size and number, vascular involvement, and extra-hepatic disease is essential to identify those patients who are most likely to benefit from long-term survival without tumor recurrence in order to make best use of the donor organ pool. In patients with no more than three small (<5 cm) tumors, survival was similar to that of patients with benign end-stage liver disease, and transplantation has become the treatment of choice for HCC in a cirrhotic liver. This experience has underpinned the development of the Milan criteria (Table 9.3) to guide the selection of patients for transplantation, which can lead to 5-year survival in excess of 70 per cent.[42] Other reports have indicated that these criteria may be extended whilst retaining good outcomes, including University California San Francisco (UCSF) criteria, the "metro ticket" system, and "up to 7" criteria.[43,44]

TABLE 9.2   **Prognostic Scoring Systems**

	Tumor Factors	**Host Factors**	**Environmental Factors**
TNM	(See text)	Nil	Nil
Child–Pugh	Nil	Bilirubin, albumin, INR, ascites, encephalopathy	Nil
Okuda	Tumor size	Bilirubin, albumin, ascites	Nil
CLIP	Morphology (uni-/multi-nodular) AFP, portal vein thrombosis	Child–Pugh score	Nil
CUPI	TNM, AFP	Bilirubin, ascites, alkaline phosphate, symptoms	Nil
BCLC	Tumor size, symptoms morphology, extra-hepatic disease	Portal hypertension, Child–Pugh score, bilirubin, performance status, co-morbidity	Surgery, ablation, TACE, sorafenib, trials, supportive care

Abbreviations: CLIP, Cancer of the Liver Italian Programme; CUPI, Chinese University Prognostic Index; BCLC, Barcelona Clinic Liver Cancer; AFP, alpha-fetoprotein; INR, international normalized ratio; TACE, transarterial chemoembolization.

TABLE 9.3 First-Line Clinical Trials of Systemic Therapy for Advanced HCC

	SHARP, 2007	REFLECT, 2018	CHECKMATE, 2019	IMbrave 150, 2019
Placebo	7.9 months			
Sorafenib	10.7 months	12.3 months	14.7 months	13.2 months
Lenvatinib		13.6 months		
Nivolumab			16.4 months	
Atezolizumab + bevacizumab				Not reached
HR (95% CI)	0.69 (0.55–0.87)	0.92 (0.79–1.06)	0.85 (0.72–1.02)	0.58 (0.42–0.79)
Statistical analysis plan	Superiority endpoint met	Non-inferiority endpoint met Superiority endpoint not met	Superiority endpoint not met Non-inferiority analysis not pre-specified	Superiority endpoint met

A further consequence of the short supply of donor organs is the resultant period, of uncertain duration, between listing and transplantation, with the risk that the tumor will grow beyond the indications for transplant.[45] For this reason, in North America, the scoring systems used to allocate donor organs equitably are weighted to prioritize patients with HCC for transplant.[46] Dropout (i.e. disease progression to a level at which transplantation is no longer appropriate whilst awaiting a donor liver) may be best reduced by increasing the number/availability of donor organs, and this may be helped by the use of living donors. Early data indicate similar results to those achieved with cadaveric organs if the Milan criteria are followed, with low mortality amongst donors.[47] Many transplant units employ "bridging" therapies (commonly chemoembolization or radiofrequency ablation) to reduce the risk of progression whilst awaiting transplantation. Although there are no data from randomized controlled trials, retrospective data suggest this approach to be beneficial if transplant waiting times exceed 6 months' duration. Some units utilize surgical resection as a bridge to transplantation with the proposed advantage that histological examination of the resected tumor may inform decision-making for subsequent transplantation.[48]

Local ablation: Percutaneous ethanol injection and radiofrequency ablation

Image-guided ablation is regarded as the best therapeutic option for patients with small HCC not suitable for resection or transplantation. Treatment is usually performed percutaneously under ultrasound or CT guidance. Several methods for tumor destruction have been used, the most widely studied being percutaneous ethanol injection (PEI) and radiofrequency ablation (RFA). The injection of 90 per cent ethanol under ultrasound guidance is technically straightforward, inexpensive, safe, and results in 5-year survival of 50 per cent in Child A, 30 per cent in Child B, but less than 10 per cent in Child C cirrhotics.[49] Complete tumor necrosis is achieved in 70 per cent of tumors less than 3 cm in diameter, but this falls with increasing size (50 per cent in lesions 3–5 cm), probably due to the inability of the injected volume to disperse evenly throughout larger tumors that may contain fibrous septae. Radiofrequency ablation is a localized thermal treatment producing tumor destruction by heating a probe inserted into the tumor to temperatures exceeding 50°C, which can be performed percutaneously under image guidance, laparoscopically or at laparotomy.

Several randomized studies have compared RFA with PEI. A study in patients with tumors up to 4 cm demonstrated that RFA was superior in terms of tumor necrosis and survival, with 3-year survival of 74 per cent vs. 51 per cent.[50] Further studies have demonstrated similar advantages for RFA in treating smaller tumors (<3 cm).[51,52] In general, RFA was associated with fewer sessions to achieve complete tumor necrosis and with no significant differences in morbidity and a likely improvement in survival. It is generally considered that RFA is superior to PEI for larger lesions.

Randomized trials have compared RFA with surgical resection, suggesting similar outcomes, although such studies have proven difficult to recruit to in a timely fashion and have generally been underpowered.[53]

Other locally ablative techniques are commonly used, including microwave ablation and irreversible electroporation.[54,55] Whilst different techniques may have technical or anatomical advantages and operators may have individual preferences, there are no adequately powered randomized trials to guide choice of one technique over another.

To date, there are no conclusive data indicating that any adjuvant treatment can decrease the risk of tumor recurrence after either surgery or local ablation. The largest randomized, double-blind, placebo-controlled phase III study in this context evaluated the safety and efficacy of sorafenib (see below) vs. placebo after potentially curative treatment with surgical resection or local ablation, taken continuously for up to 4 years. As well as the risk of disease recurrence through micrometastases (which may conceivably be eradicated by an active systemic therapy) there is also a risk of *de novo* tumor formation in the remaining diseased liver. It is for this reason that a four-year duration of therapy was selected in this trial, although to date there is no evidence that sorafenib may prevent the progression of pre-malignant lesions to invasive cancer. This study demonstrated no benefit for sorafenib in the adjuvant setting.[56]

Locoregional therapies: Transarterial chemoembolization and radioembolization

Hepatocellular carcinomas are highly vascularized, predominantly via the hepatic artery. In contrast, 75 per cent of normal liver parenchyma derives its blood supply from the portal vein. Thus the hepatic artery provides the potential for tumor-selective targeting of drugs and a rationale for arterial obstruction as a therapeutic approach. Transarterial chemoembolization (TACE) utilizes super-selective catheterization of the hepatic artery to deliver regional chemotherapy and embolize tumor-feeding arteries (Figure 9.4). Chemotherapy is first injected, mixed with lipiodol, an oily compound that tends to accumulate in tumors, probably via enhanced permeability of leaky tumor vasculature and retention due to impaired lymphatic drainage, with the aim of also retaining the chemotherapy to increase tumor concentration and reduce systemic exposure. For chemoembolization to be performed

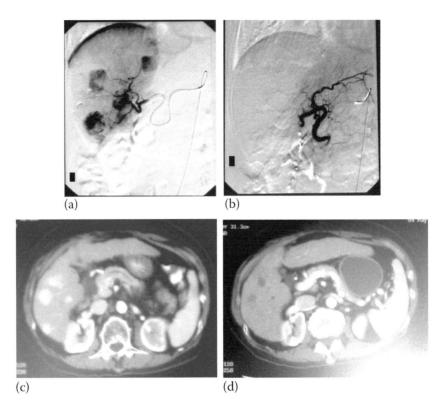

(a)   (b)

(c)   (d)

FIGURE 9.4   Hepatic arterial angiogram (a and b) and contrast-enhanced CT scan (c and d) before and after chemoembolization (non-lipiodol) in a patient with multi-focal hepatocellular carcinoma. (a) and (c) tumors are characterized by hypervascular lesions in arterial phase. (b) and (d) post-chemoembolization. (b) angiogram demonstrating occlusion of right hepatic artery. (d) hypodense lesions on CT.

safely, there must be adequate blood supply to the non-tumorous liver via the portal vein, and therefore it is contraindicated in the presence of main portal vein thrombosis. Other contraindications include extra-hepatic disease, advanced cirrhosis, and poor performance status. Embolization frequently causes a characteristic syndrome of abdominal pain, fever, and nausea, which is normally self-limiting within 2–4 days, although occasionally patients go on to develop liver abscess and, rarely, liver failure.[57]

Two small randomized trials have shown survival benefit from chemoembolization[58,59] (Figure 9.5) and a meta-analysis of 7 trials, incorporating 545 patients, confirmed improved survival compared to supportive care or systemic therapy.[60] The general applicability of this meta-analysis is, however, limited in view of its relatively small size, the heterogeneity of the patient populations and of the techniques used, and differences in the choice of chemotherapeutic agent, embolic agent, and the use of lipiodol. The key to successful chemoembolization is patient selection with the ideal candidate having well-preserved liver function and small tumor volume.

Irrespective of the approach used, the major limitation of all these loco-regional approaches is disease recurrence. The risk of recurrence is conventionally related to tumor size, the rate increasing in direct relation to tumor size. In fact, it is probably the presence or absence of vascular invasion (micro- or macro-) that really defines the risk of recurrence, but since the former cannot readily be determined prior to treatment, and correlates well with tumor size, tumor size is the more convenient parameter. A number of prognostic scoring systems have been developed with the aim of guiding selection of patients most likely to benefit from TACE and those who have undergone TACE may benefit from repeat TACE.[61–64]

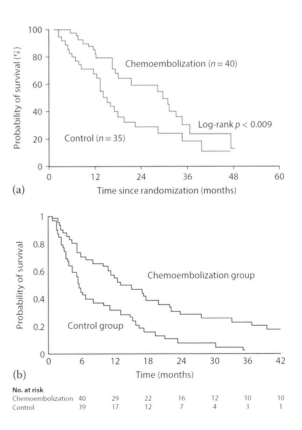

FIGURE 9.5   Survival curves comparing transarterial chemoembolization against best supportive therapy. (a, from reference 60, with permission; b, from reference 59 with permission.)

Since TACE induces acute hypoxia, a potential mechanism of treatment failure is the induction of angiogenic cytokines, notably vascular endothelial growth factor (VEGF), that may stimulate revascularization and progression of disease. This underpins the rationale for the combination of systemic therapies targeting angiogenesis through VEGF inhibition with TACE. A number of large, randomized placebo-controlled trials have investigated sorafenib and other anti-angiogenic drugs with TACE, all demonstrating no benefit for this strategy and, in the case of bevacizumab, a potential detrimental effect.[65–69]

Systemic therapies

The majority of patients with HCC have multi-focal disease, bilobar disease, extra-hepatic disease, and/or underlying cirrhosis, such that surgery, embolization, or ablation is not indicated. For these patients, systemic therapy is required.

Response rates for single-agent chemotherapy are low and significant durable remission is rare. The most widely used single cytotoxic agent has been doxorubicin.[70,71] However, in systematic reviews of randomized trials of doxorubicin therapy, no significant survival effect was discernable.[72] Combination chemotherapy may induce a higher response rate, although again the duration of remission is usually short and toxicity high. In general, even for well-selected patients, the expected objective response rate is only around 20–30 per cent.[73] A phase II study of a four-drug systemic combination regimen—cisplatin, recombinant interferon alpha-2b, doxorubicin, and 5-fluorouracil (PIAF)—was encouraging, showing that although the response rate was not high (25 per cent), 9 of the 13 partial responders had their disease rendered resectable.[74] However, a prospective randomized study comparing PIAF to conventional systemic doxorubicin suggested that any benefit in terms of increased survival was counteracted by increased toxicity.[75] A recent randomized phase III trial has compared the combination of oxaliplatin, leucovorin, and infusional 5-FU (FOLFOX4) with doxorubicin. Three hundred and seventy-one patients with predominantly hepatitis B-related HCC from China, Taiwan, Korea, and Thailand were recruited. Although there was a trend towards improved survival with combination chemotherapy (median 6.4 vs. 4.97 months; hazard ratio 0.8), this difference was not statistically significant ($p = 0.07$).[76]

Endocrine manipulation has been studied in advanced HCC based on reports of estrogen receptor expression in some HCCs. Early small studies with anti-estrogenic and anti-androgenic agents showed some promise.[77] However, recent large-scale prospective controlled studies have refuted any role for hormonal agents, including tamoxifen and the androgen receptor inhibitor enzalutamide.[78,79]

HCC is a highly vascular tumor and the elucidation of the molecular mechanisms mediating tumor angiogenesis, notably the contribution of VEGF signaling, has provided pharmacological targets. Phase II trials of bevacizumab, a humanized monoclonal antibody against VEGF ligand, have demonstrated activity against HCC, although there are concerns regarding the risk of GI bleeding, and recent studies have mandated prophylactic treatment of varices prior to treatment.[80]

Sorafenib is a small molecule inhibitor of the serine–threonine kinases Raf-1 and B-Raf and the receptor tyrosine kinase activity of VEGF receptors 1, 2, and 3 and platelet-derived growth factor receptor β (PDGFR-β). A large phase III, double-blind, placebo-controlled trial in a predominantly European population demonstrated a median survival of 10.7 months in the sorafenib group and 7.9 months in the placebo group (hazard ratio 0.69;

$p < 0.001$).[81] A parallel study conducted in patients from the Asia-Pacific region with predominantly HBV-driven cancers also showed a survival benefit for sorafenib (median 6.5 months vs. 4.2 months, hazard ratio 0.68, $p = 0.014$).[82] On this basis, sorafenib has become established as the standard of care for patients with advanced HCC, good performance status, and compensated liver disease. There remain limited data on the safety and efficacy of sorafenib in patients with Child–Pugh class B or C cirrhosis. In the phase II trial, 38 of the 137 patients had Child–Pugh B cirrhosis, and their survival was worse than those with Child–Pugh A liver disease (median overall survival 14 weeks vs. 41 weeks), and further prospective evaluation in this group is required.[83]

To date, other drugs or combinations have failed to improve upon sorafenib. Despite encouraging phase II data, sunitinib was significantly inferior to sorafenib (median survival 7.9 vs. 10.2 months, HR 1.3; $p = 0.001$) in a large phase III trial.[84] The failure of sunitinib, despite its more potent inhibition of VEGFR than sorafenib, may be attributable to greater toxicity and, consequently, reduced dose intensity, or may suggest the importance of raf inhibition in the efficacy of sorafenib. Negative results have also emerged from a large phase III trial of the potent VEGFR inhibitor, linifanib, which was terminated early due to toxicity, again reflecting the challenges of investigating systemic therapies in patients with HCC and underlying cirrhosis.[85]

A number of studies have explored sorafenib in combination with other agents based on rational pre-clinical data. Pre-clinical models suggest that EGFR signaling is a pre-requisite for angiogenesis in HCC via up-regulation of VEGF.[86] A phase II trial has investigated the combination of bevacizumab with erlotinib, with an objective response rate of 25 per cent (including one complete response), median progression-free survival of 9 months, and median survival 15.6 months.[87] However, a randomized phase III trial of erlotinib in combination with sorafenib reported no significant survival benefit and greater toxicity compared with sorafenib alone.[88] There is also pre-clinical evidence of synergy between doxorubicin and raf inhibition. In a vascular endothelial model, resistance to doxorubicin is, at least in part, mediated via FGF-mediated raf-dependent survival signals, and can be overcome by inhibition of raf, providing rationale for combining doxorubicin with sorafenib or inhibitors of FGFR such as brivanib.[89] A randomized phase II study has investigated the combination of sorafenib and doxorubicin compared to doxorubicin alone.[90] The overall survival in the combination arm was more than double the control arm (13.7 months compared to 6.5 months, HR 0.45). However, these data were not reproduced in the phase III trial, which reported no survival benefit and, again, additional toxicity, for the addition of doxorubicin to sorafenib.[91]

Since FGF is an important alternative pathway of angiogenesis, it may contribute to resistance to VEGF-targeted drugs and thus brivanib, a VEGF and FGF receptor tyrosine kinase inhibitor, may have the potential to delay the emergence of such resistance. A large phase III trial of this drug also failed to improve outcomes compared with sorafenib.[92] However, lenvatinib, another drug predominantly targeting VEGFRs and FGFRs, has been shown to be statistically non-inferior (but not superior) to sorafenib in terms of overall survival in a large phase III trial, such that lenvatinib has now also been approved as a standard of care for patients with advanced HCC (see Table 9.2).[93] Although lenvatinib had superior efficacy for secondary outcome measures such as radiological response rate, progression-free survival, and time to progression, these did not appear to translate into measurable benefits in terms of quality of life, and there are currently no clear criteria to guide the choice between sorafenib and lenvatinib for individual patients. This study raises important questions for clinical trial design in advanced HCC in terms of the significance of secondary outcomes as surrogates of overall survival, the potential impact of post-progression therapy on OS as primary endpoint in an era of active second-line treatments (see below), and statistical design particularly in relation to non-inferiority as a pre-planned analysis.

A better understanding of the mechanisms of resistance to VEGF-targeted therapies may help improve therapeutic strategies. For example there is evidence that hepatocyte growth factor (HGF) signaling through its receptor, c-met, may play a role in mediating such resistance and, indeed, may contribute to the emergence of a more aggressive phenotype during anti-VEGF therapy. This suggests a potential role for c-met inhibition as a second-line strategy, or in combination with anti-angiogenic therapy. The c-met inhibitor tivantinib has been investigated in a randomized phase II trial for patients with HCC and significantly prolonged time to progression, the primary endpoint of the study, compared with best supportive care (HR 0.64). An exploratory analysis of survival according to c-met expression assessed by immunohistochemistry on tumor biopsies suggested that c-met was an adverse prognostic factor and that patients with high c-met may derive greatest benefit.[94] However, a prospective phase III trial enrolling patients with high c-met expression failed to demonstrate a survival benefit in this population.[95] Conversely, a phase III placebo-controlled trial of cabozantinib, which also inhibits c-met (as well as other targets), did demonstrate a survival benefit in patients previously treated with anti-angiogenic drugs (largely sorafenib) without any biomarker selection.[96]

Two further positive placebo-controlled trials in the second-line setting have been reported. The first investigated regorafenib, a molecule similar to sorafenib but with more potent inhibition of a broader range of kinases, in a selected population who had progressed on sorafenib but had been able to tolerate at least 400 mg sorafenib daily for 21 of the 28 days preceding progression.[97] A subsequent analysis of the effect of sequential treatment with sorafenib followed by regorafenib reported a median survival of 26 months from the time of commencing first-line systemic therapy in this select population who remain sufficiently well to receive second-line therapy after progression on sorafenib.[98]

The second trial investigated ramucirumab, a monoclonal antibody targeting VEGFR2. Subgroup analysis of an initial negative trial suggested potential benefit for ramucirumab in patients with elevated baseline serum AFP >400 ng/ml.[99] This observation has been confirmed in a prospective second-line trial enrolling patients with AFP >400 ng/ml.[100]

Immunotherapy for HCC

HCC possesses characteristics that render it a good target for immunotherapy. There is an active recruitment of lymphocytes suggesting potential for cytotoxic effector cell activation. Tumor-infiltrating lymphocytes (TILs) derived from HCC and then expanded *ex vivo* in the presence of IL-2 are able to lyse autologous but not allogeneic tumors, indicating that cytotoxic T lymphocytes (CTL) can recognize tumor-specific antigens in HCC. There is also evidence from early-phase clinical trials that clinical and immune responses to adoptive immunotherapy with dendritic cells can be elicited.[101] However, TILs in HCC proliferate only at very low level and fail to kill tumor cells unless activated by IL-2 *in vitro* suggesting that immunosuppressive mechanisms prevent CTL maturation into useful anti-tumor effectors. A number of mechanisms contribute to an immunosuppressive tumor micro-environment. These include failure of effective T cell

activation and T cell exhaustion through T cell checkpoint signaling. Effective T cell activation requires antigen presentation to the T cell receptor associated with appropriate co-stimulatory signals including, for example, engagement of the CD28 receptor on T cells by its ligand B7. However, engagement of B7 by an alternative T cell receptor, CTLA4, results in T cell inactivation and anergy. Sustained T cell activation is regulated through the PD1 (programmed death-1) receptor on T cells interacting with its ligands PD-L1 and PD-L2. Thus, expression of these ligands on tumor cells (and other cell types within the tumor micro-environment) contributes to immunosuppression.

Monoclonal antibodies that interfere with these T cell checkpoints (checkpoint inhibitors, CPI) have demonstrated clinical efficacy in a number of other tumor types. Early-phase trials of the CPIs nivolumab and pembrolizumab in patients with advanced HCC have shown encouraging evidence of significant efficacy and tolerability leading to accelerated FDA approval.[102,103] However, randomized phase III trials in the first line (nivolumab vs. sorafenib) and second line (pembrolizumab vs. placebo) both failed to meet their primary endpoints of improved overall survival.[104,105] Both studies are likely to have been affected by post-progression therapy and, in the case of nivolumab, since the study was designed to demonstrate superiority over sorafenib, non-inferiority cannot be confirmed despite an apparently favorable toxicity profile since this was not a pre-specified analysis. Notably, survival in the sorafenib control arm of first-line phase III studies has improved in recent years (Table 9.3), likely due in part to more selective eligibility criteria and to post-progression therapy, again highlighting challenges for future clinical trial design for advanced HCC with implications for overall survival as primary endpoint and the need for validated surrogates.

Early-phase trials investigating the combination of CPIs with VEGF inhibitors have reported encouraging radiological response rates, including complete and durable responses, presumed to be mediated by the immunomodulatory effects of VEGF inhibition (e.g. the anti-PD1 antibody, atezolizumab, with the anti-VEGF antibody, bevacizumab; and pembrolizumab with lenvatinib). A phase III trial of atezolizumab with bevacizumab compared with sorafenib has met its co-primary endpoints of improved overall and progression-free survival, as well as meeting secondary endpoints including radiological responses and delayed deterioration of quality of life.[106] The hazard ratio for overall survival is 0.58 (95% CI 0.42, 0.79, $p = 0.0006$). The median survival for the sorafenib-treated patients was 13.2 months but has not yet been reached for the experimental arm. Further follow-up is required to allow the survival data to mature.

Systemic therapy in patients with Child–Pugh B cirrhosis

Although data from randomized controlled trials are limited, it is evident that the survival benefits of systemic therapy are significantly reduced in Child–Pugh B cirrhosis. In a meta-analysis of trials on the use of sorafenib and the sorafenib post-registration study GIDEON, approximately 30 per cent of patients had Child–Pugh (C–P) B cirrhosis. While toxicity in C–P A and B patients was similar, survival in C–P B patients was significantly shorter (approx. 4–5 months, compared with 10–11 months for C–P A).[107] Similarly, in a cohort of patients with C–P B7 and B8 cirrhosis in the Checkmate 040 study investigating the T-cell checkpoint inhibitor nivolumab in various cohorts of patients with advanced HCC, whilst response rates and toxicity were similar, survival was again significantly shorter (approx. 7 months compared with 15 months for C–P A patients).[108] This

TABLE 9.4   Outcomes for Randomized Controlled Trials of SIRT vs. Sorafenib in Advanced HCC

		Median OS (Months) ITT	HR (95% CI) p Value	Media OS (Months) per Protocol	HR (95% CI) p Value
SARAH	SIRT	8.0	1.15 (0.94–1.4) $p = 0.18$	9.9	0.99 (0.79–1.24) $p = 0.39$
	Sorafenib	9.9		9.9	
SIRveNIB	SIRT	8.8	1.12 (0.9–1.4) $p = 0.36$	11.3	0.86 (0.7–1.1) $p = 0.27$
	Sorafenib	10.0		10.4	

emphasizes the need to preserve liver function in order to benefit from systemic therapy and the judicious timing of when to switch from TACE to systemic therapy before irreparable liver damage occurs.

Radiation therapy

The use of external-beam radiotherapy was previously limited by the radiosensitivity of normal hepatocytes, with normal tissue tolerance 25–30 Gy.[109] Higher doses are associated with increasing risk of radiation hepatitis. Further, in patients with cirrhosis, the liver may be even less tolerant of radiotherapy. The use of conformal techniques allows tumor doses up to 72 Gy without severe hepatitis and with evidence of objective responses.[110] Radiation techniques that allow tumor-directed delivery appear promising, with evidence of anti-tumor activity, although to date the impact on survival and the niche in which radiotherapy may be effective have not been defined.[111]

Radio-isotopes can be delivered via the hepatic artery using yttrium-90-labeled microspheres, so-called selective internal radiotherapy (SIRT). Yttrium-90 is a beta emitter with short tissue penetration, which may reduce the risk of radiation hepatitis. In patients receiving doses in excess of 120 Gy, median survival was 15 months, with no evidence of radiation hepatitis, even in cirrhotic patients.[112] These procedures are associated with a risk of lung toxicity if there is extensive arteriovenous shunting in patients with cirrhosis, and an assessment of the degree of shunting should be made prior to treatment.

Two randomized trials have compared SIRT with sorafenib in patients with inoperable HCC (SARAH and SIRVENIB). Of note, up to a third of patients randomized to SIRT did not receive it (due to lung shunting or disease progression during work up) although in both the intention to treat and the per protocol populations, SIRT was not superior to sorafenib (Table 9.4).[113] Like nivolumab (see above), since it was not pre-specified in the statistical analysis plan, non-inferiority cannot be claimed in these trials. A further study of SIRT in combination with sorafenib (SORAMIC) also failed to demonstrate improvement in survival compared with sorafenib alone for patients with advanced HCC. In all these studies, patients typically had advanced-stage HCC, which due to the loco-regional nature of SIRT, may have contributed to their failure.

Key learning points

- Identification of the major risk factors (chronic liver disease, chronic HBV and/or HCV infection, and aflatoxin exposure) for HCC has laid the basis for screening and prevention.
- Hepatocellular carcinoma presents with the triad of pain, hepatomegaly, and weight loss, or decompensation of pre-existing chronic liver disease, although with screening, pre-symptomatic diagnosis is becoming more common.

- The diagnosis of HCC can often be established without recourse to biopsy by characteristic features on CT and MRI scanning, serum AFP estimation, and the presence of underlying chronic liver disease.
- Surgical resection, liver transplantation, and ablative techniques (such as PEI and RFA) offer the possibility of "cure" for smaller tumors, but as tumor size increases, so does the rate of recurrence.
- Chemoembolization may offer useful palliation in a small subset of patients with excellent liver function and minimal symptoms. Statistical models may help guide patient selection and decisions to re-treat.
- Sorafenib and lenvatinib are standards of care for patients with advanced HCC, good PS, and compensated liver disease. The combination of atezolizumab with bevacizumab has met its primary endpoints of superiority over sorafenib for overall and progression-free survival and may become a new standard of care.

References

1. Parkin DM, Bray F, Ferlay J, Pisani P. Global cancer statistics, 2002 CA. *Cancer J Clin.* 2005; 55:74–108.
2. El-Serag HB, Mason AC. Rising incidence of hepatocellular carcinoma in the United States. *N Engl J Med.* 1999; 340:745–50.
3. Willis RA. Secondary tumours of the liver. *Postgraduate Medical Journal.* 1952: 178.
4. Beasley RP. Hepatitis B virus. The major etiology of hepatocellular carcinoma. *Cancer.* 1988; 61(10):1942–56.
5. Chang MH, Chang MH, Chen CJ et al. Universal hepatitis B vaccination in Taiwan and the incidence of hepatocellular carcinoma in children. *N Engl J Med.* 1997; 336:1855–9.
6. Liaw YF, Sung JJ, Chow WC et al. Lamivudine for patients with chronic hepatitis B and advanced liver disease. *N Engl J Med.* 2004; 351(15):1521–31.
7. Colombo M. Hepatitis C virus and hepatocellular carcinoma. *Semin Liver Dis.* 1999; 19(3):263–9.
8. Davila JA, Morgan RO, Shaib Y et al. Hepatitis C infection and the increasing incidence of hepatocellular carcinoma: A population-based study. *Gastroenterology.* 2004; 127:1372–80.
9. Bourlière M, Gordon SC, Flamm SL et al. POLARIS-1 and POLARIS-4 Investigators. Sofosbuvir, velpatasvir, and voxilaprevir for previously treated HCV infection. *N Engl J Med.* 2017; 376(22):2134–46.
10. Van Rensburg SJ, Cook-Mozaffari P, Van Schalkwyk DJ et al. Hepatocellular carcinoma and dietary aflatoxin in Mozambique and Transkei. *Br J Cancer.* 1985; 51(5):713–26.
11. Groopman JD, Wild CP, Hasler J et al. Molecular epidemiology of aflatoxin exposures: Validation of aflatoxin-N7-guanine levels in urine as a biomarker in experimental rat models and humans. *Environ Health Perspect.* 1993; 99:107–13.
12. Ross RK, Yu MC, Henderson BE et al. Aflatoxin biomarkers. *Lancet.* 1992; 340(8811):119.
13. Kensler TW, Egner PA, Wang JB et al. Chemoprevention of hepatocellular carcinoma in aflatoxin endemic areas. *Gastroenterology.* 2004; 127(5 Suppl. 1):S310–18.
14. Turner PC, Sylla A, Gong YY et al. Reduction in exposure to carcinogenic aflatoxins by postharvest intervention measures in West

Africa: A community-based intervention study. *Lancet.* 2005; 365(9475):1950–6.

15. Johnson PJ, Williams R. Cirrhosis and the aetiology of hepatocellular carcinoma. *J Hepatol.* 1987; 4(1):140–7.

16. Bismuth H. Surgical anatomy and anatomical surgery of the liver. *World J Surg.* 1982; 6(1):3–9.

17. Melia WM, Wilkinson ML, Portmann BC et al. Hepatocellular carcinoma in the non-cirrhotic liver: A comparison with that complicating cirrhosis. *QJM* (New Series LIII). 1984; 211:391–400.

18. Lai EC, Lau WY. Spontaneous rupture of hepatocellular carcinoma: A systematic review. *Arch Surg.* 2006; 141(2):191–8.

19. Bruix J, Sherman M. Practice Guidelines Committee, American Association for the Study of Liver Diseases. Management of hepatocellular carcinoma. *Hepatology.* 2005; 42(5):1208–36.

20. Bhattacharjya S, Bhattacharjya T, Quaglia A et al. Liver transplantation in cirrhotic patients with small hepatocellular carcinoma: An analysis of pre-operative imaging, explant histology and prognostic histologic indicators. *Dig Surg.* 2004; 21(2):152–9; discussion 159–60.

21. Johnson PJ. The role of serum alpha-fetoprotein estimation in the diagnosis and management of hepatocellular carcinoma. *Clin Liver Dis.* 2001; 5(1):145–59.

22. Sakon M, Monden M, Gotoh M et al. The effects of vitamin K on the generation of des-gamma-carboxy-prothrombin (PIVKA-II) in patients with hepatocellular carcinoma. *Am J Gastroenterol.* 1991; 86:339–43.

23. Chen JG, Parkin DM, Chen QG et al. Screening for liver cancer: Results of a randomised controlled trial in Qidong, China. *J Med Screen.* 2003; 10(4):204–9.

24. Sherman M. Hepatocellular carcinoma: Epidemiology, risk factors, and screening. *Semin Liver Dis.* 2005; 25(2):143–54.

25. Craig JR, Peters RL, Edmondson HA, Omata M. Fibrolamellar carcinoma of the liver: A tumor of adolescents and young adults with distinctive clinico-pathologic features. *Cancer.* 1980; 46(2):372–9.

26. Katzenstein HM, Krailo MD, Malogolowkin MH et al. Fibrolamellar hepatocellular carcinoma in children and adolescents. *Cancer.* 2003; 97(8):2006–12.

27. Okuda K. Natural history of hepatocellular carcinoma including fibrolamellar and hepato-cholangiocarcinoma variants. *J Gastroenterol Hepatol.* 2002; 17(4):401–5.

28. Johnson PJ, Pirrie SJ, Cox TF et al. The detection of hepatocellular carcinoma using a prospectively developed and validated model based on serological biomarkers. *Cancer Epidemiology, Biomarkers, & Prevention.* 2014; 23(1):144–53.

29. Yang JD, Addissie BD, Mara KC et al. GALAD score for hepatocellular carcinoma detection in comparison with liver ultrasound and proposal of GALADUS score. *Cancer Epidemiology, Biomarkers, & Prevention.* 2019; 1;28(3):531–8.

30. Geddes EW, Falkson G. Malignant hepatoma in the Bantu. *Cancer.* 1970; 25(6):1271–8.

31. Llovet JM, Bustamante J, Castells A et al. Natural history of untreated nonsurgical hepatocellular carcinoma: Rationale for the design and evaluation of therapeutic trials. *Hepatology.* 1999; 29(1):62–7.

32. Palmer DH, Johnson PJ. Hepatocellular carcinoma. In: Gospodarowicz MK, O'Sullivan B, Sobin LH (eds.), *Prognostic Factors in Cancer* 3rd ed. Hoboken, NJ: Wiley-Liss, 2006, pp. 143–146.

33. Ebara M, Ohto M, Shinagawa T et al. Natural history of minute hepatocellular carcinoma smaller than three centimeters complicating cirrhosis. A study in 22 patients. *Gastroenterology.* 1986; 90(2):289–98.

34. Wayne JD, Lauwers GY, Ikai I et al. Preoperative predictors of survival after resection of small hepatocellular carcinomas. *Ann Surg.* 2002; 235(5):722–30; discussion 730–1.

35. Poon RT, Ng IO, Fan ST et al. Clinicopathologic features of long-term survivors and disease-free survivors after resection of hepatocellular carcinoma: A study of a prospective cohort. *J Clin Oncol.* 2001; 19(12):3037–44.

36. Sobin LH, Gospodarowicz MK, Wittekind CH (eds.). *UICC: TNM Classification of Malignant Tumors* 7th ed. New York: Wiley, 2011.

37. Prospective validation of the CLIP score: A new prognostic system for patients with cirrhosis and hepatocellular carcinoma.

The Cancer of the Liver Italian Program (CLIP) Investigators. *Hepatology.* 2000; 31(4):840–5.

38. Leung TW, Tang AM, Zee B et al. Construction of the Chinese University Prognostic Index for hepatocellular carcinoma and comparison with the TNM staging system, the Okuda staging system, and the Cancer of the Liver Italian Program staging system: A study based on 926 patients. *Cancer.* 2002; 94(6):1760–9.

39. European Association for the Study of the Liver. Electronic address: easloffice@easloffice.eu; European Association for the Study of the Liver. EASL Clinical Practice Guidelines: Management of hepatocellular carcinoma. *J Hepatol.* 2018; 69(1):182–236.

40. Farmer DG, Rosove MH, Shaket A, Busuttil RW. Current treatment modalities for hepatocellular carcinoma. *Ann Surg.* 1994; 219:236–47.

41. Vauthey JN, Klimstra D, Franceschi D et al. Factors affecting long term outcome after hepatic resection for hepatocellular carcinoma. *Am J Surg.* 1995; 169:28–34.

42. Mazzaferro V, Regalia E, Doci R et al. Liver transplantation for the treatment of small hepatocellular carcinomas in patients with cirrhosis. *N Engl J Med.* 1996; 334(11):693–Yao FY, Ferrell L, Bass NM et al. Liver transplantation for hepatocellular carcinoma: Expansion of the tumor size limits does not adversely impact survival. *Hepatology.* 2001; 33(6):1394–403.

43. Mazzaferro V, Llovet JM, Miceli R et al. Predicting survival after liver transplantation in patients with hepatocellular carcinoma beyond the Milan criteria: A retrospective, exploratory analysis. *Lancet Oncol.* 2009; 10:35–43.

44. Yao FY, Bass NM, Nikolai B et al. A follow-up analysis of the pattern and predictors of dropout from the waiting list for liver transplantation in patients with hepatocellular carcinoma: Implications for the current organ allocation policy. *Liver Transpl.* 2003; 9(7):684–92.

45. United Network for Organ Sharing. www.unos.org.

46. Gondolesi GE, Roayaie S, Munoz L et al. Adult living donor liver transplantation for patients with hepatocellular carcinoma: Extending UNOS priority criteria. *Ann Surg.* 2004; 239(2):142–9.

47. Belghiti J, Fuks D. Liver resection and transplantation in hepatocellular carcinoma. *Liver Cancer.* 2012; 1(2):71–82.

48. Livraghi T, Giorgio A, Marin G et al. Hepatocellular carcinoma and cirrhosis in 746 patients: Long-term results of percutaneous ethanol injection. *Radiology.* 1995; 197(1):101–8

49. Shiina S, Teratani T, Obi S et al. A randomized controlled trial of radiofrequency ablation with ethanol injection for small hepatocellular carcinoma. *Gastroenterology.* 2005; 129(1):122–30.

50. Lencioni R, Cioni D, Crocetti L et al. Early-stage hepatocellular carcinoma in patients with cirrhosis: Long-term results of percutaneous image-guided radiofrequency ablation. *Radiology.* 2005; 234(3):961–7.

51. Livraghi T, Goldberg SN, Lazzaroni S et al. Small hepatocellular carcinoma: Treatment with radio-frequency ablation versus ethanol injection. *Radiology.* 1999; 210(3):655–61.

52. Izumi N, Hasegawa K, Nishioka Y et al. A multicenter randomized controlled trial to evaluate the efficacy of surgery vs. radiofrequency ablation for small hepatocellular carcinoma (SURF trial). *J Clin Oncol.* 2019 37:(15_suppl):4002.

53. Poggi G, Tosoratti N, Montagna B, Picchi C. Microwave ablation of hepatocellular carcinoma. *World J Hepatol.* 2015; 7(25): 2578–89.

54. Zimmerman A, Grand D, Charpentier KP. Irreversible electroporation of hepatocellular carcinoma: Patient selection and perspectives. *J Hepatocell Carcinoma.* 2017; 4:49–58.

55. Bruix J, Takayama T, Mazzaferro V et al. Adjuvant sorafenib for hepatocellular carcinoma after resection or ablation (STORM): A phase 3, randomised, double-blind, placebo-controlled trial. *Lancet Oncol.* 2015; 16(13):1344–54.

56. Brown DB, Geschwind JF, Soulen MC et al. Society of Interventional Radiology position statement on chemoembolisation for hepatic malignancies. *J Vasc Interv Radiol.* 2006; 17:217–23.

57. Llovet JM, Bruix J. Systematic review of randomized trials for unresectable hepatocellular carcinoma: Chemoembolization improves survival. *Hepatology.* 2003; 37(2):429–42.

58. Lo CM, Ngan H, Tso WK et al. Randomized controlled trial of transarterial lipiodol chemoembolization for unresectable hepatocellular carcinoma. *Hepatology*. 2002; 35(5):1164–71.

59. Llovet JM, Real MI, Montana X et al. Barcelona Liver Cancer Group. Arterial embolisation or chemoembolisation versus symptomatic treatment in patients with unresectable hepatocellular carcinoma: A randomised controlled trial. *Lancet*. 2002; 359(9319): 1734–9.

60. Kadalayil L, Benini R, Pallan L et al. A simple prognostic scoring system for patients receiving transarterial embolisation for hepatocellular cancer. *Ann Oncol*. 2013; 24(10):2565–70.

61. Sieghart W, Hucke F, Pinter M et al. The ART of decision making: Retreatment with transarterial chemoembolization in patients with hepatocellular carcinoma. *Hepatology*. 2013; 57(6): 2261–73.

62. Han G, Berhane S, Toyoda H et al. Prediction of survival among patients receiving transarterial chemoembolization for hepatocellular carcinoma: A response-based approach. *Hepatology*. 2019. Nov 7. doi:10.1002/hep.31022

63. Adhoute X, Penaranda G, Naude S et al. Retreatment with TACE: The ABCR SCORE, an aid to the decision-making process. *J Hepatol*. 2015; 62(4):855–62.

64. Lencioni R, Llovet JM, Han G et al. Sorafenib or placebo plus TACE with doxorubicineluting beads for intermediate stage HCC: The SPACE trial. *J Hepatol*. 2016; 64(5):1090–8.

65. Meyer T, Fox R et al. Sorafenib in combination with transarterial chemoembolization in patients with unresectable hepatocellular carcinoma (TACE 2): A randomised placebo- controlled, double-blind, phase 3 trial. *Lancet Gastroenterol Hepatol*. 2017; 2:565–75.

66. Kudo M, Imanaka K, Chida N et al. Phase III study of sorafenib after transarterial chemoembolisation in Japanese and Korean patients with unresectable hepatocellular carcinoma. *Eur J Cancer*. 2011; 47(14):2117–27.

67. Kudo M, Han G, Finn RS et al: Brivanib as adjuvant therapy to transarterial chemoembolization in patients with hepatocellular carcinoma: A randomized phase III trial. *Hepatology*. 2014; 60: 1697–707.

68. Pinter M, Ulbrich G, Sieghart W et al. Hepatocellular carcinoma: A phase II randomized controlled double-blind trial of transarterial chemoembolization in combination with biweekly intravenous administration of Bevacizumab or a Placebo. *Radiology*. 2015; 277(3):903–12.

69. Olweny CL, Toya T, Katongole-Mbidde E et al. Treatment of hepatocellular carcinoma with adriamycin. Preliminary communication. *Cancer*. 1975; 36(4):1250–7.

70. Johnson PJ, Williams R, Thomas H et al. Induction of remission in hepatocellular carcinoma with doxorubicin. *Lancet*. 1978; 1(8072):1006–9.

71. Simonetti RG, Leberati A, Angiolini C et al. Treatment of hepatocellular carcinoma: A systematic review of randomized controlled trials. *Ann Oncol*. 1997; 8:117–36.

72. Leung TW, Johnson PJ. Systemic therapy for hepatocellular carcinoma. *Semin Oncol*. 2001; 28:514–20.

73. Leung TW, Patt YZ, Lau WY et al. Complete pathological remission is possible with systemic combination chemotherapy for inoperable hepatocellular carcinoma. *Clin Cancer Res*. 1999; 5(7): 1676–81.

74. Yeo W, Mok TS, Zee B et al. A randomized phase III study of doxorubicin versus cisplatin/interferon alpha-2b/doxorubicin/fluorouracil (PIAF) combination chemotherapy for unresectable hepatocellular carcinoma. *J Natl Cancer Inst*. 2005; 97(20):1532–8.

75. Qin S, Bai Y, Lim HY et al. Randomized, multicenter, open-label study of oxaliplatin plus fluorouracil/leucovorin versus doxorubicin as palliative chemotherapy in patients with advanced hepatocellular carcinoma from Asia. *J Clin Oncol*. 2013; 31(28):3501–8.

76. Farinati F, De Maria N, Fornasiero A et al. Prospective controlled trial with antiestrogen drug tamoxifen in patients with unresectable hepatocellular carcinoma. *Dig Dis Sci*. 1992; 37(5):659–62.

77. CLIP Group (Cancer of the Liver Italian Programme). Tamoxifen in treatment of hepatocellular carcinoma: A randomised controlled trial. *Lancet*. 1998; 352(9121):17–20.

78. Chow PK, Tai BC, Tan CK et al. Asian–Pacific Hepatocellular Carcinoma Trials Group. High-dose tamoxifen in the treatment of inoperable hepatocellular carcinoma: A multicenter randomized controlled trial. *Hepatology*. 2002; 36(5):1221–6.

79. Siegel AB, Cohen EI, Ocean A et al. Phase II trial evaluating the clinical and biologic effects of bevacizumab in unresectable hepatocellular carcinoma. *J Clin Oncol*. 2008; 26(18):2992–8.

80. Llovet JM, Ricci S, Mazzaferro V et al. Sorafenib in advanced hepatocellular carcinoma. *N Engl J Med*. 2008; 359(4):378–90.

81. Cheng AL, Kang YK, Chen Z et al. Efficacy and safety of sorafenib in patients in the Asia-Pacific region with advanced hepatocellular carcinoma: A phase III randomised, double-blind, placebo-controlled trial. *Lancet Oncol*. 2009; 10(1):25–34.

82. Abou-Alfa GK, Schwartz L, Ricci S et al. Phase II study of sorafenib in patients with advanced hepatocellular carcinoma. *J Clin Oncol*. 2006; 24(26):4293–300.

83. Cheng AL, Kang YK, Lin DY et al. Sunitinib versus sorafenib in advanced hepatocellular cancer: Results of a randomized phase III trial. *J Clin Oncol*. 2013; 31(32):4067–75.

84. Cainap C, Qin S, Huang WT et al. Linifanib versus Sorafenib in patients with advanced hepatocellular carcinoma: Results of a randomized phase III trial. *J Clin Oncol*. 2015; 33(2):172–9.

85. Thomas MB, Morris JS, Chadha R et al. Phase II trial of the combination of bevacizumab and erlotinib in patients who have advanced hepatocellular carcinoma. *J Clin Oncol*. 2009; 27(6):843–50.

86. Zhu AX, Rosmorduc O, Evans TR et al. SEARCH: A phase III, randomized, double-blind, placebo-controlled trial of sorafenib plus erlotinib in patients with advanced hepatocellular carcinoma. *J Clin Oncol*. 2015; 33(6):559–66.

87. Alavi AS, Acevedo L, Min W, Cheresh DA. Chemoresistance of endothelial cells induced by basic fibroblast growth factor depends on Raf-1-mediated inhibition of the proapoptotic kinase, ASK1. *Cancer Res*. 2007; 67(6):2766–72.

88. Abou-Alfa GK, Johnson P, Knox JJ et al. Doxorubicin plus sorafenib vs. doxorubicin alone in patients with advanced hepatocellular carcinoma: A randomized trial. *JAMA*. 2010; 304(19): 2154–60.

89. Abou-Alfa GK, Shi Q, Knox JJ et al. Assessment of treatment with sorafenib plus doxorubicin vs. sorafenib alone in patients with advanced hepatocellular carcinoma: Phase 3 CALGB 80802 randomized clinical trial. *JAMA Oncol*. 2019; 5(11):1582–8.

90. Johnson PJ, Qin S, Park JW et al. Brivanib versus sorafenib as first-line therapy in patients with unresectable, advanced hepatocellular carcinoma: Results from the randomized phase III BRISK-FL study. *J Clin Oncol*. 2013; 31(28):3517–24.

91. Kudo M, Finn RS, Qin S et al. Lenvatinib versus sorafenib in first-line treatment of patients with unresectable hepatocellular carcinoma: A randomised phase 3 non-inferiority trial. *Lancet*. 2018; 391(10126):1163–73.

92. Santoro A, Rimassa L, Borbath I et al. Tivantinib for second-line treatment of advanced hepatocellular carcinoma: A randomised, placebo-controlled phase 2 study. *Lancet Oncol*. 2013; 14(1): 55–63.

93. Rimassa L, Assenat E, Peck-Radosavljevic M et al. Tivantinib for second-line treatment of MET-high, advanced hepatocellular carcinoma (METIV-HCC): A final analysis of a phase 3, randomised, placebo-controlled study. *Lancet Oncol*. 2018; 19(5):682–693.

94. Abou-Alfa GK, Meyer T, Cheng AL et al. Cabozantinib in patients with advanced and progressing hepatocellular carcinoma. *N Engl J Med*. 2018; 379(1):54–63.

95. Bruix J, Qin S, Merle P et al. Regorafenib for patients with hepatocellular carcinoma who progressed on sorafenib treatment (RESORCE): A randomised, double-blind, placebo-controlled, phase 3 trial. *Lancet*. 2017; 389(10064):56–66.

96. Finn RS, Merle P, Granito A et al. Outcomes of sequential treatment with sorafenib followed by regorafenib for HCC: Additional analyses from the phase III RESORCE trial. *J Hepatol*. 2018; 69(2):353–358.

97. Zhu AX, Park JO, Ryoo BY et al. Ramucirumab versus placebo as second-line treatment in patients with advanced hepatocellular carcinoma following first-line therapy with sorafenib (REACH):

A randomised, double-blind, multicentre, phase 3 trial. *Lancet Oncol.* 2015; 16(7):859–70.

98. Zhu AX, Kang YK, Yen CJ et al. Ramucirumab after sorafenib in patients with advanced hepatocellular carcinoma and increased α-fetoprotein concentrations (REACH-2): A randomised, double-blind, placebo-controlled, phase 3 trial. *Lancet Oncol.* 2019; 20(2):282–296.

99. Palmer DH, Midgley RS, Mirza N et al. A phase II study of adoptive immunotherapy using dendritic cells pulsed with tumor lysate in patients with hepatocellular carcinoma. *Hepatology.* 2009; 49(1):124–32.

100. El-Khoueiry AB, Sangro B, Yau T et al. Nivolumab in patients with advanced hepatocellular carcinoma (CheckMate 040): An open-label, non-comparative, phase 1/2 dose escalation and expansion trial. *Lancet.* 2017; 389(10088):2492–2502.

101. Zhu AX, Finn RS, Edeline J et al. Pembrolizumab in patients with advanced hepatocellular carcinoma previously treated with sorafenib (KEYNOTE-224): A non-randomised, open-label phase 2 trial. *Lancet Oncol.* 2018; 19(7):940–52.

102. Yau T, Park JW, Finn RS et al. CheckMate 459: A randomized, multi-center phase 3 Study of Nivolumab (NIVO) vs. Sorafenib (SOR) as First-Line (1L) Treatment in Patients (pts) with advanced hepatocellular carcinoma (aHCC). ESMO, 2019 LBA38.

103. Finn RS, Ryoo BY, Merle P et al. Pembrolizumab as second-line therapy in patients with advanced hepatocellular carcinoma in KEYNOTE-240: A randomized, double-blind, phase III trial. *J Clin Oncol.* 2020; 38(3):193–202.

104. Cheng A-L, Qin S, Ikeda M et al. IMbrave150: Efficacy and safety results from a ph III study evaluating atezolizumab (atezo) + bevacizumab (bev) vs. sorafenib (Sor) as first treatment (tx) for patients (pts) with unresectable hepatocellular carcinoma (HCC). *Annals Oncol.* 2019; 30(Suppl 9):LBA 3.

105. Marrero JA, Kudo M, Venook AP et al. Observational registry of sorafenib use in clinical practice across Child-Pugh subgroups: The GIDEON study. *J Hepatol.* 2016; 65(6):1140–1147.

106. Kudo M, Matilla A, Santoro A et al. Checkmate-040: Nivolumab (NIVO) in patients (pts) with advanced hepatocellular carcinoma (aHCC) and Child-Pugh B (CPB) status. *J Clin Oncol.* 2019; 37(4_suppl):327–327.

107. Hawkins MA, Dawson LA. Radiation therapy for hepatocellular carcinoma: From palliation to cure. *Cancer.* 2006; 106(8):1653–63.

108. Robertson JM, Lawrence TS, Dworzanin LM et al. Treatment of primary hepatobiliary cancers with conformal radiation therapy and regional chemotherapy. *J Clin Oncol.* 1993; 1(7):1286–93.

109. Raoul JI, Bretagne JF, Caucanas JP et al. Internal radiation therapy for hepatocellular carcinoma. Results of a French multicenter phase II trial of transarterial injection of iodine 131-labeled lipiodol. *Cancer.* 1992; 69(2):346–52.

110. Salem R, Lewandowski RJ, Atassi B et al. Treatment of unresectable hepatocellular carcinoma with use of 90Y microspheres (TheraSphere): Safety, tumor response, and survival. *J Vasc Interv Radiol.* 2005; 16(12):1627–39.

111. Vilgrain V, Pereira H, Assenat E et al. Efficacy and safety of selective internal radiotherapy with yttrium-90 resin microspheres compared with sorafenib in locally advanced and inoperable hepatocellular carcinoma (SARAH): An open-label randomised controlled phase 3 trial. *Lancet Oncol.* 2017; 18(12):1624–36.

112. Chow PKH, Gandhi M, Tan SB et al. Selective internal radiation therapy versus sorafenib in Asia-Pacific patients with hepatocellular carcinoma. *J Clin Oncol.* 2018; 36(19):1913–1921.

113. Ricke J, Klümpen HJ, Amthauer H et al. Impact of combined selective internal radiation therapy and sorafenib on survival in advanced hepatocellular carcinoma. *J Hepatol.* 2019; 71(6):1164–74.

10 PANCREATIC CANCER

Kulbir Mann, Andrea Sheel, and Paula Ghaneh

Incidence, epidemiology, and etiology

Pancreatic cancer is still associated with a poor outcome, with the number of annual deaths from the disease expected to exceed that of breast cancer in Europe.[1] Across the world, the incidence of pancreatic cancer was 458,918 in 2018 with 432,242 mortalities, giving an age standardized incidence rate of 5.5 per 100,000 and a mortality rate of 4.8 per 100,000.[2] It predominately occurs across Asia and Europe with incidence proportions of 46.7% and 28.9%, respectively.[2] There is a slight male preponderance compared with females, with incidence rates per 100,000 of 5.5 and 4.0, respectively.[2] The 5-year survival rates range between 3% and 9% across the world.[3–5]

The risk factors for pancreatic cancer are listed in Table 10.1, and it is important to note that there is no single predisposing factor. Genetic risks are responsible for 10% of all pancreatic cancers and are covered later in the chapter.[4] Pancreatic malignancy is more likely to occur in older patients, with 80% arising in patients aged 60–80. Half of these patients are over the age of 70, and it is unlikely to occur under 40 years of age.[3]

There have been many studies describing an alcohol dose–dependent increased risk of pancreatic cancer. A recent meta-analysis found that high alcohol intake, defined as >24 g a day, gave a relative risk ratio of 1.15, and no association with low or moderate alcohol intake was recorded.[6] Smoking may act as an associated factor and increase risk with a low to moderate alcohol intake.[5] Multiple studies and meta-analyses have reviewed cigarette smoking as a risk factor alone and pooled up to 80 studies, including case-control studies and cohorts, to give a relative risk of 1.66–1.77.[7,8] Smoking one pack per year raises the risk of pancreatic cancer by 1%, and the risk remains at this level until 10 years of smoking cessation is achieved.[4,7,8]

Obesity has been shown by many studies to increase the risk of pancreatic cancer. A cohort study of over 14,000 patients discovered a robust association between increased body mass and pancreatic cancer. An odds ratio of 1.34 for every standard deviation increase in body mass index was reported, and they also noted an odds ratio of 1.66 for increased fasting insulin levels but not diabetes.[9] A recent meta-analysis reviewed 13 studies and found a hazard ratio of 1.06 and 1.31 in overweight and obese patients, respectively. This finding has not been shown in Asia-Pacific populations.[10] Sarcopenia is emerging as a risk factor for survival in many different cancers, including colorectal and ovarian.[11–14] A similar association has been found in pancreatic cancer, with odds ratios of 1.67 and 2.58 in overweight and obese patients.[15] A meta-analysis reviewed 11 studies, revealing that sarcopenic and sarcopenic obese patients had increased hazard ratios of 1.49 and 2.01, respectively.[12]

With respect to dietary factors, there have been many studies reviewing the risk of red meat consumption for pancreatic cancer.[16] A study of 11 case-control studies found that red meat intake increased the risk of pancreatic cancer by 48%, and the intake of vegetables and fruits reduced it by 38%.[17] Two further meta-analyses have found similar risks from the consumption of 100–120 g of red meat a day, with a relative risk of 1.13 of developing pancreatic malignancy.[18,19] The EPIC European prospective group undertook one of the largest cohort studies, and they found no association amongst red meat and processed meat consumers and pancreatic cancer (relative risk [RR] = 1.03 and 0.93, respectively).[20] There is insufficient evidence to reliably state that red meat consumption increases the risk of pancreatic cancer.

Genetic aspects of disease

It is estimated that approximately 10% of pancreatic ductal adenocarcinoma (PDAC) cases may be familial in origin. With a rapidly ageing population, the incidence and frequency of PDAC will increase in turn. Several genetic mutations and familial cancer syndromes are believed to confer a significantly increased risk of developing PDAC. It can be further refined if an individual has undergone specific genetic testing to identify mutations in known pancreatic cancer susceptibility genes. Several germline gene mutations have been identified, including PALB2, ATM, STK11/LKB1 (Peutz–Jeghers disease, RR = 132), p16/CDKN2A (familial atypical multiple mole melanoma [FAMMM], RR = 20–34), PRSS1 (hereditary pancreatitis [HP], RR = 50–80), and DNA mismatch repair genes along with certain BRCA2 (RR = 3.5–10) mutations.[21] Familial pancreatic cancer (FPC) is characterized by an autosomal dominant pattern of inheritance of PDAC. The underlying genetic mechanisms responsible for FPC are not yet fully understood. Attempts to further understand FPC have led to the identification of additional novel genes, which confer an increase in risk but do not explain the phenomenon fully.

Pancreatitis

Approximately 1% of all cases of pancreatitis have an underlying inherited cause. A number of genetic mutations are recognized in their association with HP and idiopathic pancreatitis. HP is characterized by recurrent attacks of acute pancreatitis, which progresses to chronic pancreatitis. There is a family history of pancreatitis consistent with an autosomal dominant inheritance pattern and/or the presence of a proven known genetic mutation in the cationic trypsinogen gene (PRSS1) and high penetrance of approximately 80%. Typically, symptoms of malabsorption and diabetes mellitus commence at a younger age in HP than in other causes of chronic pancreatitis, and the cumulative rate of both endocrine and exocrine failure is higher.[22]

In addition to the familial cancer syndromes described, the reported cumulative PDAC risk in HP varies between 60- and 100-fold, with a lifetime risk of around 40%.[23,24] Tobacco smoking can further increase this risk, and smokers were seen to develop PDAC 20 years earlier than non-smokers, reflecting findings in the general population.[25] There is ample epidemiological evidence that chronic pancreatitis increases the risk of pancreatic cancer, and in addition, there is a solid theoretical basis for a link between cancer and inflammation. There is, however, currently no evidence to support screening in the presence of sporadic or alcohol-related chronic pancreatitis.

TABLE 10.1 **Major Risk Factors for Pancreatic Cancer**

High Risk (RR >2.0)	Moderate Risk (RR 1.5–2.0)	Low Risk (RR <1.5)
Inherited syndromes	Family history	Excess body weight
Hereditary pancreatitis (PRSS1)	Tobacco smoking	Low physical activity
Hereditary non polyposis colorectal cancer (MSH2 MLH1)	Long term diabetes	Metabolic syndrome
Hereditary breast & ovarian cancer (BRCA1 BRCA2)		O blood group (protective)
Familial atypical multiple mole melanoma syndrome (p16)		Atopic allergy (protective)
Peutz–Jeghers syndrome (STK11)		*Helicobacter pylori*
Ataxia-telangiectasia (ATM)		Hepatitis B infection
Familial adenomatous polyposis		Dietary factors
Familial pancreatic cancer		High alcohol intake (>30 g/day)
Von Hippel–Lindau syndrome (VHL)		High red meat consumption
Li–Fraumeni syndrome (p53)		High processed meat consumption
Fanconi Anaemia (FANC)		Low fruit, vegetable & dietary folate
ABO SNPs rs9543324/rs401681		
Chronic pancreatitis		

Source: Reproduced from Ilic and Ilic, 2016. Open access.

Pathology and staging

The pathology of the majority of pancreas tumors is ductal adenocarcinoma, which accounts for over 85%. Table 10.2 lists the other types of tumors arising from the pancreas. For lesions that obstruct the distal bile duct, clinical presentation and investigations are the same and often lead to identical surgical management. The differential includes distal cholangiocarcinoma, duodenal carcinoma, and peri-ampullary malignancy, which may be of intestinal or pancreatic type. The size of the tumor and the extent of local invasion and distant metastatic spread are of paramount importance in determining management strategies, especially with the advent of neoadjuvant clinical trials. The staging process of pancreatic cancer is through the TNM classification of malignant tumors maintained by the Union of International Cancer Control. It is depicted in Table 10.3.

Clinical diagnosis

Signs and symptoms

The retroperitoneal location of the pancreas reduces the effect a mass has on the gastrointestinal tract, and lesions become quite sizeable before they cause any symptoms. If they occur at the head of the pancreas, the first noticeable symptom may be jaundice as the distal bile duct becomes obstructed. This partly explains why only 10% of patients are able to undergo curative surgery.[26] Patients complain of non-specific symptoms of weight loss, change in appetite, early satiety, and vague back pain. Specific complications of the disease include obstructive jaundice, malabsorption, and late onset diabetes.[27] Patients may present with gastrointestinal bleeding from an invasive tumor or even a degree of gastric outlet obstruction. Examination findings are often vague, with some signs of weight loss or cachexia. Jaundice may be apparent from the sclera to the skin, and a mass may be palpable, which represents the tumor itself or a distended gallbladder (Courvoisier's sign).

Serum investigations may yield deranged liver function tests, but other standard markers are indicators of progressive deterioration but not specific to pancreatic cancer. The use of carbohydrate antigen nineteen nine (CA19-9) as a diagnostic marker has become standard across the world, with a specificity and sensitivity of 80% and 75–80%, respectively.[28,29] CA19-9 is a cell surface antigen glycoprotein expressed on pancreatic cancer cells

TABLE 10.2 **Pathology of Pancreatic Cancer**

Pancreatic cancer pathology
Pancreatic ductal carcinoma
Adenosquamous carcinoma
Mucinous non cystic (colloid) carcinoma
Mucinous cystic neoplasms
Intraductal papillary mucinous neoplasm with an associated invasive carcinoma
Solid pseudopapillary neoplasm
Acinar cell carcinoma
Pancreatoblastoma
Serous cystadenocarcinoma
Undifferentiated anaplastic carcinoma
Signet ring cell carcinoma
Giant cell carcinoma

Source: Parks, 2018. With permission.

TABLE 10.3 **TNM Staging of Pancreatic Cancer**

Tumor			Nodes		Metastases	
1	a Tumor <0.5 cm b Tumor 0.5–1 cm c Tumor 1–2 cm	0	No nodes	0	No metastases	
2	Tumor 2–4 cm	1	1-3 nodes involved	1	Distant metastases	
3	Tumor >4 cm	2	4 or more involved nodes			
4	Tumor involves coeliac axis, superior mesenteric artery/common hepatic artery					

Stage	Gradings			
Ia	T1		N0	M0
Ib	T2		N0	M0
IIa	T3		N0	M0
IIb	T1, T2, T3		N1	M0
III	T1, T2, T3		N2	M0
	T4		Any N	M0
IV	Any T		Any N	M1

Source: Brierley et al., 2016. With permission.

but is also raised in other conditions such as acute and chronic pancreatitis, obstructive jaundice, cholangitis, liver cirrhosis, and bile duct malignancy.[30] In addition, Lewis negative blood type Caucasians do not produce CA19-9, and it can be raised in obstructive jaundice, contributing to the low positive predictive value of 0.5–0.9%.[30,31] Despite this, there has been some evidence that it can be used as a prognostic marker pre-operatively with respect to extent of disease and post-operatively in relation to overall survival.[27,31–35] A multiple and diverse set of biomarkers are currently being studied, including micro-RNAs and also those that select for chemotherapy and potential immunomodulatory treatments.[30,36]

Investigations

Cross-sectional imaging forms the mainstay of diagnosis and allows an assessment of staging through multi-disciplinary meetings, determining the optimal management strategy of pancreatic lesions.[37] Though most patients with vague symptoms and red flag suspicions for malignancy will undergo a contrast enhanced computed tomography (CT), patients with presentations of deranged liver function tests will merit an ultrasound first line. The absence of gallstones and presence of dilated ducts is the main stimulus for cross-sectional imaging, especially as the pancreas is often obscured by gas. The sensitivity has been reported as 50–90% and is very dependent upon the user.[38]

Multi-detector CT (MD-CT) is the single most important imaging modality for pancreatic cancer, specifically assessing not only the anatomical location of the tumor and its surrounding structures but also distant disease. With a sensitivity of 76–100%, a specificity of 72%, and a positive predictive value of 89%, it is recommended by many guidelines for diagnosis and staging.[38–40] The classic finding is that of hypoattenuating pancreatic mass associated with duct dilatation and atrophy of the upstream pancreas. It has excellent spatial resolution and provides reconstructed three-dimensional images to delineate vascular involvement.[41] MD-CT is less effective at picking up small lesions or peritoneal nodules but can be used as surveillance post chemotherapy.[41] The definitions of borderline resectability of pancreatic cancer, devised by the National Comprehensive Cancer Network, are focused around triphasic, 1–2 mm MD-CT images.[42]

Magnetic resonance imaging has a sensitivity of 83–93.5% and heightened soft tissue contrast enabling better views of small lesions, isoattenuating lesions, and hypertrophied pancreas tissue.[38,41] It may serve as an adjunct to MD-CT but is not a routine part of staging. It is useful for lesions not visible on MD-CT and indeterminate liver lesions as well as visualizing the pancreatic and biliary ductal system, and morphological changes to the parenchyma and gallstones.[38,41] It has a role in determining resectability when liver metastases are confirmed.[41]

Positron emission tomography (PET) utilizes the radiotracer ^{18}F-fluoro-2-deoxy-D-glucose (FDG), which builds up in cells with high metabolism. Its sole role in diagnosis is not as a substitute for MD-CT, as it has reduced spatial resolution and a poor false-positive rate.[38,41] The sensitivity of PET-CT has been reported as 84.4–96.8%, but it is important for detecting extra-pancreatic disease. In combination with MD-CT, there is an anatomical and functional element to staging pancreatic cancer. PET-PANC was a multicenter prospective accuracy and clinical value study of PET-CT in patients with pancreatic cancer. In a cohort of 589 patients, a maximum standardized uptake value of 7.5 provided a significant increase in sensitivity over MD-CT. The clinical impact of this was more pertinent, as it stopped 58 patients from having surgery due to inappropriate staging and

influenced management in 250 patients.[43] This incremental diagnostic benefit has led to PET-CT being recommended by the National Institute for Health and Care Excellence (NICE) as part of the routine staging process.[40]

The combination of endoscopic ultrasound (EUS) and fine needle aspiration (FNA) is being more often utilized to produce high-resolution images, especially with lesions smaller than 3 cm. It has the ability to obtain anatomically accurate tissue for pathological analysis. In many centers, it is being used in preference to cytological brushings obtained from endoscopic retrograde cholangiopancreatography (ERCP).[38,41] There are fewer complications and a sensitivity of 86.8% and specificity of 95.8% for pancreatic malignancy.[41,44] Unfortunately, the sensitivity drops when attempting to differentiate a malignant lesion from chronic inflammation (76%). Contrasted enhanced EUS and elastography are techniques that may enhance the diagnostic accuracy, and a systematic review of two papers demonstrated their utility over other imaging modalities post MD-CT.[38,45]

The use of ERCP as a diagnostic tool has been mentioned; however, its importance as an intervention for biliary drainage remains a controversial topic with conflicting research. It has been reported that jaundice has adverse effects on post-operative complications and survival in pancreatic cancer, advocating the need for endoscopic decompression prior to surgery.[46,47] A multicenter randomized control trial of 202 patients from 2010 found that routine use of endoscopic decompression increased post-operative infectious complications.[48] This has been confirmed by a number of other studies, including a meta-analysis of over 6000 patients.[49–53] It has led to some institutions in the United Kingdom developing a fast track pathway for pancreatoduodenectomy for pancreatic and ampullary cancers.[54,55] Though the effect of post-operative morbidity has been studied, the effect on survival is less clear. A review of Surveillance, Epidemiology, and End Results (SEER) data in the United States found no difference between preoperative decompression and early surgery with respect to survival in 16,670 patients.[56] NICE guidance has suggested that patients who have obstructive jaundice secondary to malignancy should have early resection providing they are fit for surgery.[40] The effects of jaundice and ERCP are apparent with respect to post-operative complications but not necessarily survival, and there is an important role for endoscopic decompression in certain subsets of patients.

Staging laparoscopy has been advocated for resectable pancreatic cancer for a number of years, but its exact use has not been fully established. It was reported that a CA19-9 level of 150 kU/l was the threshold for patients to have a staging laparoscopy based upon a single center practice, with a sensitivity of 52% and a specificity of 93%.[57] Since then, multiple studies and reviews have advocated this threshold as well as tumor size of greater than 3 cm.[57–59] A Cochrane review analyzed 16 studies to assess the use of laparoscopy post CT in the resectability of pancreatic cancer. It summarized that if a patient had a resectable lesion on cross-sectional imaging, then a laparoscopy would determine that it was unresectable in 20% of cases compared with 41% when only CT was employed.[60]

Management

Surgery and peri-operative principles

Though there are promising studies trialing neoadjuvant chemotherapy for pancreatic cancer, surgical resection is the mainstay of curative management. Even so, only 10% of patients had surgery in 2013–2014 in the United Kingdom, predominately Stage 1 and 2.[61] The median survival of patients undergoing curative surgery is 11–23 months, and 10–27% are alive at 5 years.[27]

The choice of surgery approach is dependent on the location of the mass and its relationship to the local vasculature. For lesions at the tail of the pancreas, a radical left pancreatectomy is performed, which involves a splenectomy and local nodal excision. For pancreatic head lesions, a pancreatoduodenectomy is performed, which was first described by Walter Kausch in 1912.[62] He resected the majority of the duodenum and head of pancreas, but it was Allen Whipple who excised the whole duodenum, developed reconstructions, and published them in 1946.[62] The principle of the procedure involved resection of the head of the pancreas together with the duodenum/pylorus and the main portion of the bile duct. A reconstruction is created employing a Roux-en-Y bypass, with a hepatico-jejunostomy and a pancreato-jejunostomy forming a bilopancreatic limb. A pylorus preserving version of the procedure is commonly performed using a single limb (Figure 10.1).

Resectability is dependent upon tumor involvement of the superior mesenteric vein (SMV) and portal vein and any major arterial vessels. The definitions of borderline resectability (BR) have been established by an international consensus in 2016 order to standardize reporting and multi-disciplinary team (MDT) decision making.[42] They defined BR with respect to anatomical, biological, and conditional factors and extended features of the disease to incorporate additional factors that make surgery high risk. These are focused upon studies that have demonstrated poor perioperative survival and incorporate TMN staging and anesthetic fitness.[42] The anatomical factors are listed in Table 10.4 and are focused upon MD-CT and the relationship of the lesion around the superior mesenteric artery or the coeliac axis.[42] The concerning features are stenosis, deformity, and narrowing or occlusion of major vessels without extension beyond the inferior border of the duodenum. The biological features are those of particular suspicion of metastatic disease and lymph node disease. Serum CA 19-9 levels of greater than 500 units/ml and suspicious regional nodes on MD-CT and PET imaging are

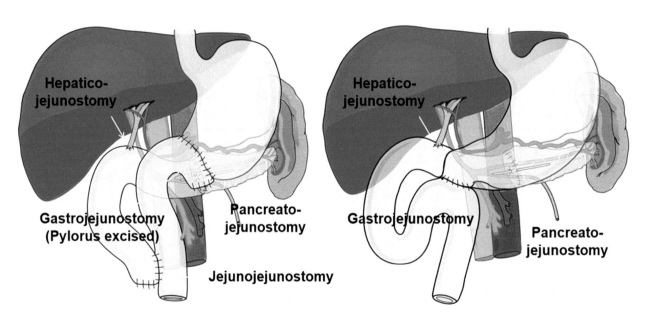

FIGURE 10.1   (Left) Kausch Whipple; (right) pylorus preserving Kausch Whipple.

TABLE 10.4   International Consensus of Classification of BR PDAC Based on Anatomical Definition Using MD-CT

Resectable	• SMV/PV: no tumor contact or unilateral narrowing
	• SMA, CA, CHA: no tumor contact
Borderline resectable *BR-PV (SMV/PV involvement) BR-A (arterial involvement)*	Subclassified according to SMV/PV involvement alone or arterial invasion
	• SMV/PV: tumor contact 180 or greater or bilateral narrowing/occlusion, not exceeding the inferior border of the duodenum
	• SMA, CA, CHA: no tumor contact/invasion
	• SMA, CA: tumor contact of less than 180 without showing deformity/stenosis.
	• CHA: tumor contact without showing tumor contact of the PHA and/or CA.
	• (The involvement of the aorta is categorized as unresectable. Presence of variant arterial anatomy is not taken into consideration)
Unresectable *Locally advanced Metastatic*	Subclassified according to the status of distant metastasis
	• SMV/PV: bilateral narrowing/occlusion, exceeding the inferior border of the duodenum.
	• SMA, CA: tumor contact/invasion of 180 or more degrees.
	• CHA: tumor contact/invasion showing tumor contact/invasion of the PHA and/or CA.
	• AO: tumor contact or invasion
	• Distant metastasis

Source: Isaji et al., 2018. With permission.

concerning for resectability, and these nodes may require FNA under EUS. The final parameters are with respect to patient factors and focus around the performance status of the patient.[63] The tumor may be resectable, but the patient may be high risk for surgery and require more extensive preoperative investigations and consideration of prehabilitation.[64] This has become a fundamental principle in enhanced recovery, which will be discussed later.

The role of vascular resection and extended pancreatectomy operations has been extensively reviewed for borderline resectable lesions and those invading other organs. The 1 mm resection margin clearance is key for disease free and overall survival in pancreatic cancer, and so extra-pancreatic visceral resections may improve survival.[65,66] There have been many reviews analyzing data from retrospective cohort series that have shown improved survival in patients who have had a pancreatoduodenectomy together with a vascular resection or another organ resected.[67] Many have shown an increase in median survival over palliative bypass operations, with results more favorable in benign disease.[67–69] Operating times, blood loss, and morbidities are significantly higher with this patient cohort, and these operations should only be performed at a high-volume center in order to ensure long-term survival.[69–71]

The main complications of a pancreatoduodenectomy are pancreatic fistula (11.2%) and delayed gastric emptying (DGE) (27.7%).[72,73] These are the common causes of failure to return to enteral nutrition and delay discharge. Significant perioperative improvements have reduced the in-hospital mortality post pancreatoduodenectomy to 1–6%.[74–77] The operation still carries a significant degree of morbidity with rates up to 20–40%.[74,77,78] There are many aspects of the perioperative care of a patient that may have an impact on outcomes; the most pertinent features follow.

Post-operative pancreatic fistula (POPF) is a term that was used inconsistently for many years in the literature until the International Study Group of Pancreatic Surgery (ISGPS) created definitions and grades. The clinically relevant grades are B and C, which often mean that the patient requires persistent drainage after 3 weeks and may require further intervention due to sepsis.[79] This has afforded precise definitions, and newer studies are able to be compared easily at a standard baseline.[80]

The left sided pancreatectomy has POPF as its major morbidity, with fistula rates of approximately 30%.[81,82] Multiple risk factors have been reviewed, and it has been suggested that obesity, blood loss, and non-ligation of the pancreatic duct may increase fistula rates.[81] Multiple remnant ligation techniques have been described, including hand-sewn sutures, stapler techniques, anastomoses, bio-sealants, and autologous patches. From multiple studies, trials, and meta-analyses, there has been no clear answer to which technique is best, and the two common suture and staple techniques are equivalent.[81–85] A recent meta-analysis discovered that specific suture ligation of the pancreatic duct may reduce the incidence of a severe POPF, but further trials are still required.[83]

A pancreatoduodenectomy involves a pancreatic anastomosis, and reducing the risk of a fistula incorporates different strategies compared with a left pancreatectomy. A meta-analysis has been recently carried out that compared an anastomosis of the pancreas remnant to the posterior wall of the stomach with the traditional pancreatojejunostomy. There was no significant difference in POPF rates between the two techniques, but there were more hemorrhagic complications with the pancreatogastrostomy.[86] A Cochrane review analyzed 10 randomized

control trials and made similar findings.[77] Other strategies to reduce POPF include the routine use of somatostatin analogues such as octreotide. Initial meta-analyses demonstrated some benefit, in that it reduces length of stay and POPF rates, but later studies refuted this, and now it is not recommended, though it is still used.[87–90] The ISGPS released a position statement stating that there is no specific technique that can reduce the rate of POPF.[91]

DGE has an incidence of 11–51% and is the most common complication post pancreatoduodenectomy.[72,92,93] It has been reported that in the absence of intra-abdominal complications and POPF, the incidence is at the lower aspects of this range. This American study reviewed 10,500 patients in the National Surgical Quality Improvement Program and found independent risk factors for DGE to be age >75, male sex, pylorus preserving, or a prolonged operating time.[94] There have been many studies reviewing anatomical reconstructive variations to reduce the risk, and preservation of the pylorus was one of the initial techniques. Unfortunately, though some studies suggested it does affect DGE, many others, including a meta-analysis, have found no association.[72,94–96] Techniques such as a pancreaticogastrostomy vs. pancreatojejunostomy or a retrocolic vs. antecolic anastomosis for the gastrojejunostomy have also shown limited findings.[93,97,98]

Minimally invasive surgery is rapidly becoming the gold standard for some sub-specialty cancer resections, but its progress in pancreatic cancer is slow. This is due to the technical nature of the resection with the potential for locally advanced disease and the intricacies of the multiple anastomoses. The published reports are all retrospective case series, and the minimally invasive approach is carefully selected for in particular patients.[99] There have certainly been some suggestions that minimally invasive surgery in the form of laparoscopic and robotic pancreatoduodenectomy provides at least similar long-term outcomes but shorter lengths of stay and reduced blood loss compared with open surgery.[99–103] The time factor is more problematic in robotic surgery, with specialized equipment needing close monitoring with low technical failure rates as compared with laparoscopic procedures.[99–103] There is clearly a steep learning curve, and multiple reviews and meta-analyses have stated that minimally invasive pancreatic resection is a technically feasible, oncologically sound procedure that takes longer to perform and may reduce post-operative complications.[99–104] The heterogeneity of studies and a weak methodology make more definitive conclusions difficult to achieve at this time.

The Enhanced Recovery After Surgery (ERAS) society published guidelines on pancreatoduodenectomy in 2012, indicating that there was a strategy to follow the well-established protocols in other surgical specialties. Table 10.5 demonstrates the basic principles that have evolved over the years with a continued focus on preoperative counseling, lifestyle modification, and nutrition.[105] There have been multiple studies that have reviewed the use of ERAS principles but are largely retrospective and inconsistent in terms of baseline.[106,107] They have shown faster recovery times and reduced length of stay, demonstrating the benefits of ERAS. Further studies are needed to critically review principles such as operative techniques, pain relief strategies, and management of complications.[106,107] Prompt removal of nasogastric tubes, catheters, and intra-abdominal drains together with early reinstigation of nutrition and mobilization are crucial to enhanced recovery.[105] A recent study has suggested that patients can be discharged on Day 5, showing that there are still advancements to be made.[108]

TABLE 10.5   Current ERAS Recommendations with Evidence Base Assessment

Item	Recommendation	Evidence base
Preoperative counselling	Patients should receive dedicated counselling routinely	Low evidence, strong recommendation
Perioperative biliary drainage	This should not be undertaken routinely in patients with a serum bilirubin <250 µmol/L	Moderate evidence, weak recommendation
Preoperative smoking and alcohol consumption	For alcohol abusers, 1 month of abstinence before is beneficial and should be attempted. For daily smokers, 1 month of abstinence before surgery is beneficial. For appropriate group, both should be attempted	Alcohol abstention: low evidence, strong recommendation Smoking cessation: moderate evidence, strong recommendation
Preoperative nutrition	Routine use is not warranted but significantly malnourished patients should be optimised orally or enterally pre-operatively	Very low evidence, weak recommendation
Perioperative oral immunonutrition (IN)	Balance of evidence suggests that IN for 5–7 days perioperatively may be considered to reduce infectious complications	Moderate evidence, weak recommendation
Oral bowel preparation	Extrapolating from colorectal studies, this should not be used	Moderate evidence, weak recommendation
Preoperative fasting and treatment with carbohydrates	Intake of clear fluids up to two hours before anaesthesia does not increase gastric residual volume. Extrapolating data from colorectal studies suggests oral carbohydrate therapy be used in patients without diabetes	Fluid intake: high evidence Solid intake: low evidence Carbohydrate: low evidence Strong recommendations
Preanaesthetic medication	No clinical benefit from pre-operative use of long-acting sedatives, short acting anxiolytics may be used for smaller anaesthetic procedures	Moderate evidence, weak recommendation
Anti-thrombolytic prophylaxis	Low molecular weight heparin reduces risk of thromboembolic complications and should be continued for 4 weeks after hospital discharge	High evidence, strong recommendation
Antimicrobial prophylaxis and skin preparation	Prevents surgical site infections and used in a single dose manner 30–60 minutes before skin incision.	High evidence, strong recommendation
Epidural analgesia	Mid thoracic epidurals are recommended based on evidence that it is superior to intravenous opioids with a reduced incidence of respiratory complications	Pain: high evidence Respiratory complications: moderate evidence Weak evidence
Intravenous analgesia	Some evidence supports PCA or IV lidocaine methods, insufficient evidence	PCA: low evidence Lidocaine: moderate evidence Weak recommendations
Transverse abdominis plane block/ infusions	Conflicting and variable results but some evidence is in support of wound catheters or TAP blocks	Wound catheters: moderate evidence TAP blocks: moderate evidence
Postoperative nausea and vomiting	There are benefits to using multimodal pharmacological agents depending on patient's history	Low evidence, strong recommendation
Incision	At the discretion of surgeon	Very low evidence, strong recommendation
Avoiding hypothermia	Intraoperative patient warming should be used by forced air or circulating water garments	High evidence, strong recommendation
Postoperative glycaemic control	Insulin resistance and hyperglycaemia are strongly associated with morbidity and mortality. Intravenous insulin may be used but close monitoring as to avoid hypoglycaemia is essential	Low evidence, strong recommendation
Nasogastric intubation	Does not improve outcomes, not warranted routinely	Moderate evidence, strong recommendation
Fluid balance	Near zero fluid balance and avoiding overload of electrolytes and water improves outcomes. Intraoperative monitoring of stroke volume with a transoesophageal Doppler is recommended. Balanced crystalloid solutions are preferred to 0.9% saline	Fluid balance: moderate evidence, strong recommendation Balanced crystalloids: moderate evidence Strong recommendations
Perianastomotic drain	Early removal after 72 hrs in patients that are low risk for developing a pancreatic fistula (Drain amylase <5000 U/L).	High evidence, strong recommendation
Somatostatin analogues	Somatostatin & its analogues show no benefit on outcomes	Moderate evidence, strong recommendation
Urinary drainage	Transurethral catheters can be removed safely on postoperative day 1 or 2 unless otherwise indicated	High evidence, strong recommendation
Delayed gastric emptying	No acknowledged strategy	Very low evidence, weak recommendation
Stimulation of bowel movement	Oral laxatives and chewing gum given postoperatively are safe, and may accelerate gastrointestinal transit	Low evidence, weak recommendation
Postoperative artificial nutrition	Allow a normal diet after surgery without restrictions. Begin carefully and increase intake depending on tolerance. Enteral feeding should be given for specific indications and parenteral should not be used routinely	Moderate evidence, strong recommendation
Early and scheduled mobilisation	Mobilise actively from morning of first postoperative day and encourage to meet daily targets	Very low evidence, strong recommendation
Audit	Systematic improves compliance and clinical outcomes	Low evidence, strong recommendation

Abbreviations: PCA: Patient-controlled analgesis; IV: intravenous; TAP: transverse abdominus plane.
Source: Lassen et al., 2013. With permission.

Adjuvant and neoadjuvant therapy

Resectable disease

Over the past 20 years, multicenter randomized control trials have been the mainstay of pancreatic cancer research and have been practice changing. The European Study Group for Pancreatic Cancer (ESPAC) has delivered multiple randomized trials, beginning with ESPAC-1, published in 2004. In this trial, 289 patients were randomized into four groups receiving chemoradiotherapy, chemotherapy, both chemotherapy and chemoradiotherapy, and observation alone. Adjuvant chemotherapy led to a 5-year survival of 21% compared with 10% receiving chemoradiotherapy and 8% in the observation group.[109] The ESPAC-3 trial demonstrated that adjuvant gemcitabine was similar in survival to 5-fluorouracil/folinic acid but had a lower toxicity profile, becoming the standard of care for a long period of time.[110] ESPAC-4 randomized 732 patients into two treatment groups: gemcitabine vs. gemcitabine and capecitabine (GEMCAP). They found a median survival advantage of 28 months over 25.5 months in the GEMCAP group.[111] This study was particularly important, as it confirmed the superiority of combination chemotherapy over single agent therapy for pancreatic cancer. A Canadian and French group performed a multicenter randomized control trial reviewing gemcitabine with a modified dose combination of fluorouracil, leucovorin, irinotecan, and oxaliplatin (FOLFIRINOX) in 493 resected pancreatic cancers. They discovered a median survival of 54.4 months compared with 35 months in the FOLFIRINOX group. Unfortunately, there was a greater proportion of serious adverse events, 75.9% compared with 52.9% with FOLFIRINOX and gemcitabine, respectively.[112] Currently, NICE U.K. guidelines recommend GEMCAP and for those not well enough to tolerate combined treatment, gemcitabine monotherapy as adjuvant therapy for patients who have undergone resection for pancreatic cancer. FOLFIRINOX is recommended in patients with metastatic disease who have a performance status of 0–1.[40] The American Society of Clinical Oncology recently updated its guidelines and stated that a modified dose of FOLFIRINOX should be offered to patients who have had resected pancreatic adenocarcinoma.[113] It is worth noting that the JASPAC-1 trial was a randomized trial in 385 Japanese resected pancreatic cancer patients, treating them with either gemcitabine or S-1. This trial found a 5-year survival of 24.4% with gemcitabine and 44.1% in the S-1 group.[114] Though a major adjuvant treatment in Japan, these findings have not been confirmed in a randomized trial in a Western population. Chemoradiation is not recommended as routine management for adjuvant therapy in current management guidelines.[40]

Borderline resectable and locally advanced disease

There have been multiple trials reviewing the impact of FOLFIRINOX on patients with locally advanced cancer and BR

disease, and its role as a neoadjuvant treatment is being evaluated. Two studies from Italy and Germany have demonstrated the resectability of tumors post FOLFIRINOX treatment.[115,116] In a cohort of 575 patients in Germany with locally advanced pancreatic cancer, a successful resection was achieved in 50.8%, with a median overall survival of 15.3 months compared with 8.5 months in the non-resected group.[115] In a cohort of 680 patients in Italy, there was a resection rate of 15.1% in patients who initially had locally advanced/unresectable disease treated with neoadjuvant chemotherapy. Median survival was 35.4 months and 41.8 months in patients who were initially locally advanced and BR, respectively.[116] These studies show great promise, with increased rates of resection and extended median survival time. There have been several meta-analyses that highlight areas of further research.[117–119] Schorn et al. reviewed 35 studies and stated that 40% of all neoadjuvant patients remain unresectable, but patients who are resected have genuine down-staging of the tumor and higher rates of R0 resection.[117] Versteijne et al. reviewed 38 studies and found that in all patients (borderline or resectable) treated with neoadjuvant therapy, fewer patients were resected compared with the upfront surgery group (66% vs. 81.3%, $p < 0.001$). There was a greater overall median survival despite this: 18.8 months in the neoadjuvant group and 14.8 months in the upfront surgery group.[119] This has led to the conclusion that neoadjuvant treatment with FOLFIRINOX does lead to increased survival and improved histological outcomes in patients with locally advanced or unresectable pancreatic cancer.[117,120,121] There has yet to be a Phase III randomized control trial to evaluate this treatment strategy; however, ESPAC-5 is aiming to develop this evidence base. It is currently recruiting patients with borderline resectable disease to be treated with upfront surgery compared with GEMCAP, FOLFIRINOX, or chemoradiotherapy[122] (Tables 10.6 and 10.7).

The use of chemoradiotherapy in the neoadjuvant setting in patients with borderline/locally advanced pancreatic cancer has been investigated in many Phase II trials throughout the world. They have all suggested that further development into a Phase III trial is needed.[123–126] Jang et al. found that there were more R0 resections with locally advanced pancreatic cancer patients who had neoadjuvant chemoradiation in comparison to upfront surgery.[124] A Dutch multicenter trial reviewing neoadjuvant chemoradiotherapy against immediate surgery for borderline resectable disease (PREOPANC-1) presented short-term results of 142 patients revealing higher overall median survival of 17.1 vs. 13.5 months (chemoradiotherapy vs. upfront surgery) and higher R0 resection rates of 65% vs. 35%, respectively.[127] The only Phase III trial that has completed is the LAP07 trial, which was an international multicenter Phase III randomized trial reviewing 449 locally advanced pancreatic cancer patients, who were treated in two stages. The initial randomization consisted of gemcitabine alone or in combination with erlotinib, and after 4 months, a

TABLE 10.6 **Pancreatic Cancer Learning Points**

Learning points
- One should have a low clinical suspicion for patients with insidious upper abdominal symptoms.
- Key staging investigations include serum CA19-9 levels, MD-CT, and PET-CT.
- One should have a holistic awareness of borderline resectability and not only focus upon imaging.
- Neoadjuvant treatment is slowly becoming more utilized in borderline disease and may be a feasible option for clinical trials.
- Pancreatoduodenectomy and distal pancreatectomy are both developing minimal access strategies and should incorporate enhanced recovery principles.
- Multimodal adjuvant chemotherapy is crucial to longer-term survival.
- A personalized approach to treatment is likely to be the future of pancreatic cancer management.

TABLE 10.7   **Current Trials in Progress Listed with the ISRCTN Registry**

Name of study	Intervention	Aims
SharkBITE Study	Performing a randomized study of FNA or a Sharkcore biopsy for pancreatic lesions	The aim of this study is to compare the performance of a standard fine needle aspiration needle and the Sharkcore biopsy needle in endoscopic ultrasound guided pancreatic tissue sampling
Precision Panc	Patients with suspected pancreatic cancer will have extra core biopsies to allow molecular profiling together with additional blood samples	To establish a mechanism and framework to recruit and screen patients with pancreatic cancer to perform molecular profiling and evaluation of circulating biomarkers and allow enrolment to Precision Panc PRIMUS studies
Primus 001 and 002	A Phase II study reviewing FOLFOX or nab-paclitaxel and gemcitabine use in patients with resectable (002 non-randomized) and metastatic disease (001 randomized). Both studies will have tissue samples collected from the patients at baseline under the Precision Panc Master Protocol	Primus 001: Progression free survival from the date of randomization to progression or death Primus 002: That biomarker positive patients will respond better to FOLFOX-A treatment than biomarker negative patients in the neoadjuvant setting
Distal pancreatectomy, minimally invasive or open for malignancy (DIPLOMA) AND Comparison of laparoscopic and open distal pancreatectomy	Patients who have suspected PDAC in the body or tail of the pancreas are randomized into minimally invasive surgery or open resection	To determine whether minimally invasive (laparoscopic and robot-assisted) distal pancreatectomy (MIDP) provides similar oncologic efficacy to open distal pancreatectomy (ODP)
NEOPA: Sequential NEOadjuvant chemoradiotherapy (CRT) followed by curative surgery vs. primary surgery alone for resectable, non-metastasized Pancreatic Adenocarcinoma	A randomized Phase III study of resectable pancreatic cancer patients randomized into neoadjuvant chemoradiotherapy followed by surgery group or upfront surgery and adjuvant chemoradiotherapy	Aiming to assess efficacy of neoadjuvant and adjuvant chemoradiotherapy on 3-year survival
ESPAC-5F: European Study group for Pancreatic Cancer—Trial 5F	A four-arm, prospective, multicenter, randomized feasibility trial of immediate surgery compared with neoadjuvant chemotherapies (FOLFIRINOX and GEMCAP) and neoadjuvant chemoradiotherapy	To compare neoadjuvant chemotherapy or chemoradiotherapy with immediate surgery. All patients who undergo resection will also receive adjuvant chemotherapy as standard
ALLIANCE Trial (North America)	A two-arm prospective multicenter Phase II randomized trial reviewing FOLFIRINOX and FOLFIRINOX combined with stereotactic body radiation therapy	To compare 18-month overall survival between treatment arms and the R0 resection rate

second randomization to continued chemotherapy as per initial regimen or chemoradiation with 54 Gy and capecitabine. The trial stopped early with the criteria for futility being fulfilled. They found no difference in median survival (16.5 vs. 15.2 months, gemcitabine vs. gemcitabine and erlotinib) in the initial randomization and no difference in survival with the second randomization. There was a reduced local progression rate of 32% compared with 46%, chemoradiation vs. chemotherapy. Overall, they concluded that there was no benefit to overall survival from utilizing chemoradiation.[128] The role of chemoradiation is still being investigated, and the final results of PREOPANC-1 together with ESPAC-5 will provide a strong evidence base on the question of the use of chemoradiation in the management of pancreatic cancer.

The use of neoadjuvant S-1 has been reviewed in multiple Phase II trials in Japan, often with concurrent use of radiotherapy in patients with locally advanced and borderline disease. The only study investigating neoadjuvant S1 without radiotherapy reviewed 24 patients with borderline/locally advanced pancreatic cancer. It found a response rate of 17.4% and a disease control rate of 87%. There was a resection rate of 60.9% and an R0 resection rate of 76.5%.[129] The JASPAC-05 study was recently completed and further reviewed the use of S-1 and radiotherapy in borderline pancreatic cancer. The study recruited 50 patients and had an overall median survival of 25.8 months and median progression

free survival of 6.7 months, and a Phase III trial is currently ongoing. It also reported an R0 resection rate of 52% with Grade III/IV complication rate of 43%.[130] Two further Japanese Phase II trials reviewed the use of neoadjuvant and hypofractionated/intensity-modulated radiotherapy in borderline pancreatic cancer. They reported resection rates of 96% and 70% and low toxicity profiles, indicating that Phase III studies are needed to investigate these treatment regimens further.[131,132] There is a clear benefit of S-1 and potentially radiotherapy in the Japanese population, but the lack of Phase III trials weakens the evidence base, and the effects are confined to Eastern populations.

Nab-paclitaxel is an albumin bound taxane drug showing promise in treating pancreatic cancer. Its role in metastatic pancreatic cancer is described later, but with borderline disease, there has been some early promise with a couple of small Phase II trials.[133,134] In an American study, 32 locally advanced/borderline patients who were ineligible for FOLFORINOX were treated with gemcitabine and nab-paclitaxel. The study found a 19% R0 resection rate and 15% showing a partial response, demonstrating a potential benefit of nab-paclitaxel in borderline disease.[135] A further American study reviewed second-line use of nab-paclitaxel as a neoadjuvant treatment for locally advanced cancer post FOLFIRINOX. It found that 52% of patients reached resection and recommended that nab-paclitaxel and gemcitabine be used as rescue therapy.[136] A further retrospective single-institution study reviewed 193 patients with resectable or BR pancreatic cancer treated with neoadjuvant FOLFIRINOX or gemcitabine and nab-paclitaxel. It found similar R0 resection rates of 80% but significantly less lymph node involvement in the FOLFIRINOX group and an increase of median overall survival of 4.9 months compared with gemcitabine and nab-paclitaxel.[137] Unfortunately, as the study was non-randomized, there were younger patients with fewer co-morbidities receiving FOLFIRINOX. An Italian study randomized 54 patients with locally advanced or BR pancreatic cancer into two treatment arms receiving nab-paclitaxel and gemcitabine (AG) or nab-paclitaxel, gemcitabine, cisplatin, and capecitabine (PAXG). They found similar tumor resection rates of 31% and 32%, PAXG vs. AG, and overall survival at 18 months of 69% and 54%, respectively.[133] There is clearly a role for neoadjuvant gemcitabine nab-paclitaxel in the borderline/locally advanced setting, but Phase III trials are required to further explore this treatment option.

Metastatic pancreatic cancer

The latest guidance has suggested that nab-paclitaxel plus gemcitabine and FOLFIRINOX are the regimens recommended for metastatic pancreatic cancer. Many studies have been performed using FOLFIRINOX in metastatic disease, but the PRODIGE4/ACCORD 11 and MPACT were Phase III trials comparing both recommended agents with gemcitabine.[138] The PRODIGE4/ACCORD 11 enrolled 342 patients across 48 centers in France and compared FOLFIRINOX and gemcitabine. The median overall survival was significantly improved with FOLFIRINOX at 11.1 months vs. 6.8 months with gemcitabine. There were greater but manageable toxicities in the former group, with 45.7% developing neutropenia, 12.7% diarrhea, and 11.4% alopecia. A quality of life analysis of this cohort of patients demonstrated worse survival for patients who spent "quite a bit" or "very much" time in a chair or bed during the day.[138] The impact on survival is clear with FOLFIRINOX, but the effect on quality of life can be quite substantial.

In patients with metastatic pancreatic cancer, using nab-paclitaxel combined with gemcitabine gave a median survival advantage of approximately 2 months compared with gemcitabine alone.[139] The only Phase III trial, MPACT, was performed as a multicenter study of 861 metastatic pancreatic patients comparing nab-paclitaxel and gemcitabine with gemcitabine monotherapy. They found increased survival in the nab-paclitaxel group of 8.5 months compared with 6.7 months with gemcitabine alone.[140,141] A Phase II study from France reviewed 114 patients with metastatic disease and combined nab-paclitaxel with either gemcitabine or leucovorin and fluorouracil. The aim of the study was to review 4-month recurrence free survival with continued treatment until unacceptable toxicity. They found promising results in the leucovorin and fluorouracil group, with over 50% of patients demonstrating progression free survival at the 4-month end point and a tolerable toxicity profile.[134] This suggests that Phase III trials would be a feasible future direction. These studies have led these agents to be incorporated into Cochrane reviews, American guidelines, and NICE guidance for metastatic pancreatic cancer.[40,121,142] There is clearly a need to stratify patients according to performance status in order to manage potential side-effects.

Palliation

The World Health Organization definition of palliative care focuses upon patients with non-curable disease having measures in place for pain control and psychological, social, and spiritual care.[27] There are specific considerations that need to be addressed with pancreatic cancer. The interventions that may be required are for the management of obstructive jaundice and gastric outlet obstruction. Many patients present with biliary obstruction and are often stented at the ERCP procedure. Multiple randomized control trials have been performed reviewing the use of plastic and self-expandable metal stents (SEMS) for malignant obstruction.[143] A recent meta-analysis all of these trials found that metal stents, though providing no benefit to survival, had higher symptom free survival (odds ratio [OR] 5.96), lower complication rates (OR 0.43), fewer occlusions (OR 0.11) and interventions (weighted mean difference [WMD] −0.83), and longer patency rates.[143,144] If unresectable disease is found at laparotomy, then there is evidence that a hepaticojejunostomy may be performed, but it is dependent on the patient's symptoms and quality of life at the time of the procedure.[144] A retrospective U.K. study suggested that a single bypass procedure and an SEMS stent has fewer complications and readmissions compared with a double bypass procedure, and another Swedish study stated that "wait and see" is reasonable.[145,146]

It has been reported that 10–25% of patients with pancreatic cancer will exhibit symptoms of gastric outlet obstruction prior to death.[144] Many may experience nausea due to cachexia associated with malignancy leading to malnutrition, but a proportion of these will have luminal narrowing. It has long been thought that a surgical retrocolic gastrojejunostomy to the posterior wall of the stomach is the best management strategy, but often, it depends on the disease progression. DGE remains a complication.[144] Endoscopic palliation using an SEMS stent has been reported on extensively with comparable outcomes compared with a surgical bypass and a quicker return to oral intake and shorter admission times.[147,148] There are still complications of perforation, hemorrhage, aspiration pneumonia, and stent migration/failure in 26% of patients.[144] A randomized multicenter study from the Netherlands found better short-term outcomes with stenting but longer-term patency in patients with surgical gastrojejunostomy. They recommended that for patients expected to survive longer than 2 months, a surgical bypass should be performed.[149]

Laparoscopic gastrojejunostomy has also been reported in a number of small cohort studies, which have all reported technical success with comparable co-morbidities to other strategies. Its acceptance as a standard strategy remains to be seen, especially as prospective research studies are few in number.[144,150]

Future aspects of management

Early detection remains the critical aspect of pancreatic cancer research, which would afford more curative resections. CA19-9 remains the only suitable biomarker, but it has low sensitivity and specificity and is not suitable as a screening tool but more as a monitoring marker. Many serum and tumor biological markers have been investigated with little clinical success. There have been gene mutations detected in pancreatic cancer: genetic, epigenetic, non-coding RNA, metabolomics, and microbiomics.[151] Chromosomal structural variations have been studied, and the rearrangements, deletions, and amplifications have been categorized into stable, locally rearranged, scattered, and instable subtypes.[152] It has been theorized that responses to chemotherapy may vary according to these groups. Ultimately, pancreatic cancer is a complicated disease with an average of 63 genetic mutations per cancer, and thus, subclass classifications may be a novel approach.[151]

With the advent of multiple chemotherapy regimens that improve survival, with the associated morbidities, there is an onus on tailoring specific therapies to the individual patient. An example is that low serum hENT1 (human equilibrative nucleoside transporter 1) has been associated with a poor response to gemcitabine monotherapy.[153,154] A recent Cochrane review suggested that for advanced cancer, combination chemotherapy confers most benefit, and biomarker development is essential for personalized selection for patients.[121] The Precision Panc project aims to molecularly profile all patients with pancreatic cancer, both resectable and advanced disease, in association with clinical trials with differing chemotherapy arms. The results of these studies will provide valuable information for the future of pancreatic cancer management.

References

1. Ferlay J, Partensky C, Bray F. More deaths from pancreatic cancer than breast cancer in the EU by 2017. *Acta Oncol.* 2016; 55(9–10):1158–60.
2. Bray, F, Ferlay J, Soerjomataram I et al. Global cancer statistics 2018: GLOBOCAN estimates of incidence and mortality worldwide for 36 cancers in 185 countries. *CA Cancer J Clin.* 2018; 68(6):394–424.
3. Ilic M, Ilic I. Epidemiology of pancreatic cancer. *World J Gastroenterol.* 2016; 22(44):9694–705.
4. Maisonneuve P. Epidemiology and burden of pancreatic cancer. *Presse Med.* 2019; 48(3 Pt 2):e113–23.
5. Rawla P, Sunkara T, Gaduputi V. Epidemiology of pancreatic cancer: Global trends, etiology and risk factors. *World J Oncol.* 2019; 10(1):10–27.
6. Wang YT, Gou YW, Jin WW et al. Association between alcohol intake and the risk of pancreatic cancer: A dose-response meta-analysis of cohort studies. *BMC Cancer.* 2016; 16:212.
7. Iodice S, Gandini S, Maisonneuve P et al. Tobacco and the risk of pancreatic cancer: A review and meta-analysis. *Langenbecks Arch Surg.* 2008; 393(4):535–45.
8. Korc M, Jeon CY, Edderkaoui M et al. Tobacco and alcohol as risk factors for pancreatic cancer. *Best Pract Res Clin Gastroenterol.* 2017; 31(5):529–36.
9. Carreras-Torres R, Johansson M, Gaborieau V et al. The role of obesity, Type 2 diabetes, and metabolic factors in pancreatic cancer: A mendelian randomization study. *J Natl Cancer Inst.* 2017; 109(9):djx012.
10. Majumder K, Gupta A, Arora N. Premorbid obesity and mortality in patients with pancreatic cancer: A systematic review and meta-analysis. *Clin Gastroenterol Hepatol.* 2016; 14(3):355–68 e; quiz e32.
11. Mei KL, Batsis JA, Mills JB et al. Sarcopenia and sarcopenic obesity: Do they predict inferior oncologic outcomes after gastrointestinal cancer surgery? *Perioper Med.* 2016; 5:30.
12. Mintziras I, Miligkos M, Waechter S et al. Sarcopenia and sarcopenic obesity are significantly associated with poorer overall survival in patients with pancreatic cancer: Systematic review and meta-analysis. *Int J Surg.* 2018; 59:19–26.
13. Rutten IJ, Ubachs J, Kruitwagen RF et al. The influence of sarcopenia on survival and surgical complications in ovarian cancer patients undergoing primary debulking surgery. *Eur J Surg Oncol.* 2017; 43(4):717–24.
14. Vashi PG, Gorsuch K, Wan L et al. Sarcopenia supersedes subjective global assessment as a predictor of survival in colorectal cancer. *PLoS One.* 2019; 14(6):e0218761.
15. Li D, Morris JS, Liu J et al. Body mass index and risk, age of onset, and survival in patients with pancreatic cancer. *JAMA.* 2009; 301(24):2553–62.
16. Beaney AJ, Banim PJ, Luben R et al. Higher meat intake is positively associated with higher risk of developing pancreatic cancer in an age-dependent manner and are modified by plasma antioxidants: A prospective cohort study (EPIC-Norfolk) using data from food diaries. *Pancreas.* 2017; 46(5):672–8.
17. Paluszkiewicz P, Smolińska K, Dębińska I et al. Main dietary compounds and pancreatic cancer risk. The quantitative analysis of case-control and cohort studies. *Cancer Epidemiol.* 2012; 36(1):60–7.
18. Larsson SC, Wolk A. Red and processed meat consumption and risk of pancreatic cancer: Meta-analysis of prospective studies. *Br J Cancer.* 2012; 106(3):603–7.
19. Zhao Z, Yin Z, Pu Z et al. Association between consumption of red and processed meat and pancreatic cancer risk: A systematic review and meta-analysis. *Clin Gastroenterol Hepatol.* 2017; 15(4):486–493.
20. Rohrmann S, Linseisen J, Nöthlings U et al. Meat and fish consumption and risk of pancreatic cancer: Results from the European Prospective Investigation into Cancer and Nutrition. *Int J Cancer.* 2013; 132(3):617–24.
21. Brand RE, Lerch MM, Rubinstein WS et al. Advances in counselling and surveillance of patients at risk for pancreatic cancer. *Gut.* 2007; 56(10):1460–9.
22. Howes N, Lerch MM, Greenhalf W et al. Clinical and genetic characteristics of hereditary pancreatitis in Europe. *Clin Gastroenterol Hepatol.* 2004; 2(3):252–61.
23. Lowenfels AB, Maisonneuve P, Whitcomb, DC. Risk factors for cancer in hereditary pancreatitis. International Hereditary Pancreatitis Study Group. *Med Clin North Am.* 2000; 84(3):565–73.
24. Lowenfels AB, Maisonneuve P, DiMagno EP. Hereditary pancreatitis and the risk of pancreatic cancer. International Hereditary Pancreatitis Study Group. *J Natl Cancer Inst.* 1997; 89(6):442–6.
25. Lowenfels AB, Maisonneuve P, Whitcomb DC. Cigarette smoking as a risk factor for pancreatic cancer in patients with hereditary pancreatitis. *JAMA.* 2001; 286(2):169–70.
26. Allemani C, Matsuda T, Di Carlo V et al. Global surveillance of trends in cancer survival 2000-14 (CONCORD-3): Analysis of individual records for 37 513 025 patients diagnosed with one of 18 cancers from 322 population-based registries in 71 countries. *Lancet.* 2018; 391(10125):1023–75.
27. Parks RW. *Hepatobiliary and Pancreatic Surgery* (6th ed.). Edinburgh, NY: Elsevier, 2018.
28. Huang Z, Liu, F. Diagnostic value of serum carbohydrate antigen 19–9 in pancreatic cancer: A meta-analysis. *Tumour Biol.* 2014; 35(8):7459–65.
29. Xing H, Wang J, Wang Y et al. Diagnostic value of CA 19–9 and carcinoembryonic antigen for pancreatic cancer: A meta-analysis. *Gastroenterol Res Pract.* 2018; 2018:8704751.
30. Hasan S, Jacob R, Manne U. Advances in pancreatic cancer biomarkers. *Oncol Rev.* 2019; 13(1):410.
31. Ballehaninna UK, Chamberlain RS. The clinical utility of serum CA 19–9 in the diagnosis, prognosis and management of pancreatic adenocarcinoma: An evidence based appraisal. *J Gastrointest Oncol.* 2012; 3(2):105–19.
32. Smith RA, Bosonnet L, Ghaneh P et al. Preoperative CA19-9 levels and lymph node ratio are independent predictors of survival in patients with resected pancreatic ductal adenocarcinoma. *Dig Surg.* 2008; 25(3):226–32.
33. Kondo N, Murakami Y, Uemura K et al. Comparison of the prognostic impact of pre- and post-operative CA19-9, SPan-1, and DUPAN-II levels in patients with pancreatic carcinoma. *Pancreatology.* 2017; 17(1):95–102.
34. Distler M, Pilarsky E, Kersting S et al. Preoperative CEA and CA 19–9 are prognostic markers for survival after curative resection for ductal adenocarcinoma of the pancreas–A retrospective tumor marker prognostic study. *Int J Surg.* 2013; 11(10):1067–72.
35. Ferrone CR, Finkelstein DM, Thayer SP et al. Perioperative CA19-9 levels can predict stage and survival in patients with resectable pancreatic adenocarcinoma. *J Clin Oncol.* 2006; 24(18):2897–902.
36. Chantrill LA, Nagrial AM, Watson C et al. Precision medicine for advanced pancreas cancer: The individualized molecular pancreatic cancer therapy (IMPaCT) trial. *Clin Cancer Res,* 2015; 21(9):2029–37.
37. Brierley JD, Gospodarowicz MK, Wittekind C. *TNM Classification of Malignant Tumours* (8th ed.). Hoboken, NJ: Wiley-Blackwell, 2016.

38. Lee ES, Lee JM. Imaging diagnosis of pancreatic cancer: A state-of-the-art review. *World J Gastroenterol.* 2014; 20(24):7864–77.

39. Zamboni GA, Kruskal JB, Vollmer CM et al. Pancreatic adenocarcinoma: Value of multidetector CT angiography in preoperative evaluation. *Radiology.* 2007; 245(3):770–8.

40. Pancreatic Cancer in Adults: Diagnosis and management. NICE Guideline [NG 85]. https://www.nice.org.uk/guidance/ng85

41. Chu LC, Goggins MG, Fishman EK. Diagnosis and detection of pancreatic cancer. *Cancer J.* 2017; 23(6):333–42.

42. Isaji S, Mizuno S, Windsor JA et al. International consensus on definition and criteria of borderline resectable pancreatic ductal adenocarcinoma 2017. *Pancreatology.* 2018; 18(1):2–11.

43. Ghaneh P, Hanson R, Titman A et al. PET-PANC: Multicentre prospective diagnostic accuracy and health economic analysis study of the impact of combined modality 18fluorine-2-fluoro-2-deoxy-d-glucose positron emission tomography with computed tomography scanning in the diagnosis and management of pancreatic cancer. *Health Technol Assess.* 2018; 22(7):1–114.

44. Puli SR, Bechtold ML, Buxbaum JL et al. How good is endoscopic ultrasound-guided fine-needle aspiration in diagnosing the correct etiology for a solid pancreatic mass?: A meta-analysis and systematic review. *Pancreas.* 2013; 42(1):20–6.

45. Tamburrino D, Riviere D, Yaghoobi M et al. Diagnostic accuracy of different imaging modalities following computed tomography (CT) scanning for assessing the resectability with curative intent in pancreatic and periampullary cancer. *Cochrane Database Syst Rev.* 2016; 9:CD011515.

46. Smith RA, Dajani K, Dodd S et al. Preoperative resolution of jaundice following biliary stenting predicts more favourable early survival in resected pancreatic ductal adenocarcinoma. *Ann Surg Oncol.* 2008; 15(11):3138–46.

47. Strasberg SM, Gao F, Sanford D et al. Jaundice: An important, poorly recognized risk factor for diminished survival in patients with adenocarcinoma of the head of the pancreas. *HPB,* 2014; 16(2):150–6.

48. van der Gaag NA, Rauws EA, van Eijck CH et al. Preoperative biliary drainage for cancer of the head of the pancreas. *N Engl J Med.* 2010; 362(2):129–37.

49. Chen Y, Ou G, Lian G et al. Effect of preoperative biliary drainage on complications following pancreatoduodenectomy: A meta-analysis. *Medicine.* 2015; 94(29):e1199.

50. Ng ZQ, Suthananthan, AE, Rao S. Effect of preoperative biliary stenting on post-operative infectious complications in pancreaticoduodenectomy. *Ann Hepatobiliary Pancreat Surg.* 2017; 21(4):212–16.

51. Liu C, Lu JW, Du ZQ et al. Association of preoperative biliary drainage with postoperative morbidity after pancreaticoduodenectomy. *Gastroenterol Res Pract.* 2015; 2015:796893.

52. Arkadopoulos N, Kyriazi MA, Papanikolaou IS et al. Preoperative biliary drainage of severely jaundiced patients increases morbidity of pancreaticoduodenectomy: Results of a case-control study. *World J Surg.* 2014; 38(11):2967–72.

53. di Mola FF, Tavano F, Rago RR et al. Influence of preoperative biliary drainage on surgical outcome after pancreaticoduodenectomy: Single centre experience. *Langenbecks Arch Surg.* 2014; 399(5):649–57.

54. Roberts KJ, Prasad P, Steele Y et al., A reduced time to surgery within a "fast track" pathway for periampullary malignancy is associated with an increased rate of pancreatoduodenectomy. *HPB.* 2017; 19(8):713–20.

55. Shin SH, Han IW, Ryu Yet al. Optimal timing of pancreaticoduodenectomy following preoperative biliary drainage considering major morbidity and postoperative survival. *J Hepatobiliary Pancreat Sci.* 2019; 26(10):449–458.

56. Rustgi SD, Amin S, Yang A et al. Preoperative endoscopic retrograde cholangiopancreatography is not associated with increased pancreatic cancer mortality. *Clin Gastroenterol Hepatol.* 2019; 17(8):1580–6.

57. Halloran CM, Ghaneh P, Connor S et al. Carbohydrate antigen 19.9 accurately selects patients for laparoscopic assessment to determine resectability of pancreatic malignancy. *Br J Surg.* 2008; 95(4):453–9.

58. De Rosa A, Cameron IC, Gomez D. Indications for staging laparoscopy in pancreatic cancer. *HPB.* 2016; 18(1):13–20.

59. Connor S, Bosonnet L, Alexakis N et al. Serum CA19-9 measurement increases the effectiveness of staging laparoscopy in patients with suspected pancreatic malignancy. *Dig Surg.* 2005; 22(1–2):80–5.

60. Allen VB, Gurusamy KS, Takwoingi Y et al. Diagnostic accuracy of laparoscopy following computed tomography (CT) scanning for assessing the resectability with curative intent in pancreatic and periampullary cancer. *Cochrane Database Syst Rev,* 2016; 7:CD009323.

61. Cancer Research UK. Pancreatic cancer statistics. 2019 [cited 2019 01/08/2019]; Available from: https://www.cancerresearchuk.org/health-professional/cancer-statistics/statistics-by-cancer-type/pancreatic-cancer.

62. Are C, Dhir M, Ravipati L. History of pancreaticoduodenectomy: Early misconceptions, initial milestones and the pioneers. *HPB.* 2011; 13(6):377–84.

63. Oken MM, Creech RH, Tormey DC et al. Toxicity and response criteria of the Eastern Cooperative Oncology Group. *Am J Clin Oncol.* 1982; 5(6):649–55.

64. Dunne DF, Jack S, Jones RP et al. Randomized clinical trial of prehabilitation before planned liver resection. *Br J Surg.* 2016; 103(5):504–12.

65. Ghaneh P, Kleeff J, Halloran CM et al. The impact of positive resection margins on survival and recurrence following resection and adjuvant chemotherapy for pancreatic ductal adenocarcinoma. *Ann Surg.* 2019; 269(3):520–9.

66. Campbell F, Smith RA, Whelan P et al. Classification of R1 resections for pancreatic cancer: The prognostic relevance of tumour involvement within 1 mm of a resection margin. *Histopathology.* 2009; 55(3):277–83.

67. Hartwig W, Vollmer CM, Fingerhut A et al. Extended pancreatectomy in pancreatic ductal adenocarcinoma: Definition and consensus of the International Study Group for Pancreatic Surgery (ISGPS). *Surgery.* 2014; 156(1):1–14.

68. Mitra A, Pai E, Dusane R et al. Extended pancreatectomy as defined by the ISGPS: Useful in selected cases of pancreatic cancer but invaluable in other complex pancreatic tumors. *Langenbecks Arch Surg.* 2018; 403(2):203–12.

69. Wang X, Demir IE, Schorn S et al. Venous resection during pancreatectomy for pancreatic cancer: A systematic review. *Transl Gastroenterol Hepatol.* 2019; 4:46.

70. Hartwig W, Gluth A, Hinz U et al. Outcomes after extended pancreatectomy in patients with borderline resectable and locally advanced pancreatic cancer. *Br J Surg.* 2016; 103(12):1683–94.

71. Kaiser J, Hackert T, Buchler MW. Extended pancreatectomy: Does it have a role in the contemporary management of pancreatic adenocarcinoma? *Dig Surg.* 2017; 34(6):441–6.

72. Panwar R, Pal S. The International Study Group of Pancreatic Surgery definition of delayed gastric emptying and the effects of various surgical modifications on the occurrence of delayed gastric emptying after pancreatoduodenectomy. *Hepatobiliary Pancreat Dis Int.* 2017; 16(4):353–3.

73. McMillan MT, Zureikat AH, Hogg ME et al. A propensity score-matched analysis of robotic vs. open pancreatoduodenectomy on incidence of pancreatic fistula. *JAMA Surg.* 2017; 152(4):327–5.

74. Cusworth BM, Krasnick BA, Nywening TM et al. Whipple-specific complications result in prolonged length of stay not accounted for in ACS-NSQIP Surgical Risk Calculator. *HPB.* 2017; 19(2):147–53.

75. DeOliveira ML, Winter JM, Schafer M et al. Assessment of complications after pancreatic surgery: A novel grading system applied to 633 patients undergoing pancreaticoduodenectomy. *Ann Surg.* 2006; 244(6):931–7; discussion 937–9.

76. Relles DM, Burkhart RA, Pucci MJ et al. Does resident experience affect outcomes in complex abdominal surgery? Pancreaticoduodenectomy as an example. *J Gastrointest Surg.* 2014; 18(2):279–85; discussion 285.

77. Cheng Y, Briarava M, Lai M et al. Pancreaticojejunostomy versus pancreaticogastrostomy reconstruction for the prevention of

postoperative pancreatic fistula following pancreaticoduodenectomy. *Cochrane Database Syst Rev.* 2017; 9:CD012257.

78. Mogal HD, Fino N, Clark C, Shen P. Comparison of observed to predicted outcomes using the ACS NSQIP risk calculator in patients undergoing pancreaticoduodenectomy. *J Surg Oncol.* 2016; 114(2):157–62.

79. Bassi C, Dervenis C, Butturini G et al. Postoperative pancreatic fistula: An international study group (ISGPF) definition. *Surgery.* 2005; 138(1):8–13.

80. Bassi C, Dervenis C, Butturini G et al. The 2016 update of the International Study Group (ISGPS) definition and grading of postoperative pancreatic fistula: 11 Years after. *Surgery.* 2017; 161(3): 584–91.

81. Tieftrunk E, Demir IE, Schorn S et al. Pancreatic stump closure techniques and pancreatic fistula formation after distal pancreatectomy: Meta-analysis and single-center experience. *PLoS One.* 2018; 13(6):e0197553.

82. Diener MK, Seiler CM, Rossion I et al. Efficacy of stapler versus hand-sewn closure after distal pancreatectomy (DISPACT): A randomised, controlled multicentre trial. *Lancet.* 2011; 377(9776):1514–22.

83. Kollar D, Huszár T, Pohárnok Z et al. A review of techniques for closure of the pancreatic remnant following distal pancreatectomy. *Dig Surg.* 2016; 33(4):320–8.

84. Probst P, Huettner FJ, Klaiber U et al. Stapler versus scalpel resection followed by hand-sewn closure of the pancreatic remnant for distal pancreatectomy. *Cochrane Database Syst Rev.* 2015; (11):CD008688.

85. Zhang H, Zhu F, Shen M et al. Systematic review and meta-analysis comparing three techniques for pancreatic remnant closure following distal pancreatectomy. *Br J Surg.* 2015; 102(1):4–15.

86. Lyu Y, Li T, Cheng Y et al. Pancreaticojejunostomy Versus pancreaticogastrostomy after pancreaticoduodenectomy: An up-to-date meta-analysis of RCTs applying the ISGPS (2016) criteria. *Surg Laparosc Endosc Percutan Tech.* 2018; 28(3):139–46.

87. Gurusamy KS, Koti R, Fusai G, Davidson BR. Somatostatin analogues for pancreatic surgery. *Cochrane Database Syst Rev.* 2013; (4):CD008370.

88. Jin K, Zhou H, Zhang J et al. Systematic review and meta-analysis of somatostatin analogues in the prevention of postoperative complication after pancreaticoduodenectomy. *Dig Surg.* 2015; 32(3):196–207.

89. Garg PK, Sharma J, Jakhetiya A, Chishi N. The role of prophylactic octreotide following pancreaticoduodenectomy to prevent postoperative pancreatic fistula: A meta-analysis of the randomized controlled trials. *Surg J (N Y).* 2018; 4(4):e182–7.

90. Han X, Xu Z, Cao S, Zhao Y, Wu W. The effect of somatostatin analogues on postoperative outcomes following pancreatic surgery: A meta-analysis. *PLoS One.* 2017; 12(12):e0188928.

91. Shrikhande SV, Sivasanker M, Vollmer CM et al. Pancreatic anastomosis after pancreatoduodenectomy: A position statement by the International Study Group of Pancreatic Surgery (ISGPS). *Surgery.* 2017; 161(5):1221–34.

92. Parmar AD, Sheffield KM, Vargas GM et al. Factors associated with delayed gastric emptying after pancreaticoduodenectomy. *HPB.* 2013; 15(10):763–72.

93. Vandermeeren C, Loi P, Closset J. Does pancreaticogastrostomy decrease the occurrence of delayed gastric emptying after pancreatoduodenectomy? *Pancreas.* 2017; 46(8):1064–68.

94. Ellis RJ, Gupta AR, Hewitt DB et al. Risk factors for post-pancreaticoduodenectomy delayed gastric emptying in the absence of pancreatic fistula or intra-abdominal infection. *J Surg Oncol.* 2019; 119(7):925–31.

95. Glowka TR, Webler M, Matthaei H et al. Delayed gastric emptying following pancreatoduodenectomy with alimentary reconstruction according to Roux-en-Y or Billroth-II. *BMC Surg.* 2017; 17(1):24.

96. Klaiber U, Probst P, Strobel O et al. Meta-analysis of delayed gastric emptying after pylorus-preserving versus pylorus-resecting pancreatoduodenectomy. *Br J Surg.* 2018; 105(4):339–49.

97. Imamura M, Kimura Y, Ito T et al. Effects of antecolic versus retrocolic reconstruction for gastro/duodenojejunostomy on delayed

gastric emptying after pancreatoduodenectomy: A systematic review and meta-analysis. *J Surg Res.* 2016; 200(1):147–57.

98. Hanna MM, Gadde R, Alllen CJ et al. Delayed gastric emptying after pancreatoduodenectomy. *J Surg Res.* 2016; 202(2):380–8.

99. Liu M, Ji S, Xu W et al. Laparoscopic pancreaticoduodenectomy: Are the best times coming? *World J Surg Oncol.* 2019; 17(1):81.

100. Torphy RJ, Friedman C, Halpern A et al. Comparing short-term and oncologic outcomes of minimally invasive versus open pancreaticoduodenectomy across low and high volume centers. *Ann Surg.* 2018; 270(6):1147–1155.

101. Wang S, Shi N, You L, Dai M, Zhao Y. Minimally invasive surgical approach versus open procedure for pancreaticoduodenectomy: A systematic review and meta-analysis. *Medicine.* 2017; 96(50):e8619.

102. Pedziwiatr M, Małczak P, Pisarska M et al. Minimally invasive versus open pancreatoduodenectomy-systematic review and meta-analysis. *Langenbecks Arch Surg.* 2017; 402(5):841–51.

103. Chen K, Pan Y, Liu XL et al. Minimally invasive pancreaticoduodenectomy for periampullary disease: A comprehensive review of literature and meta-analysis of outcomes compared with open surgery. *BMC Gastroenterol.* 2017; 17(1):120.

104. Poves I, Burdío F, Morató O et al. Comparison of perioperative outcomes between laparoscopic and open approach for pancreatoduodenectomy: The PADULAP randomized controlled trial. *Ann Surg.* 2018; 268(5):731–9.

105. Lassen K, Coolsen MM, Slim K et al. Guidelines for perioperative care for pancreaticoduodenectomy: Enhanced Recovery After Surgery (ERAS(R)) Society recommendations. *World J Surg.* 2013; 37(2):240–58.

106. Pecorelli N, Nobile S, Partelli S et al. Enhanced recovery pathways in pancreatic surgery: State of the art. *World J Gastroenterol* 2016; 22(28):6456–68.

107. Xu X, Zheng C, Zhao Y, Chen W, Huang Y. Enhanced recovery after surgery for pancreaticoduodenectomy: Review of current evidence and trends. *Int J Surg.* 2018; 50:79–86.

108. Daniel SK, Thornblade LW, Mann GN, Park JO, Pillarisetty VG. Standardization of perioperative care facilitates safe discharge by postoperative day five after pancreaticoduodenectomy. *PLoS One.* 2018; 13(12):e0209608.

109. Neoptolemos JP, Stocken DD, Friess H et al. A randomized trial of chemoradiotherapy and chemotherapy after resection of pancreatic cancer. *N Engl J Med.* 2004; 350(12):1200–10.

110. Neoptolemos JP, Moore MJ, Cox TF et al. Effect of adjuvant chemotherapy with fluorouracil plus folinic acid or gemcitabine vs. observation on survival in patients with resected periampullary adenocarcinoma: The ESPAC-3 periampullary cancer randomized trial. *JAMA.* 2012; 308(2):147–56.

111. Neoptolemos JP, Palmer DH, Ghaneh P et al. Comparison of adjuvant gemcitabine and capecitabine with gemcitabine monotherapy in patients with resected pancreatic cancer (ESPAC-4): A multicentre, open-label, randomised, phase 3 trial. *Lancet,* 2017; 389(10073):1011–24.

112. Conroy T, Hammel P, Hebbar M et al. FOLFIRINOX or gemcitabine as adjuvant therapy for pancreatic cancer. *N Engl J Med.* 2018; 379(25):2395–406.

113. Khorana AA, McKernin SE, Berlin J et al. Potentially curable pancreatic adenocarcinoma: ASCO clinical practice guideline update. *J Clin Oncol.* 2019; 37(23):2082–8.

114. Uesaka K, Boku N, Fukutomi A et al. Adjuvant chemotherapy of S-1 versus gemcitabine for resected pancreatic cancer: A phase 3, open-label, randomised, non-inferiority trial (JASPAC 01). *Lancet.* 2016; 388(10041):248–57.

115. Hackert T, Sachsenmaier M, Hinz U et al. Locally advanced pancreatic cancer: Neoadjuvant therapy with FOLFIRINOX results in resectability in 60% of the patients. *Ann Surg.* 2016; 264(3):457–63.

116. Maggino L, Malleo G, Marchegiani G et al. Outcomes of primary chemotherapy for borderline resectable and locally advanced pancreatic ductal adenocarcinoma. *JAMA Surg.* 2019; 154(10): 932–942.

117. Schorn S, Demir IE, Reyes CM et al. The impact of neoadjuvant therapy on the histopathological features of pancreatic ductal adenocarcinoma—A systematic review and meta-analysis. *Cancer Treat Rev.* 2017; 55:96–106.

118. Suker M, Beumer BR, Sadot E et al. FOLFIRINOX for locally advanced pancreatic cancer: A systematic review and patient-level meta-analysis. *Lancet Oncol.* 2016; 17(6):801–10.

119. Versteijne E, Vogel JA, Besselink MG et al. Meta-analysis comparing upfront surgery with neoadjuvant treatment in patients with resectable or borderline resectable pancreatic cancer. *Br J Surg.* 2018; 105(8):946–58.

120. Scheufele F, Hartmann D, Friess H. Treatment of pancreatic cancer-neoadjuvant treatment in borderline resectable/locally advanced pancreatic cancer. *Transl Gastroenterol Hepatol.* 2019; 4:32.

121. Chin V, Nagrial A, Sjoquist K et al. Chemotherapy and radiotherapy for advanced pancreatic cancer. *Cochrane Database Syst Rev.* 2018; 3:CD011044.

122. Registry I. ESPAC-5F: European Study group for Pancreatic Cancer - Trial 5F. 2019 [cited 2019 01/08/2019]; Available from: https://doi.org/10.1186/ISRCTN89500674.

123. Fiore M, Ramella S, Valeri S et al. Phase II study of induction chemotherapy followed by chemoradiotherapy in patients with borderline resectable and unresectable locally advanced pancreatic cancer. *Sci Rep.* 2017; 7:45845.

124. Jang JY, Han Y, Lee H et al. Oncological benefits of neoadjuvant chemoradiation with gemcitabine versus upfront surgery in patients with borderline resectable pancreatic cancer: A prospective, randomized, open-label, multicenter phase 2/3 trial. *Ann Surg.* 2018; 268(2):215–22.

125. Katz MH, Shi Q, Ahmad SA et al. Preoperative modified FOLFIRINOX treatment followed by capecitabine-based chemoradiation for borderline resectable pancreatic cancer: Alliance for clinical trials in oncology trial A021101. *JAMA Surg.* 2016; 151(8):e161137.

126. Murphy JE, Wo JY, Ryan DP et al. Total neoadjuvant therapy with FOLFIRINOX followed by individualized chemoradiotherapy for borderline resectable pancreatic adenocarcinoma: A phase 2 clinical trial. *JAMA Oncol.* 2018; 4(7):963–69.

127. Tienhoven VG, Suker M, Groothuis KBC et al. Preoperative chemoradiotherapy versus immediate surgery for resectable and borderline resectable pancreatic cancer (PREOPANC-1): A randomized, controlled, multicenter phase III trial(18). *J Clin Oncol.* 2018; 38(16):1763–1773.

128. Hammel P, Huguet F, van Laethem JL et al. Effect of chemoradiotherapy vs. chemotherapy on survival in patients with locally advanced pancreatic cancer controlled after 4 months of gemcitabine with or without erlotinib: The LAP07 randomized clinical trial. *JAMA.* 2016; 315(17):1844–53.

129. Saito K, Isayama H, Sakamoto Y et al. A phase II trial of gemcitabine, S-1 and LV combination (GSL) neoadjuvant chemotherapy for patients with borderline resectable and locally advanced pancreatic cancer. *Med Oncol.* 2018; 35(7):100.

130. Takahashi S, Ikeda M, Konishi M et al. Final results of JASPAC05: Phase II trial of neoadjuvant S-1 and concurrent radiotherapy followed by surgery in borderline resectable pancreatic cancer. *J Clin Oncol.* 2019; 37(15):4127.

131. Nagakawa Y, Hosokawa Y, Nakayama H et al. A phase II trial of neoadjuvant chemoradiotherapy with intensity-modulated radiotherapy combined with gemcitabine and S-1 for borderline-resectable pancreatic cancer with arterial involvement. *Cancer Chemother Pharmacol.* 2017; 79(5):951–7.

132. Okano K, Suto H, Oshima M et al. A prospective phase II trial of neoadjuvant S-1 with concurrent hypofractionated radiotherapy in patients with resectable and borderline resectable pancreatic ductal adenocarcinoma. *Ann Surg Oncol.* 2017; 24(9):2777–84.

133. Reni M, Zanon S, Balzano G et al. A randomised phase 2 trial of nab-paclitaxel plus gemcitabine with or without capecitabine and cisplatin in locally advanced or borderline resectable pancreatic adenocarcinoma. *Eur J Cancer.* 2018; 102:95–102.

134. Bachet JB, Hammel P, Desramé J et al. Nab-paclitaxel plus either gemcitabine or simplified leucovorin and fluorouracil as first-line therapy for metastatic pancreatic adenocarcinoma (AFUGEM GERCOR): A non-comparative, multicentre, open-label, randomised phase 2 trial. *Lancet Gastroenterol Hepatol.* 2017; 2(5):337–46.

135. Peterson SL, Husnain M, Pollack T et al. Neoadjuvant nab-paclitaxel and gemcitabine in borderline resectable or locally advanced unresectable pancreatic adenocarcinoma in patients who are ineligible for FOLFIRINOX. *Anticancer Res.* 2018; 38(7):4035–9.

136. Vreeland TJ, McAllister F, Javadi S et al. Benefit of gemcitabine/nab-paclitaxel rescue of patients with borderline resectable or locally advanced pancreatic adenocarcinoma after early failure of FOLFIRINOX. *Pancreas.* 2019; 48(6):837–43.

137. Dhir M, Zenati MS, Hamad A et al. FOLFIRINOX versus gemcitabine/nab-paclitaxel for neoadjuvant treatment of resectable and borderline resectable pancreatic head adenocarcinoma. *Ann Surg Oncol.* 2018; 25(7):1896–903.

138. Lambert A, Gavoille C, Conroy T. Current status on the place of FOLFIRINOX in metastatic pancreatic cancer and future directions. *Therap Adv Gastroenterol.* 2017; 10(8):631–45.

139. Von Hoff DD, Ervin T, Arena FP et al. Increased survival in pancreatic cancer with nab-paclitaxel plus gemcitabine. *N Engl J Med.* 2013; 369(18):1691–703.

140. Young R, Mainwaring P, Clingan P et al. nab-Paclitaxel plus gemcitabine in metastatic pancreatic adenocarcinoma: Australian subset analyses of the phase III MPACT trial. *Asia Pac J Clin Oncol.* 2018; 14(5):e325–31.

141. Tabernero J, Kunzmann V, Scheithauer W et al. nab-Paclitaxel plus gemcitabine for metastatic pancreatic cancer: A subgroup analysis of the Western European cohort of the MPACT trial. *Onco Targets Ther.* 2017; 10:591–6.

142. Sohal DP, Mangu PB, Laheru D. Metastatic pancreatic cancer: American society of clinical oncology clinical practice guideline summary. *J Oncol Pract.* 2017; 13(4):261–64.

143. Almadi MA, Barkun A, Martel M. Plastic vs. self-expandable metal stents for palliation in malignant biliary obstruction: A series of meta-analyses. *Am J Gastroenterol.* 2017; 112(2):260–73.

144. Perone JA, Riall TS, Olino K. Palliative care for pancreatic and periampullary cancer. *Surg Clin North Am.* 2016; 96(6):1415–30.

145. Angelico R, Khan S, Dasari B et al. Is routine hepaticojejunostomy at the time of unplanned surgical bypass required in the era of self-expanding metal stents? *HPB.* 2017; 19(4):365–70.

146. Williamsson C, Wennerblom J, Tingstedt B et al. A wait-and-see strategy with subsequent self-expanding metal stent on demand is superior to prophylactic bypass surgery for unresectable periampullary cancer. *HPB.* 2016; 18(1):107–12.

147. Uemura S, Iwashita T, Iwata K et al. Endoscopic duodenal stent versus surgical gastrojejunostomy for gastric outlet obstruction in patients with advanced pancreatic cancer. *Pancreatology.* 2018;.

148. Yoshida Y, Fukutomi A, Tanaka M et al. Gastrojejunostomy versus duodenal stent placement for gastric outlet obstruction in patients with unresectable pancreatic cancer. *Pancreatology.* 2017; 17(6):983–89.

149. Jeurnink SM, Steyerberg EW, van Hooft JE et al. Surgical gastrojejunostomy or endoscopic stent placement for the palliation of malignant gastric outlet obstruction (SUSTENT study): A multicenter randomized trial. *Gastrointest Endosc.* 2010; 71(3):490–9.

150. Manuel-Vazquez A, Latorre-Fragua R, Ramiro-Pérez C et al. Laparoscopic gastrojejunostomy for gastric outlet obstruction in patients with unresectable hepatopancreatobiliary cancers: A personal series and systematic review of the literature. *World J Gastroenterol.* 2018; 24(18):1978–88.

151. Zhou B, Xu JW, Cheng YG et al. Early detection of pancreatic cancer: Where are we now and where are we going? *Int J Cancer.* 2017; 141(2):231–41.

152. Waddell N, Pajic M, Patch AM et al. Whole genomes redefine the mutational landscape of pancreatic cancer. *Nature.* 2015; 518(7540):495–501.

153. Greenhalf W, Ghaneh P, Neoptolemos JP et al. Pancreatic cancer hENT1 expression and survival from gemcitabine in patients from the ESPAC-3 trial. *J Natl Cancer Inst.* 2014; 106(1):djt347.

154. Nordh S, Ansari D, Andersson R. hENT1 expression is predictive of gemcitabine outcome in pancreatic cancer: A systematic review. *World J Gastroenterol.* 2014; 20(26):8482–90.

11 BILIARY TRACT CANCER

Hemant M. Kocher, Vincent S. Yip, and Ajit T. Abraham

Tumors of the bile duct (cholangiocarcinoma)

Incidence

Tumors of the biliary tract can be divided into those of the intra-hepatic bile ducts, peri-hilar bile ducts and distal bile duct, and gall bladder. For most epidemiological studies, peri-hilar cholangiocarcinomas (which are anatomically extra-hepatic) are considered, perhaps mistakenly due to anomalies in coding, as intra-hepatic.

Biliary tract tumors account for 10%–15% of all primary hepatobiliary cancers and 3% of all gastrointestinal cancers worldwide. There is a suggestion that intra-hepatic cholangiocarcinomas may be rising in incidence, whereas extra-hepatic cholangiocarcinomas show an opposite trend. However, there is concern that this may be due to errors in the International Classification of Diseases (C22-C24) in cancer registries.[1–4] Age-standardized rates in England and Wales vary from 1.08 to 1.25 per 100,000 population. These figures are in remarkable contrast to those reported from some other areas of the world, notably northeast Thailand, where age-standardized annual incidence rates of 41.5 per 100,000 men and 16.6 per 100,000 women have been reported.[5] Other high-risk areas include Japan, Korea, and Eastern Europe (European Russia, Czech Republic, and Poland), and American Indians have an age-adjusted incidence rate of 4–12 per 100,000 women. In most areas, biliary tumors (except gall bladder cancers) have a slightly higher incidence in men than in women (2.2 to 1.5:1).

Etiology

Environmental, genetic, and anatomic predisposing factors have been associated with the development of cholangiocarcinomas. Anatomic factors include the presence of fibrocystic disease of the liver (Caroli's disease),[6] choledochal cysts,[7] and biliary papillomatosis and abnormal pancreatico-biliary duct junction.[8] Environmental factors include exposure to toxins such as Thorotrast (a radiologic material used in the 1950s)[9] and industrial toxins such as dioxins and polyvinyl chloride.[10,11] Infestations of liver flukes such as *Opisthorchis viverrini* in Thailand, Laos, and Cambodia[12] and *Clonorchis sinensis* in China and Korea[13] are associated with a high incidence of intra-hepatic cholangiocarcinomas in those areas. Smoking and alcohol consumption further increase the risk in these ethnic groups.[14] Hepatitis C seems to have a causative epidemiologic link (and may explain the rise in cholangiocarcinomas in the West), but a link with hepatitis B remains to be proved.[15] Underlying cirrhosis increases the risk of intra-hepatic cholangiocarcinomas.[16]

In the West, the best known predisposing factor is primary sclerosing cholangitis (PSC), which carries a lifetime risk of 9%–23%.[17–20] However, screening and surveillance in this group, with the current tools, have proved to be less than successful.[21] In the Far East, hepatolithiasis is a known predisposing factor, and a stepwise progression from hyperplasia, dysplasia, carcinoma in situ, and adenocarcinoma has been shown in patients with hepatolithiasis.[22,23] Biliary-enteric anastomosis (done mostly for choledochal cysts) is also a putative, though unproven etiological factor. Previous cholecystectomy,[24] thalassaemia,[25] and prior external-beam radiotherapy[26] may increase the risk of cholangiocarcinoma, but so far the evidence is anecdotal. Obesity is considered to be a risk factor, at least in the Western population.[27]

Molecular biology and genetics

A multi-hit hypothesis has been suggested for carcinogenesis in the bile ducts.[28,29] It has been suggested that this may occur in many stages, such as predisposition and risk factors of biliary cancer, such as anatomic abnormalities increasing the exposure to genotoxic events usually due to chemical carcinogens leading to specific DNA damage and mutation patterns, which in turn lead to alterations in microenvironment, such as inflammatory and fibrotic repair mechanisms, which are harnessed by cancer cells to drive tumor growth. Further dysregulation of DNA-repair mechanisms and apoptosis, as well as epigenetic changes permit survival of mutated cells, leading to morphological evolution from pre-malignant biliary lesions to cholangiocarcinoma. A recent multi-omic analysis of nearly 489 cholangiocarcinomas from 10 countries with whole-genome, targeted/exome, copy-number, gene expression, and DNA methylation information, leading to integrative clustering, defined 4 distinct clusters.[30] There were two fluke-positive CCAs (clusters 1/2) which are enriched in ERBB2 amplifications, with cluster 2 being additionally enriched in TP53 mutations. There were two fluke-negative CCAs (clusters 3/4) exhibiting either high copy-number alterations (cluster 3) associated with PD-1/PD-L2 expression, or epigenetic mutations (IDH1/2, BAP1) and FGFR/PRKA-related gene rearrangements. There were new insights into noncoding promoter mutations such as histone H3K27me3-associated as well as distinct DNA hypermethylation patterns. These insightful results demonstrate that integration of different -omics approaches can identify new driver genes, noncoding promoter mutations, and structural variants, which may in turn identify different extrinsic and intrinsic carcinogenic processes, and are agnostic of anatomic sub-types or geographic location. This comprehensive study identifies new potential therapeutic strategies such as FGFR and IDH targeting as well as immune-oncology options for a fraction of patients.

Anatomy and lymphatic drainage

The difficult tumors at the confluence of the right and left ducts are sometimes eponymously referred to as Klatskin tumors, after Klatskin's report of 13 cases in 1965.[31] Intra-hepatic cholangiocarcinomas could be histologically classified as mass-forming, peri-ductal infiltrating, intraductal, or mixed, which may be related to their prognosis as well as getting a R0 resection.[32] Bile duct tumors spread to the lymph node groups along the proper and common hepatic arteries; coeliac nodes; and, for distally placed lesions, retropancreatic and superior mesenteric nodes. It is important to sample lymph nodes when considering curative resection and when resecting tumors to skeletonize the hepatic artery and remove all lymphatic tissues and associated neural tissue. These tumors have a propensity for spread along the sub-epithelial planes and for longitudinal perineural and lympho-vascular invasion, both proximally and distally. Such invasion has a negative impact on survival.[32,33] This histological feature presents challenges in pre- and intra-operative diagnosis, as choledochoscopic biopsies may underestimate the extent of tumor. Bile duct cancer may give rise to very well-differentiated nests of biliary epithelial cells within lymph nodes. Lymph node metastases have been seen to the left supraclavicular lymph nodes (Virchow's sign).

Staging

The type of staging and potential surgical intervention is dependent on the level of biliary tree involvement. In general, cholangiocarcinoma is divided into intrahepatic (iCC), peri-hilar (pCC), and distal cholangiocarcinoma (dCC). For the purpose of this chapter, we will focus on pCC and dCC.

For the 8th edition of AJCC TNM staging (2018) pCC, pTis includes pre-neoplastic lesions termed BilIN or biliary intra-epithelial neoplasia. pT1 is often confirmed only on histology as confined to the wall of bile duct. T2 can be divided into T2a; infiltrating adipose tissue and T2b as infiltrating hepatic parenchyma. T3 lesions involve the unilateral branch of the portal vein or the hepatic artery, on the same side of the tumor (biliary involvement), if unilateral biliary involvement is present, and can be confirmed radiologically and would not preclude surgery. The T4 category includes involvement of main portal vein of common hepatic artery or both their branches or second-order biliary radicles with contralateral hepatic artery or portal vein. However, its use is limited by a lack of correlation of T stages to outcomes after resection, and also its need for microscopic evaluation of tumor invasion depth. The 8th edition of TNM stage distinguishes N1 (where <3 nodes are involved) from N2 (where ≥3 nodes are involved based on sampling of at least 15 nodes). This has a prognostic impact.

The Bismuth classification is a practical and commonly used surgical classification of hilar tumors based on the extent and location of ductal involvement.[34] However, this does not take into account of radial tumor growth, vascular involvement, and lobar atrophy and so is not truly indicative of tumor staging or resectability. Generally accepted criteria for unresectability of hilar cholangiocarcinomas include vascular involvement in terms of hepatic artery involvement, complete occlusion or encasement of the main portal vein proximal to the bifurcation, or bilateral involvement of the hepatic arteries; distant spread with extra-hepatic invasion, nodal metastases beyond the hepatoduodenal ligament, or disseminated disease; and extensive local disease with bilateral involvement of hepatic ducts beyond the level of secondary biliary radicles, atrophy of one liver lobe with encasement of the contralateral portal vein branch, or atrophy of one liver lobe with contralateral secondary biliary radicle involvement.[35,36] However, with the advancement of surgical techniques and intensive care support, some of these are relative rather than absolute contraindication.

Formal pathological staging for cholangiocarcinoma is based on the TNM system, which is of limited clinical value in the pre-operative situation. A modified version of preoperative T staging for tumors of the biliary confluence has been proposed which takes into account the degree of tumor extension to second-order biliary radicles and ipsilateral or contralateral portal venous involvement as well as hepatic atrophy.[37] For patients being considered for resection, ceCT of the chest, abdomen, and pelvis should be carried out to exclude metastatic disease.

Natural history

Untreated, most patients with bile duct cancer die within 6 months to 1 year of diagnosis from a combination of local tumor spread, jaundice, and cholangitis. Direct spread to the liver is the rule, but distant involvement of intra-hepatic bile radicles may also be found and may represent a field change. Metastasis occurs to the liver, lymph nodes, lung, bone, and rarely to the brain.

Pathology

Partly described above, three histological sub-types have been described. Mass forming is usually more central with typically sclerosing, scirrhous appearance, and extensive desmoplastic stroma whilst periductal infiltrating is usually more peripheral with extensive infiltration along intrahepatic portal structures. Lastly, intraductal or mixed are usually observed in the large bile ducts with papillary architecture, which, in turn, may be related to a better prognosis as well as getting a R0 resection.[32] More rarely, a mixed cholangiocellular carcinoma type is noted with hepatocellular and cholangiocellular features. Extrahepatic cholangiocarcinomas typically form firm, infiltrating, ill-defined lesions at the hilum (Klatskin) or along the extrahepatic bile duct.

Mucin-secreting cholangiocarcinomas have acinar histology with mucin lakes which may help to distinguish cholangiocarcinomas from hepatocellular carcinoma at the liver hilum. A dense fibrous reaction surrounds the hilar tumors, which may be indistinguishable from the tumors radiologically and even at operation. Histological differentiation of this desmoplastic reaction from tumor requires careful and experienced examination of multiple sections. Invasion of nerve trunks occurs in 80% of cases. Biliary intra-epithelial neoplasia (BilIN), intraductal papillary neoplasia of the bile duct (IPNB), and the rarer intraductal tubulopapillary neoplasms of the bile duct (ITPN) are considered precursor lesions in the multistep progression to invasive cholangiocarcinoma.[38–40] Immunocytochemical staining is positive for monoclonal carcinoembryonic antigen (mCEA) in up to 75% of CCs, with strong cytokeratin (CK)7 and CK19 positivity in most cases, but usually negative for α-fetoprotein and HepPAR1.

Symptoms and presentation

Cholangiocarcinoma rarely occurs in individuals under the age of 40. Presenting features are determined by the tumor location. Patients with extra-hepatic bile duct or hilar cholangiocarcinomas usually present with unremitting painless jaundice and pruritus, dark urine, and pale stools. Prior abdominal pain consistent with a biliary origin may be present in up to 40% of patients. Cholangitis may occur and is suggested by pain in the right hypochondrium, fever, and rigors. Weight loss and anorexia are late symptoms. Intra-hepatic cholangiocarcinoma needs to be considered as a possibility in patients presenting with an unknown primary and suspected liver metastasis. Peripheral cholangiocarcinomas may present with pain, malaise, and weight loss, and an elevated alkaline phosphatase because of sectoral or lobar biliary obstruction, prior to actual involvement of the confluence by the tumor causing jaundice.

Patients known to have primary sclerosing cholangitis who develop cholangiocarcinoma may present with worsening cholestasis and rapid deterioration in their Child–Pugh scores and performance status. Occasionally, asymptomatic patients with the disease may be identified during investigation for unexplained increases in cholestatic enzymes. The differential diagnosis for cholangiocarcinoma includes pancreatic, biliary, and other pathologies such as malignancy of pancreatic head, peri-ampullary area and duodenum, chronic pancreatitis, stones in the common bile duct, primary sclerosing cholangitis, recurrent pyogenic cholangitis, iatrogenic injuries to the bile duct, parasitic infestations, and porta hepatis lymph node metastases. Rarely, hepatitis can masquerade as obstructive jaundice. Hepatomegaly may be present in up to 75% of patients, and ascites may be seen in advanced tumors. Virchow's node (metastasis to the left supraclavicular lymph node) should be looked for, as its confirmation with fine-needle aspiration or biopsy indicates advanced metastatic disease.

Diagnosis

Most patients with cholangiocarcinoma present with hilar strictures and cholestatic jaundice. However, histological confirmation of the diagnosis can prove difficult. A high index of suspicion and a multidisciplinary investigative approach are required, especially in patients with PSC who already have dominant biliary strictures and deranged liver function with secondary biliary cirrhosis. These patients do not always develop significant intra-hepatic biliary dilatation due to pre-existing biliary fibrosis. Obstructive jaundice manifests with an elevation in total (and direct) serum bilirubin and derangement of the liver enzymes alkaline phosphatase and γ-glutamyl transpeptidase. Hepatic transaminases may also be elevated. Tumor markers have a limited value, as none is specific for cholangiocarcinoma. Carbohydrate antigen (CA) 19-9 may be elevated in cholangiocarcinoma but is also raised in other cancers, including pancreatic, colorectal, gastric, and gynecological malignancies; in cholangitis; in benign cholestasis; and following liver injury. Whilst elevation of CA19-9 is not useful in making the diagnosis of cholangiocarcinoma, it may have a prognostic impact.[41] CA-125 and CEA may help in making decisions on resectability and long-term prognosis of patients, especially when they are not jaundiced.[42] No reliable novel tumor markers have been useful in enabling diagnostic certainty over the last four decades.[43] Immunoglobulin G4 (IgG4) cholangiopathy can mimic cholangiocarcinoma. It is part of a multisystem inflammatory disorder characterized by a lymphoplasmacytic infiltrate rich in IgG4-positive cells in the affected organs. Serum IgG4 can be tested if IgG4-related sclerosing cholangitis is in the differential diagnosis.[44]

Accurate imaging is essential for the diagnosis, staging, and planning of treatment. Ultrasound is the initial diagnostic investigation of choice. It is highly sensitive for biliary duct dilatation and may localize the site of obstruction, showing intra-hepatic dilatation only in cases of hilar obstruction and both intra-hepatic and extra-hepatic dilatation in more distal lesions. Ultrasound may also suggest alternative diagnoses such as gallstones. Extensive ductal dilatation may not be a feature in PSC because of ductal fibrosis. Doppler ultrasound may suggest vascular encasement or thrombosis. Contrast-enhanced, triple-phase helical computed tomography (ceCT) can detect ductal dilatation and intra-hepatic mass lesions greater than 1 cm as well as the level of biliary obstruction, presence of lymphadenopathy, and vascular involvement. The hepatic atrophy–hypertrophy complex may be seen in patients with cholangiocarcinoma where tumors obstruct a single hepatic lobe, with ipsilateral portal vein invasion resulting in ipsilateral hepatic lobar atrophy and contralateral hypertrophy. Computed tomography may only help determine resectability in 60% of cases. Magnetic resonance imaging (MRI) is perhaps the most useful single investigation for cholangiocarcinoma and is rapidly becoming the imaging modality of choice. It can delineate the extent of tumor and invasion of adjacent hepatic parenchyma

by hilar cholangiocarcinoma and can also detect intra-hepatic cholangiocarcinoma, local lymphadenopathy, and vascular involvement but without excluding extra-hepatic distant metastases. Magnetic resonance cholangiopancreatography (MRCP) using non-invasive three-dimensional biliary reconstruction provides a road map for the biliary anatomy above and below the stricture. Magnetic resonance angiography (MRA) helps to clarify vascular anatomy, which has many normal variants. With the advent of MRA, the role of traditional invasive angiography is limited, although it is still occasionally indicated in selected cases considered for radical resection. MRCP is superior to endoscopic retrograde cholangiopancreatography (ERCP) in defining biliary anatomy and resectability as it allows visualization of undrained bile ducts. Being non-invasive, it also avoids the risk of cholangitis. However, correlation with the extent of resected cholangiocarcinoma suggests that MRCP underestimates the extent of disease in up to 20% of malignant hilar strictures. In most tertiary referral centers, patients usually undergo combined MRI plus MRCP as well as ceCT.[45–48]

ERCP and percutaneous trans-hepatic cholangiography (PTC) are invasive modalities that allow therapeutic drainage and washings, brushings, and even intraductal biopsies to be obtained for cytopathological analysis. The diagnostic yield is low, although sensitivity may be increased by techniques such as fluorescent in situ hybridization. The choice between PTC and ERCP is usually determined by local expertise, availability, and failure of one or the other technique, usually ERCP. PTC is preferable for more proximal strictures, and at times a combination of both procedures is required. These invasive techniques carry the risk of procedural complications (up to 9%), including bleeding, biliary leakage, pancreatitis, cholangitis, and duodenal perforation.[49] Per-oral cholangioscopy, also called SpyGlass cholangioscopy as well as PTC cholangioscopy, is performed in specialized centers, where biopsy can be obtained under direct vision.[50–52]

Laparoscopy can detect small-volume peritoneal disease or liver secondaries missed in cross-sectional imaging, although it is less accurate for vascular invasion, lymph node involvement, and extent of biliary spread. The combination of laparoscopy with laparoscopic ultrasound may prevent unnecessary laparotomy in up to a third of patients with hilar or gall bladder cancer deemed resectable radiologically, with an accuracy of 48% for hilar cholangiocarcinomas.[53]

Histological and cytological confirmation is necessary for the definitive diagnosis of cholangiocarcinoma. Brush cytology is positive only in about 30% of cases, but combining cytology with endoscopic biopsy may enable correct diagnosis in 40–70% of cases of cholangiocarcinoma.[45,51] Immunohistochemical markers such as CA19-9 and CA50 may distinguish cholangiocarcinoma from hepatocellular carcinoma (positive for HepPar1), and staining with anti-cytokeratin type-1 (monoclonal antibody AE1) could distinguish a biliary tract rather than hepatocyte origin. Histological diagnosis is not mandatory prior to surgical exploration.

Positron emission tomography (PET) using the nucleotide tracer 18-F-fluorodeoxyglucose can detect mass-like nodular cholangiocarcinoma lesions[80] as well as the presence of distant metastases. This ability of PET to detect distant metastases may alter surgical management in up to 30% of cases. PET is less useful for patients with infiltrating lesions and those with stents in situ or background primary sclerosing cholangitis.[48]

Endoscopic ultrasound (EUS) increasingly plays a role in the diagnosis of cholangiocarcinoma and can detect duct dilatation and lymphadenopathy and also guide fine-needle aspiration for cytological diagnosis. EUS-guided fine-needle aspiration is reported to have greater sensitivity than ERCP brushings for detecting malignancy.[50]

Treatment

The treatment options for cholangiocarcinoma are determined by the stage of the disease in terms of local extent, vascular involvement, and presence or absence of metastases; whereas the type of surgical intervention is dependent on the level of biliary tree involvement.

Surgery

Complete surgical resection with histologically negative (R0) resection margins offers the only potentially curative treatment for cholangiocarcinoma. Unfortunately, most patients (80%) present with unresectable disease at diagnosis. The few patients considered suitable for surgery must be medically fit, with no metastases, and have local disease that can be resected with clear margins.[37,54,55] Patients with poor performance status, major cardiovascular disease, or Child–Pugh–Turcotte stage B or C liver cirrhosis are not candidates for surgery. Sepsis, severe jaundice, and malnutrition also predict poor outcomes but may be corrected to an extent prior to surgery.

Preoperative biliary drainage (PBD)

PBD has not been shown to significantly decrease morbidity or mortality, but is still controversial.[56] It increases the risk of cholangitis and increases hospital stay, but it must be considered in patients with severe cholestasis who otherwise run the risk of liver failure and with existing suspected cholangitis. In general, it is now accepted that in the majority of cases, proximal biliary obstruction that is suitable for major hepatic resection requires PBD; whereas middle-distal obstruction might not require routine biliary drainage, if curative surgery can be performed in a timely manner.[57] Despite that, one of the most recent meta-analyses reaffirmed that preoperative drainage seems to be associated with higher postoperative morbidity.[58] However, it is important to note that all studies included in the meta-analysis were retrospective series, and are therefore not the best evidence.

Another controversy in biliary drainage for hilar cholangiocarcinoma is the modality of the drainage procedure. One of the most recent multi-center randomized controlled trials had to be closed earlier than anticipated due to the higher morbidities associated with percutaneous biliary drainage group vs. the endoscopic drainage group.[58,59] However, the authors in the trial urged for careful interpretation of the results due to small sample sizes. Nevertheless, it offers some of the best evidence available at present.

Type of surgery

The type and extent of surgery depend on the location of the cancer within the liver or the biliary tract. Extra-hepatic cholangiocarcinomas of the common bile duct (Bismuth types I and II) require excision of the extra-hepatic bile duct and regional hepatoduodenal lymphadenectomy with Roux-en-Y biliary reconstruction. Tumors involving the confluence (Bismuth type III) require additional partial hepatectomy, and type IV tumors need an extended right or left hepatectomy to achieve negative margins. Caudate lobe (segment 1) excision is generally accepted as part of the routine for type II, III, and IV tumors where hepatectomy is indicated. Caudate lobe bile duct involvement with

cholangiocarcinoma has been suggested to range between 43% and 98%.[60] Distal cholangiocarcinomas should be managed with pancreatico-duodenectomy (pylorus-preserving or standard Kausch–Whipple pancreatico-duodenectomy) just as per ampullary or pancreatic head cancers, with the aim once again to achieve an R0 resection margin.

Portal vein embolization (PVE)

One of the main challenges for treating pCC is preserving adequate future liver remnant (FLR) following hepatectomy. Selective ipsilateral PVE can induce compensatory hypertrophy of the FLR and reduce the risk of hepatic dysfunction following liver resections in patients with a predicted FLR less than 25% to 30%.[61–63] Preoperative biliary drainage of the obstructed FLR prior to contralateral PVE may aid hypertrophy after PVE. Further controlled studies are required to determine the role of PVE and preoperative biliary drainage.[64]

The majority of Western series report a resectability rate of 15–35% for cholangiocarcinoma.[65–68] Although the adoption of a more aggressive policy in terms of en-bloc resection with vascular reconstruction leads to higher resectability rates of 35–66% in the West,[66,69] the Japanese series report even higher resectability rates of 52–92%.[70–73] The adoption of an increasingly aggressive resection policy and achievement of higher R0-negative resection margin rates correlate with a significant trend towards prolonged survival, with 40–60% 3-year survival rates in most series. However, the more extensive resections are associated with a higher mortality of around 10% and significant post-operative morbidity up to 40%.[61,74] Reported overall 5-year survival rates for hilar cholangiocarcinoma range from 11% to 40%.[55,61,75]

Neo- and adjuvant therapy

Evidence for neoadjuvant chemoradiotherapy for resectable pCC and dCC is sparse. For borderline resectable cholangiocarcinoma, retrospective series suggested the neoadjuvant treatment may allow tumor downstaging and therefore improve resectability, but not necessarily offering survival benefit.[76,77] However, this approach of upfront chemotherapy is limited by the presence of obstructive jaundice, failure to secure a tissue diagnosis, or poor performance status in many patients.

The BILCAP multicenter randomized clinical trial confirmed the survival benefit of using capecitabine as adjuvant chemotherapy in cholangiocarcinoma after curative surgical resection. The median overall survival was increased from 36 months to 53 months in capecitabine arm vs. control, and is now the standard of treatment in the UK.[78] Following the success of the BILCAP trial, ACTICCA is currently recruiting to investigate the combination of gemcitabine and cisplatin vs. capecitabine after curative intent resection of cholangiocarcinoma. There is currently no good clinical evidence suggesting that adjuvant chemoradiation provides a long-term survival benefit. The evidence for its use is mostly derived from retrospective case series.[79–82]

Liver transplantation

Early results of orthotopic liver transplantation (OLT) for cholangiocarcinoma were disappointing. Pichlmayr et al. found no difference in 1-year and 5-year survival for patients with proximal bile duct cancer undergoing either surgical resection or OLT. Meyer et al.[83,84] found a tumor recurrence rate of 51% for patients undergoing OLT for hilar and intra-hepatic cholangiocarcinoma, with survival after recurrence rarely exceeding 1 year. Liver transplantation was, until recently, contraindicated for unresectable hilar cholangiocarcinoma because of the unacceptably high recurrence rate of up to 90% within 2 years.[84,85] But excellent outcomes of neoadjuvant chemoradiation and liver transplantation for unresectable perihilar cholangiocarcinoma from the Mayo Clinic have given rise to second thoughts. A recent paper analyzed data from 1993 to 2010 (n = 287) provided by 12 large-volume transplant centers in the United States.[86] These were patients with perihilar cholangiocarcinoma treated with neoadjuvant therapy, followed by liver transplantation. The neoadjuvant treatments included external radiation (99%), brachytherapy (75%), radiosensitizing therapy (98%), and/or maintenance chemotherapy (65%). Of the total number, 71 (11.5%) patients dropped out before liver transplantation. Intent-to-treat survival rates were 68% and 53% at 2 and 5 years after therapy, respectively; the post-transplant, recurrence-free 5-year survival rate was 65%. Most patients came from 1 center (n = 193), but the other 11 centers had similar survival times. In the UK, OLT is not the standard of care for patient with cholangiocarcinoma, apart from patients with primary sclerosing cholangitis, where OLT is indicated due to its progressive idiopathic structuring of the biliary system leading to liver cirrhosis.

Palliation

Endoscopic and radiological biliary stenting

Patients with unresectable cholangiocarcinomas have a median survival of 3 months without, and 6 months with, biliary drainage.[87] Endoscopic or percutaneous palliative stenting for biliary drainage seeks to relieve jaundice and pruritus, prevent cholangitis, avoid liver failure, and improve quality of life.[88] Endoscopic stenting is suitable for distal cholangiocarcinomas, whereas percutaneous trans-hepatic insertion of stents may be preferable for hilar tumors.[88] Both plastic and self-expanding mesh metal stents are available for biliary drainage. The choice of stent must be tailored to the individual patient. Overall, self-expanding metal stents offer the more cost-effective treatment for patients likely to survive longer than 3–6 months. Although more expensive, they have a larger diameter and longer patency rates (6–12 months) compared to plastic stents (3–6 months)[89] and are associated with shorter hospital stays, fewer repeat procedures, and reduced duration of antibiotic treatment. Covered metal stents may last even longer than uncovered (bare) metal stents by preventing tumor ingrowth and occlusion.[90]

A more recent multicenter RCT comparing bilateral vs. unilateral placement of metal stents for inoperable malignant hilar biliary stricture suggested that bilateral drainage resulted in fewer re-interventions and more durable stent patency (252 vs. 139 days), despite a similar technical success rates for both of them.[91] Tissue confirmation of cancer and a careful assessment of resectability is essential prior to the insertion of metal stents, especially uncovered ones, which tend to become embedded in the bile duct wall and can only be removed at operation. A prospective randomized comparison of endoscopically placed covered and uncovered stents revealed no significant differences in stent patency time, patient survival, or complication rates. Covered stents migrated significantly more often than uncovered stents, and tumor ingrowth was more frequent with uncovered stents.[92]

Surgical palliation

Surgical palliation with biliary-enteric bypass (usually, segment 3 hepatico-jejunostomy) is now rarely done, following the introduction of percutaneous and endoscopic stenting. However, surgical bypass can still provide effective palliation in fit patients found to have unresectable dCC on exploratory laparotomy. Although surgical biliary drainage procedure is more durable, morbidity is greater with surgery, and there are longer times to recovery and higher costs. Neurolytic coeliac plexus blockade can be considered at the same setting for unremitting pain.[55]

Palliative chemotherapy and radiotherapy

Until recently, chemotherapy for cholangiocarcinoma had poor results. But the UK NCRI ABC-02 trial in 2010 was a large randomized phase III study (n = 410) that changed this perception.[93] Patients with locally advanced or metastatic cholangiocarcinoma or gall bladder or ampullary cancer were randomized to receive 24 weeks of either cisplatin plus gemcitabine (CisGem) or only gemcitabine (Gem). Median overall survival was 11.7 months for the CisGem group and 8.1 months for the Gem group, and hazard ratio (HR) was 0.64 (95% confidence interval [CI], 0.52 to 0.80; p < 0.001). The median progression-free survival was 8.0 months for the CisGem group vs. 5.0 months for the Gem group (p < 0.001). Patients in the CisGem group had a significantly improved tumor control rate (81.4% vs. 71.8%; p = 1/40.049). Toxicity was similar between the arms, with a slight excess in clinically non-significant hematological toxicities for the CisGem group. Patients with performance status 2 did not gain a survival advantage. There was no clear advantage for patients with ampullary cancer. However, patients with gall bladder cancer (about 30% of the total cohort and balanced well between the arms) derived as much benefit as the patients with cholangiocarcinoma. Following the success of ABC-02, ABC-06 trial was conducted and recently completed to find out whether mFOLFOX should be used when patients become resistant to CisGem treatment. The result was recently reported in ASCO 2019,[94] and demonstrated an improvement of survival in the mFOLFOX arm compared with the active symptom control arm (6.2 vs. 5.3 months).

There is currently no evidence to support the routine use of radiotherapy post-operatively or for unresectable disease. Radiotherapy may have palliative value, for example, for localized metastases or uncontrolled bleeding. External-beam radiotherapy and local radiation techniques such as intra-operative radiotherapy or intraductal brachytherapy have been used at times in conjunction with surgery, and with stenting, with the suggestion in some instances of survival benefit.[95,96]

Photodynamic therapy

Photodynamic therapy (PDT) involves the intravenous administration of a photosensitizer such as sodium porfimer, which localizes preferentially in tumor tissue over 24–48 hours. Subsequent endoscopic laser illumination of the tumor bed with a specific wavelength of light activates the porfimer, generating oxygen free radicals and causing cancer-cell death. One prospective randomized trial of 39 patients comparing stenting plus PDT vs. stenting alone showed increased median survival (493 vs. 98 days), improved stabilization of Karnofsky performance status, less cholestasis, and better quality of life scores.[97] But the larger UK Photostent-02 trial with 92 patients showed a shorter overall survival with PDT plus stenting compared to stenting alone (6.2 vs. 9.8 months; HR, 1.56; p = 0.048). Fewer patients (20%) in the PDT/stenting arm received subsequent chemotherapy than in the stenting alone arm (41%). Although overall survival was significantly improved among those who had chemotherapy compared with those who did not, adjusting for this does not completely explain the excess risk from PDT.[98] Other local ablation strategies such as radiofrequency ablation and ethanol injection are unproven. Loco-regional therapies such as irreversible electroporation, transcatheter arterial chemoembolization, and radioembolization with[91] Y microspheres need further evaluation with randomized trials.

Authors' view on surgery

In summary, it is the authors' policy to carry out aggressive surgical resection for cholangiocarcinomas whenever possible, as surgery offers the only potentially curative option. Cholangiocarcinoma is a complex disease, and all patients should be treated in a tertiary center with specific interest in hepatobiliary and pancreas surgical oncology. All patients undergo intensive investigation including computed tomography (CT) and MRI plus MRCP (and PET, EUS, and laparoscopy as required) for accurate staging and assessment of resectability, with preoperative biliary drainage and PVE when indicated. Surgery may include extended resection of the liver, biliary tree, portal vein, and lymph nodes to achieve negative resection margins and is warranted despite high morbidity and not insignificant mortality. For young and fit patients with unresectable lesions or patients found at exploration to be unresectable, a biliary-enteric bypass is the treatment of choice for distal cholangiocarcinoma. For most others, percutaneous trans-hepatic or endoscopic stent placement is preferred depending on the availability of local expertise. The choice of plastic stents or self-expanding metal stents is based on estimated survival.

Gall bladder cancer

Epidemiology

Gall bladder cancer is the most common biliary malignancy in Central and South America (Native American Indians and Hispanics), Central and Eastern Europe (Poland, Czech Republic, and Slovakia), the Far East (Korea and Japan), and parts of northern and north-eastern India, Bangladesh, and Pakistan.[99–104] Underlying genetic predisposition or dietary factors may explain this segregation of cases. American Indians, especially women in southern Chile, have a very high incidence of gall bladder cancer.[105,106]

Etiology

Gallstones are perhaps the single most important risk factor for gall bladder cancer, although the etiologic link is unclear. All the other risk factors associated with gallstone disease are also associated with gall bladder cancer, such as elevated body mass index, high caloric and carbohydrate intake, female sex, high parity and young age at first childbirth, and estrogen exposure. The association with gender varies with geography (female to male ratios can exceed 5:1 in northern India but are close to 1:1 in Korea and Japan) and ethnicity (female to male ratios are high in Hispanic whites and American Indians but not so among African Americans or Caucasians). Calcifications in the wall of gall bladder, such as porcelain gall bladder, may predispose to gall bladder cancer risk, especially in younger patients.[107] Chronic *Salmonella* infection, which predisposes to gallstone formation, also predisposes to gall bladder cancer risk, perhaps due to chronic inflammation.[108] Similarly, *Helicobacter* colonization has been suggested to predispose to gall bladder cancer, but these claims have not been substantiated by recent studies.[109] Single, large (>1 cm) sessile polyps are more likely to be malignant.[110,111] Environmental and dietary factors may also predispose to the disease; however, the causal evidence is weak.[100,102,112]

Molecular biology and genetics

Recent whole exome sequencing has identified the importance of ERBB2/3 gene mutations in addition to TP53 and K-Ras mutations, suggesting new potential therapeutic targets.[113–115]

Anatomy and lymphatic drainage

The lymphatic drainage follows the arterial supply and therefore the cancer spread is commonly to the cystic lymph node, pancreatico-duodenal lymph nodes (superior and posterior), and coeliac lymph nodes. Para-aortic and aorto-caval lymph nodes are also involved in advanced cases. Gall bladder cancer can invade adjacent organs, most commonly the liver, duodenum, and the transverse colon with omental seedlings being very common.

Natural history

The natural progression is similar to extra-hepatic cholangiocarcinomas. The commonest mode of spread for gall bladder cancer is contiguous spread to the liver, bile ducts, stomach, colon, and duodenum, in that order. Distant metastasis occurs to lymph nodes, liver, peritoneum, and lungs. Usually, patients succumb to the locally advanced disease rather than to distant metastasis.[105]

Pathology

Most cancers are adenocarcinomas, but adenosquamous and squamous-cell carcinomas are also seen. Most tumors are of the flat, infiltrating variety, but polypoid and nodular tumors are also seen. Lymphatic spread depends on tumor stage, with T1 tumors having no lymphatic spread and T3 and T4 tumors having up to 75% lymphatic spread. Neuro-endocrine differentiation is frequently seen.[116]

Symptoms and presentation

The commonest presentation for gall bladder cancers is pain, anorexia and weight loss, and obstructive jaundice. A gall bladder mass may be palpable in half the patients on presentation. Incidental, suspicious gall bladder lesions or masses may increasingly be picked up on work up for suspected gallstones or other abdominal pathology.[117]

Staging

The TNM v8 classification is the most commonly used staging tool for gall bladder cancers. Tis or carcinoma in situ, and T1 (T1a invading lamina propria and T1b invading muscle) are usually not diagnosed on imaging and therefore are pathological diagnosis. T shows invasion into perimuscular connective tissue (T2a invades peritoneal side whilst T2b invades liver aspect). T3 lesions invade the liver or breach the peritoneal margin of liver into surrounding organs, and T4 lesions invade the portal vein, hepatic artery, or more than two extra-hepatic organs. N staging is similar to cholangiocarcinoma but requires a minimum of six nodes to be sampled.

Investigations

Apart from baseline blood investigations including liver function tests, serum levels of the tumor markers CEA and CA19-9 should be measured. CEA and CA19-9 may be elevated in a minority of patients, and may be useful in monitoring progress or identifying recurrence after therapy, only if elevated at baseline.

The first imaging investigation is ultrasound of the liver and biliary tract. Ultrasound detects thickening of the wall of the gall bladder (the differential diagnosis being inflammation), but polypoid lesions in the gall bladder may also be detected. Ultrasound also gives an estimate of the degree of bile duct and liver involvement, and with duplex scanning it may give an estimate of vascular involvement.

Spiral CT scan probably gives the best estimate of the locoregional disease. However, MRI gives images with equally high resolutions, with the additional benefit of providing an MRCP. Nevertheless, most patients undergo an ERCP after ultrasound to relieve the obstructive jaundice and, therefore, ERCP provides information on ductal involvement. In cases in which it is difficult to cannulate the bile duct from below, PTC may be helpful. CT and MRI usually give adequate information about the local vascular anatomy, and hepatic angiography is rarely indicated. EUS is used only occasionally. Fine-needle aspiration cytology is not recommended as routine because of the risk of peritoneal or needle-tract seeding in curable cases (although the instances are anecdotal), but it is perfectly acceptable in unresectable cases that are considered for palliative therapy. The differential diagnosis on imaging is essentially stone disease and its sequelae. Xanthogranulomatous cholecystitis, adenomyomatosis of the gall bladder, and stone disease causing Mirizzi's syndrome can be quite difficult to distinguish from gall bladder carcinoma.[45]

Treatment

Surgery

There are three groups of patients that warrant discussion:

1. Patients with the incidental finding of a gall bladder polyp on imaging
2. Patients in whom a hitherto unsuspected gall bladder carcinoma is found at the time of cholecystectomy for gallstone disease, or on subsequent histological assessment of the gall bladder after cholecystectomy
3. Symptomatic patients in whom gall bladder carcinoma is suspected or diagnosed on imaging

Gall bladder polyps are often discovered incidentally on imaging, and not all of them warrant a cholecystectomy. Polyps that are sessile, solitary, and 1 cm or more in diameter should be deemed highly suspicious. Also, polyps that have developed in older patients (over the age of 50 years) and developed in association with stones or are associated with symptoms are at a higher risk of being malignant or subsequently turning malignant.[118–120] Laparoscopic cholecystectomy is the treatment of choice in these patients (unless the suspicion of malignancy is high, in which case surgical exploration and intra-operative frozen section are preferable, with preparation for extended resection if necessary). A consensus guideline by radiological, gastrointestinal, and surgical societies based on a series of Delphi questionnaires and a seven-point Likert scale was published in 2017, which formulated a management algorithm for gallbladder polyps according to risk factors.[110]

If a surgeon suspects gall bladder carcinoma at the time of cholecystectomy for stone disease, it is reasonable to take tissue samples for histology and then terminate the operation, with the intention of subsequently referring the patient to a specialist Hepatobiliary Multi-Disciplinary Team for further management, after full cross-sectional imaging as part of the staging process.

If gall bladder carcinoma is found on histological assessment after cholecystectomy, the depth of tumor invasion through the gall bladder wall (T stage) and the involvement of surgical margins should be carefully assessed, as these are the two major determinants of prognosis. Although the presence of lymph node metastasis and perineural invasion is also highly relevant, this does not preclude the patient from further extended cholecystectomy with curative intent. Gall bladder perforation at the time of the cholecystectomy greatly increases the chances of recurrence.[121]

Simple cholecystectomy is adequate for mucosal or T1a lesions (where only the lamina propria has been invaded), and further surgery is not necessary. For T1b tumors (where the muscle layer has been invaded but not breached), there is evidence to suggest that a simple cholecystectomy is adequate, especially if the surgical margins are clear, there is no evidence of lymph node spread, and the gall bladder was not perforated at the time of surgery.[122,123] Increasingly surgery is recommended for T1b disease to ensure the lymph nodes have been fully sampled. For T2 tumors (which have invaded the perimuscular connective tissue but where there is no extension beyond the serosa or into the liver) and T1b tumors where the surgical resection margins are involved or the cystic lymph node is involved, a second radical operation should be performed. This should involve a hepatic resection in the form of an extended cholecystectomy (excision of the gall bladder bed) or a formal excision of liver segments 4b and 5, with regional lymphadenectomy and excision of the extra-hepatic bile duct with biliary reconstruction. The laparoscopic port site resection was not associated with improved outcome, rather the presence of port site disease is the surrogate marker for peritoneal metastasis.[124]

Gall bladder cancers that have caused symptoms and then been identified on imaging are already quite advanced. For T3 and T4 lesions, the prognosis is poor, and the majority of patients would have unresectable disease. But radical resection offers the only chance of cure or prolongation of survival time, and a specialist surgical opinion should be sought in all patients who do not have distant metastases. A diagnostic laparoscopy prior to laparotomy may be useful in further staging the extent of disease. If the possibility of benign disease is being considered, a laparotomy and frozen-section confirmation of the nature of the disease should be the first step. Radical excision involves a liver resection of at least segments 4b and 5, but a wide central resection of segments 4, 5, and 8 or, in some instances, even a trisegmentectomy may be necessary for disease clearance, depending on the extent of liver involvement.

Lymphadenectomy

Most patient will have metastases to regional lymph nodes. A complete staging and management would include regional portal lymphadenectomy.[125] This is combined with regional lymphadenectomy (removal of nodes in the hepatoduodenal ligament, posterosuperior pancreato-duodenal nodes, and nodes along the hepatic artery) and excision of the extra-hepatic bile duct with creation of a Roux-loop hepatico-jejunostomy. A formal pancreato-duodenectomy and/or portal vein resection may be necessary in some instances to achieve complete excision. If the para-aortic or retropancreatic nodes are involved, radical excision and regional lymphadenectomy provide no survival benefit, and frozen-section assessment of these nodes may be useful before commencing a radical resection to minimize surgical morbidities.[126] To summarize, T3 and N1 disease should be seriously assessed with a view to resection; T4 disease may still be occasionally resectable, but para-aortic or retropancreatic node involvement or M1 disease should be considered unresectable.[126–130] Cytoreductive surgery does not increase survival, and is therefore not indicated.[131] Following surgical resection with clear margins, 5-year survivals of 62–100% have been reported in patients with T2 lesions and 20–50% in patients with more advanced lesions.[132] As part of the BILCAP trial discussed under "neo and adjuvant therapy," capecitabine given as adjuvant treatment is the standard care after extended cholecystectomy. We are currently awaiting the completion of the ACTICAA-1 trial, which compares survival of the CisGem vs. the capecitabine regime. There has been no proven benefit for adjuvant radiation to improve the survival outcome. It has been suggested that adjuvant radiation be reserved only for patients with positive surgical margins post-resection.[133]

Palliative radiotherapy

Gall bladder cancer is generally considered relatively radioresistant. Patients with advanced disease do have some survival benefit from radiotherapy, but the studies are too few and too small to allow any effective judgment of the value of various types of radiotherapy, for example, intra-operative or brachytherapy and conformal post-operative external-beam radiotherapy.[134,135]

Palliative chemotherapy

The ABC-02 study in 2010 demonstrated an improvement in survival with cisplatin plus gemcitabine in unresectable cholangiocarcinomas, and mFOLFOX is now the second-line chemotherapy for the CisGem-resistant group following the ABC-06 trial (see "Palliative Chemotherapy and Radiotherapy"). The patients with gall bladder cancer (about 30% of the total cohort) derived as much survival benefit as the patients with cholangiocarcinoma.[93]

Future trends

Cancers of the bile duct and gall bladder remain difficult tumors to diagnose and treat effectively. Improvements in the outcome of surgical resection have caused this approach to be re-evaluated. The use of interventional radiology and endoscopy has considerably improved our ability to obtain successful biliary drainage in these patients. The addition of chemotherapy, and internal radiotherapy, to this may produce valuable increases in survival over the next decade. Although they still pose formidable surgical problems, much of the nihilistic thinking about these cancers has been replaced by a more aggressive and somewhat optimistic outlook.

Key learning points

- Cancers of bile duct and gall bladder are often diagnosed late.
- Management of cancers of bile duct and gall bladder should take place in multi-disciplinary teams consisting of oncologists, interventional radiologists, endoscopists, hepatologists, and surgeons, all with specialist interests in biliary tract disease.
- Research into personalized management based on "-omics" data holds great promise, but requires concerted global effort due to the relative rarity of this disease.

References

1. Bridgewater J, Galle PR, Khan SA et al. Guidelines for the diagnosis and management of intrahepatic cholangiocarcinoma. *J Hepatol.* 2014; 60(6):1268–89.
2. Rizvi S, Khan SA, Hallemeier CL et al. Cholangiocarcinoma—evolving concepts and therapeutic strategies. *Nat Rev Clin Oncol.* 2018; 15(2):95–111.
3. Uhlig J, Sellers CM, Cha C et al. Intrahepatic cholangiocarcinoma: socioeconomic discrepancies, contemporary treatment approaches and survival trends from the National Cancer Database. *Ann Surg Oncol.* 2019; 26(7):1993–2000.
4. Konfortion J, Coupland VH, Kocher HM et al. Time and deprivation trends in incidence of primary liver cancer subtypes in England. *J Eval Clin Pract.* 2014; 20(4):498–504.
5. Yeesoonsang S, McNeil E, Virani S et al. Trends in incidence of two major subtypes of liver and bile duct cancer: 1989–2030. *J Cancer Epidemiol.* 2018; 2018:8267059.
6. Fozard JB, Wyatt JI, Hall RI. Epithelial dysplasia in Caroli's disease. *Gut.* 1989; 30(8):1150–3.
7. Voyles CR, Smadja C, Shands WC, Blumgart LH. Carcinoma in choledochal cysts. Age-related incidence. *Arch Surg.* 1983; 118(8):986–8.
8. Ohta T, Nagakawa T, Ueno K et al. Clinical experience of biliary tract carcinoma associated with anomalous union of the pancreaticobiliary ductal system. *Jpn J Surg.* 1990; 20(1):36–43.
9. Sharp GB. The relationship between internally deposited alpha-particle radiation and subsite-specific liver cancer and liver cirrhosis: an analysis of published data. *J Radiat Res.* 2002; 43(4):371–80.
10. Bond GG, McLaren EA, Sabel FL et al. Liver and biliary tract cancer among chemical workers. *Am J Ind Med.* 1990; 18(1):19–24.
11. Walker NJ, Crockett PW, Nyska A et al. Dose-additive carcinogenicity of a defined mixture of "dioxin-like compounds". *Environ Health Perspect.* 2005; 113(1):43–8.
12. Kurathong S, Lerdverasirikul P, Wongpaitoon V et al. *Gastroenterology.* 1985; 89(1):151–6.
13. Choi Blcrsak, Han JK, Hong ST, Lee KH. Clonorchiasis and cholangiocarcinoma: etiologic relationship and imaging diagnosis. East Asia. A large and compelling body of evidence links clonorchiasis and pathognomonic for clonorchiasis since they reflect the unique pathological changes of this disorder. These radiological examinations currently play in the treatment of cholangiocarcinoma. The morphological features and radiological findings of clonorchiasis-associated cholangiocarcinoma are essentially combinations of the findings for the two diseases. The morphological cholangiocarcinoma. In patients diagnosed with or suspected to have cholangiocarcinoma. 2004.
14. Mitacek EJ, Brunnemann KD, Hoffmann D et al. Volatile nitrosamines and tobacco-specific nitrosamines in the smoke of Thai cigarettes: a risk factor for lung cancer and a suspected risk factor for liver cancer in Thailand. *Carcinogenesis.* 1999; 20(1):133–7.
15. Wang Z, Sheng YY, Dong QZ, Qin LX. Hepatitis B virus and hepatitis C virus play different prognostic roles in intrahepatic cholangiocarcinoma: A meta-analysis. *World J Gastroenterol.* 2016; 22(10):3038–51.
16. Sorensen HT, Friis S, Olsen JH et al. Risk of liver and other types of cancer in patients with cirrhosis: a nationwide cohort study in Denmark. *Hepatology.* 1998; 28(4):921–5.
17. Farrant JM, Hayllar KM, Wilkinson ML et al. Natural history and prognostic variables in primary sclerosing cholangitis. *Gastroenterology.* 1991; 100(6):1710–7.
18. Broome U, Olsson R, Loof L et al. Natural history and prognostic factors in 305 Swedish patients with primary sclerosing cholangitis. *Gut.* 1996; 38(4):610–5.
19. Kornfeld D, Ekbom A, Ihre T. Survival and risk of cholangiocarcinoma in patients with primary sclerosing cholangitis. A population-based study. *Scand J Gastroenterol.* 1997; 32(10):1042–5.
20. Bergquist A, Glaumann H, Persson B, Broome U. Risk factors and clinical presentation of hepatobiliary carcinoma in patients with primary sclerosing cholangitis: a case-control study. *Hepatology.* 1998; 27(2):311–6.
21. Hamaoka M, Kozaka K, Matsui O et al. Early detection of intrahepatic cholangiocarcinoma. *Jpn J Radiol.* 2019; 1(10):019–00860.
22. Ohta G, Nakanuma Y, Terada T. Pathology of hepatolithiasis: cholangitis and cholangiocarcinoma. *Prog Clin Biol Res.* 1984; 152:91–113.

23. Terada T, Nakanuma Y. Pathological observations of intrahepatic peribiliary glands in 1,000 consecutive autopsy livers. II. A possible source of cholangiocarcinoma. *Hepatology*. 1990; 12(1):92–7.

24. Ekbom A, Hsieh CC, Yuen J et al. Risk of extrahepatic bileduct cancer after cholecystectomy. *Lancet*. 1993; 342(8882):1262–5.

25. Insiripong ST, Thaisamakr S, Amatachaya C. Hemoglobin typing in cholangiocarcinoma. *Southeast Asian J Trop Med Public Health*. 1997; 28(2):424–7.

26. Burmeister BH, Turner SL. External beam radiation therapy as an agent in the aetiology of carcinoma of the bile duct: a report on two patients. *Clin Oncol (R Coll Radiol)*. 1995; 7(1):48–9.

27. Li L, Gan Y, Li W, Wu C, Lu Z. *Obesity*. 2016; 24(8):1786–802.

28. Fouassier LF, Marzioni M, Afonso MBP et al. Signalling networks in cholangiocarcinoma: Molecular pathogenesis, targeted therapies and drug resistance. *Liver Int*. 2019; 39(Suppl 1):43–62.

29. Labib PLpluau, Goodchild G, Pereira SP. Molecular pathogenesis of cholangiocarcinoma. *BMC Cancer*. 2019; 19(1):185.

30. Jusakul A, Cutcutache I, Yong CH et al. Whole-genome and epigenomic landscapes of etiologically distinct subtypes of cholangiocarcinoma. *Cancer Discov*. 2017; 7(10):1116–35.

31. Klatskin G. Adenocarcinoma of the hepatic duct at its bifurcation within the porta hepatis. An unusual tumor with distinctive clinical and pathological features. *Am J Med*. 1965; 38:241–56.

32. Guglielmi A, Ruzzenente A, Campagnaro T et al. Intrahepatic cholangiocarcinoma: prognostic factors after surgical resection. *World J Surg*. 2009; 33(6):1247–54.

33. Suzuki S, Shimoda M, Shimazaki J et al. Number of positive lymph nodes and lymphatic invasion are significant prognostic factors after pancreaticoduodenectomy for distal cholangiocarcinoma. *Clin Exp Gastroenterol*. 2019; 12:255–62.

34. Bismuth H, Majno PE. Biliary strictures: classification based on the principles of surgical treatment. *World J Surg*. 2001; 25(10):1241–4.

35. Ebata T, Kosuge T, Hirano S et al. Proposal to modify the International Union Against Cancer staging system for perihilar cholangiocarcinomas. *Br J Surg*. 2014; 101(2):79–88.

36. Patel T. Cholangiocarcinoma. *Nat Clin Pract Gastroenterol Hepatol*. 2006; 3(1):33–42.

37. Jarnagin WR, Conlon K, Bodniewicz J et al. A clinical scoring system predicts the yield of diagnostic laparoscopy in patients with potentially resectable hepatic colorectal metastases. *Cancer*. 2001; 91(6):1121–8.

38. Nakanuma Y, Jang KT, Fukushima N et al. A statement by the Japan-Korea expert pathologists for future clinicopathological and molecular analyses toward consensus building of intraductal papillary neoplasm of the bile duct through several opinions at the present stage. *J Hepatobiliary Pancreat Sci*. 2018; 25(3):181–7.

39. Zaccari P, Cardinale V, Severi C et al. Common features between neoplastic and preneoplastic lesions of the biliary tract and the pancreas. *World J Gastroenterol*. 2019; 25(31):4343–59.

40. Zarei M, Shasaeefar A, Kazemi K et al. Biliary intraepithelial neoplasia in non-biliary cirrhosis-report from 100 explanted livers: a single center experience. *Clin Pathol*. 2019; 12:2632010X19876934.

41. Bergquist JR, Ivanics T, Storlie CB et al. Implications of CA19-9 elevation for survival, staging, and treatment sequencing in intrahepatic cholangiocarcinoma: A national cohort analysis. *J Surg Oncol*. 2016; 114(4):475–82.

42. Fang T, Wang H, Wang Y et bal. Clinical significance of preoperative serum CEA, CA125, and CA19-9 levels in predicting the resectability of cholangiocarcinoma. *Dis Markers*. 2019; 2019:6016931.

43. Wang B, Chen L, Chang HT. Potential diagnostic and prognostic biomarkers for cholangiocarcinoma in serum and bile. *Biomark Med*. 2016; 10(6):613–9.

44. Swensson J, Tirkes T, Tann M, Cui E, Sandrasegaran K. Differentiating IgG4-related sclerosing cholangiopathy from cholangiocarcinoma using CT and MRI: experience from a tertiary referring center. *Abdom Radiol (NY)*. 2019; 44(6):2111–5.

45. Krampitz GW, Aloia TA. Staging of biliary and primary liver tumors: Current recommendations and workup. *Surg Oncol Clin N Am*. 2019; 28(4):663–83.

46. D'Antuono F, De Luca S, Mainenti PP et al. Comparison between multidetector CT and high-field 3T MR imaging in diagnostic and tumour extension evaluation of patients with cholangiocarcinoma. *J Gastrointest Cancer*. 2019; 29(10):019-00276.

47. Joo I, Lee JM, Yoon JH. Imaging diagnosis of intrahepatic and perihilar cholangiocarcinoma: Recent advances and challenges. *Radiology*. 2018; 288(1):7–13.

48. Hu JH, Tang JH, Lin CH et al. Preoperative staging of cholangiocarcinoma and biliary carcinoma using 18F-fluorodeoxyglucose positron emission tomography: a meta-analysis. *J Investig Med*. 2018; 66(1):52–61.

49. Roy M, Kyaw Tun J, Banerjee A, Mohandas S, Abraham AT, Hutchins RR, Bhattacharya S, Renfrew I, Low D, Fotheringham T, Kocher HM. Factors affecting length of stay after percutaneous biliary interventions. *Br J Radiol*. 2018 Oct 25:20180814. doi: 10.1259/bjr.20180814. PubMed PMID: 30359118.

50. Yeo SJ, Cho CM, Jung MK et al. Comparison of the diagnostic performances of same-session endoscopic ultrasound- and endoscopic retrograde cholangiopancreatography-guided tissue sampling for suspected biliary strictures at different primary tumor sites. *Korean J Gastroenterol*. 2019; 73(4):213–8.

51. Parsa N, Khashab MA. The role of peroral cholangioscopy in evaluating indeterminate biliary strictures. *Clin Endosc*. 2019; 16(011):011.

52. Weber A, Schmid RM, Prinz C. Diagnostic approaches for cholangiocarcinoma. *World J Gastroenterol*. 2008; 14(26):4131–6.

53. Arumugam P, Balarajah V, Watt J et al. Role of laparoscopy in hepatobiliary malignancies. *Indian J Med Res*. 2016; 143(4):414–9.

54. Burke EC, Jarnagin WR, Hochwald SN et al. Hilar cholangiocarcinoma: patterns of spread, the importance of hepatic resection for curative operation, and a presurgical clinical staging system. *Ann Surg*. 1998; 228(3):385–94.

55. Jarnagin WR, Shoup M. Surgical management of cholangiocarcinoma. *Semin Liver Dis*. 2004; 24(2):189–99.

56. Farges O, Regimbeau JM, Fuks D et al. Multicentre European study of preoperative biliary drainage for hilar cholangiocarcinoma. *Br J Surg*. 2013; 100(2):274–83.

57. Iacono C, Ruzzenente A, Campagnaro T et al. Role of preoperative biliary drainage in jaundiced patients who are candidates for pancreatoduodenectomy or hepatic resection: highlights and drawbacks. *Ann Surg*. 2013; 257(2):191–204.

58. Celotti A, Solaini L, Montori G et al. Preoperative biliary drainage in hilar cholangiocarcinoma: Systematic review and meta-analysis. *Eur J Surg Oncol*. 2017; 43(9):1628–35.

59. Coelen RJS, Roos E, Wiggers JK et al. Endoscopic versus percutaneous biliary drainage in patients with resectable perihilar cholangiocarcinoma: a multicentre, randomised controlled trial. *Lancet Gastroenterol Hepatol*. 2018; 3(10):681–90.

60. Sugiura Y, Nakamura S, Iida S et al. Extensive resection of the bile ducts combined with liver resection for cancer of the main hepatic duct junction: a cooperative study of the Keio Bile Duct Cancer Study Group. *Surgery*. 1994; 115(4):445–51.

61. Nimura Y, Kamiya J, Kondo S et al. Aggressive preoperative management and extended surgery for hilar cholangiocarcinoma: Nagoya experience. *J Hepatobiliary Pancreat Surg*. 2000; 7(2):155–62.

62. Hemming AW, Reed AI, Howard RJ et al. Preoperative portal vein embolization for extended hepatectomy. *Ann Surg*. 2003; 237(5):686–91; discussion 91–3.

63. Abdalla EK, Barnett CC, Doherty D et al. Extended hepatectomy in patients with hepatobiliary malignancies with and without preoperative portal vein embolization. *Arch Surg*. 2002; 137(6):675–80; discussion 80–1.

64. Khan SA, Thomas HC, Davidson BR, Taylor-Robinson SD. Cholangiocarcinoma. *Lancet*. 2005; 366(9493):1303–14.

65. Blumgart LH, Hadjis NS, Benjamin IS, Beazley R. Surgical approaches to cholangiocarcinoma at confluence of hepatic ducts. *Lancet*. 1984; 1(8368):66–70.

66. de Groen PC, Gores GJ, LaRusso NF et al. Biliary tract cancers. *N Engl J Med*. 1999; 341(18):1368–78.

67. Pinson CW, Rossi RL. Extended right hepatic lobectomy, left hepatic lobectomy, and skeletonization resection for proximal bile duct cancer. *World J Surg*. 1988; 12(1):52–9.

68. Longmire WP, McArthur MS, Bastounis EA, Hiatt J. Carcinoma of the extrahepatic biliary tract. *Ann Surg.* 1973; 178(3):333–45.

69. Launois B, Campion JP, Brissot P, Gosselin M. Carcinoma of the hepatic hilus. Surgical management and the case for resection. *Ann Surg.* 1979; 190(2):151–7.

70. Tsuzuki T, Ogata Y, Iida S et al. Carcinoma of the bifurcation of the hepatic ducts. *Arch Surg.* 1983; 118(10):1147–51.

71. Mizumoto R, Kawarada Y, Suzuki H. Surgical treatment of hilar carcinoma of the bile duct. *Surg Gynecol Obstet.* 1986; 162(2):153–8.

72. Nagino M, Nimura Y, Kamiya J et al. Segmental liver resections for hilar cholangiocarcinoma. *Hepatogastroenterology.* 1998; 45(19):7–13.

73. Nimura Y, Hayakawa N, Kamiya J et al. Hepatic segmentectomy with caudate lobe resection for bile duct carcinoma of the hepatic hilus. *World J Surg.* 1990; 14(4):535–43; discussion 44.

74. Ebata T, Mizuno T, Yokoyama Y et al. Surgical resection for Bismuth type IV perihilar cholangiocarcinoma. *Br J Surg.* 2018; 105(7):829–38.

75. Jarnagin WR, Fong Y, DeMatteo RP et al. Staging, resectability, and outcome in 225 patients with hilar cholangiocarcinoma. *Ann Surg.* 2001; 234(4):507–17; discussion 17–9.

76. Jung JH, Lee HJ, Lee HS et al. Benefit of neoadjuvant concurrent chemoradiotherapy for locally advanced perihilar cholangiocarcinoma. *World J Gastroenterol.* 2017; 23(18):3301–8.

77. Wagner A, Wiedmann M, Tannapfel A et al. Neoadjuvant downsizing of hilar cholangiocarcinoma with photodynamic therapy—Long-term outcome of a phase II pilot study. *Int J Mol Sci.* 2015; 16(11):26619–28.

78. Primrose JN, Fox RP, Palmer DH et al. Capecitabine compared with observation in resected biliary tract cancer (BILCAP): a randomised, controlled, multicentre, phase 3 study. *Lancet Oncol.* 2019; 20(5):663–73.

79. Hughes MA, Frassica DA, Yeo CJ et al. Adjuvant concurrent chemoradiation for adenocarcinoma of the distal common bile duct. *Int J Radiat Oncol Biol Phys.* 2007; 68(1):178–82.

80. Kim TH, Han SS, Park SJ et al. Role of adjuvant chemoradiotherapy for resected extrahepatic biliary tract cancer. *Int J Radiat Oncol Biol Phys.* 2011; 81(5):e853–9.

81. Nelson JW, Ghafoori AP, Willett CG et al. Concurrent chemoradiotherapy in resected extrahepatic cholangiocarcinoma. *Int J Radiat Oncol Biol Phys.* 2009; 73(1):148–53.

82. Sagawa N, Kondo S, Morikawa T et al. Effectiveness of radiation therapy after surgery for hilar cholangiocarcinoma. *Surg Today.* 2005; 35(7):548–52.

83. Jeyarajah DR, Klintmalm GB. Is liver transplantation indicated for cholangiocarcinoma? *J Hepatobiliary Pancreat Surg.* 1998; 5(1):48–51.

84. Meyer CG, Penn I, James L. Liver transplantation for cholangiocarcinoma: results in 207 patients. *Transplantation.* 2000; 69(8):1633–7.

85. Pichlmayr R, Weimann A, Klempnauer J et al. Surgical treatment in proximal bile duct cancer. A single-center experience. *Ann Surg.* 1996; 224(5):628–38.

86. Darwish Murad S, Kim WR et al. Efficacy of neoadjuvant chemoradiation, followed by liver transplantation, for perihilar cholangiocarcinoma at 12 US centers. *Gastroenterology.* 2012; 143(1):88–98 e3; quiz e14.

87. Farley DR, Weaver AL, Nagorney DM. "Natural history" of unresected cholangiocarcinoma: Patient outcome after noncurative intervention. *Mayo Clinic Proceedings.* 1995; 70(5):425–9.

88. Abu-Hamda EM, Baron TH. Endoscopic management of cholangiocarcinoma. *Semin Liver Dis.* 2004; 24(2):165–75.

89. Kaassis M, Boyer J, Dumas R et al. Plastic or metal stents for malignant stricture of the common bile duct? Results of a randomized prospective study. *Gastrointest Endosc.* 2003; 57(2):178–82.

90. Isayama H, Komatsu Y, Tsujino T et al. A prospective randomised study of "covered" versus "uncovered" diamond stents for the management of distal malignant biliary obstruction. *Gut.* 2004; 53(5):729–34.

91. Lee TH, Kim TH, Moon JH et al. Bilateral versus unilateral placement of metal stents for inoperable high-grade malignant hilar biliary strictures: a multicenter, prospective, randomized study (with video). *Gastrointest Endosc.* 2017; 86(5):817–27.

92. Kullman E, Frozanpor F, Soderlund C et al. Covered versus uncovered self-expandable nitinol stents in the palliative treatment of malignant distal biliary obstruction: results from a randomized, multicenter study. *Gastrointest Endosc.* 2010; 72(5):915–23.

93. Valle J, Wasan H, Palmer DH et al. Cisplatin plus gemcitabine versus gemcitabine for biliary tract cancer. *N Engl J Med.* 2010; 362(14):1273–81.

94. Lamarca A. *Active Symptom Control Alone or With mFOLFOX Chemotherapy for Locally Advanced/ Metastatic Biliary Tract Cancers (ABC06).* NCT01926236. https://clinicaltrials.gov/ct2/show/NCT01926236.

95. Valek V, Kysela P, Kala Z et al. Brachytherapy and percutaneous stenting in the treatment of cholangiocarcinoma: a prospective randomised study. *Eur J Radiol.* 2007; 62(2):175–9.

96. Shinohara ET, Mitra N, Guo M, Metz JM. Radiotherapy is associated with improved survival in adjuvant and palliative treatment of extrahepatic cholangiocarcinomas. *Int J Radiat Oncol Biol Phys.* 2009; 74(4):1191–8.

97. Ortner ME, Caca K, Berr F et al. Successful photodynamic therapy for nonresectable cholangiocarcinoma: a randomized prospective study. *Gastroenterology.* 2003; 125(5):1355–63.

98. Pereira SP, Jitlal M, Duggan M et al. PHOTOSTENT-02: porfimer sodium photodynamic therapy plus stenting versus stenting alone in patients with locally advanced or metastatic biliary tract cancer. *ESMO Open.* 2018; 3(5):e000379.

99. Miquel JF, Covarrubias C, Villaroel L et al. Genetic epidemiology of cholesterol cholelithiasis among Chilean Hispanics, Amerindians, and Maoris. *Gastroenterology.* 1998; 115(4):937–46.

100. Nogueira L, Foerster C, Groopman J et al. Association of aflatoxin with gallbladder cancer in Chile. *JAMA.* 2015; 313(20):2075–7.

101. Mhatre SS, Nagrani RT, Budukh A et al. Place of birth and risk of gallbladder cancer in India. *Indian J Cancer.* 2016; 53(2):304–8.

102. Navarro Rosenblatt D, Duran Aguero S. Gallbladder cancer and nutritional risk factors in Chile. *Nutr Hosp.* 2016; 33(1):105–10.

103. Hori M, Saito E. Gallbladder cancer incidence rates in the world from the Cancer Incidence in Five Continents XI. *Jpn J Clin Oncol.* 2018; 48(9):866–7.

104. Wang CC, Tsai MC, Wang SCT et al. Favorable gallbladder cancer mortality-to-incidence ratios of countries with good ranking of world's health system and high expenditures on health. *BMC Public Health.* 2019; 19(1):1025.

105. Gourgiotis S, Kocher HM, Solaini L et al. Gallbladder cancer. *Am J Surg.* 2008; 196(2):252–64.

106. Hariharan D, Saied A, Kocher HM. Analysis of mortality rates for gallbladder cancer across the world. *HPB.* 2008; 10(5):327–31.

107. Schnelldorfer T. Porcelain gallbladder: a benign process or concern for malignancy? *J Gastrointest Surg.* 2013; 17(6):1161–8.

108. Koshiol J, Wozniak AC, Cook P et al. Salmonella enterica serovar Typhi and gallbladder cancer: a case-control study and meta-analysis. *Cancer Med.* 2016; 5(11):3310–235.

109. Tsuchiya Y, Mishra K, Kapoor VK et al. Plasma *Helicobacter pylori* antibody titers and *Helicobacter pylori* infection positivity rates in patients with gallbladder cancer or cholelithiasis: a hospital-based case-control study. *Asian Pac J Cancer Prev.* 2018; 19(7):1911–5.

110. Wiles R, Thoeni RF, Barbu ST et al. Management and follow-up of gallbladder polyps: Joint guidelines between the European Society of Gastrointestinal and Abdominal Radiology (ESGAR), European Association for Endoscopic Surgery and other Interventional Techniques (EAES), International Society of Digestive Surgery—European Federation (EFISDS) and European Society of Gastrointestinal Endoscopy (ESGE). *Eur Radiol.* 2017; 27(9):3856–66.

111. Heitz L, Kratzer Wwku-ud, Grater T, Schmidberger J. Gallbladder polyps—a follow-up study after 11 years. *BMC Gastroenterol.* 2019; 19(1):42.

112. Stepien M, Hughes DJ, Hybsier S et al. Circulating copper and zinc levels and risk of hepatobiliary cancers in Europeans. *Br J Cancer.* 2017; 116(5):688–96.

113. Li M, Zhang Z, Li X et al. Whole-exome and targeted gene sequencing of gallbladder carcinoma identifies recurrent mutations in the ErbB pathway. *Nat Genet.* 2014; 46(8):872–6.

114. Iyer PI, Shrikhande SV, Ranjan MI et al. ERBB2 and KRAS alterations mediate response to EGFR inhibitors in early stage gallbladder cancer. *Int J Cancer.* 2019; 144(8):2008–19.

115. Li M, Liu F, Zhang F et al. Genomic ERBB2/ERBB3 mutations promote PD-L1-mediated immune escape in gallbladder cancer: a whole-exome sequencing analysis. *Gut.* 2019; 68(6):1024–33.

116. Iype S, Mirza TA, Propper DJ et al. Neuroendocrine tumours of the gallbladder: three cases and a review of the literature. *Postgrad Med J.* 2009; 85(1002):213–8.

117. Solaini L, Sharma A, Watt J et al. Predictive factors for incidental gallbladder dysplasia and carcinoma. *J Surg Res.* 2014; 189(1):17–21.

118. Chattopadhyay D, Lochan R, Balupuri S et al. Outcome of gall bladder polypoidal lesions detected by transabdominal ultrasound scanning: a nine year experience. *World J Gastroenterol.* 2005; 11(14):2171–3.

119. Lee KF, Wong J, Li JC, Lai PB. Polypoid lesions of the gallbladder. *Am J Surg.* 2004; 188(2):186–90.

120. Sun XJ, Shi JS, Han Y et al. Diagnosis and treatment of polypoid lesions of the gallbladder: report of 194 cases. *Hepatobiliary Pancreat Dis Int.* 2004; 3(4):591–4.

121. Z'Graggen K, Birrer S, Maurer CA et al. Incidence of port site recurrence after laparoscopic cholecystectomy for preoperatively unsuspected gallbladder carcinoma. *Surgery.* 1998; 124(5):831–8.

122. Yamaguchi K, Chijiiwa K, Saiki S et al. Retrospective analysis of 70 operations for gallbladder carcinoma. *Br J Surg.* 1997; 84(2):200–4.

123. Wakai T, Shirai Y, Yokoyama N et al. Early gallbladder carcinoma does not warrant radical resection. *Br J Surg.* 2001; 88(5):675–8.

124. Ethun CG, Postlewait LM, Le N et al. Routine port-site excision in incidentally discovered gallbladder cancer is not associated with improved survival: A multi-institution analysis from the US Extrahepatic Biliary Malignancy Consortium. *J Surg Oncol.* 2017; 115(7):805–11.

125. Jensen EH, Abraham A, Jarosek S et al. Lymph node evaluation is associated with improved survival after surgery for early stage gallbladder cancer. *Surgery.* 2009; 146(4):706–11; discussion 11–3.

126. Kondo S, Nimura Y, Hayakawa N et al. Regional and para-aortic lymphadenectomy in radical surgery for advanced gallbladder carcinoma. *Br J Surg.* 2000; 87(4):418–22.

127. Todoroki T, Takahashi H, Koike N et al. Outcomes of aggressive treatment of stage IV gallbladder cancer and predictors of survival. *Hepatogastroenterology.* 1999; 46(28):2114–21.

128. Kondo S, Nimura Y, Hayakawa N et al. Extensive surgery for carcinoma of the gallbladder. *Br J Surg.* 2002; 89(2):179–84.

129. Chijiiwa K, Noshiro H, Nakano K et al. Role of surgery for gallbladder carcinoma with special reference to lymph node metastasis and stage using western and Japanese classification systems. *World J Surg.* 2000; 24(10):1271–6; discussion 7.

130. Bartlett DL, Fong Y, Fortner JG et al. Long-term results after resection for gallbladder cancer. Implications for staging and management. *Ann Surg.* 1996; 224(5):639–46.

131. Misra S, Chaturvedi A, Misra NC, Sharma ID. Carcinoma of the gallbladder. *Lancet Oncol.* 2003; 4(3):167–76.

132. Yip VS, Gomez D, Brown S et al. Management of incidental and suspicious gallbladder cancer: focus on early referral to a tertiary centre. *HPB.* 2014; 16(7):641–7.

133. Shroff RT, Kennedy EB, Bachini M et al. Adjuvant therapy for resected biliary tract cancer: ASCO clinical practice guideline. *J Clin Oncol.* 2019; 37(12):1015–27.

134. Mehta A, Bahadur AK, Aranya RC, Jain AK. Role of radiation therapy in carcinoma of the gall bladder—a preliminary indian experience. *Trop Gastroenterol.* 1996; 17(1):22–5.

135. Houry S, Haccart V, Huguier M, Schlienger M. Gallbladder cancer: role of radiation therapy. *Hepatogastroenterology.* 1999; 46(27):1578–84.

12 GASTRIC CANCER

Mark A. Baxter and Russell D. Petty

Incidence

Gastric cancer accounts for approximately 2% of new cancer cases and 3% of all cancer deaths in the United Kingdom, a percentage that comprises over 5000 people per year. Within Europe, there are approximately 140,000 new cases each year, and although the mortality from gastric cancer is reducing worldwide, it remains the second most common cause of cancer death. There are dramatic geographical variations in the incidence of gastric cancer characterized by reducing rates in westernized countries such as the United Kingdom (current incidence 9.6/100,000), whereas countries such as Japan, Brazil, Portugal, and Lithuania continue to have a high incidence of the disease (50–100/100,000). The pattern of the disease also differs between countries; in Western countries, tumors of the proximal stomach and gastro-esophageal junction (GEJ) are increasing and now outnumber antral cancers. This change in position of the tumors is not observed to the same extent in high-incidence regions. Gastric cancer in eastern populations tends to occur at a younger age, and patients present at an earlier stage and generally have fewer co-morbid medical conditions. Because of these epidemiological, clinical, and pathological differences, there has been speculation regarding biological differences between eastern and western patients, although no biological or molecular differences have been identified. In all regions, gastric cancer is rare before the age of 40 but thereafter rises steadily and peaks in the seventh decade of life.

Etiology

It is likely that there is an interaction between genetic and environmental factors in the development of most gastric cancers. First-generation migrants from high-incidence to low-incidence areas retain the risk of their native country, but subsequent generations acquire the risk of their new country, suggesting that overall environmental factors are more important. Most gastric cancers are sporadic, but a familial inherited component may be responsible for up to 10% of cases. Germ-line mutations in the E-cadherin gene (*CDH-1*) resulting in disruption of the normal E-cadherin–catenin complex required to maintain intercellular adhesion is associated with an autosomal dominant predisposition to gastric cancer of the diffuse histological sub-type. The penetrance is 70%, and overall, this accounts for between 1% and 3% of gastric cancers. Prophylactic gastrectomy is advocated for individuals with *CDH-1* mutations from affected kindreds. Younger age at diagnosis and the diffuse histological sub-type are more commonly found in familial cases, and it remains important to determine the role of germ-line mutations other than *CDH-1* in these patients.

In regions with a high incidence of gastric cancer, it is the intestinal pattern of the tumor that predominates, frequently associated with a high incidence of *Helicobacter pylori* infection. Epidemiological studies indicate that *H. pylori* infection is associated with a three to eight times increased incidence of gastric cancer. However, even in high-incidence regions of the world, the majority of patients infected with *H. pylori* do not develop gastric cancer, and the interaction between different strains of *H. pylori* and the individual is critical. *H. pylori* strains are divided according to their ability to express *CagA* (cytotoxin-associated gene) and to secrete VacA (vacuolating cytotoxin), and this may determine their pathogenicity. Gastric atrophy and intestinal metaplasia, both regarded as pre-malignant conditions, are more likely in patients infected with CagA positive strains of *H. pylori* that incite an intense inflammatory response. The role of VacA in gastric carcinogenesis appears to be more complex, but strains of *H. pylori* expressing this protein do appear to be associated with severe gastritis. Individual responses to infecting agents may also vary in that patients with gastritis limited to the gastric antrum appear to produce excess acid and are at risk of duodenal ulceration, whereas those with an extensive response in the body of the stomach develop gastric atrophy, achlorhydria, and intestinal metaplasia and are at the highest risk of gastric cancer. Genetic heterogeneity in the cytokine response to infection may determine the pattern of disease observed in individuals. Other infective agents have also been implicated in the carcinogenesis of gastric cancer, including the Epstein–Barr virus.

H. pylori eradication has been demonstrated to reverse many of the findings regarded as pre-malignant in the stomachs of infected individuals. There is, however, only indirect evidence that eradication may prevent gastric cancer. Other interventional studies have looked at increasing dietary antioxidants and cyclo-oxygenase 2 (COX2) inhibitors in at-risk populations, but such studies have had inconclusive results to date. Dietary risk factors include a low intake of animal fat and protein, a high intake of complex carbohydrates, nitrate, or salt, and a low intake of salads, fresh greens, and fruit. When the pH of the stomach is higher than usual, bacteria can survive and may reduce dietary nitrate to nitrite to form *N*-nitroso compounds through nitrosation of dietary amines. *N*-nitroso compounds are known to be carcinogenic in animals. The source of dietary nitrites is preservatives and coloring agents, especially in home-cured meats, dried fish, and sausages. Nitrates are found in crop fertilizers and recycled sewage, and they can be converted to nitrites by bacterial action in the food or in the stomach. The protective effect of greens may be explained by the possibility that ascorbic acid may increase gastric acidity and block the bacterial conversion of ingested nitrate to nitrite, thereby decreasing the concentration of nitrosanes. This may also explain the role of diffuse *H. pylori* infections associated with achlorhydria. Other conditions associated with reduced gastric acid production, such as pernicious anemia and previous gastric surgery, have also been linked with a higher incidence of gastric cancer.

Diagnosis

In Britain, 1 in 50 patients presenting to their general practitioner for the first time with dyspepsia will have gastric cancer. Up until 1980, only 1% of cases in this country were diagnosed at an early stage—carcinoma confirmed within the sub-mucosa. Conversely, the higher incidence of the disease in Japan has encouraged screening of the population, which resulted in an increase in the proportion of early diagnoses from 2% in 1955 to

30% in 1978. The Japanese mass screening was by indirect radiology. In Britain, an improvement in the proportion of early tumors was seen when British dyspeptic patients over the age of 40 were referred for endoscopy following the first consultation with their general practitioner; 26% of the gastric cancers found were early, and 63% of the cases were operable. The importance of detecting the disease at an early stage is emphasized by 5-year survival figures following surgical resection of 82% for those tumors confined to the mucosa (pT1a; for the American Joint Committee on Cancer/Union for International Cancer Control [AJCC/UICC] eighth edition, see "Staging") and 76% for those confined to the sub-mucosa (pT1), compared with 56% for those that have penetrated the muscularis propria (pT2) and 38% for those that have penetrated the sub-serosa connective tissue (pT3), and in western populations.[1,2]

The importance of detecting gastric cancer at an early stage is undeniable, but there is controversy on the merits of open-access endoscopy in low-incidence countries such as the United Kingdom. There is also debate regarding the routine endoscopy of patients with dyspeptic symptoms. It is clear that the detection rate of early gastric cancer in patients with uncomplicated dyspepsia under the age of 50 years is very low. This has led many to advocate screening for *H. pylori* in such patients and treating accordingly, with endoscopy reserved only for those whose symptoms fail to settle. Although this may be a cost-effective policy, it ignores the potential impact of the occasional early tumor detected in a young patient, which may not be cured with such a conservative policy.

Pathology

A total of 96%–97% of gastric cancers are adenocarcinomas. The other 3%–4%—sarcomas and lymphomas—will not be discussed in this chapter. Several different histological sub-classifications of adenocarcinoma are recognized. The intestinal and diffuse varieties were originally described by Lauren and are widely accepted with concordance of approximately 80% among pathologists. This sub-classification has proven useful to identify distinct epidemiological patterns in disease incidence, distinct clinical and pathological correlations, and distinct precursor lesions. The intestinal type occurs predominantly in the body and fundus, and tumor cells adhere to each other to form gland-like structures; it is more likely to ulcerate and is more common in high-incidence areas. In the diffuse type that occurs more frequently in younger patients, there is less cohesion between malignant cells, which infiltrate and thicken the stomach wall and may extend to involve the whole stomach and lead to "linitis plastica." The World Health Organization (WHO) sub-classification describes five histological subtypes—adenocarcinoma (intestinal and diffuse), papillary, tubular, mucinous, and signet ring cell—and also assigns grades to adenocarcinoma based on the degree of resemblance to metaplastic intestinal tissue.

A macroscopic classification by Borman—polypoid (I), ulcerating (II), combined (III), and infiltrating (IV) growth patterns—predates Lauren and has found use in modern clinical practice, as they are easily recognized on endoscopy. The Japanese have added early gastric cancer, which is also an endoscopic diagnosis, made on the discovery of discrete single or multiple lesions confined to the mucosa.

More recently, advances in the understanding of the molecular pathogenesis of gastric cancer are starting to provide a new molecular sub-classification of gastric cancers, which may have distinct vulnerabilities to different systemic therapies. Four

molecular subtypes identified are Epstein–Barr Virus (EBV), microsatellite instability (MSI), genomically stable (GS), and chromosomal instability (CIN).[3] The clinical significance of these sub-groups for treatment direction is under investigation.

Molecular pathogenesis

Elucidation of the molecular pathogenesis of gastric cancer has provided targets for novel rationally designed targeted anti-cancer drugs. A key breakthrough in translational cancer research has been recognition that tumors in individual patients can become "addicted" to or dependent on continued signaling from individual molecules—in such cases, developing targeted drugs against these molecules, especially receptor tyrosine kinases (RTKs), has proven successful.

The paradigm that has emerged is the use of a predictive biomarker assay, which identifies that the growth of a particular patient's tumor is dependent on the activation of a particular molecule, and then the use of an agent against this target in that patient. This paradigm was successfully applied to gastric cancer with the demonstration of the effectiveness of trastuzumab, a monoclonal antibody against HER2, in "HER2-positive" gastric cancers. Between 7% and 17% of gastric cancers have either high expression of the HER2 protein (assessed by immunohistochemistry, 3+ score) or *HER2* gene amplification, which are the clinically useful predictive biomarker assays for HER2 growth dependence.[4] This sub-group in gastric cancer is fairly typical of the proportional size of biomarker-defined sub-groups that have emerged for targeted therapies in other cancer types so far.

Amplification of other so-called "druggable" RTKs, for example epidermal growth factor receptor (EGFR), fibroblast growth factor receptor 2 (FGFR2), and met proto-oncogene (MET), occur in a significant proportion of gastric cancer. Targeted agents exist against these RTKs. However, in contrast to HER2 clinical trials, the use of these RTK inhibitors, including in selected patients with RTK amplification and/or overexpression, has not shown great benefit in trials performed so far, but more recent advances in the molecular pathogenesis of gastric cancer provide expansions for these clinical results and a way forward for improved targeting and patient selection for treatment.[5-7] In particular, more recent large-scale genomic landscaping studies of gastric cancer have revealed a complex molecular pathogenesis with high levels of genetic heterogeneity.[8] The presence of heterogeneity provides understanding as to why previous biomarker-directed targeted therapies have failed. For example, co-amplification of RTKs appears to be more common than previously indicated. New molecular classifications of gastric cancer have emerged from these large-scale genomic landscaping studies, and gastric cancer molecular sub-groups have been proposed with specific actionable genomic aberrations and therapeutic vulnerabilities, which will be evaluated in future precision medicine trials, for example EBV, MSI, GS, and CIN sub-groups.[3,9]

Staging

As in other tumors, the stage of disease at diagnosis is relevant both to the plan of management and to the prognosis.

Computed tomography (CT) of the chest, abdomen, and pelvis is a standard staging investigation, which permits visualization of gastric lumen, wall, and adjacent structures to provide a comprehensive picture of the disease, including the detection of distant metastases. However, CT scanning is limited in its ability to detect peritoneal metastases.

Endoscopic ultrasonography (EUS) provides accurate T staging and in particular, can accurately predict mucosal and sub-mucosal invasion of gastric cancer. Accordingly, EUS is useful in identifying early gastric lesions, which are suitable for endoscopic treatments, and in distinguishing such cases from those that require surgical resection with or without neo-adjuvant therapy. EUS can also be useful to assess regional lymph-node involvement, and fine needle aspiration can be performed if there is doubt. The advantage of EUS over high-resolution CT for staging of regional lymph nodes is less certain.

Laparoscopy of the peritoneal cavity is useful in the detection of peritoneal disease and allows direct assessment of fixation to adjacent organs. Diagnostic laparoscopy is usually considered a prerequisite before determining that a tumor is resectable.

Fluorodeoxyglucose-positron emission tomography (FDG-PET) and FDG-PET CT are useful for detecting distant metastatic disease and detect distant metastases, which are not evident on CT, in approximately 10% of patients.

For patients with early gastric cancers (limited to the mucosa and sub-mucosa), the gross appearance, described by experienced endoscopists, may allow analysis of the extent of disease. Subdivisions are:

I. Protruding type
II. Superficial; A elevated, B flat, C depressed
III. Excavated

Types IIB and IIC predominate and are associated with a 95% 5-year survival rate, possibly related to the fact that the lymphatic channels are very rarely found in the gastric mucosa and superficial sub-mucosa. In more advanced cases, the preferred staging in the United Kingdom is the AJCC/UICC system, and this was recently revised in 2017.[2,10] The latest (eighth) edition involves several changes. There is segregation of N3 disease into N3a (metastasis to 7–15 lymph nodes) and N3b (metastasis to more than 16 lymph nodes). Incorporation of N3a and N3b separately in the eighth edition resulted in T1–T3 disease being grouped as a higher stage when it had 16 or more lymph nodes than if it had 7–15 positive nodes. It also resulted in T4aN3a disease being downstaged to IIIB instead of IIIC. Other changes included T4bN0 and T4aN2 being reclassified from IIIB to IIIA and T4aN2 being reclassified from IIIB to IIIA. The largest validation cohort in a western population was performed by In et al. in 2017 on 12,041 patients.[10] These patients had gastric cancer resected without neo-adjuvant therapy. The 5-year overall survival was 81% for Stage 1A, 68.5% for Stage 1B, 59.3% for Stage 2A, 46.4% for Stage 2B, 30.5% for Stage 3A, 20.1% for Stage 3B, 8.3% for Stage 3C, and 5.6% for Stage 4.

Treatment

Surgery

In patients with tumors limited to the gastric mucosa (T1a), endoscopic mucosal resection (EMR) has been demonstrated to be an effective treatment. Clearly, such treatment avoids both the immediate and the long-term morbidity of surgery. It is important to select patients carefully, as there is an increasing incidence of lymph-node involvement when tumors invade into the sub-mucosa—up to 20%. Most authorities would limit EMR to endoscopic type I and II lesions (see the "Staging" section) and those without ulceration and to patients in whom there was pathological confirmation of tumor clearance. Recently, endoscopic sub-mucosal dissection was introduced in Japan as an alternative

technique, which allows *en bloc* resection of larger lesions (>2 cm) and possibly those with ulceration and may offer advantages in terms of histological clear margins and recurrence rates but at the expense of higher rates of perforation.

The cornerstone of treatment for gastric cancer remains surgical resection, but meaningful long-term survival is only achieved in patients in whom it is possible to achieve complete macroscopic and microscopic clearance of their tumor (R_0 resection). Traditionally, resection was performed as an open procedure, but minimally invasive approaches are becoming more commonplace.

The poor prognosis of patients with residual microscopic (R_1) or macroscopic tumor (R_2) after resection is highlighted by many authors. As a result, there is a trend towards a more conservative approach to offering patients surgery. Akoh and McIntyre in a review of 100 English language papers on the treatment of gastric cancer reported that the number of patients operated fell from 92% before 1970 to 71% by 1990, but the proportion of operated patients undergoing resection increased from 37% to 48% in the same period, suggesting an improvement in patient selection. Better staging and selection procedures, perhaps in combination with improved operative techniques, resulted in a larger proportion of operated patients being thought suitable for curative or radical resection (9% before 1970 vs. 31% by 1990). These rates of curative resection have remained more or less static since this time, with data from the National Oesophago-gastric Cancer Audit in England and Wales 2018 reporting that 31% of gastric cancer patients underwent curative resection.

There is an inverse relationship between surgical volume in a center and surgical outcomes, which has driven a move in many countries towards centralization of gastroesophageal surgery.[11] Historically, there have been several problems associated with the surgery for gastric cancer in the Western hemisphere. Previously, accurate surgical staging was often not carried out, resections were not standardized, and there was frequently a lack of pathological data in the reporting of the surgical specimens. Peri-operative mortality was frequently excessive, and even after surgical procedures that were thought to be curative, the local regional relapse rate was around 85%. This is in contrast to series from Japan and East Asia, which have consistently reported operative mortality rates below 3% and disease-free survival rates above 60% at 5 years. Although there are potentially many reasons for these differences, it is clear that a structured approach to surgery, as laid down by the Japanese Society for Gastric Cancer, does lead to a more uniform approach.

The National Oesophago-gastric Cancer Audit England and Wales 2018 demonstrates how a more uniform approach to patient staging and assessment for surgery benefits patients with improved peri-operative morbidity and mortality in particular (90-day mortality from gastrectomy between 2015 and 2017 was 3.3% compared with 4.1% between 2013 and 2015).

Perhaps the area of greatest controversy in the surgical management of patients with potentially curative gastric cancer is the extent of surgical resection required to achieve this goal. Most authorities would now agree that total gastrectomy is not always required if sufficient tumor clearance is possible without removal of the whole stomach. Similarly, routine removal of adjacent organs is only indicated where there is direct tumor extension into these, and even then, the increased surgical morbidity must be balanced against the limited benefits in patients with such extensive disease. The upper gastrointestinal tract (GI) surgical community is, however, divided in the attitude towards the extent of lymphadenectomy required in curative resections of the stomach. Meticulous mapping of lymph-node involvement for tumors in different anatomical locations within the stomach led to the concept of systematic lymph-node dissection in Japan.

In non-randomized series in both Japan and Europe, it has been shown that extended lymphadenectomy (D2 resection) improves disease-free survival in selected patients compared with historical controls. Two large European randomized, controlled trials in the United Kingdom and the Netherlands failed to show any benefit to extended lymph-node dissection compared with limited dissection (D1), and both demonstrated excess morbidity and mortality with the more extensive dissection. Both trials have been heavily criticized, because much of the morbidity in the D2 arms of the trials was due to the routine removal of the spleen and pancreatic tail. As discussed earlier, the routine removal of adjacent organs is no longer recommended for tumor clearance. Furthermore, in both trials, surgeons were being asked to perform procedures with which they were unfamiliar; this may have been a cause for the increased morbidity in the D2 arms, and there may have been wide variations in surgical quality. More recently, a randomized trial from Taiwan demonstrated improved survival with D2 lymphadenectomy compared with D1, without increases in morbidity.[12] In addition, long-term 15-year follow-up of the Dutch trial[13] has recently been published and shows a survival advantage for D2 lymphadenectomy, albeit with increased peri-operative morbidity and mortality, as reported earlier. Taken together, this suggests that D2 lymphadenectomy offers advantages but only if performed by experienced surgeons and in appropriately selected patients. These trials also highlight the importance of surgical quality control and standardization not only in clinical practice but also in clinical trials. This is an important issue when considering the results of neo-adjuvant and adjuvant trials.

There is further controversy regarding intra-operative lymph-node mapping. If lessons are to be learned from the controversy of lymphadenectomy in gastric cancer, it is clear that these techniques should be subjected to rigorous scientific scrutiny from the outset. Similarly, minimally invasive and hybrid techniques for resection have been developed and appear safe, and these may offer advantages in terms of peri-operative morbidity and mortality, but they require evaluation in randomized trials.

In the surgical management of locally advanced disease, where by definition, there are involved regional lymph nodes, adjacent tissues, or organs that preclude resection *en bloc*, the median survival is 5 months with all patients dead by 2 years. The poor figures belie the symptomatic benefit enjoyed by many patients who obtain relief from obstruction bleeding or pain associated with their tumor pre-operatively. In fitter patients, downstaging with chemotherapy may be appropriate, as discussed later in the section "Neo-adjuvant chemotherapy." For those unsuitable for chemotherapy, resection should be considered wherever possible, because this confers both a greater palliative relief from GI symptoms and an improved survival rate. Total gastrectomy is not recommended as a palliative procedure because of the significant morbidity and high mortality from the procedure in this setting. For tumors of the GEJ, however, esophagogastrectomy is the treatment of choice for fit patients. Although palliative gastrostomy and jejunostomy are practiced in some centers, the poor response and high complication rates make these unattractive options in the majority of cases. The high morbidity and mortality associated with endoscopic insertion of a prosthetic stent make it a procedure suitable only for those with a very poor prognosis who are unfit for surgery but who require palliation of salivary aspiration.

The conclusion on surgical management of gastric cancer is that only complete resection can currently offer a cure for the disease, and the trend towards more careful selection of patients suitable for curative resection must be welcomed. Meticulous documentation of the extent of disease by surgeons and pathologists will aid in determining what constitutes a curative procedure, and specialization of surgeons will also help to reduce operative mortality. As always, entering patients into trials for gastric cancer will expedite the accumulation of knowledge of the optimum treatment for different disease stages. In the palliative setting, development of non-invasive techniques and improvement of those that are currently available will ensure maximum benefit with minimum morbidity for people with unresectable tumors.

Adjuvant and neo-adjuvant treatment

High rates of both loco-regional and distant recurrence after surgical resection have led to the evaluation of adjuvant and neo-adjuvant therapies with chemotherapy, and concurrent chemoradiotherapy. Several large randomized trials have been completed, which establish neo-adjuvant and adjuvant chemotherapy, and adjuvant concurrent chemoradiotherapy, as reasonable standards of care (Table 12.1). Randomized trials are underway to compare these different modalities of adjuvant therapy for resectable gastric cancer, which will establish their relative effectiveness. Until these trials report, neo-adjuvant chemotherapy, adjuvant chemotherapy, and adjuvant concurrent chemoradiotherapy remain reasonable standards of care for patients with resectable gastric cancer, but there are specific limitations to the evidence base provided by randomized trials for each of these modalities, which need to be taken into account when considering the choice of adjuvant therapy in individual cases (Table 12.1). In particular, the importance of surgical quality control in trials of adjuvant therapy has been recognized. Note must also be made that the emergence of immune checkpoint inhibitors (ICIs) is likely to change the current standard of care regimes significantly in the near future.

Adjuvant chemoradiotherapy

The intergroup trial 0116 (INT-0116) randomized 556 patients with resected gastric cancer ($\geq$T3 and/or node-positive that had a R0 resection) to observation or post-operative chemoradiotherapy comprising 45 Gy in 25 fractions over 5 weeks with bolus fluorouracil (5FU).[18] A survival advantage was demonstrated with median survival 27 months in the surgery-alone group as compared with 36 months in the chemoradiotherapy group; the hazard ratio for death was 0.75 (95% confidence interval [CI], 0.60 to 0.94; $p = 0.005$). This study established adjuvant chemoradiotherapy as a standard of care, and this remains the most common practice in North America. Recently, long-term follow-up for INT-0116 has been reported,[19] and these survival benefits for concurrent chemoradiotherapy are maintained. In a sub-group analysis of the long-term follow-up data, the benefit of adjuvant chemoradiotherapy is seen across all subsets (sex, race, T stage, N stage, extent of lymphadenectomy, Maruyama index, and intestinal histology) except diffuse histology. Notwithstanding the caveats that these subset analyses were not pre-specified and some sub-groups were small—for example, only 54 patients had D2 lymphadenectomy—this analysis suggests that chemoradiotherapy effects are consistent across all patient sub-groups except those patients with diffuse histology. Importantly, this addresses to a certain degree criticisms of INT-0116 regarding the quality of surgical resection. The majority (54%) of patients received less than a D1 resection, and only 10% received a D2 resection, so the

TABLE 12.1 Key Published Randomized Trials of Neo-adjuvant and Adjuvant Treatment of Gastric Cancer

Study	Patient Numbers and Type	Stage Inclusion	D2 Lymphadenectomy (%)	Treatment Arms	Median Survival	Overall Survival	HR (95% CI)	Notes
INT-0116[6,7]	557 Gastric	IB, II, III, and IV (M0)	10	Surgery / Surgery and adjuvant chemoradiotherapy (45 Gy/25# with 5FU)	27 months / 36 months	3 years 41% / 3 years 50%	0.75 (0.60–0.94) p = 0.005	R0 resection required. Sub-group analysis shows no differential effect according to extent of lymphadenectomy
MAGIC[8]	372 Gastric, 187 GEJ, 73 esophageal	II and III	51	Surgery / Peri-operative chemotherapy (three cycles ECF pre- and post-operatively)	NR / NR	5 years 23% / 5 years 36%	0.75 (0.60–0.93) p = 0.009	Sub-group analysis demonstrates similar survival benefit for chemotherapy in gastric, GEJ, and esophageal
CLASSIC[10]	1035 Gastric	II and III	100	Surgery / Adjuvant chemotherapy (eight cycles oxaliplatin and capecitabine)	NR / NR	3 years 78% / 3 years 78%	0.72 (0.5–1.0) p = 0.0049	R0 resection required
ACTS-GC[9]	1059 Gastric	II and III	100	Surgery / Surgery and adjuvant chemotherapy (1 year oral S1)	NR / NR	3 year 78% / 3 year 78%	0.68 (0.52–0.8) p = 0.003	R0 resection required
ARTIST[14]	458 Gastric	II and III	100	Surgery and adjuvant chemotherapy (six cycles cisplatin and capecitabine (XP)) / Surgery and chemoradiotherapy (two cycles XP, 45 Gy with capecitabine, two cycles XP)	NR / NR	3 year disease-free survival 74.2% / 3 year disease-free survival 77.5% (p = 0.0862)	NR	R0 resection required. Sub-group analysis shows disease-free survival advantage for chemoradiotherapy in node-positive patients (hazard ratio, 0.69; 95% CI, 0.47–0.91, p = 0.0471)
ARTIST-2[15]	538 Gastric	II and IIINode positive	100%	Surgery and chemoRT (S-1 plus oxaliplatin, 45 Gy) / Surgery and adjuvant chemotherapy (1 year of S-1) / Surgery and adjuvant chemotherapy (6 months of S-1 and oxaliplatin)	NR / NR / NR	3 year disease-free survival 73% / 3 year disease-free survival 65% (p = 0.057) / 3 year disease-free survival 78% (p = 0.667)	SOX vs. S-1 (HR 0.617, p = 0.016)	
FLOT[16]	318 Gastric233 GEJ Siewert Type 2165 GEJ Siewert Type 1	T2+ and/or node positive	55%	Surgery plus peri-operative chemotherapy (four cycles of FLOT pre- and post-operatively) / Surgery plus peri-operative chemotherapy (four cycles of ECF/ECX pre- and post-operatively)	Median DFS 30 months; Median OS 50 months / Median DFS 18 months (p = 0.0036); Median OS 35 months (p = 0.012)		DFS HR 0.75 (95% CI 0.62-0.91); OS HR 0.77 (95% CI 0.63–0.94)	Hospitalization for toxicity occurred in 94 patients (26%) in the ECF/ECX group and 89 patients (25%) in the FLOT group.
CRITICS[17]	653 Gastric135 GEJ	IB-IVA	5%	Surgery plus peri-operative chemotherapy (three cycles ECX/ EOX pre-operatively and three cycles post-operatively) / Surgery, pre-operative chemotherapy (three cycles EP/OX), post-operative ChemoXRT 45 Gy with CX)	Median OS 43 months / Median OS 37 months		OS HR 1.01 (95% CI 0.84–1.22); DFS HR 0.99 (95% CI 0.82–1.19)	Poor post-operative patient compliance in both groups

Abbreviations: NR = Not reached; DFS = Disease free survival; OS = Overall survival; HR = Hazard ratio; CI = Confidence intervals; OX = Oxaliplatin; XP = Capecitabine plus cisplatin; ChemoXRT = Chemoradiotherapy; RT = Radiotherapy high rate of D0 resections has led to the criticism that adjuvant chemoradiotherapy was compensating for inadequate surgery. The data from the long-term follow-up of INT-0116 shows that the survival benefit associated with post-operative chemoradiotherapy does not vary according to the extent of lymphadenectomy.

More recently, in a randomized trial in North America (CALGB 80101, n = 546), adding post-operative adjuvant chemotherapy with epirubicin, cisplatin, and 5FU (ECF) before and after concurrent chemoradiotherapy as per the INT-0116 protocol was not found to be beneficial.[20]

Neo-adjuvant chemotherapy

The MAGIC trial[21] randomized 503 patients with resectable gastric cancer (n = 372), GEJ adenocarcinomas (n = 580), and lower esophageal adenocarcinoma (n = 73) to surgery alone or surgery and neo-adjuvant and adjuvant chemotherapy with three cycles of ECF given pre- and post-operatively. There was a survival benefit for the addition of ECF in this trial to surgery (hazard ratio for death, 0.75; 95% CI, 0.60 to 0.93; p = 0.009; 5-year survival rate, 36% vs. 23%). This survival advantage was evident across gastric, GEJ, and lower esophageal sub-groups. This trial established the so-called "peri-operative chemotherapy" approach as a standard of care and is the most common practice in the United Kingdom for patients with resectable gastric cancer. Pre-operative neo-adjuvant chemotherapy was well tolerated by patients in the MAGIC study, with 86% completing three cycles or 9 weeks of pre-operative ECF. However, the MAGIC trial highlighted issues with the tolerance of post-operative adjuvant chemotherapy in particular and also post-operative adjuvant treatment for gastric cancer more generally. Only 55% started the post-operative ECF in the MAGIC trial, and 42% completed three cycles of post-operative ECF. Tolerance of adjuvant therapy was limited by post-operative complications and associated morbidity, which is significant following gastrectomy. Accordingly, reserving adjuvant therapy until after surgery results in a clinically significant proportion of patients not being able to receive it at all or to receive full protocol treatment, which arguably disadvantages this group and highlights the potential importance and advantage of pre-operative neo-adjuvant therapy.

More recently, a new peri-operative treatment regime has been adopted following the publication of the FLOT study.[16] In this study, 716 patients with gastric or GEJ adenocarcinomas were randomly assigned to three cycles of pre- and post-operative ECF/epirubicin, cisplatin, and capecitabine (ECX) or four cycles of pre- and post-operative FLOT (5-fluorouracil, leucovorin, oxaliplatin, docetaxel). This approach was adopted due to the sensitivity of advanced disease to docetaxel. Similar rates proceeded to surgery (95% and 97%, respectively) with more patients allocated to FLOT completing all allocated cycles of treatment (37% vs. 46%). There was a significant overall survival benefit with FLOT (hazard ratio 0.77, p = 0.0162) and an estimated 5-year survival of 45% compared with 36% with ECX/ECF. FLOT has now been adopted in the United Kingdom and Europe as standard of care.

Adjuvant chemotherapy

More recent trials from Asia have demonstrated the efficacy of adjuvant chemotherapy. The Japanese ACTS-GC[22] randomized 1059 patients to surgery or 1 year of adjuvant chemotherapy with S1 and demonstrated an improvement in overall survival for S1 (hazard ratio, 0.68; 95% CI, 0.52–0.80; p = 0.0003). S1 is an oral fluoropyrimidine that until recently was not available

in Europe or North America, and the European license for S1 is for advanced gastric cancer only at present. The CLASSIC trial[23] in South Korea, Japan, and Taiwan randomized 1035 patients to surgery or adjuvant chemotherapy with 6 months of oxaliplatin and capecitabine and demonstrated a survival benefit for the adjuvant chemotherapy (hazard ratio, 0.72; 95% CI, 0.50–1.00; p = 0.0493). In both trials, patients were Stage II or III and had an R0 resection. Importantly, there was strict surgical quality control in both of these trials, and patients were required to have undergone a D2 lymphadenectomy. These studies importantly demonstrate the efficacy of adjuvant chemotherapy in patients who have had D2 lymphadenectomy, but whether the same advantages would be observed in patients who have D1 or D0 lymphadenectomies, which are more common at present in the West, is less certain and has led to some questioning of the generalizability of these data. In addition, the epidemiological and demographic differences between eastern and western gastric cancer populations has led to some concern about the application of these trials to western patients. Nevertheless, the ACTS-GC and CLASSIC trials establish adjuvant chemotherapy as a reasonable standard of care for patients who have R0 resected gastric cancer and who have had a D2 lymphadenectomy.

The ARTIST trial[14] randomized 458 patients from South Korea with gastric cancer, who had undergone an R0 resection and D2 lymphadenectomy for a Stage II or III tumor, to post-operative chemotherapy with capecitabine and cisplatin (XP) six cycles or to two cycles of XP adjuvant chemotherapy followed by concurrent chemoradiotherapy (45 Gy over 5 weeks) with capecitabine and then two further cycles of XP. No survival advantage was demonstrated for the addition of the concurrent chemoradiotherapy to adjuvant chemotherapy overall, but a sub-group analysis suggested that patients with node-positive disease experience superior disease-free survival.

On the basis of the sub-group analysis from ARTIST, the ARTIST-2 trial compared post-operative adjuvant chemotherapy alone (S-1 or SOX) with post-operative chemoradiotherapy (SOXRT) in node-positive gastric cancer patients. Results presented in abstract format report that in patients with curatively D2-resected, Stage II/III, node-positive gastric cancer, adjuvant SOX or SOXRT was equally effective in prolonging DFS and superior to S-1 chemotherapy alone. These findings were confirmed by the CRITICS trial.[17] The CRITICS trial compared pre-operative neo-adjuvant ECX followed post-operatively by randomization to adjuvant ECX or concurrent chemoradiotherapy. It found that post-operative chemoradiotherapy did not improve overall survival compared with post-operative chemotherapy in patients with resectable gastric cancer treated with adequate pre-operative chemotherapy and surgery.

Ongoing adjuvant therapy trials

A number of ongoing trials have been designed to address the important question of the comparative efficacy of different modality adjuvant and neo-adjuvant therapies when used in combination with ICIs. These are yet to report but involve the use of PD-1, PD-L1, CTLA-4, and Lag-3 inhibitors. Trials include KEYNOTE-585 (comparing peri-operative cisplatin plus 5-FU/capecitabine with pembrolizumab/placebo), VESTIGE (comparing post-operative immunotherapy in the form of ipilimumab and nivolumab with standard chemotherapy), ICONIC (peri-operative FLOT with avelumab), and PANDA (neo-adjuvant capecitabine, oxaliplatin, docetaxel, and atezolizumab).

Treatment of advanced disease

In the Western world, 60%–70% patients with gastric cancer are diagnosed with advanced disease, and the majority who undergo initial curative treatment will ultimately relapse. Accordingly, palliative treatment represents the only treatment option for the majority of patients with gastric cancer. Cytotoxic chemotherapy provides an effective treatment option for patients who are fit enough to receive it, and more recently, the addition of targeted agents to cytotoxic chemotherapy has been evaluated in randomized trials. Evidence is now emerging for the utility of second-line systemic therapy in selected patients.

First-line systemic therapies

Cytotoxic chemotherapy is an effective palliative treatment for advanced gastric cancer, providing symptomatic and quality-of-life benefits and prolongation of survival. Randomized trials in the 1980s demonstrated the benefit of cytotoxic chemotherapy over supportive care, and subsequent randomized trials have demonstrated the increased efficacy of combination chemotherapy over single agents.[24]

The REAL2 trial[25] involved 1002 patients with advanced gastro-esophageal cancer (383 with gastric cancer and 318 with GEJ adenocarcinoma) randomized with a two-by-two design to one of four regimens—ECF, EC with capecitabine (ECX), E oxaliplatin F (EOF), and E oxaliplatin capecitabine (EOX). Equivalent efficacy was demonstrated for infusion 5FU with capecitabine and for oxaliplatin and cisplatin. This study has led to the adoption of EOX as the standard regimen for the first-line treatment of advanced disease in the United Kingdom. The use of capecitabine as an oral therapy removes the requirement for indwelling venous line insertion, and the shorter infusion time and greater utility in patients with mild renal impairment for oxaliplatin are perceived as advantageous without compromising the efficacy of treatment.

Epirubicin adds toxicity, and in light of this, the incremental benefit of adding epirubicin to cisplatin or oxaliplatin and capecitabine has been questioned by some researchers, but no adequately powered definitive randomized trials have been performed to address this. Similarly, the V325 randomized trial demonstrated that although adding docetaxel to cisplatin and 5FU increased efficacy, the advantage was marginal, and docetaxel greatly increased toxicity.[26] This has led to some authors advocating platinum doublets comprising cisplatin or oxaliplatin with capecitabine or 5FU as the optimal first-line cytotoxic therapy—balancing efficacy and toxicity—for advanced gastric cancer.

In those unable to tolerate platinums or who are not felt to be suitable for a platinum agent, an irinotecan regime may be an alternative option. A recent meta-analysis suggests that irinotecan combinations are non-inferior first-line.[27]

As mentioned earlier, toxicity plays a significant role in treatment. This is particularly important as patients with gastric cancer are often frail and may not be able to tolerate full dose combination treatment. The GO-2 study, which has recently been presented in abstract form, looked at reducing chemotherapy dose in this group of frailer patients. Patients were given a combination of oxaliplatin and capecitabine at either 100%, 80%, or 60% dose. The trial found that 60% dose was non-inferior in overall survival to 100% with reduced toxicity. This suggests that in frailer populations, chemotherapy dose can be reduced without affecting efficacy. Discussions regarding the optimal cytotoxic chemotherapy in advanced disease have taken on further relevance in recent years as the addition of targeted therapies to cytotoxic regimens has been evaluated, and in some cases, difficulties with toxicity

have been encountered when adding a targeted agent to platinum triplets.

The ToGA trial[4] represents a landmark study in the palliative management of advanced gastric cancer, demonstrating for the first time the efficacy of addition of a targeted agent to cytotoxic chemotherapy and also providing the first biomarker-directed therapy for the disease. In ToGA, 594 patients with advanced gastric or GEJ adenocarcinoma (478 with gastric cancer) who were HER2 positive (defined as HER2 amplification by fluorescence in-situ hybridization [FISH] and/or strong overexpression of HER2 protein by immunohistochemistry—IHC 3+) were randomized to cisplatin and 5FU or capecitabine or the same regimen plus trastuzumab. A survival advantage was demonstrated for the addition of trastuzumab. Median overall survival was 13.8 months in those assigned to trastuzumab plus chemotherapy compared with 11.1 months in those assigned to chemotherapy alone (hazard ratio, 0·74; 95% CI, 0·60–0·91; p = 0.0046). In addition, sub-group analysis demonstrated that the greatest benefit was seen in patients who were HER2 IHC 3+, with median survival of 17.9 months with the addition of trastuzumab compared with 12.3 months with chemotherapy alone (hazard ratio, 0.58; 95% CI, 0.40–0.81). Patients with HER2 IHC 2+ tumors with HER amplification by FISH also benefited, but patients who were IHC 1+ did not benefit. Patients with HER IHC 3+ tumors or IHC 2+ with HER2 amplification by FISH had a median survival of 16.0 months with the addition of trastuzumab compared with 11.8 months with chemotherapy alone (hazard ratio, 0.65; 95% CI, 0.51–0.83), and those with HER2 IHC 0 or 1+ with or without HER2 amplification by FISH did not benefit from addition of trastuzumab (median survival for trastuzumab was 10.0 months compared to 8.7 months for chemotherapy alone; hazard ratio, 1.07; 95% CI, 0.70–1.62). This trial has established cisplatin and 5FU or capecitabine combined with trastuzumab as the standard of care for gastric and GEJ adenocarcinomas that are HER2 IHC 3+ or HER2 amplified by FISH. Non-randomized Phase II trials have demonstrated similar benefits for oxaliplatin with 5FU or capecitabine and trastuzumab combinations in HER2-positive advanced gastric cancer, and therefore oxaliplatin is a suitable alternative to cisplatin in this setting if there are specific contraindications or concerns regarding the use of cisplatin.[28]

More recently, two large randomized trials (EXPAND and REAL 3) have failed to demonstrate a benefit for the addition of EGFR-targeting agents to chemotherapy in advanced gastric cancer. EXPAND[29] randomized 904 patients with advanced gastric cancer to cisplatin and 5FU or capecitabine alone or with cetuximab. Median survival was not significantly different. REAL3[30] randomized 553 patients with advanced gastro-esophageal adenocarcinoma to EOX or EOX plus panitumumab (EOX+P). Because of toxicity, the doses of EOX had to be modified, and modified EOX plus panitumumab was inferior to EOX (median survival for EOX was 11.3 months compared with 8.8 months in modified EOX+P; hazard ratio, 1.37; 95% CI, 1.07–1.76; p = 0.013). These studies suggest that addition of EGFR-targeted therapy to chemotherapy is not effective in advanced gastric cancer.

Other studies of targeted therapies have also had limited success. The LOGiC trial[7] randomized 545 patients with advanced gastric cancer who were HER2 positive (defined as IHC2+ and FISH amplified, or IHC 3+) to cisplatin and 5FU or capecitabine alone or with the dual EGFR/HER2 tyrosine kinase inhibitor lapatinib. Although the response rate was significantly higher, no survival benefit was demonstrated for the addition of lapatinib. The AVAGAST[6] study randomized 774 patients with advanced gastric cancer to cisplatin and 5FU or capecitabine alone or with the vascular endothelial growth factor (VEGF) monoclonal antibody bevacizumab. No survival advantage was demonstrated for the addition of bevacizumab. Likewise, the recently published RAINFALL study looked at the addition of the VEGFR2 antagonist ramucirumab to first-line chemotherapy in 645 patients and found no overall survival advantage.[5] The RILOMET-1 study[31] looked at the addition of rilotumumab (a MET pathway ligand antagonist) to chemotherapy in MET-positive advanced gastric or GEJ cancer. The study was stopped early due to inferiority.

In summary, platinum (oxaliplatin or cisplatin) plus fluoropyrimidine (5FU or capecitabine) chemotherapy, with or without trastuzumab depending on HER2 status, remains standard of care in first-line advanced gastric cancer. Adding epirubicin to the platinum fluoropyrimidine doublet in HER2-negative (IHC score 0 or 1+, or IHC score 2+/FISH negative) is an option, but consideration should be given to the balance of increased toxicity versus clinical benefit in individual patients.

Second-line and subsequent therapies

The median survival for patients who have progressed after second-line treatment in the supportive care arms of randomized trials is about 3 months. This indicates the poor prognosis for this group of patients and the care needed to avoid toxicity with second-line systemic treatments. Several randomized trials have demonstrated a small benefit for second-line treatment versus best supportive care.

A German trial[32] and the recent COUGAR-02 trial[33] demonstrate efficacy from cytotoxic agents such as irinotecan and docetaxel, respectively. However, the benefits of these treatments are small and the toxicity significant. Overall, irinotecan and docetaxel are reasonable options for a selected sub-group of patients in the second-line setting.

The REGARD[34] trial demonstrated a survival benefit of 1.4 months for the vascular endothelial growth factor receptor (VEGFR) monoclonal antibody ramucirumab over supportive care. Although this benefit is small, the toxicity profile of ramucirumab is very favorable, making this a more feasible option for subsequent therapy. The RAINBOW trial subsequently looked at ramucirumab in addition to paclitaxel in the second-line setting compared with paclitaxel alone.[35] The addition of ramucirumab significantly improved overall survival (9.6 months vs. 7.4 months, $p = 0.017$) with only a small increase in toxicity. These trials provide a range of second-line therapy options.

Beyond second line, the recently published TAGS trial[36] has shown a 2.1-month survival advantage for Lonsurf (Trifluridine/tipiracil) when compared with supportive care. Lonsurf has now been licensed in the third-line setting in the United Kingdom.

There has been limited success with other targeted therapies. The GRANITE study[37] randomized patients to everolimus versus supportive care; no survival benefit was demonstrated. The SHINE study[38] was an open-label study of the FGFR2 inhibitor AZD4547 in FGFR2 amplified patients. When compared with paclitaxel, there was no improvement in progression-free survival.

In the absence of other options, many oncologists have re-challenged patients with the same first-line platinum combination regimen. Although there is no randomized evidence to support this, large observational cohorts suggest that this may be an option for patients who have good and durable responses in the first-line setting. Overall, as all patients will progress after first-line palliative therapy, there remains a need to develop further effective second and subsequent therapy options for patients with advanced gastric cancer.

Immune checkpoint inhibitors in advanced disease

ICIs have shown some promising activity in gastric cancer. Response rates in unselected pretreated gastric cancer patients range from 10% to 17%, but when responses do occur, they often prove to be durable. The ATTRACTION-2 study in biomarker unselected patients demonstrated a small overall survival advantage for nivolumab (1.18 months) compared with supportive care in pretreated gastric cancer patients (hazard ratio 0.63, $p < 0.0001$); however, 12-month survival was 26.2% compared with 10.9%, suggesting a significant benefit and durable responses for a sub-group of patients.[28]

KEYNOTE-061[39] compared pembrolizumab with paclitaxel in the second-line setting. Although there was no significant survival advantage, the survival curves crossed, and in those who responded to treatment, response duration was significantly longer for pembrolizumab than for paclitaxel (18.0 months vs. 5.2 months), again suggesting durable responses to immune checkpoint blockade in a sub-group of patients. Patients in this study with a PD-L1 CPS (combined positivity score) ≥10 appeared more likely to benefit. In the first-line setting in advanced HER2-negative GEJ, KEYNOTE 062[40] demonstrated non-inferiority for platinum fluoropyrimidine chemotherapy versus pembrolizumab monotherapy in patients with PD-L1 CPS ≥1, with a more favorable toxicity profile for pembrolizumab versus chemotherapy and superior survival for pembrolizumab over chemotherapy in those with PD-L1 CPS ≥10. This suggests a possible role for ICIs in the first-line setting in HER2-negative GOA, but there was no survival benefit for the addition of pembrolizumab to chemotherapy over chemotherapy alone. In the first-line setting in HER2-positive advanced GOA patients, the ongoing KEYNOTE 811 study randomizes patients to platinum fluoropyrimidine chemotherapy and trastuzumab plus pembrolizumab or placebo (NCT03615326).

Overall, these trials with ICIs suggest promising activity but also indicate that the majority of patients with gastric cancer do not benefit from treatment and highlight the need for a predictive biomarker to identify the minority sub-group of gastric cancer patients who have durable responses to ICIs. Nevertheless, the emerging results from these trials suggest it is likely that the landscape of gastric cancer treatment will change dramatically over the course of the next decade.

Predictive biomarkers

ICIs are associated with durable responses in a minority subset of patients with gastric cancer, highlighting the need for biomarkers that will enable these patients to be identified, and this is a current active focus of research. There are several candidates that are being investigated in solid tumors, including gastric cancer. The marker most commonly used at present is PD-L1 (Programmed Death Ligand-1). Expression level is calculated using the tumor proportionality score or combined positivity score. Improved outcome with ICIs has been associated with higher expression of PD-L1.[39] EBV positivity is associated with PD-L1 overexpression and dense tumor immune infiltrate, suggesting that EBV positivity could be a useful predictive biomarker in itself.[41]

Another proposed biomarker for response to ICIs is MSI. Nivolumab has been licensed pan-cancer by the Food and Drug Administration (FDA) for MSI-high (MSI-H) tumors. In gastric cancer, response rates in deficient mismatch repair (dMMR) or MSI-H patients in the Phase I/II CheckMate-032 trial[42] to combination ipilimumab and nivolumab were 50% compared with 19% in non-MSI-H.

MSI and other deficits in DNA repair result in a higher tumor mutational burden (TMB). This in turn results in increased tumor antigens and increased immune cell infiltrate. As a result, TMB has also been proposed as another emerging biomarker,[43] although it is yet to be validated in gastric cancer. As translational research on completed trials emerges, the role of biomarkers in prediction of response will become better defined.

Future directions

The development of a precision medicine approach to systemic therapy by identifying predictive biomarkers for chemotherapy, targeted therapies, and immunotherapies is a key aim of future research. The proof of principle that this is effective in gastric cancer has been demonstrated with HER2 and trastuzumab in the ToGA trial. The more recent negative trials of other receptor tyrosine kinase inhibitors and targeted agents, even in biomarker selected patients, have revealed a more complex molecular pathogenesis characterized by high levels of genomic heterogeneity.

This has highlighted the importance of new data from large-scale genomic landscaping studies in gastric cancer, which have provided key understandings into why previous precision medicine approaches failed and enabled a new level of precision in our biological understanding of gastric cancer. This understanding includes mechanisms of targeted therapy resistance; when seen in the context of previous clinical trial results, this has paved the way for a new approach to identifying actionable subtypes with specific therapeutic vulnerabilities.

ICIs have shown promising activity, with durable responses seen in a subset of patients with advanced gastric cancer in recent clinical trials. Together, this body of clinical and translational research is providing a comprehensive molecular classification of gastric cancer, which will be evaluated in future trials and may form the basis for a widely applicable precision medicine strategy in gastric cancer with predictive biomarker–directed systemic therapy selection in individual patients, including chemotherapy, targeted therapy, and immune-oncology monotherapies or combinations.

The successes with ICIs and targeted agents in advanced-stage disease have led to ongoing translation of this approach into early stages of the disease in the neo-adjuvant and adjuvant setting and could provide improved cure rates for gastric cancer.

Although earlier stage at diagnosis would improve outcomes significantly, clinical tools for screening that are feasible and cost effective in lower-incidence western populations are not yet available, but these remain an area for much-needed development.

Key learning points

- Outcomes for operable gastric cancer have been significantly improved following the positive results of the recent FLOT4 Phase III randomized trial establishing peri-operative chemotherapy with the FLOT regimen as a new standard of care with estimated 5-year survival reported as 45%.
- Post-operative chemoradiotherapy may have a benefit in node-positive gastric cancer after D2 lymphadenectomy but is not yet established as a standard of care, and prospective randomized trials are ongoing.
- In palliative treatment, in the first-line setting, platinum fluoropyrimidine chemotherapy remains the standard of care for HER2-negative gastric cancer, with the addition of trastuzumab offering benefit in HER2-positive patients.

Ramucirumab as monotherapy or in combination with paclitaxel has an established role in the second-line setting, and the ICIs pembrolizumab and nivolumab have established benefit over supportive care alone in the third-line setting.

- MSI-H is emerging as a potentially useful predictive biomarker for ICIs in gastric cancer, and in the first palliative setting, it may identify a sub-group that can be treated and achieve durable disease control with ICIs alone without chemotherapy.
- Genomic landscaping studies have provided a molecular classification of gastric cancer, and precision medicine trials evaluating targeted therapies and immunotherapy directed by molecular classification are in progress.
- High degrees of molecular heterogeneity are evident in gastric cancer and have presented a challenge to the development of effective precision medicine strategies.

References

1. Reim D, Loos M, Vogl F et al. Prognostic implications of the seventh edition of the international union against cancer classification for patients with gastric cancer: the Western experience of patients treated in a single-center European institution. *Am. J. Clin. Oncol.* 2013; 31(2):263–71.
2. Liu J-Y, Peng C-W, Yang X-J et al. The prognosis role of AJCC/UICC 8(th) edition staging system in gastric cancer, a retrospective analysis. *Am J Transl Res.* 2018; 10(1):292–303.
3. Cancer Genome Atlas Research Network. Comprehensive molecular characterization of gastric adenocarcinoma. *Nature* 2014; 513(7517):202–9.
4. Bang YJ, Van Cutsem E, Feyereislova A et al. Trastuzumab in combination with chemotherapy versus chemotherapy alone for treatment of HER2-positive advanced gastric or gastro-oesophageal junction cancer (ToGA): a phase 3, open-label, randomised controlled trial. *Lancet* 2010; 376(9742):687–97.
5. Fuchs CS, Shitara K, Di Bartolomeo M et al. Ramucirumab with cisplatin and fluoropyrimidine as first-line therapy in patients with metastatic gastric or junctional adenocarcinoma (RAINFALL): a double-blind, randomised, placebo-controlled, phase 3 trial. *Lancet Oncol.* 2019; 20(3):420–35.
6. Ohtsu A, Shah MA, Van Cutsem E et al. Bevacizumab in combination with chemotherapy as first-line therapy in advanced gastric cancer: a randomized, double-blind, placebo-controlled phase III study. *Am. J. Clin. Oncol.* 2011; 29(30):3968–76.
7. Hecht JR, Bang YJ, Qin SK et al. Lapatinib in combination with capecitabine plus oxaliplatin in human epidermal growth factor receptor 2-positive advanced or metastatic gastric, esophageal, or gastroesophageal adenocarcinoma: TRIO-013/LOGiC—A randomized phase III trial. *Am. J. Clin. Oncol.* 2016; 34(5):443–51.
8. Alsina M, Gullo I, Carneiro F. Intratumoral heterogeneity in gastric cancer: a new challenge to face. *Ann Oncol.* 2017; 28(5):912–13.
9. Cancer Genome Atlas Research Network. Integrated genomic characterization of oesophageal carcinoma. *Nature.* 2017; 541(7636):169–75.
10. In H, Solsky I, Palis B et al. Validation of the 8th edition of the AJCC TNM staging system for gastric cancer using the national cancer database. *Ann. Surg. Oncol.* 2017; 24(12):3683–91.
11. Claassen YHM, van Sandick JW, Hartgrink HH et al. Association between hospital volume and quality of gastric cancer surgery in the CRITICS trial. *Br J Surg.* 2018; 105(6):728–35.
12. Wu CW, Hsiung CA, Lo SS et al. Nodal dissection for patients with gastric cancer: a randomised controlled trial. *Lancet Oncol.* 2006; 7(4):309–15.
13. Songun I, Putter H, Kranenbarg EM et al. Surgical treatment of gastric cancer: 15-year follow-up results of the randomised nationwide Dutch D1D2 trial. *Lancet Oncol.* 2010; 11(5):439–49.
14. Park SH, Sohn TS, Lee J et al. Phase III trial to compare adjuvant chemotherapy with capecitabine and cisplatin versus concurrent

chemoradiotherapy in gastric cancer: Final report of the adjuvant chemoradiotherapy in stomach tumors trial, including survival and subset analyses. *Am. J. Clin. Oncol.* 2015; 33(28):3130–6.

15. Park SH, Zang DY, Han B et al. ARTIST 2: Interim results of a phase III trial involving adjuvant chemotherapy and/or chemoradiotherapy after D2-gastrectomy in stage II/III gastric cancer (GC). *J Clin Oncol.* 2019; 37(15_suppl):4001–01.

16. Al-Batran SE, Homann N, Pauligk C et al. Perioperative chemotherapy with fluorouracil plus leucovorin, oxaliplatin, and docetaxel versus fluorouracil or capecitabine plus cisplatin and epirubicin for locally advanced, resectable gastric or gastro-oesophageal junction adenocarcinoma (FLOT4): a randomised, phase 2/3 trial. *Lancet* 2019; 393(10184):1948–57.

17. Cats A, Jansen EPM, van Grieken NCT et al. Chemotherapy versus chemoradiotherapy after surgery and preoperative chemotherapy for resectable gastric cancer (CRITICS): an international, open-label, randomised phase 3 trial. *Lancet Oncol.* 2018; 19(5):616–28.

18. Macdonald JS, Smalley SR, Benedetti J et al. Chemoradiotherapy after surgery compared with surgery alone for adenocarcinoma of the stomach or gastroesophageal junction. *N Engl J Med.* 2001; 345(10):725–30.

19. Smalley SR, Benedetti JK, Haller DG et al. Updated analysis of SWOG-directed intergroup study 0116: a phase III trial of adjuvant radiochemotherapy versus observation after curative gastric cancer resection. *Am. J. Clin. Oncol.* 2012; 30(19):2327–33.

20. Fuchs CS, Niedzwiecki D, Mamon HJ et al. Adjuvant chemoradiotherapy with epirubicin, cisplatin, and fluorouracil compared with adjuvant chemoradiotherapy with fluorouracil and leucovorin after curative resection of gastric cancer: Results from CALGB 80101 (Alliance). *Am. J. Clin. Oncol.* 2017; 35(32):3671–77.

21. Cunningham D, Allum WH, Stenning SP et al. Perioperative chemotherapy versus surgery alone for resectable gastroesophageal cancer. *N Engl J Med.* 2006; 355(1):11–20.

22. Sakuramoto S, Sasako M, Yamaguchi T et al. Adjuvant chemotherapy for gastric cancer with S-1, an oral fluoropyrimidine. *N Engl J Med.* 2007; 357(18):1810–20.

23. Bang YJ, Kim YW, Yang HK et al. Adjuvant capecitabine and oxaliplatin for gastric cancer after D2 gastrectomy (CLASSIC): a phase 3 open-label, randomised controlled trial. *Lancet* 2012; 379(9813):315–21.

24. Wagner AD, Grothe W, Haerting J et al. Chemotherapy in advanced gastric cancer: a systematic review and meta-analysis based on aggregate data. *Am. J. Clin. Oncol.* 2006; 24(18):2903–9.

25. Cunningham D, Starling N, Rao S et al. Capecitabine and oxaliplatin for advanced esophagogastric cancer. *N Engl J Med.* 2008; 358(1):36–46.

26. Van Cutsem E, Moiseyenko VM, Tjulandin S et al. Phase III study of docetaxel and cisplatin plus fluorouracil compared with cisplatin and fluorouracil as first-line therapy for advanced gastric cancer: a report of the V325 Study Group. *Am. J. Clin. Oncol.* 2006; 24(31):4991–7.

27. Wagner AD, Syn NL, Moehler M et al. Chemotherapy for advanced gastric cancer. *Cochrane Database Syst Rev.* 2017; 8:Cd004064.

28. Kang YK, Boku N, Satoh T et al. Nivolumab in patients with advanced gastric or gastro-oesophageal junction cancer refractory to, or intolerant of, at least two previous chemotherapy regimens (ONO-4538-12, ATTRACTION-2): a randomised, double-blind, placebo-controlled, phase 3 trial. *Lancet.* 2017; 390(10111): 2461–71.

29. Lordick F, Kang YK, Chung HC et al. Capecitabine and cisplatin with or without cetuximab for patients with previously untreated advanced gastric cancer (EXPAND): a randomised, open-label phase 3 trial. *Lancet Oncol.* 2013; 14(6):490–9.

30. Waddell T, Chau I, Cunningham D et al. Epirubicin, oxaliplatin, and capecitabine with or without panitumumab for patients with previously untreated advanced oesophagogastric cancer (REAL3): a randomised, open-label phase 3 trial. *Lancet Oncol.* 2013; 14(6):481–9.

31. Catenacci DVT, Tebbutt NC, Davidenko I et al. Rilotumumab plus epirubicin, cisplatin, and capecitabine as first-line therapy in advanced MET-positive gastric or gastro-oesophageal junction

cancer (RILOMET-1): a randomised, double-blind, placebo-controlled, phase 3 trial. *Lancet Oncol.* 2017; 18(11):1467–82.

32. Thuss-Patience PC, Kretzschmar A, Bichev D et al. Survival advantage for irinotecan versus best supportive care as second-line chemotherapy in gastric cancer—a randomised phase III study of the Arbeitsgemeinschaft Internistische Onkologie (AIO). *Eur J Cancer.* 2011; 47(15):2306–14.

33. Ford HE, Marshall A, Bridgewater JA et al. Docetaxel versus active symptom control for refractory oesophagogastric adenocarcinoma (COUGAR-02): an open-label, phase 3 randomised controlled trial. *Lancet Oncol.* 2014; 15(1):78–86.

34. Fuchs CS, Tomasek J, Yong CJ et al. Ramucirumab monotherapy for previously treated advanced gastric or gastro-oesophageal junction adenocarcinoma (REGARD): an international, randomised, multicentre, placebo-controlled, phase 3 trial. *Lancet* 2014; 383(9911):31–39.

35. Wilke H, Muro K, Van Cutsem E et al. Ramucirumab plus paclitaxel versus placebo plus paclitaxel in patients with previously treated advanced gastric or gastro-oesophageal junction adenocarcinoma (RAINBOW): a double-blind, randomised phase 3 trial. *Lancet Oncol.* 2014; 15(11):1224–35.

36. Shitara K, Doi T, Dvorkin M et al. Trifluridine/tipiracil versus placebo in patients with heavily pretreated metastatic gastric cancer (TAGS): a randomised, double-blind, placebo-controlled, phase 3 trial. *Lancet Oncol.* 2018; 19(11):1437–48.

37. Ohtsu A, Ajani JA, Bai YX et al. Everolimus for previously treated advanced gastric cancer: results of the randomized, double-blind, phase III GRANITE-1 study. *Am. J. Clin. Oncol.* 2013; 31(31):3935–43.

38. Van Cutsem E, Bang YJ, Mansoor W et al. A randomized, open-label study of the efficacy and safety of AZD4547 monotherapy versus paclitaxel for the treatment of advanced gastric adenocarcinoma with FGFR2 polysomy or gene amplification. *Ann Oncol.* 2017; 28(6):1316–24.

39. Shitara K, Ozguroglu M, Bang YJ et al. Pembrolizumab versus paclitaxel for previously treated, advanced gastric or gastro-oesophageal junction cancer (KEYNOTE-061): a randomised, open-label, controlled, phase 3 trial. *Lancet.* 2018; 392(10142):123–33.

40. Tabernero J, Cutsem EV, Bang Y-J et al. Pembrolizumab with or without chemotherapy versus chemotherapy for advanced gastric or gastroesophageal junction (G/GEJ) adenocarcinoma: The phase III KEYNOTE-062 study. *J Clin Oncol.* 2019; 37(18_suppl):LBA4007-LBA07.

41. Kelly RJ. Immunotherapy for esophageal and gastric cancer. *Am Soc Clin Oncol Educ Book.* 2017; (37):292–300.

42. Janjigian YY, Bendell J, Calvo E et al. CheckMate-032 study: Efficacy and safety of nivolumab and nivolumab plus ipilimumab in patients with metastatic esophagogastric cancer. *Am. J. Clin. Oncol.* 2018; 36(28):2836–44.

43. Chan TA, Yarchoan M, Jaffee E et al. Development of tumor mutation burden as an immunotherapy biomarker: utility for the oncology clinic. *Ann Oncol.* 2018; 30(1):44–56.

Useful websites

www.esmo.org/Guidelines-Practice/Clinical-Practice-Guidelines/Gastrointestinal-Cancers/Gastric-Cancer

www.esmo.org/Guidelines-Practice/Clinical-Practice-Guidelines/Sarcoma-and-GIST/Gastrointestinal-Stromal-Tumours

www.cancer.gov/cancertopics/types/stomach

www.cancer.gov/cancertopics/types/gastrointestinalcarcinoid

http://seer.cancer.gov/statfacts/html/stomach.html

www.ncin.org.uk/cancer_type_and_topic_specific_work/cancer_type_specific_work/upper_gi_cancers/

http://pathways.nice.org.uk/pathways/gastrointestinal-cancers?fno=1#content=view-node%3Anodes-gastric-and-duodenal-cancer

www.cancerresearchuk.org/cancer-help/type/stomach-cancer/

www.cancer.net/cancer-types/stomach-cancer

www.nostomachforcancer.org

13 BLADDER CANCER

Robert Huddart and Pradeep Kumar

Introduction

Bladder cancer is a disease with significant heterogeneity of outcome, ranging from tumors involving mucosa, in which metastatic disease is rare, to muscle-invasive disease with poor prognosis. Management is further complicated as bladder cancer often occurs in the elderly, who frequently suffer concurrent medical conditions (often related to smoking) and may be of poor performance status, thus limiting treatment options.

Management of bladder cancer, in particular, remains an area of controversy, with significant variability in management worldwide. Over recent years there have been significant advances in operative technique and technical radiotherapy, in the administration of chemotherapy, and the advent of immune check point-targeted therapy. This has resulted in attendant reduction in treatment-related morbidity and improvements in survival in patients suitable for radical treatment. In addition, advances in molecular biology have provided us with further insights into the mechanism of bladder cancer pathogenesis, invasion, and metastasis from which new targets for therapy may be derived.

Epidemiology

Bladder cancer is the seventh most commonly diagnosed cancer in the UK,[1] affecting in 2010 10,000 individuals each year and causing around 4,900 deaths. The disease is commonest in men with a male:female ratio of 2.6:1.0.[1] Incidence rose during the twentieth century in developed countries, including the UK, to reach a peak in the late 1980s but has since been declining, though changes in coding and classification practices affecting the definition of carcinoma of the bladder make trends difficult to interpret.[2] Internationally the incidence rate of bladder cancer among men varies more than ten-fold with high rates occurring in Western Europe and North America while the disease is less common in Eastern Europe and Asia. It is a disease mainly of older adults, and 80% of diagnoses are in those >65 years.[1] Survival rates are improving for individuals in affluent groups and, in contrast to most other common malignancies, show a consistent survival advantage for men over women.[3] The decline in death rate for men has been significant, falling from 12.2 to 8.7 per 100,000 in the year 2003. For women however the rates have changed little from around 3.3 in the early 1970s to 3.1 in 2003 resulting in a male:female ratio of 3.7:1 in 1979 to 2.8:1 in 2003.

Etiology

The development of bladder cancer has been associated with a number of etiological risk factors which are summarized in Table 13.1. The risk factor with the highest attributable risk is smoking. Industrial exposure was a major risk in the past but since control measures have been instituted the attributable risk is now small.

Biology of bladder cancer

In recent years, driven by the Cancer Genome Research Network, there has been a significant broadening of the understanding of the genetic mechanisms underlying muscle invasive bladder cancer and increasing appreciation of the heterogeneity of the illness. An initial study of 131 samples has been expanded to over 400 samples in a 2017 publication.[4]

Bladder cancer has a high mutation rate with TCGA reporting a median of 5.8 mutations per megabase. An analysis of mutation signatures suggested that around 67% of mutations were due to APOBEC mutagenesis. Other mutations were associated with 5-methylcytosine deamination, POLE, and ERCC2 mutations. Patients with a high mutation burden and APOBEC signature seemed to have better prognosis.

Fifty-eight significantly mutated genes have been identified; the main features are summarized in Figure 13.1. TP53 and cell cycle genes were mutated in 89% of tumors including TP53 in 48%, MDM2 over-expression in 25%, and RB mutations 17%, CDKN2a mutation/deletion 22%, CDKN1A in 11%. RAS/PI3K pathway was also frequently mutated (in ~70%). An unexpected major feature has been the frequency of chromatin remodeling genes with ten genes mutated at >5% frequency and occurring in over 50% of tumors, the significance of which is unclear. DNA repair genes are also found to be mutated in around 16% cases including ATM (14%), ERCC2 (9%), and RAD51 (2%). FGFR2/3 mutations have reported to occur in 15–20% of cases with the frequency being higher in lower-stage lower-grade tumors.

A number of groups, including the TCGA, have reported outcomes of mRNA expression arrays which have shown that bladder cancers can be subdivided into subgroups based on their mRNA expression patterns, similar to that seen on other cancers.[5] Details vary from study to study with varying numbers of subgroups reported. The main divide is between "luminal" subtypes and basal/squamous subtypes and possibly a "neuronal" (neuroendocrine) subtype. These have provoked interest as prognosis and response to systemic therapies (chemotherapy and immunotherapy) vary between groups. For instance the "luminal papillary" group may be characterized by a better prognosis, a preponderance of FGFR mutations, but poor immunotherapy response whereas basal subtype has a poorer prognosis but greater benefit from neoadjuvant chemotherapy.[6]

Pathology

In Europe and the USA, more than 90% of tumors are of urothelial (transitional cell) origin and approximately 5% are squamous-cell carcinomas, except in areas where schistosomiasis is endemic (where they constitute up to 80% of all urothelial malignancy). Primary adenocarcinoma of the bladder may arise from the urachal remnant or in bladder exstrophy; the remainder are rare tumors such as small-cell carcinoma, sarcoma, lymphoma, and melanoma.

In the UK around 70% of newly diagnosed bladder cancers are, at least initially, non-muscle invasive (NMIBC). Prognostic differences exist between tumors confined by the basement membrane (Ta tumors) and T1 tumors which invade the lamina propria and according to tumor grade. Historically tumors have been graded on a scale of 1–3, with G3 tumors representing those with the most aggressive features at pathological analysis. In 2004 the grading system was adjusted to address the ambiguity in the

TABLE 13.1   **Summary of Key Risk Factors for the Development of Bladder Cancer**

Risk Factor	Commentary
Smoking	Key current risk factor with 40% of male and 10% female cases attributed to smoking. Smokers have a 3-fold increased risk with clear dose response and risks declines with cessation.
Industrial carcinogens	Dye stuffs and rubber industries[6,7] associated with a 10–50-fold increased risk of bladder cancer, primarily attributed to exposure to the aromatic amines, 2-Napthylamine and Benzedine[6,8,9] but up to 40 chemicals are implicated. The risk of death increases with young age at first exposure and increasing duration of employment, and mortality decreases with increasing time from last exposure. Reduced bladder cancer risk was demonstrated following the introduction of protective measures.
Drugs	Cytotoxic drugs such as the alkylating agent cyclophosphamide and its metabolites are carcinogenic. The carcinogenic effect is dose-dependent, with bladder cancer risk increasing with dose delivered. Phenacetin is linked to carcinoma of both the upper and lower urinary tracts.
Radiation	Therapeutic pelvic radiotherapy for both benign (e.g., dysfunctional uterine bleeding) and malignant disorders (e.g., cervical cancer) increases bladder cancer risk with relative risks up to 8.7. Similarly, post-radioactive iodine (iodine-131) treatment for thyroid cancer and in the survivors of the atomic bombs of Hiroshima and Nagasaki is associated with increased risk.
Infection/ inflammation	Chronic or repeated urinary tract infections, developmental abnormalities of the bladder, bladder diverticulae, chronic bladder stones, or indwelling catheters which to urinary stasis and/or chronic inflammation increase the risk of bladder carcinoma. Schistosoma Haematobium, which is endemic in developing countries and associated with high incidence of squamous cell carcinoma (SCC).
Genetic predisposition	Studies have shown an increased relative risk for developing bladder cancer in the relatives of bladder cancer patients. Large-scale genome-wide association studies have identified a number of single nucleotide polymorphisms associated with increased risk of bladder cancer. Patients with hereditary nonpolyposis colon cancer (Lynch syndrome) and mutations in mismatch repair genes, (*MSH2*). Patients with deficient detoxification mechanisms, e.g., slow acetylator phenotype (mutated gene [NAT 2]) absence of human glutathione transferase M1 (GSTM1) gene are at increased risk of bladder cancer.

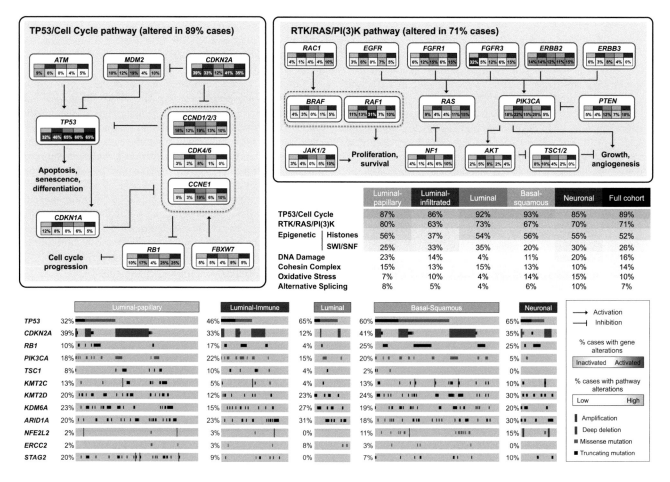

FIGURE 13.1   Somatic alterations in signaling pathways across mRNA expression subtypes in muscle invasive bladder cancer. The table shows the fraction of samples with alterations in selected signaling pathways. In the pathway diagrams, edges show pairwise molecular interactions; boxes outlined in red denote alterations leading to pathway activation, while boxes outlined in blue denote predicted pathway inactivation. The oncoprint at bottom illustrates type and frequency of alteration, as well as patterns of co-occurrence, for selected genes from the pathways highlighted in the table for each expression subtype. (Reproduced with permission from Robertson et al., 2017.)

intermediate (G2) subgroup by assigning them as high- or low-risk tumors.

Bladder carcinoma *in situ* (CIS) is highly malignant sub-category of NMIBC with a high propensity for progression. It can be diffuse or focal, symptomatic or asymptomatic, and may or may not be associated with other non-muscle or muscle invasive tumors. Macroscopically, lesions may appear as raised red "velvety" patches or be indistinguishable from adjacent urothelium.

Muscle invasive bladder cancer (MIBC) ranges in appearance at cystoscopy from papillary tumors through solid masses to ulcerated lesions of the bladder wall. MIBC are usually high-grade and may contain foci of glandular or squamous differentiation or atypical spindle cells that mimic sarcomas.

Pure squamous-cell carcinomas of the bladder vary in morphological appearance but are usually large and deeply invasive. Adenocarcinoma is generally of poor prognosis, with tumors arising from urachal remnants having the best outlook and signet-ring carcinomas (accounting for 3–5% of tumors) the worst. The mucosa is usually edematous and ulcerated in most cases of adenocarcinoma; some develop diffuse fibrosis and mural thickening similar to linitis plastica of the stomach. Small-cell carcinoma is microscopically similar to its lung counterpart and carries a similarly poor prognosis.

Clinical presentation and investigation

Approximately 80% of bladder cancers present with hematuria, which is usually painless and intermittent and either visible (macroscopic) or detected on urinalysis (microscopic). Detection rates of bladder cancer in UK series vary between 12 and 20% of those presenting to a hematuria clinic.[7] Storage type urinary symptoms, including urinary frequency, urgency, and dysuria, may be associated with both CIS and invasive bladder tumors. Patients with advanced or metastatic disease often suffer constitutional symptoms, including anorexia, weight loss, and pain arising from sites of metastasis such as bone. Physical examination may be unremarkable in these patients; a careful pelvic examination can determine whether a mass is palpable or to assess the fixity of tumor to adjacent organs. Urine microscopy and culture should be performed and, if negative, repeated in view of the intermittent nature of the hematuria.

Management of hematuria

Urological opinion should be sought in any case of macroscopic hematuria or persistent microscopic hematuria. Presence of a proven urinary tract infection does not remove the need to investigate hematuria as the detection rate of urological malignancy is similar to that in those without UTI in patients presenting to a hematuria clinic.[8] Current recommendations include CT urogram or urinary tract ultrasound, urine for culture and sensitivity, and cystoscopy. When cystoscopy detects a bladder tumor, ipsilateral hydronephrosis on concurrent imaging is associated with muscle-invasive bladder carcinoma (approximately 90% of cases) and its presence should prompt rigorous investigation.

The use of urinary cytology is debated, though it is frequently positive, in high-grade tumors and CIS there remains a 20% false-negative rate and it is usually negative in low-grade tumors. A number of urinary tests (e.g. the urinary nuclear matrix protein NMP22) are commercially available but to date problems of false-negatives and false-positives mean that they are not routinely recommended.[9] A new generation of tests based on detecting genetic abnormalities are under development but have yet to establish a clear role.[10]

The initial examination for patients with hematuria is often by flexible cystoscopy under local anesthetic. Abnormal findings are confirmed under general anesthetic, with bimanual examination to confirm the presence, extent, and fixity of any palpable bladder mass. Biopsy or resection of a tumor is performed accompanied by directed biopsies of adjacent and normal-appearing bladder mucosa.

Following diagnosis patients are staged according to the current TNM staging system (Table 13.2, Figure 13.2).

TABLE 13.2 **UICC 2018 TNM Staging System for Bladder Carcinoma**

Primary Tumor (T)	
TX	Primary tumor cannot be assessed
T0	No evidence of primary tumor
TA	Non-invasive papillary carcinoma
Tis	CIS: flat tumor
T1	Invades subepithelial connective tissue
T2A	Superficial (inner half) muscle invasion
T2B	Deep (outer half) muscle invasion
T3A	Microscopically invades perivesical tissue
T3B	Macroscopically invades perivesical tissue
T4A	Invades prostate, uterus, or vagina
T4B	Invades pelvic or abdominal wall
Lymph nodes	
NX is regional lymph, nodes cannot be assessed	
N0	No regional node involvement
N1	A single node in the true pelvis
N2	Multiple nodes in the true pelvis
N3	Metastasis in common iliac lymph nodes
Metastasis	
M0	No metastasis
M1	Distant metastasis

Note: Suffix "m" should be added to the appropriate "T" to indicate multiple tumors. Suffix "IS" may be added to any T to indicate the presence of associated CIS. Add "p" before T to distinguish pathological staging.

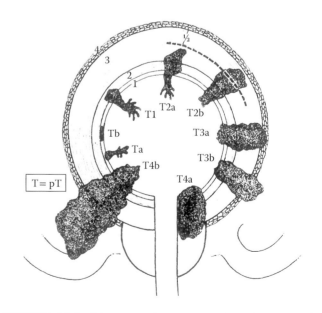

FIGURE 13.2 Diagrammatic representation of tumor node metastasis (TNM) 2011 classification for local staging. 1. Epithelium. 2. Subepithelial connective tissue. 3. Muscle. 4. Perivesical fat.

Imaging of bladder cancer

Accurate staging of bladder cancer is important both to determine prognosis and for treatment decision-making. The mainstay of pelvic staging has been computerized tomography (CT). CT can identify tumors that extend into the bladder lumen and perivesical tissue, and the presence of bladder wall thickening. However, these findings may reflect inflammatory processes rather than tumor infiltration which along with the inability to distinguish between individual layers of the muscle wall limit the value of CT scans in defining depth of invasion and consequently local stage of disease. Nodes of greater than 1–1.5 cm in diameter are considered abnormal with a resulting sensitivity of between 50 and 85%. However, nodal enlargement may result from other causes resulting in false-positives, such that specificity rates lie between 67 and 100%.[11]

[18]FDG PET-CT[12] has been shown to improve accuracy over CT alone. Though it improves the specificity of nodal disease detection, its sensitivity is still limited in the precystectomy setting. Despite this, recent studies have shown the use of FDG PET CT can change management in up to 40% of cases. Its precise role in management is still being identified but its use in locally advanced patients has been recommended by NICE.[13]

Magnetic resonance imaging (MRI) is generally thought to offer advantages over CT in the staging of bladder cancer. MRI is superior to CT in the delineation of organ-confined tumor, due to an increased ability to differentiate between the various layers of the bladder wall. However, the ability of MRI to distinguish between T2a and T2b tumors is still limited. Recently a new scoring system (VI-RADs) has been proposed that provides diagnostic criteria for describing muscle wall invasion that may facilitate this.[14] The facility for multiplanar imaging is also particularly advantageous in the assessment of tumors of the bladder base close to the trigone. Recent reviews have suggested that diffusion-weighted MR imaging (DWI) and other quantitative parameters can distinguish tumors from associated fibrosis/inflammation[15] and might aid response assessment.[16]

Management

The main division in management is between tumors that invade muscle, where patients are at substantial risk of local and distant recurrence, and those that are restricted to the superficial lamina propria with a good prognosis. We will therefore consider management in three groups: Low-grade non-muscle invasive disease, high-grade non-muscle invasive disease (including CIS), and muscle-invasive carcinoma (see Table 13.3).

Low-grade non-muscle invasive bladder cancer

Surgery

The vast majority of NMIBC are amenable to transurethral resection (TUR). Full clinical staging (with contrast-enhanced CT scan including a urographic phase) is ideally undertaken prior to resection in order to avoid localized artefact due to the procedure itself. Resection involves removal of all macroscopic evidence of tumor and separate biopsies of deep detrusor muscle in order to accurately inform T stage.

Recurrent low-grade papillary tumors may be treated by thermo-coagulation using a neodymium-Yag (Nd-Yag) laser where no specimen is required for pathological analysis.[17] Where high-grade disease or deep invasion is suggested by a more sessile appearance, electrocautery resection is preferable, as an adequate

TABLE 13.3 Guidelines for the Treatment of Patients with Superficial Bladder Cancer Adapted from European Association of Urology Guidelines 2013

Risk Group	Definition	Recommended Adjuvant Treatment
Low	Primary, solitary, Ta G1/G2 (low grade) <3 cm no CIS	Single dose post-operative Mitomycin C
Intermediate	Not low or high risk	Single dose post-operative Mitomycin C plus course of Mitomycin C (6–12 months)
High	Any grade 3 or CIS, T1(G2), multiple and recurrent and large other tumors	BCG induction and maintenance or radical cystectomy
Very high risk	T1G3 with CIS Multiple and/or large T1G3 Recurrent T1G3 T1 G3 with CIS in prostatic urethra Unusual histology	Consider primary cystectomy or BCG plus maintenance if refuses

Source: Adapted from Babjuk et al., 2017.

specimen containing detrusor muscle for histological examination can be more readily assured.

Attempts have been made to improve the efficiency of local resection by using fluorescence endoscopy. Fluorescence endoscopy is based on using a fluorochrome, such as 5-amino laevulinic acid (ALA) or its ester derivative, which is then visualized by light of appropriate wavelength (a blue light for ALA). Tumors emit light of a different wavelength (red for ALA). A number of studies have demonstrated enhanced sensitivity for tumor detection, with sensitivities of 70–75% for standard resection compared to more than 95% for fluorescence endoscopy, with detection of CIS being of particular value.[18] Using "narrow band imaging" can also increase the sensitivity of cystoscopy and may provide many of the potential benefits of fluorescence cystoscopy.[19]

What is debated is the long-term effect on recurrence and progression, though in 1 randomized trial of 191 patients, Filbeck et al. showed that fluorescence endoscopy improved 4-year recurrence-free survival from 60.7% to 85%,[20] although the long-term impact on progression is unclear.[19]

Predicting recurrence in patients with superficial tumors

The initial management of all patients with superficial bladder cancer involves complete resection of the tumor, with subsequent treatment being dependent on the predicted risks of recurrence and progression. Predictive factors have been reported in a number of studies, the most widely used being from the European Organisation for Research and Treatment for Cancer (EORTC) database of patient randomized into trials of intra-vesical chemotherapy (see below).[21,22] Although generalizations from these data must be interpreted with care, as only patients fulfilling the entry criteria for the studies are included, several important prognostic factors have been identified, as shown in Table 13.4. The grade and tumor number at presentation, as well as the outcome of 3-month cystoscopy are highlighted as predictors of subsequent recurrence. These data are supported by subsequent data incorporating patients receiving BCG (e.g. from Spanish co-operative group CUETO).[23] Disease recurrence at cystoscopy continues to

TABLE 13.4 **Prognostic Factors for Superficial Bladder Cancer**

EORTC Trials			MRC trial
Time to First Recurrence (Univariate)	Recurrence Rate/Year (Multivariate)	Time to Invasion (Multivariate)	Recurrence Rate at 2 Years (Univariate)
Number of tumors[a]	Recurrence at 3 months	Recurrence at 3 months	Result of 3-month cystoscopy[b]
Grade[b]	Prior recurrence	Grade	Number of tumors[b]
Prior recurrence[b]	Number of tumors at entry	Prior recurrence	Grade[b]
Time from diagnosis[b]	Grade	Site of tumor	Maximum size[b]
Site of tumor[b]		Size of tumor	Site of tumor
		Sex	

[a] Included in multivariate analysis if site is excluded.
[b] Positive on multivariate analysis.

be highly predictive of future recurrence, with the probability of developing recurrence decreasing with each negative cystoscopy, reaching 8% at 5 years and 0% at 10 years.[21] In these studies, T stage (Ta versus T1) was not a strong predictor for recurrence, but it is likely, as shown by Kurth et al., that T stage does predict risk of progression.

Intra-vesical therapy: Chemotherapy

Intra-vesical therapy can be given in the prophylactic, or adjuvant, setting, where it is intended to prevent recurrence after endoscopic resection of all visible tumors, or as definitive therapy where it is designed to treat unresectable papillary tumors, or CIS. The advantages of the intra-vesical route are that high concentrations of agent are in contact with tumor-bearing mucosa or bladder epithelium at risk with little or no systemic toxicity. Disadvantages include the local side effects in the bladder due to high local drug concentrations and the need for transurethral manipulation. A variety of drugs of similar efficacy and toxicity have been tested but mitomycin-C is most commonly used currently.

Most randomized trials show adjuvant treatment following TUR results in decreased recurrence rate or prolonged disease-free interval.[24] A meta-analysis[25] has confirmed the favorable impact on disease-free interval in these patients. However, no long-term benefit could be demonstrated in terms of increasing time to progression to invasive disease, duration of survival, or progression-free survival.

The benefit of early versus more delayed chemotherapy as well as short (sometimes single-instillation) chemotherapy versus long-term adjuvant therapy has also been studied. Three trials investigating a single instillation of mitomycin-C (MMC) (40 mg in 40 mL saline) or epirubicin (80 mg in 40 mL saline) given within 24 hours of TUR demonstrated[26] a 40–50% reduction of risk of recurrence compared with TUR alone. This treatment has minimal toxicity and, as even the best prognostic groups have a 30% risk of recurrence, these results suggest that a single instillation of mitomycin-C (or epirubicin) may be advantageous at diagnosis. However, the potentially devastating complication of extravasation of chemotherapeutic agent through an undetected bladder perforation contraindicates its use in those who have undergone deep resection or who have continued heavy hematuria postoperatively.

Trials comparing single and more prolonged treatments suggest that additional benefit may be gained by repeated instillation of intra-vesical chemotherapy, although the majority of the benefit is gained from an early postoperative treatment. Such treatment is therefore advised for patients at high risk of recurrence at presentation or first cystoscopy (Table 13.2), patients with

multiple tumors, or frequently relapsing patients. A number of different regimes have been investigated, but there is little clear evidence that one regime is superior to another, and a common pragmatic regime is to treat with mitomycin-C (40 mg in 40 mL saline) weekly for 6 weeks (side effects allowing).[27]

One potential problem with mitomycin-C is variable drug delivery. Decreasing urine volume (by pre-treatment dehydration and reducing administration volume) and urine alkalinization has been shown to result in a longer time to recurrence and recurrence-free fraction.[28] An alternative technique, electromotive drug delivery, is to externally apply a potential difference across the bladder wall by a pulsed electric current. This has been reported to improve drug absorption and increase time to recurrence in one small randomized trial.[29] Likewise, improved results have been reported for combining mitomycin with hyperthermia[30,31,32] either by heating the bladder with microwave probes or by preheating the mitomycin-C.

Intra-vesical Bacillus Calmette–Guérin (BCG) in low-grade NMIBC can also reduce the risk of recurrence versus TURBT alone, but seems no more effective that MMC at preventing recurrence in lower-risk disease.[33] However, when maintenance BCG is used[34] it may reduce progression risk. As the majority of this patient group have a low risk for progression and recurrence, it would seem reasonable to use intra-vesical chemotherapy as first-line treatment and reserve BCG (with its higher toxicity) for patients with poor-risk disease and a high risk of progression (including high grade and CIS), or for chemotherapy failures.

High-grade non-muscle invasive bladder cancer

High-grade NMIBC and CIS have high rates of progression if untreated, for instance a third of T1 tumors progress to muscle invasive disease within 3 years. A proposed management pathway is shown in Figure 13.3.

CIS may not be visible endoscopically, and even if lesions are seen, ill-defined disease margins make complete resection difficult. This, in association with the frequency of concomitant invasive carcinoma and high risk of progression to invasive disease described above, has resulted in a historical preference for cystectomy for patients with high-grade NMIBC. However, the results of immediate cystectomy are not superior to those of cystectomy performed after failure of intra-vesical treatment[35] which has led to a more widespread adoption of an organ-preserving approach.

Intra-vesical therapy for carcinoma *in situ* is attractive as close contact between agent and the tumor can be achieved. Bacillus Calmette–Guérin is an active intra-vesical immunotherapy agent for bladder cancer, although its precise mechanism of action is not well-understood. It is likely that BCG activates dendritic cells

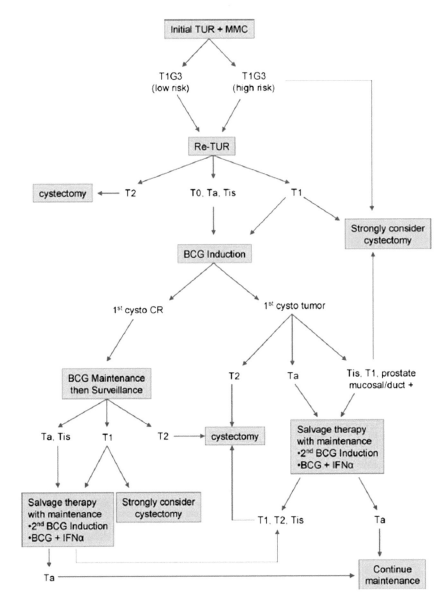

FIGURE 13.3 Treatment algorithm for high-grade T1 G3 disease; management decisions are outlined in boxes. BCG Bacillus Calmette–Guérin, MMC mitomycin-C, TUR transurethral resection, INF-α interferon alpha. (Reproduced with permission from Kulkarni et al., 2010.)

(DCs) in a non-specific manner and that potent anti-tumor Th1 responses are generated. A significant reduction in tumor recurrence and progression is noted in most prospective controlled studies comparing BCG with TUR alone.[33] A meta-analysis of these studies shows that, compared to intra-vesical treatment, BCG improves complete response rate (68% versus 51.5%) and long-term control (46.7% versus 26.2%, odds ratio 0.41, $p <$ 0.0001). Patients on BCG with maintenance had an OR of 0.57 (p = 0.04) for progression.[36]

Primary CIS (no previous TCC), secondary CIS (occurring after previous TCC), and concurrent CIS (associated with superficial TCC) respond similarly to BCG treatment, and today BCG is recommended as first-line therapy for this disease.

Initial induction therapy usually consists of once-weekly instillations for 6 weeks with subsequent maintenance therapy usually consisting of repeated 3-week courses at 3 months, 6 months, and 6 monthly for 3 years; this generally has greater effect on disease

progression in the meta-analyses compared to induction BCG alone.[34,36] This is now regarded as the optimal schedule for BCG. It has to be accepted that this is at the cost of significantly increased toxicity which often results in early cessation of treatment.

The alternative is to repeat the 6-week course at time of treatment failure, as tested by Catalona et al.[37]

BCG produces a profound inflammatory reaction in bladder mucosa and results in more pronounced local toxicity than chemotherapy. Serious systemic symptoms are uncommon but do occur, and as many as 25% of patients have an influenza-like syndrome lasting between 12 and 24 hours after installation. Those patients suspected of contracting systemic tuberculosis are usually successfully treated with anti-tuberculous therapy. However, following intra-vesical treatment, a number of deaths have been reported related to bladder trauma, either secondary to traumatic instillation or when the instillation has occurred immediately after TURBT. The use of prophylactic isoniazid prior to BCG treatment has shown no benefit in terms of local or systemic side effects.[38] The use of BCG is contraindicated in immunocompromised patients such as those with HIV infection, patients undergoing immunosuppressive therapy, patients with coexistent malignancy such as leukemia or Hodgkin disease, and pregnant or lactating women.[39]

Intra-vesical BCG produces high and durable response rates in CIS; however 25% of patients fail to respond to first-line treatment, whilst a further 25% achieving a complete response with initial induction therapy relapse within 5 years. Overall, only 31% of patients treated with BCG for CIS remain tumor-free at 10 years.[36] A considerable proportion of the failure is related to extra-vesical progression of disease, either to the lower ureters or prostatic urethra. In the literature, reports of prostatic urethral involvement after BCG range from 1.5% to 6.3%, which is lower than that for chemotherapy (33–37%).[40]

The treatment of refractory CIS that incompletely responds or recurs after BCG is debatable. Generally, immediate cystectomy is considered the treatment of choice, especially when CIS is associated with high-grade disease (T1G3). However, many patients with relatively asymptomatic CIS may prefer to retain normal bladder function even after relapse following BCG; the fact that progression usually occurs after 2 years means that in many cases a trial of second-line therapy is reasonable. Reports suggest that up to 25% of patients respond to a second course of BCG, especially if maintenance has not been used.[37] The addition of interferon to BCG, techniques to improve intra-vesical drug delivery such as electromotive mitomycin-C and intra-vesical hyperthermia/chemotherapy, new intra-vesical agents such as gemcitabine, and photodynamic therapy are all being tested in this setting.[41]

Radiotherapy and systemic treatments for superficial disease

Radiotherapy is usually considered ineffective in superficial disease; although it is effective in eradicating the primary, it has little impact on preventing recurrence. However, there has been some experience with T1G3 disease. Rodel et al. treated 74 patients with T1G3 tumors with radiotherapy ± concomitant chemotherapy (median dose 54 Gy, 45–60 Gy).[42] A complete remission at restaging was achieved in 83.7%, 47% remained disease-free, with 77% of surviving patients retaining their bladder at 5 years. Its role in this context has been tested in a randomized MRC trial in which radiotherapy was compared to TUR alone (solitary disease) or BCG (multiple tumors).[43] This study showed no advantage for radiotherapy (hazard ratio 1.16 [in favor of control], 95% CI 0.7–1.92, $p = 0.552$). It would suggest that radiotherapy should not be used routinely for T1G3 disease but may be an alternative for those who have failed other conservative treatments and are unable to undergo cystectomy.

As intra-vesical treatment is an attractive alternative for superficial disease, little exploration of systemic therapies in the prevention of recurrence has been undertaken. Small studies of retinoids and high-dose vitamins, including vitamin A, have shown reduction in recurrence,[44] but concerns about overall efficacy and toxicity have meant they are rarely used.

COX2 over-expression has been associated with bladder cancer, and the use of the COX2 inhibitor, Celecoxib, has been tested in a UK randomized trial (BOXIT trial). This study showed Celecoxib improved time to recurrence of pT1G3 tumors but did not improve overall recurrence, progression rates, or overall survival. As there were more cardiovascular events in the Celecoxib arm this approach isn't recommended.[45] Recently, the development of immune check point inhibitors in metastatic bladder cancer has led them to be studied in BCG refractory muscle invasive disease. A number of studies have been launched but definitive results are awaited. The current guidelines for the treatment of patients with superficial bladder cancer are outlined in Table 13.3.

Management of invasive bladder cancer

Prognostic factors

Stage and grade remain the most important prognostic factors for invasive disease, with the presence of extra-vesical extension[46] and lymph-node positivity[47] having the greatest impact on survival. The extent of lymph-node involvement is also of prognostic significance, with survival decreasing with increasing number of positive nodes.[47]

A number of potential biological prognostic markers have also been investigated in invasive bladder cancer; however none to date has made it to routine use. Evaluation of this area has been inhibited by a general lack of robust prospective evaluation in large groups of patients.

Neoadjuvant chemotherapy

Neoadjuvant chemotherapy aims to treat micrometastatic disease present at the time of initial diagnosis. The largest trial of neoadjuvant combination chemotherapy has been the EORTC/MRC study of three cycles of cisplatin, methotrexate, and vinblastine (CMV) followed by either radical radiotherapy or cystectomy; 976 patients were randomized. An updated analysis[48] with median follow-up of 7 years has shown that neoadjuvant chemotherapy was associated with improvement in metastasis-free survival (54% versus 45%, $p = 0.002$) and in overall survival (56.5% versus 50.0%, $p = 0.03$).

The phase III Intergroup Trial in the USA evaluated three cycles of neoadjuvant M-VAC chemotherapy.[49] Three hundred and seven patients were randomized to cystectomy alone or cystectomy after neoadjuvant M-VAC. Thirty-eight percent of patients on the chemotherapy arm had no residual disease in the cystectomy specimen (15% if no chemotherapy was given). The median survival for patients receiving chemotherapy was longer, at 77 months compared with 46 months, which was statistically significant on unstratified two-sided log rank analysis ($p = 0.05$) and of borderline significance after stratifying for age and tumor stage ($p = 0.06$). This equated to a disease-specific hazard ratio of 1.66 (95% CI 1.22–2.45, $p = 0.002$).

The international data on neoadjuvant chemotherapy were included in an individual patient data meta-analysis (Figure 13.4). This confirmed that multi-agent chemotherapy reduced the risk of death by about 13% (hazard ratio 0.87, 95% CI 0.78–0.97, $p = 0.016$), equating to a 5% absolute improvement in survival at 5 years, and for platinum-based combination chemotherapy there was a significant disease-free survival benefit of 9%.[50]

On the basis of these data most guidelines recommend this treatment should be offered to eligible patients[13] (www.nice.org.uk/guidance/ng2).[51]

Adjuvant chemotherapy

Advocates of adjuvant chemotherapy indicate the benefits of immediate definitive therapy of the known localized disease

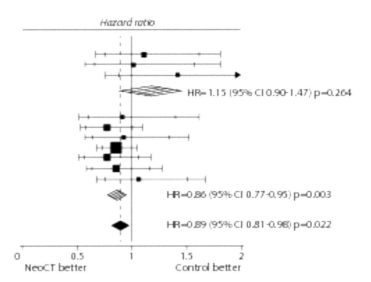

| | (no. events/no. entered) | | | |
	CT	Control	O-E	Variance
Single agent platinum				
Wallace [2]	50/83	50/76	2.74	27.18
Martinez-Pineiro [3]	43/62	38/59	0.33	20.11
Raghavan [2]	34/41	37/55	5.85	16.51
Sub-total	136/186	125/190	8.92	63.80
Platinum-based combinations				
Cortesi unpublished	43/82	41/71	-1.87	20.84
Grossman [9]	98/158	106/159	-13.61	51.00
Bassi [5]	53/102	60/104	-1.95	28.13
MRC/EORTC [6]	275/491	301/485	-23.69	143.61
Malmstrom [8]	68/151	84/160	-0.97	37.94
Sherif [8]	79/158	90/159	-6.37	42.18
Sengelev [7]	70/78	60/75	1.79	31.96
Sub-total	686/1220	744/1213	-55.67	355.65
Total	822/1406	869/1403	-46.75	419.45

HR= 1.15 (95% CI 0.90-1.47) p=0.264

HR=0.86 (95% CI 0.77-0.95) p=0.003

HR=0.89 (95% CI 0.81-0.98) p=0.022

NeoCT better — Control better

FIGURE 13.4 Meta-analysis of randomized trials of neoadjuvant chemotherapy in bladder carcinoma. HR plot for overall survival: Each trial is represented by a square, the center of which gives the HR for that trial; size of the square is proportional to the information; ends of horizontal bars denote the 99% CI, and inner bars mark the 95% CI; the shaded diamonds denote the HRs for the trial groups. CT, chemotherapy; O-E, observed minus expected events. (Reproduced from Advanced Bladder Cancer (ABC), 2005. With permission.)

and, in the setting of cystectomy, the ability to stage accurately and thus judge the indication for chemotherapy more precisely. Unfortunately,[52] most trials have been underpowered often due to recurrent issues of recruitment after cystectomy for a number of reasons and some have used questionable techniques of analysis. The largest adjuvant trial was performed by the EORTC. Despite failing to meet recruitment targets, it randomized 284 patients to either immediate or deferred (gemcitabine/cisplatin or MVAC) chemotherapy. Immediate chemotherapy improved progression-free survival (HR 0.54, 95% CI 0.4–0.73, $p < 0.0001$), but failed to confirm an overall survival benefit even though there was a trend towards improvement (adjusted HR 0.78, 95% CI 0.56–1.08; $p =$ 0.13).[52] These results are similar to what was reported in an earlier meta-analysis of older adjuvant trials[50] that showed an absolute reduction of risk of death of 11% at 3 years for trials using cisplatin-based combination chemotherapy. Though we can't be entirely certain the evidence generally supports adjuvant treatment being offered to patients who either cannot have neoadjuvant chemotherapy or who have had cystectomy for non-muscle invasive disease and are upstaged but should not replace neoadjuvant therapy.

Surgical treatment

Radical cystectomy remains the treatment associated with highest local cure, with pelvic recurrence rates of less than 10% in node-negative tumors and 10–20% in patients with resected pelvic nodal metastases.[53] A review comparing outcomes of surgery in National Cancer Institute (NCI) cancer centers ($n = 2,977$) with those in other American hospitals ($n = 2,566$) included patients over 65 years of age on the Medicare database treated for cancer by cystectomy in cancer centers between 1994 and 1999.[54] As illustrated in Figure 13.5a, there was no significant difference between the two hospital groups, with 5-year survival of approximately 38%. In the past, cystectomy was associated with significant morbidity and high mortality, but improvements

in operative technique have seen the perioperative complication rate fall from approximately 35% prior to 1970 to less than 10% reported currently. In the UK, combined with centralization surgery this has resulted in a fall in operative mortality from nearly 20% to 3% and improvement in 5-year survivals (Figure 13.5b).[54,55]

Radical cystectomy involves en-bloc removal of bladder, prostate, and seminal vesicles in the male, or bladder, urethra, uterus, cervix, fallopian tubes, ovaries, and anterior vaginal wall in the female with surrounding perivesical fat, pelvic visceral peritoneum, and lymph nodes. Following cystectomy, the urine is most commonly diverted into an incontinent stoma via an ileal conduit, and formation of a uretero-ileal anastomosis. This is associated with a lower incidence of long-term metabolic disturbance and renal deterioration than its predecessor, the ureterosigmoidostomy. However, it is associated with significant physical and psychological morbidity and is therefore being superseded by continent diversions or orthotopic bladder substitutes.

The continent urinary diversion is an intra-abdominal urinary reservoir, which is catheterizable or has an outlet controlled by the anal sphincter. The reservoir is usually fashioned from stomach, ileum, or part of the large bowel, with formation of some form of mechanism to prevent reflux of urine to the kidneys. Probably the best studied ileal continent diversion is the Kock pouch.[56]

This technique has been adapted for use as an orthotopic bladder substitute.[57] Here, a bladder is constructed using loops of ileum and re-anastomosed onto the urethra. The drawback of this approach is the longer operating time, with high complication and re-operation rates and a high incidence of urinary incontinence. This, in combination with the age and performance status of the average bladder cancer patient, means that this procedure is only suitable in a minority of cases. It has been suggested that orthotopic bladder substitutes have a higher risk of chronic renal damage than an ileal conduit.[58]

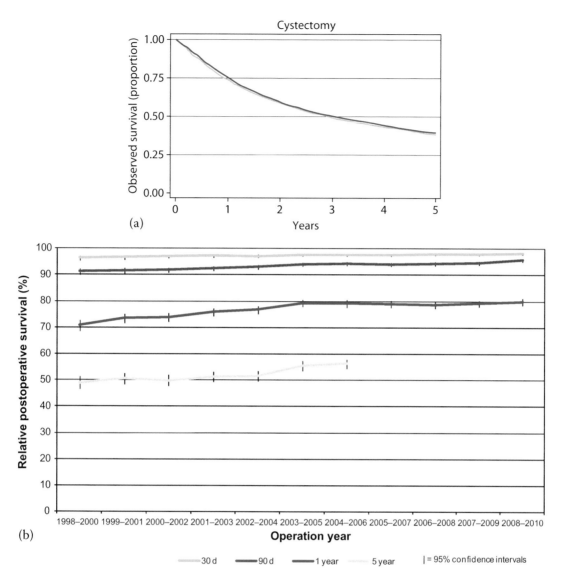

FIGURE 13.5 (a) Survival following cystectomy in NCI and non-NCI surgical centers in the USA, 1994–1991 (reproduced from Birkmeyer et al., 2005 ref 54 with permission); (b) trends in overall survival after radical cystectomy outcomes in UK from 1998 to 2010. (Reproduced from Hounsome et al., 2015. With permission.)

More recently minimally invasive techniques have been introduced which may reduce peri-operative morbidity but as yet to date have not been clearly proven to improve outcomes over open surgery.[59]

Other technical developments include the development of a nerve-sparing technique in the male, which has resulted in the preservation of sexual potency,[60] and the urethra-sparing procedure in the female.[61] By using a selective approach to urethrectomy, continence should be possible with an orthotopic bladder replacement, provided meticulous follow-up is employed to ensure the early detection of recurrence. However, urethral preservation should be avoided in patients with multiple papillary tumors, tumors involving the bladder neck or posterior urethra, and in the presence of CIS.

Bladder-preserving surgery results in the retention of physiological bladder function, continence, potency, and the ability to sample regional pelvic lymph nodes. Partial cystectomy alone is only suitable for a minority of patients with invasive bladder cancer. Suitable patients have a solitary muscle-invasive primary

that is amenable to complete excision and biopsy, proven absence of cellular atypia, or CIS, in the remaining bladder. High recurrence rates (38–78%) have been reported in unselected cases,[62] but 5-year survival figures comparable to those of contemporary series of radical cystectomy can be achieved in carefully selected patients.[62]

Bladder preservation rates of 53–77% with an overall survival of approximately 80% have been reported following radical TUR alone. However, these were small studies in highly selected patients.[63] The primary should be solitary and organ confined, with a maximum diameter of 2–3 cm at the base and located at a fixed portion of the bladder. The completeness should be confirmed by repeat TUR with biopsy and cytology. Though long-term control rates can be achieved, it is probably best to reserve such approaches, if possible supported by the use of chemotherapy[64] and/or radiotherapy in combination with radical TUR, for patients who are not fit enough or who are unable to have local radical treatment. This is discussed below.

Radiotherapy in the management of muscle-invasive bladder cancer

Radiotherapy has been used in the successful treatment of bladder cancer, for many years, to achieve bladder preservation. The lack of well-executed trials comparing radical radiotherapy to cystectomy has limited its uptake. Comparisons between institutional studies and non-randomized data have consistently shown a higher local control rate for cystectomy and have led to fears of disease progression prior to salvage surgery, with a possible compromise in survival. However, when the effects of selection bias (e.g. fitter patients being selected for surgery), stage migration due to clinical versus pathological staging, and differences in prognostic factors between patients selected for radiotherapy or surgery are taken into consideration, there is little evidence from the current data that overall survival is compromised when these factors are taken into account.[65] Ideally the two modalities should be compared in a randomized controlled trial. To date these have been unsuccessful due to patient and physician choice making randomization of patients very difficult. The latest such trial (SPARE trial) closed due to poor recruitment and is unlikely to be repeated in the near future. The small numbers recruited and protocol violations make this trial difficult to interpret but despite a higher local recurrence rate in the radiotherapy arm there is no obvious survival difference.[66]

If relapse does occur after radiotherapy, the patient will require surgery in addition to radiotherapy, and this post-radiation cystectomy is a more difficult operation and associated with greater morbidity with little possibility of reconstructive surgery. All patients undergoing attempted bladder-preserving treatment should be counselled accordingly before commencing treatment. Despite these problems, the improved results seen with concomitant chemotherapy, development of image guidance, and the use of selective bladder preservation are likely to lead to the more widespread use of radiotherapy.

Case selection for radiotherapy

In deciding to attempt bladder preservation using radiotherapy, case selection is required as there are several situations in which primary cystectomy may be preferred. This is clearly the case where pelvic radiotherapy is contraindicated (e.g. inflammatory bowel disease, previous radiotherapy). Patients whose disease has resulted in irretrievable loss of bladder function will gain little benefit from bladder preservation. Radiotherapy does not improve incontinence or the capacity of a bladder damaged by previous interventions, and will exacerbate symptoms arising from a severely irritable bladder.

Finally, patients whose pattern of disease suggests a lower possibility of control with radiotherapy alone should be considered for surgery. These include those who have undergone multiple resections for or multiple courses of chemotherapy/BCG or resection for recurrent superficial tumors, patients with diffuse malignant involvement, large tumors with extra-vesical masses >5 cm, and tumors of squamous or adenocarcinoma histology. There are conflicting views as to the influence of coexistent CIS to local tumor control following radiotherapy.[67]

Selective bladder preservation

An approach to seeking the advantages of bladder preservation with the efficacy of cystectomy has been to select for preservation using the criterion of initial response, an important indication of prognosis. When survival data from 125 patients treated with neoadjuvant chemotherapy and cystectomy were analyzed, 91% of down-staged patients survived, as opposed to only 37% of those with persisting muscle-invasive disease.[68] This approach was developed by Shipley and colleagues whose protocol required complete TUR followed by neoadjuvant and concomitant platinum chemo-radiation to a limited dose. At this time, cystoscopic reassessment is undertaken and patients in remission are selected for complete radiotherapy and organ conservation, whereas those with persisting tumors have cystectomy. In a series of 348 patients over 70% were able to retain their bladders with good urinary function and survival similar to that seen in cystectomy series.[69] The response to neoadjuvant chemotherapy has also been assessed as a predictive marker. In a series at the Royal Marsden 78/89[70] patients were judged to be responders and received radiotherapy of whom 82% attained bladder preservation at last follow-up. Patients who achieved durable response had a median survival of 90 months (95% CI 64.7, 115.9) compared with 16 months (95% CI 5.4, 27.4; $p < 0.001$) in poor responders. The overall conclusion of this study is that chemotherapy response may be prognostic rather than predictive.

An alternative approach would be to have a genetic or imaging biomarker to predict which patients would do well or otherwise on radiotherapy treatment. There has been interest in expression of DNA repair markers and in particular MRE11. A study of MRE11 in patients treated by radiotherapy or cystectomy showed that patients with high MRE11 expression had better outcomes after radiotherapy than both patients with low expression and those treated by surgery.[71] Low MRE11 expressors had better outcomes from surgical treatment. In this study MRE11 behaved as a predictive factor but validation to date has not been possible.[72]

Preoperative and adjuvant radiotherapy

Preoperative radiotherapy prior to cystectomy could prevent the intra-operative seeding of tumor cells and sterilize microscopic tumor deposits. Retrospective studies have suggested a benefit for preoperative radiotherapy over cystectomy alone. Data from the few small randomized trials conducted suggest a possible benefit[73] but it is probably best to conclude that the case for preoperative radiotherapy is not proven.

Examination of postoperative treatment has been hindered by concerns over a high risk of bowel toxicity.[74] Interest in this area has been sparked by the advent of intensity-modulated treatment which makes radiotherapy more viable and appreciation of the risk of isolated pelvic recurrence in patients with pT3 and/or node-positive disease.[75,76] The RTOG has provided guidelines for administration of therapy which has facilitated delivery of postoperative treatment.[77] A small randomized trial from Egypt has also reported a significant 25% improvement in local relapse-free survival (HR, 0.08; 95% CI, 0.02–0.39; $p < 0.01$) and an 11% (HR, 0.61; 95% CI, 0.33–1.11; $p = 0.11$) increase in survival compared to patients receiving adjuvant chemotherapy alone.[78] Additional randomized trials are underway.

Radiotherapy technique

Standard radiotherapy techniques utilize CT-scan-associated planning to visualize the bladder. The target volume comprises the empty bladder (to minimize the irradiated volume) and any extra-vesical disease with a 1.5–2 cm margin (to allow for microscopic disease and organ movement). In most instances, an anterior and two lateral treatment fields encompass this. Whether to include the pelvis is debated as it adds to treatment toxicity without any clear evidence for improved pelvic control.[79]

Studies comparing the CT-planned target volume before and during radiotherapy demonstrate that changes in position and shape of target volume are common and lead to geographical misses despite the use of substantial margins.[80,81]

Recently development of the use of fiducial markers and in particular online soft tissue imaging such as cone beam CT means that daily assessment of bladder position can be made and errors corrected. The UK's National Radiotherapy imaging group now recommend the imaging of soft tissue to ensure the bladder is adequately covered. It is also recognized that for some patients the large margins used in an attempt to cover variation can lead to excessive normal tissue irradiation. This has led a number of investigators to investigate "adaptive" radiotherapy. Most commonly an approach termed "plan of the day" has been explored. A series of plans of varying sizes are designed before treatment and the best fitting plan is selected each day by using online imaging. The number of plans and how they are defined have varied between studies, but this approach consistently improves coverage and reduces volumes irradiated.[82] Phase II data are promising, but prospective studies are required to confirm this increased complexity delivers better results.

The predominant acute symptoms are radiation cystitis associated with urinary frequency, urgency and dysuria, proctitis, and lethargy. In the long term, bladder function may deteriorate as a result of organ shrinkage related to fibrosis. Superficial telangiectasia in the bladder may give rise to hematuria, and late bowel damage may result in bleeding, which may occasionally be profound and require operative intervention. Impotence may also occur, although the precise incidence is not well-documented.

There is a clear dose–effect relationship for radiotherapy,[83,84] so on this basis, doses in the region of 64 Gy in 2-Gy fractions are used at the Royal Marsden. Elsewhere in the UK, shorter fractionation schemes, such as 55 Gy in 20 fractions, are used, which, although not tested against standard fractionation schedules, are thought to be of equivalent efficacy. The results of radical radiotherapy at the Royal Marsden Hospital are shown in Figure 13.6 in terms of survival according to stage and lymphnode status.

Significant proportions of patients are too frail or old to tolerate a standard course of radiotherapy and in such patients local control can be achieved by using weekly 6-Gy fractions to 30–36 Gy.[85] This regime appears well-tolerated, with acceptable levels of late toxicity. This sort of schema can also be useful for the control of local symptoms in patients with metastatic disease. A similar regime of 21 Gy in 3 fractions in 1 week has been tested in this setting and 35 Gy in 10 fractions in a multicenter MRC trial of 500 patients. The results demonstrated no difference in efficacy, toxicity, or survival between the two arms.[86]

Prognostic factors for local control after radiotherapy treatment

A favorable response to radiotherapy may be expected in small-volume T2 (rather than T3/4 patients), in the absence of ureteral obstruction[87] in papillary rather than sessile tumors[87] with normal hemoglobin levels above 13 g[88] and following a good response to the first 40 Gy of radical radiotherapy.[69] De-bulking of the tumor prior to radiotherapy also improves local control; however, it is unclear if the benefits of debulking could be partly attributed to case selection (i.e. tumors are small enough to be de-bulked) rather than to the surgery itself.

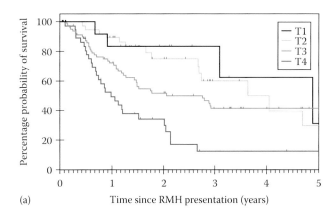

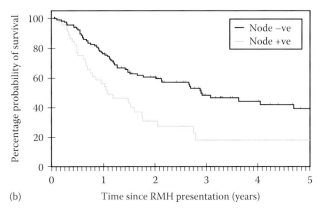

FIGURE 13.6 Results of radiotherapy at the Royal Marsden hospital according to: (a) T stage; (b) nodal status.

Improving the results of radical radiotherapy

Altered fractionation

Following the observation that treatment breaks are associated with impaired outcome and that bladder cancer has a short potential doubling time, accelerated fractionation (AF) has been explored. However, a randomized trial of 60.8 Gy in 32 fractions over 4 weeks treating twice daily versus a standard treatment of 64 Gy in 32 daily fractions over 6.5 weeks has failed to show survival benefit from AF[89] and late radiation toxicity equivalent to RTOG grade 2 was greater in AF patients. Thus, it was considered that CF should remain the standard of care.

Modifying hypoxia

Radiation resistance may be related to tumor hypoxia. Historical data suggest that reversal of this using hyperbaric oxygen can improve local control.[88] The use of carbogen (95% O_2, 5% CO_2) in combination with nicotinamide to improve tumor oxygenation has been tested in a randomized trial of 333 patients. Though there was no significant difference in the primary endpoint (6-month cystoscopic control) there was a trend to improve relapse-free survival for patients receiving CON and RT (54% for RT+CON versus 43% for RT alone [$p = 0.06$]) and significant improvement in three-year estimates of overall survival (59% RT +CON versus 46% for RT alone [$p = 0.04$]).[90] The benefit was predominantly seen in patients with necrosis on histological examination or having a hypoxia gene signature.[91,92]

Radiation dose escalation

Increased radiation dose could improve local control, but the challenge is to maintain acceptable local morbidity. Interstitial radiotherapy has been used to achieve this, most frequently in combination with TUR and low-dose external-beam radiotherapy (usually up to 30 Gy).[93] Impressive local control rates in excess of 80% are reported, with acceptable toxicity levels, although the impact of case selection on these results is difficult to assess.[94] The need for the surgical placement of the implant has restricted its use to a few specialist centers.

The dose of external-beam radiotherapy is limited by the tolerance of normal tissues, and in the bladder retrospective data suggest that radiation tolerance is a function of the volume irradiated; the tolerance of part of the bladder is greater than that of the whole bladder. Though two prospective studies[95] have been unable to demonstrate reduced toxicity. Both studies pre-date adaptive/image-guided radiotherapy treatment and use large margins. Dose escalation phase I–II studies have shown that using adaptive radiotherapy, a tumor boost approach dose of 68–70 Gy in 32 fractions can be applied without excessive toxicity and excellent local control.[96,97] This approach is being tested in an international randomized phase II trial RAIDER

Concurrent chemotherapy and radiotherapy

To improve the therapeutic ratio of radiotherapy, concurrent chemotherapy has been investigated as a radiosensitizer. A large number of phase II studies have been performed, the majority utilizing cisplatin alone or in combination with 5-fluorouracil (5-FU), which have demonstrated high complete responses, with bladder preservation in more than 60% of patients. Two randomized trials have been performed. The National Cancer Institute of Canada[98] randomized 99 patients to receive or not receive cisplatin 100 mg/m² every 2 weeks during radiotherapy. Despite the lack of power of this small study, it demonstrated improved recurrence-free survival for the chemotherapy group and a non-significant trend to improved overall survival. The absolute difference in pelvic relapse-free survival was 20% ($p = 0.038$). Cisplatin is not necessarily the ideal agent in this group of patients, who are often elderly and have renal impairment. The BC2001 trial tested a non-cisplatin regimen, randomizing 360 patients to infusional 5 FU 500 mg/m² given in the first and fourth week of radiotherapy and mitomycin-C 12 mg/m² on day 1 versus radiotherapy alone.[99] Patients were treated with 64 Gy in 32 fractions or 55 Gy in 20 fractions. After median follow-up of 69 months, patients receiving concomitant chemotherapy had a significantly improved survival without pelvic disease progression (chemoradiotherapy 67% (95% confidence interval [CI], 59 to 74); radiotherapy alone 54% (95% CI, 46 to 62) (hazard ratio 0.68; 95% CI, 0.48 to 0.96; $p = 0.03$), largely due to reduction in invasive recurrences (hazard ratio, 0.57; 95% CI, 0.37 to 0.90; $p = 0.01$)) (Figure 13.7). Five-year rates of overall survival were 48% (95% CI, 40 to 55) in the chemoradiotherapy group and 35% (95% CI, 28 to 43) in the radiotherapy group (hazard ratio, 0.82; 95% CI, 0.63 to 1.09; $p = 0.16$). The benefit in local control was seen equally for patients receiving both radiotherapy fractionations and was also beneficial for the 25% of patients who received neoadjuvant chemotherapy. Concomitant chemotherapy was associated with some increase in acute bowel toxicity but no increase in late toxicity.

Low-dose gemcitabine has also been tested in a number of non-randomized studies. A recent overview of 8 studies reported a complete response rate of 93% with <20% reporting a bladder recurrence and a 93% 5-year cystectomy-free survival rate.[100]

Based on these data concomitant chemotherapy (or hypoxic sensitization) is recommended to be used when radical bladder radiotherapy is being used.

Recommended management pathways for locally advanced non-metastatic muscle invasive bladder cancer are shown in Figure 13.8.

Management of advanced disease

Despite the recognized chemo-sensitivity and radio-sensitivity of TCC of the bladder, more than 5,000 deaths are attributable to

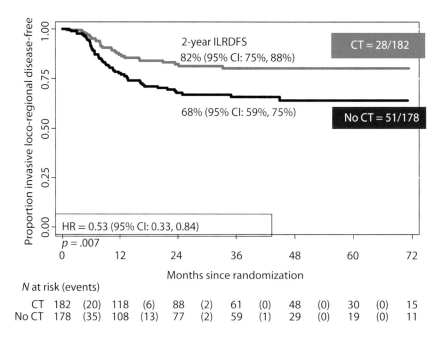

FIGURE 13.7 Invasive local recurrence-free survival (ILRDFS) in BC2001 trial comparing radiotherapy alone versus radiotherapy and concomitant 5-Fluoro-uracil/mitomycin chemotherapy. (Modified from James et al., 2012. With permission.)

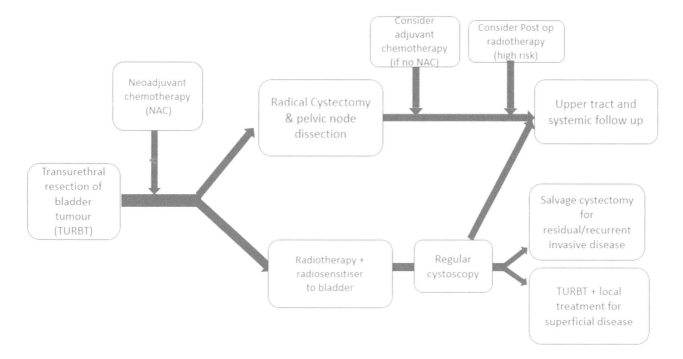

FIGURE 13.8 Proposed management pathway for locally advanced non-metastatic muscle invasive bladder cancer.

the disease in the UK each year. Approximately 50% of patients with muscle invasion ultimately succumb to metastatic disease. The commonest sites of metastasis include the regional lymph nodes, bone, lung, skin, and liver, and, less frequently, brain and meninges and the organs within the peritoneal cavity. The distribution of metastasis is important when considering treatment, as the site(s) of involvement correlate with prognosis, with improved survival in those with disease confined to the lymph nodes or skin, and with a substantially worse prognosis with liver and bone metastases.[89] Consideration of these factors and other prognostic factors, especially performance status,[101] is important when comparing the results of clinical trials in this setting.

Chemotherapy

Until recently systemic chemotherapy has been the mainstay for patients with metastatic disease. Single-agent chemotherapy yields objective responses of the order of 15–20%, with complete responses of 5–10% but with limited response duration of only 4–6 months. The most active agents in these historical studies included cisplatin, doxorubicin, mitomycin-C, and methotrexate and then the vinca alkaloids and 5-FU and more recently gemcitabine and taxanes.

The development of multi-drug combinations increased response rates and survival. MVAC and CMV regimes[102] incorporate methotrexate, vinblastine, and cisplatin (with or without doxorubicin), described in Table 13.5. Both attain high response rates, including a significant complete response rate. Typically in an average patient population response rates of 40–50% with a 10% complete response rate were more common.[103] These schedules improve median survival of patients with metastatic urothelial cancer from around 3–6 months, to around 9–12 months with treatment.[102,104,105] Though not tested against best supportive care, there is improved survival compared to single-agent or less intensive schedules.[104,105] Toxicities include significant rates of mucositis (40%), renal toxicity (31%), and neutropenic sepsis

TABLE 13.5 Summary of the Chemotherapy Regimes Used in the Treatment of Muscle Invasive Bladder Cancer

CMV	Methotrexate 40 mg/m^2 days 1 and 8
	Vinblastine 5 mg/m^2 days 1 and 8
	Cisplatin 100 mg/m^2 day 2
	Cycle repeated every 21 days
MVAC	Methotrexate 30 mg/m^2 days 2, 15, and 22
	Vinblastine 3 mg/m^2 days 2, 15, and 22
	Adriamycin 30 mg/m^2 day 2
	Cisplatin 70 mg/m^2 day 2
	Cycle repeated every 28 days
Accelerated MVAC	Methotrexate 30 mg/m^2 day 1
	Vinblastine 3 mg/m^2 day 1
	Adriamycin 30 mg/m^2 day 1
	Cisplatin 70 mg/m^2 day 1
	GCSF days 4–11
	Cycle repeated every 14 days
GC	Gemcitabine 1,000 mg/m^2 days 1, 8, and 15
	Cisplatin 70 mg/m^2 day 2
	Cycle repeated every 28 days
	Or every 21 days with day 15 gemcitabine omitted

Abbreviation: GCSF, granulocyte colony-stimulating factor.

(20%), with a toxic death rate of 4%.[102] An accelerated MVAC schedule administered on a 2-week cycle supported by granulocyte colony-stimulating factor (GCSF) was shown to achieve more complete responses (21% versus 12%) with some borderline evidence of benefit in long-term survival (24.6% versus 13.2%, borderline statistical significance) in EORTC randomized trial.[106] As there were similar or lower levels of toxicity and treatment is completed more quickly this would be the preferred way to administer MVAC.

Gemcitabine, an analogue of cytosine arabinoside, has also showed significant single-agent and combination response rates. A trial of the gemcitabine/cisplatin doublet (GC) versus MVAC found that survival was similar in both arms (median 14 months for GC and 15 months for MVAC, 5-year survival 13.0% and 15.3% respectively).[107] The better toxicity profile of GC has led to GC being widely adopted as first-line therapy.

Adding paclitaxel to cisplatin/gemcitabine (GCP) achieved a high response rate of 76% in phase II studies. Despite a randomized EORTC trial showing a higher response rate for GCP (57% versus 46%; *p* = 0.02), there was no statistically significant difference in survival (hazard ratio [HR], 0.85; *p* = 0.075)[108] and thus it has not moved into routine practice.

Many patients are either too frail or have inadequate renal function to tolerate cisplatin-based treatment. The cisplatin analogue, carboplatin, in this setting has confirmed activity, but with a tendency for lower efficacy.[109] The best evidence for its use comes from an EORTC randomized trial that compared carboplatin with gemcitabine and carboplatin with methotrexate and vinblastine (M-CAVI) in patients unfit for cisplatin. Gemcitabine and carboplatin were less toxic and had better response rates than M-CAVI (41% versus 30%) though both achieved similar survival rates with median overall survival rates of 9.3 months.[110] It was noteworthy that patients with both impaired renal function and impaired performance status had more severe toxicity, lower response rates, and lower survival than patients entered into the trial with one of the factors, questioning the value of chemotherapy in those patients.

The role of second-line chemotherapy is debated. Patients who respond to first-line therapy and remain of good performance status may achieve reasonable response rates when retreated with the same chemotherapy or an alternative first-line therapy. For instance, in a French report, accelerated MVAC after first-line gemcitabine/platinum achieved response rates of over 50% though at the cost of significant toxicity including treatment deaths.[111] (A number of other combinations such as gemcitabine/paclitaxel and paclitaxel/carboplatin have[112] been tested in phase II studies and have achieved response rates of around 20–30% and median progression-free survival of around 4–6 months.) The only randomized trial in second-line therapy tested the third-generation vinca alkaloid, vinflunine, against best supportive care. Median survival was non-significantly improved from 4.6 months on best supportive care to 6.9 months with vinflunine (HR 0.88 CI 0.69–1.12; *p* = 0.29).[113] This result was significant in the eligible patient population and on this basis is the first treatment licensed for use as second-line treatment. Recent interest has centered on emerging data on antibody conjugated therapy such as enfortumab vedotin which is targeted against nectin-4 that is expressed on most bladder cancers. A phase II trial reported a 44% ORR as third-line therapy.[114]

Immune check points inhibitors

Following initial reports of activity of the PDL1 inhibitor, atezolizumab, in platinum refractory urothelial cancer,[115] this class of drugs has rapidly entered into clinical practice with three agents approved in Europe (atezolizumab, nivolumab, and pembrolizumab) and these three agents plus two others (durvalumab and avelumab) are approved in the US. PD1 is a negative regulator of T effector cells, and these agents block the interaction of PD1 (on T effector cells) and PDL1 (on tumor cells), abrogating the tumor-induced negative effect on T effector cells and thus enabling a better immune response to be mounted against the tumor. Large phase I/II studies of the 5 PD1/PDL1 inhibitors tested to date have confirmed response rates of 15–20% in platinum refractory patients with a trend of patients who have immunohistochemical evidence of PDL1 staining achieving higher response rates.[116]

Median overall survival varies widely across these studies being in the order of 6–12 months. The most remarkable feature has been the long median duration of response in responders and a significant proportion of patients alive 2 years after commencing treatment. Two phase III studies have been reported in this setting. Keynote 045 tested pembrolizumab versus second-line taxane or vinflunine chemotherapy.[117] Pembrolizumab significantly improved median OS compared with those treated with chemotherapy (HR = 0.73; 95% CI 0.59–0.91; *p* = 0.002), from around 7.3 months to around 10.3[118] regardless of PD-L1 expression. ORR was significantly higher in the pembrolizumab group versus the chemotherapy group (*p* = 0.001), and responses in the pembrolizumab group were durable. Overall, treatment-related AEs of any grade and grade ≥3 were more common in the chemotherapy arm. Immune-mediated AEs were observed in 45 (16.9%) patients in the pembrolizumab arm and 19 (7.5%) patients in the chemotherapy arm.[119] A similar study testing atezolizumab was reported as negative in the PDL1 positive cohort that was the primary endpoint but had a similar benefit in an exploratory all-patient intention to treat cohort (HR = 0.85; 95% CI 0.73–0.99; *p* = 0.038).[120]

PD1/PDL1 inhibitors have also been tested in two large phase II studies in the first-line cisplatin-ineligible population. Atezolizumab and pembrolizumab achieved ORR of 23% and 28% respectively and median survivals of 15.9 and 11.3 months in unselected patients.[121] In a PDL1-positive population, pembrolizumab achieved a 47% response rate and a median survival of 18.5 months. These results compare favorably to carboplatin-based chemotherapy. These studies lead to these drugs being licensed for this indication both in Europe and the US, though as yet unpublished data subsequently led to restriction in the license to the biomarker-positive cohort. Development of these agents is a rapidly evolving area with many trials underway testing neoadjuvant, adjuvant, and combinations which are likely to report in the next 1–2 years and perhaps lead to further shifts in the treatment paradigm.

Targeted agents

As identified by the TCGA, a significant proportion of urothelial cancers have mutations that could potentially be targeted. HER2 was targeted in a study of trastuzumab combined with paclitaxel, gemcitabine, and carboplatin which reported a response rate of 70% and median survival of 9 months in patients with HER2-positive tumors, though in this single-arm study it is unclear if this is any better than chemotherapy alone.[122] The UK LAMB study tested maintenance with lapatinib in HER1/HER2-positive tumors, which respond to first-line chemotherapy, but found no evidence of significant benefit.[123]

A number of studies have investigated vascular-targeted agents such as sunitinib and pazopanib as single agents which have low response rates and have proven toxic when used in combination with chemotherapy.[124,125] A UK trial of pazopanib showed it was inferior to weekly paclitaxel in second-line therapy.[126] A phase III study of docetaxel with or without the vascular agent ramucirumab showed the combination could improve progression-free survival at the cost of increased toxicity but didn't improve overall d.[127]

Approximately 15–20% of patients with metastatic urothelial cancer harbor mutations of amplifications in FGFR2 or FGFR3. A molecularly targeted phase II study of the FGFR2/3 inhibitor, erdafitinib, has reported a 40% ORR and median duration of overall survival of 13.8 months in mutation carriers and has now entered phase III testing.[128]

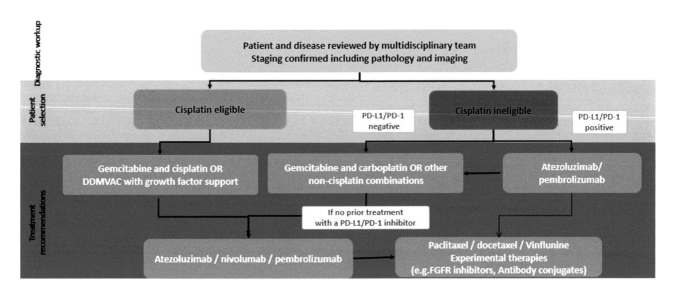

FIGURE 13.9   Proposed management pathway for metastatic muscle invasive bladder cancer.

A current schema for managing metastatic bladder cancer is shown in Figure 13.9.

Radiotherapy and surgery in the palliation of advanced disease

In patients with symptomatic advanced local disease, surgery and radiotherapy may be needed when conservative measures fail. When patients with urinary fistulae/leakage cannot be managed by simple conservative measures such as catheterization, supravesical bladder diversions (and occasionally cystectomy) can be an effective maneuver, particularly in patients of good performance status and reasonable life expectancy, to relieve the problems of bladder irritability and perineal excoriation caused by constant urinary leakage

Palliative radiotherapy may be very effective in controlling the bleeding using hypofractionation.[86,129] Radiotherapy may also provide benefit for those patients with obstructive nephropathy, urinary incontinence, and bone or brain metastases. In all cases the expected benefit of any intervention in the palliative setting must be carefully weighed against its morbidity. Although treatment with surgery and multi-agent chemotherapy may result in excellent palliation for some patients, it must be remembered that this may be at the expense of significant toxicity. Most are too frail, and simple conservative measures or palliative radiotherapy in the setting of multidisciplinary care may be most appropriate.

Future perspectives

After years of relatively little progress in the management of bladder cancer the recent progress has seen significant developments in treatment, and it can be anticipated that further progress will be made in the near future.

Improved surgical, radiotherapy treatments, and treatment approaches in NMIBC have all had an impact, but it is anticipated that future change will be fueled by the advent of systemic immune therapy, improved imaging and biological biomarkers, plus the development and implementation of targeted therapies. A vision for the care of these patients is shown in Figure 13.10.

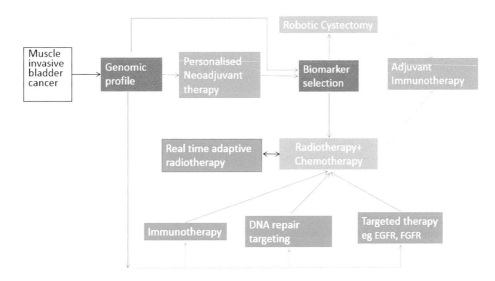

FIGURE 13.10   A vision for the management of MIBC in 2025.

Immune therapies currently are used largely in second-line metastatic disease. It is not unreasonable to expect them to move earlier into treatment as neoadjuvant or adjuvant therapies, either alone or in combinations. A large proportion of bladder cancers have potentially targetable mutations including in tyrosine kinases and DNA repair genes. Along with emerging data on biological predictors of response to neoadjuvant chemotherapy and response to radiotherapy in MIBC it is entirely possible that biological selection of patients to follow individualized pathways may emerge.

Bringing systemic therapies into NMIBC may revolutionize care though there are formidable logistical and ethical concerns to overcome.

The pace of recent change in systemic therapy has been rapid, and there is no sense this will slow. These developments now need testing in well-designed clinical studies.

Key learning points

- Bladder cancer is the fifth commonest cancer in the UK, causing 5,400 deaths per year.
- The risk of developing bladder cancer is increased by exposure to environmental carcinogens (tobacco smoking, aromatic amines), drugs, radiation, and factors leading to chronic irritation of the bladder.
- The majority of bladder cancers present with painless macroscopic hematuria and in the UK are largely transitional-cell carcinoma subtypes.
- Superficial (non-invasive) tumors carry a good prognosis and can usually be controlled by local resections.
- Recurrence of superficial disease is common following local treatment, especially if tumors are multiple or high-grade. Risk of recurrence is reduced by intra-vesical chemotherapy or immunotherapy.
- Invasive disease carries a worse prognosis. Radical cystectomy and radiotherapy (with salvage cystectomy for relapse or persistent disease) are alternative strategies with similar long-term survival outcomes.
- Adding concomitant chemotherapy or carbogen to radiotherapy significantly improves results.
- Neoadjuvant chemotherapy confers a survival benefit of about 5%; further trials are needed to confirm the possible benefit of adjuvant chemotherapy.
- Metastatic disease carries a poor prognosis. Multi-agent platinum-based chemotherapy is useful palliative treatment and carries survival and quality-of-life benefits.
- Check point inhibitors are active in bladder cancer and may add to survival and quality of life.

References

1. Office for National Statistics. Cancer statistics registrations: Registrations of cancer diagnosed in 2001, England. National Statistics: London. 2004; Series MB1(No.32).
2. Anderson, Stephenson J. UKACR comparison of cancer registrations. Bladder Tumours Internal Report. 2004;Report No.3.
3. Coleman M, Babb P, Damiecki P et al. Cancer survival trends in England and Wales 1971–1995 deprivation and NHS Region. The Stationary Office. 1999.
4. Robertson AG, Kim J, Al-Ahmadie H et al. Comprehensive molecular characterization of muscle-invasive bladder cancer. *Cell*. 2017; 171(3):540–56 e25.
5. Choi W, Ochoa A, McConkey DJ et al. Genetic alterations in the molecular subtypes of bladder cancer: Illustration in the cancer genome atlas dataset. *Eur Urol*. 2017; 72(3):354–65.
6. Seiler R, Ashab HAD, Erho N et al. Impact of molecular subtypes in muscle-invasive bladder cancer on predicting response and survival after neoadjuvant chemotherapy. *Eur Urol*. 2017; 72(4):544–54.
7. Blick CG, Nazir SA, Mallett S et al. Evaluation of diagnostic strategies for bladder cancer using computed tomography (CT) urography, flexible cystoscopy and voided urine cytology: results for 778 patients from a hospital haematuria clinic. *BJU Int*. 2012; 110(1):84–94.
8. Vasdev N, Thorpe AC. Should the presence of a culture positive urinary tract infection exclude patients from rapid evaluation hematuria protocols? *Urol Oncol*. 2013; 31(6):909–13.
9. Gopalakrishna A, Longo TA, Fantony JJ et al. The diagnostic accuracy of urine-based tests for bladder cancer varies greatly by patient. *BMC Urol*. 2016; 16(1):30.
10. Tan WS, Feber A, Dong L et al. DETECT I & DETECT II: a study protocol for a prospective multicentre observational study to validate the UroMark assay for the detection of bladder cancer from urinary cells. *BMC Cancer*. 2017; 17(1):767.
11. MacVicar D, Husband JE. Radiology in the staging of bladder cancer. *Br J Hosp Med*. 1994; 51(9):454–8.
12. Zattoni F, Incerti E, Dal Moro F et al. (18)F-FDG PET/CT and urothelial carcinoma: Impact on management and prognosis—A multicenter retrospective study. *Cancers*. 2019; 11(5).
13. National Institute for Health and Care Excellence. Bladder Cancer: Diagnosis and Management (Internet). [London]: NICE; 2015 [published 2015 Feb; cited 2020 Jul 10]. (Clinical guideline [NG2]). Available from: https://www.nice.org.uk/guidance/ng2
14. Panebianco V, Narumi Y, Altun E et al. Multiparametric magnetic resonance imaging for bladder cancer: Development of VI-RADS (vesical imaging-reporting and data system). *Eur Urol*. 2018; 74(3):294–306.
15. Rosenkrantz AB, Haghighi M, Horn J et al. Utility of quantitative MRI metrics for assessment of stage and grade of urothelial carcinoma of the bladder: preliminary results. *AJR Am J Roentgenol*. 2013; 201(6):1254–9.
16. Hafeez S, Huddart R. Advances in bladder cancer imaging. *BMC Med*. 2013; 11:104.
17. Hofstetter A, Frank F, Keiditsch E, Bowering R. Endoscopic neodymium-YAG laser application for destroying bladder tumors. *Eur Urol*. 1981; 7(5):278–82.
18. Mowatt G, Zhu S, Kilonzo M et al. Systematic review of the clinical effectiveness and cost-effectiveness of photodynamic diagnosis and urine biomarkers (FISH, ImmunoCyt, NMP22) and cytology for the detection and follow-up of bladder cancer. *Health Technol Assess*. 2010; 14(4):1–331, iii–iv.
19. Zheng C, Lv Y, Zhong Q et al. Narrow band imaging diagnosis of bladder cancer: systematic review and meta-analysis. *BJU Int*. 2012; 110(11 Pt B):E680–7.
20. Filbeck T, Pichlmeier U, Knuechel R et al. [Reducing the risk of superficial bladder cancer recurrence with 5-aminolevulinic acid-induced fluorescence diagnosis. Results of a 5-year study]. *Urologe A*. 2003; 42(10):1366–73.
21. Kurth KH, Denis L, Bouffioux C et al. Factors affecting recurrence and progression in superficial bladder tumours. *Eur J Cancer*. 1995; 31A(11):1840–6.
22. Sylvester RJ, van der Meijden AP, Oosterlinck W et al. Predicting recurrence and progression in individual patients with stage Ta T1 bladder cancer using EORTC risk tables: a combined analysis of 2596 patients from seven EORTC trials. *Eur Urol*. 2006; 49(3):466–5; discussion 75–7.
23. Fernandez-Gomez J, Madero R, Solsona E et al. Predicting non-muscle invasive bladder cancer recurrence and progression in patients treated with bacillus Calmette-Guerin: the CUETO scoring model. *J Urol*. 2009; 182(5):2195–203.
24. Kurth K, Tunn U, Ay R et al. Adjuvant chemotherapy for superficial transitional cell bladder carcinoma: long-term results of a European Organization for Research and Treatment of Cancer randomized trial comparing doxorubicin, ethoglucid and transurethral resection alone. *J Urol*. 1997; 158(2):378–84.
25. Pawinski A, Sylvester R, Kurth KH et al. A combined analysis of European Organization for Research and Treatment of

Cancer, and Medical Research Council randomized clinical trials for the prophylactic treatment of stage TaT1 bladder cancer. European Organization for Research and Treatment of Cancer Genitourinary Tract Cancer Cooperative Group and the Medical Research Council Working Party on Superficial Bladder Cancer. *J Urol.* 1996; 156(6):1934–40, discussion 40–1.

26. Sylvester RJ, Oosterlinck W, Holmang S et al. Systematic review and individual patient data meta-analysis of randomized trials comparing a single immediate instillation of chemotherapy after transurethral resection with transurethral resection alone in patients with stage pTa-pT1 urothelial carcinoma of the bladder: Which patients benefit from the instillation? *Eur Urol.* 2016; 69(2):231–44.

27. Tolley DA, Parmar MK, Grigor KM et al. The effect of intravesical mitomycin C on recurrence of newly diagnosed superficial bladder cancer: a further report with 7 years of follow up. *J Urol.* 1996; 155(4):1233–8.

28. Au JL, Badalament RA, Wientjes MG et al. Methods to improve efficacy of intravesical mitomycin C: results of a randomized phase III trial. *J Natl Cancer Inst.* 2001; 93(8):597–604.

29. Di Stasi SM, Giannantoni A, Stephen RL et al. Intravesical electromotive mitomycin C versus passive transport mitomycin C for high risk superficial bladder cancer: a prospective randomized study. *J Urol.* 2003; 170(3):777–82.

30. Sooriakumaran P, Chiocchia V, Dutton S et al. Predictive factors for time to progression after hyperthermic mitomycin C treatment for high-risk non-muscle invasive urothelial carcinoma of the bladder: An observational cohort study of 97 patients. *Urol Int.* 2016; 96(1):83–90.

31. de Jong JJ, Hendricksen K, Rosier M et al. Hyperthermic intravesical chemotherapy for BCG unresponsive non-muscle invasive bladder cancer patients. *Bladder Cancer.* 2018; 4(4):395–401.

32. Sousa A, Inman BA, Pineiro I et al. A clinical trial of neoadjuvant hyperthermic intravesical chemotherapy (HIVEC) for treating intermediate and high-risk non-muscle invasive bladder cancer. *Int J Hyperthermia.* 2014; 30(3):166–70.

33. Shelley MD, Wilt TJ, Court J et al. Intravesical bacillus Calmette-Guerin is superior to mitomycin C in reducing tumour recurrence in high-risk superficial bladder cancer: a meta-analysis of randomized trials. *BJU Int.* 2004; 93(4):485–90.

34. Bohle A, Bock PR. Intravesical bacille Calmette-Guerin versus mitomycin C in superficial bladder cancer: formal meta-analysis of comparative studies on tumor progression. *Urology.* 2004; 63(4):682–6; discussion 6–7.

35. Lamm DL, Blumenstein BA, Crawford ED et al. A randomized trial of intravesical doxorubicin and immunotherapy with bacille Calmette-Guerin for transitional-cell carcinoma of the bladder. *N Engl J Med.* 1991; 325(17):1205–9.

36. Sylvester RJ, van der Meijden AP, Witjes JA, Kurth K. Bacillus calmette-guerin versus chemotherapy for the intravesical treatment of patients with carcinoma in situ of the bladder: a meta-analysis of the published results of randomized clinical trials. *J Urol.* 2005; 174(1):86–91; discussion–2.

37. Catalona WJ, Hudson MA, Gillen DP et al. Risks and benefits of repeated courses of intravesical bacillus Calmette-Guerin therapy for superficial bladder cancer. *J Urol.* 1987; 137(2):220–4.

38. van der Meijden AP, Brausi M, Zambon V et al. Intravesical instillation of epirubicin, bacillus Calmette-Guerin and bacillus Calmette-Guerin plus isoniazid for intermediate and high risk Ta, T1 papillary carcinoma of the bladder: a European Organization for Research and Treatment of Cancer genito-urinary group randomized phase III trial. *J Urol.* 2001; 166(2):476–81.

39. Lamm DL, van der Meijden PM, Morales A et al. Incidence and treatment of complications of bacillus Calmette-Guerin intravesical therapy in superficial bladder cancer. *J Urol.* 1992; 147(3):596–600.

40. Schelhammer P. *Intravesical BCG Treatment Superficial Transitional Cell Carcinoma of the Bladder and Prostatic Urethra BCG Immunotherapy in Superficial Bladder Cancer.* Pagano FP, editor: Cleup, Badova; 1994.

41. Joudi FN, O'Donnell MA. Second-line intravesical therapy versus cystectomy for bacille Calmette-Guerin (BCG) failures. *Curr Opin Urol.* 2004; 14(5):271–5.

42. Rodel C, Dunst J, Grabenbauer GG et al. Radiotherapy is an effective treatment for high-risk T1-bladder cancer. *Strahlenther Onkol.* 2001; 177(2):82–8; discussion 9.

43. Harland SJ, Kynaston H, Grigor K et al. A randomized trial of radical radiotherapy for the management of pT1G3 NXM0 transitional cell carcinoma of the bladder. *J Urol.* 2007; 178(3 Pt 1):807–13; discussion 13.

44. Lamm DL, Riggs DR, Shriver JS et al. Megadose vitamins in bladder cancer: a double-blind clinical trial. *J Urol.* 1994; 151(1):21–6.

45. Kelly JD, Tan WS, Porta N et al. BOXIT-A randomised phase III placebo-controlled trial evaluating the addition of celecoxib to standard treatment of transitional cell carcinoma of the bladder (CRUK/07/004). *Eur Urol.* 2019; 75(4):593–601.

46. Shelley MD, Wilt TJ, Barber J, Mason MD. A meta-analysis of randomised trials suggests a survival benefit for combined radiotherapy and radical cystectomy compared with radical radiotherapy for invasive bladder cancer: are these data relevant to modern practice? *Clin Oncol (R Coll Radiol).* 2004; 16(3):166–71.

47. Skinner DG, Daniels JR, Russell CA et al. The role of adjuvant chemotherapy following cystectomy for invasive bladder cancer: a prospective comparative trial. *J Urol.* 1991; 145(3):459–64; discussion 64–7.

48. International Collaboration of Trialists, Medical Research Council Advanced Bladder Cancer Working Party, European Organisation for Research and Treatment of Cancer Genito-Urinary Tract Cancer Group et al. International phase III trial assessing neoadjuvant cisplatin, methotrexate, and vinblastine chemotherapy for muscle-invasive bladder cancer: Long-term results of the BA06 30894 trial. *J Clin Oncol.* 2011;29(16):2171–7.

49. Grossman HB, Natale RB, Tangen CM et al. Neoadjuvant chemotherapy plus cystectomy compared with cystectomy alone for locally advanced bladder cancer. *N Engl J Med.* 2003; 349(9):859–66.

50. Advanced Bladder Cancer (ABC) Meta-analysis Collaboration. Adjuvant chemotherapy in invasive bladder cancer: a systematic review and meta-analysis of individual patient data Advanced Bladder Cancer (ABC) Meta-analysis Collaboration. *Eur Urol.* 2005; 48(2):189–99; discussion 99–201.

51. Babjuk M, Burger M, Zigeuner R et al. EAU guidelines on non-muscle-invasive urothelial carcinoma of the bladder: update 2013. *Eur Urol.* 2013; 64(4):639–53.

52. Sternberg CN, Skoneczna I, Kerst JM et al. Immediate versus deferred chemotherapy after radical cystectomy in patients with pT3-pT4 or N+ M0 urothelial carcinoma of the bladder (EORTC 30994): an intergroup, open-label, randomised phase 3 trial. *Lancet Oncol.* 2015; 16(1):76–86.

53. Roehrborn CG, Sagalowsky AI, Peters PC. Long-term patient survival after cystectomy for regional metastatic transitional cell carcinoma of the bladder. *J Urol.* 1991; 146(1):36–9.

54. Birkmeyer NJ, Goodney PP, Stukel TA et al. Do cancer centers designated by the National Cancer Institute have better surgical outcomes? *Cancer.* 2005; 103(3):435–41.

55. Hounsome LS, Verne J, McGrath JS, Gillatt DA. Trends in operative caseload and mortality rates after radical cystectomy for bladder cancer in England for 1998–2010. *Eur Urol.* 2015; 67(6):1056–62.

56. Kock NG, Hulten L, Myrvold HE. Ileoanal anastomosis with interposition of the ileal "Kock pouch." Preliminary results. *Dis Colon Rectum.* 1989; 32(12):1050–4.

57. Kock NG, Ghoneim MA, Lycke KG, Mahran MR. Replacement of the bladder by the urethral Kock pouch: functional results, urodynamics and radiological features. *J Urol.* 1989; 141(5):1111–6.

58. Song C, Kang T, Hong JH et al. Changes in the upper urinary tract after radical cystectomy and urinary diversion: a comparison of antirefluxing and refluxing orthotopic bladder substitutes and the ileal conduit. *J Urol.* 2006; 175(1):185–9; discussion 9.

59. Rai BP, Bondad J, Vasdev N et al. Robotic versus open radical cystectomy for bladder cancer in adults. *Cochrane Database Syst Rev.* 2019; 4:CD011903.

60. Schoenberg MP, Walsh PC, Breazeale DR et al. Local recurrence and survival following nerve sparing radical cystoprostatectomy for bladder cancer: 10-year followup. *J Urol.* 1996; 155(2):490–4.

61. Coloby PJ, Kakizoe T, Tobisu K, Sakamoto M. Urethral involvement in female bladder cancer patients: mapping of 47 consecutive cysto-urethrectomy specimens. *J Urol.* 1994; 152(5 Pt 1): 1438–42.

62. Sweeney P, Kursh ED, Resnick MI. Partial cystectomy. *Urol Clin North Am.* 1992; 19(4):701–11.

63. Kondas J, Szentgyorgyi E. Transurethral resection of 1250 bladder tumours. *Int Urol Nephrol.* 1992; 24(1):35–42.

64. Thomas DJ, Roberts JT, Hall RR, Reading J. Radical transurethral resection and chemotherapy in the treatment of muscle-invasive bladder cancer: a long-term follow-up. *BJU Int.* 1999; 83(4):432–7.

65. Vashistha V, Wang H, Mazzone A et al. Radical cystectomy compared to combined modality treatment for muscle-invasive bladder cancer: A systematic review and meta-analysis. *Int J Radiat Oncol Biol Phys.* 2017; 97(5):1002–20.

66. Huddart RA, Birtle A, Maynard L et al. Clinical and patient-reported outcomes of SPARE—a randomised feasibility study of selective bladder preservation versus radical cystectomy. *BJU Int.* 2017; 120(5):639–50.

67. Fung CY, Shipley WU, Young RH et al. Prognostic factors in invasive bladder carcinoma in a prospective trial of preoperative adjuvant chemotherapy and radiotherapy. *J Clin Oncol.* 1991; 9(9):1533–42.

68. Splinter TA, Scher HI, Denis L et al. The prognostic value of the pathological response to combination chemotherapy before cystectomy in patients with invasive bladder cancer. European Organization for Research on Treatment of Cancer--Genitourinary Group. *J Urol.* 1992; 147(3):606–8.

69. Efstathiou JA, Spiegel DY, Shipley WU et al. Long-term outcomes of selective bladder preservation by combined-modality therapy for invasive bladder cancer: the MGH experience. *Eur Urol.* 2012; 61(4):705–11.

70. Hafeez S, Horwich A, Omar O et al. Selective organ preservation with neo-adjuvant chemotherapy for the treatment of muscle invasive transitional cell carcinoma of the bladder. *Br J Cancer.* 2015; 112(10):1626–35.

71. Choudhury A, Nelson LD, Teo MT et al. MRE11 expression is predictive of cause-specific survival following radical radiotherapy for muscle-invasive bladder cancer. *Cancer Res.* 2010; 70(18):7017–26.

72. Walker AK, Karaszi K, Valentine H et al. MRE11 as a predictive biomarker of outcome after radiation therapy in bladder cancer. *Int J Radiat Oncol Biol Phys.* 2019; 104(4):809–18.

73. McAlpine K, Fergusson DA, Breau RH et al. Radiotherapy with radical cystectomy for bladder cancer: A systematic review and meta-analysis. *Can Urol Assoc J.* 2018; 12(10):351–60.

74. Reisinger SA, Mohiuddin M, Mulholland SG. Combined pre- and postoperative adjuvant radiation therapy for bladder cancer—a ten year experience. *Int J Radiat Oncol Biol Phys.* 1992; 24(3):463–8.

75. Reddy AV, Pariser JJ, Pearce SM et al. Patterns of failure after radical cystectomy for pT3-4 bladder cancer: Implications for adjuvant radiation therapy. *Int J Radiat Oncol Biol Phys.* 2016; 94(5): 1031–9.

76. Baumann BC, Sargos P, Eapen LJ et al. The rationale for post-operative radiation in localized bladder cancer. *Bladder Cancer.* 2017; 3(1):19–30.

77. Baumann BC, Bosch WR, Bahl A et al. Development and validation of consensus contouring guidelines for adjuvant radiation therapy for bladder cancer after radical cystectomy. *Int J Radiat Oncol Biol Phys.* 2016; 96(1):78–86.

78. Zaghloul MS, Christodouleas JP, Smith A et al. Adjuvant sandwich chemotherapy plus radiotherapy vs. adjuvant chemotherapy alone for locally advanced bladder cancer after radical cystectomy: A randomized phase 2 trial. *JAMA Surg.* 2018; 153(1):e174591.

79. Tunio MA, Hashmi A, Qayyum A et al. Whole-pelvis or bladder-only chemoradiation for lymph node-negative invasive bladder cancer: single-institution experience. *Int J Radiat Oncol Biol Phys.* 2012; 82(3):e457–62.

80. Lalondrelle S, Huddart R, Warren-Oseni K et al. Adaptive-predictive organ localization using cone-beam computed tomography for improved accuracy in external beam radiotherapy for bladder cancer. *Int J Radiat Oncol Biol Phys.* 2011; 79(3):705–12.

81. Turner SL, Swindell R, Bowl N et al. Bladder movement during radiation therapy for bladder cancer: implications for treatment planning. *Int J Radiat Oncol Biol Phys.* 1997; 39(2):355–60.

82. McDonald F, Lalondrelle S, Taylor H et al. Clinical implementation of adaptive hypofractionated bladder radiotherapy for improvement in normal tissue irradiation. *Clin Oncol (R Coll Radiol).* 2013; 25(9):549–56.

83. Morrison R. The results of treatment of cancer of the bladder—a clinical contribution to radiobiology. *Clin Radiol.* 1975; 26(1):67–75.

84. Parsons JT, Million RR. Planned preoperative irradiation in the management of clinical stage B2-C (T3) bladder carcinoma. *Int J Radiat Oncol Biol Phys.* 1988; 14(4):797–810.

85. Hafeez S, McDonald F, Lalondrelle S et al. Clinical outcomes of image guided adaptive hypofractionated weekly radiation therapy for bladder cancer in patients unsuitable for radical treatment. *Int J Radiat Oncol Biol Phys.* 2017; 98(1):115–22.

86. Duchesne G, Bolger J, Griffiths G et al. A randomized trial of hypofractionated schedules of palliative radiotherapy in the management of bladder carcinoma: results of Medical Research Council Trial BA09. *Int J Radiol Oncol Biol Phys.* 2000; 47(2):379–88.

87. Shipley WU, Rose MA, Perrone TL et al. Full-dose irradiation for patients with invasive bladder carcinoma: clinical and histological factors prognostic of improved survival. *J Urol.* 1985; 134(4):679–83.

88. Overgaard J, Horsman MR. Modification of hypoxia-induced radioresistance in tumors by the use of oxygen and sensitizers. *Semin Radiat Oncol.* 1996; 6(1):10–21.

89. Horwich A, Dearnaley D, Huddart R et al. A randomised trial of accelerated radiotherapy for localised invasive bladder cancer. *Radiother Oncol.* 2005; 75(1):34–43.

90. Hoskin PJ, Rojas AM, Bentzen SM, Saunders MI. Radiotherapy with concurrent carbogen and nicotinamide in bladder carcinoma. *J Clin Oncol.* 2010; 28(33):4912–8.

91. Yang L, Taylor J, Eustace A et al. A gene signature for selecting benefit from hypoxia modification of radiotherapy for high-risk bladder cancer patients. *Clin Cancer Res.* 2017; 23(16):4761–8.

92. Eustace A, Irlam JJ, Taylor J et al. Necrosis predicts benefit from hypoxia-modifying therapy in patients with high risk bladder cancer enrolled in a phase III randomised trial. *Radiother Oncol.* 2013; 108(1):40–7.

93. Pernot M, Hubert J, Guillemin F et al. Combined surgery and brachytherapy in the treatment of some cancers of the bladder (partial cystectomy and interstitial iridium-192). *Radiother Oncol.* 1996; 38(2):115–20.

94. Aluwini S, van Rooij PH, Kirkels WJ et al. Bladder function preservation with brachytherapy, external beam radiation therapy, and limited surgery in bladder cancer patients: Long-term results [corrected]. *Int J Radiat Oncol Biol Phys.* 2014; 88(3):611–7.

95. Cowan RA, McBain CA, Ryder WD et al. Radiotherapy for muscle-invasive carcinoma of the bladder: results of a randomized trial comparing conventional whole bladder with dose-escalated partial bladder radiotherapy. *Int J Radiat Oncol Biol Phys.* 2004; 59(1):197–207.

96. Hafeez S, Warren-Oseni K, McNair HA et al. Prospective study delivering simultaneous integrated high-dose tumor boost (<= 70 Gy) with image guided adaptive radiation therapy for radical treatment of localized muscle-invasive bladder cancer. *Int J Radiat Oncol Biol Phys.* 2016; 94(5):1022–30.

97. Murthy V, Gupta P, Baruah K et al. Adaptive radiotherapy for carcinoma of the urinary bladder: Long-term outcomes with dose escalation. *Clin Oncol (R Coll Radiol).* 2019; 31(9):646–52.

98. Coppin CM, Gospodarowicz MK, James K et al. Improved local control of invasive bladder cancer by concurrent cisplatin and preoperative or definitive radiation. The National Cancer Institute of Canada Clinical Trials Group. *J Clin Oncol.* 1996; 14(11):2901–7.

99. James ND, Hussain SA, Hall E et al. Radiotherapy with or without chemotherapy in muscle-invasive bladder cancer. *N Engl J Med.* 2012; 366(16):1477–88.

100. Caffo O, Thompson C, De Santis M et al. Concurrent gemcitabine and radiotherapy for the treatment of muscle-invasive bladder

cancer: A pooled individual data analysis of eight phase I-II trials. *Radiother Oncol.* 2016; 121(2):193–8.

101. Hoskin PJ, Saunders MI, Dische S. Hypoxic radiosensitizers in radical radiotherapy for patients with bladder carcinoma: hyperbaric oxygen, misonidazole, and accelerated radiotherapy, carbogen, and nicotinamide. *Cancer.* 1999; 86(7):1322–8.

102. Sternberg CN, Yagoda A, Scher HI et al. Methotrexate, vinblastine, doxorubicin, and cisplatin for advanced transitional cell carcinoma of the urothelium. Efficacy and patterns of response and relapse. *Cancer.* 1989; 64(12):2448–58.

103. Geller NL, Sternberg CN, Penenberg D et al. Prognostic factors for survival of patients with advanced urothelial tumors treated with methotrexate, vinblastine, doxorubicin, and cisplatin chemotherapy. *Cancer.* 1991; 67(6):1525–31.

104. Mead GM, Russell M, Clark P et al. A randomized trial comparing methotrexate and vinblastine (MV) with cisplatin, methotrexate and vinblastine (CMV) in advanced transitional cell carcinoma: results and a report on prognostic factors in a Medical Research Council study. MRC Advanced Bladder Cancer Working Party. *Br J Cancer.* 1998; 78(8):1067–75.

105. Loehrer PJ, Sr., Einhorn LH, Elson PJ et al. A randomized comparison of cisplatin alone or in combination with methotrexate, vinblastine, and doxorubicin in patients with metastatic urothelial carcinoma: a cooperative group study. *J Clin Oncol.* 1992; 10(7):1066–73.

106. Sternberg CN, de Mulder P, Schornagel JH et al. Seven year update of an EORTC phase III trial of high-dose intensity M-VAC chemotherapy and G-CSF versus classic M-VAC in advanced urothelial tract tumours. *Eur J Cancer.* 2006; 42(1):50–4.

107. von der Maase H, Sengelov L, Roberts JT et al. Long-term survival results of a randomized trial comparing gemcitabine plus cisplatin, with methotrexate, vinblastine, doxorubicin, plus cisplatin in patients with bladder cancer. *J Clin Oncol.* 2005; 23(21):4602–8.

108. Bellmunt J, von der Maase H, Mead GM et al. Randomized phase III study comparing paclitaxel/cisplatin/gemcitabine and gemcitabine/cisplatin in patients with locally advanced or metastatic urothelial cancer without prior systemic therapy: EORTC Intergroup Study 30987. *J Clin Oncol.* 2012; 30(10):1107–13.

109. Petrioli R, Frediani B, Manganelli A et al. Comparison between a cisplatin-containing regimen and a carboplatin-containing regimen for recurrent or metastatic bladder cancer patients—A randomized phase II study. *Cancer.* 1996; 77(2):344–51.

110. De Santis M, Bellmunt J, Mead G et al. Randomized phase II/III trial assessing gemcitabine/carboplatin and methotrexate/carboplatin/vinblastine in patients with advanced urothelial cancer who are unfit for cisplatin-based chemotherapy: EORTC study 30986. *J Clin Oncol.* 2012; 30(2):191–9.

111. Edeline J, Loriot Y, Culine S et al. Accelerated MVAC chemotherapy in patients with advanced bladder cancer previously treated with a platinum-gemcitabine regimen. *Eur J Cancer.* 2012; 48(8):1141–6.

112. Vaughn DJ, Malkowicz SB, Zoltick B et al. Paclitaxel plus carboplatin in advanced carcinoma of the urothelium: an active and tolerable outpatient regimen. *J Clin Oncol.* 1998; 16(1):255–60.

113. Bellmunt J, Fougeray R, Rosenberg JE et al. Long-term survival results of a randomized phase III trial of vinflunine plus best supportive care versus best supportive care alone in advanced urothelial carcinoma patients after failure of platinum-based chemotherapy. *Ann Oncol.* 2013; 24(6):1466–72.

114. Rosenberg JE, O'Donnell PH, Balar AV et al. Pivotal trial of enfortumab vedotin in urothelial carcinoma after platinum and anti-programmed death 1/programmed death ligand 1 therapy. *J Clin Oncol.* 2019; 37(29):2592–600.

115. Powles T, Eder JP, Fine GD et al. MPDL3280A (anti-PD-L1) treatment leads to clinical activity in metastatic bladder cancer. *Nature.* 2014; 515(7528):558–62.

116. Hussain SA, Birtle A, Crabb S et al. From clinical trials to real-life clinical practice: The role of immunotherapy with PD-1/PD-L1 inhibitors in advanced urothelial carcinoma. *Eur Urol Oncol.* 2018; 1(6):486–500.

117. Bellmunt J, de Wit R, Vaughn DJ et al. Pembrolizumab as second-line therapy for advanced urothelial carcinoma. *N Engl J Med.* 2017; 376(11):1015–26.

118. Bellmunt J, de Wit R, Vaughn DJ et al. Pembrolizumab as second-line therapy for advanced urothelial carcinoma. *N Engl J Med.* 2017; 376(11):1015–26.

119. Plimack ER, Bellmunt J, Gupta S et al. Safety and activity of pembrolizumab in patients with locally advanced or metastatic urothelial cancer (KEYNOTE-012): a non-randomised, open-label, phase 1b study. *Lancet Oncol.* 2017; 18(2):212–20.

120. Powles T, Duran I, van der Heijden MS et al. Atezolizumab versus chemotherapy in patients with platinum-treated locally advanced or metastatic urothelial carcinoma (IMvigor211): a multicentre, open-label, phase 3 randomised controlled trial. *Lancet.* 2018; 391(10122):748–57.

121. Balar AV, Galsky MD, Rosenberg JE et al. Atezolizumab as first-line treatment in cisplatin-ineligible patients with locally advanced and metastatic urothelial carcinoma: a single-arm, multicentre, phase 2 trial. *Lancet.* 2017; 389(10064):67–76.

122. Hussain MH, MacVicar GR, Petrylak DP et al. Trastuzumab, paclitaxel, carboplatin, and gemcitabine in advanced human epidermal growth factor receptor-2/neu-positive urothelial carcinoma: results of a multicenter phase II National Cancer Institute trial. *J Clin Oncol.* 2007; 25(16):2218–24.

123. Powles T HR, Elliott T, Sarker SJ et al. Phase III, double-blind, randomized trial that compared maintenance lapatinib versus placebo after first-line chemotherapy in patients with human epidermal growth factor receptor 1/2-positive metastatic bladder cancer. *J Clin Oncol.* 2017; 35:48–55.

124. Galsky MD, Hahn NM, Powles T et al. Gemcitabine, cisplatin, and sunitinib for metastatic urothelial carcinoma and as preoperative therapy for muscle-invasive bladder cancer. *Clin Genitourin Cancer.* 2013; 11(2):175–81.

125. Geldart T, Chester J, Casbard A et al. SUCCINCT: an open-label, single-arm, non-randomised, phase 2 trial of gemcitabine and cisplatin chemotherapy in combination with sunitinib as first-line treatment for patients with advanced urothelial carcinoma. *Eur Urol.* 2015; 67(4):599–602.

126. Jones RJ, Hussain SA, Protheroe AS et al. Randomized phase II study investigating pazopanib versus weekly paclitaxel in relapsed or progressive urothelial cancer. *J Clin Oncol.* 2017; 35(16):1770–7.

127. Petrylak DP, de Wit R, Chi KN et al. Ramucirumab plus docetaxel versus placebo plus docetaxel in patients with locally advanced or metastatic urothelial carcinoma after platinum-based therapy (RANGE): a randomised, double-blind, phase 3 trial. *Lancet.* 2017; 390(10109):2266–77.

128. Loriot Y, Necchi A, Park SH et al. Erdafitinib in locally advanced or metastatic urothelial carcinoma. *N Engl J Med.* 2019; 381(4):338–48.

129. Jose CC, Price A, Norman A et al. Hypofractionated radiotherapy for patients with carcinoma of the bladder. *Clin Oncol (R Coll Radiol).* 1999; 11(5):330–3.

14 PROSTATE CANCER

Malcolm Mason and Howard Kynaston

Introduction

Prostate cancer is a uniquely challenging disease. At the heart of the challenge is the disparity between the mortality rate (around 47 deaths per 100,000 men per annum in the United Kingdom) and the incidence of the disease (around 171 cases per 100,000 men per annum in the United Kingdom).[1] This disparity is not because of successful treatment. Indeed, the incidence figures underestimate the true "biological" prevalence of the disease; post-mortem studies indicate that around 5% of men aged 30 and 60% of men by the age of 80 harbor foci of prostate cancer.[2] Rather, it is because in the overwhelming majority of men in the population, prostate cancer is an indolent, even harmless disease. Our challenges are first, correctly to identify those men whose cancer threatens their health and second, to identify the best treatment for such men at an early stage. W. Whitmore's dictum, written in 1990[3] and paraphrased here, still encapsulates the challenge that this chapter attempts to address:

Is treatment possible for those in whom it is necessary?
Is treatment necessary for those in whom it is possible?

Epidemiology and etiology

There is a striking geographical variation in the incidence of prostate cancer, with high levels in Western countries and low levels in Asia and the Far East. However, prostate cancer is the most frequently diagnosed cancer in 105 countries, with an estimated 1.3 million new cases in 2018 globally, and the fifth most frequent cause of cancer death.[4] The rates are highest among men of African descent in the United States and the Caribbean, reflecting ethnic and genetic predisposition. As with breast cancer, the changing incidence in migrants from low-incidence to high-incidence regions also suggests a dietary or other environmental component. However, despite years of research, it is difficult to pin down exactly which components of a "Western diet" might enhance the risk of prostate cancer or conversely, which components of an "Eastern diet" might protect against it. A compelling hypothesis, which links breast and prostate cancer risks to focal inflammation induced by carcinogens in cooked meat, deserves to be further debated.[5] Specific "healthy" diets, such as the Mediterranean diet, might have some modest benefits for disease behavior.

Prostate cancer is generally a disease of old age. Its age-specific incidence curve shows a steady rise, with most cases diagnosed in 60- and 70-year-old men.

A genetic component to the etiology is suggested by the increased risk of the disease in first-degree relatives, especially when multiple cases are affected at a young age (<60 years), and candidate gene regions are being sought. Recent studies of single nucleotide polymorphisms indicate that multiple genes, each conferring a small or modestly increased risk, may combine to confer a substantially increased risk in some men.[6] Some single gene mutations confer substantially increased risk, notably in families carrying mutations of the *BRCA-1* and *BRCA-2* genes,[7] which in turn might implicate a wider role for variations in *ATM* gene polymorphisms in the wider population. Genetic factors may be one of several that contribute to an increased risk of the disease in some races, most notably among black Americans, who are more likely to present with high-grade disease.[8]

There are very few well-documented additional risk factors for the development of prostate cancer, although obesity is associated with higher-risk disease.[9]

Prevention and screening

There is no topic in medicine as controversial as prostate cancer screening, and this remains so even after the publication of the long-awaited randomized trials. To the layman, it seems obvious that early detection must lead to better outcomes, and the path to early detection of prostate cancer is through screening. This is reinforced by public health messages about screening for hypertension, or cervical cancer, or breast cancer, or diabetes. How could it be different for prostate cancer?

The advent of prostate-specific antigen (PSA) testing in the late 1980s promised a simple way of screening for prostate cancer, but conflicting data from observational studies made this a controversial subject. The European Randomised Trial of Screening for Prostate Cancer (ERSPC) recruited 182,000 men between the ages of 50 and 74, who were randomly allocated PSA screening every 4 years or no screening.[10] Long-term follow-up at 13 years found that screening was associated with a 21% reduction in the odds of death from prostate cancer, with an absolute risk reduction of 0.11 per 1000 person-years or 1.28 per 1000 men randomized. This translates into a need to screen 781 men and to treat 27 men to prevent one death from prostate cancer.[11] It is recognized that at the same time, screening results in an unacceptable rate of overdiagnosis and overtreatment, while many men otherwise destined to die of prostate cancer will still do so. The PLCO (Prostate, Lung, Colon, and Ovary) program also published the results of its PSA screening in 76,693 men, randomized to annual PSA testing or to usual care, and no differences in prostate cancer mortality were observed.[12] However, there was a high rate of contamination in this trial, with many men in the control arm receiving PSA testing. Finally, in the United Kingdom, the Prostate testing for cancer and Treatment (ProtecT)[13] study has a companion study (the comparison arm for Protec-T [CAP] study), which compared prostate cancer mortality between men who were invited to have a single PSA test and those who were not, having randomized primary-care providers to participate or not to participate, and found no difference in outcome at 10 years.[14] The ProtecT study is discussed in more detail later.

Can prostate cancer be prevented? Dietary modification would seem to be one means of achieving this. Components of the Asian/Far Eastern diet might also help to prevent prostate cancer, for example, soy isoflavonoids. The potential for anti-oxidants to reduce prostate cancer risk has also been long debated, but a randomized trial of dietary selenium or vitamin E supplementation (the selenium and vitamin E cancer prevention trial [SELECT] trial) disappointingly showed no evidence of benefit (indeed, vitamin E may actually increase the risk.[15] Nonetheless, it is possible that certain dietary components, such as lycopenes (from cooked or processed tomatoes) and green tea, may have a protective effect. A randomized trial of the 5-alpha reductase inhibitor, finasteride, as a possible chemo-preventative agent (acting by preventing the conversion of testosterone to the active dihydrotestosterone) did, indeed, show a reduction in the incidence of prostate cancer in the treated group. However, it appeared to show an increased proportion of high-risk disease in those who did develop prostate cancer, a finding that continues to excite much debate, although these concerns do not appear to have been borne out with longer term follow-up.[16] Patients who remained prostate cancer free at the end of the study (7 years) were biopsied. Prostate cancer was detected in a staggering 24% of the men in the control arm of the study, which must represent the best demonstration yet of our ability to over-diagnose prostate cancer using current methods. If this does not eloquently warn of the dangers of unnecessarily diagnosing and treating men for innocent prostate cancers, nothing will! A second, similar study (the REDUCE trial), using dutasteride, also reported a reduction in biopsy proven prostate cancer after 4 years of treatment.[17]

Pathogenesis

Prostatic intra-epithelial neoplasia (PIN) was so named because it was presumed to be the precursor of prostate cancer in the same way as cervical intra-epithelial neoplasia (CIN) is of cervical cancer. It was graded according to the degree of cellular atypia but is generally referred to simply as low-grade PIN or high-grade PIN.[18] However, its relationship to invasive prostate cancer is much less clear than is the case with CIN and cervical cancer. Any relationship that exists is likely to be predominantly in high-grade and not in low-grade PIN. On the other hand, it is equally clear that not all men with high-grade PIN will go on to develop invasive prostate cancer, and it may be that it is a marker of common risk factors rather than a true biological precursor per se. A second condition, termed atypical small acinar proliferation (ASAP), was thought to progress to frank carcinoma more than does high-grade PIN, but this is unlikely to represent an entity in its own right; rather, it is simply another way of saying "suspicious for low-grade adenocarcinoma."

The other condition that could be a precursor to prostate cancer is proliferative inflammatory atrophy.[19] This is more difficult to see in needle-biopsy specimens (as opposed to whole-organ mounts from radical prostatectomy specimens). In fact, contrary to expectations, cell turnover in regions of inflammatory atrophy is extremely high, explaining why such an association would make sense. Moreover, such lesions express high levels of glutathione-S-transferase, an enzyme involved in the detoxification of polycyclic aromatic hydrocarbons, consistently with the relationship to inflammation.

Prostate cancer is androgen dependent; that is to say, it does not develop in the absence of testosterone (for example, it is exceedingly rare in eunuchs), and growth control, mediated by the androgen receptor, is key to the pathogenesis of the disease. At the same time, other growth factors are of importance, including epidermal growth factor (EGF) and insulin-like growth factor-1 (IGF-1), and circulating levels of these can in turn be influenced by diet. In understanding the development of prostate cancer, it is a mistake to consider the prostatic epithelium in isolation; the prostate is an example *par excellence* of an organ in which the behavior of the epithelium is governed by the stroma, and vice versa. Prostatic stromal fibroblasts and tumor cells secrete a number of growth factors that impact on the development and progression of prostate cancer, including fibroblast growth factors

(FGF), vascular-endothelial growth factor (VEGF), transforming growth factor beta (TGF-β), and hepatocyte growth factor (HGF).

It is possible that prostate cancers, like other types of cancer, originate in stem cells. Stem cells are rare components of the prostatic epithelium, are situated in the basal layer, and are thought to give rise to luminal epithelial cells, luminal secretory cells, and neuro-endocrine cells. The phenotypic markers that describe these cell lineages are currently being described. A prostate cancer stem cell has also recently been described, and an understanding of its biology may yield new insights and new targets for cancer therapy.[20]

Pathology and staging

Nearly all prostate cancers are adenocarcinomas.

The Gleason grading system is now almost universally employed for prostatic adenocarcinomas. In its original form, it took as its starting premise that histologically, there was a major pattern and a minor pattern in prostate cancers. Gleason ascribed a score of 1–5 to each pattern, and the Gleason sum score simply adds them together.[21] For example, a Gleason sum score of 3 + 3 = 6 implies a score of 3/5 for the major pattern and 3/5 for the minor pattern, making a sum score of 6. In the years following its first description, there was a relatively even spread of Gleason scores among diagnosed prostate cancers, but there was also wide inter-observer variation in ascribing a score to an individual tumor. In recent years, this variability has lessened considerably, together with an interesting decline in the number of cases that are ascribed a Gleason sum score of less than 6. Indeed, in the Cardiff practice, Gleason 3 + 3 = 6 is the most commonly found sum score following review in a specialist prostate cancer multidisciplinary team (MDT) meeting (Figure 14.1). Care is needed in comparing outcomes in a contemporary series of patients with those in a historical series. The most striking indication of this stage shift is seen in the re-analysis of the Connecticut series of patients managed by "watchful waiting"—the contemporary histological assessment (which was blinded with respect to the original assessment) shows that Gleason scores 2–5, which were well represented in the original analysis, have now become uncommon, with the majority of cases now being graded as Gleason 3 + 3 = 6, *even though the analysis has been done on the same series of patients.*[22]

The World Health Organization (WHO) has also described a grading system, which is less often used now than it was formerly (when the Gleason system was less established). Tumors are graded I, II, and III (corresponding roughly to Gleason scores 2–4, 5–7, and 8–10, respectively), equivalent to well-differentiated, moderately differentiated, and poorly differentiated tumors. More recently, however, there has been widespread adoption of a more patient-centric grading system, resulting in five grade groups (1 to 5).[23]

Immunohistochemical stains used to identify prostate cancers include PSA, cytokeratins, and more recently, alpha-methylacyl-CoA-racemase (AMACR), which appears to be a particularly promising marker for distinguishing prostate cancer from benign prostatic disease.

Rare tumors of the prostate include small-cell carcinomas, which behave in a similar fashion to small-cell carcinomas at other sites, and which show features of neuro-endocrine differentiation. Others, such as sarcomas and lymphomas, are managed according to the principles adopted for those tumors at other anatomical sites. Transitional-cell carcinomas (TCCs) can arise from the prostatic urethra and are more likely to behave like muscle-invasive bladder cancers. TCC can also involve the prostate due to local spread from a bladder tumor, and more rarely, the prostate

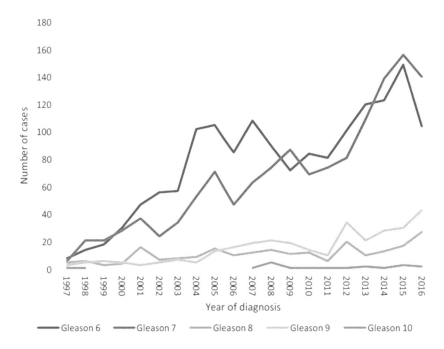

FIGURE 14.1 Gleason scores by year of diagnosis. (Cardiff MDT 1997–2016.)

can be involved in local spread from other pelvic tumors, such as from the rectum or sigmoid colon.

Adenocarcinomas typically spread locally, involving the periprostatic tissues or the seminal vesicles, and to regional lymph nodes in the pelvis. The distribution of lymph node metastases has been mapped out using nanoparticle-enhanced magnetic resonance imaging (MRI) after pathological confirmation and shows quite extensive variation; this is an important consideration in therapeutic nodal irradiation[24] (Figure 14.2). Subsequent spread to para-aortic and on occasions, to supra-diaphragmatic lymph nodes can occur. One of the most striking features of prostate cancer, however, is its peculiar propensity to bone metastases, which are typically osteoblastic, in contrast to the lytic metastases seen, for example, in multiple myeloma or (less strikingly) in breast cancer. This clinical feature must be a reflection of an important biological feature of prostate cancers, and it is clear that there are important interactions between bone cells—especially osteoblasts and to a lesser extent, osteoclasts—and prostate cancer cells, with the latter secreting a number of factors, including bone morphogenetic proteins and osteoprotegerin. Bone metastases are seen particularly in the axial skeleton, in the pelvis, and in the proximal femora, and the anatomical distribution was ascribed to the rich venous drainage from the prostate into Batson's vertebral plexus. This is likely to be only part of the story, however, given the biological aspects of "soil and seed," and bone metastases can also occur elsewhere, notably in the base of the skull. It is, however, almost forgotten that previous generations of pathologists, who carried out meticulous post-mortem examinations, recognized that despite the *clinical* dominance of bone metastases, *pathologically*, visceral metastases do, in fact, occur more widely than is supposed today.

The TNM staging system, either from the Union for International Cancer Control (UICC) or American Joint Committee on Cancer (AJCC), is the one most widely in use in clinical practice (Box 14.1). It is important to be clear about which

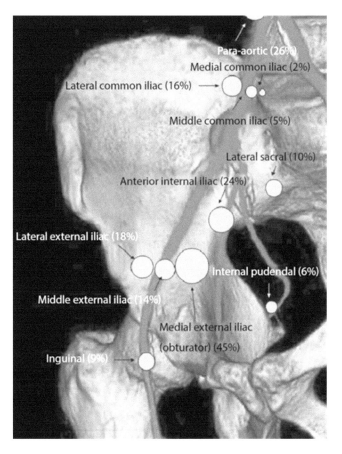

FIGURE 14.2 Incidence of lymph node metastases by site based on pathological staging in patients with locally advanced disease. (From Shih et al., 2005. With permission.)

system is being used, particularly with regard to staging the primary tumor, as the classifications do change.

BOX 14.1 TNM CLASSIFICATION OF PROSTATE CANCER

PRIMARY TUMOR (T)

Tx   Primary tumor cannot be assessed
T0   No evidence of primary tumor
T1*   Clinically inapparent tumor not palpable or visible by imaging
   T1a*   Tumor incidental histological finding in 5% or less of tissue resected
   T1b*   Tumor incidental histological finding in more than 5% of tissue resected
   T1c*   Tumor identified by needle biopsy (e.g. because of elevated PSA)**
T2   Tumor confined within prostate
   T2a   Tumor involves one half of one lobe or less
   T2b   Tumor involves more than half of one lobe, but not both lobes
   T2c   Tumor involves both lobes
T3   Tumor extends through the prostate capsule***
   T3a   Extraprostatic extension (unilateral or bilateral) including microscopic bladder neck involvement
   T3b   Tumor invades seminal vesicle(s)
T4   Tumor is fixed or invades adjacent structures other than seminal vesicles, for example the external sphincter, rectum, levator muscles, or pelvic wall

*The pT and pN categories correspond to the T and N categories. However, there is no pT1 category because there is insufficient tissue to assess the highest pT category.

**Tumor found in one or both lobes by needle biopsy, but not palpable or visible by imaging, is classified as T1c.

***Invasion into the prostatic apex or into (but not beyond) the prostatic capsule is not classified as T3, but as T2.

REGIONAL LYMPH NODES (N)

NX   Regional lymph nodes cannot be assessed
N0   No regional lymph node metastasis
N1   Regional lymph node metastasis

DISTANT METASTASIS (M)

M0   No distant metastasis
M1   Distant metastasis
   M1a   Non-regional lymph node(s)
   M1b   Bone(s)
   M1c   Other site(s)

STAGE GROUPING

Stage I	T1, T2a	N0	M0
Stage II	T2b, T2c	N0	M0
Stage III	T3, T4	N0	M0
Stage IV	Any T	N1	M0
	Any T	Any N	M1

(From Brierley et al., 2017, with permission.[25])

Clinical features

Symptoms and signs

Early, organ-confined prostate cancer is entirely asymptomatic. There is something uncomfortable in today's public health "message," at least in the way in which it is interpreted by the public, which essentially asserts that lower urinary tract symptoms (LUTS) should lead to immediate referral and investigation so that an underlying prostate cancer can be picked up as early as possible. The best reason for prompt assessment of LUTS is that the underlying condition, most commonly benign prostatic hypertrophy (BPH), can be effectively treated and symptoms improved. Men with a predisposition to prostate cancer, such as those carrying a germ-line BRCA-1 or -2 mutation, might prove to be a special category, and a low threshold for investigation and treatment in such men is reasonable.

Digital rectal examination (DRE) is an important part of the assessment of a patient with suspected prostate cancer but by itself is often inaccurate. The TNM staging may be based on the DRE assessment of clinical stage, although this is often supplemented with information from other investigations. A nodule may be palpable, and extension of the disease beyond the prostate gland or into the seminal vesicles may also be noted.

Bulky local or locally advanced disease can give rise to LUTS or more rarely, to other pelvic symptoms such as rectal pain, bleeding or constipation due to rectal involvement, and deep perineal discomfort due to peri-prostatic soft-tissue involvement. The last-mentioned seems to be a feature of "PSA-negative" prostate cancers, i.e. those that produce lower amounts of PSA, such that serum PSA levels are disproportionately low for the stage of disease. Hemospermia is more common as a symptom of locally advanced disease than is recognized, but most cases of hemospermia have causes other than prostate cancer.

Lymph node metastases may give rise to lymphoedema in the lower limbs and genitalia, and occasionally, peripheral lymphadenopathy may be palpable in the groins or in the neck.

Bone metastases may be asymptomatic in the early stages but ultimately give rise to bone pain or to other complications—typically pathological fractures and spinal cord compression. The latter is a potentially disastrous complication, and the clinician should be perpetually alert to this possibility. Hypercalcemia is relatively less common in prostate cancer than in breast cancer, reflecting a lower degree of bone resorption (although increased bone resorption due to increased osteoclast activity most definitely *does* occur in prostate cancer). When hypercalcemia does occur, it may be a reflection of a paraneoplastic syndrome with ectopic parathyroid hormone production.

Prostate-specific antigen

PSA has evolved from humble beginnings[26] to become arguably the most successful tumor marker in the entire field of oncology. It is produced by more than 95% of all prostate cancers, mirrors disease activity extraordinarily well, and provides a sensitive guide to disease recurrence many years before it becomes clinically apparent. For patients who have had complete ablation of the prostate (i.e., after radical prostatectomy), the PSA will fall to undetectable limits, although ultra-sensitive assays enable the detection of disease recurrence with PSA levels as low as 0.1 ng/L. Variations of a one-off, total PSA measurement in managing men with established disease includes making use of PSA kinetics. These can aid clinical decision-making, for example in an older man with a very long PSA doubling time, which can give some rationale to deferring or avoiding treatment.

Where PSA has been less successful and more controversial is in the diagnosis of prostate cancer. This is principally due to its lack of specificity, in that most men with a raised PSA have BPH rather than prostate cancer. Furthermore, some men whose PSA is in the "normal" range have prostate cancer on biopsy (maybe not surprisingly, given the incredibly high biological prevalence of the disease). In trying to overcome this, studies have asked whether any other features of PSA might improve its sensitivity/specificity profile. Two facets in particular have been postulated: the free:total ratio, or absolute levels of "free" PSA—because a higher risk of prostate cancer is associated with lower levels of "free" as opposed to "complexed" PSA—and the PSA doubling time. A third profile—the PSA density, which relates the PSA level to the prostatic volume—is becoming more important with the advent of MRI in the diagnostic pathway, as prostate volume estimation is more accurately measured with this technique.[27]

Other tumor markers

An older tumor marker—prostatic acid phosphatase—is occasionally helpful, for example in immunochemistry. Two other potential tissue markers, used in research, are prostate membrane-specific antigen (PSMA) and prostate stem-cell antigen (PSCA). At the moment, they are not useful in routine clinical practice. More recently, the PC3a test, which directly measures genes identified in prostate cancer cells from a urine specimen, has been investigated to determine whether its use in combination with PSA might improve diagnostic sensitivity and specificity. It has not yet found widespread adoption, however.

Diagnosis and staging

A histological diagnosis is usually made following a transrectal ultrasound (TRUS)-guided biopsy. Prostate cancer may be suspected on a TRUS on the basis of a hypo-echogenic area, particularly if it is in the peripheral zone, the most usual site for prostate cancers. If an abnormal region is seen, targeted biopsies can be performed. If not, a series of biopsies is taken (usually five to six from each side, although this varies from one center to another), and even if targeted biopsies are taken, additional samples will also be taken from elsewhere in the gland. Prostate template biopsy, where large numbers of transperineal biopsies are taken under general anesthetic using a rigid grid similar to that used for brachytherapy, may be used for more thorough histological assessment of the whole gland and would be practical if it were possible to accurately define those patients most likely to benefit from it. More recently, pre-biopsy MRI, using the additional sequences of diffusion weighting and gadolinium infusion (multiparametric MRI), has proven to be more accurate in diagnosing significant prostate cancer than TRUS biopsy alone and to reduce the detection of non-significant disease.[28,29] However, the addition of gadolinium increases the cost considerably, and biparametric MRI, using diffusion weighting in addition to T2 sequences, is more likely to achieve widespread acceptability worldwide. In addition, MRI provides better tumor staging than computed tomography (CT), such as extension of disease beyond the capsule or into the seminal vesicles. Either CT or MRI may be used to detect lymph node spread. Their contribution is limited to a description of the size and shape of lymph nodes; as yet, they can say little about nodal architecture. The combination of MRI with microscopic super-paramagnetic nanoparticles, which are taken up in lymph nodes, has not yet progressed due to adverse effects.

Technetium-99 bone scanning is a sensitive means of detecting bone metastases, the likelihood of metastases being greater, the higher the PSA. Conversely, patients with a PSA below 20 ng/mL have a rate of positive bone scans of less than 1%, and many centers therefore omit bone scanning in patients with a PSA in this range unless they have Gleason Grade Group 3 or higher on biopsy.[30] Indeed, the relatively low rate of detection of metastatic disease in general in today's patient population argues that a more risk-based approach to staging investigations might be justified.

Alternatives to bone scanning include MRI of the spine to detect bony lesions and more recently, positron emission tomography (PET) scanning using tracers such as choline and PSMA to detect metastatic disease, which may be equivocal on standard imaging.[31] However, PET scanning is currently not widely available for routine use in most centers.

Is a histological diagnosis always required? It is a good oncological principle that it is, wherever possible. However, in the case of a patient with radiologically demonstrable sclerotic bone metastases, a clinically malignant prostate gland on rectal examination, and a PSA of over 100 ng/mL, the diagnosis of metastatic prostate cancer is almost incontrovertible. Sometimes, such patients can be treated on the basis of a clinical diagnosis alone and spared the indignity and discomfort of a TRUS-guided biopsy. Usually, though, a histological diagnosis will be required, especially if the patient is to be entered into a clinical trial.

Principles of management

The major distinction—in terms of management philosophy—is between organ-confined disease, locally advanced disease, and metastatic disease. The management of more advanced disease is discussed later, but some preliminary remarks are useful before considering organ-confined disease.

The incredibly high prevalence of prostate cancer has already been stressed. One consequence of this is that the majority of men diagnosed with early (organ-confined) disease could actually have insignificant disease. On the other hand, by definition, those men who die of prostate cancer have significant disease, and a number of these men will have originally been diagnosed with (apparently) organ-confined disease. The problem is that there is currently no reliable way of distinguishing between the two–the "tiger," which has the potential to metastasize and cause death, and the "pussycat," which if left alone, will cause no clinical problems during a patient's lifetime.

Patients are usually stratified by "risk," the d'Amico classification[32] being especially popular, where low risk comprises T1–T2a, Gleason ≤6, and PSA <10; intermediate risk comprises T2b and either Gleason 7 and/or PSA 10–20; and high risk >T2b, Gleason ≥8, and/or PSA >20. This is a useful basis for clinical decision-making, but it is too often forgotten that this form of assessment is a *guide to the probability of disease being significant* and not a measure of whether the disease is *actually* significant.

Management of organ-confined disease

Can we tame the tiger without drowning the pussycat?

There are three broad strategies for the management of localized (T1–2) prostate cancer: active surveillance (manifestly distinct from "watchful waiting"), radiotherapy (by external beam or brachytherapy), and surgery (by open, laparoscopic, or robotic radical prostatectomy). For the asymptomatic patient diagnosed solely on the basis of a raised PSA, with organ-confined disease, especially of the most common Gleason score of 3 + 3 = 6, *there is no evidence that any one of these approaches is superior in terms of prolonging life.* This statement needs to be made clearly and uncategorically. Selecting the "right" treatment for an individual patient is a complex process, which has been plagued by a number of problems, including the tendency for specialists to recommend their own modality of treatment. Different specialists asserting that their own treatment is "best," and the "hype" around newer treatment modalities confuse patients, and the major impact of case selection is often ignored. However, to patients, it seems self-evident that excellent results are due to an excellent treatment, especially if this view is reinforced by the specialist. Unrandomized comparisons overestimate the efficacy of a treatment modality.

In the United Kingdom, the ProtecT study randomized 1643 men, diagnosed with organ-confined prostate cancer following an invitation to over 230,000 men to attend for PSA testing, between active surveillance, radical prostatectomy, and radical radiotherapy.[13] This trial found no difference in prostate-specific survival between the three arms, although the two treatment arms of radiotherapy and surgery equally reduced the risk of progression and metastases at 10-year follow-up.[33] This trial also documented the treatment-related effects on quality of life[34] and is an important step in informing decision-making for men diagnosed on the basis of a raised PSA.

Active surveillance and "watchful waiting"

In the late 1980s and 1990s, outcomes from patients managed conservatively began to appear in the literature, indicating that a substantial proportion would remain alive and well despite not having been treated initially by surgery or radiotherapy.[35] For some patients, the terminology itself ("watchful waiting" was coined in the 1980s) was unacceptable ("you watch, while I wait to die").

There are two different scenarios that determine the philosophy and hence, the policy. For a patient with low-risk disease who is elderly and/or has significant co-morbidity, the aim of management is to avoid treatment insofar as this is possible, and it is likely that any treatment given will be palliative or at least, will be given in response to symptoms. This is the philosophy of "watchful waiting." For a younger patient with no symptoms who has low-risk disease, active surveillance implies that treatment will be given in response to evidence of disease progression, which might consist of a rising PSA or a higher Gleason score on a subsequent re-biopsy (a procedure that would never be done in the first scenario). Furthermore, such treatment would be radical in intent, assuming that the patient is still suitable for such treatment. There are now a number of published studies of active surveillance, which have recently been reviewed. A policy of active surveillance can avoid radical therapy in up to two-thirds of patients, with very low (<1%) death rates from prostate cancer, with a median follow-up of around 7 years.

There is no universal agreement on the optimum follow-up schedule or even the appropriate "trigger" for re-investigation and/or treatment. Many, but not all, centers will perform a repeat biopsy after 2 years of surveillance. In the future, repeat biopsy in selected patients with functional MRI might provide further refinements to the process.

Radical prostatectomy

Open radical prostatectomy involves the removal of the prostate, seminal vesicles, and pelvic lymph nodes. The bladder neck is then re-anastomosed to the urethra, and a catheter is placed in situ for around 10 days. In experienced hands, blood loss is usually below the threshold for transfusion, and the length of hospital stay, particularly with robotic-assisted laparoscopic prostatectomy (RALP), is on average 1 day. Postoperative mortality is exceedingly low. There is undoubtedly a "learning curve," the best results depending on experience and also on the numbers of patients treated by the center. The main risks following radical prostatectomy are incontinence and erectile dysfunction. Following a classical open radical prostatectomy, the incidence of erectile failure is between 90% and 100%, but in recent years, it has been possible to perform a nerve-sparing procedure on appropriately selected patients, which is said to preserve potency in up to 80% of patients. Significant incontinence rates are usually of the order of around 1%–2%, but more minor degrees of leakage might occur in around 9% of men, particularly in the first year after surgery.

Newer surgical techniques, such as laparoscopic and robotic techniques, offer the potential for advantages in terms of pain, time to recovery, blood loss, and ability to perform nerve-sparing surgery.[36] Indeed, robotic surgery is now the predominant surgical approach for prostate cancer in the United States and the United Kingdom. One randomized trial that compared open prostatectomy and RALP[37] found similar functional outcomes at 2 years post-surgery but better biochemical recurrence rates for RALP, although longer follow-up was required. A limitation of this study was the very high experience of the robotic surgeon in the study, again highlighting the role of experience in this surgery. Essentially, open and robotic surgery are more dependent on surgeon experience than on precise technique, but allowing for this, RALP is equivalent to or better than open surgery, and in many countries, open surgery is so infrequently performed that experience in the technique is falling.

The results of two randomized trials comparing surgery with conservative management in early-stage prostate cancer have now been reported. The Scandinavian Prostate Cancer Study Group performed a randomized trial comparing radical prostatectomy with watchful waiting; 695 men were randomized between 1989 and 1999. At a median follow-up of 18 years, 200 men in the prostatectomy group had died, compared with 247 men in the watchful-waiting group.[38] This is the first Level 1 evidence that radical treatment might improve survival in some men with prostate cancer. There are important differences between the patients enrolled into this study and contemporary patients, as they were diagnosed somewhat later in the course of their disease. The majority had T2 tumors, only around 5% having been diagnosed by PSA screening, and 17%–20% having had a PSA level of more than 20 ng/mL at diagnosis. Furthermore, watchful waiting, rather than active monitoring, was performed. It has been estimated that if applied to a contemporary series of patients, the true benefits of surgery in terms of survival might not become apparent for a substantial number of years, based on the time taken for the survival curves to separate in this study, plus the inevitable lead time achieved with PSA screening compared with symptomatic presentation. Is there a survival benefit for much earlier surgery (i.e., at the time of diagnosis of a PSA-detected cancer) compared with delayed surgery (based on active monitoring)?

The second randomized trial compared radical prostatectomy and observation. In this study, 731 men were randomized between the two options, but after a median of 12 years' follow-up, there was no significant difference in either overall survival or prostate cancer–specific survival.[39]

Radiotherapy

Radiotherapy has been used to treat primary prostate cancer since the pioneering work of Bagshaw, beginning in the 1960s. Most initial work, summarizing retrospective studies from this period, used external-beam radiotherapy (EBRT). More recently, prostate brachytherapy has become popular, with the potential to deliver very high doses of radiation to the prostate with an almost ideal dose distribution.

External-beam radiotherapy (EBRT)

Patients treated with EBRT should be treated with intensity-modulated radiotherapy, since there is evidence that this approach reduces treatment complications and side effects and also allows dose escalation, which cannot be performed safely with conventional open collimators. There has been a steady trend towards ever-increasing doses of EBRT over the last 15 years or so, most recently achieved with the use of high-precision intensity-modulated radiotherapy or image-guided radiotherapy. High-dose EBRT has been tested in five randomized studies and is now firmly established as the reference standard if conventional 1.8–2 Gy fractions are used (for example, in the recent CHHIP trial, discussed later.[40]) To date, however, none of these trials has shown an overall survival benefit. It is likely that the use of neoadjuvant/adjuvant hormone therapy plus a lower dose of radiotherapy (e.g., 74 Gy) may be equivalent to a higher dose (e.g., 80 Gy) without hormone therapy. However, there is evidence that additional hormone therapy does not benefit men with low-risk disease.[41] The usefulness of hormone therapy in patients with earlier-stage disease has been tested by the European Organisation for Research and Treatment of Cancer (EORTC) 22991 study, in which 819 patients with localized intermediate or high-risk disease were randomized to radiotherapy plus no androgen deprivation therapy (ADT) or to radiotherapy plus 6 months' treatment with androgen deprivation. Biochemical progression was significantly reduced in the group receiving ADT, but the study is not yet mature enough in terms of overall survival.[42] Another randomized trial has suggested that 18 months of hormone therapy is adequate for men with intermediate-/high-risk but localized disease.[43] However, there is also evidence for long-term hormone therapy in patients with high-risk disease,[44] and a duration of 2–3 years would be regarded as standard. The approach to adjuvant/neoadjuvant hormone therapy recommended by the UK National Institute for Health and Care Excellence is that patients with intermediate- and high-risk disease should be offered radiotherapy plus ADT, but low-risk patients could be offered radiotherapy alone.[45]

In some centers, a high dose per fraction (e.g. a dose of 55 Gy in 20 fractions) has been standard. However, a radiobiological argument states that an even higher dose per fraction might be advantageous for the treatment of prostate cancer, as it might have the characteristics associated with a "late-reacting" tissue and a low alpha:beta ratio. Recent trials are evaluating the prospects for getting the best of both worlds: escalating the total radiation dose beyond 55 Gy and towards a target of around 70 Gy, but doing so with larger (>2 Gy) doses per fraction. The UK CHHIP trial[40] recruited 3216 men with T1b–T3a disease, who were randomized to 74 Gy in 37 fractions, 57 Gy in 19 fractions, or 60 Gy in 30 fractions. At 5 years of follow-up, the 60 Gy arm was shown to be non-inferior to the 74 Gy arm and has therefore been recommended

for practice. However, the 57 Gy arm outcome was shown to be inferior and this dose is therefore not recommended. There were no differences in late toxicity between the three arms.[40] Recent early results from the PACE-B trial suggest that extreme hypofractionation using stereotactic body radiotherapy given in five fractions over 1–2 weeks did not increase acute gastrointestinal or urinary toxicity. However, long-term efficacy and toxicity data are awaited.[46]

EBRT for prostate cancer should be CT or MRI planned with the patient supine and having a full bladder. In the CHHIP study, the definitions of target volumes and dose constraints have also been published, and these serve as an exemplar of radiotherapy planning techniques for IMRT. Two risk groups are defined, based on studies from the Radiation Therapy Oncology Group (RTOG), and used in the CHHIP protocol:

> Group L (low risk of seminal vesicle involvement): Clinical stages T1b/c or T2a with (PSA + [(Gleason score − 6) × 10]) <15
> Group M (moderate or high risk of seminal vesicle involvement): Clinical stages T1b/c or T2a with (PSA + [(Gleason score − 6) × 10]) ≤15

The prostate gland is capable of a substantial degree of movement, which could affect the accuracy of treatment delivery, and image-guided radiotherapy (IGRT) can ameliorate this. It has been suggested that there is a small increased risk of rectal cancer following prostate radiotherapy, and patients should be counselled about this, though the risk is not considered high enough to obviate radiotherapy as a safe and tested treatment option.

Following high-dose conformal radiotherapy, the incidence of significant/severe (RTOG Grade III/IV) late bowel toxicity is of the order of 1%–2%.[40] Erectile function can be preserved in around 60% of patients who are potent before treatment, but some suggest that this figure declines with time. Incontinence is uncommon unless the patient has already had other surgical procedures such as a transurethral resection of the prostate. Patient-reported outcomes comparing toxicity after EBRT and surgery were reported in the ProtecT trial and indicate comparable overall levels, though with more bowel toxicity after radiotherapy, compared with more urinary and sexual toxicity after radical prostatectomy.[47]

Brachytherapy

Brachytherapy offers the ideal of a very high radiation dose to the prostate with a rapid fall-off in dose beyond the prostate (due to the inverse square law). Patients have a planning TRUS scan performed under general anesthetic in the lithotomy position. At a second procedure, also under general anesthetic, permanent radioactive seeds, usually made of iodine-125 or palladium-103, are implanted into the prostate. Their distribution is guided by meticulous planning based on the planning TRUS scan and information from prior CT scanning. A grid system in a perineal mount is used to guide the insertion of radioactive seeds into the prostate. Seeds are usually placed in tandem and are linked to prevent seed migration. Doses can be manipulated in order to spare the urethra, which may go some way towards reducing urinary complications. Treatment is usually very well tolerated, requiring minor analgesics, and the reported outcomes are excellent. The main side effects are urinary, with dysuria and frequency, sometimes even amounting to acute retention due to urethral inflammation and edema. After an onset after a few weeks, it is maximal around 6–8 weeks later, and generally subsides thereafter, although it can sometimes persist to a degree for several months.

Brachytherapy is reported to produce potency rates that are as good as, or better than, those with EBRT and has a very low incidence of rectal complications. However, it has not been compared with EBRT in a randomized trial, and a single trial comparing it with surgery has not yielded interpretable results. The evidence is summarized in Chin et al.[48]

A variation of permanent, low-dose-rate brachytherapy as discussed in the previous paragraph is the use of high-dose-rate brachytherapy, which involves a similar planning technique, but in place of permanent seeds, temporary tubes are inserted into the prostate and are then afterloaded in the same way as for gynecological and other cancers. This can be performed either as monotherapy or in combination with EBRT and/or ADT.[45]

Novel forms of therapy

Several alternative forms of local treatment to the prostate gland have emerged in recent years. Cryotherapy involves the insertion of a thermal probe transperineally into the prostate, analogously to the brachytherapy technique discussed above, and the creation of a region of thermal injury due to the formation of an ice ball around the probe. As yet, this should not be offered as a standard curative option outside a formal study setting. It may have a role to play in the management of locally recurrent disease following radiotherapy. In its early years, cryotherapy was associated with substantial complications, most severely, the development of a rectourethral fistula. This is now less common with better control of the ice probe and better selection of patients, although complication rates are high when it is used as salvage therapy compared as primary therapy.

High-intensity focused ultrasound (HIFU) is another non-invasive technique, which uses an ultrasound probe in the rectum that can be focused to a specific region of the prostate and generate a thermal injury. The extent of injury induced by the probe can be visualized under ultrasound control, and the procedure can be computer controlled. Typically, the procedure, done under a general anesthetic, involves the creation of a "mosaic" of thermal burns that cover the entire prostate or the region required. There may be more potential for control of the ultrasound distribution and even for sparing the neurovascular bundle. There is a growing body of data from well-structured but unrandomized studies of HIFU, but more information is needed before this technique can be recommended outside a study setting.

The same applies to photodynamic therapy (PDT), in which there has been a resurgence of interest with the development of better light sources and better photo-sensitizers. A review of the evidence led the European Association of Urology (EAU) Guidelines Group to regard all forms of focal therapy as being unsuitable for use outside a formal study setting.[49]

Proton beam therapy has been used for prostate cancer for over 40 years, mainly in the US. Clinical trial data is confusing and there is no intrinsic reason why protons should have any increased cure rate. The ability to reduce the rectal dose using the physical properties of the Bragg peak should, in theory, result in lower levels of late toxicity. Similarly, the dose to the other two main organs at risk, the bladder and small intestine, should be lower. The main troublesome long-term side effects of protons are bowel and bladder disturbances, as well as impotence.

A careful search of the literature shows there is little well-documented evidence of the benefits of protons compared with well-delivered IMRT.[50] However, it seems self-evident that there would be a group of patients whose anatomy favors the abrupt fall off

of radiation dose with protons.[51] Where both IMRT and protons are available, double planning with both proton and photon fields would seem to be the gold standard for proceeding to radical radiation for this common disease followed by treatment with whichever modality gives the best dose distribution. It is unlikely that sufficient quality randomised trials will ever be carried out. The development of hypo-fractionated regimens—for example, seven fractions in 10 days—seems to be the most convenient way forward for this common clinical problem. The use of a balloon rectal spacer is another development that needs further study, though it is used in a number of centers.

Management of locally advanced disease

EBRT is the mainstay of management for locally advanced (T3 to T4) disease. A classic EORTC study demonstrated that for patients with locally advanced disease who were being managed by EBRT, overall survival and disease-free survival were significantly better with additional adjuvant ADT for 3 years, starting on the last day of radiotherapy.[52] Not surprisingly, this led to the standard use of some form of ADT in this setting. The story might have ended there but for a number of outstanding questions. What is the optimum scheduling of ADT? What is its optimum duration? What is the optimum dose of radiotherapy? In the EORTC trial, the dose was between 65 and 69 Gy. Additionally, a few patients had organ-confined disease (T2) but with other unfavorable factors, such as a high histological grade.

In the absence of other data, it might have been argued that the benefits of combined radiotherapy and ADT were due to the ADT alone. However, there have now been three published randomized trials, which report substantial benefits for EBRT. Patients with, predominantly, locally advanced disease were randomized to ADT alone or ADT plus EBRT.[53–55] In the largest of these, the intergroup PR3/PR07 study, 1205 patients were entered, and the final analysis, at a median follow-up time of 8 years, demonstrates a 54% reduction in the odds of death from prostate cancer, absolute 10 year disease-specific death rates being 15% with and 26% without radiotherapy.

In locally advanced disease, radiotherapy to the prostate and the seminal vesicles is uncontroversial. Whether or not the pelvic lymph nodes should be irradiated has been a matter of debate. Two RTOG randomized trials failed to show a significant benefit for whole pelvic radiotherapy (though one is claimed to show some benefits on subgroup analysis), and undoubtedly, such an approach increases toxicity compared with treatment confined to the prostate alone. The same is true of irradiation of the para-aortic nodes. In the future, developments in radiotherapy treatment such as IMRT could allow treatment of regional lymph nodes to a far higher dose than previously, and this may yet completely change the management of this disease by radiotherapy. Indeed, two randomized trials addressing this question are currently in progress. A secondary analysis of data from the U.K. Medical Research Council (MRC) STAMPEDE trial (discussed later) suggests improved outcomes with pelvic radiotherapy, which argues for using it in fit patients and even in patients with clinically involved pelvic nodes.

There has been much recent interest in surgery for selected patients with locally advanced disease, and indeed, in experienced hands and with very careful selection, the results appear to be excellent. However, there are no Level 1 data comparing surgery with radiotherapy, and such a study, if achievable, is badly needed, but it is doubtful whether this can now be performed.

Management of recurrent disease after radical local therapy

Most patients who relapse after radical local therapy (radical prostatectomy or radiotherapy) will do so with a rising PSA as their first, and usually only, indication of disease. For patients relapsing after radiotherapy, the next line of treatment is usually with ADT. Before embarking on this, it is worth making some assessment of the rate of PSA climb (e.g., using the PSA doubling time). Occasionally, patients may relapse with a very slow PSA doubling time, and in such patients, it is important to weigh up any benefits from early hormone therapy against the adverse effects, particularly against the background of the PSA doubling time and the patient's age and general fitness, as well as his own personal wishes. It is possible that novel therapy such as HIFU or cryotherapy might have a role in the management of patients relapsing with local disease following previous radiotherapy, and more data are needed on this.

For patients relapsing after radical prostatectomy, the situation is a little different. Following a radical prostatectomy, the expectation is that the PSA will fall to undetectable levels. The definition of what constitutes "undetectable" obviously depends on the sensitivity of the PSA assay, but in most modern centers, ultra-sensitive assays are performed with a lower limit of detection of up to 0.01 ng/mL. This extremely sensitive assay allows the identification of patients relapsing biochemically after radical prostatectomy at a very early stage. Prior to the use of such sensitive assays, the recommendations might have been somewhat different. Three randomized trials assigned patients treated by radical prostatectomy and with histological evidence of disease at the resection margins to immediate postoperative radiotherapy to the prostate bed or to no immediate treatment.[56–58] These studies have all indicated a benefit for patients treated with radiotherapy in terms of biochemical progression-free survival but only one indicated benefit in terms of overall survival.[58] There are issues with these studies. Two of the three studies included men with persistent, as opposed to recurrent, PSA after surgery, and just one study[57] was in men with recurrent disease only. For men with undetectable PSA post radical prostatectomy, but with unfavorable features such as pathological T3 disease, a recent meta-analysis of three randomized trials (GETUG-17, RAVES, and RADICALS) has shown that adjuvant radiotherapy offers no benefits compared with early salvage therapy but does significantly increase toxicity.[59,60] Offering surveillance and early salvage to those men who develop PSA recurrence will spare more than half of all such men from undergoing radiotherapy.

Management of metastatic disease

First-line therapy

It was through the dramatic effects of orchidectomy, and hormone therapy with estrogens in patients with metastatic prostate cancer, that the exquisite sensitivity to androgen deprivation was first demonstrated in the 1940s. The overall response rate to first-line ADT is of the order of 85%. Subsequent studies by the Veterans Administration in the United States confirmed these high response rates, but the use of stilbestrol in relatively high doses was associated with an unacceptably high rate of deaths from cardiovascular disease. The mainstay of ADT remained surgical orchidectomy until the introduction in the 1980s of LHRH agonists, which are now the most commonly used form of ADT.

The LHRH agonists are associated with an initial tumor "flare" in response to a transient rise in serum testosterone, which can be prevented using short-term oral anti-androgens (for, say, 3 weeks). Untreated, the consequences for patients with metastatic disease could be severe—incipient renal obstruction becomes renal failure, and incipient spinal cord compression becomes paraparesis. Recently, a new LHRH antagonist, degarelix, which avoids the need for "flare" protection, has been tested in Phase III trials. Whatever form of hormone therapy is used, there is a risk of reduced bone density, which can lead to pathological fractures, and this should be monitored in all patients. There is Level 1 evidence that the routine use of bisphosphonates protects against loss of bone mineral density.[61]

Three recent, large randomized trials—the STAMPEDE, LATTITUDE, and CHAARTED trials—have changed the paradigm for metastatic, hormone-sensitive disease. They have all compared the standard of care (long-term hormone therapy) with standard of care plus additional systemic treatment in the form of docetaxel chemotherapy. The results have been summarized in a series of meta-analyses.[62] These trials have all demonstrated an improvement in overall survival with additional systemic therapy, using either docetaxel chemotherapy or abiraterone, of up to 20 months, and hormone therapy alone should no longer be regarded as the standard of care. However, neither the meta-analysis nor a within-trial comparison in STAMPEDE definitively shows one agent to be superior to the other.[62,63] In addition, the STAMPEDE trial and a second trial (HORRAD) have shown that for men with limited-volume metastatic disease, local radiotherapy to the prostate also confers a survival advantage compared with hormone therapy, and these are summarized in a further meta-analysis.[64] Intermittent hormone therapy has been studied in several Phase III trials. While it appears to be a safe option in patients with biochemical relapse after radical curative therapy, there is more uncertainty about its efficacy in the metastatic setting, and for now, continuous ADT remains the standard option, especially as the landscape has changed with additional systemic therapy.

Systemic therapy in castrate refractory disease

With current therapy, patients with M1 disease can expect a period of disease control for around 3 years before they experience disease progression. At that stage, the disease—formerly classified as "hormone refractory"—is now more properly described as "castrate refractory" (CRPC), a term almost universally hated by patients. This major new insight came from Phase III studies of abiraterone acetate, a drug that potently inhibits androgen synthesis. Two pivotal trials (one in patients naïve to chemotherapy and another in patients previously treated with docetaxel) demonstrated significant responses with associated improvements in symptoms and quality of life plus significant prolongation of overall survival. These studies were followed by others of similar design using enzalutamide, an agent that not only blocks androgen binding to the androgen receptor but also blocks translocation of the androgen receptor to the nucleus. As with abiraterone, the AFFIRM trial of enzalutamide in patients post-docetaxel indicated a significant prolongation of survival. However, the optimum use of these agents in patients who have previously received them in their hormone-sensitive phase remains unclear.

In the current era, many men demonstrate the onset of CRPC on the basis of a rising PSA without evidence of metastatic disease. Recent randomized trials have shown that novel anti-androgens such as apalutamide and enzalutamide confer a progression-free and overall survival benefit if used early,[65,66] and it is likely that this will become the standard of care.

Currently, in addition to abiraterone and enzalutamide, several other systemic therapies have also been shown in Phase III trials to prolong survival in metastatic CRPC, albeit by a modest few months. Not all of these agents are universally available as yet. Cabazitaxel is a novel taxane, which showed a survival benefit compared with mitoxantrone in patients progressing during or soon after docetaxel therapy. Although the duration of survival benefit has been insufficient for its approval in the National Health Service, it was striking to see such activity in such a poor-risk group of patients.[67] Sipuleucel-T is a complex immunotherapy delivered by treating autologous dendritic cells *ex-vivo* with a combination of prostatic acid phosphatase and granulocyte-macrophage colony-stimulating factor, following which they are re-infused. Published evidence from the main Phase II trial indicates that this, too, prolongs survival in metastatic CRPC. The logistics of delivering this treatment have precluded its widespread use outside the United States, but this is likely to change in the next few years. Another recent development has been the report of a Phase III, placebo-controlled trial of radium-223 (an alpha emitter) in patients with symptomatic bone metastases, which has demonstrated a significant overall survival benefit.[68]

Other options include bisphosphonates. In metastatic disease affecting bone, there is every reason to expect that these agents should be beneficial, since there is a very clear element of bone resorption (osteoclastic) in prostate cancer patients, despite the overall picture of osteoblastic (sclerotic) metastatic disease. A placebo-controlled randomized trial of zoledronic acid has, however, shown a significant delay in time to a skeletal-related event (radiotherapy for bone pain, pathological fracture, spinal cord compression, or hypercalcemia) in patients with hormone refractory disease. Interestingly, a significant component of this benefit is the reduction in risk of pathological fractures. Similarly, the humanized monoclonal antibody to the RANK-ligand, denosumab (another means of targeting the osteoclast), has been evaluated in a placebo-controlled randomized trial, and patients with high-risk but M0 disease allocated to the active agent showed prolonged time to bone metastasis.

The next era in the development of novel treatments for prostate cancer will surely be marked by biologically targeted agents. One such agent, the PARP inhibitor olaparib, has already been shown to yield responses in CRPC, particularly in disease characterized by defects in DNA repair.[69]

Growth areas and major ongoing clinical trials

- Radioactive lutetium-PSMA targeted therapy is currently under investigation in ongoing clinical trials.
- The STAMPEDE trial is continuing, with current arms investigating the use of metformin and estradiol patches.
- The MRC Add-aspirin trial is testing the efficacy of aspirin in preventing disease progression following curative treatment in intermediate-risk localized disease.
- The hormone duration arms of the RADICALS trial are awaiting maturity and analysis, and will inform on the need for, and optimum duration of, hormone therapy in patients undergoing salvage radiotherapy following previous radical prostatectomy.
- The RE-IMAGINE study is testing the addition of biomarkers to MRI as a possible route to prostate cancer screening.

- Other biomarker studies including urinary biomarkers such as EV-RNA are under evaluation.[70]
- A randomized trial of partial-gland focal therapy versus conventional whole-gland therapy is expected to be launched in 2020.
- Immunotherapy for advanced disease is promising, with a recent study of pembrolizumab suggesting a small subgroup of patients who respond well, but further studies are needed.

Key learning points

- One-off, PSA-based screening for prostate cancer is ineffective. Repeated rounds do reduce mortality, but at the expense of overdiagnosis and overtreatment, and this has precluded formal uptake into national screening programs.
- Multiparametric MRI helps to select patients with a raised PSA who are most likely to harbor significant disease.
- There are no differences at 10 years in prostate cancer–specific mortality for surgery, radiotherapy, or active monitoring in patients with organ-confined disease. However, progression rates are higher with active monitoring, and 20 year outcomes are awaited.
- Locally advanced disease should be treated with either surgery, probably combined with radiotherapy, or radiotherapy plus 2–3 years of hormone therapy.
- Hormone-naïve patients with metastatic disease should be treated with a combination of hormone therapy and either docetaxel chemotherapy or abiraterone.
- Patients with low-volume metastatic disease should additionally receive radiotherapy to the prostate.
- Patients with castrate refractory disease should be treated with a novel anti-androgen if they have no evidence of metastatic disease.

References

1. Cancer Research UK. UK Prostate Cancer Statistics. ttp://info.cancerresearchuk.org/cancerstats/types/prostate/.
2. Bell KJL, Del Mar C, Wright G et al. Prevalence of incidental prostate cancer: A systematic review of autopsy studies. *Int J Cancer.* 2015; 137:1749–57.
3. Whitmore WF, Jr. Natural history of low-stage prostatic cancer and the impact of early detection. *Urol Clin North Am.* 1990; 17: 689–97.
4. Bray F, Ferlay J, Soerjomataram I et al. Global cancer statistics 2018: GLOBOCAN estimates of incidence and mortality worldwide for 36 cancers in 185 countries. *Cancer J Clin.* 2018; 68:394–424.
5. Coffey DS. Similarities of prostate and breast cancer: Evolution, diet, and estrogens. *Urology.* 2001; 57 Supplement 1:31–8.
6. Eeles RA, Olama AA, Benlloch S et al. Identification of 23 new prostate cancer susceptibility loci using the iCOGS custom genotyping array. *Nat Gen.* 2013; 45(4):385–91, 91e1–2.
7. Liede A, Karlan BY, Narod SA. Cancer risks for male carriers of germline mutations in BRCA1 or BRCA2: A review of the literature. *J Clin Oncol.* 2004; 22:735–42.
8. Thompson IM, Ankerst DP, Chi C et al. Assessing prostate cancer risk: Results from the prostate cancer prevention trial. *J Natl Cancer Inst.* 2006; 98:529–34.
9. Bray F, Kiemeney L. Epidemiology of prostate cancer in Europe: patterns, trends and determinants. In: Bolla M, van Poppel H (eds). *Management of Prostate Cancer: A Multidisciplinary Approach.* Berlin: Springer-Verlag; 2017. pp. 1–11
10. Schroeder FH, Hugosson J, Roobol MJ et al. Screening and prostate-cancer mortality in a randomized European study. *N Engl J Med.* 2009; 360(13):1320–8.

11. Schröder FH, Hugosson J, Roobol MJ et al. Screening and prostate cancer mortality: results of the European randomised study of screening for prostate cancer (ERSPC) at 13 years of follow-up. *Lancet* 2014; 384:2027–35.

12. Andriole GL, Grubb RL, III, Buys SS et al. Mortality results from a randomized prostate-cancer screening trial. *N Engl J Med.* 2009; 360(13):1310–9.

13. Donovan J, Hamdy F, Neal D et al. Prostate testing for cancer and treatment (ProtecT) feasibility study. *Health Technol Assess.* 2003; 7:1–88.

14. Martin RM, Donovan JL, Turner EL et al. Effect of a low-intensity PSA-based screening intervention on prostate cancer mortality: The CAP randomized clinical trial. *JAMA.* 2018; 319(9):883–95.

15. Lippman SM, Klein EA, Goodman PJ et al. Effect of selenium and vitamin E on risk of prostate cancer and other cancers: the selenium and vitamin E cancer prevention trial (SELECT). *JAMA.* 2009; 301(1):39–51.

16. Goodman PJ, Tangen CM, Darke AK et al. Long-term effects of finasteride on prostate cancer mortality. *N Engl J Med.* 2019; 380:393–4.

17. Andriole GL, Bostwick D, Brawley O et al. Effect of dutasteride on the risk of prostate cancer. *N Engl J Med.* 2010; 362:1192–202.

18. Bostwick DG, Qian J. High-grade prostatic intraepithelial neoplasia. *Mod Pathol.* 2004; 17:360–79.

19. De Marzo AM, Marchi VL, Epstein JI, Nelson WG. Proliferative inflammatory atrophy of the prostate: Implications for prostatic carcinogenesis. *Am J Pathol.* 1999;155:1985–92.

20. Collins AT, Berry PA, Hyde C et al. Prospective identification of tumorigenic prostate cancer stem cells. *Cancer Res* 2005; 65:10946–51.

21. Gleason DF. The Veteran's administration cooperative urologic research group: Histological grading and clinical staging of prostatic carcinoma. In: Tannenbaum M (ed.) *Urologic Pathology: The Prostate.* Philadelphia, PA: Lea and Febiger, 1977. pp. 171–98.

22. Albertsen PC, Hanley JA, Barrows GH et al. Prostate cancer and the Will Rogers phenomenon. *J Natl Cancer Inst.* 2005; 97:1248–53.

23. Kryvenko ON, Epstein JI. Changes in prostate cancer grading: Including a new patient-centric grading system. *Prostate.* 2016; 76(5):427–33.

24. Shih HA, Harisinghani M, Zietman AL et al. Mapping of nodal disease in locally advanced prostate cancer: Rethinking the clinical target volume for pelvic nodal irradiation based on vascular rather than bony anatomy. *Int J Radiat Oncol Biol Phys.* 2005; 63:1262–9.

25. Brierley JD, Gospodarowicz MK, Wittekind C (eds). *TNM Classification of Malignant Tumours.* 8th ed. Oxford, UK: Wiley-Blackwell, 2017.

26. Ablin RJ, Pfeiffer L, Gonder MJ, Soanes WA. Precipitating antibody in the sera of patients treated cryosurgically for carcinoma of the prostate. *Exp Med Surg.* 1969; 27:406–10.

27. Stephan C, Stroebel G, Heinau M et al. The ratio of prostate-specific antigen (PSA) to prostate volume (PSA density) as a parameter to improve the detection of prostate carcinoma in PSA values in the range of <4 ng/mL. *Cancer.* 2005; 104:993–1003.

28. Ahmed HU, Bosaily AE, Brown LC et al. Diagnostic accuracy of multi-parametric MRI and TRUS biopsy in prostate cancer (PROMIS): a paired validating confirmatory study. *Lancet.* 2017; 389:815–22.

29. Kasivisvanathan V, Rannikko AS, Borghi M et al. MRI-targetted or standard biopsy for prostate-cancer diagnosis. *N Eng J Med.* 2018; 378: 1767–77.

30. KandaSwamy GV, Bennett A, Narahari K et al. Establishing the pathways and indications for performing isotope bone scans in newly diagnosed intermediate-risk localized prostate cancer—results from a large contemporaneous cohort. *BJU Int.* 2017; 120: E59–63.

31. Yaxley JW, Raveenthiran S, Nahaud F-X et al. Risk of metastatic disease on 68gallium-prostate specific membrane antigen positron emission tomography/computed tomography scan for primary staging of 1253 men at the diagnosis of prostate cancer. *BJU Int.* 2019; 124: 401–7.

32. D'Amico AV, Whittington R, Malkowicz SB et al. Biochemical outcome after radical prostatectomy, external beam radiation therapy, or interstitial radiation therapy for clinically localized prostate cancer. *JAMA* 1998; 280:969–74.

33. Hamdy FC, Donovan JA, Lane M et al. 10-year outcomes after monitoring, surgery, or radiotherapy for localized prostate cancer. *N Engl J Med.* 2016; 375:1415–24.

34. Donovan JL, Hamdy FC, Lane JA et al. Patient-reported outcomes after monitoring, surgery, or radiotherapy for prostate cancer. *N Engl J Med.* 2016; 375:1425–37.

35. Albertsen PC, Hanley JA, Fine J. 20-year outcomes following conservative management of clinically localized prostate cancer. *JAMA* 2005; 293:2095–101.

36. Robertson C, Close A, Fraser C et al. Relative effectiveness of robot-assisted and standard laparoscopic prostatectomy as alternatives to open radical prostatectomy for treatment of localised prostate cancer: A systematic review and mixed treatment comparison meta-analysis. *BJU Int.* 2013; 112(6):798–812.

37. Coughlin GD, Yaxley JW, Chambers SK et al. Robot-assisted laparoscopic prostatectomy versus open retropubic prostatectomy: 24-month outcomes from a randomized controlled study. *Lancet Oncol.* 2018; 19:1051–60.

38. Bill-Axelson A, Holmberg L, Garmo H et al. Radical prostatectomy or watchful waiting in early prostate cancer. *N Engl J Med.* 2014; 370: 932–42.

39. Wilt TJ, Brawer MK, Jones KM et al. Radical prostatectomy versus observation for localized prostate cancer. *N Engl J Med.* 2012; 367(3):203–13.

40. Dearnaley D, Syndikus I, Mossop H et al. Conventional versus hypofractionated high-dose intensity-modulated radiotherapy for prostate cancer: 5-year outcomes of the randomised, non-inferiority, phase 3 CHHiP trial. *Lancet Oncol.* 2016; 17(8):1047–60.

41. Jones CU, Hunt D, McGowan DG et al. Radiotherapy and short-term androgen deprivation for localized prostate cancer. *N Engl J Med.* 2011; 365:107–18.

42. Bolla M, Maingon P, Carrie C et al. Short androgen suppression and radiation dose escalation for intermediate- and high-risk localized prostate cancer: Results of EORTC trial 22991. *J Clin Oncol.* 2016; 34:1748–56.

43. Nabid A, Carrier N, Martin AG et al. Duration of androgen deprivation therapy in high-risk prostate cancer: A randomized phase III trial. *Eur Urol.* 2018; 74:432–41.

44. Bolla M, de Reijke TM, Van Tienhoven G et al. Duration of androgen suppression in the treatment of prostate cancer. *N Engl J Med.* 2009; 360:2516–27.

45. Prostate cancer: diagnosis and management [NICE guideline NG131] Published date: May 2019. https://www.nice.org.uk/guidance/ng131

46. Brand, H, Tree A, Ostler P et al. Intensity-modulated fractionated radiotherapy versus stereotactic body radiotherapy for prostate cancer (PACE-B): acute toxicity findings from an international, randomised, open-label, phase 3, non-inferiority trial. *Lancet Oncol.* 2019. published online Sept 17, 2019.

47. Donovan JL, Hamdy FC, Lane JA et al. Patient-reported outcomes after monitoring, surgery, or radiotherapy for prostate cancer. *N Engl J Med.* 2016; 375(15):1425–37.

48. Chin J, Rumble RB, Kollmeier M et al. Brachytherapy for patients with prostate cancer: American society of clinical oncology/cancer care ontario joint guideline update. *J Clin Oncol (JCO).* 2017; 35:1737–43.

49. van der Poel HG, van den Bergh RCN, Briers E et al. Focal therapy in primary localised prostate cancer: The European association of urology position in 2018. *Eur Urol.* 2018; 74(1):84–91.

50. Royce TJ, Efstathiou JA. Proton therapy for prostate cancer: a review of the rationale, evidence, and current state. *Urologic Oncology: Seminars and Original Investigations.* 2019 Sep 1; 37(9):628–636. Elsevier.

51. Wang T, Zhou J, Tian S et al. A planning study of focal dose escalations to multiparametric MRI-defined dominant intraprostatic lesions in prostate proton radiation therapy. *The British Journal of Radiology.* 2020 Mar; 93(1107):20190845.

52. Bolla M, Van Tienhoven G, Warde P et al. External irradiation with or without long-term androgen suppression for prostate cancer with high metastatic risk: 10-year results of an EORTC randomised study. *Lancet Oncol.* 2010; 11:1066–73.

53. Mason MD, Parulekar WR, Sydes MR. Final report of the intergroup randomized study of combined androgen-deprivation therapy plus radiotherapy versus androgen-deprivation therapy alone in locally advanced prostate cancer. *J Clin Oncol.* 2015 Jul 1;33(19):2143.

54. Sargos P, Mottet N, Bellera C et al. Long-term androgen deprivation, with or without radiotherapy, in locally-advanced prostate cancer: updated results from a phase III randomized trial. *BJU Int.* 2019 Apr 4.

55. Fosså SD, Wiklund F, Klepp O et al. Ten- and 15-yr prostate cancer-specific mortality in patients with nonmetastatic locally advanced or aggressive intermediate prostate cancer, randomized to lifelong endocrine treatment alone or combined with radiotherapy: Final results of the scandinavian prostate cancer group-7. *Eur Urol.* 2016; 70(4):684–91.

56. Bolla M, van Poppel H, Tombal B et al. Postoperative radiotherapy after radical prostatectomy for high-risk prostate cancer: Long-term results of a randomised controlled trial (EORTC trial 22911). *Lancet* 2012; 380(9858):2018–27.

57. Wiegel T, Bottke D, Steiner U et al. Phase III postoperative adjuvant radiotherapy after radical prostatectomy compared with radical prostatectomy alone in pT3 prostate cancer with postoperative undetectable prostate-specific antigen: ARO 96–02/AUO AP 09/95. *J Clin Oncol.* 2009; 27(18):2924–30.

58. Thompson IM, Tangen CM, Paradelo J et al. Adjuvant radiotherapy for pathological T3N0M0 prostate cancer significantly reduces risk of metastases and improves survival: Long-term followup of a randomized clinical trial. *J Urol.* 2009; 181(3):956–62.

59. Vale C, ARTISTIC meta-analysis of RAVES, GETUG-17 and RADICALS *Proc ESMO* 2019.

60. Parker C. Results of RADICALS radiotherapy timing. *Proc ESMO* 2019.

61. Smith MR, Eastham J, Gleason DM, et al. Randomized controlled trial of zoledronic acid to prevent bone loss in men receiving androgen deprivation therapy for nonmetastatic prostate cancer. *J Urol.* 2003; 169:2008–12.

62. Vale CL, Fisher DJ, White IR et al. What is the optimal systemic treatment of men with metastatic, hormone-naive prostate cancer? A STOPCAP systematic review and network meta-analysis. *Ann Oncol.* 2018; 29:1249–57.

63. Sydes MR, Spears MR, Mason MD et al. Adding abiraterone or docetaxel to long-term hormone therapy for prostate cancer: directly randomised data from the STAMPEDE multi-arm, multi-stage platform protocol. *Ann Oncol.* 2018; 29:1235–48.

64. Burdett S, Boevé LM, Ingleby FC et al. Prostate Radiotherapy for metastatic hormone-sensitive prostate cancer: A STOPCAP systematic review and meta-analysis. *Eur Urol.* 2019; 76:115–24.

65. Small EJ, Saad F, Chowdhury S et al. Apalutamide and overall survival in non-metastatic castration-resistant prostate cancer. *Ann Oncol.* 2019 Nov 1;30(11):1813–20.

66. Hussain M, Fizazi K, Saad F et al. Enzalutamide in men with non-metastatic, castration-resistant prostate cancer. *N Engl J Med.* 2018; 378:2465–74.

67. de Bono JS, Oudard S, Ozguroglu M et al. Prednisone plus cabazitaxel or mitoxantrone for metastatic castration-resistant prostate cancer progressing after docetaxel treatment: A randomised open-label trial. *Lancet* 2010; 376(9747):1147–54.

68. Parker C, Nilsson S, Heinrich D et al. Alpha emitter radium-223 and survival in metastatic prostate cancer. *N Engl J Med* 2013; 369(3):213–23.

69. Mateo J, Carreira S, Sandhu S et al. DNA-repair defects and olaparib in metastatic prostate cancer. *N Engl J Med.* 2015; 373:1697–708.

70. Connell SP et al. A four-group urine risk classifier for predicting outcomes in patients with prostrate cancer. *BJUI* 2919: 124:609–620.

15 COLORECTAL CANCER

Harpreet Wasan and Richard Adams

Introduction

Colorectal cancer (CRC) remains a major cause of cancer mortality in developed countries with an incidence ranking of third in women and men. There have been significant advances in risk prediction, molecular characterization, bowel cancer screening, surgery (including surgery for liver metastases), radiotherapy, and systemic treatments, including novel biological targeted approaches, reflected in improvements in cure and survival rates. Many patients with advanced incurable disease now live for over 2 years, and the options for multi-modal treatment approaches are reflected in the complexity of treatment choices. The next decade will further optimize personalized treatment with molecular and clinical biomarker-driven methods.

Incidence

In the United Kingdom, over 250,000 individuals are living with CRC, and 42,000 new cases are diagnosed annually, with a slight sex bias in males. Just under half die of the disease. The lifetime incidence is 1 in 18 for men and 1 in 20 for women, increasing exponentially with age, with nearly 85% of cases diagnosed in people aged 60 years or more. CRC incidence has slowly decreased, with European rates decreasing from 1% to 2% between 1998 and 2017. Survival rates have more than doubled over the last 30 years with diagnosis and treatment advances. About a quarter of CRC patients present with advanced incurable or metastatic disease, while another quarter will develop metastatic disease after presenting with local disease only. Once metastases develop, only 7% will survive 5 years or more.[1]

Genetic damage accumulation

CRC results from the gradual accumulation of aberrant genetic changes in colonic epithelial cells. As most epithelial cells are shed frequently by apoptosis (also acting as a protective measure against accumulating damage), the accrual is potentially detrimental in putative stem cells residing within the colonic crypt bases. This helps explain the increasing incidence with age and the relative rarity of incidence before 40 years in sporadic cases.[2]

The familial inheritance of specific single-gene defects accounts for a minority of cases (around 5%) in recognized family cancer syndromes and results in both polyps and carcinoma at an earlier age, usually before 50 years. This follows Knudson's "two-hit" hypothesis in that the familial component is present at birth in crucial genes, and the subsequent accumulation of genetic damage required for carcinogenesis is significantly accelerated. This leads to particular clinical phenotypes, described later (see "Associated predisposing conditions"). The key molecular genetic changes by which colonic mucosa progresses through the normal–adenoma–carcinoma sequence (genotype–phenotype correlation) have been extensively described by Fearon and Vogelstein.[3]

Environmental influences (diet and lifestyle)

The association between the environment and the incidence of CRC has long been postulated but has been difficult to quantify in terms of risk individually. More consistency is found in the association of low incidence epidemiologically with high fruit and vegetable intake. A diet high in red meat[4] and saturated fat[5] is associated with increased risk of CRC, as are physical obesity and reduced physical exercise. Risk increases by around 15% in overweight and 33% in obese people. Risk is also associated with "metabolic syndrome" (relative insulin resistance, diabetic risk, hypertension, and hyperlipidemia).

The difficulty of a reductionist approach in identifying specific risk factors within the environment is that evidence from prospective trials does not always confirm the link. Even though a meta-analysis of over 60 human observational dietary studies supports the high-fiber hypothesis,[9] prospective interventional studies of high-fiber supplements have not borne this out. The same reductionist approach to vitamin A, C, and E supplementation as protective antioxidants in lung cancer studies surprisingly led to *increased*, not decreased, risk of cancer in two independent studies.[10,11] Thus, it is not likely that micronutrients in larger than physiological quantities are protective, and they may even be harmful.

The use of non-steroidal anti-inflammatory drugs, including regular aspirin consumption, has been consistently shown in epidemiological studies to confer a reduced CRC risk, although the exact dosage and duration are unknown and must be balanced against the possible side effects of hemorrhagic complications, especially stroke and gastrointestinal ulceration.[12] Intriguingly, recent data have emerged that suggest a specific beneficial interaction between aspirin use and specific mutations (*PIK3CA*) in CRC.[13] A large randomized trial, "Add Aspirin," is testing this hypothesis in four cancers, including CRC, and definitive results should be available by 2022.

Diagnosis and the multidisciplinary team

Presentation of persistent symptoms like change in bowel habit, rectal bleeding (especially altered blood), mucus in the stool, abdominal pain, tenesmus, weight loss, or symptoms/signs of an iron-deficiency anemia should lead to rectal digital examination (PR), proctoscopy, and colonoscopy. The whole colon must be examined if a carcinoma is located in the lower bowel in case of a synchronous tumor elsewhere in the colon. In the elderly or frail, the use of air-contrast computed tomography (CT) colonography is a sensitive and specific alternative, but they will frequently require a pathological biopsy.[14]

Once confirmed, CT of the abdomen, pelvis, and thorax provides the most accurate and rapid practical staging investigation. Serum carcinoembryonic antigen (CEA) should be measured as a potentially helpful indicator and for monitoring if it is elevated at the outset. Magnetic resonance imaging (MRI) is mandatory in planning treatment modalities and sequence in rectal cancer, which is anatomically differentiated from CRC as it requires more complex and skilled treatment strategies. MRI can also be helpful in imaging potentially operable suspected liver metastases.

Modern management of CRC is rapidly increasing in complexity and encompasses the full patient pathway, including diagnosis, staging, and treatment, and managing potential medical and psychological complications. It thus compels a multidisciplinary or team approach. Throughout a patient's cancer journey, the central tenet for the team is providing continuous and optimal care. About one-third of patients present with incurable disease and have higher needs from an extended team at the outset. The challenge is for each clinical case to be analyzed systematically in detail by the colorectal multidisciplinary team (MDT) and to use a contemporaneous evidence-based approach to facilitate the stepwise clinical interventions appropriate by consensus. Recommendations must be made in the best interest of the patient with the primary aim of increasing the probability of disease and symptom control. The team structure includes a core or essential team and an extended team, allowing super-specialist input.

The core team should include:

1. Minimum two specialist surgeons trained and with a special interest in modern techniques in CRC surgery and who have high skill levels in this area. Each surgeon should do at least 20 colorectal resections with curative intent annually. Patients with primary rectal cancer often need complex surgical decisions or interventions, and rectal cancer surgery is rapidly becoming a sub-specialization.
2. Gastroenterologists with expert endoluminal and colonoscopic training. Skilled colonoscopists may be of any discipline (surgeon, physician, or specialist nurse). The criteria for assessing skill in colonoscopy, audits, and training must be agreed by the MDT.
3. Minimum one oncologist. A specialist colorectal (or gastrointestinal) medical oncologist is central in the MDT, with access to clinical trials and expertise in new therapies. Whenever elective surgery is considered for patients with rectal cancer, a radiation oncologist should be involved in discussions before and after surgery.
4. Diagnostic radiologist with gastrointestinal expertise. Training in modern imaging methods such as rectal MRI interpretation and preoperative staging is essential.
5. Histopathologist, preferably with a gastrointestinal specialization, who can report minimum specific datasets for colon and particularly rectal cancer.
6. Advanced nurse practitioners (ANPs) and clinical nurse specialists (CNSs) to provide support, assistance, information, and independent advice to patients. They should have expertise in CRC and be trained in communication skills and counselling. The nurses should ensure that patients' information and support needs are met and link with specialists to provide psychosocial support.
7. Palliative care specialist (doctor or nurse) to work with palliative care services in the community.
8. Meeting coordinator to take responsibility for the administrative processes in organizing MDT meetings. The coordinator should ensure that extended team members such as social workers and psychologists are available when required. The coordinator should also be responsible for feedback about patients referred to more specialized teams and their return to the local CRC MDT. Ideally, an MDT secretary will provide clerical support, recording all team decisions and promptly communicating appropriate written information.

Extended and specialist teams ideally include:

1. Liver/hepatic surgeons who are members of a liver resection MDT and can advise the CRC MDT. They should be embedded within specialist liver treatment centers due to the complexity of care of hepatic interventions.
2. Thoracic surgeon with expertise in lung resection.
3. Interventional radiologist with expertise in liver and vascular staging technologies and interventions, direct tumor targeting (such as radiofrequency ablation [RFA]), and insertion of intestinal stents (although this can also be done by other members of the specialist team).
4. General practitioners/primary care or community linked teams.
5. Dietitian.
6. Liaison psychiatrist/clinical psychologist.
7. Social worker.
8. Clinical geneticist/genetics counsellor.
9. Clinical trials coordinator or research nurse.

Pathology of colorectal tumors

Polyps

Normal large-bowel epithelium has a turnover of approximately 6 days. The proliferative compartment is restricted to the lower third of the crypt. As cells divide and migrate from this zone, they differentiate and lose the ability to divide. In adenomatous lesions, the proliferative compartment enlarges, so the entire crypt and surface may be involved, which, combined with increased longevity of the cells/reduced cell death, results in crypt extension and branching, producing a tubular architecture. In lesions with mesenchymal proliferation, a villous architecture results in a tubulovillous adenoma. A polyp is a protrusion of a circumscribed lesion into a hollow viscus.

Colorectal polyps may be classified according to their architecture and degree of dysplasia, or their origin: epithelial (adenomatous and hyperplastic), hamartomatous (e.g., Peutz–Jeghers and juvenile polyps), inflammatory, lymphoid, and mesenchymal (e.g. lipomas) polyps. The commonest polyps reported by pathologists are adenomatous and hyperplastic lesions. Adenomatous polyps are dysplastic by definition. Whereas many polyps are stalked, some are sessile lesions. Tubular adenomas are composed of greater than 75% tubular glands, villous lesions greater than 50% villous architecture, and tubulovillous adenomas 25–50% villous pattern.[15] The degree of dysplasia is classified as mild, moderate, or severe, based on the cytological features of the lining epithelial cells and an assessment of the neoplastic architecture. Thus, severely dysplastic adenomas show loss of polarity, nuclear enlargement, prominent nucleoli, numerous mitoses, and an often complex branching and cribriform pattern of the glands.[16]

Adenomas are thus benign neoplasms with malignant potential and so are precursor lesions. The risk of invasive malignancy is related to size, architectural subtype, degree of dysplasia, and number of adenomatous lesions in any one patient, although not all adenomas will transform, and the exact risk and time course are not known.[17] Adenomas less than 1 cm in maximal dimension have less than 1% risk of invasive malignancy, compared with 10% for adenomas between 1 and 2 cm in diameter and 50% for adenomas larger than 2 cm.[18] Increasing malignant potential is noted for lesions with a villous architecture and severe dysplasia—the latter is associated with a greater incidence of aneuploidy.[19] Polyps removed endoscopically should always be submitted for histological examination. Adenomatous polyps should be categorized by the pathologist in terms of architecture and dysplasia. Completeness of excision cannot always be evaluated due to poor orientation and fragmentation of the sample.

Typical invasive CRCs develop through the normal–adenoma–carcinoma sequence: a morphological corollary of the multistep theory of neoplasia. Evidence supporting this includes:

- Subjects with familial adenomatous polyposis (FAP) syndrome develop adenomas at an earlier age than is the case with carcinoma.
- Adenomas are six times more common in CRC resections than in control subjects without carcinoma (matched for age, sex, and segment).[20]
- Adenomas are found in 75% of resection specimens for synchronous cancers,[21] and patients with previous adenomas have a greater risk of metachronous cancer development.[22]
- Residual adenomatous change may be found adjacent to invasive carcinoma. This is unusual when examining large tumors histologically, presumably reflecting the destruction of the parent adenoma by the infiltrating tumor edge.

Hyperplastic polyps are not neoplastic and result from a defect in epithelial cell maturation, producing their characteristic histological appearance. These are distinct from serrated adenomas (originally called mixed hyperplastic adenomatous polyps), which combine the low-power architectural appearance of a hyperplastic polyp with the cytological atypia of an adenoma. Longacre and Fenoglio-Preiser[23] described malignant transformation in 10% of serrated adenomas. These were often described as "intramucosal carcinomas" (a controversial term not recognized by all pathologists but equivalent to severe dysplasia in general nomenclature).

Associated predisposing conditions (high risk)

Any insult—genetic or environmental—that leads to damage (including chronic inflammation) of the colonic crypt epithelium can lead to a higher incidence of CRC.

Ulcerative colitis

Tumors in patients with early-onset, longstanding, and extensive ulcerative colitis (UC) are multifocal, flat with a diffusely infiltrating edge, and poorly differentiated.[24] Over 95% of dysplasia occurs in endoscopically normal areas or foci with ill-defined velvety nodular mucosal thickening, distinct from adenomatous polyps in the non-colitis population.[25] Microscopically, mucosal areas are flat or have mixed villiform and tubular architecture and are lined by variably dysplastic epithelium. A confident dysplasia diagnosis is difficult: atypical areas often arise in the bowel involved in active inflammation. Regenerative epithelial atypia may mimic dysplasia, and pathologists must review multiple re-biopsies. Unequivocal high-grade dysplasia should prompt consideration of subtotal colectomy. Fewer than 5% of patients with UC can develop polypoid dysplasia (dysplasia-associated lesion or mass [DALM]). These are endoscopically complex villiform mucosal lesions, distinct from adenomatous polyps. Histologically, they are characterized by a complex arborizing villiform and tubular structure lined by variably dysplastic epithelium. DALM carries an ominous prognosis—Blackstone et al.[26] described coexistent carcinoma in 67% of patients with DALM—requiring urgent extensive colectomy.

Hereditary non-polyposis colorectal cancer

Hereditary non-polyposis colorectal cancer (HNPCC) is an autosomal dominant disorder. The loss of function of DNA mismatch repair deficiency genes (mainly *hMSH2*, *hMLH1*, *hPMS1*, and *hPMS2*) is responsible for a predisposition to increased risk of multiple polyps and CRC. The average age of diagnosis is 45 years, and the overall lifetime risk is 80% in gene carriers.[27] Although the disorder is not associated with the almost carpeting of adenomas seen in FAP (hence the comparative label [but a misnomer] "non-polyposis"), the tumors still arise through the adenoma–carcinoma sequence, but the adenomas appear more "aggressive," with a higher incidence of larger size, abnormal villous architecture, and severe dysplasia.[28] Additionally, the resultant invasive carcinoma is often right-sided, with mucinous differentiation and tumor-infiltrating lymphocytes microscopically, which in young patients, should suggest HNPCC.[29]

HNPCC is associated with other malignancies. Muir–Torre syndrome is a variant in which CRC is associated with sebaceous tumors and keratoacanthomas.[30] The value of the proposed diagnostic criteria in identifying subjects with mutations in HNPCC-associated mismatch repair genes has been evaluated by Syngal et al.[31] (Table 15.1). In practice, patients with suspected HNPCC should be referred for genetic counselling and possible gene testing.

Familial adenomatous polyposis coli

FAP is an autosomal dominant inherited disorder characterized by mutations in the tumor suppressor gene *APC*, located on chromosome 5.[32] The function of the adenomatous polyposis coli (APC) protein is unknown, although it does interact with the cell adhesion molecule catenin.[30] *APC* gene mutation is an early and critical event in the development of CRC. The study of this gene has led to our major understanding of the molecular pathogenesis of the common (i.e., non-hereditary) forms of CRC (see "Molecular pathogenesis" section). In FAP, the colorectum is carpeted with hundreds to thousands of adenomatous polyps occurring at a mean age of 16 years, and unless prophylactic colectomy supervenes, 90% will have one or more invasive cancers by 45 years.[33] In Gardner's syndrome, colorectal adenomatous polyps are associated with osteomas and desmoid tumors. Turcot's syndrome colonic polyposis is associated with central nervous system tumors; one-third of subjects have mutations in DNA mismatch repair genes and develop glioblastoma multiforme.[34] Attenuated FAP is a variant of FAP characterized by far fewer adenomas, which are typically right-sided and relate to mutations in the first hundred or so codons of the gene. This is one of the first known examples of phenotypic–genotypic correlations in molecular genetics.[35]

Most CRCs occur in families with no known inherited gene defect and unaffected by polyposis syndromes. There is a two- to fourfold increased risk if a first-degree relative has CRC,[33,36] which is further increased if more than one first-degree relative is affected and they are under 50 years. Specific genetic mutations are not known. Pilot studies in CRC patients under 30 years have shown that 41% have *MMR* gene mutations.[37] The risks for people with these mutations of developing CRC by the age of 70 are approximately 91% for men and 69% for women.[39] A number of polymorphisms with a moderate effect on risk have also been described, including variants in the *APC*, *HRAS1-VNTR*, and *MTHFR* genes.[40]

Molecular pathogenesis

The histological progression of normal large-bowel mucosa through adenoma to carcinoma[41] is the commonest (80%) type of CRC development. The earliest mutation is *APC*. Wild-type *APC*

TABLE 15.1 Clinical Criteria for HNPCC

Name	Criteria
Amsterdam[a]	Three relatives with CRC, one of whom is a first-degree relative (FDR) of the other two; CRC involving at least two generations; one or more CRC cases diagnosed before the age of 50
Amsterdam I[b]	1. Very small families, which cannot be further expanded, can be considered as Lynch (HNPCC) even if only two CRCs in FDRs; CRC must involve at least two generations, and one or more CRC cases must be diagnosed under age 55
	or
	2. In families with two FDRs affected by CRC, the presence of a third relative with an unusual early-onset neoplasm or endometrial cancer is sufficient
Amsterdam II	Three relatives with an HNPCC-associated tumor (CRC, endometrial, small bowel, ureter, or renal pelvis), one of whom is an FDR of the other two; involving at least two generations; one or more cases diagnosed before the age of 50
Revised Bethesda criteria[b38]	CRC in patients <50 years of age
	A pt with two primaries (synchronous/metachronous CRCs or two Lynch-related cancers)
	CRC with MSI or histological features of Lynch in a pt <60
	Two or more pts—one with CRC and the other an FDR with a Lynch-related tumor, at least one diagnosed <50
	Three or more pts—two with CRC, and a third with a Lynch-related tumor, at any age
	CRC in a pt <50
	Lynch-related tumors include CRC, small-bowel cancer, endometrial and renal tract plus ovarian, gastric, pancreas, biliary tract, and primary brain (especially glioblastoma), sebaceous adenoma, and keratoacanthoma

Source: Syngal et al., 2000.
Note: HNPCC is now termed Lynch.
[a] All criteria must be met.
[b] Meeting all the features listed under any of the numbered criteria is sufficient.

encodes a cytoplasmic protein found in the highest density in the upper portion of crypt epithelium. It interacts with β-catenin and is thought to be important in the transmission of contact inhibition stimuli into cells.[42] *APC* is a tumor suppressor gene and therefore acts in a recessive manner. FAP subjects inherit a germline mutation of one *APC* allele. The mutant *APC* gene protein product may form a heterodimer with the *APC* gene protein product from the unaffected allele, preventing normal function. This mechanism occurs in sporadic CRC cases following a somatic mutation of one allele. Mutation of one *APC* gene allele can be followed by deletion of the normal allele. This may be a consequence of genomic instability with flawed segregation of chromosomal material during mitosis. This loss of heterozygosity (LOH) results in loss of normal tumor suppressor function with clonal expansion and proliferation. *APC* mutations have been found in adenomas less than 1 cm in size, and the rate of mutation is similar in adenomas and carcinomas, further endorsing the role of *APC* as the initial critical "gatekeeper" step in tumorigenesis.[43] The *KRAS* oncogene then mutates. The wild-type gene encodes a protein with GDP/GTP-binding domains and is important in intracellular signal transduction.[44] As oncogenes act in a dominant manner, mutation in only one allele is required to inhibit normal function. The enlarging adenomas can then develop further mutations in the *P53* gene and including deletions in DCC. The *DCC* tumor suppressor gene region (containing the SMAD family of genes), located on chromosome 18, encodes a transmembrane protein with structural homologies to the cell adhesion molecule NCAM.[45] Mutation in this gene confers a metastatic capacity to the tumor cells.[41,45] Wild-type *P53* is the most widespread mutation in human cancers.[46] It is located on the short arm of chromosome 17 and is important in the control of the cell cycle, programmed cell death, and DNA repair and synthesis.[47] Thus, *P53* mutation allows unregulated cell growth. Genetic studies indicate that *P53* loss is a late event, occurring after mutations within the *DCC* region and corresponding histologically to the development of invasive carcinoma in an adenomatous polyp.[48]

BRAF oncogene mutations are exclusively associated with serrated polyp morphology and may account for a significant subset of CRC (10–20%). These tumors tend to be the most aggressive of all CRCs with a poor prognosis (see "Treatment" section). BRAF mutant polyps and cancers commonly methylate a defined subgroup of CpG islands, a phenomenon called CpG island methylator phenotype (CIMP). Conversely, CRC tumors with mismatch repair instability (microsatellite instability [MSI] or microsatellite deficient) have a good prognosis, with higher cure rates (prognostically better) but interestingly, with less cytotoxic chemosensitivity in the adjuvant setting.

Pathology of invasive colorectal cancers

Macroscopic appearance

The gross morphology of CRCs may be polypoid, fungating, ulcerative, or diffusely infiltrating.

Microscopic appearance

Scattered neuroendocrine and Paneth cells may occasionally be evident. Mucinous carcinomas are characterized by strips and sheets of neoplastic glandular epithelium bathed in lakes of mucin (the latter being >50% of the tumor). Undifferentiated carcinomas are characterized by sheets of undifferentiated malignant cells with vesicular nuclei and prominent nucleoli typically located in the caecum. Cancers can have (mixed) small components of rarer variants, including small-cell carcinoma and primary colorectal signet-cell carcinoma. The former is an aggressive tumor, histologically indistinguishable from its pulmonary counterpart and biologically similar.[54] Some 50 cases have been reported in the literature of primary colorectal signet-cell carcinoma.[55] Gastric signet-cell carcinoma or breast lobular carcinoma should be excluded before confirming a primary diagnosis of CRC. Goblet-cell tumors are rare and predicting their behavior remains uncertain; they have also been classified as "carcinoid," but these tumors do not behave like classical carcinoids (or neuroendocrine tumors) of the gastrointestinal tract and are never secretory.

Prognostic factors

Staging

The mucosal origin of bowel cancers allows tumors to infiltrate circumferentially or longitudinally along the bowel. Typically, macroscopic assessment correlates well with microscopic spread, and a 2 cm distal margin of excision is adequate, as the risk of undetectable tumor growth beyond this is negligible.[56] Complete circumferential excision for rectal tumors is important and represents a successful total mesorectal excision (TME). The circumferential margin (CRM) is the area below the peritoneal reflection anteriorly, continues to the posterior wall, and extends superiorly into the triangular "bare area" up to the sigmoid mesocolon. Pathologically, the CRM is involved if tumor is less than 1 mm from it.[56] Positive CRM involvement determines local recurrence and predicts poorer overall survival.[57] The 5-year survival rate of rectal carcinoma is 40–70%, mainly due to local recurrence rates of 5–40% even in curative procedures.[58]

High–spatial resolution MRI of the rectum is the best method for local staging.[59]

Most of the colon and the anterior wall of the rectum are covered by serosa. Ulceration of this by tumor constitutes a breach of the peritoneum and a route for the dissemination of malignant cells into the abdominal cavity. Colonic tumors with microscopic serosal surface ulceration by tumor resulted in peritoneal recurrence in 50% of cases.[60] Although typically, metastases involve nodes sequentially corresponding to the anatomical sequence of drainage, in advanced carcinomas, node blockage "upstream" by tumor can result in retrograde lymph-node spread. The 5-year survival for Dukes' C (Stage III) with one node positive is 63.6%, but falls to 2.1% when more than 10 nodes are involved. At least 12 lymph nodes are needed for accurate staging.[61] The routine analysis of hematoxylin and eosin sections of nodes is as sensitive as ancillary techniques in identifying tumor involvement compared with using additional CEA and epithelial membrane antigen (EMA) immunohistochemical techniques (Table 15.2).[62] Studies that have re-staged patients after additional immunohistochemical examination for micro-metastases have failed to show any difference in predicting 5-year survival.[63] Furthermore, tumor may disseminate via the portal venous system to the liver and in low rectal carcinomas, via the inferior hemorrhoidal veins directly to the lungs. Prognosis is adversely affected when thicker-walled-caliber extramural veins are involved.[64] Similarly, newer technologies in routine detection of circulating tumor cells (CTCs) or residual postoperative total circulating free DNA thought to be shed from residual cancer cells (ct- or cf-DNA) have suggested additional prognostic value, but are rarely used in routine clinical practice to guide clinical decision making.

Dukes' staging (tumor, node, metastasis [TNM]) remains the most important prognostic indicator. Dukes' A tumors infiltrate into the submucosa or muscularis propria, do not breach the bowel wall, and are without lymph-node metastases (90–95% 5-year survival); Dukes' B tumors extend further into mesorectal or pericolic fat but without lymph-node involvement (45–80% 5-year survival); Dukes' C tumors have loco-regional lymph-node involvement (23–50% 5-year survival).[66] Dukes' C is subdivided into C1 (apical node-negative) and C2 (apical node-positive) with 5-year survival rates of 40.9% and 13.6%, respectively.[61] Dukes' D represents distant metastases.[67]

The American staging system classifies CRC as Stages I to IV, broadly correlating with Dukes' A to D (Box 15.1). The American Joint Commission on Cancer (AJCC) and Union Internationale Contre Cancer developed TNM and assessed CRCs by the extent of local invasion, lymph-node status, and presence or absence of distant metastases.[68] The AJCC[69,70] regularly updates after multidisciplinary consensus conferences to develop a progressive classification system of prognostic markers and so keeps updating the exact classification.

BOX 15.1   CORRELATION OF STAGING SYSTEMS

Stage	T (Primary tumor)		N (Node metastases)	M (Distant metastases)	Dukes classification
Stage 0	Tis	Carcinoma in situ	N0	M0	
Stage I	T1 or T2	Invades submucosa or muscularis propria	N0	M0	A
ᵃStage II	T3	Invades through the muscularis propria into subserosa or into non-peritonealized pericolic or perirectal tissues	N0	M0	B
	T4ₐ ₒᵣ ᵦ	Perforates visceral peritoneum (T4a) or directly invades or adherent to other organs / structures (T4b)ᵃ	N0	M0	
*Stage III	Any T		N1	M0	C
	Any T		N2, N3	M0	
Stage IV	Any T		Any N	M1	D

Notes: Dukes B and C are both composites of better and worse prognostic groups.

*   AJCC (2018) subdivides both Stages II and III into A to C.[170]

Abbreviations: N1, Metastasis in 1–3 pericolic/perirectal nodes; N2, Metastasis in 4+ pericolic/perirectal lymph nodes; N3, Metastasis in any lymph node along course of named vascular trunk.

See further: Dukes and Bussey, 1958; O'Dwyer et al., 2001.

Prognostic factors

Different countries use variations of the AJCC system. The AJCC Working Party recommends TNM groups be stratified with the presence/absence of elevated serum levels of CEA ($\geq$5 ng/mL) on preoperative examination. Additionally, appendiceal carcinoma should be excluded from CRC staging because of fundamental differences in natural history. In 2017, the U.K. National Institute for Health and Care Excellence (NICE) mandated that every patient *must* have molecular markers assessed to detect and refer all cases of suspected HNPCC as a means of cancer prevention in families.

TABLE 15.2   **Incidence of Positive Tumor Markers at Different Stages of Disease**

Dukes' stage	5-Year survival (%)	Raised CEA (%)	Raised CA19-9 (%)
A	80	4	11
B	50	26	31
C	30	44	26
Distant metastases	<5	65	49

Abbreviation: CA19-9, carbohydrate antigen 19-9.

Treatment

Surgery

For tumors involving the caecum and ascending colon, the ileocolic, right colic, and right branch of the middle colic arteries are divided at their origins. The mesocolon is dissected from the right ureter, duodenum, pancreas, and gonadal vessels, and the entire right colon and the greater omentum are removed. An anastomosis is formed between the terminal ileum and the mid-transverse colon. Similar principles are used for transverse and descending colon tumors, the anastomosis being made between ascending and descending colon or transverse and sigmoid colon, respectively. In the sigmoid colon, the inferior mesenteric artery is ligated at its origin with the aorta, and the anastomosis is made, after mobilization of the splenic flexure, between the descending colon and the rectum.

The principles applied to curative surgery for rectal cancer are governed by the blood supply to the rectum from the inferior mesenteric artery, the middle rectal branches of the internal iliac artery laterally, and the pudendal vessels. Anal sphincter function must be preserved whenever possible and damage avoided to the parasympathetic pelvic nerves, which would cause impotence and bladder dysfunction.

Tumors above the levator ani muscle and anal sphincter are resected by anterior restorative resection through the abdomen. The inferior mesenteric artery is ligated and the rectum and mesorectum removed, but without node dissection on the lateral pelvic wall. Local recurrence is minimized by TME, although fecal continence may be impaired if the anastomosis is very low.[71] A colonic reservoir immediately proximal to the anastomosis may improve functional results,[72] although there may be some difficulty in spontaneous defecation after this modification. The rectum is divided at least 1 cm[73] below the tumor and anastomosis made between the sigmoid colon and the rectum or anal canal. Most surgeons use a circular stapler to achieve a secure low colorectal or colo-anal anastomosis, although excellent results can be achieved by hand-sewn anastomosis.[74] The place of protective colostomy or ileostomy after low anastomosis remains contentious. There appears to be little evidence that either the incidence of anastomotic leakage or the mortality following such a leakage is improved, but it is likely that pelvic floor contamination may impair later continence.

Laparoscopic-assisted surgery for CRC has been widely adopted, and data from large-scale randomized trials supporting its use been extensively published. In the Medical Research Council (MRC) CLASSICC trial,[75] apart from patients undergoing laparoscopic anterior resection for rectal cancer, rates of positive resection margins were similar between treatment groups. Patients requiring conversion to open surgery had raised complication rates. Leung et al.[76] investigated patients with the more difficult anatomical location of recto-sigmoid carcinomas and found that laparoscopic resection did not jeopardize survival (5-year survivals for the laparoscopic and open resection groups were 76.1% [SE, 3.7%] and 72.9% [SE, 4.0%], respectively). The probabilities of being disease free at 5 years were 75.3% (SE, 3.7%) and 78.3% (SE, 3.7%), respectively. Appropriate patient selection, surgical training, and a need for further information about long-term outcomes are ongoing issues.

Low rectal carcinomas

Rectal cancers adjacent to or invading the levator ani and anal sphincter muscles can only be cured by removing these structures.

Abdominoperineal excision (APE) surgery is identical to anterior restorative resection as far as the abdominal part of the operation is concerned. Synchronously, the anal canal, the contents of the ischiorectal fossa, and the entire levator ani muscle are removed by a perineal approach, often referred to as extralevator APE (ELAPE). ELAPE is an anatomical concept, and although popularized to be performed in the prone position by Holm et al.[77] (2007), it may be adequately completed in the supine Lloyd–Davis position.[78] One aspect of an ELAPE is the larger perineal defect, and either a surgical flap or a biological mesh is considered to result in optimal wound healing. A permanent colostomy is constructed, usually in the left iliac fossa, but preoperative fitting is essential so that the precise position of the stoma can be tailored to the patient's needs.

Locally extensive tumors

About 10% of large-bowel tumors, particularly pelvic, are adherent to adjacent organs due to either inflammatory fibrosis or malignancy. Resection of adjacent organs is achieved with reasonable safety in non-metastatic disease, and survival results are comparable to those for tumors confined to the rectum or colon.[79,80] Complete pelvic exenteration for primary or recurrent local disease has a high morbidity and mortality, but careful selection may occasionally achieve worthwhile survival times.[81] Preoperative radiotherapy allows the removal of advanced tumors, potentially converting CRM-positive tumors into margin-negative resections with reduced morbidity[82] and with a lower incidence of local recurrence.[83]

Incompletely resectable tumors

Controversy exists in terms of a resectable but asymptomatic primary tumor in the face of incurable metastatic disease. Clinical trials to define optimum care have proved difficult to recruit to, although case series suggest potential survival advantages to resection. Endoscopic stenting of distal colonic (non-rectal) tumors may provide adequate immediate palliation in certain symptomatic incurable cases but in the longer term, is associated with increased morbidity with its own complications.[84,85] Endoscopic laser ablation[86] may also potentially relieve obstruction. Routinely symptomatic primary tumors should be bypassed or removed if they do not benefit from radiotherapy or systemic chemotherapeutic approaches.

Operative mortality and morbidity

Operative mortality for non-emergency resections of potentially curable cancers is less than 5%. Sepsis predominates the common surgical complications. The rate of anastomotic leakage among surgeons is 1–10%. Temporary and rarely, permanent impotence in male patients may occur if there is damage to the pelvic parasympathetic nerves, and both sexes may suffer bladder dysfunction.

Obstructing and perforating cancers

Emergency operations in this setting have significantly higher peri-operative mortality and worse long-term survival.[87] National Bowel Cancer Audit (NBOCAP) data indicate that emergency surgery occurs in 10–13% of all CRC patients in the United Kingdom.[171] The 30- and 90-day mortality figures, for elective/scheduled surgery were 2.6% and 3.8%, respectively, versus 8.6% and 13.4% for emergency surgery. The management of obstructing or perforated carcinoma of the left colon is controversial: some prefer staged resection and others primary resection and anastomosis. In the United Kingdom, the St. Mary's Hospital Large Bowel

Cancer Project[88] included 713 patients with malignant large-bowel obstruction. Immediate anastomosis in the obstructed left colon had a high clinical leak rate, but the mortality of primary resection was no greater than the cumulative mortality of the staged procedure. Primary resection has the advantage of a much-reduced hospital stay.[89–91] Better results are achieved by more experienced surgeons whichever policy is adopted.[92–94]

Local recurrence

Although the place of routine follow-up after surgery for CRC has been questioned,[95] there is evidence that an aggressive approach and attempted surgical resection of any local recurrence can be worthwhile.[96,97] A rise in CEA level above the baseline level established after a primary resection[98,99] seems to be a sensitive indicator of recurrence (local or systemic). Not all tumors secrete CEA, however.

Local or anastomotic recurrence often presents with recurrent bleeding, tenesmus, pain, incontinence, and eventual obstruction. If the initial procedure was an anterior restorative resection, treatment can be with abdominoperineal (AP) resection,[100] but often, further radical surgery is impossible.[101] Small recurrences may be palliated with the NdYAG laser.[102]

Radiotherapy

The potential clinical indications for radiotherapy (often with radiosensitizing chemotherapy) are to:

- Enhance the outcome of operable disease in local control and to improve survival
- Facilitate potentially difficult surgery
- Treat extensive inoperable disease:
  - rendering it operable
  - obtaining long-term local control or possibly eradication
  - controlling symptoms
- Conserve anal function as:
  - an adjunct to surgery
  - exclusive treatment

These are achieved by:
- tumor mass reduction
- local elimination of small-volume disease to reduce local recurrence/a source of potential metastasis
- local elimination of disease allowing a watch-and-wait non-surgical approach
- elimination of micro-metastases

See Table 15.3.

Rectal carcinoma

Radiotherapy with surgery

Reviewing results for the likelihood of recurrence, Hager et al.[103] found that patients with only mucosal involvement had a local recurrence rate of 8%, with a 90% 5-year survival. Patients with muscular invasion had a recurrence rate of 15% with a 58% 5-year survival. A high-risk group with incomplete resection had a recurrence rate of 24%, with 61% surviving at 4 years. Other studies show similar results. Approximately one-third of patients have Dukes' A (T1N0 and T2N0) tumors, for which the local recurrence rate is less than 5%. For non-adherent Dukes' B (about one-third of cases), the recurrence rate is approximately 10%, and for adherent tumors or node-positive tumors (Dukes' B3 and C), approximately the remaining one-third of cases, recurrence rates are 20–70%. The desired effect of adjuvant treatment is to reduce local recurrence and increase survival. The former can be achieved, but the latter has proved more elusive.

Preoperative radiotherapy

Data show that preoperative radiotherapy reduces local recurrence rates compared with surgery alone. There is less clarity on whether radiotherapy improves overall survival, as most trials have failed to show any difference.[104–109] A consensus has been published that aimed to establish the risks and benefits of preoperative radiotherapy followed by TME, using the Delphi technique, in the United Kingdom, the Netherlands, and Sweden. Major and minor complication criteria, including, for example, anastomotic leak, hemorrhage, fistula, and sepsis, which would lead them to reconsider preoperative radiotherapy, were suggested by colorectal surgeons.[109] The aim of these criteria is to allow a risk–benefit assessment of the application of preoperative radiotherapy and therefore to evaluate treatment.

A meta-analysis involving 22 randomized trials and 8507 patients reported that the yearly risks of local recurrence were 46%, and 37% lower in those who had preoperative (biologically effective dose ≥30 Gy) and postoperative radiotherapy, respectively, compared with surgery alone. However, there was no significant difference in overall survival among those who had received radiotherapy (62% died) versus surgery alone (63% died).[110] However, the preoperative group did have a reduced cancer-related mortality of 45% compared with 50%. The aim is to increase sphincter preservation, especially in low rectal tumors, and therefore avoid AP resection. Overall, these data show that preoperative radiotherapy reduces local recurrence rates compared with surgery alone. There is less clarity on whether

TABLE 15.3   Applications of Radiotherapy

	Location in rectum	Preoperative RT, short-course	Preoperative RT, long course or chemo/RT	Postoperative chemo/RT	RT	Chemotherapy alone or chemo/RT	Surgery
Low-risk T1, T2, operable	High rectal						+
Low-risk T1, T2, operable	Low rectal	?+			?		+
(Tethered) T2, T3, operable	High rectal					+	+
(Tethered) T2, T3, operable	Low rectal	++				+	+
Inoperable/CRM involved	Any		++			+	?
Macroscopic or microscopic residual tumor (R1/R2)				+			+
Recurrence			++				+
Node positive			++	?		+	+

Abbreviations: RT, radiotherapy; chemo, chemotherapy.

radiotherapy improves overall survival, as most trials have failed to show any difference, including CRO7.

Chemoradiation: Preoperative versus postoperative

In a 2012 Phase III randomized trial, 805 patients were allocated to preoperative arm 50.4 Gy in 28 fractions with 5-day infusional 5-fluorouracil (5-FU) on weeks 1 and 5, followed by maintenance chemotherapy, or the same regimen to the postoperative group with a further 5.4 Gy boost (Sauer et al.[111]). The acute toxicity was tolerated well in both groups, with the postoperative period having complications of 12% in both instances. The overall survival data were 76% versus 74% for the preoperative and postoperative arms, respectively ($p = 0.80$), and 5-year disease-free survival of 68% versus 65% (Sauer et al.[111]). Although no survival benefit was achieved, there was again minimal difference in surgical morbidity in both groups. The adapted surgery data, potentially based on tumor shrinkage after neoadjuvant chemoradiation, in this trial are particularly interesting to many. Surgeons were asked to indicate their surgical operation preference for the individual patient prior to randomization, and this was compared with the actual surgery performed. In the neoadjuvant group, 40% of patients initially assessed as requiring an APE underwent a sphincter-sparing procedure compared with fewer than 20% in the postoperative (adjuvant) group. Follow-up revealed local recurrence rates of 7.1% versus 10.1% in favor of the preoperative group and 10-year overall survival rates of 59.6% versus 59.9%, suggesting that such adaptive surgery in selected patients may be feasible and safe.[111]

Capecitabine use in chemoradiation

Whereas 5-FU has been the mainstay of treatment, oral preparations of fluoropyrimidines are increasingly used. The oral pro-drug capecitabine is part of the management in adjuvant and metastatic settings. A German Phase III trial compared adjuvant 5-FU plus radiotherapy with adjuvant capecitabine plus radiotherapy. The 5-year overall survival rates were 66.6% and 75.7%, respectively.

A further preoperative Phase II trial[112] gave capecitabine (825 mg/m^2 twice a day on days 1–14 and 22–35) and oxaliplatin (initial dose 50 mg/m^2 on days 1, 8, 22, and 29, which was then escalated in steps of 10 mg/m^2) concurrently with 50.4 Gy in 28 fractions of radiotherapy. Patients had T3–4 adenocarcinoma of the rectum, tumors close to the levator sling, any T stage with M1 disease requiring surgery to primary tumor, or locally recurrent disease. The dose-limiting toxicity of diarrhea occurred at 60 mg/m^2, so the oxaliplatin dose was capped at this level. Surgery was measured at 6 weeks following completion of chemoradiotherapy. Primary endpoints included downstaging (59%), negative lymph nodes (68%), and pathological complete response (CR) at the resection margin (19%), suggesting significant tumor reduction, which facilitated sphincter-preserving surgery in 36% of cases. Oxaliplatin toxicity included sensory neuropathy and Grade 2 leucopenia. Compliance was noted in 89%, and all patients received full-dose radiation. The regimen was well tolerated, and the results suggest that the combination may have a role in future management.

Preoperative radiotherapy for anus preservation

Preoperative radiotherapy for low and/or locally advanced (T3 and T4) tumors results in anal sphincter preservation in about 80% of cases and a 5-year survival of about 80%. Chemoradiation may be even more effective.

Dose response to radiotherapy

Low doses are generally ineffective compared with higher doses. In one report, the relapse rate was only 10% if the radiotherapy dose was equal to or greater than 45 Gy but 50% if the dose was lower than 40 Gy.[117] There seems little doubt that there is a dose–response effect.[114] However, at doses beyond 50–54 Gy for external-beam radiotherapy, toxicities rapidly increase without significant evidence of additional benefit or tumor downstaging. More conformal radiotherapy with intensity-modulated radiotherapy is beginning to enter clinical practice without a significant evidence base and is likely to result in lower toxicity acutely. However, it remains to be seen whether this will alter late toxicities. Such techniques will generally result in a lower dose of radiotherapy to the small bowel but will not generally reduce doses to anal sphincters and levator muscles.

Timing of surgery following radiotherapy

It is important to leave at least 4–6 weeks for regression of bulk tumor to occur. However, some have favored surgery at 7–10 days post-radiation, when tissues are relatively easy to dissect. The earlier timing ensures that any residual tumor is seen and resected. The Stockholm studies[104] recommend surgery less than a week from radiotherapy completion. Conversely, many surgeons prefer to operate once the reaction has settled and the tumor has shrunk further. Recent trials have explored a greater delay before surgical resection. The only trial (Lyon R90-01) to report at the time of writing on the optimal interval post-radiotherapy randomized between under 2 weeks and 6–8 weeks, demonstrating an increase in T and N downstaging in those undergoing a longer deferral; retrospective series appear to concord.

A treatment deferral or "watch-and-wait" policy has been used to closely monitor patients who may not require surgical intervention. As many as one-fifth of patients have high-quality radiological and pathological responses to neoadjuvant radiotherapy. These patients generally have good oncological remissions. This strategy may be useful in patients deemed by the MDT to be elderly, less fit or high-comorbidity. However, longer delays in treating some patients post-radiotherapy may allow progression and proliferation of clonogenic cells and reduced efficacy for adjuvant therapy if metastases become more deeply rooted. International registries look at outcomes and surveillance of these patients, and early data suggests that even with local recurrence, most patients can be salvaged by delayed surgery. There is significant heterogeneity of patients selected for this approach and of methods employed to identify them, so it cannot be recommended as a standard of routine care. A U.K. prospective randomized clinical trial comparing 6 versus 12 weeks is accruing at the time of writing to definitively address this issue.

Localized inoperable tumors

This includes patients with previously untreated primary advanced disease and those with recurrent disease who have received either surgery alone or surgery and radiotherapy or all three modalities, and the approach depends on the treatment already given, disease extent, and the general patient status. Supraradical surgery with extended dissections can be attempted to excise extensive tumor, and long-term control may be achieved.

Radical radiotherapy

Radiotherapy alone may be as effective as surgery in controlling disease if major surgery is contraindicated. In one retrospective report of patients with recurrent disease, both time to recurrence and overall survival were similar in both groups.

Preoperative radiotherapy and chemoradiation for localized inoperable tumors

Doses of 45 Gy or more have been used, allowing resection in 50–75% of cases, but long-term control is only achieved in 25–35%. Mendenhall et al.,[118] using 33–60 Gy, reported that resection became possible in most cases (37 out of 42); half were complete and half incomplete, resulting in 5-year survivals of 14% in those with incomplete resection and 29% with complete resection. Most would now use chemoradiation in this situation.

Intraoperative radiotherapy

The Mayo Clinic[119] used 45–55 Gy given by external radiotherapy and an intraoperative boost of 10–20 Gy. There was a local failure rate of 17%, and the overall 5-year survival rate of 25% was not greatly enhanced compared with the previous studies of preoperative external-beam therapy alone. Likewise, the Massachusetts General Hospital reported using 50.4 Gy in 5.5 weeks with an intraoperative boost of 10–20 Gy. In this study, 70% of patients went on to achieve complete surgical clearance, and the early report of 3-year survival was 60%.[120] Both studies had worse results with recurrent disease than with primary locally advanced disease. More recent studies combined chemoradiation as primary treatment with intraoperative radiotherapy and reported improved overall survival.

Postoperative radiotherapy for residual macroscopic disease and/or recurrent inoperable disease

Where residual disease remains apparent and preoperative radiotherapy has not been given, radiotherapy can be offered. There are no randomized studies. Local recurrence rates vary from 15% to 76%, but 5-year survival is more consistent at around 25%.[121]

Perhaps the most promising approach remains with preoperative radiotherapy and chemotherapy, but randomized studies are needed to establish this.

Locally advanced disease: Palliative radiotherapy

Patients with relapsed locally advanced disease may still achieve good local response and good palliation. Even patients who were previously irradiated will tolerate up to 30 Gy.

Advances in radiotherapy and chemoradiotherapy

To date, the use of additional chemotherapy to 5-FU or capecitabine as radiosensitizers has not shown clear overall benefits: acute toxicities have been severe. Cetuximab (immunoglobulin G1) monoclonal antibody (mAb) to the epidermal growth factor receptor (EGFR) ligand-binding domain and bevacizumab (vascular endothelial growth factor [VEGF] inhibitor) are being assessed in clinical trials but are not recommended outside research settings.

Radiotherapy techniques

Principles of radiotherapy

The treatment volume and dose given depend on the amount of tumor present and/or the risk of tumor recurrence, and normal-tissue tolerance. For "standard" preoperative radiotherapy, a uniform dose to the whole pelvis has been used. With a bulky or inoperable tumor, a proportionally higher dose may be needed for the tumor itself, achieved using a shrinking volume technique. Likewise, if surgery cannot be contemplated, a shrinking volume technique is again appropriate.

For postoperative radiotherapy, treatment can be tailored to the operative findings. Where excellent local clearance is achieved, a uniform field to the pelvis, to include the tumor bed and pelvic nodes at risk, is appropriate, but if there is an area of high risk of local recurrence, this can be boosted by the shrinking volume technique.

For palliative radiotherapy, lower doses, such as 3000 cGy in 10 fractions or 2000 cGy in five fractions, can be given by the simple technique of anterior and posterior fields.

For the treatment of colonic carcinoma, similar principles apply, although in general, it is difficult to avoid the small bowel, and therefore, either reduced doses or a reduced margin to the tumor must be used to limit the exposure of the small bowel, but small-bowel problems are likely in some 5% of patients.[122]

Regions at risk and tissue tolerance

The use of anterior and posterior fields for postoperative radiotherapy at the MD Anderson Cancer Center, with the upper margin of the fields extending up to L2, resulted in a 17.5% incidence of small-bowel obstruction compared with only 5% in those who had surgery alone. When the fields were altered to an upper limit of just below L5, the incidence dropped to below 10%.[123] In practice, therefore, the paraaortic and high pelvic nodes are seldom included unless there are special indications.

The internal iliac and presacral nodes are at high risk of metastatic involvement and should be included in the radiotherapy field. External iliac nodes are not usually involved unless there has been invasion of pelvic organs such as the prostate, bladder, vagina, or uterus.

Recommended treatment volume

To cover the regional nodes, the pelvic volume extends from the bottom of L5 to the upper side of the anal canal for high tumors and includes the anal canal for lower tumors. The perineum need only be included if it is at special risk or after an AP resection. Bolus may help to make the dose more uniform. Posteriorly, the field includes the sacrum, thus encompassing the presacral nodes and the sacral canal. Anteriorly, the margin may be more difficult to define with a plain film only. If the anterior margin is taken to just behind the symphysis pubis, this will cover the primary lesion, the adjacent prostate, base of bladder, vagina, and internal iliac nodes, although to include the external iliac nodes, the field would need to come to the front of the symphysis pubis.

If a high-risk area requires an additional dose over and above the small-bowel tolerance of 40–50 Gy, or if palliative radiotherapy is the objective, where minimal bowel toxicity is required, the reduced high-dose volume is best planned by CT.

Inclusion of the perineum adds considerably to the acute morbidity, but there has not been a reported increase in chronic complications. After AP resection without radiotherapy, a perineal recurrence rate as high as 23% has been reported, but following radiotherapy including the perineum, the incidence was only 2% at the Mayo Clinic.

Radiotherapy planning, field arrangements, and doses

Localization may be achieved by simulator or CT planning. The patient is best treated prone, and the bladder should be full to minimize small bowel in the pelvis. A marker wire is placed over the lower anal margin to help identify the anal canal. On the lateral projection, the rectum is generally clearly outlined by the normal rectal air, although a contrast tampon in the vagina may be a useful aid. Immobilization body molds also help with accuracy, and small-bowel contrast helps identify small bowel where a large amount of small bowel is potentially being irradiated.

TABLE 15.4 Factors Potentially Increasing Normal-Tissue Damage from Radiation

Radiotherapy related	Non-radiotherapy related
Total dose	Pelvic inflammatory disease
Large fraction size	Hypertension
Short overall treatment time	Diabetes mellitus
Low radiation energy	Obesity
Large treatment volume	Concomitant chemotherapy or biological therapy
Prior pelvic irradiation	Immunocompromise (primary or secondary)
	Genetic disorders, e.g., Li Fraumeni, ataxia telangiectasia

A direct posterior field and two lateral fields are commonly used, or two post-oblique fields may be used. Lateral fields allow perhaps a slightly easier assessment of shielding of normal tissues. Areas prone to a brisk reaction and delayed healing include the natal cleft and perineum, and provided these areas are not at risk, they can be easily shielded by appropriate leading of the lateral fields.

Using fractionated radiotherapy, doses of 40 Gy in 20 fractions to 50 Gy in 30 fractions are used, to which a boost to a reduced volume of a further 10–20 Gy may be added, provided small bowel is excluded from the field.

Complications of radiotherapy

Perhaps the most common and serious complications of radiotherapy are to the small bowel, although reactions occur in the perineum also (Table 15.4).

Acute reactions include the small-bowel symptoms of diarrhea and abdominal cramps, and the large-bowel effects of acute proctitis with urgency and frequency, tenesmus, and occasionally a bloody or mucous discharge. Urinary frequency and dysuria may occur. Skin erythema may be particularly troublesome in the skinfolds of the natal cleft and perineum. Acute effects occur 2–3 weeks into a course of fractionated radiotherapy, generally resolving within a few weeks of stopping the treatment.

Delayed reactions may persist in carrying on from acute reactions or may develop after a latent period of 6–18 months (Box 15.2). In one retrospective study, ileus occurred in 8% of cases without radiotherapy but in 23% with radiotherapy, and surgery was required in only 4% of those without radiotherapy versus 21% in those receiving radiotherapy.[124] Infertility is inevitable if the gonads are included in the radiation field and may occur even if they are close to the edge of the field.

BOX 15.2 LATE RADIATION COMPLICATIONS

- Chronic diarrhea
- Proctitis
- Rectal blood loss
- Rectal pain
- Small-bowel obstruction
- Small-bowel perforation
- Perineal and scrotal tenderness
- Delayed perineal healing
- Bladder atrophy and bleeding
- Sacral necrosis
- Infertility

To minimize the risk of reactions, the factors listed in Table 15.4 should be taken into account. Total dose is the ultimate criterion, but for maximum therapeutic benefit and minimum toxicity, fractions should probably be 200 cGy or less. A linear accelerator with 8–15 MV electrons is optimal, and the treatment volume should be carefully assessed, being planned by computer to avoid hot spots and to limit the amount of bowel in the field. The other non-radiotherapy-related factors and medical conditions are difficult to quantify, but some allowance may need to be made.

Where radiation tissue damage has developed, a conservative approach is often successful. For radiation proctitis with troublesome intermittent bleeding, which may demand recurrent transfusions, local instillation of formalin has been reported to be effective (and simple) in controlling the bleeding.[125] If surgery has to be embarked upon, fresh tissues are needed to assist healing, such as un-irradiated omentum or full-thickness pedicle skin flaps.

Chemotherapy

The same principles as for colon cancer apply to patients with rectal cancer who have not undergone chemoradiation. (In patients who have received chemoradiation, the role of adjuvant chemotherapy remains unclear.)

Adjuvant chemotherapy

Adjuvant chemotherapy in CRC is given to eliminate micro-metastatic residual disease in order to reduce the risk of recurrence and improve survival. Until recently, 5-FU formed the mainstay of adjuvant treatment. More recently, capecitabine, oxaliplatin, and irinotecan have been studied for adjuvant treatment of colon cancer.

Dukes' stage C. The first large study reporting a significant benefit of adjuvant chemotherapy with 5-FU in patients with Dukes' stage C colon carcinoma was reported in 1990 by Moertel et al.[126,127] The 5-days–4-weekly schedule used has since been shown to be more toxic than other schedules but was confirmed efficacious in the large QUASAR Colorectal Cancer Group Study,[128] although the comparison was non-randomized. Less toxicity and equal efficacy were found with an infusional regimen of 5-FU/folinic acid (FA) over 2 days every 2 weeks.[129] Capecitabine, a 5-FU pro-drug given orally, is convenient and has comparable efficacy.[130] The addition of oxaliplatin to 5-FU/FA for adjuvant treatment was investigated in the pivotal MOSAIC trial. In this trial, the combination was reported to improve disease-free survival significantly in patients with Dukes' stage C cancer.[131,132] Peripheral sensory neuropathy is a common side effect of oxaliplatin. Although it is reversible in most patients, 1% of patients experienced persistent Grade 3 peripheral sensory neuropathy 1 year after completion of treatment. Improvement of 3-year disease-free survival with 5-FU/FA and oxaliplatin was confirmed in a second U.S. trial using a weekly bolus regimen.[133] In contrast to oxaliplatin, the addition of irinotecan to 5-FU failed to reveal a significant improvement in disease-free survival.[134,135] This has led to the recommendation to offer oxaliplatin routinely to Dukes' C, node-positive cancer patients.

Dukes' stage B. Dukes' stage B has been included in several randomized trials of adjuvant chemotherapy, along with stage C. However, proving unequivocal benefit and the magnitude of the benefit has been difficult. The benefit of adjuvant treatment in Dukes' stage B cancer is supported by two meta-analyses. The National Surgical Adjuvant Breast and Bowel Project (NSABP) investigators[137] analyzed four trials, including 1565 patients with Dukes' B tumors. They compared the patient groups receiving the best regimen (usually 5-FU and FA) with the patients with the worst outcome (either no treatment or other chemotherapy regimens). The cumulative odds of death in the Dukes' B group were 0.7, which was statistically significant. The IMPACT B2 investigators pooled data from five trials with 1016 patients.[138] At a median follow-up of 5.75 years, they found hazard ratios for event-free survival and overall survival of 0.83 and 0.86, respectively, but this benefit did not reach statistical significance. In addition, results from the MOSAIC trial showed a small and statistically non-significant improvement in disease-free survival in higher risk, Dukes' stage B disease. Although adjuvant treatment for all Dukes' stage B cancers still remains contentious for all patients, there is increasing evidence of benefit for patients with adverse prognostic features, including bowel obstruction and perforation, so its use in these cases should be considered, since this group of patients has a worse prognosis than some Dukes' stage C patients.

Unfortunately, other newer doublet combinations with 5-FU, such as irinotecan and triplets, with the addition of biological agents (the anti-EGFR antibody cetuximab and the anti-VEGF antibody bevacizumab, which are also discussed under metastatic tumor therapy), have disappointingly not shown any additional benefits over MOSAIC in large randomized studies. Thus, the standard of care for adjuvant chemotherapy remains FA, 5-FU, and oxaliplatin (FOLFOX) (or its equivalent, oxaliplatin and capecitabine [CAPOX]) for Dukes' C colon cancer. For Dukes' B cancer, the risk assessment can favor no adjuvant treatment versus monotherapy with capecitabine or 5-FU, or in higher-risk patients (at the potential expense of a risk of permanent neuropathy), FOLFOX or CAPOX. For the latter, there has been no prospective randomized study unequivocally demonstrating the additional benefit of oxaliplatin, even in the higher-risk Dukes' B patients. Newer risk assessment tools using molecular signatures are now available, and some trials have validated them retrospectively, but the cost-benefit analysis for their use is not generally accepted.

Since the pivotal MOSAIC trial, no further progress in improving overall survival in unselected Dukes' B and C patients has been made. The addition of a third agent to FOLFOX, either cetuximab or bevacizumab, was not superior. Neither was their equivalence when switching from oxaliplatin to irinotecan. However, approaches to reduce treatment toxicity and improve the quality of life in patients by giving shorter-duration FOLFOX or CAPOX chemotherapy have been successfully tested. In the United Kingdom, the SCOT trial, which was also part of a larger global initiative (the IDEA collaboration), demonstrates that 3 months duration versus the standard 6 months, in most subsets of patients, is a non-inferior approach with a significant reduction in neuropathy risk, improved quality of life, and improved health economics.[180]

Another major advance in adjuvant therapy is only within the subset of patients whose tumors have MSI, including Lynch syndrome. The strongest evidence is for patients with Dukes' B/ Stage II–MSI, in that they have *no* benefit from adjuvant chemotherapy, so this can be avoided. Indeed, these patients have a better prognosis after curative surgery alone than their commoner equivalent non-MSI (microsatellite stable [MSS]) counterparts. It is postulated that MSI tumors engender random immune activation as a mechanism of eliminating tumor cells, as they are hypermutated, and generate epitopes that are then distinguished as foreign (non-self).

Metastatic and locally recurrent tumors

Choice of treatment: chemotherapy, radiotherapy, and palliative treatment (best or active supportive care)

Chemotherapy forms the mainstay of treatment for inoperable metastatic colon and rectal cancer (mCRC). A Cochrane collaborative meta-analysis of a subset of trials that provided individual patient data compared palliative treatment with chemotherapy with 5-FU. Chemotherapy with 5-FU resulted in a median survival of 11.7 months, compared with 8 months in the control group, and improved survival at 6 and 12 months by 16%.[139] The systemic treatment options for patients with mCRC have evolved considerably following the introduction of new drugs in the 1990s, including the pairing of 5-FU with the cytotoxics oxaliplatin and irinotecan. The addition of targeted biological agents incorporated into triplet (three drug) regimens was the second major stepwise improvement in mCRC. The anti-EGFR antibody cetuximab (Figure 15.1) and panitumumab and the anti-VEGF antibody bevacizumab are now incorporated into the standard of care as the first choice for many patients. In parallel, more convenient oral analogues of 5-FU, notably capecitabine, are now frequently incorporated. It then became evident that anti-EGFR

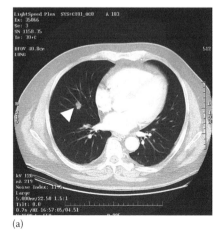
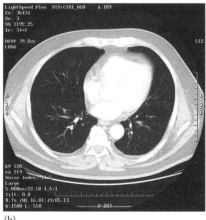

(a)   (b)

FIGURE 15.1   Response of recurrent rectal carcinoma to cetuximab and irinotecan after becoming refractory to irinotecan, fluorouracil, and folinic acid. The arrow shows a lung metastasis, which was no longer detectable after treatment.

antibodies only had efficacy in tumors without constitutive activation of the RAS-RAF-MEK oncogenic pathway, so that in mCRC with mutations in KRAS, NRAS, and BRAFV600E their activity is so significantly reduced or absent as to make them ineffectual. With these agents, the average survival of mCRC improved to 2–2.5 years.

In the last decade, the development of the new active oral agents trifluridine-tipiracil and the tyrosine kinase inhibitor regorafenib has allowed over half of patients to receive third and fourth lines of treatment after the failure of two lines of systemic therapy, and the survival of mCRC patients has overall improved further to the 2.5- to 3.5-year range, with the greatest benefit in cancers without any mutations in RAS and BRAFV600E genes. Superimposed on this is better selection of patients for the right therapy integrated with smaller subsets that benefit from integrated strategies for oligo-metastatic or liver-confined metastases, so that around 10% of patients can now survive 5 years.

Since 2018, there is evidence of potential personalized benefits in small, selected subgroups with rarer molecular characterization, including immunotherapy with checkpoint inhibitors in: MSI tumors (<4%), those with HER2 inhibition (<2%), NTRK (<1%), and BRAFV600E inhibition (<10%). The last is discussed later as representing a potential paradigm shift.[140]

The role of EBRT is limited in metastatic disease, but patients with relapsed locally advanced disease may still achieve a good local response and good symptom palliation.

Chemotherapy regimens are summarized in Box 15.3.

BOX 15.3 COMMONEST CHEMOTHERAPY REGIMENS (*N.B. ALL 5-FU/CAPECITABINE REGIMENS SHOULD IDEALLY BE PRE-TESTED FOR DPYD DEFICIENCY*)

MODIFIED DEGRAMONT (5-FU) 14-DAY CYCLE

FA 350 mg (flat dose) intravenous (i.v.) in 250 mL 0.9% sodium chloride over 2 h
5-FU 400 mg/m² i.v. bolus then 5-FU 2400 mg/m² i.v. via infusion pump over 46 h

FOLFIRI OR IRMDG 14-DAY CYCLE

Irinotecan 180 mg/m² i.v. in 250 mL 0.9% sodium chloride over 60 minutes with Modified DeGramont (acute cholinergic symptoms [diarrhea, abdominal cramps, sweating, salivation/lacrimation] atropine 0.25 mg subcutaneously)

FOLFOX OR OXMDG 14-DAY CYCLE

Oxaliplatin 85 mg/m² i.v. in 250 mL 5% dextrose over 2 h with modified DeGramont
Capecitabine (oral 5-FU equivalent) monotherapy 21-day cycle 1250 mg/m² b.d. PO for 14 days
Capecitabine can be combined with both Oxaliplatin or Irinotecan as CAPOX or CAPIRI
There are 21- and 14-day regimens. The most commonly used is CAPOX 21 days
Oxaliplatin 130 mg/m² i.v. in 500 mL dextrose 5% over 2 h with Capecitabine 1000–1250 mg/m² b.d. days 1–14
Cetuximab (EGFR inhibitor) monotherapy weekly (if no mutations in RAS)
Pre-meds Chlorphenamine 10 mg i.v. bolus and Dexamethasone 8 mg i.v. bolus

Cycle 1 Loading dose: cetuximab 400 mg/m² i.v. 2 h. *N.B.*: Infusion rate must not exceed 10 mg/min
Cycle 2 *onwards* cetuximab 250 mg/m² i.v. 1 h
Cetuximab is usually combined as a triplet regimen every 14 days with either FOLFIRI or FOLFOX as earlier, allowing 1 h gap after the cetuximab infusion, i.e., Cetuximab–oxaliplatin–5-FU (cetuximab-OxMdG) and Cetuximab–irinotecan–5-FU (cetuximab-IrMdG)
Bevacizumab (VEGF inhibitor) is usually combined as a triplet regimen every 14 days with either FOLFIRI or FOLFOX as earlier, i.e., Bevacizumab–oxaliplatin–5-/FU (Bev-OxMdG) and bevacizumab–irinotecan–MdG (Bev-IrMdG). The first infusion of bevacizumab is infused over 90 min. If well tolerated, it is reduced to 60 then 30 min
FOLFOXIRI—three cytotoxics combined at 14-day intervals: Oxaliplatin 85 mg/m², Irinotecan 165 mg/m², Leucovorin 200 mg/m², and 5-fluorouracil 3200 mg/m² infusion over 46 hours
FOLFOXIRI, with the addition of Bevacizumab at 5 mg/kg at 14-day intervals

Trifluridine-tipiracil: 35 mg/m² PO BD on Days 1–5 and Days 8–12: 28-day cycle (not to exceed 80 mg/dose)

Regorafenib: 160 mg PO OD days 1–21: 28-day cycle

Only for Braf mutation in mCRC (second line)
Encorafenib 300 mg PO once daily and Cetuximab (standard weekly dosing as earlier)

Nivolumab and Pembrolizumab: Immune checkpoint inhibitors approved in some countries for dMMR/MSI–high mCRC

Fluoropyrimidines. 5-FU is the mainstay of almost all CRC chemotherapy and inhibits the enzyme thymidilate synthetase (TS), which leads to the depletion of deoxythymidine triphosphate, thus interfering with DNA synthesis and repair. An enhancement of this effect is seen when 5-FU is combined with FA, which prolongs the inhibition of TS activity and hence, the interference of DNA synthesis produced by 5-FU, through stabilization of the ternary complex of 5,10-methylene tetrahydrofolic acid with the 5-FU metabolite FdUMP and TS. Response rates with 5-FU bolus alone are low (10–15%). The effect is dose and schedule related, with infusions over a minimum of 24 h associated with increased response rates. Biomodulation with FA also increases response rates and can improve symptom control in more patients. Meta-analysis has confirmed a twofold increase in tumor response of 21% compared with 11% and a small but statistically significant overall survival benefit of 11.7 compared with 10.5 months.[141] The side effects of 5-FU and FA include mucositis; this manifests principally as diarrhea, which may be severe and even life threatening, particularly in patients with congenital variants in reduced 5-FU degradation. It should be treated promptly with high-dose loperamide and dehydration avoided. Subsequent dose reductions will normally prevent recurrence. Myelosuppression is uncommon in infusional regimens. Most patients become fatigued during chemotherapy lasting over 3–6 months. Infusion of 5-FU is associated with a dermatitis involving the hands and feet (palmar–plantar syndrome or erythrodysesthesia), which is now known *not* to be relieved, as originally thought, with oral pyridoxine supplements. The potential life-threatening cardiac ischemia (angina) of 5-FU, due to a vasospasm-inducing 5FU-metabolite, indicates the need for caution and patient guidance, as it is often idiosyncratic (occurring in patients without pre-existing heart disease) and rapidly reversible on stopping the drug.

Raltitrexed is a more potent TS inhibitor and can be given at 3-weekly intervals due to its pharmacokinetics. One trial was terminated early due to an unexpectedly high treatment-related death rate.[142] Because of this, there are reservations about the use of this drug, as there are reasonable alternatives in the form of 5-FU and FA and capecitabine. However, it remains available as an alternative to 5-FU or capecitabine in patients who develop angina (coronary vasospasm) on fluoropyrimidines, which is a serious, potentially fatal, and under-recognized serious side effect (in up to 3% of patients).

Oral fluoropyrimidines. 5-FU is absorbed erratically (0–80%) and is thus not useful by this route. *Capecitabine* and, less commonly used, *UFT* (uracil and tegafur) have been developed to give sustained and predictable serum levels after oral administration. Capecitabine is an orally bioavailable pro-drug of 5-FU. Thymidine phosphorylase is required for activation, and this enzyme is also overexpressed in some CRCs, particularly in response to tumor hypoxia. Treatment with capecitabine in mCRC has been shown to be equally effective compared with 5-FU/FA.[143] Myelotoxicity was found to occur with lower intensity than with 5-FU/FA, but diarrhea and palmar–plantar syndrome were experienced more frequently. On the basis of these data, capecitabine is increasingly replacing 5-FU because of greater patient convenience and reduced hospital costs.

Irinotecan is a topoisomerase-I inhibitor with SN-38 as the active moiety. It blocks DNA replication mediated by the enzyme and induces single-strand DNA breaks, which inhibit replication. Treatment with this topoisomerase-I inhibitor alone produced response rates of 11–23% in Phase II studies of patients with CRC whose tumors were resistant to 5-FU. A further 40% of patients showed stabilization of tumor for a median of 5 months.[143] The most common adverse effects include diarrhea, nausea and vomiting, myelosuppression, asthenia, alopecia, and cholinergic syndrome; the last effect occurs at the time of administration and can be mitigated by atropine.

Two randomized trials of irinotecan have shown survival benefit, with the 1-year survival being increased by 13% and 22.4% compared with palliative therapy[144] and 5-FU infusion, respectively.[145] Patients whose tumors progressed within 6 months of 5-FU showed a significant, though small, survival advantage following treatment with irinotecan.

Combinations of irinotecan with 5-FU and FA showed synergy in pre-clinical studies, and clinical combination regimens were developed and have become a standard of care globally. Randomized comparison of the combination with 5-infusional FU and FA showed significantly higher response rates for the combination in two trials[146,147] and a survival improvement of 17.4 versus 14.1 months. A 2-weekly combination with infusional 5-FU/FA (FOLFIRI) is favored over the original 3-weekly irinotecan monotherapy due to increased diarrheal toxicity with the latter.

Oxaliplatin belongs to a group of platinum compounds synthesized to include the 1,2-diaminocyclohexane-carrier ligand. Oxaliplatin intercalates in DNA to cause bulkier adducts than cisplatin and is effective in cisplatin-resistant cell lines, possibly through greater resistance to DNA repair. Low single-agent response rates of 10–20% were reported, and in Phase I trials, a unique reversible cold-related peripheral neuropathy was dose limiting, but the ototoxicity and renal toxicity seen with cisplatin were largely absent. Synergy with TS inhibitors and with topoisomerase-I, reported in pre-clinical studies, led to subsequent clinical trials of oxaliplatin in combination with 5-FU and FA, with higher response rates of 40–50% in previously untreated patients and 20–40% in patients who had relapsed after 5-FU/FA. In randomized controlled trials, oxaliplatin with 5-FU/FA (FOLFOX) demonstrated significantly higher response rates, of 51% versus 22%, and a disease-free survival of 9 versus 6.2 months compared with 5-FU/FA alone. However, the number of CRs remained low (for a review, see the study by Raymond et al.[148]). There is Phase II evidence that oxaliplatin given for metastases confined to the liver may increase survival when combined with subsequent resection of liver metastases.[149]

Choice, timing and sequencing of first-line chemotherapy in advanced disease

With both oxaliplatin and irinotecan combinations showing efficacy in colon cancer, the question of which of these doublets should be used as first choice has been tested in a sequencing Phase III trial by Tournigand et al.[150] This compared oxaliplatin and 5-FU followed by irinotecan and 5-FU with the reverse sequence and found no significant difference in median survival. A larger trial in the United States showed modest superiority for oxaliplatin in terms of response rate and time to progression; however, the availability of second-line chemotherapy was imbalanced.[151] It appears, therefore, that the choice of drug for first-line treatment remains a question of patient preference after discussing the different toxicity profiles with their oncologist, and that after 4 months of oxaliplatin use, many patients develop a persistent neuropathy, which is irreversible in some.

Triplet combinations with or without biological agents

After over 40 years of frustratingly slow progress with conventional cytotoxics, the last 15 years have been remarkable due to the realization of new active agents of different biological mechanisms of action with specific molecular targets, which have incrementally improved response rates and overall survival over and above 5-FU and best supportive care (BSC) alone. The chemotherapeutic agents irinotecan and oxaliplatin now form part of the doublet chemotherapy approach (with 5-FU/LV) in the majority of patients worldwide, in the form of FOLFOX (or CAPOX) or FOLFIRI. There has also been a recent resurgence of using three cytotoxic agents combined: FOLFOX plus irinotecan (FOLFOXIRI regimen; see later).

Two targeted biological agents that are more cancer-mechanism specific, with less conventional toxicity profiles, are also now used additionally (although they are limited in some countries due to their high cost). These are an anti-VEGF mAb, bevacizumab, and the human EGFR (HER-1 or EGFR)-targeted mAb, cetuximab (and subsequently, panitumumab). However, as the number of available agents and the survival increase, choosing the most effective treatment strategy becomes increasingly complex and progressively more expensive, as more lines of therapy are being offered in palliative situations as sequential combinations. The expertise required to choose the best pathway for the patient requires both significant experience in mCRC and the support of the MDT.

Inhibiting angiogenesis in mCRC: VEGF: Bevacizumab, a VEGF inhibitor, in combination with cytotoxic chemotherapy (but not alone) in the first- and second-line settings in patients with mCRC has significant additional activity. In a pivotal study, over 900 patients were randomized to one of three treatments with bolus 5-FU: Irinotecan+5FU/leucovorin (IFL)+placebo, IFL+bevacizumab, or FU/LV+bevacizumab. The addition of bevacizumab to IFL resulted in a significantly increased response rate, duration of response, and progression-free survival and improved overall survival by almost 5 months (20.3 vs. 15.6 months; $p < 0.001$). For the subgroup of patients who received second-line therapy with oxaliplatin-containing regimens, overall survival times were 25.1 and 22.2 months for the IFL/bevacizumab and IFL/placebo arms, respectively.[140] There are similar second-line survival benefit data with oxaliplatin–5-FU and bevacizumab combinations. Chemotherapy with bevacizumab is generally well tolerated, with few, if any, overlapping toxicities with cytotoxics. Adverse events include bleeding, thrombosis, proteinuria, and hypertension, which are generally manageable. However, a low percentage of patients (~2%) have serious gastrointestinal events, including bowel perforation, thrombosis, or bleeding. Also, there has to be caution with respect to healing following VEGF inhibitors (and chemotherapy), especially in complex multidisciplinary pathways requiring liver, vascular, or surgical intervention.

Two new agents with anti-angiogenesis activity gained registration after 2012 for second-line use with FOLFIRI chemotherapy after positive results from large-scale (Phase III) randomized studies as alternatives to bevacizumab. Aflibercept was the most attractive in principle of all the VEGF inhibitors because of its wide-ranging activity in multiple parts of the angiogenesis pathway. Aflibercept is formed from the fusion protein of key domains from human VEGF receptors 1 and 2 with human IgG Fc1 and blocks all human VEGF-A isoforms, VEGF-B, and placental growth factor (PlGF)-2; indeed, at such high affinity that it binds VEGF-A and PlGF more tightly compared with the native receptors. Mechanistically, aflibercept is a VEGF trap as opposed to a pure VEGF ligand inhibitor such as bevacizumab. The Phase III VELOUR study of aflibercept and FOLFIRI in second line (after failure of an oxaliplatin regimen) showed a significant survival advantage, even in patients showing resistance after prior bevacizumab exposure. However, it has a more toxic profile than bevacizumab and so has gradually fallen out of favor. The second agent, ramicirumab, is more specific for VEGF-R2 inhibition and also demonstrated survival advantage in a Phase 3 study with FOLFIRI in second line and is very well tolerated, like bevacizumab.

Inhibiting the HER-1/EGFR signaling pathway in mCRC: The EGFR-RAS-RAF-MEK growth pathway is thought to play a pivotal role in tumor growth and progression of colorectal and other cancers, where EGFR overexpression is correlated with disease progression, poor prognosis, and reduced sensitivity to chemotherapy. EGFR belongs to the HER family of receptors. These receptors are transmembrane glycoproteins with an extracellular ligand-binding domain and an intracellular tyrosine kinase (TK) domain. Ligands that bind to the HER-1/EGFR extracellular domain induce receptor homo- or heterodimerization with other HER-1/EGFR receptor or family members. This results in activation of the receptor's TK activity, initiating a downstream signaling cascade that ultimately leads to tumor cell proliferation, migration, inhibition of apoptosis, and angiogenesis. Cetuximab was the first antibody with potent EGFR-inhibitory activity. Demonstrable activity with cetuximab plus irinotecan chemotherapy in patients with irinotecan-refractory

CRC showed response rates of around 23%.[148] Unfortunately, responses did not correlate with the degree of EGFR expression as predicted by pre-clinical studies. First-line randomized trials with cetuximab combinations with irinotecan (FOLFIRI regimen in the CRYSTAL study) have now established this as a standard of care. More importantly, the clinical–translational work arising led to the first definitive molecular biomarker of non-response to EGFR inhibitors in mCRC. Thus, mutation detection within the important *RAS* oncogene, common in CRC (50–60%), leads to resistance to the effects of cetuximab and thus predicts for non-response and is therefore of no benefit in the majority of mCRC patients. Conversely, where there is no RAS mutation, cetuximab shows significantly higher response rates than combinations with bevacizumab. This makes triplet combinations with EGFR inhibitors a very attractive, if not the *de facto*, option in neoadjuvant therapy for potentially operable metastatic disease (i.e., downsizing of inoperable liver metastases to operable ones; see later). Cetuximab's most common Grade 3/4 adverse events are hypersensitivity, asthenia, fatigue, malaise, and lethargy. More curiously, an acne-like rash typically associated with HER-1/EGFR inhibition is also observed. Panitumumab is another equivalent humanized version of cetuximab developed later and in clinical use. Testing for RAS mutations on diagnosis of mCRC is thus essential to optimize the best first treatment choices for patients.

Randomized studies comparing strategies of VEGF vs. EGFR inhibition, such as the FIRE-3 study, as the superior option suggest that in RAS wild-type mCRC, EGFR inhibition, especially in left-sided colon cancers (see later), conveys the largest overall survival benefit of up to 7.5 months over first-line VEGF inhibition strategies.

Drugs used in third-line or later lines of therapy in mCRC

About 30–40% of patients who do not have mutations in the RAS oncogene, and have not had prior exposure to EGFR inhibition in earlier lines, will potentially gain benefit in tumor shrinkage and overall survival with either cetuximab or panitumumab as monotherapy. More recently, it appears that if there has been around 12 months or more of a treatment interval after prior first-line exposure of cetuximab, which was beneficial (i.e., and then no exposure to EGFR inhibition in second line), then re-challenge with EGFR inhibition can be successful for a few months in third line or later. This is due to a "resetting" of the tumor biology of emergent resistant RAS clones (detectable in blood as ctDNA on using EGFR inhibitors), which rise during EGFR-treatment selection pressure and then reduce again on stopping treatment.

For patients with RAS mutant tumors, or patients who are RAS wild type and who progress on third-line EGFR inhibition, there are two conventional oral treatment options developed after 2015: *Trifluridine-tipiracil (TAS-102)* and *regorafenib*. For both, their positive benefits were confirmed in two separate Phase III double-blind trials in mCRC, compared with placebo, but they have never been compared with each other, and it is unknown whether they still convey benefit if both are used sequentially. Trifluridine-tipiracil is a combination of a thymidine-based nucleic acid analog, trifluridine, and a thymidine phosphorylase inhibitor, tipiracil hydrochloride. Trifluridine is the active cytotoxic component of TAS-102; its triphosphate form is incorporated into DNA, instigating antitumor effects. Tipiracil hydrochloride prevents rapid degradation of the trifluridine, allowing maintenance of adequate plasma levels of the active drug. In the pivotal Phase III RECOURSE trial with refractory colorectal cancer, the median overall survival improved from 5.3 months with placebo to 7.1 months with TAS-102, and the hazard ratio for death in the TAS-102 group versus the placebo group was 0.68 (95% confidence interval [CI], 0.58 to 0.81; $p < 0.001$).

Regorafenib is an oral multi-kinase inhibitor predominately of the angiogenesis pathway and has shown a significant survival advantage, after failure of all known chemotherapy (i.e., in the salvage setting), compared with BSC in the CORRECT trial. Interestingly, all patients had received prior bevacizumab, and the median overall survival improved to 6.4 months for regorafenib vs. 5.0 months on placebo (hazard ratio [HR]: 0.77; $p = 0.0052$). The response rate was under 2%.

Thus, both these oral agents only work in a small minority (fewer than 20%) of patients and stabilize disease with very low response rates for a few months. Trifluridine-tipiracil has a better tolerability profile but is more myelosuppressive than regorafenib, which has more symptomatic toxicities, particularly hand-foot syndrome and fatigue, which can be a challenge to manage in patients with poorer performance status.

Quadruplet regimens (four drug combinations) of FOLFOXIRI plus bevacizumab have also been shown to have significant efficacy with proven benefit in overall survival in Phase III trials with very high response rate but at the expense of significant toxicity. Patients, especially with RAS mutant tumors, who are fit with many symptoms and high disease burden may benefit from this approach. The TRIBE and TRIBE-2 studies have studied the relative benefit of this approach, but the incremental value of the bevacizumab component has not been clearly established, and the future options following the failure of these four drugs are limited. Thus, the majority of mCRC patients will receive a doublet or triplet as the first-line standard of care. An understanding of the principles of systemic chemotherapy and rapidly evolving standards of care generated from Level 1 evidence (adequately powered randomized Phase III multicenter trials) is very important in the context of a starting framework in the MDT discussion on mCRC, especially if it is planned to integrate multiple interventions, as certain sequences of treatment may be better tolerated as well as being more efficacious.

Prediction of response to chemotherapy: CRC biomarkers and application in practice

The development of high-throughput techniques such as whole genome and exon next generation sequencing (NGS), which can give results within hours both in tissue and increasingly, in small blood samples (cell-free[cfDNA] or circulating tumor DNA [tDNA]), has led to the first steps of a personalized approach to predicting and treating CRC. RAS, BRAF, and MSI are the minimum pre-requisites that need to be known via these methods (and including immunohistochemistry) before a treatment can be initiated. The application of more complex signals with DNA microarray expression or transcriptomic profiling, proteomic profiling, comparative genomic hybridization analysis, and metabolomics will also eventually (but currently only as research tools) significantly enhance the potential of predicting patient outcomes and response to treatment.

Historically, initial studies focused on the effect of assaying proteins in relation to predicting 5-FU efficacy, as this was the only active mCRC drug. Tumor TS quantification and subsequently, expression were studied, with high levels of TS found to predict poor response to treatment with 5-FU,[152,153] and in a number of studies, high levels of TS predicted worse survival for Dukes' stage B and C patients.[152,154] A subset of patients have been described with low TS expression who do not respond to 5-FU

and for whom a different mechanism of resistance appears likely. TS gene polymorphisms were also investigated for the prediction of outcome and toxicity, since this could affect transcription and translation of the TS gene.[155] Dihydropyrimidine dehydrogenase (DPD) catalyzes the rate-limiting step in the catabolism of 5-FU, and tumor levels of DPD have also been reported to determine response.[156] Patients with genetic variants determining DPD deficiency experience profound systemic toxicity, including death after small doses of 5-FU or capecitabine in homozygotes. In practice, TS levels have not been reliable in predicting response and have fallen out of favor, especially as combination therapy has made single-drug biomarkers less relevant. Routine blood DPD testing, however, has gained traction in some European countries in predicting and avoiding rare lethal 5-FU (and capecitabine) drug toxicities, as has testing in the United States for UGT1A polymorphisms for irinotecan toxicity. RAS mutations are prognostic and predict for poorer overall survival; they are now tested routinely in mCRC to identify early which patients will and will not derive benefits from EGFR inhibition (as discussed earlier in this chapter).

Genomic instability (MSI) leading to hypermutation and BRAFV600E mutations: Paradigm shifts

Genetic instability at the DNA level, which includes MSI and Lynch syndrome, occurs as a result of DNA replication errors. Mutations with functional effects in any of the complex genomic replication, detection, and repair systems that are responsible for ensuring that replicated DNA is of perfect fidelity can lead to DNA errors and eventually, a hypermutated genome. MSI (also known as mismatch repair-deficient [dMMR]) is found in 15–20% of primary colonic cancers, but in metastatic disease, it is less common at around 4%, as MSI tumors relapse less frequently. Microsatellites are sections of DNA in which a short sequence of DNA is repeated multiple times. MSI is classified when a microsatellite has gained or lost repeat units and has undergone a change in length, which results in frame-shift mutations or base-pair mutations, or both. It is typically associated with DNA mismatch repair defects, in particular mutations in the mismatch repair genes *MLH1*, *MSH2*, *MSH6*, and *PMS2*. Studies exploring the correlation of MSI with response to chemotherapy in MCRC are controversial but increasingly suggest no, or poor, response to conventional cytotoxic chemotherapy. In the adjuvant Dukes' B setting, chemotherapy confers no benefit; MSI is both prognostic and predictive of non-response and a favorable prognostic factor and should be tested routinely.[157,158]

High somatic mutation loads or high tumor mutation burden (TMB) leads to immune activation in tumors with MSI, and this has translated into encouraging efficacy of single-agent programmed cell death protein 1 (PD1) checkpoint inhibitors in mismatch repair-deficient CRC, in contrast to lack of efficacy in unselected mismatch repair-proficient or stable (MSS) populations. Hypermutation rates are not exclusively found in tumors with MSI. DNA polymerase-ε (*POLE*)-mutated tumors that show microsatellite stability, for example, also harbor high neoantigen loads, immune stimulation, and tumor-infiltrating lymphocytes in their microenvironment. To avoid immune attack, multiple immune checkpoint receptors are adaptively hijacked by *POLE*-mutated tumor cells and upregulate PD-L1, supporting the use of PD1 mAb as therapy. Pembrolizumab is a humanized IgG4 monoclonal antibody that binds to PD-1 with high affinity, preventing its interaction with PD-L1 and PD-L2. It was investigated in this regard in a pivotal Phase II study in 11 patients with MSI/

dMMR colorectal cancer, 21 patients with MMR-proficient/MSS mCRC, and nine patients with MSI/dMMR rarer metastatic non-colorectal cancers. The response rates were remarkable at 40%, 0%, and 71%, respectively. MSI is thus a powerful predictive marker for the effectiveness of PD1 mAb therapy across tumor types. Similar results have been seen with other immune checkpoint strategies such as nivolumab (humanized IgG4 PD-1 blocking antibody). When nivolumab was combined with a second immune-stimulation agent, ipilimumab (CTLA-4 inhibitor), in MSI mCRC, the early results are more impressive, although at the expense of increased toxicity.

Larger clinical trials are ongoing to confirm the benefit of these drugs in both the adjuvant and the mCRC setting.

Although immune checkpoint inhibitors are generally well tolerated, serious adverse reactions, specifically immune-mediated, occur in 20% to 45% of patients, especially to the skin, liver, kidneys, gastrointestinal tract, lungs, and endocrine systems. Pneumonitis, potentially leading to fatality, occurs in around 5% of patients on pembrolizumab or nivolumab. Immune therapies can thus be transformational for some patients who achieve high-quality tumor responses.[172]

As alluded to in other sections of this chapter, mutations in CRC of the BRAF gene are developmentally important in a subset of CRC and occur in around 10% of patients, invariably with mutations at codon 600 (or V600EBRAF). This results in a substitution to glutamic acid from the native valine, which functionally, constitutively activates downstream MEK phosphorylation and thus, continuous activation of the MAPK (RAS/RAF/MEK/ERK), NF-kB, and PI3K/AKT signaling pathways. RAS and V600EBRAF mutations are consequently mutually exclusive. They correlate with specific clinicopathologic characteristics, notably arising from serrated adenomas, and tend to occur more frequently in females aged more than 60 years; they have a right-sided preponderance, high-grade histology, more frequent peritoneal metastases, and a higher frequency (10–25%) of MSI. In advanced disease, V600EBRAF denotes the subsets with the poorest outcomes as well as the highest resistance to conventional therapies, with no prospective trial clearly demonstrating any significant survival advantage of a specific combination of conventional therapies, as outlined earlier in this chapter. Most patients with mCRC harboring V600EBRAF survive on average 6–18 months less than their non-V600EBRAF counterparts, and although also RAS wild type, response to anti-EGFR therapies is short-lived. Non-V600E BRAF mutations, which are very rare, appear to behave differently; most can have a significantly better (rather than worse) prognosis and so are functionally very different. V600EBRAF is also commonly found in melanoma, and using selective oral V600EBRAF inhibitor therapy rapidly became a standard of care in combination with dual MEK inhibition. Intuitively, inhibition of two nodes in the same pathway could be more effective in maximizing the degree of ERK inhibition as well as overcoming potential adaptive resistance mechanisms or alternatively, could be redundant therapeutically. Furthermore, BRAF inhibitor monotherapy also activates ERK signaling in normal (non-cancerous) cells, which have wild-type BRAF, and this phenomenon is thought to be responsible for the increased incidence of keratoacanthomas and squamous cell carcinomas in patients treated with BRAF inhibitors due to activation of ERK signaling in normal skin, which can be suppressed by dual therapy with a MEK inhibitor. In mCRC, disappointingly, unlike in melanoma, V600EBRAF inhibitor monotherapy alone was ineffective due to a feedback loop further activating EGFR. Thus, strategies for dual inhibition of V600EBRAF in combination with cetuximab and in parallel,

triple inhibition with V600EBRAF, EGFR, and MEK inhibition were tested in a randomized Phase III study. In 2019, these results led to a paradigm shift in the treatment of V600EBRAF mCRC, as those patients who had the double and triple inhibition with encorafenib, binimetinib, and cetuximab (triplet), and encorafenib and cetuximab (doublet), survived approximately twice as long as those who had conventional control treatments. The value of the additional MEK inhibition (triplet with binimetinib) remains questionable, as although there was an increased response rate, there appears to be equivalent survival with or without the addition of the binimetinib. The safety and tolerability profile of both combinations allowed the maintenance of high dose intensity for most patients, and overall quality of life was preserved and better than with the control chemotherapy. This is thus the first ever evidence of survival benefit for a chemotherapy-free targeted treatment regimen in a prospective biomarker-defined Phase III trial in metastatic CRC.[173]

Clinical biomarkers remain powerful and simple predictive and prognostic tools:

The functional status of mCRC patients objectified as a performance status score (ECOG, WHO, or Karnofsky) and the serum albumin remain potent predictors of patient outcomes, with practical dynamic utility and simplicity. Other simple to test pathology values, such as the serum c-reactive protein (crp) and neutrophil to lymphocyte ratio, also appear consistently in studies as negative prognostic markers but have not been used universally. Since 2001, a theme has emerged that the anatomic locations of the right and the left side of the colon were also behaving differently in advanced colorectal cancer studies. This has evolved into one of the most commonly used simple predictive and prognostic tools despite remaining scientifically enigmatic. Right-sided (RS) colon carcinomas are located within the colon derived from the embryologic midgut, which encompasses the proximal two-thirds of the transverse colon, ascending colon, and caecum, while left-sided (LS) colon carcinomas lie within the colon derived from the embryologic hindgut, which includes the distal third of the transverse colon, splenic flexure, descending colon, sigmoid colon, and rectum. Differences in outcomes between mCRC arising as primary tumors from the RS and the LS colon were first observed in 2001, when O'Dwyer and colleagues reported that median survival was 15.8 months in LS patients versus 10.9 months in RS (mortality HR 1.5 for RS versus LS, $p = 0.0001$) based on 1120 patients with histologically confirmed metastatic, residual, or recurrent adenocarcinoma of the colon or rectum.[174]

This simple and intriguing consideration has continued to prove accurate throughout the development of newer, more effective and biologically targeted agents to this day, in that almost all subsequent large randomized studies in mCRC have shown RS and LS to be both prognostic and predictive. Tumors arising from the RS overall do significantly worse and are less responsive to all known therapies compared with LS tumors. "Sidedness" is thus a powerful factor that always needs to be taken into account and predicts for poorer survival independently of treatment and all other clinical and molecular biomarkers, including the RAS mutation status. Studies with chemotherapy combined with EGFR inhibitors in RAS wild-type mCRC as first-line treatment suggest that RS tumors have poorer responses and less beneficial outcomes with EGFR inhibitors than their LS counterparts. Thus, in mCRC, the patients with the best survival and best treatment outcomes tend to have LS metastatic tumors, which are intrinsically more treatment responsive, as yet for unknown reasons. RS tumors are also more frequently associated with mutations in BRAF, TGFβR2, and PI3KCA, while amplification of EGFR and HER2, overexpression of EGFR ligands, and chromosomal instability are more common in LS tumors. However, these and other currently identified molecular factors to date have not been able to elucidate the significant RS vs. LS differential.[175,176]

More complex compound expression biomarkers remain evolving research tools despite early promise of utility:

As molecular technologies have evolved, whole genome sequencing and gene expression arrays have become powerful research tools that can be assessed in tumor samples from patients, including in randomized clinical trials, in search of reliable and consistent tests that can be more powerfully prognostic and predictive in mCRC patients. In practice, they have not been useful as yet, but they are to be considered the first step in our understanding of the complexities of the fundamental driving biological forces in mCRC on an individual basis, personalized treatment choices, and possibly, prevention and potentially targeted therapeutic strategies. The current best molecular sub-classification that is being investigated has been developed by the Colorectal Cancer Subtyping Consortium. Expression arrays for unsupervised clustering of genes for molecular subtypes in independent datasets have led to the consensus molecular subtypes (CMS). Four homogeneous (with a fifth, as yet unclassified) diverse groups are now described: CMS1—MSI Immune; CMS2—Canonical; CMS3—Metabolic; and CMS4—Mesenchymal. As yet, they have had no practical applications and cannot and do not either explain, or co-segregate individually or collectively with, the potent LS vs. RS conundrum.[140,177]

Potentially curative liver surgery and oligometastatic disease in Stage IV mCRC

The overall 5-year survival of all patients with Stage IV disease remains at around 10% (most with disease). The challenge is thus to develop multidisciplinary combination treatment pathways, for appropriately clinically and molecularly selected patients, that increase the probability of 5-year survival and ultimately, lead to higher cure rates.

In CRC, there is a relatively predictable pattern of systemic metastasis development (for unclear reasons) in a significant subset (15–25%) of patients. This is unlike the patterns seen in other common cancers, where metastases represent widespread and disseminated incurable disease. Thus, at first presentation of CRC (synchronous) or 1–5 years after resection of the primary tumor (metachronous), metastatic disease commonly develops first in the liver. About 20–25% of patients have clinically detectable synchronous liver metastases at the time of initial diagnosis, and a further 40–50% of patients develop metachronous liver metastases, usually within 3 years of primary surgery. When the metastatic deposits appear confined only to the liver with modern imaging techniques (as they do in about one-third of all mCRC liver metastasis patients), in about 30–40% of these patients, the metastases can be completely resected by expert liver surgeons. Within this group, 20–25% of patients are eventually cured (survive to 10 years without recurrent disease), and an additional 10% remain as longer-term survivors at 5 years (i.e., up to 35%), despite disease recurrence. This leads to the alluring prospect for our patients that a combination of different MDT specialist approaches, surgical procedures, tools, and interventional technologies can be utilized for major overall and disease-free survival gains for individual patients.[160,161]

This process has been made significantly easier by the low and reducing morbidity and mortality (<1% currently) of liver surgery in mCRC that have been demonstrated from major liver centers around the world. Furthermore, the complex surgical techniques and approaches, including locally ablative therapies and support from complex interventional hepatic radiology, have made the technicality of almost all liver surgeries potentially feasible. Resections can extend to almost 85% of liver volumes (if residual liver function is normal), staged resections over two to three procedures over a few months, and even vascular reconstruction techniques are rapidly pushing the limits of what is possible to new, ever-expanding frontiers.

Thus, expert liver surgery offers the possibility of long-term cancer-free survival. About 8–15% of all mCRC patients are potential candidates for liver resection, of whom one-third are long-term survivors. Over the last 10 years, this proportion has been rising rapidly, as chemotherapeutic advances (as outlined earlier) can convert or "downstage" a further subset of inoperable mCRC patients, who have initially presented as clearly unresectable metastatic disease, into resectable or operable categories. This subset is frequently also referred to as "potentially operable," "potentially curable," or "potentially convertible." Increasing response rates of combination systemic therapies now approach 60–70% for modern chemotherapeutic regimens. If well-planned and managed methodically by the specialist within the extended MDT with a liver emphasis, this can select out such patients by this neoadjuvant or preoperative approach from the outset. Indeed, the challenge now, paradoxically, is to select the most appropriate patients who are deemed to potentially benefit from liver surgery, rather than choosing patients who are technically possible to resect, but. Thus, the target of the MDT discussion of liver surgical selection is clinical benefit rather than technical feasibility or safety.

Chemotherapy can induce hepatic steatosis, fibrosis, and functional liver derangements that need to be considered prospectively in the overall management planning in such scenarios. Chemotherapy, even at a minimum of 3 months' exposure with oxaliplatin regimens such as FOLFOX, does increase liver morbidity post hepatic resection. We now have randomized clinical trial data to clearly define this (as well as definitive outcomes in operable liver metastases),[162] as discussed in the next section.

There are now increasing data to support that limited (fewer than three) extra-hepatic metastases in the lung and, possibly and more rarely, isolated localized disease in the peritoneum may also potentially still lead to cure in about one-third of patients. Thus, the surgical or ablative control of liver metastases may still be desirable, even if there is limited extra-hepatic disease, as this may exploit further the synergies of local and systemic therapies. The key is to have an extended MDT discussion at the presentation of metastases and to discuss this plan regularly after each scan during chemotherapy for the optimum liver surgical plan. In deciding treatment options, the primary question is whether the patient has a technically or potentially curable malignancy. The secondary and equally important point is whether it is clinically appropriate for the patient to be subject to this potentially curative approach.

Inoperable liver metastases: Debulking strategies and the concept of "organ"-directed therapy approaches

When curative resection is not possible, patients may benefit from palliative resection, which is becoming increasingly minimally invasive, and more alternatives, such as endoluminal stenting to temporarily relieve partial or sub-acute obstruction, are now available as means of expediting the systemic treatment.

The approach of treating metastases with systemic therapies is thus palliative in intent in the majority, whereas surgical resection of limited metastases can be curative. Unfortunately, fewer than 5% of all metastatic patients eventually fall into the latter category (even if this is not apparent at the outset), as the majority of these relapse eventually. The disappointment has been that even with the newer biological agents, complete remission rates and thus, cure rates from chemotherapy alone remain exceedingly rare. The challenge is thus to develop treatment pathways that increase the probability of longer-term disease-free survival or periods of partial remission off treatments to allow the patients to have some hospital-free time in the context of trying to lead a normal life.

The liver is a vital organ and as already discussed, is the most frequent site of colorectal metastases; it leads to organ-specific morbidity, which often translates to dominant global symptoms in terminal care, impacting both quality and quantity of life. Progress in therapies having overall impact on the patient can thus be organ directed. Rapid advances in medical technologies are enabling this and allowing evidence from trials to support this concept. More extraordinarily, focusing on one organ can often achieve better response outcomes that can translate to a bridge to curative outcomes, which is the ultimate goal of cancer research. Improved outcomes with such a multi-modality approach have already been demonstrated in rectal cancer with radiotherapy and better surgical and imaging technologies. In principle, other metastatic sites such as liver, lung, and peritoneum are developing similar paradigms.

Response rates to systemic chemotherapy over the last 20 years have been gradually improving as new active agents have been developed, but the proportional gains in terms of overall survival benefits (on the order of months) and percentages of complete responders has been disappointing. However, liver-specific response rates have major relevance if advantage can be taken of other interventional modalities at the time of maximum chemotherapy response. This has been retrospectively and comparatively demonstrated in many Phase III trials. Traditionally, the other modality has been liver surgery; but other non-operative modalities are increasingly being used, expanding the possible patient cohorts and selection criteria. Biologically, this has rationale, as residual disease post-chemotherapy will contain resistant clonal cancer-cell populations that other modalities can eradicate directly in a complementary way (i.e., potentially eliminate the putative cancer stem or key propagating cancer cells).

To summarize the current evidence:

1. A synergistic approach with systemic chemotherapy and liver surgery in operable liver metastases (one to four deposits) can improve disease-free survival outcomes.
2. In a subset of patients, chemotherapy can downstage inoperable liver metastases, enabling potentially curative surgery with similar outcomes to operable liver metastases.
3. Liver-directed chemotherapy infused via the portal vein (PV) or hepatic artery (HA) improves overall survival. A meta-analysis of six HA infusion trials has shown benefit in terms of increased response rates compared with the equivalent systemic chemotherapy and improved statistically significant overall survival advantage (14.5 vs. 10.1 months; $p = 0.0009$). However, many centers have methodological and practical problems with HA or PV infusion, making it less popular as other parallel developments have occurred in both systemic therapy and liver resection

techniques. The evidence base, however, does still prove the principle of potential benefits of organ-directed strategies.

4. A synergistic approach with systemic chemotherapy and palliative liver ablative techniques such as radio-frequency ablation (RFA) or similar ablative technologies (e.g., microwave or irreversible electroporation), traditionally considered non-curative, may improve disease-free survival outcomes or may be good surrogates to formal liver surgery where the clinical situation dictates. This has been demonstrated in the randomized CLOCC study.[178]
5. A synergistic approach with systemic chemotherapy and palliative liver-directed yttrium90-loaded particle brachytherapy (SIRT) delivered via the HA to conceptually debulk non-operable or non-ablatable liver metastases. The largest multidisciplinary trial ever performed with over a thousand patients globally (the FOXFIRE study) has shown that liver disease control can be extended by 6–10 months using this interventional procedure in addition to standard-of-care chemotherapy. Overall survival was unfortunately not impacted, although intriguingly, it appeared better in RS primary tumors treated with SIRT as compared with chemotherapy alone. Good and prolonged disease control in the liver allows synergistic benefits such as treatment-free "holidays" in a cancer patient's journey. This can allow patients valuable (treatment-free) time to achieve goals and aims in a limited–life expectancy situation. Another earlier trial using SIRT after two lines of chemotherapy also demonstrated advantages.[179]

Follow-up after initial treatment: Surveillance

After curative treatment of CRC, many patients are still at risk of developing metastatic disease, and they are also at a higher risk of developing a second primary CRC than the general population. The aim of follow-up is therefore the early detection of second primary tumors in the colon as well as of potentially resectable, and so curable, recurrent disease. Colonoscopy should be performed at least every 3–5 years after surgery, preferably lifelong. Newer non-invasive radiological technologies may complement surveillance. The exact frequency and overall benefits of surveillance remain debatable and vary significantly in different countries around the world, with an overall survival benefit difficult to consistently demonstrate. The CEA tumor marker, and sometimes the CA19-9, can also aid in surveillance, but there can be prolonged periods where patients have a rising CEA and non-detectable disease on CT. Fluorodeoxyglucose–positron emission tomography (FDG-PET) scanning can be considered. The latter appears particularly effective in locating recurrences that may be missed by CT or MRI, albeit in a small number of cases.[162,163]

If there were no effective treatment for metastases or local recurrence, it could be argued that minimal follow-up is all that is necessary and that if recurrence occurs, the symptoms should be treated palliatively. It was estimated in the 1980s[168] that as many as 20% of patients relapsing after apparently curative resection could be cured by resection of hepatic or pulmonary metastases. Advances in imaging, surgical technique, and supportive measures have probably improved this, but the exact magnitude of benefit remains controversial. Results with metachronous recurrence of liver or lung metastases are best when there is a solitary liver deposit and the time of relapse is greater than 18 months; as discussed in an earlier section, multiple deposits can be resected with long-term survival.[167,168] The survival benefits of chemotherapy for metastatic disease are also greatest when deposits are detected and treated at an early stage, although there is a lead-time bias in this argument for asymptomatic recurrences. Therefore, there is a strong case for early detection of either resectable or unresectable recurrence, and that this allows better patient informed choices for life planning is self-evident. The contrary argument is that intensive follow-up usually detects recurrence before symptoms, and if this incurable, it can lead to anxiety and lead-time treatment, which may be non-essential at the time of recurrence and can be saved for when necessary.

Summary and future developments

1. Colorectal cancer remains a major cause of cancer deaths worldwide. There have been major improvements in the outlook for patients with CRC, as many advances in surgery, radiotherapy, systemic chemotherapy, and newer molecularly targeted biological agents have improved both cure rates as well as non-curative median survivals incrementally in metastatic disease over the last 20 years. However, to effect even higher cure rates in a subset of patients (survival >5 years and above), there remains dependency on selection for liver surgical excision of residual metastases, as the complete pathological, and thus durable, response rates of systemic treatments alone remain very low.

2. The solutions are thus to have improved patient (clinical) and molecular selection, combined with expanding the populations suitable for integrated combination modalities including liver surgery, leading to complete eradication of organ-confined metastases. Rapid technological developments with reducing treatment morbidities are making this an increasing reality.

3. The expertise of the MDT, with a patient-centered focus, allows interpretation and implementation of a significant cumulative evidence base to achieve the best treatment pathway and outcomes for each individual. It thus follows from concurrent clinical trials that informed decision making about safety, efficacy, and quality of life must be allowed for better long-term qualitative and quantitative outcomes. There is increasing evidence that this multitude of technologies can be synergistic as opposed to additive if selected and tested properly. The application of an innovative multidisciplinary approach for oligometastatic disease that integrates advanced approaches (such as radioembolization [SIRT] and local ablative therapies) should ultimately allow the benefits of curative hepatic resections to be extended to a broader group of patients.

4. There may also be significant quantitative palliative benefits, hitherto ignored, if the novel concept of "vital organ" salvage develops an evidence base. That is, targeting metastases early in the treatment pathway in specific organs such as the liver may have an overall higher impact on the patient than generally controlling systemic metastatic disease in other sites.

   Current multidisciplinary approaches should be truly cross-specialty in effect, with integrated treatment options being discussed on a regular basis from the outset. They should not, as is often the case, be single-technology or single-specialty dependent or only discuss other options at the salvage (end) of the treatment pathway, when unfortunately, no realistic treatment options exist and the patient cohorts are significantly smaller and less functionally able or likely to benefit.

5. As post-genomic knowledge and integration of the molecular basis of cancer develops, there is scope for novel therapies directed against many cell surface and intracellular targets, with a reasonable prospect of useful progress in the coming decade. Several new approaches are now established, and the molecular biomarkers RAS, RAF, and MSI are now a minimum prerequisite, essential for appropriate and personalized therapies.

National health service guidelines

There are some key recommendations for CRC services:[173]

- *Patient focus.* Patients should be given full verbal and written information about their condition and about any treatment that may be offered. They should have continuing access to a member of the core team who can offer guidance and support.
- *MDTs.* Management of cancer care by MDTs, which work to agreed-on protocols, is likely to facilitate the implementation of the Clinical Outcomes Group guidelines and improve the quality and coordination of care. These teams should include clinicians with up-to-date knowledge of diagnosis and treatment of CRC and specialized nursing staff who can support and advise patients.
- *Endoscopy facilities.* Adequate endoscopy facilities should be provided to help ensure accurate and timely diagnosis. The quality of endoscopy facilities—particularly colonoscopy completion and complication rates—should be monitored and the staff given additional training when necessary to improve standards.
- *Surgery for rectal cancer.* Surgery for rectal cancer should be concentrated in the hands of surgeons who can demonstrate good results, particularly in terms of low recurrence rates. Surgeons should monitor their response by working closely with histopathologists.
- *Improved pathology reporting.* Pathology reporting should be sufficiently detailed to give comprehensive feedback on the adequacy of surgery, particularly for rectal cancer. Reports on surgical specimens should include data related to the size, type, grade, and Dukes' stage of the tumor and the involvement of lymph nodes and surgical margins. This information is important for guiding treatment decisions, routine collection of data on case mix by cancer registries, and monitoring long-term outcomes.
- *Adjuvant therapies.* Preoperative radiotherapy should be available for patients with rectal cancer. Adjuvant therapy can improve survival in some groups of patients and should be more widely available. Large-scale, nationally or internationally coordinated randomized trials should be supported to determine the best management of patients with CRC.

Conclusions

Early diagnosis through case finding and screening of high-risk groups can make it possible to treat CRC at a stage at which prognosis is good, with over half the patients now expected to be cured. Adjuvant and neo-adjuvant chemotherapy and radiotherapy and MDTs play a major role in improving survival. Particular attention should be paid to measuring quality of life in clinical trials and in routine practice. Teams including the relevant specialists are likely to be most effective in implementing these measures in an efficient and cost-effective way. The improved understanding of cancer biology and of personalized therapeutics promises continuing progress in diagnosis and management in the coming decade.

References

1. Cancer Research UK. Cancer Statistics for the UK. https://www.cancerresearchuk.org/health-professional/cancer-statistics-for-the-uk. Accessed April, 2020.
2. Cancer Statistics Registrations, England (Series MB1): https://www.cancerresearchuk.org/health-professional/cancer-statistics-for-the-uk. Accessed April, 2020.
3. Fearon ER, Vogelstein B. A genetic model of carcinogenesis. *Cell.* 1990; 61:759.
4. Giovannucci E, Rimm EB, Stampfer MJ et al. Intake of fat, meat and fiber in relation to risk of colon cancer in men. *Cancer Res.* 1994; 54:2390–7.
5. Willett WC, Stampfer MJ, Colditz GA et al. Relation of meat, fat and fiber intake to the risk of colon cancer in a prospective study amongst women. *N Engl J Med.* 1990; 323:1664–72.
6. COMA. *Nutritional Aspects of the Development of Cancer.* London: Department of Health, 1998.
7. Peipins LA, Sandler RS. Epidemiology of colorectal adenomas. *Epidemiol Rev.* 1994; 16(2):273–97.
8. Jacobs LR. Fiber and colon cancer. *Gastroenterol Clin North Am.* 1988; 17:747–60.
9. Trock B, Lanza E, Greenwald P. Dietary fibre, vegetables and colon cancer: Critical review and meta-analysis of the epidemiologic evidence. *J Natl Cancer Inst.* 1990; 82:650.
10. Gerhardsson M, Floderus B, Norell SE. Physical activity and colon cancer risk. *Int J Epidemiol.* 1989; 18(3):728–9.
11. Wasan HS, Goodlad RA. Fibre-supplemented foods may damage your health. *Lancet.* 1996; 348(9023):319–20.
12. Greenberg ER, Baron JA. Prospects for preventing colorectal cancer death. *J Natl Cancer Inst.* 1993; 85:1182–4.
13. Liao X, Lochhead P, Nishihara R et al. Aspirin use, tumor PIK3CA mutation, and colorectal-cancer survival. *N Engl J Med.* 2012; 367(17):1596–606.
14. Halligan S, Altman DG, Taylor SA et al. CT colonography in the detection of colorectal polyps and cancer: systematic review, meta-analysis, and proposed minimum data set for study level reporting. *Radiology.* 2005; 237(3):893–904.
15. Crawford JM. The gastrointestinal tract. In: Cotran RS, Kumar V, Robbins S (eds), *Robbins Pathologic Basis of Disease.* 5th ed. Philadelphia: W. B. Saunders, 1994. pp. 811–13.
16. Konishi F, Morson BC. Pathology of colorectal adenomas. *J Clin Pathol.* 1982; 35:830–41.
17. Morson BC, Bussey HJR. Magnitude of risk for cancer patients and colorectal adenomas. *Br J Surg.* 1985; 72 Suppl:523–5.
18. Muto T, Bussey HJR, Morson BC. The evaluation of cancer of the colon and rectum. *Cancer.* 1975; 36:2251–70.
19. Goh HS, Jass JR. DNA content and the adenoma-carcinoma sequence in the colorectum. *J Clin Pathol.* 1986; 39:387–92.
20. Eide TJ. Prevalence and morphological features of adenomas of the large intestine with and without colorectal carcinoma. *Histopathology.* 1986; 10:111–18.
21. Heald RJ, Lockhart-Mummery HE. The lesion of the second cancer of the large bowel. *Br J Surg.* 1972; 59:16–9.
22. Bussey HJR, Wallace MH, Morson BC. Metachronous carcinoma of the large intestine and intestinal polyps. *Proc R Soc Med.* 1967; 60:208–10.
23. Longacre TA, Fenoglio-Preiser CM. Mixed hyperplastic adenomatous polyps/serrated adenomas. *Am J Surg Pathol.* 1990; 14:524–37.
24. Lennard-Jones JE, Morson BC, Ritchie JK, Williams CB. Cancer surveillance in ulcerative colitis. Experience over 15 years. *Lancet.* 1983; 2:149–52.
25. Dhir V, Gopinath N. Endoscopic appearance of dysplasia and cancer in JBD Tytgat GNJ. *Eur J Cancer.* 1995; 31:1174–7.
26. Blackstone M, Riddell R, Gerald Rogers BH et al. Dysplasia-associated lesion or mass (DALM) detected by colonoscopy in long-standing ulcerative colitis: an indication for colectomy. *Gastroenterology.* 1981; 80:366–74.
27. Vasen HF, van der Luijt RB, Slors JF et al. Molecular genetic tests as a guide to surgical management of familial adenomatous polyposis. *Lancet.* 1996; 348(9025):433–5.
28. Jass JR, Smyrk TC, Stewart SM et al. Pathology of hereditary non polyposis colorectal carcinoma. *Anticancer Res.* 1994; 14:1631–4.
29. Jass JR. Diagnosis of hereditary non polyposis colorectal carcinoma. *Histopathology.* 1998; 32:491–7.
30. Burt RW. Familial risk and colorectal cancer. *Gastroenterol Clin North Am.* 1996; 25:793–803.
31. Syngal S, Fox EA, Eng C et al. Clinical criteria for HNPCC (Amsterdam II, Sensitivity and specificity of clinical criteria for hereditary non-polyposis colorectal cancer associated mutations in MSH2 and MLH1Sapna). *J Med Genet.* 2000; 37:641–5.
32. Hamilton SR. Colon cancer testing and screening. *Arch Pathol Lab Med.* 1999; 123(11):1027–9.
33. Burt RW, Di Sario JA, Cannon-Albright L. Genetics of colon cancer: impact of inheritance on colon cancer risk. *Annu Rev Med.* 1995; 46:371–9.
34. Hamilton SR, Liu B, Parsons RE et al. The molecular basis of "Turcot syndrome". *N Engl J Med.* 1995; 332:839–47.
35. Spirio L, Olschwang S, Groden J et al. Alleles of the APC gene: an attenuated form of familial polyposis. *Cell.* 1993; 75:951–7.
36. Fuchs CS, Giovannucci E, Colditz GA et al. A prospective study of family history and the risk of colorectal cancer. *N Engl J Med.* 1994; 331:1669–94.
37. Dunlop MG, Farrington SM, Carothers AD et al. Cancer risk associated with germline DNA mismatch repair gene mutations. *Hum Mol Gen.* 1997; 6(1):105–10.
38. Umar A, Boland CR, Terdiman JP et al. Revised Bethesda Guidelines for hereditary nonpolyposis colorectal cancer (Lynch syndrome) and microsatellite instability. *J Natl Cancer Inst.* 2004; 96(4):261–8.
39. Houlston RS, Tomlinson IP. Polymorphisms and colorectal tumor risk. *Gastroenterology.* 2001; 121(2):282–301.
40. Fearnhead NS, Wilding JL, Bodmer WF. Genetics of colorectal cancer: hereditary aspects and overview of colorectal tumorigenesis. *Br Med Bull.* 2002; 64:27–43.
41. Vogelstein B, Fearon ER, Hamilton SR et al. Genetic alterations during colorectal tumour development. *N Engl J Med.* 1988; 319:525–32.
42. Rubinfeld B, Souza B, Albert I et al. Association of the APC gene product with β catenin. *Science.* 1993; 262:1731–4.
43. Powell SM, Zilz N, Beazer-Barclay Y et al. APC mutations occur early during colorectal tumourigenesis. *Nature.* 1992; 359:235–7.
44. Barbacid M. Ras genes. *Annu Rev Biochem.* 1987; 56:779–827.
45. Fearon ER, Cho KR, Nigro JM. Identification of a chromosome 18q gene that is altered in colorectal cancers. *Science.* 1990; 247: 49–58.
46. Greenblatt MS, Bennett WP, Hollstein M et al. Mutations in the P53 tumour suppressor gene: clues to cancer etiology and molecular pathogenesis. *Cancer Res.* 1994; 54:4855–78.
47. Lane DP. Cancer, P53, guardian of the genome. *Nature.* 1992; 358:15–16.
48. Boland SR, Sato J, Appelman HD et al. Microallelotyping defines the sequence and tempo of allelic losses at tumour suppressor gene loci during colorectal cancer progression. *Nat Med.* 1995; 1:902–9.
49. http://www.ncbi.nlm.nih.gov/entrez/query.fcgi?db=Snp.
50. http://www.ncbi.nlm.nih.gov/entrez/query.fcgi?db=OMIM.
51. Chung CH, Bernard PS, Perou CM. Molecular portraits and the family tree of cancer. *Nat Genet.* 2002; 32 Supplement:533–40.
52. Ramaswamy S, Ross KN, Lander ES, Golub TR. A molecular signature of metastasis in primary solid tumors. *Nat Genet.* 2002; 33:49–54.
53. Slater GI, Haber RH, Aufses AH. Changing distribution of carcinoma of the colon and rectum. *Surg Gynaecol Obstet.* 1984; 158:716–18.
54. Mills SE, Allen MS Jr, Cohen AR. Small cell undifferentiated carcinoma of the colon. *Am J Sur Pathol.* 1983; 7:643–51.

55. Sasaki O, Atkin WS, Jass JR. Mucinous carcinoma of the rectum. *Histopathology.* 1987; 11:259–72.

56. Quirke P, Williams GT (coordinators). *Standards and Minimum Datasets for Reporting Common Cancers. Minimum Dataset for Colorectal Cancer Histopathology Reports.* London: Royal College of Pathologists, 1998.

57. Adam IJ, Mohamdee MO, Martin IG et al. Role of circumferential margin involvement in the local recurrence of rectal carcinoma. *Lancet.* 1994; 344:707–10.

58. Quirke P. Assessing the quality of rectal surgery. *Bulletin Royal College of Pathologists* 1998; 104: Abstract VII.

59. Brown G. Thin section MRI in multidisciplinary pre-operative decision making for patients with rectal cancer. *Br J Radiol.* 2005; 78 Spec No 2:S117–27.

60. Shepherd NA, Baxter K, Love S. The prognostic importance of peritoneal involvement in colonic carcinoma: A prospective evaluation. *Gastroenterology.* 1997; 112:1096–102.

61. Dukes CE, Bussey HJR. The spread of rectal cancer and its effect on prognosis. *Br J Cancer.* 1958; 12:309–20.

62. O'Brien MJ, Zamcheck N, Burke B et al. Immunocytochemical localisation of carcinoembryonic antigen in benign and malignant colorectal tissues. *Am J Clin Pathol.* 1981; 75:283–90.

63. Cutait, R, Alvee VAF, Lopes LC et al. Restaging of colorectal carcinoma based on the identification of lymph node micrometastases through immunoperoxidase staining of CEA and cytokeratins. *Dis Colon Rectum.* 1991; 34:917–20.

64. Jass JR, Atkin WS, Cuzick J et al. The grading of rectal carcinoma. Historical perspectives and a multi variate analysis of 447 cases. *Histopathology.* 1986; 10:437–59.

65. Dukes CE. The classification of cancer of the rectum. *J Pathol Bacteriol.* 1932; 35:373.

66. Dukes CE. Cancer of the rectum: an analysis of 1000 cases. *J Pathol Bacteriol.* 1940; 50:527–39.

67. Turnbull RB, Kyle K, Watson FR et al. Cancer of the rectum. The influence of the no touch isolation technique on survival rates. *Ann Surg.* 1967; 166:420–7.

68. Beahrs ON, Henson DE, Hutter RVP et al. *Manual for Staging of Cancer.* 4th ed. Philadelphia: JB Lippincott, pp. 69–73.

69. Compton C, Fenoglio-Preiser CM, Pettigrew N, Fielding LP. AJCC, American Joint Committee on cancer prognostic factors consensus conference: Colorectal working group. *Cancer.* 2000; 88:1739–57.

70. Colon and rectum. In: Edge SB, Byrd DR, Compton CC, et al. (eds). *AJCC Cancer Staging Manual.* 7th ed. New York, NY: Springer, 2010. pp. 143–64.

71. Karanjia ND, Schache DJ, Heald RJ. Function of the distal rectum after low anterior resection for carcinoma. *Br J Surg.* 1992; 79:114–6.

72. Dehni N, Tiret E, Singland JD et al. Long-term functional outcome after low anterior resection: comparison of low colorectal anastomosis and colonic J-pouch-anal anastomosis. *Dis Colon Rectum.* 1998; 41(7):817–22; discussion 822–3.

73. Williams NS, Dixon MF, Johnston D. Reappraisal of the 5 centimetre rule of distal excision for carcinoma of the rectum: a study of distal intramural spread and of patients survival. *Br J Surg.* 1983; 70:150–4.

74. Matheson NA, McIntosh CA, Krukowski Z. Continuing experience with single layer appositional anastomosis in the large bowel. *Br J Surg.* 1985; 72 Supplement:S104–6.

75. Guillou PJ, Quirke P, Thorpe H et al. Short-term endpoints of conventional versus laparoscopic-assisted surgery. *Lancet.* 2005; 365(9472):1718–26.

76. Leung KL, Kwok SP, Lam SC et al. Laparoscopic resection of rectosigmoid carcinoma: prospective randomised trial. *Lancet.* 2004; 363(9416):1187–92.

77. Holm T, Ljung A, Híggmark T et al. Extended abdominoperineal resection with gluteus maximus flap reconstruction of the pelvic floor for rectal cancer. *Br J Surg.* 2007; 94:232–8.

78. Moore TJ, Moran BJ. Precision surgery, precision terminology: the origins and meaning of ELAPE. *Colorectal Dis.* 2012; 14(10):1173–4.

79. Izbicki JR, Hosch SB, Knoefel WT et al. Extended resections are beneficial for patients with locally advanced colorectal cancer. *Dis Colon Rectum.* 1995; 38(12):1251–6.

80. Poeze M, Houbiers JG, van de Velde CJ et al. Radical resection of locally advanced colorectal cancer. *Br J Surg.* 1995; 82(10):1386–90.

81. Shirouzu K, Isomoto H, Kakegawa T. Total pelvic exenteration for locally advanced colorectal carcinoma. *Br J Surg.* 1996; 83(1):32–5.

82. Saito N, Sarashina H, Nunomura M et al. Clinical evaluation of nerve-sparing surgery combined with preoperative radiotherapy in advanced rectal cancer patients. *Am J Surg.* 1998; 175(4):277–82.

83. Marsh PJ, James RD, Schofield PF. Adjuvant preoperative radiotherapy for locally advanced rectal carcinoma. Results of a prospective, randomized trial. *Dis Colon Rectum.* 1994; 37(12):1205–14.

84. Ptok H, Meyer F, Marusch F et al. Palliative stent implantation in the treatment of malignant colorectal obstruction. *Surg Endosc.* 2006; 20(6):909–14.

85. Carne PW, Frye JN, Robertson GM, Frizelle FA. Stents or open operation for palliation of colorectal cancer: a retrospective, cohort study of perioperative outcome and long-term survival. *Dis Colon Rectum.* 2004; 47(9):1455–61.

86. Daneker GWJ, Carlson GW, Hohn DC et al. Endoscopic laser recanalization is effective for prevention and treatment of obstruction in sigmoid and rectal cancer. *Arch Surg.* 1991; 126:1348–52.

87. Garcia Valdecasas JC, Llovera JM, deLacy AM et al. Obstructing colorectal carcinomas. Prospective study. *Dis Colon Rectum.* 1991; 34:759–62.

88. Phillips RKS, Hittinger R, Fry JS et al. Malignant large bowel obstruction. *Br J Surg.* 1985; 72:296–302.

89. Ross S, Krukowski ZH, Munro A, Russel IT. Single-stage treatment for malignant left-sided colonic obstruction: a prospective randomized clinical trial comparing subtotal colectomy with segmental resection following intraoperative irrigation. The SCOTIA study group. Subtotal colectomy versus on-table irrigation and anastomosis. *Br J Surg.* 1995; 82(12):1622–7.

90. Lopez-Kostner F, Hool GR, Lavery IC. Management and causes of acute large-bowel obstruction. [Review]. *Surg Clin North Am.* 1997; 77(6):1265–90.

91. Poon RT, Law WL, Chu KW, Wong J. Emergency resection and primary anastomosis for left-sided obstructing colorectal carcinoma in the elderly. *Br J Surg.* 1998; 85(11):1539–42.

92. Anderson JH, Hole D, McArdle CS. Elective versus emergency surgery for patients with colorectal cancer. *Br J Surg.* 1992; 79:706–9.

93. Sjodahl R, Franzen T, Nystrom PO. Primary versus staged resection for acute obstructing colorectal carcinoma. *Br J Surg.* 1992; 79:685–8.

94. Deans GT, Krukowski ZH, Irwin ST. Malignant obstruction of the left colon. [Review]. *Br J Surg.* 1994; 81(9):1270–6.

95. Bohm B, Schwenk W, Hucke HP et al. Does methodic long-term follow-up affect survival after curative resection of colorectal carcinoma? *Dis Colon Rectum.* 1993; 36:280–6.

96. Abulafi AM, Williams NS. Local recurrence of colorectal cancer: The problem, mechanisms, management and adjuvant therapy. [Review]. *Br J Surg.* 1994; 81:7–19.

97. Pietra N, Sarli L, Costi R et al. Role of follow-up in management of local recurrences of colorectal cancer: a prospective, randomized study. *Dis Colon Rectum.* 1998; 41(9):1127–133.

98. Chu DZ, Erickson CA, Russell MP et al. Prognostic significance of carcinoembryonic antigen in colorectal carcinoma. Serum levels before and after resection and before recurrence. *Arch Surg.* 1991; 126:314–6.

99. Rocklin MS, Senagore AJ, Talbott TM. Role of carcinoembryonic antigen and liver function tests in the detection of recurrent colorectal carcinoma. *Dis Colon Rectum.* 1991; 34:794–7.

100. Rodriguez Bigas MA, Stulc JP et al. Prognostic significance of anastomotic recurrence from colorectal adenocarcinoma. *Dis Colon Rectum.* 1992; 35:838–42.

101. Killingback MJ. Indications for local excision of rectal cancer. *Br J Surg.* 1985; 72 Supplement:S54–6.

102. Bright N, Hale P, Mason R. Poor palliation of colorectal malignancy with the neodymium yttrium-aluminium-garnet laser. *Br J Surg.* 1992; 79:308–9.

103. Hager, TH, Gall FP, Hermanek P. Local excision of cancer of the rectum. *Dis Colon Rectum*. 1983; 26:149.

104. Stockholm Rectal Cancer Study Group. Preoperative short-term radiation therapy in operable rectal cancer: A randomized trial. *Cancer*. 1990; 66:49–55.

105. Sebag-Montefiore D, Stephens RJ, Steele R et al. Preoperative radiotherapy versus selective postoperative chemoradiotherapy in patients with rectal cancer (MRC CR07 and NCIC-CTG C016): A multicentre, randomised trial. *Lancet*. 2009; 373(9666):811–20.

106. Quirke P, Steele R, Monson J, Grieve R et al. MRC CR07/NCIC-CTG CO16 Trial Investigators; NCRI colorectal cancer study group. Effect of the plane of surgery achieved on local recurrence in patients with operable rectal cancer: A prospective study using data from the MRC CR07 and NCIC-CTG CO16 randomised clinical trial. *Lancet*. 2009; 373(9666):821–8.

107. Peeters KCMJ, van de Velde CJH, Leer JWH et al. Late side effects of short-source preoperative radiotherapy combined with total mesorectal excision for rectal cancer: Increased bowel dysfunction in irradiated patients—A Dutch Colorectal Cancer Group Study. *J Clin Oncol*. 2005; 23:6199–206.

108. Stephens RJ, Thompson LC, Quirke P et al. Impact of short-course preoperative radiotherapy for rectal cancer on patients' quality of life: Data from the Medical Research Council CR07/National Cancer Institute of Canada Clinical Trials Group C016 randomized clinical trial. *J Clin Oncol*. 2010; 28(27):4233–9.

109. Bakx R, Emous M, Legemate DA et al. Categorization of major and minor complications in the treatment of patients with resectable rectal cancer using short-term pre-operative radiotherapy and total mesorectal excision: A Delphi round. *Colorectal Dis*. 2006; 8(4):302–8.

110. Colorectal Cancer Collaborative Group. Adjuvant radiotherapy for rectal cancer: A systematic overview of 8,507 patients from 22 randomised trials. *Lancet*. 2001; 358:1291–4.

111. Sauer R, Liersch T, Merkel S et al. Preoperative versus postoperative chemoradiotherapy for locally advanced rectal cancer: results of the German CAO/ARO/AIO-94 randomized phase III trial after a median follow-up of 11 years. *J Clin Oncol*. 2012; 30(16):1926–33.

112. Bozzetti F, Baratti D, Andreola S et al. Preoperative radiation therapy for patients with T2-T3 carcinoma of the middle-to-lower rectum. *Cancer*. 1999; 86(3):398–404.

113. Mohiuddin M, Regine WF, Marks GJ, Marks JW. High-dose preoperative radiation and the challenge of sphincter-preservation surgery for cancer of the distal 2 cm of the rectum. *Int J Radiat Oncol Biol Phys*. 1998; 40(3):569–74.

114. Ahmad NR, Nagle D. Long-term results of preoperative radiation therapy alone for stage T3 and T4 rectal cancer. *Br J Surg*. 1997; 84(10):1445–8.

115. Wagman R, Minsky BD, Cohen AM et al. Sphincter preservation in rectal cancer with preoperative radiation therapy and coloanal anastomosis: long term follow-up. *Int J Radiat Oncol Biol Phys*. 1998; 42(1):51–7.

116. Rosenthal SA, Yeung RS, Weese JL et al. Conservative management of extensive low-lying rectal carcinomas with transanal local excision and combined preoperative and postoperative radiation therapy. A report of a phase I–II trial. *Cancer*. 1992; 69(2):335–41.

117. Brizel HE, Tepperman BS. Postoperative adjuvant irradiation for adenocarcinoma of the rectum and sigmoid. *Am J Clin Oncol*. 1984; 28:3.

118. Mendenhall WM, Bland KI, Copeland EM et al. Does preoperative radiation therapy enhance the probability of local control and survival in high risk distal rectal cancer? *Ann Surg*. 1992; 215:696–705.

119. Gunderson LK, Martin JK, Beart RW et al. Intraoperative and external beam irradiation for locally advanced colorectal cancer. *Ann Surg*. 1988; 207:52.

120. Tepper JE, Cohen AM, Wood WC et al. Intraoperative electron beam radiotherapy in the treatment of unresectable rectal cancer. *Arch Surg*. 1986; 121:421.

121. Whiting JF, Howes A, Osteen RT. Preoperative irradiation for unresectable carcinoma of the rectum. *Surg Gynaecol Obstet*. 1993; 176:203–7.

122. Duttenhaver JR, Hoskins RB, Gunderson LK et al. Adjuvant postoperative radiation therapy in the management of adenocarcinoma of the colon. *Cancer*. 1986; 57:955.

123. Withers HR, Cuasay L, Mason KA et al. Elective radiation therapy in the curative treatment of cancer of the rectum and rectosigmoid colon. In: Stroehlein JR, Romsdahl MM (eds), *Gastrointestinal Cancer*. New York: Raven Press, 1981. p351.

124. Els M, Gross T, Ackermann C, Tondelli P. Incidence of ileus after rectal resection for rectal carcinoma, with and without adjunctive radiation therapy. *Schweiz Med Wochenschr*. 1992; 122:745–7.

125. Seow Choen F, Goh HS, Eu KW et al. A simple and effective treatment for hemorrhagic radiation proctitis using formalin. *Dis Colon Rectum*. 1993; 36:135–8.

126. Moertel CG, Fleming TR, Macdonald JS et al. Levamisole and fluorouracil for adjuvant therapy of resected colon carcinoma. *N Engl J Med*. 1990; 322(6):352–8.

127. Wolmark N, Rockette H, Mamounas E et al. Clinical trial to assess the relative efficacy of fluorouracil and leucovorin, fluorouracil and levamisole, and fluorouracil, leucovorin, and levamisole in patients with Dukes' B and C carcinoma of the colon: results from National Surgical Adjuvant Breast and Bowel Project C-04. *J Clin Oncol*. 1999; 17(11):3553–9.

128. Kerr DJ, Gray R, McConkey C, Barnwell J. Adjuvant chemotherapy with 5-fluorouracil, L-folinic acid and levamisole for patients with colorectal cancer: non-randomised comparison of weekly versus four-weekly schedules—less pain, same gain. QUASAR Colorectal Cancer Study Group. *Ann Oncol*. 2000; 11(8):947–55.

129. Andre T, Colin P, Louvet C et al. Semimonthly versus monthly regimen of fluorouracil and leucovorin administered for 24 or 36 weeks as adjuvant therapy in stage II and III colon cancer: results of a randomized trial. *J Clin Oncol*. 2003; 21(15):2896–903.

130. Twelves C, Wong A, Nowacki MP et al. Capecitabine as adjuvant treatment for stage III colon cancer. *N Engl J Med*. 2005; 352(26):2696–704.

131. Andre T, Boni C, Mounedji-Boudiaf L et al. Oxaliplatin, fluorouracil, and leucovorin as adjuvant treatment for colon cancer. *N Engl J Med*. 2004; 350(23):2343–51.

132. De Gramont A, Boni C, Navarro M et al. Oxaliplatin/5FU/LV in the adjuvant treatment of stage II and stage III colon cancer: efficacy results with a median follow-up of 4 years. *J Clin Oncol*. 2005; 23(16S):246.

133. Wolmark N, Wieand HS, Kuebler JP et al. A phase III trial comparing FULV to FULV + oxaliplatin in stage II or III carcinoma of the colon: results of NSABP protocol C-07. *J Clin Oncol*. 2005; 23(16S):246.

134. Van Cutsem E, Labianca R, Hossfeld D et al. PETACC 3 randomized phase III trial comparing infused irinotecan/5-fluorouracil (5-FU)/folinic acid (IF) versus 5-FU/FA (F) in stage III colon cancer patients (pts). (PETACC 3). *J Clin Oncol*. 2005; 23(16S):3.

135. Ychou M, Raoul J, Douillard J et al. for the GI Group of the FNCLCC and the FFCD. A phase III randomized trial of LV5FU2+CPT-11 vs. LV5FU2 alone in adjuvant high risk colon cancer (FNCLCC Accord02/FFCD9802). *J Clin Oncol*. 2005; 23(16S):246.

136. Gray RG, Barnwell J, Hills R et al. QUASAR: a randomised study of adjuvant chemotherapy (CT) vs. observation including 3238 colorectal cancer patients. *J Clin Oncol*. 2004; 22(14S):245.

137. Mamounas E, Wieand S, Wolmark N et al. Comparative efficacy of adjuvant chemotherapy in patients with Dukes' B versus Dukes' C colon cancer: results from four National Surgical Adjuvant Breast and Bowel Project adjuvant studies (C-01, C-02, C-03, and C-04). *J Clin Oncol*. 1999; 17(5):1349–55.

138. Impact B2 investigators. International multicentre pooled analysis of B2 colon cancer trials. Efficacy of adjuvant fluorouracil and folinic acid in B2 colon cancer. *J Clin Oncol*. 1999; 17:1356–63.

139. Cochrane review. Colorectal meta-analysis collaboration: palliative chemotherapy for advanced or metastatic colorectal cancer (Cochrane Review). The Cochrane Library, Issue 2. Oxford: Update Software, 2000.

140. Stebbing J, Wasan HS. Decoding metastatic colorectal cancer to improve clinical decision making (Editorial). *J Clin Oncol*. 2019; 37(22):1847–50.

141. Thirion P, Michiels S, Pignon JP et al. Modulation of fluorouracil by leucovorin in patients with advanced colorectal cancer: An updated meta-analysis. *J Clin Oncol.* 2004; 22(18):3766–75.

142. Maughan TS, James RD, Kerr D et al. Preliminary results of a multicentre randomised trial comparing 3 chemotherapy regimens (de Gramont, Lokich and Raltitrexed) in metastatic colorectal cancer. *J Clin Oncol.* 1999; 18:262.

143. Von Hoff DD, Rothenberg ML, Pitot HC. Irinotecan therapy for patients with previously treated metastatic colorectal cancer. Overall results of FDA approved pivotal US clinical trials. *J Clin Oncol.* 1997; 16:803.

144. Cunningham G, Pyrhonen S, James R et al. Randomised trial of irinotecan versus supportive care alone after fluorouracil failure for patients with metastatic colorectal cancer. *Lancet.* 1998; 352:1407–12.

145. Rougier P, Van Cutsem E, Bajetta E et al. Randomised trial of irinotecan versus fluorouracil by continuous infusion after fluorouracil failure in patients with metastatic colorectal cancer. *Lancet.* 1998; 352(9138):1407–12.

146. Saltz LB, Cox JV, Blanke C et al. Irinotecan plus fluorouracil and leucovorin for metastatic colorectal cancer. Irinotecan Study Group. *N Engl J Med.* 2000; 343(13):905–14.

147. Douillard JY, Cunningham D, Roth AD et al. Irinotecan combined with fluorouracil combined with fluorouracil alone as first line treatment for metastatic colorectal cancer: a multicentre randomised trial. *Lancet.* 2000; 355:1041–7.

148. Raymond E, Chaney SG, Taamma A, Cvitkovic E. Oxaliplatin: a review of preclinical and clinical studies. *Ann Oncol.* 1998; 9(10):1053–71.

149. Giacchetti S, Itzhaki M, Gruia G et al. Long-term survival of patients with unresectable colorectal cancer liver metastases following infusional chemotherapy with 5-fluorouracil, leucovorin, oxaliplatin and surgery. *Ann Oncol.* 1999; 10(6):663–9.

150. Tournigand C, Andre T, Achille E et al. FOLFIRI followed by FOLFOX6 or the reverse sequence in advanced colorectal cancer: A randomized GERCOR study. *J Clin Oncol.* 2004; 22(2):229–37.

151. Goldberg RM, Sargent DJ, Morton RF et al. A randomized controlled trial of fluorouracil plus leucovorin, irinotecan, and oxaliplatin combinations in patients with previously untreated metastatic colorectal cancer. *J Clin Oncol.* 2004; 22(1):23–30.

152. Johnston PG, Fisher ER, Rockette HE et al. The role of thymidylate synthase expression in prognosis and outcome of adjuvant chemotherapy in patients with rectal cancer. *J Clin Oncol.* 1994; 12(12):2640–7.

153. Lenz HJ, Danenberg KD, Leichman CG et al. p53 and thymidylate synthase expression in untreated stage II colon cancer: associations with recurrence, survival, and site. *Clin Cancer Res.* 1998; 4(5):1227–34.

154. Edler D, Hallstrom M, Johnston PG et al. Thymidylate synthase expression: an independent prognostic factor for local recurrence, distant metastasis, disease-free and overall survival in rectal cancer. *Clin Cancer Res.* 2000; 6(4):1378–84.

155. Kawakami K, Omura K, Kanehira E, Watanabe Y. Polymorphic tandem repeats in the thymidylate synthase gene is associated with its protein expression in human gastrointestinal cancers. *Anticancer Res.* 1999; 19(4B):3249–52.

156. Salonga D, Danenberg KD, Johnson M et al. Colorectal tumors responding to 5-fluorouracil have low gene expression levels of dihydropyrimidine dehydrogenase, thymidylate synthase, and thymidine phosphorylase. *Clin Cancer Res.* 2000; 6(4):1322–27.

157. Liang JT, Huang KC, Lai HS et al. High-frequency microsatellite instability predicts better chemosensitivity to high-dose 5-fluorouracil plus leucovorin chemotherapy for stage IV sporadic colorectal cancer after palliative bowel resection. *Int J Cancer.* 2002; 101(6):519–25.

158. Ribic CM, Sargent DJ, Moore MJ et al. Tumor microsatellite-instability status as a predictor of benefit from fluorouracil-based adjuvant chemotherapy for colon cancer. *N Engl J Med.* 2003; 349(3):247–57.

159. Kemeny N, Fata F. Arterial, portal, or systemic chemotherapy for patients with hepatic metastasis of colorectal carcinoma. *J Hepatobiliary Pancreas Surg.* 1999; 6:39–49.

160. Seifert JK, Junginger T, Morris DL. A collective review of the world literature on hepatic cryotherapy. *Br J Coll Surg Edinb.* 1998; 43:141–54.

161. Ogunbiyi OA, Flanagan FL, Dehdashti F et al. Detection of recurrent and metastatic colorectal cancer: comparison of positron emission tomography and computed tomography. *Ann Surg Oncol.* 1997; 4(8):613–20.

162. Nordlinger et al. Perioperative chemotherapy with FOLFOX4 and surgery versus surgery alone for resectable liver metastases from colorectal cancer (EORTC Intergroup trial 40983): a randomised controlled trial. *Lancet.* 2008; 371(9617):1007–16.

163. Taylor I. Liver metastases from colorectal cancer: lessons from past and present clinical studies. *Br J Surg.* 1996; 83(4):456–60.

164. 168 Millikan KW, Staren ED, Doolas A. Invasive therapy of metastatic colorectal cancer to the liver. *Surg Clin North Am.* 1997; 77(1):27–48.

165. NHS. Cancer guidance subgroup of the clinical outcomes group 1997. *BMJ.* 1997; 315:1485

166. Amin MB, Edge SB, Greene FL, et al. eds. *AJCC Cancer Staging Manual.* 8th ed. New York: Springer; 2017.

167. National Bowel Cancer Audit: www.hscic.gov.uk/bowel

168. Le DT, Uram JN, Wang H, et al. PD-1 blockade in tumors with mismatch-repair deficiency. *N Engl J Med.* 2015; 372:2509–20.

169. Kopetz S, Grothey A, Yaeger R et al. Encorafenib, binimetinib, and cetuximab in BRAF V600E-mutated colorectal cancer. *N Engl J Med.* 2019; 381(17):1632–43.

170. O'Dwyer PJ, Manola J, Valone FH et al: Fluorouracil modulation in colorectal cancer: Lack of improvement with N -phosphonoacetyl-l -aspartic acid or oral leucovorin or interferon, but enhanced therapeutic index with weekly 24-hour infusion schedule—An Eastern Cooperative Oncology Group/Cancer and Leukemia Group B Study. *J Clin Oncol.* 2001; 19:2413–21.

171. Loupakis F, Yang D, Yau L, et al. Primary tumor location as a prognostic factor in metastatic colorectal cancer. *J Natl Cancer Inst.* 2015; 107(3).

172. Arnold D, Lueza B, Douillard JY et al. Prognostic and predictive value of primary tumour side in patients with RAS wild-type metastatic colorectal cancer treated with chemotherapy and EGFR directed antibodies in six randomized trials. *Ann Oncol.* 2017; 28(8):1713–29.

173. Guinney J, Dienstmann R, Wang X et al. The consensus molecular subtypes of colorectal cancer. *Nat Med.* 2015; 21(11):1350–6.

174. Ruers T, Van Coevorden F, Punt CJ et al. Local treatment of unresectable colorectal liver metastases: Results of a randomized phase II trial. *J Natl Cancer Inst.* 2017; 109(9):djx015.

175. Wasan HS, Gibbs P, Sharma NK et al. First-line selective internal radiotherapy plus chemotherapy versus chemotherapy alone in patients with liver metastases from colorectal cancer (FOXFIRE, SIRFLOX, and FOXFIRE-Global): a combined analysis of three multicentre, randomised, phase 3 trials. *Lancet Oncol.* 2017. pii: S1470–2045(17)30457-6.

176. Iveson TJ, Kerr RS, Saunders MP et al. 3 versus 6 months of adjuvant oxaliplatin-fluoropyrimidine combination therapy for colorectal cancer (SCOT): an international, randomised, phase 3, non-inferiority trial. *Lancet Oncol.* 2018; 19(4):562–78.

Useful websites

www.esmo.org/Guidelines-Practice/Clinical-Practice-Guidelines/Gastrointestinal-Cancers/

www.cancer.gov/cancertopics/types/colon-and-rectal

http://seer.cancer.gov/statfacts/html/colorect.html

www.ncin.org.uk/cancer_type_and_topic_specific_work/cancer_type_specific_work/colorectal_cancer/

www.lifemath.net/cancer/coloncancer/outcome/index.php

http://pathways.nice.org.uk/pathways/colorectal-cancer/colorectal-cancer-overview

www.cancerresearchuk.org/cancer-help/type/bowel-cancer/

www.cancer.net/cancer-types/colorectal-cancer

www.bowelcanceruk.org.uk

www.beatingbowelcancer.org

16 ANUS

Bernard J. Cummings and James D. Brierley

Anatomy

The "anus" is a general term for the outlet of the bowel and includes both the anal canal and peri-anal skin. The canal is 3–4 cm long, the superior limit being the palpable upper border of the anal sphincters and puborectalis muscles of the anorectal ring, and the distal limit, or anal verge, is the level at which the walls of the canal come into contact in their normal resting state. The peri-anal area, sometimes called the anal margin, is the skin within a 5 cm radius of the anal verge.

There are three major lymphatic pathways. Lymphatics from the uppermost part of the canal drain predominantly to the peri-rectal and superior hemorrhoidal nodes of the inferior mesenteric system. Those from the area around and above the dentate line flow to the internal pudendal, hypogastric, and obturator nodes of the internal iliac system. Lymphatics from the distal canal, anal verge, and peri-anal skin drain to the superficial inguinal nodes, and occasionally to the femoral nodes, of the external iliac system. There are numerous lymphatic connections between the various levels of the canal and the peri-anal skin close to the anal verge.

The veins from the inferior anal canal communicate mainly with the systemic venous system and those from the upper canal predominantly with the portal system.

Pathology

The World Health Organization (WHO) histological classification of anal tumors describes intra-epithelial and invasive neoplasms.[1] The term "anal intra-epithelial neoplasia" (AIN) is applied to pre-cancerous changes in the epithelium of the anal canal and peri-anal skin. The term "squamous cell carcinoma" is applied to all the various subtypes previously used, including basaloid, cloaco-genic, and large-cell keratinizing and non-keratinizing. About 85–90% of primary anal canal cancers are squamous cell type, and 10–15% are adenocarcinomas, most of which arise from anal glands. Adenocarcinomas from rectal-type mucosa in the proximal canal are usually classified as primary rectal cancers. About 5% are rare variants, including squamous cell carcinoma with mucinous microcysts, small-cell, and undifferentiated cancers.

Primary cancers of the peri-anal skin are similar to cancers of the skin arising in other sites. Most are squamous cell cancers, with occasional basal-cell cancers and skin adnexal adenocarcinomas.

Many reports do not clearly separate squamous cell cancers of the anal canal from those arising in the peri-anal skin. In this chapter, they are referred to collectively as anal squamous cell cancer (ASCC).

Epidemiology and risk factors

Cancers of the anal region are about 1/10th as common as cancers of the rectum, although there is considerable international geographic variation. Malignant tumors arise in the canal about four times as frequently as in the peri-anal skin. The incidence of ASCC has been increasing in many countries over the past 30 years.[2–4] The incidence rate in England in males rose from 0.43/100,000 in 1990–1994 to 0.73 in 2006–2010 and in females from 0.50 to 1.13.[2]

Epidemiological studies have identified a number of factors associated with ASCC, although no unequivocal etiologic pathway. Benign conditions such as fistulae, fissures, and hemorrhoids do not predispose to anal cancer, nor do inflammatory bowel diseases such as Crohn's disease and ulcerative colitis.[5] Sexually transmitted factors are thought to be a significant cause of cancers of the anogenital area. The risk of ASCC is increased in men, and to a lesser extent in women, who give a history of anoreceptive intercourse,[6,7] likely related to sexually transmitted viral infection.[6] Other significant factors include multiple sexual partners and a history of cancer or intra-epithelial neoplasia of the vulva, vagina, or cervix.[8] Compromised cell-mediated immunity in patients infected with human immunodeficiency virus (HIV) is associated with an increased risk of ASCC, although anal cancer is not AIDS-defining.[9] Other risk factors include cigarette smoking,[7] and iatrogenic immunosuppression, typically following organ transplant.[10]

The sexually transmissible agent implicated as the most likely basis for these various epidemiological observations is human papillomavirus (HPV). Eighty-five percent or more of anal canal and peri-anal cancers are HPV positive, the percentage depending on the sensitivity of the tests used. Frequencies are higher in anal canal than in peri-anal cancers, in women, and in patients who are HIV positive or immunosuppressed. Type 16 is the most commonly found genotype (in about 75%), followed by HPV 18 (about 5%) and types 6, 11, and 31 (<5%).[9] There is some geographical variation in the prevalence of the HPV types identified in anal cancer tissue.[11]

Presentation

Most symptoms are non-specific. Bleeding, discharge, and anal discomfort are reported by about half the patients with cancers of the canal, and about a quarter are aware of a mass. A palpable mass, discomfort, and discharge are the most common presenting features of peri-anal tumors. A few asymptomatic primary cancers are found during physical examinations for other conditions or during investigation of an enlarged inguinal node. Unsuspected superficial cancer or high-grade intra-epithelial neoplasia is sometimes found on histological examination of hemorrhoidectomy specimens or peri-anal condylomata. Gross fecal incontinence due to sphincter destruction or vaginal fistula formation occurs in fewer than 5%, even in neglected cancers, which may reach a considerable size. Fecal incontinence should be distinguished from the more common fecal-stained discharge.

Diagnostic work-up and staging

Anal canal cancers

The features of greatest prognostic significance for survival are, in ascending order of seriousness, the size of the primary cancer, spread to regional lymph nodes, and extrapelvic metastases.

The primary tumor should be biopsied, if necessary under general anesthesia. Since non-specific or reactive enlargement of inguinal nodes is common, metastasis should be confirmed by fine-needle aspiration or excision biopsy. About half of all pelvic node metastases are less than 0.5 cm in size and may not be identified reliably by any available imaging modality, although fluorodeoxyglucose positron emission tomography (FDG-PET) offers some help.[12] Magnetic resonance imaging (MRI) is the preferred pelvic imaging study. Abdominal and pelvic computed tomography (CT) scans will disclose liver and large nodal metastases, and thoracic CT is favored to screen for pulmonary metastases. Localized skeletal symptoms should be evaluated radiologically. Full blood count, renal and liver function tests, and if risk factors are present, HIV antibody tests should be performed. Inguinal sentinel node biopsy is of uncertain value.[13,14] FDG-PET/CT is used frequently, although it is not yet shown to add definitively to MRI in assessment of pelvic nodes; it may have greater utility in disclosing the infrequent, and otherwise undiagnosed, extrapelvic metastases at presentation.

The current (eighth edition)[15] and previous (seventh edition)[16] Union for International Cancer Control (UICC) staging systems are shown in Table 16.1. The most significant changes in the eighth edition relate to the combining of cancers of the anal canal and peri-anal skin into a single staging system, the definition of the extent of the peri-anal skin, the addition of external iliac nodes to the regional node groups, simplification of the categorization of lymph node metastases (essentially to lymph node positive [N1] versus negative [N0], though subdivisions are defined if desired), and reworking of stage groupings.

Potential prognostic and predictive markers. A variety of tumor marker, cellular, molecular, and histopathological features have been studied,[17] although none has yet been incorporated into daily clinical practice.

Recent analyses of retrospective data indicate the possible value of readily available markers for stratifying patients and for the study of different treatment approaches.[17–19] The potential usefulness of identifying the presence of tumor HPV and p16 overexpression (both are more useful than one) was described in a systematic review of retrospective cohort studies of patients

TABLE 16.1   UICC TNM Classification of Malignant Tumors

Tumor		2009	2017		
TX	Primary tumor cannot be assessed	TX	Same		
T0	No evidence of primary tumor	T0	Same		
Tis	Carcinoma in situ, Bowen disease, HSIL, anal intra-epithelial neoplasia II-III (AIN II-III)	Tis	Same		
T1	Tumor 2 cm or less in greatest dimension	T1	Same		
T2	Tumor more than 2 cm but not more than 5 cm in greatest dimension	T2	Same		
T3	Tumor more than 5 cm in greatest dimension	T3	Same		
T4	Tumor of any size invades adjacent organs, e.g. vagina, urethra, or bladder (direct invasion of the rectal wall, perianal skin, subcutaneous tissue, or the sphincter muscle[s] alone is not classified as T4)	T4	Same		
Regional Nodes					
NX	Regional lymph nodes cannot be assessed	NX	Same		
N0	No regional lymph node metastasis	N0	Same		
N1	Metastasis in perirectal lymph nodes	N1	Metastasis in regional lymph node(s)		
N2	Metastases in unilateral internal iliac and/or unilateral inguinal lymph nodes	N1a	Metastases in inguinal, mesorectal, and/or internal iliac nodes		
		N1b	Metastases in external iliac nodes		
N3	Metastases in perirectal and inguinal lymph nodes and/or bilateral internal iliac nodes, and/or bilateral inguinal lymph nodes	N1c	Metastases in external iliac and in inguinal, mesorectal, and/or internal iliac nodes		
Metastases					
MX	Distant metastasis cannot be assessed	MX	–		
M0	No distant metastasis	N0	Same		
M1	Distant metastasis	M1	Same		

Stage Grouping 2009				**Stage Grouping 2017**			
Stage 0	Tis	N0	M0	Stage 0	Tis	N0	M0
Stage I	T1	N0	M0	Stage I	T1	N0	M0
Stage II	T2, T3	N0	M0	Stage IIA	T2	N0	M0
				Stage IIB	T3	N0	M0
Stage IIIA	T1, T2, T3	N1	M0	Stage III A	T1, T2	N1	M0
	T4	N0	M0				
Stage IIIB	T4	N1	M0	Stage IIIB	T4	N0	M0
	Any T	N2, N3	M0	Stage IIIC	T3, T4	N1	M0
Stage IV	Any T	Any N	M1	Stage IV	Any T	Any N	M1

Abbreviation: HSIL: high grade squamous intraepithelial lesion.
Sources: Adapted from Shiels et al. 2015; Frisch et al., 1994; Sobin et al., 2009; Brierley et al., 2017.

treated by chemoradiotherapy (ChRT).[19] HPV positivity (HPV+ve) and p16 overexpression (p16+ve) each showed a statistically significant association ($p < 0.05$) with better locoregional control, overall survival (OS), and disease-free survival (DFS). HPV+ve/ p16+ve tumors had improved OS when compared with HPV−ve/ p16−ve tumors but not with HPV−ve/p16+ve tumors. In one of the larger series, 87% (93 of 107) of tumors were HPV+ve, and all were p16+ve; 13% were HPV−ve, with 9% HPV−ve/ p16−ve and 4% HPV−ve/p16+ve.[18] HPV16+ve head and neck cancer cell lines have greater intrinsic sensitivity to radiation,[20] and it has been suggested that this phenomenon is present in all HPV-related squamous cell cancers.

One of the first identified potential prognostic biomarkers suggested for ASCC was p53. Disruptive mutations in p53 were associated with worse outcomes after ChRT. Such mutations are more common in HPV-ve/p16-ve tumors.[18]

Studies of tumor genome profiling have shown high expression of epidermal growth factor receptor (EGFR) (>80%).[21,22] However, mutations of EGFR, KRAS, and BRAF genes are infrequent (<5%) in ASCC.[23] Gene mutations were found in P1K3CA in about 40% and other mutations in smaller numbers.[21,22] In these studies, there was no correlation between molecular abnormalities and clinical outcome.

High levels of tumor infiltrating lymphocytes (TIL) were associated with improved outcomes in HPV+ve tumors in some series.[17,24] It has been postulated that infection with HPV may support greater anti-tumor immunological responses.[20]

In a study of 174 patients, elevated levels of serum squamous cell carcinoma antigen prior to treatment correlated with lower complete response rate (86% versus 95%, $p = 0.05$) and worse OS and DFS rates.[25]

Peri-anal cancers

As with cancers of the canal, the strongest prognostic factors for survival are the size of the primary tumor and the presence of inguinal node or more distant metastases. Inguinal node metastases are found in no more than 5 to 10% and should be confirmed histologically. The same panel of imaging and blood tests as for anal canal cancer should be used.

The staging system for peri-anal cancers has now been combined with that for anal canal cancer.[15]

Management

Anal canal cancers

Combined-modality radiation and chemotherapy, with radical surgery reserved for the management of recurrent cancer, is firmly established as the initial treatment of choice for ASCC. The combination recommended in 2019 is radiation with concurrent mitomycin C (MMC) and 5-fluorouracil (5FU) (or capecitabine).[26,27] Comparison of these guidelines showed that although they were not completely concordant, differences were minor.[28]

Prior to the adoption of combined-modality treatment, most patients were treated by radical surgery such as abdominoperineal resection, although some centers had favored radiation therapy alone. Radiation-based treatment permits the preservation of anorectal function in the majority of patients. Radical resection has not been compared with radiation alone or with combined-modality treatment in formal randomized trials, but reviews of published results indicate that cure rates are comparable.[29]

Following the initial description in 1974 by Nigro, Vaitkevicius, and Considine of the ability of concurrent radiation, 5FU, and MMC, a protocol designed as preoperative adjuvant therapy, to produce complete regression of ASCC,[30] a series of similar favorable reports, often using higher doses of radiation than the 30 Gy in 3 weeks in the original protocol, led to the widespread adoption of combined-modality treatment without planned surgery. Several randomized trials, systematically reviewed by Lim and Glynne-Jones[31] and Spithoff et al.,[32] established that delivering 5FU and MMC concurrently with radiation resulted in outcomes superior to those achieved by the same schedule of radiation alone,[33,34] radiation and 5FU alone,[35] or radiation with 5FU and cisplatin (CDDP).[36,37] Further, neither neoadjuvant (induction) nor adjuvant 5FU and CDDP improved locoregional control or survival rates.[35–38] A trial in which higher radiation doses were compared with lower doses did not show significant advantages to the higher doses.[38] There is considerable variation in most aspects of these randomized trials, including primary endpoints.[31,32] A set of core outcome research measures for anal cancer studies has been proposed.[39]

Long-term results (>5 years) have been published for only the first UK Coordinating Committee for Cancer Research (UKCCCR) Trial (ACT I)[40] (Table 16.2).

In Table 16.3, several of the most clinically meaningful outcomes are shown, indicating the superior treatment. An outcome is described as "better" as determined by statistical significance ($p < 0.05$, according to the statistical test applied by the authors of the trial report); similarly, a "trend" is said to be present if $p < 0.1$ and ≥ 0.05.

In the most recent trial in North America, RTOG 9811, which included 644 patients, 5FU and CDDP as neoadjuvant (induction) treatment, coupled with 5FU-CDDP concurrently with radiation, were compared with radiation and 5FU-MMC without neoadjuvant treatment.[36,41] Patients received a minimum of 45 Gy in 5 weeks at 1.8 Gy per fraction to the primary cancer and involved nodes. Patients with T3–4N+ disease and T2 patients with residual tumor after 45 Gy received an additional 10 to 14 Gy in 2 Gy fractions in 2 weeks. Chemotherapy in the standard arm consisted of concurrent 5FU (1000 mg/m²/day) by continuous intravenous infusion (contiv) on days 1 to 4 and 29 to 32, plus MMC 10mg/m² intravenous bolus (ivb) injection on days 1 and 29; radiation started on day 1. In the experimental arm, patients received 5FU in the same dose as in the standard arm on days 1 to 4, 29 to 32, 57 to 60, and 85 to 88 plus CDDP (75mg/m² ivb injection) on days 1, 29, 57, and 85 with the same 45 to 59 Gy radiation schedule (start day 57). Acute Grade 3 or 4 non-hematologic toxicity rates were 75% in each arm, but

TABLE 16.2   UK CCR: ACT 1, 5- and 10-Year Results

	RT (N = 285)		RT–5FU-MMC (N = 292)		
Time (years)	5	10	5	10	*p* value
Locoregional relapse rate (%)	57.1	59.1	32.8	33.8	<.001
Colostomy-free survival rate (%)	33.7	23.5	46.6	36.2	.004
Anal cancer death rate (%)	41.8	47.7	30.5	35.3	.004
Overall survival rate (%)	53.0	35.8	58.1	41.5	.12

Source: Adapted from Northover et al., 2010.
Abbreviations: 5FU: 5-Fluorouracil; MMC: mitomycin C; RT: radiation.

TABLE 16.3   **Anal Cancer Randomized Trials**

Trials (references)	Treatments	OS	DFS/RFS/TFS/RFS	LRControl	Colostomy
ACT I [33]	(A) RT, 5FU, MMC vs. (B) RT	5 years N.D	(RFS) (A) Better	(A) Better	(CFS) (A) Better
EORTC [34]	(A)RT, 5FU, MMC vs. (B) RT	5 years N.D	(RFS) (A) Better	(A) Better	(CFS) (A) Better
RTOG 8704 [35]	(A)RT, 5FU, MMC vs. (B) RT, 5FU	4 years N.D	(DFS) (A) Better	(A) Better	(CFS +CRate) (A) Better
RTOG 9811 [36]	(A)RT, 5FU, MMC vs. (B) Neoadjuvant, 5FU, CDDP + RT, 5FU, CDDP	5 years (A) Better	(DFS) (A) Better	(A) Trend	(CFS +CRate)(A) Trend
ACT II [37]	(A)RT, 5FU, MMC vs. (B) RT, SFU, CDDP	5 years N.D	N.R	N.R	(CFS + CRate) N.D
ACT II	In cCR responders (C) No adjuvant (D) Adjuvant 5FU, CDDP	5 years N.D	(TFS) N.D	N.R	N.R
ACCORD-03 [38]	RT, 5FU, CDDP (A) Low-dose RT 45 Gy + 15 Gy vs. (B) High-dose RT 45 Gy + 20–25 Gy	5 years N.D	(TFS) N.D	N.D	(CFS) (B) Trend
	(C) No neoadjuvant vs. (D) neoadjuvant 5FU, CDDP	5 years N.D	(TFS) N.D	N.D	(CFS) N.D

Abbreviations: RT = Radiation; 5FU = 5 Fluorouracil; MMC = Mitomycin C; CDDP = Cisplatin; N.D: No difference (p > 0.05); Trend: (p<1.0 ≥ 0.05); Better: (p<0.05); N.R: Not reported; cCR: complete clinical response; OS: overall survival; DFS: disease free survival; RFS: recurrence free survival; TFS: tumour free survival; CFS: colostomy free survival; CRate: colostomy rate

hematologic toxicity was higher in those who received MMC (62% versus 42%, $p < 0.001$). Severe long-term toxicity was similar in each group (13% MMC versus 11% CDDP, $p = 0.35$). The 5-year colostomy (12% versus 17%, $p = 0.074$) and locoregional failure (20% versus 26%, $p = 0.087$) rates showed trends in favor of radiation with 5FU-MMC. The 5-year DFS (68% versus 58%, $p = 0.004$) and OS (78% versus 71%, $p = 0.021$) rates significantly favored radiation, 5FU, and MMC. The authors recommended that radiation with concurrent 5FU and MMC remain the standard treatment.

A 2×2 factorial design randomized trial (ACCORD-03) conducted in France, of treatment with or without neoadjuvant 5FU and CDDP, failed to show any difference in 5-year locoregional control, DFS, or OS rates.[38] In this trial, all patients received 5FU and CDDP concurrently with radiation. The second randomization was to different doses of radiation, which also did not result in any significant differences.

The second UK Anal Cancer Trial (ACT II) was a randomized 2×2 factorial design, intended to study the combinations of radiation plus 5FU-MMC, and radiation plus 5FU-CDDP, with or without two courses of maintenance adjuvant 5FU and CDDP.[37] Nine hundred and forty patients were randomly assigned to one of four groups to receive either MMC (12 mg/m^2 ivb on day 1) or CDDP (60 mg/m^2 ivb on days 1 and 29) with 5FU (1000 mg/m^2 contiv on days 1–4 and 29–32) and radiation (50.4 Gy in 28 treatments of 1.8 Gy over 5.5 weeks, start day 1), with or without two courses of maintenance chemotherapy (5FU and CDDP) at weeks 11 and 14. The primary endpoints were complete response at 26 weeks, acute toxicity (for chemoradiation), and progression-free survival (PFS) (for maintenance chemotherapy). Complete clinical (cCR) response at 26 weeks was 90.5% in the MMC group and 89.6% in the CDDP group, $p = 0.64$. After 5.1 years' median follow-up, 3-year progression-free survival rates were 74% maintenance chemotherapy versus 73% no maintenance, $p = 0.70$. Colostomy-free survival (CFS) rates were not significantly different and at 3 years, were from 72% to 75% for the four treatment arms. Three-year OS rates ranged between 82% and 86% (not significant, either separately, or MMC versus CDDP, or maintenance versus no maintenance). Overall, acute toxic effects were similar, with about 70% experiencing any Grade 3 or 4 toxicity. Neutropenia was more common with MMC (24% versus 12%) but was not associated with increased rates of febrile neutropenia (3% in each group). This trial was not designed as a non-inferiority

study. The authors concluded that standard practice in the United Kingdom should be 5FU and MMC concurrently with 50.4 Gy in 28 daily treatments over 5.5 weeks.

The prolonged period of assessments, without early surgical intervention for a residual mass, for up to 26 weeks from the start of ChRT in the ACT II trial is unique among the randomized trials.[37,42] In other randomized trials, assessment without intervention has been recommended for no more than 6 to 16 weeks. Analysis of the data from ACT II showed that cCR rose from 64% at 11 weeks, to 81% at 18 weeks, and to 85% at 26 weeks. One hundred and fifty-one (72%) of 209 patients not in cCR at 11 weeks had achieved cCR by 26 weeks. The results were similar when nodal status was included in the 26-week assessment. Survival outcomes (OS and PFS) were independent of when cCR was achieved.[42] Complete tumor regression over even longer periods, up to nearly 12 months, has been seen in some case series,[43] but this length of observation of residual masses has not been tested in randomized studies.

Assessments in ACT II did not include elective biopsies of either the site of the primary tumor or residual mass. Protocol-mandated biopsies 4 to 6 weeks after treatment with radiation, 5FU, and MMC in RTOG 8704 were negative in 92%.[35] Biopsies have been shown to yield both false positives and false negatives.[44,45] Biopsy is indicated when tumor progression is suspected, and pathologic confirmation of residual potentially viable cancer should be obtained before salvage surgery.

Some have suggested that changes in FDG-PET prior to, during, and after treatment may provide prognostic information predictive of failure.[46,47]

The success of radiation, 5FU, and MMC has allowed substantial numbers of patients to retain anorectal function. However, in general, the randomized trials and institution-based studies did not include detailed prospective evaluation of late toxicity or the quality of anorectal function. A systematic review of papers published from 1980 to 2018, which described late gastrointestinal toxicity after radiotherapy for anal cancer, found a wide range in overall incidence (7% to 65%), with severe toxicity (considered Grade 3 or worse) in up to 33%.[48] The most common toxicities were fecal incontinence (up to 44%), diarrhea (up to 27%), and ulceration (up to 23%). Low-grade chronic bleeding was reported in up to 35%, anal stricture in up to 8%, and pelvic or perineal fibrosis in as many as 50%. Numerous other adverse symptoms were described. Many patients had multiple toxicities. Late

Grade 3 or worse toxicities of any type were recorded in 10–13% in the recent trials, ACT II[37] and RTOG 8411.[36] Colostomy due to severe anal canal dysfunction was reported in from 0.5% to 11% in the publications reviewed by Pan et al.[48] However, in ACT II, following 50.4 Gy in 5.5 weeks, only 1.7% (15 of 884 patients) had treatment-related colostomies, possibly reflecting the use of lower radiation doses than in some other series.[49] Even with total doses ranging from 60 to 80 Gy, the rate of treatment-related colostomy was only 3% (9 of 307) in the ACCORD-03 trial.[38] The majority of the papers reviewed by Pan et al.[48] described treatment with ChRT in which most investigators had used two-dimensional or three-dimensional planned external beam radiation techniques. There are as yet few reports of long-term outcomes from currently favored intensity-modulated radiation therapy (IMRT) techniques, although Grade 3 and 4 anal and sexual organ toxicities were still frequent in one prospective single center series.[50]

Patient-reported quality of life (QoL) has been recognized increasingly as an important measure of clinical outcome. Fecal incontinence, diarrhea, and buttock pain were associated with lower scores in QoL scales in several studies.[48,51,52] A health-related QoL measure specific to anal cancer, to supplement questionnaires such as EORTC QLQ–C30, has been developed and pilot tested.[53]

In order to attempt to preserve anorectal function, defunctioning ileostomies or colostomies prior to treatment are sometimes required in order to allow delivery of ChRT in patients who present with severe pain, anorectal obstruction, or significantly compromised anal sphincter function. These patients have been excluded from some trials. In the ACT II trial, for which such patients were eligible, these stomas were later closed in only 17% (20 of 118 patients).[49]

The reported effectiveness of surgical salvage of residual cancer varies considerably. Survival rates are best if microscopically complete (R0) resection is achieved. A systematic review of 39 observational studies (1388 patients) who underwent salvage surgery found a pooled 5-year OS rate of about 45% and DFS of about 40%.[54] There were no differences between patients with residual and those with recurrent cancer. Major postoperative complications and perineal wound complications were common (about 28% and 33%, respectively), but postoperative mortality was rare (2%).[54] Clinical and technical features important in assessing a patient for salvage surgery have been described.[55]

Surgical salvage for nodal recurrences after radiation and chemotherapy has not been discussed extensively. However, inguinal node dissection may be effective, as may abdominoperineal resection for the infrequently diagnosed perirectal node recurrences. Recurrences in pelvic side wall nodes are not usually amenable to surgical salvage.

Efforts have been made to improve local control rates by intensifying treatment, particularly radiation therapy. The primary tumor site has been the most common site of failure, and the great majority of these failures were in-field.[50,57] Radiation schedules can be intensified by increasing total dose and/or shortening the overall time in which treatment is delivered. Neither the randomized trials described earlier nor the numerous non-randomized studies have established the optimum schedules. When combined with 5FU and MMC, radiation doses of as low as 30 Gy in 15 fractions in 3 weeks are capable of eradicating up to about 90% of anal cancers 3 cm or less in size. Higher doses, from 45 Gy in 25 fractions in 5 weeks to 54 Gy in 30 fractions in 6 weeks, sometimes supplemented by further radiation after an interval of 4 to 8 weeks to a total of 60 to 65 Gy, have controlled from 55% to 65% of primary tumors larger than 4 cm. A randomized

trial in which all patients received 5FU/CDDP concurrently with the first phase of radiation compared 45 Gy in 25 treatments followed 3 weeks later by a 15 Gy boost (either external beam or brachytherapy) with 45 Gy plus 20 to 25 Gy.[38] Although the authors reported a trend towards better 5-year CFS rates (78% versus 74%, $p = 0.067$) from the higher dose, there was no difference in local control rates. A prospective non-randomized study of ChRT found local failure in 42% (14 of 33) patients with category T3 and T4 tumors treated with image-guided IMRT to 63 Gy/35 fractions/7 weeks.[50]

Escalation of radiation dose will likely be limited by the functional tolerance of the anal tissues. The radiation tolerance of the anal mucosa and sphincters has been discussed principally for males treated for prostate cancer.[58] In one typical study, the risk of higher-grade loss of sphincter control was >10% after a mean dose to the anal surface of about 45 Gy and to the anal sphincters of about 47 Gy (conformal radiation to prostate; doses of 64 or 74 Gy/2 Gy fractions). Most patients irradiated for prostate cancer receive higher doses to only the upper anal canal. The tolerance and function of the anal canal in patients with ASCC are affected in so-far unquantifiable ways by tumor infiltration into the mucosa and sphincters and by post-treatment fibrosis at the tumor site. Anal function is known to deteriorate naturally with age, making the age at which function is assessed an important variable.

There is interest both in reducing radiation dose for smaller tumors and in increasing dose for more advanced tumors. The UKCCCR is currently conducting a series of trials (PLATO), opened in 2016, to evaluate several radiation dose levels, in combination with chemotherapy, in different clinical scenarios[59] (Table 16.4).

Interruptions in the delivery of radiation, either elective or clinically necessary, are common in the treatment of anal cancer. Shorter interruptions, usually up to about 2 weeks, are related principally to the pain associated with acute dermatitis and anoproctitis. Longer intervals, up to 8 weeks, have been introduced where decisions regarding further treatment are predicated on the extent of clinical or histopathological response to the initial phase of combined radiation and chemotherapy. In the ACT II trial, in which there was no planned interruption in radiation and IMRT was not used, approximately 90% of patients received the full planned dose of 50.4 Gy in 5.5 weeks, with about 80% treated to full dose with no interruption.[42] Breaks in radiation treatments run counter to radiobiological theory, in that extended overall time of radiation may increase the risk of cancer re-growth. Anal cancers appear to have a short potential doubling time of about 4 days (range 1 to 30 days, $n = 26$),[60] a finding that would argue against interruptions and prolonged treatment times. When overall treatment time has been considered in multivariate analyses of risk factors for failure, most have found that shorter treatment times are to be preferred.[61,62]

Most protocols use radiation techniques that encompass the whole lower pelvis and inguinal regions initially in order to include regional lymph nodes and the primary cancer. Volumes are later reduced after the dose chosen to irradiate uninvolved nodes electively is reached, and higher doses are then delivered to the primary tumor and any involved nodes. The radiation strategies of the randomized trials have been reviewed elsewhere.[63] There is some evidence that both acute and late morbidity are influenced by technique as well as by radiation dose-time–fractionation parameters, and the ideal technique has not yet been established.

In the ACT II trial, patients were treated by a two-phase technique.[37] In Phase 1, 30.6 Gy in 17 daily fractions, five fractions per

TABLE 16.4   PLATO—*PersonaLizing Anal cancer radioTherapy dOse*

ACT 3—Low risk—non-randomized Phase II
  Early, small tumors–surgery
  Margins >1 mm. No further treatment
  Margins ≤1 mm. RT + chemotherapy
  PTV_P 41.4 Gy/23/4.5 weeks plus chemotherapy
  No elective RT to nodes

ACT 4—Intermediate risk—randomized Phase II
    T1, or T2 up to 4 cm, N0 or NX
Standard dose: PTV_P 50.4 Gy/28/5.5 weeks plus chemotherapy
              PTV_EN 40.0 Gy/28/5.5 weeks
Reduced dose: PTV_P 41.4 Gy/23/4.5 weeks plus chemotherapy
              PTV_EN 34.5 Gy/23/4.5 weeks

ACT 5—High risk—randomized pilot / Phase II / Phase III
  T2 >4 cm, or T3, or T4, NX, N0, N1, N2, N3
  Standard dose: PTV_P 53.2 Gy/28/5.5 weeks plus chemotherapy
  ($N \leq 3$ cm) PTV_N 50.4 Gy/28/5.5 weeks
  ($N > 3$ cm) PTV_N 53.2 Gy/28/5.5 weeks
  PTV_EN 40.0 Gy/28/5.5 weeks

		ARM 1	ARM 2
Dose escalation:		PTV_P 53.2 Gy/28/5.5 weeks	53.2 Gy/28/5.5 weeks
		PTV_Boost 58.8 Gy/28/5.5 weeks	61.6 Gy/28 /5.5 weeks
($N \leq 3$ cm)		PTV_N 53.2 Gy/28/5.5 weeks	Same
($N > 3$ cm)		PTV_N 53.2 Gy/28/5.5 weeks	Same
		PTV_EN 40.0 Gy/28/5.5 weeks	Same

Chemotherapy	
ACT 3	MMC 12 mg/m^2 D1; capecitabine 825 mg/m^2 p.o b.d. 5 days/week (on days of RT) for 23 days
ACT 4	As for ACT 3, for 28 days in standard arm and for 23 days in reduced dose arm
ACT 5	(center choice)
	As for ACT 3, for 28 days
	Or MMC 12 mg/m^2 day 1: 5FU 1000 mg/m^2 continuous IV Infusion days 1–4 and days 29–32

  Primary endpoint for all trials: locoregional failure.
  Secondary endpoints: multiple—see reference 59.

Abbreviations: 5FU = 5 Fluorouracil; CDDP: cisplatin; MMC: mitomycin C; PTV_EN: PTV Elective nodes; PTV_N: PTV Metastatic node; PTV_P: PTV Primary Tumor.

week, was delivered to the ICRU point (International Commission of Radiological Units [ICRU] Report 50) using non-conformal rectangular parallel-opposed fields intended to treat all pelvic nodes except the common iliac. Phase 2 employed conformal volumes planned using CT imaging; 19.8 Gy in 11 daily fractions was delivered to the ICRU point to encompass the primary tumor and the whole anal canal, with a 3 cm margin around all macroscopic tumor defining the field size.

Techniques such as IMRT have been shown to reduce the severity of toxicity and facilitate uninterrupted treatment to 50.4 to 54 Gy in 6 weeks with concurrent chemotherapy. A recent Phase II trial of IMRT combined with 5FU and MMC (RTOG 0528) showed a reduction in acute Grade 2 hematologic, Grade 3+ gastrointestinal, and Grade 3+ dermatologic toxicity compared with historical controls, although treatment interruptions were still necessary in half those treated.[64] Doses in this study were adjusted according to cancer stage, with up to 54 Gy in 30 fractions over 6 weeks to large tumor volumes and 45 Gy in 30 fractions to elective node volumes. Effective IMRT requires careful attention to contouring of target volumes, and in this centrally reviewed study, planning revisions were required in fully 81% of 52 cases.[64] The current UKCCCR PLATO Trial requires use of IMRT, for which guidelines have been developed and tested.[65]

Other guidelines for the contouring of pelvic organs are available also.[66,67] Acute side effects reported with IMRT techniques vary from study to study, suggesting inconsistency in the application of toxicity scales and ambiguity in some items.[68] A detailed report of late toxicity from a prospective institutional series treated with ChRT, using image-guided RT/IMRT, described predominantly abnormal anal function, worse in those who were treated with doses from 54 to 63 Gy at 1.8 Gy per fraction compared with patients with smaller tumors treated to 54 Gy.[50] Interstitial brachytherapy is not currently used extensively for the treatment of anal cancer, although some consider it superior to external beam therapy for local boost treatment of the primary cancer.[69]

Concurrent radiation and chemotherapy has become the standard for treatment of ASCC. Full and clear explanations for the superiority of this approach have not been elucidated. There is laboratory evidence, some of it conflicting, of synergistic interaction between radiation and 5FU and between radiation and CDDP, but neither these interactions nor the mechanism by which MMC enhances outcomes has been examined in detail in clinical studies of ASCC.

The dose intensity of chemotherapy may affect outcome.[70] The randomized trials described earlier used short continuous infusions of 5FU, similar to those in the original protocol described by Nigro et al.[30] These 4-day or 5-day infusions of 750 to 1000 mg/m^2 per day generally deliver more 5FU in the same overall time period (and with much higher short-term serum and tissue levels) than infusions continued throughout the several weeks of radiation. Extended infusions, typically of about 225 mg/m^2 per day for 5 weeks, are favored by those who argue that it is desirable to seek a potentially synergistic radio-sensitizing interaction with 5FU for every radiation fractional treatment.[71] In the ACT II trial, about 20% (MMC, 5FU) to 30% (CDDP, 5FU) had delay or dose reduction or both in chemotherapy during radiation.[42] A recent study of compliance and toxicity of either 5FU or capecitabine with MMC and radiation (50.4 to 54 Gy in 1.8 Gy fractions) found that fewer patients who received MMC/capecitabine experienced Grade 3 hematologic toxicity, but a lower proportion of patients received their planned chemotherapy dose. Overall, no significant difference was seen in Grade 3/4 toxicities between the two chemotherapy schedules.[72] Administration of capecitabine on each day of radiation is in accord with theory that this will enhance the effect of each radiation fraction. Oral capecitabine (825mg/m^2 b.i.d.) on each day of radiation (commonly 28 treatments, each of 1.8 Gy, 5 days per week), together with MMC ivb on day 1 (and in some series on day 29 also), has appeared tolerable, although in non-randomized comparisons, modification of the dose of capecitabine due to toxicity appeared more frequent than alteration in the dose of 5FU (where omission of the second course was the most common modification). Mitomycin doses in the randomized trials have ranged from 10 to 15 mg/m^2, with 10 and 12 mg/m^2 the most common. In a non-randomized institutional study in which choice of chemotherapy was at the treating oncologist's discretion, local tumor control and other oncological endpoints appeared similar following one or two doses of MMC; acute hematologic and skin toxicities were worse in those who received two doses, and there were 4.5% (3 of 63) toxicity-related deaths in that group.[73] Some trial protocols, although not ACT II[37] or PLATO,[59] included MMC with each of the two courses of 5FU given concurrently with radiation.

The cytotoxic drugs that have received the greatest attention are 5-FU, MMC, and CDDP. Bleomycin was given concurrently with radiation in Sweden, but the results of non-randomized studies did not suggest benefit.[74] The EORTC 22011 Phase II trial compared single-dose MMC and weekly CDDP given concurrently with radiation (59.4 Gy, split course over 8.5 weeks) with MMC plus prolonged continuous infusion of 5FU given concurrently with radiation.[75] In that trial, radiation and MMC/CDDP appeared superior, but this regimen has not been taken into Phase III studies. A pilot study in the United Kingdom in which 5-FU, MMC, and CDDP were all given concurrently with radiation was abandoned because of toxicity.[76] Several other cytotoxic drugs, such as combined capecitabine and oxaliplatin (CapeOx) (Table 16.5), have been studied in combination with radiation but have not been compared with 5FU/MMC.

Initial studies of targeted agents, particularly those designed to bind with the EGFR to inhibit activation of EGF, have been completed. EGFR is overexpressed in most ASCC.[17] Published studies include two Phase II trials of radiation, 5-FU, CDDP, and cetuximab, the first in HIV-negative patients,[77] and the other in HIV-positive patients.[78] In both studies, there was suggestion of improved locoregional control compared with historical controls, but there was significant Grade 4 toxicity in 26 to 32%, and small numbers of treatment-associated deaths occurred in both trials. A Phase I trial of radiation, 5FU, and MMC plus cetuximab reported good tumor response, but the maximum tolerated doses of 5FU and MMC were lower than those used in trials without cetuximab.[79] Other anti-EGFR agents studied include nimotuzomab and panitumamab.[80] The addition of targeted agents to the standard treatment of radiation, 5FU, and MMC is not recommended outside clinical trials.

Lymph node metastases

Metastases in regional lymph nodes can be eradicated by the same chemotherapy and radiation schedules used to treat the primary anal cancer. When patients diagnosed with primary anal canal cancers were treated with radical surgery, pelvic node metastases were found in about 30% and inguinal node metastases in about 15%.[81,82] A comprehensive review of lymph node positivity in 62 publications over 3 decades of treatment with ChRT found increases in the reported incidence from an estimated mean of 15.3% (95% confidence interval [CI] 10.5–20.1) in 1980 to 37.1% (34.0–41.3) in 2012 ($p < 0.0001$).[83] This was thought likely to be related to progress in imaging. The proportions of patients with locally advanced cancers (Stages T3 or T4), in which staging is less dependent on imaging, did not change over time (41.3% in 1990

TABLE 16.5 Selected Clinical Trials in Progress

Registration	Phase(s)/Centers	Summary
ISRCTN88455282	ACT 3/ACT 4/ACT 5 II/III Multicenter	PLATO. Evaluate lower RT doses in early ASCC and higher doses in locally advanced ASCC
NCT 02051868	II Multicenter	Compare 5FU/CDDP versus carboplatin/taxol in advanced, metastatic ASCC
NCT 03690921	II Single center	Evaluate proton (IMPT) radiation plus concurrent 5FU/CDDP in Stages II–III ASCC
NCT 00093379	II Single center	Evaluate capecitabine/oxaliplatin with concurrent RT in Stages II–III ASCC
NCT 02865135	I/II Single center	Evaluate DPXE7 (experimental therapeutic vaccine) in incurable HPV-related cancer
NCT 03386500	I Single center	Evaluate effect of BMX-001 (radioprotector) on toxicity rates from RT, 5FU, and MMC

Abbreviations: ISRCTN: International Standard Randomized Controlled Trials Number icrtn.com www.who.int/ictrp/network/icrctn2/en/
NCT National Clinical Trial https://clinicaltrials.gov/
5FU: 5 Fluorouracil; ASCC: anal squamous cell cancer; CDDP: cisplatin; IMPT: intensity-modulated proton therapy; MMC: mitomycin C; RT: radiation.

and 38.9% in 2012). The authors found an increase in OS rates in both node-positive and node-negative patients with increasing observed lymph node positivity (the "Will Rogers" effect).[84] Ideally, histologic confirmation of node positivity by fine-needle biopsy would be sought, but logistics and potential morbidity are prohibitive. Some centers have used sentinel node biopsy,[13,14] but this is applicable to only the inguinal nodes. At present, it does not seem possible to know the "true" rate of node positivity. It is prudent to continue to treat "positive" nodes, detected by whatever means, to higher radiation doses and node fields considered at risk to elective doses.

The probability of control of node metastases is similar to that of the primary cancer, although some consider it preferable locally to excise inguinal node metastases prior to radiation and chemotherapy.[43] Radical dissection of the inguino-femoral nodes either prior to or following high-dose radiation treatment should be avoided if possible because of the risk of poor healing and persistent lower limb edema. Most centers have applied the same radiation doses to lymph node masses as to primary tumors of comparable size. Although relapse of treated node masses is uncommon, with local nodal control rates of 80% to 90% or better, patients with nodal metastases at presentation are at increased risk of extrapelvic metastases, and 5-year OS rates are usually 10% to 20% lower than in patients who do not have demonstrable inguinal node or pelvic node metastases.

Late failure in inguinal nodes that were not abnormal at the time of first presentation has been reported in 15% to 25% of patients whose primary cancer was treated by surgery,[81,85] or in whom inguinal node basins were not irradiated electively.[86] Elective irradiation of clinically normal inguino-femoral nodes reduces the risk of late recurrence in these nodes to less than 5%.[86] Occasional authors prefer not to treat clinically negative inguinal nodes electively but to reserve treatment for node metastases diagnosed later.[87] The ideal dose for elective nodal irradiation (EN) is not known. Doses in the randomized trials ranged from 30.6 to 45 Gy, usually at 1.8 Gy per fraction; failures in EN volumes were not described in detail.

Outcome and clinical prognostic factors

Analyses of the larger randomized trials have consistently identified size of the primary tumor and the presence of lymph node metastases as major prognostic factors. Although other factors such as male gender and hemoglobin level at presentation have been significant factors in some studies, only the primary tumor size is a factor common to all studies, with lymph node metastasis also a factor in most studies.

In the RTOG 9811 trial, after a median follow-up of 2.2 years, a primary tumor ≤5 cm without node metastases was associated with a crude colostomy rate of 11% and an actuarial OS rate of 86%, compared with 9% and 75% if nodes were involved. If the primary tumor was >5 cm, without node metastases, the corresponding rates were 17% and 75%; for a tumor >5 cm with node metastases, the rates were 24% and 63%.[88–90] In the ACT II trial, the 3-year PFS was 81% in patients with primary tumors <5 cm but only 63% in patients with T3 or T4 cancers and nodal metastases.[37]

In a study of 19,199 patients with squamous cell cancer of the anal canal diagnosed between 1985 and 2000 and recorded in the U.S. National Cancer Data Base, the overall 5-year survival was 58%.[91] Patients were staged according to the American Joint Committee on Cancer (AJCC) Cancer Staging Manual, sixth edition, 2002. Twenty-five percent (25.3%) were Stage I,

51.8% Stage II, 17.1% Stage III, and 5.7% Stage IV. Those with distant metastases had a 5-year survival of 18.7% versus 59.4% for those without metastases (the surprisingly good outcome for those with metastases may reflect the categorization of external and common iliac node metastases as "distant metastases" as required by the staging rules used. These nodes are readily encompassed in radiation volumes. External iliac node metastases are considered regional nodes in the most recent staging categorization (Table 16.1)). Patients with regional node metastases had a 5-year survival of 37.4% versus 62.9% in node-negative patients. Five-year survival rates by T category were T1: 68.5%, T2: 58.9%, T3: 43.1%, and T4: 34.3%. The survival rates by AJCC stage were Stage I: 69.5%, Stage II: 59.0%, Stage III: 40.6%,and Stage IV: 18.7%.

In contrast to the 58% OS rate in the registry-based study described previously,[91] the 5-year OS rates in the Phase III trials of patients treated with radiochemotherapy (RCT) improved with time from about 60% [33,34] to about 70–80%, [36,37] likely reflecting differences in trial eligibility criteria, stage distribution, and other less clearly identifiable factors, since there have not been substantial changes in 5FU or MMC doses or in radiation doses, techniques, and volumes. In 40 non-randomized institutional-based series, each of which included more than 50 patients, and in which all patients were treated by combined radiation and doublet chemotherapy (most commonly 5FU/MMC or 5FU/CDDP), there was a wide range of survival rates with little evidence of improvement over time; 5-year OS averaged 70% (unweighted average; range 58% to 84%) in eight studies in which most patients were treated prior to about 1990). In 32 studies in which the majority were treated after 1990, the average 5-year OS was 72% (range 52% to 86%); (study details in Sekhar et al. [83]).

Extrapelvic metastases

Extrapelvic metastases occur at some time in the history of from 10% to 20% of patients. Fewer than 5% have clinically apparent metastases at first presentation. Rates in randomized trials often reflect the practice of reporting only the site of first failure. In the first UKCCCR trial (ACT I), distant metastases were the only recognized site of first failure in 10% (29 of 292) of those treated with radiation, 5FU, and MMC and in 7.4% of those treated with radiation alone.[40] In ACCORD-03, metastases were found in 4% (12 of 307).[38] First failure sites were recorded in RTOG 8411 and showed 5-year rates of distant metastases of 15% in the 5FU/MMC arm and 19% in the 5FU/CDDP arm.[41] Most metastases were found within 2 years of initial treatment.

The median survival time after the diagnosis of metastases in several small series ranged from about 8 to 36 months.

Treatment of extrapelvic metastases is unsatisfactory; it has been approached by analogy with treatment of localized pelvic disease and with other metastatic squamous cell cancers. Cisplatin and 5FU produce responses more often than other drugs, although these responses are usually partial and short lived. Combinations of radiation, 5FU, and MMC or radiation, 5FU, and CDDP appear relatively ineffective when used to treat metastases. The doublet 5FU/MMC is not used because of the risk of toxicity from cumulative MMC doses. In patients treated with chemotherapy only, 5FU/CDDP appeared possibly better than carboplatin/paclitaxel in a non-randomized institution-based study (response rates 57% versus 33%)[93]; these cytotoxic doublets are now being compared in an international multi-institutional Phase II trial[94] (Table 16.5). Two courses of 5FU and CDDP given as either neoadjuvant[36,38] or adjuvant[37] treatment did not alter failure patterns significantly. Other drug combinations have been studied in small series, but none appear better than 5FU and CDDP.

Genomic profiling studies on metastatic ASCC may guide treatment in the future.[95] There have been reports of responses to targeted agents such as cetuximab and bevacizumab, either alone or combined with chemotherapy.[93] Immune checkpoint blockade agents such as nivolumab[96] and pembrolizumab[97] have also been tested. Other approaches, for example, therapeutic vaccines (Table 16.5), are also being studied. None of these treatments is yet considered standard.

Radiation alone may be effective for painful metastases. Stereotactic body radiation therapy (SBRT) or metastatectomy may be considered for selected patients.

Radiation therapy alone

Combined-modality treatment has largely supplanted the use of radiation therapy alone for primary anal cancer. Combined-modality protocols produce higher control rates than radiation alone for all sizes of anal canal tumors treated by the radiation schedules tested. However, radical radiation alone (typically equivalent to 50 Gy in 4 weeks or 60 to 65 Gy in 6 to 8 weeks) resulted in overall local control in about 65% in several large institutional series (70% in tumors up to about 4 cm and 40% to 50% in larger cancers), with maintenance of anal function in 55–70% and 5-year OS rates of about 60%.[43,98,99] Late treatment-related toxicity and resultant colostomy rates were frequently higher than those seen in randomized trials of ChRT in which patients received lower doses of radiation.

Radiation alone should be considered when chemotherapy is contraindicated, since survival rates are comparable to those of surgery, and anorectal function can often be preserved. The most common contraindications to standard doses of chemotherapy are co-morbid conditions or concern about treatment-related toxicities. Some authors use modified doses[100] rather than withhold chemotherapy altogether.[101]

Surgery

The main roles of surgery currently are as salvage following unsuccessful radiation with/without chemotherapy (described earlier) and as treatment for radiation-induced toxicity not relieved by conservative measures.

Surgery is often appropriate for those patients who have small cancers amenable to wide local excision without compromise of anal sphincter function. Surgery is more expedient than radiation or ChRT and possibly more economical.[102] Superficial well-differentiated squamous cell cancers up to about 2 to 3 cm in size that have not penetrated the sphincter muscles are associated with a less than 10% risk of nodal metastases.[82] Locoregional control rates of small tumors in several surgical series were 90%.

Surgery as initial treatment is indicated for patients with larger tumors who cannot receive pelvic radiation, most commonly because of previous pelvic radiation treatment for another malignancy. Those few patients who present with incontinence due to destruction of the anal sphincters or to vaginal fistula are probably best managed surgically. Preoperative or postoperative adjuvant radiation with/without chemotherapy should be considered to reduce the risk of pelvic recurrence. In series managed exclusively by surgery, 5-year survival rates ranged from about 50% to 70%, with locoregional recurrence rates of 25–35%.[82,103–105] Most patients required excision of the anorectum and permanent colostomy. It was the high rate of pelvic recurrence following radical surgery that prompted Nigro and his colleagues to investigate preoperative adjuvant ChRT.[30]

Peri-anal cancer

Local excision, sometimes coupled with skin graft or rotation flap, is the preferred treatment of all histological subtypes of invasive peri-anal cancer when an adequate margin (usually considered to be not less than 0.5 or 1 cm) can be achieved without compromising anal function. This preference for surgery is based on expediency[102] and the risk of long-term morbidity in irradiated skin and anal tissues.[106] The high local recurrence rates reported by some authors[107] following resection of peri-anal squamous cell cancers are probably due to failure to achieve clear resection margins and/or to multi-centric intra-epithelial neoplasia. Further local excision of recurrence may be sufficient to effect local control.[107]

Radiation therapy is indicated when surgery would compromise anorectal function. Whereas radiation therapy alone is effective for both limited and extensive squamous cell cancers,[108–110] some centers prefer protocols of combined radiation and chemotherapy identical to those used for anal canal cancer. The U.K. randomized trials (both ACT I and ACT II) included patients with cancers of the canal or anal margin (the latter when local excision was not possible).[33,37] Results by site of origin were not reported, but site was said not to be a prognostic factor; local control and cause-specific survival rates favored combined-modality treatment over radiation alone.[3] Anal margin (peri-anal) cancers are also included in the PLATO trial.[59]

Inguinal node metastases are uncommon and may be managed by the same principles as node metastases from anal canal cancer. Elective treatment of the groin nodes is favored by some when the primary tumor is larger than 2 cm or poorly differentiated. Death from peri-anal cancer is uncommon and is generally associated with large and deeply infiltrating primary cancers or with distant metastases, the latter often preceded by involvement of inguinal nodes.

Patients with HIV infection

HIV infection causes immunosuppression, and a greater susceptibility to HPV infection, which leads in turn to higher risk of ASCC. In the United States, about 28% of men and 1% of women with ASCC are HIV-infected.[4]

The role of HIV in malignant transformation of HPV-infected cells in ASCC is reviewed elsewhere.[9]

Comparison of the types of cancer among HIV-infected persons with those in the general population in the United States for the period 1992 to 2003, which extended before, during, and after the availability of highly active antiretroviral therapy (HAART), found that anal cancer was the only cancer type that increased both in incidence among HIV-infected persons and in relative incidence compared with the general population over time (standardized incidence rate per 100,000 person-years in the HIV-infected population 19.0 in 1992–1995 versus 78.2 in 2000–2003 [linear trend $p < 0.001$] and among the general population 1.0 versus 1.3 [$p = 0.02$] for the same time periods).[111] This was thought to be because HAART does not alter the incidence or progression of AIN; hence, persons who are successfully treated with HAART but are co-infected with HIV and HPV are expected to remain at greater risk for anal cancer, and incidence rates are expected to increase as HIV-infected persons live longer.[9,111] A systematic review of publications from 1991 to 2017 identified 40 studies in which HIV+ve patients with ASCC were treated with ChRT (3720 patients overall, 1298 HIV+ve).[112] HIV+ve patients had a worse 3-year OS rate (relative risk [RR] 1.77, 95% CI 1.35–2.32, $p < 0.001$); worse 3-year DFS rate (RR 1.32, 1.01–1.74, $p = 0.043$); and higher risk of Grade ≥3 cutaneous toxicities, leukopenia, and thrombocytopenia. In that review, clinical outcomes in the HAART era (after 1996) were conflicting. Cancer-specific survival rates for 14 cancers occurring from 1996 to 2010 in the United States were studied by linking cancer and HIV/AIDS registries in six states.[113] In three cancers (anal cancer, Hodgkin lymphoma, and diffuse large B-cell lymphoma), cancer-specific mortality was not associated with HIV-status; however, about half of overall mortality in these three cancers was attributed to HIV. HIV+ve patients have not been eligible for most completed Phase III randomized trials.[32]

Current expert opinion favors treating ASCC in HIV-infected individuals with curative intent and with protocols similar to those used in immunocompetent patients. Radiation and chemotherapy doses are adjusted as needed for acute toxicity, according to individual tolerance. The management of immunodeficiency-related illness and appropriate HAART regimens in patients receiving chemotherapy are discussed elsewhere.[9]

Non-squamous cell cancers

Adenocarcinomas of the anal canal are usually managed surgically. The choice between anorectal excision and colostomy or local excision is based on the size of the cancer and general principles of oncologic surgery. Most series are small, but 5-year survival rates of less than 50%, with local recurrence rates of about 25%, are typical.[114,115] Because anal adenocarcinomas are encountered infrequently, they are often managed by the protocols in place for adenocarcinomas of the rectum, although the roles of adjuvant radiation and chemotherapy for anal adenocarcinomas are uncertain. Some centers have treated anal adenocarcinomas up to about 4 to 5 cm in size with radiation and a 5FU-based regimen, using protocols similar to those for squamous cancer, and have preserved anorectal function in some.[116,117]

Small-cell and undifferentiated cancers metastasize early. No successful approach to treatment has been devised. Systemic chemotherapy similar to that used for small-cell cancers that arise elsewhere is sometimes given but is of unproven value. The primary cancer may be managed by radiation-based protocols or by surgery.

The principles of management for adenocarcinomas and basal-cell cancers of the peri-anal skin are similar to those for squamous cell cancers. Anorectal function is preserved where possible by local excision or radiation therapy.

Summary

The standard treatment for squamous cell cancers of the anal canal and peri-anal skin is radiation with concurrent 5FU and MMC. Surgery is reserved for salvage of residual or recurrent cancers, or for those few patients who present with small tumors that can be resected without loss of anal function, or those with irreversible destruction of the anal sphincters and incontinence for whom only fecal diversion and ostomy is appropriate. Although many patients do retain anorectal function after treatment with RCT, this function is often abnormal and QoL is impaired.

This treatment paradigm has changed little over the past 30 years. Local control and cure of large anal cancers remain a

challenge, as does cure of extrapelvic metastases. Recent progress in the identification of biomarkers, and the introduction of targeted agents and immunotherapy, offers promise, but these measures have not yet entered standard practice.

Despite the relative infrequency with which these cancers occur, several groups have shown that valuable randomized trials can be performed to refine and improve outcomes.

Key learning points

- Squamous cell cancers of the anal canal and of the peri-anal skin have been combined into a single staging system (UICC Classification of Malignant Tumors, eighth edition, 2017).
- Most patients with anal cancer have good prospects for both cure and retention of anorectal function. The preferred management is based on combinations of radiation and chemotherapy, with radical surgery reserved for residual cancer.
- The standard combination is radiation with concurrent fluoropyrimidine (5FU or capecitabine) and MMC. Following treatment, patients with residual resolving or stable anal masses can be followed for up to 26 weeks before a decision need be made about further intervention.
- Anal function is frequently impaired following RCT, particularly in patients who presented with large tumors (>5 cm), but few patients require a colostomy.
- Surgery is reserved for treatment of small cancers that can be excised widely without interference with anal function; for patients who present with locally advanced cancers and in whom incontinence due to damage to the anal sphincters is considered irreversible; for management of biopsy-proven progressive residual or recurrent cancer after RCT; and for post-RCT toxicity that cannot be managed by conservative measures.
- Current research efforts are directed to improved staging, particularly the identification of small pelvic lymph node metastases; identification and verification of predictive and prognostic markers—several potential markers are available; tailoring radiation doses to each tumor, at present based on tumor size and/or invasiveness, but potentially guided by biomarkers, to reduce late toxicity and improve locoregional control rates; and to identify more effective treatments for extrapelvic metastases.

References

1. Bosman FT, Carneiro F, Hruban RH et al. *WHO Classification of Tumors of the Digestive System*. 4th ed. Lyon, France: IARC Press, 2010.
2. Wilkenson JR, Morris EJ, Downing A et al. The rising incidence of anal cancer in England 1990–2010: A population based study. *Colorectal Dis.* 2014; 16:234–9.
3. Bouvier AM, Belot A, Manfredi S et al. Trends of incidence and survival in squamous cell carcinoma of the anal canal in France: A population-based study. *Eur J Cancer Prev.* 2016;25:182–7.
4. Shiels MS, Kramer AR, Coghill AE et al. Anal cancer incidence in the United States, 1977–2011: Distinct patterns by histology and behaviour. *Cancer Epidemiol Biomarkers Prev.* 2015; 24: 1548–56.
5. Frisch M, Olsen, JH, Bautz A, Melbye M. Benign anal lesions and the risk of anal cancer. *N Engl J Med.* 1994; 331:300–2.
6. Frisch M, Glimelius B, van den Brule AJ et al. Sexually transmitted infection as a cause of anal cancer. *N Engl J Med.* 1997; 337:1350–8.

7. Daling JR, Madeleine MM, Johnson LG et al. Human papillomavirus, smoking and sexual practices in the etiology of anal cancer. *Cancer.* 2004; 101:270–80.

8. Frisch M, Olsen JH, Melbye M. Malignancies that occur before and after anal cancer: Clues to their etiology. *Am J Epidemiol.* 1994; 140:12–19.

9. Wang CJ, Sparano J, Palefsky JM. Human immunodeficiency virus/AIDS, Human papillomavirus, and anal cancer. *Surg Oncol Clin N Am.* 2017; 26:17–31.

10. Grulich AE, van Leeuwen MT, Falster MO et al. Incidence of cancers in people with HIV/AIDS compared with immunosuppressed transplant recipients: A meta-analysis. *Lancet.* 2007; 370:59–67.

11. Scholefield JH, Palmer JG, Shepherd NA et al. Clinical and pathological correlates of HPV type 16 DNA in anal cancer. *Int J Colorectal Dis.* 1990; 5:219–22.

12. Bhuva NJ, Glynne-Jones R, Sonoda L et al. To PET or not to PET? That is the question. Staging in anal cancer. *Ann Oncol.* 2012; 23:2078–82.

13. Mistrangelo DM, Bello M, Cassoni P et al. Value of staging squamous cell carcinoma of the anal margin and canal using the sentinel lymph node procedure: An update of the series and a review of the literature. *Br J Cancer.* 2013; 108:527–32.

14. Noorani A, Rabey N, Durrani A et al. Systematic review of sentinel lymph node biopsy in anal squamous cell carcinoma. *Int J Surg.* 2013; 11:762–6.

15. Brierley JD, Gospodarowicz, MK, Wittekind C (eds). *TNM Classification of Malignant Tumors.* 8th ed. Hoboken, NJ: Wiley Blackwell, 2017.

16. Sobin L, Gospodarowicz M, Wittekind C (eds.). *International Union Against Cancer (UICC) TNM Classification of Malignant Tumors.* 7th ed. Hoboken, NJ: Wiley Blackwell, 2009.

17. Jones CM, Goh V, Sebag-Montefiore D et al. Biomarkers in anal cancer: From biological understanding to stratified treatment. *Br J Cancer.* 2017; 116:156–62.

18. Meulendijks D, Tomasoa NB, Dewit L et al. HPV-negative squamous cell carcinoma of the anal canal is unresponsive to standard treatment and frequently carries disruptive mutations in TP53. *Br J Cancer.* 2015; 112:1358–66.

19. Parwaiz I, MacCabe TA, Thomas MG et al. A systematic review and meta-analysis of prognostic biomarkers in anal squamous cell carcinoma treated with primary chemoradiotherapy. *Clin Oncol.* 2019; 31:e1–13.

20. Swick AD, Chatterjee A, de Costa A-M et al. Modulation of therapeutic sensitivity by human papillomavirus. *Radiother Oncol.* 2015; 116:342–5.

21. Smaglo BG, Tesfaye A, Halfdanarson TR et al. Comprehensive multiplatform biomarker analysis of 199 anal squamous cell carcinomas. *Oncotarget,* 2015; 6:43594–604.

22. Chung JH, Sanford E, Johnson A et al. Comprehensive genomic profiling of anal squamous cell carcinoma reveals distinct genomically defined classes. *Ann Oncol.* 2016; 27:1336–41.

23. Hoff PM, Coudry R, Venchiarutti Moniz CM. Pathology of anal cancer. *Surg Oncol Clin N Am.* 2017; 26:57–71.

24. Serup-Hansen E, Linnemann D, Skovrider-Ruminski W et al. Human papillomavirus genotyping and p16 expression as prognostic factors for patients with American Joint Committee on Cancer stages I to III carcinoma of the anal canal. *J Clin Oncol.* 2014; 32:1812–7.

25. Williams M, Swampillai A, Osborne M et al. Squamous cell carcinoma antigen: A potentially useful prognostic marker in squamous cell carcinoma of the anal canal and margin. *Cancer.* 2013; 119:2391–8.

26. Glynne-Jones R, Nilsson PJ, Aschele C et al. Anal cancer: ESMO-ESSO-ESTRO clinical practice guidelines for diagnosis, treatment and followup. *Radiother Oncol.* 2014; 111:330–9.

27. NCCN Clinical Practice Guidelines in Oncology – Anal Carcinoma. Version 1.2019 – March 15, 2019. Accessed online July 2019.

28. Johnson N, Pellino G, Simillis C et al. Discrepancies between NCCN and ESMO guidelines in the management of anal cancer: A qualitative review. *Updates Surg.* 2017; 69:345–9.

29. Myerson RJ, Karnell LH, Menck HR. The National Cancer Data Base report on carcinoma of the anus. *Cancer.* 1997; 80:805–15.

30. Nigro ND, Vaitkevicius VK, Considine B Jr. Combined therapy for cancer of the anal canal: A preliminary report. *Dis Colon Rectum.* 1974; 15:354–6.

31. Lim F, Glynne-Jones R. Chemotherapy/chemoradiation in anal cancer: A systematic review. *Cancer Treat Rev.* 2011; 37:520–32.

32. Spithoff K, Cummings B, Jonker D et al. Chemoradiotherapy for squamous cell cancer of the anal canal: A systematic review. *Clin Oncol.* 2014; 26:473–87.

33. UKCCCR Working Party. Epidermoid anal cancer: Results from the UKCCCR randomised trial of radiotherapy alone versus radiotherapy, 5-fluorouracil, and mitomycin. UKCCCR Anal Cancer Trial Working Party. UK Co-ordinating Committee on Cancer Research. *Lancet.* 1996; 348:1049–54.

34. Bartelink H, Roelofsen F, Eschwege F et al. Concomitant radiotherapy and chemotherapy is superior to radiotherapy alone in the treatment of locally advanced anal cancer: Results of a phase III randomized trial of the European Organization for Research and Treatment of Cancer Radiotherapy and Gastrointestinal Cooperative Groups. *J Clin Oncol.* 1997; 15:2040–9.

35. Flam M, John M, Pajak TF et al. Role of mitomycin in combination with fluorouracil and radiotherapy, and of salvage chemoradiation in the definitive nonsurgical treatment of epidermoid carcinoma of the anal canal: Results of a phase III randomized intergroup study. *J Clin Oncol.* 1996; 14:2527–39.

36. Gunderson LL, Winter KA, Ajani, JA et al. Long-term update of US GI Intergroup RTOG 98–11 Phase III trial for anal carcinoma; survival, relapse, and colostomy failure with concurrent chemoradiation involving Fluorouracil/Mitomycin versus Fluorouracil/Cisplatin. *J Clin Oncol.* 2012; 30:4344–51.

37. James RD, Glynne-Jones R, Meadows HM et al. Mitomycin or cisplatin chemoradiation with or without maintenance chemotherapy for treatment of squamous-cell carcinoma of the anus (ACT II): A randomised, phase 3, open-label, 2x2 factorial trial. *Lancet Oncol.* 2013; 14:516–24.

38. Peiffert D, Tournier-Rangeard L, Gerard J-P et al. Induction chemotherapy and dose intensification of the radiation boost in locally advanced anal canal carcinoma: Final analysis of the randomized UNICANCER ACCORD 03 trial. *J Clin Oncol.* 2012; 30:1941–48.

39. Glynne-Jones R, Adams R, Lopes A et al. Clinical endpoints in trials of chemoradiation for patients with anal cancer. *Lancet Oncol.* 2017; 18:e218–27.

40. Northover J, Glynne-Jones R, Sebag-Montefiore D et al. Chemoradiation for the treatment of epidermoid anal cancer: 13-year follow-up of the first randomized UKCCCR Anal Cancer Trial (ACT I). *Br J Cancer.* 2010; 102:1123–8.

41. Ajani JA, Winter KA, Gunderson LL et al. Fluorouracil, mitomycin, and radiotherapy vs. fluorouracil, cisplatin and radiotherapy for carcinoma of the anal canal: A randomized controlled trial. *JAMA.* 2008; 299:1914–21.

42. Glynne-Jones R, Sebag-Montefiore D, Meadows HM et al. Best time to assess complete clinical response after chemoradiotherapy in squamous cell carcinoma of the anus (ACT II): A post-hoc analysis of a controlled phase 3 trial. *Lancet Oncol.* 2017; 18:347–56.

43. Cummings BJ, Keane TJ, O'Sullivan B, Wong CS, Catton CN. Epidermoid anal cancer: Treatment by radiation alone or by radiation and 5-fluorouracil with and without mitomycin C. *Int J Radiat Oncol Biol Phys.* 1991; 21:1115–25.

44. Nigro ND. An evaluation of combined therapy for squamous cell cancer of the anal canal. *Dis Colon Rectum.* 1984; 27:763–6.

45. Tanum G, Tveit K, Karlsen KO et al. Chemoradiotherapy of anal carcinoma: Tumor response and acute toxicity *Oncology.* 1993; 50:14–7.

46. Sadeghi R, Harsini S, Ali Qodsi Rad M et al. Prognostic significance of fluorine-18 Fluorodeoxyglucose positron emission tomography in anal squamous cell carcinoma: A systematic review and a meta-analysis. *Contrast Media Molec Imaging.* 2018; 9760492.

47. Duimering A, Riauka T, Nijjar Y et al. Prognostic utility of pre- and post-treatment FDG-PET parameters in anal squamous cell carcinoma. *Radiother Oncol.* 2019; 136:21–8.

48. Pan YB, Maeda M, Wilson A et al. Late gastrointestinal toxicity after radiotherapy for anal cancer: A systematic literature review. *Acta Oncol.* 2018; 57:1427–37.

49. Glynne-Jones R, Kadalayil, Meadows HM et al. Tumor- and treatment-related colostomy rates following mitomycin C or cisplatin chemoradiation with or without maintenance chemotherapy in squamous cell carcinoma of the anus in the ACT II trial. *Ann Oncol.* 2014; 25:1616–22.

50. Hosni A, Han K, Le LW et al. The ongoing challenge of large anal cancers: Prospective long term outcomes of intensity-modulated radiation therapy with concurrent chemotherapy. *Oncotarget.* 2018; 9:20439–50.

51. Jephcott CR, Paltiel C, Hay J. Quality of life after non-surgical treatment of anal carcinoma: A case control study in long-term survivors. *Clin Oncol.* 2004; 16:530–5.

52. Bentzen AG, Balteskard L, Wanderass EH et al. Impaired health-related quality of life after chemoradiotherapy for anal cancer: Late effects in a national cohort of 128 survivors. *Acta Oncol.* 2013; 52:736–44.

53. Sodergren SC, Johnson CD, Gilbert A et al. Phase I–III development of the EORTC QLQ-ANL27, a health-related quality of life questionnaire for anal cancer. *Radiother Oncol.* 2018; 126:222–8.

54. Cyr DP, Savage P, Theodosopoulos E et al. Outcomes of salvage surgery for anal squamous cell carcinoma: A systematic review and meta-analysis. *J Clin Oncol.* 2019; 37(Suppl):abstr 3571.

55. Sammour T, Rodriguez-Bigas MA, Skibber JM. Locally recurrent disease related to anal canal cancers. *Surg Oncol Clin N Am.* 2017; 26:115–25.

56. Chapet O, Gerard JP, Riche B et al. Prognostic value of tumor regression evaluated after first course of radiotherapy for anal canal cancer. *Int J Radiat Oncol Biol Phys.* 2005; 63:1316–24.

57. Wright JL, Patil SM, Temple LK et al. Squamous cell carcinoma of the anal canal: Patterns and predictors of failure and implications for intensity-modulated radiation treatment planning. *Int J Radiat Oncol Biol Phys.* 2010; 78:1064–72.

58. Buettner F, Gulliford SL, Webb S et al. The dose response of the anal sphincter region—an analysis of data from the MRC RT01 trial. *Radiother Oncol.* 2012; 103:347–52.

59. PLATO. Personalising anal cancer radiotherapy dose. ISRCTN88455282. Accessed online July 2019. www.hra.nhs.uk/plato-personalizing-cancer-radiotherapy-dose/.

60. Wong CS, Tsang RW, Cummings BJ et al. Proliferation parameters in epidermoid carcinomas of the anal canal. *Radiother Oncol.* 2000; 56:349–53.

61. Glynne-Jones R, Sebag-Montefiore D, Adams R et al. "Mind the gap"—The impact of variations in the duration of the treatment gap and overall treatment time in the first UK anal cancer trial (ACT I). *Int J Radiat Oncol Biol Phys.* 2011; 81:1488–94.

62. Ben-Joseph E, Moughan J, Ajani JA et al. Impact of overall treatment time on survival and local control in patients with anal cancer; A pooled data analysis of Radiation Therapy Oncology Group Study No. 8314. *J Clin Oncol.* 2010; 28:5061–6.

63. Glynne-Jones R, Lim F. Anal cancer: An examination of radiotherapy strategies. *Int J Radiat Oncol Biol Phys.* 2011; 79:1290–301.

64. Kachnic LA, Winter K, Myerson RJ et al. RTOG 0529: A phase 2 evaluation of dose-painted intensity-modulated radiation therapy in combination with 5-fluorouracil and mitomycin-C for the reduction of acute morbidity in carcinoma of the anal canal. *Int J Radiat Oncol Biol Phys.* 2013; 86:27–33.

65. Muirhead R, Adams RA, Gilbert DC et al. National Guidance for IMRT in Anal Cancer. Version 4. 07/12/2016. www.analimrtguidance.co.uk. Accessed July 2019.

66. Gay HA, Barthold HJ, O'Meara E et al. Pelvic normal tissue contouring guidelines for radiation therapy: A Radiation Therapy Oncology Group Consensus Panel atlas. *Int J Radiat Oncol Biol Phys.* 2012; 83:e353–62.

67. Ng M, Leong T, Chander S et al. Australasian Gastrointestinal Trials Group (AGITG) contouring atlas and planning guidelines for intensity-modulated radiotherapy in anal cancer. *Int J Radiat Oncol Biol Phys.* 2012; 83:1455–62.

68. Han K, Cummings BJ, Lindsay P et al. Prospective evaluation of acute toxicity and quality of life after IMRT and concurrent chemotherapy for anal canal and perianal cancer. *Int J Radiat Oncol Biol Phys.* 2014; 90:587–94.

69. Moreau-Zabotta L, Ortholan C, Hannoun-Levi J-M et al. Role of brachytherapy in the boost management of anal carcinoma with node involvement (CORS-03 Study). *Int J Radiat Oncol Biol Phys.* 2013; 85:e135–42.

70. Ceresoli GL, Ferreri AJ, Cordio S, Villa E. Role of dose intensity in conservative treatment of anal canal carcinoma. Report of 35 cases. *Oncology.* 1998; 55:525–32.

71. Rich TA, Ajani JA, Morrison WH, Ota D, Levin B. Chemoradiation therapy for anal cancer: Radiation plus continuous infusion of 5-fluorouracil with or without cisplatin. *Radiother Oncol.* 1993; 27:209–11.

72. Jones CM, Adams R, Downing A et al. Toxicity, tolerability, and compliance of concurrent and intensity modulated radiation therapy: Evaluation of a national cohort. *Int J Radiat Oncol Biol Phys.* 2018; 101:1202–11.

73. White EC, Goldman K, Aleshin A et al. Chemoradiotherapy for squamous cell carcinoma of the anal canal: comparison of one versus two cycles of mitomycin-C. *Radiother Oncol.* 2015; 117:240–5.

74. Glimelius B, Pahlman L. Radiation therapy of anal epidermoid carcinoma. *Int J Radiat Oncol Biol Phys.* 1987; 13:305–12.

75. Matzinger O, Roelofsen F, Mineur L et al. Mitomycin C with continuous fluorouracil or with cisplatin in combination with radiotherapy for locally advanced anal cancer (European Organization for Research and Treatment of Cancer phase II study 22011–40014). *Eur J Cancer.* 2009; 45:2782–91.

76. James RD, David C, Neville D et al. Chemoradiation and maintenance chemotherapy for patients with anal carcinoma: A phase II study of the UK Coordinating Committee for Cancer Research (UKCCCR) Anal Cancer Trial Working Party. *Proc Am Soc Clin Oncol.* 2000; 19:268a(abstr).

77. Garg MK, Zhao F, Sparano JA et al. Cetuximab plus chemoradiotherapy in immunocompetent patients with anal cancer: A phase II Eastern Cooperative Oncology Group—American College of Radiology Imaging Network Cancer Research Group trial (E3205). *J Clin Oncol.* 2017; 35:718–26.

78. Sparano JA, Lee JY, Palefsky J et al. Cetuximab plus chemoradiotherapy for HIV-associated anal carcinoma: A phase II AIDS Malignancy Consortium trial. *J Clin Oncol.* 2016; 35:727–33.

79. Leon O, Guren MG, Radu C et al. Phase I study of Cetuximab in combination with 5-fluorouracil, mitomycin C and radiotherapy in patients with locally advanced anal cancer. *Eur J Cancer.* 2015; 51:2740–6.

80. Feliu J, Garcia-Carbonera R, Capdevilla J et al. Phase II trial of Panitumumab, plus mitomycin C 5- profile—VITAL study, GEMCAD 09–02 clinical trial. *J Clin Oncol.* 2014; 32(Suppl):abstract4034.

81. Golden GT, Horsley JS III. Surgical management of epidermoid carcinoma of the anus. *Am J Surg.* 1976; 131:275–80.

82. Boman BM, Moertel CG, O'Connell MJ et al. Carcinoma of the anal canal. A clinical and pathologic study of 188 cases. *Cancer.* 1984;54:114–25.

83. Sekhar H, Zwahlen M, Trelle S et al. Nodal stage migration and prognosis in anal cancer: A systematic review, meta-regression and simulation study. *Lancet Oncol.* 2017; 18:1348–59.

84. Feinstein AR, Sosin DM, Wells CK. The Will Rogers phenomenon. Stage migration and new diagnostic techniques as a source of misleading statistics for survival in cancer. *N Engl J Med.* 1985; 312:1604–8.

85. Stearns MW Jr, Urmacher C, Sternberg SS, Woodruff J, Attiyeh F. Cancer of the anal canal. *Curr Probl Cancer.* 1980; 4:1–44.

86. Ortholan C, Resbeut M, Hannoun-Levi J-M et al. Anal canal cancer: Management of inguinal nodes and benefit of prophylactic inguinal irradiation (CORS-03 Study). *Int J Radiat Oncol Biol Phys.* 2012; 82:1988–95

87. Gerard JP, Chapet O, Samiei F et al. Management of inguinal lymph node metastases in patients with carcinoma of the anal canal. Experience in a series of 270 patients treated in Lyon and review of the literature. *Cancer.* 2001; 92:77–84.

88. Ajani JA, Winter KA, Gunderson LL et al. US Intergroup Anal Cancer Trial: Tumor diameter predicts for colostomy. *J Clin Oncol.* 2009; 27:1116–21.

89. Ajani JA, Winter KA, Gunderson LL et al. Prognostic factors derived from a prospective database dictate clinical biology of anal cancer. *Cancer.* 2010; 116:4007–13.

90. Gunderson LL, Moughan J, Ajani JA et al. Anal carcinoma: Impact of TN category of disease on survival, disease relapse, and colostomy failure in US Gastrointestinal Intergroup RTOG 98–11 phase 3 trial. *Int J Radiat Oncol Biol Phys.* 2013; 87:638–45.

91. Bilimoria KY, Bentrem DJ, Rock CE et al. Outcomes and prognostic factors for squamous-cell carcinoma of the anal canal: Analysis of patients from the National Cancer Data Base. *Dis Colon Rectum.* 2009; 52:624–31.

92. Greene FL, Page DL, Fleming D et al. (eds). *AJCC Cancer Staging Manual.* 6th ed. Philadelphia, PA: Lippincott Raven, 2002.

93. Morris V, Eng C. Metastatic anal cancer and novel agents. *Surg Oncol Clin N Am.* 2017; 26:133–42.

94. NIH Clinical Trials Register. https://clinicaltrials.gov/

95. Morris V, Rao X, Pickering C et al. Comprehensive genomic profiling of metastatic carcinoma of the anal canal. *Mol Cancer Res.* 2017; 15:1542–50.

96. Morris V, Salem ME, Nimeiri H et al. Nivolumab for previously treated unresectable metastatic anal cancer (NCI9673): A multicentre, single-arm, phase 2 study. *Lancet Oncol.* 2017; 18:446.

97. Ott PA, Piha-Paul SA, Munster P et al. Safety and antitumor activity of the anti-PD-1 antibody Pembrolizumab in patients with recurrent carcinoma of the anal canal. *Ann Oncol.* 2017; 28:1036–41.

98. Papillon J, Montbarbon JF. Epidermoid carcinoma of the anal canal. A series of 276 cases. *Dis Colon Rectum.* 1987; 30:324–33.

99. Touboul E, Schlienger M, Buffat L et al. Epidermoid carcinoma of the anal canal. Results of curative-intent radiation therapy in a series of 270 patients. *Cancer.* 1994; 73:1569–79.

100. Charnley N, Choudhury A, Chesser P, Cooper RA, Sebag-Montefiore D. Effective treatment of anal cancer in the elderly with low-dose chemoradiotherapy. *Br J Cancer.* 2005; 92:1221–5.

101. Chauveinc L, Buthaud X, Falcou MC et al. Anal canal cancer treatment: Practical limitations of routine prescription of concurrent chemotherapy and radiotherapy. *Br J Cancer.* 2003; 89: 2057–61.

102. Deshmukh AA, Zhao H, Das P et al. Clinical and economic evaluation of treatment strategies for T1N0 anal canal cancer. *Am J Clin Oncol.* 2018; 41:626–31.

103. Greenall MJ, Quan SH, Decosse JJ. Epidermoid cancer of the anus. *Br J Surg.* 1985; 72 Supplement:S97–103.

104. Pintor MP, Northover JM, Nicholls RJ. Squamous cell carcinoma of the anus at one hospital from 1948 to 1984. *Br J Surg.* 1989; 76:806–10.

105. Klas JV, Rothenberger DA, Wong WD, Madoff RD. Malignant tumors of the anal canal. The spectrum of disease, treatment and outcomes. *Cancer.* 1999; 85:1686–93.

106. Ortholan C, Ramaioli A, Peiffert D et al. Anal canal carcinoma: Early stage tumors ≤ 10mm (T1 or Tis): Therapeutic options and original pattern of local failure after radiotherapy. *Int J Radiat Oncol Biol Phys.* 2005; 62:479–85.

107. Greenall MJ, Quan SH, Stearns MW, Urmacher C, DeCosse JJ. Epidermoid cancer of the anal margin. Pathologic features, treatment, and clinical results. *Am J Surg.* 1985; 149:95–101.

108. Papillon J, Chassard JL. Respective roles of radiotherapy and surgery in the management of epidermoid carcinoma of the anal margin. Series of 57 patients. *Dis Colon Rectum.* 1992; 35:422–9

109. Peiffert D, Bey P, Pernot M et al. Conservative treatment by irradiation of epidermoid carcinomas of the anal margin. *Int J Radiat Oncol Biol Phys.* 1997;39:57–66.

110. Khanfir K, Ozsahin M, Bieri S et al. Patterns of failure and outcome in patients with carcinoma of the anal margin. *Ann Surg Oncol.* 2008; 15:1092–8.

111. Patel P, Hanson DL, Sullivan PS et al. Incidence of types of cancer among HIV-infected persons compared with the general population in the United States, 1992–2003. *Ann Intern Med.* 2008; 148:728–36.

112. Camandaroba, MP, Cunha de Araujo RL, Souza e Silva V et al. Treatment outcomes of patients with localized anal squamous cell carcinoma according to HIV infection: Systematic review and meta-analysis. *J Gastrointest Oncol.* 2019; 10:48–60.

113. Coghill AE, Shiels MS, Suneja G et al. Elevated cancer specific mortality among HIV-infected patients in the United States. *J Clin Oncol.* 2016; 33:2376–83.

114. Tarazi R, Nelson RL. Anal adenocarcinoma: A comprehensive review. *Semin Surg Oncol.* 1994; 10:235–40.

115. Belkacemi Y, Berger C, Poortmans P et al. Management of anal canal adenocarcinoma: A large retrospective study from the Rare Cancer Network. *Int J Radiat Oncol Biol Phys.* 2003; 56:1274–83.

116. Papagikos M, Crane CH, Skibber J et al. Chemoradiation for adenocarcinoma of the anus. *Int J Radiat Oncol Biol Phys.* 2003; 55:669–78.

117. Lukovic J, Kim J, Liu A et al. Anal adenocarcinoma: Multidisciplinary management of a rare malignancy. (submitted 2019).

17 GERM-CELL CANCER OF THE TESTIS AND RELATED NEOPLASMS

Amy Kwan and Danish Mazhar

Introduction

Germ-cell cancers are rare malignancies, predominantly occurring in males. Histologically identical neoplasms may arise in multiple sites. While the most common primary site is the testis, other recognized primary sites include the retroperitoneum, mediastinum, pineal/suprasellar area, the ovary, and (in infants) the sacro-coccygeal region. These malignancies are generally highly sensitive to chemotherapy and in some cases radiotherapy. More than 95% of the patients presenting with a germ-cell tumor can expect to be cured. This chapter focuses predominantly on male germ-cell cancers, but also includes discussion on testicular sex-cord stromal tumors.

Background

Epidemiology

Germ-cell cancers are rare malignancies making up 1% of all male cancers. They are the most common malignancy in young men, less than 35 years of age, with approximately 90% of the patients being less than 55 years.[1] Approximately 1:190 males in the United Kingdom develop a testicular germ-cell cancer in their lifetime.[1] Between 2014 and 2016, the average annual incidence of male germ-cell cancers was approximately 2400 per year in the United Kingdom.[1] Although worldwide the incidence of germ-cell tumors is low, it is estimated to have doubled in the past 40 years and there is appreciable variation between countries.[2,3] The highest rates of germ-cell cancers are reported for white Caucasian populations in industrialized countries, particularly in western and northern Europe and Australia/New Zealand.[4] The etiology of the rising trend is unclear, although there is strong evidence to suggest that sperm counts are falling, and it is hypothesized that the same etiological events underlie both abnormalities.

Germ-cell cancers of the testis are divided histologically into testicular seminoma and non-seminoma. The median age of onset of non-seminoma is 25–30 years. This is approximately a decade later for seminoma. Recent epidemiological studies have shown the median age of onset may be increasing.[5] Germ-cell tumors of the testis are rare before the age of 15 and after the age of 60.

Etiology

Known epidemiological risk factors for the development of testicular tumors are listed in Table 17.1. The most prevalent predisposing factor is testicular maldescent.[6] If either testis fails to descend normally, the incidence of testicular cancer rises approximately five-fold (both testes are at increased risk), and if both are maldescended, the incidence rises ten-fold. The cause for this relationship is not clear. Theories include gonadal dysgenesis, a systemic factor, hormonal exposure in utero, or a chromosomal abnormality.[7]

A personal history of testicular cancer also increases the risk of developing testicular cancer on the contralateral side with a 4–5% risk of developing contralateral disease.[8] All patients should

therefore be encouraged to self-examine to ensure these are diagnosed early. Familial clustering of germ-cell tumors is seen and patients with a family history of testicular germ-cell cancer (particularly siblings) have an increased risk of developing a tumor themselves approximately five-fold to ten-fold.[8,9]

Additional proposed risk factors for germ-cell cancers include Down's syndrome,[10] the presence of testicular atrophy or dysgenesis, and a previous history of mumps orchitis. Associations with these are less well-characterized.

Pathogenesis

A recognized feature of early germ-cell cancers in adults is the histological precursor of intratubular germ cell neoplasia unclassified (IGCNU)[11]—the presence of atypical intratubular germ cells (Figure 17.1). The development of IGCNU is not fully understood. It has been hypothesized that intrauterine hormonal imbalance (by intrinsic or extrinsic factors) may result in a disturbance in the fetal programming of gonadal development. Either way, the current view is that IGCNU develops early in life and factors including puberty and environmental exposure may lead to the development of cancer.[11] In adults, it can be found adjacent to recognizable cancer in the majority of resected testes containing malignant germ-cell cancer.

IGCNU is usually present throughout the testis and can be confirmed with a single biopsy. A longitudinal study on patients with this histological abnormality suggested an increasing incidence of invasive cancer with time, rising to 50% in 5 years.[12] It does not resolve spontaneously. Irradiation can lead to complete resolution of the changes[13] whereas chemotherapy may not.[14]

Tumor cytogenetics

Adult germ-cell cancers arising at any site are characterized in a high proportion of cases (approximately 80%) by the presence of an isochromosome of the short arm of chromosome 12—denoted i12p.[15] It has been suggested that i12p deletion can be tested in cases of diagnostic uncertainty. The precise role of this chromosomal abnormality in the pathogenesis of germ-cell tumors is at present unknown.[16] The same chromosomal change is also seen in IGCNU.

Analysis of markers such as M2A, C-KIT, and OCT4/NANOG suggests that the deregulation in the pluripotent program of fetal germ cells is probably responsible for the development of IGCNU and germ-cell neoplasia. There may be an overlap in the development of seminoma and embryonal carcinoma as shown by genome-wide expression analysis and detection of alpha-fetoprotein (AFP) mRNA in some atypical seminoma.[17]

Diagnosis and staging

Clinical presentation

The majority of patients present with symptoms from their testicular primary. The duration of symptoms varies from days to many years (the latter usually in patients with teratoma differentiated or seminoma). Most commonly, the diagnosis is made

TABLE 17.1 Risk Factors for the Development of Testicular Germ-Cell Tumors

Factor	Approximate Increase in Risk
Unilateral testicular maldescent	×5
Bilateral testicular maldescent	×10
Family history:	
– Brother	×10
– Father	×2–3
Contralateral testicular cancer	×10
Mumps orchitis/testicular atrophy	Unknown
Childhood inguinal hernia or hydrocoele	Unknown
Down's syndrome	Unknown

Note: Lifetime risk of testicular cancer in the United Kingdom is 1 in 190.

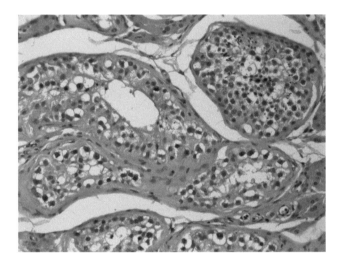

FIGURE 17.1 Intratubular germ cell neoplasia unclassified (IGCNU): several seminiferous tubules lined by atypical cells, with normal germ cells in the tubule top left. (Courtesy of Dr. A Warren, consultant histopathologist, Addenbrooke's Hospital.)

after a painless, unilateral mass in the scrotum is discovered. Other symptoms include intermittent or progressively worsening scrotal discomfort (20%), testicular shrinkage, or a change in texture of the testicle. In a handful of cases, a testicular primary can mimic an orchidoepididymitis presenting with pain, swelling, and infective symptoms; however, these symptoms do not resolve with antibiotics.[18] Finally, the presence of a testicular cancer can also manifest following trauma with associated swelling, which may have failed to settle satisfactorily. Patients with an elevated level of human chorionic gonadotrophin (hCG) commonly notice nipple tenderness, sometimes along with gynecomastia in 7%.[19]

A number of patients with germ-cell tumors present with symptoms from extra-gonadal disease. The most common symptoms in this situation are lumbar backache secondary to metastatic para-aortic lymphadenopathy. Where this disease is bulky there may be obstruction of the ureters(s) leading to hydronephrosis, bowel obstruction, or inferior vena cava occlusion (secondary to either tumor or vascular thrombus). Patients may also present with the signs and symptoms of deep vein thrombosis or pulmonary emboli. Patients with metastatic germ cell tumors (GCT) may present with lung metastases, manifested by chest pain, dyspnea, cough, or hemoptysis. Metastatic disease in the lung can be rapidly progressive, particularly in the

choriocarcinoma syndrome,[20] in which widespread vascular dissemination is common. Rarely, patients present with an inguinal lymph-node mass—usually a result of previous inguinal/scrotal surgery with resulting anomalous lymphatic drainage—or with a cervical nodal mass. Symptoms can arise due to involvement of the brain (e.g. headaches and fits) and bone (pain) though these represent a small proportion of presentations.

Testicular ultrasonography

A bilateral testicular ultrasound must be performed in all cases of suspected testicular cancer. This gives information about the size and vascularity of any mass seen within the body of the testis and can assess the size and appearance of the contralateral testis. The sensitivity of detecting a testicular tumor is approximately 100%.[21] Microlithiasis may be present in 50% of cases, although the association of microlithiasis and testicular germ-cell tumor is contentious.[22,23]

Ultrasonography should also be performed to confirm the site of primary disease in patients presenting with symptoms arising from a possible extragonadal primary. In up to 50% of the cases, ultrasound may reveal scar tissue indicating a "burnt out" testicular primary, and these cases will need an orchiectomy as part of their treatment.[24–26]

Management of the primary lesion

All patients with suspected testicular malignancy should undergo surgical exploration and orchidectomy. This should generally be via an inguinal excision. Rarely, scrotal exploration may be performed when cancer has not been considered. In these cases, the wound should be closed and inguinal orchidectomy performed.[27,28] The resection specimen should contain the tumor-bearing testicle and the spermatic cord to the level of the inguinal ring. More radical surgery is unnecessary.

Orchidectomy should be performed before further treatment as this will allow histological confirmation of the diagnosis. However, in cases of life-threatening disease with an unequivocal diagnosis (based on marker evaluation and radiological findings), orchidectomy should not delay immediate treatment with chemotherapy. Surgery to the primary should be performed at the later stage, usually after the completion of first-line chemotherapy.[29,30]

Histological assessment

It is generally recommended that histological assessment should include examination of one block per cubic centimeter of resected cancer.[21,31] The pathology report should include an assessment of gross tumor size and different histological types present, together with an assessment of their proportion.[21] Tumor extension through the tunica albuginea with involvement of the tunica vaginalis or involvement of the rete testis should be reported, as should spermatic cord or scrotal invasion. An assessment should also be made as to whether vascular/lymphatic invasion is present, and a tumor, node, metastasis (TNM) stage (see Table 17.2) should be allocated. If there is uncertainty about the histological type, immunohistochemistry should be performed. This includes staining for AFP, hCG, placental alkaline phosphatase (PLAP), c-kit, chromogranin A, and Ki-1.

Germ-cell cancers are commonly divided, for clinical purposes, into seminoma and non-seminoma germ-cell tumors. In a proportion of cases, elements of both tumor types are present in the primary. For practical purposes, these patients are managed as non-seminoma. Available pathological and clinical data suggest that occasional patients with seminoma "transform"

TABLE 17.2 TNM Classification for Testicular Cancer

pT	Primary tumor*
pTX	Primary tumor cannot be assessed
pT0	No evidence of primary tumor (e.g. histologic scar in testis)
pTis	Intratubular germ-cell neoplasia (TIN)
pT1	Tumor limited to testis and epididymis without vascular/lymphatic invasion: Tumor may invade tunica albuginea but not tunica vaginalis
pT2	Tumor limited to testis and epididymis with vascular/lymphatic invasion or tumor extending through tunica albuginea with involvement of tunica vaginalis
pT3	Tumor invades spermatic cord with or without vascular/lymphatic invasion
pT4	Tumor invades scrotum with or without vascular/lymphatic invasion
N—Regional lymph nodes clinical	
NX	Regional lymph nodes cannot be assessed
N0	No regional lymph node metastasis
N1	Metastasis with a lymph node mass <2 cm in greatest dimension or multiple lymph nodes; none <2 cm in greatest dimension
N2	Metastasis with a lymph node mass >2 cm but <5 cm in greatest dimension or multiple lymph nodes; any one mass >2 cm but <5 cm in greatest dimension
N3	Metastasis with a lymph node mass >5 cm in greatest dimension
pN—Pathologic regional lymph nodes	
pNX	Regional lymph nodes cannot be assessed
pN0	No regional lymph node metastasis
pN1	Metastasis with a lymph node mass <2 cm in greatest dimension and <5 positive nodes; none >2 cm in greatest dimension
pN2	Metastasis with a lymph node mass >2 cm but <5 cm in greatest dimension; or >5 nodes positive, none >5 cm; or evidence of extranodal extension of tumor
pN3	Metastasis with a lymph node mass >5 cm in greatest dimension
M—Distant metastasis	
MX	Distant metastasis cannot be assessed
M0	No distant metastasis
M1	Distant metastasis
M1a	Nonregional lymph node(s) or lung
M1b	Other sites
pM—Pathologic distant metastasis	
MX	Distant metastasis cannot be assessed
M0	No distant metastasis
M1	Distant metastasis
M1a	Nonregional lymph node(s) or lung
M1b	Other sites
S—Serum tumor markers	
Sx	Serum markers studies not available or not performed
S0	Serum marker study levels within normal limits

LDH, U/l	hCG, mlU/ml	AFP, ng/ml
S1 <1.5 × N and	<5000 and	<1000
S2 1.5–10 × N or	5,000–50,000 or	1000–10,000
S3 >10 × N or	>50,000 or	>10,000

Source: Brierley et al., 2016. With permission.

Note: Except for pTis and pT4, where radical orchidectomy is not always necessary for classification purposes, the extent of the primary tumor is classified after radical orchidectomy; see pT. In other circumstances, TX is used if no radical orchidectomy has been performed.

Abbreviations: LDH, lactate dehydrogenase; N, upper limit of normal for the LDH assay; hCG, human chorionic gonadotrophin; AFP, α-fetoprotein.

histologically into non-seminomas—particularly of yolk-sac type.[32]

The current ESMO guidelines recommend a pathological classification modified from the 2016 version of the World Health Organization (WHO) guidelines.[33,34] This has been revised from previous guidelines to separate germ cell neoplasia which has derived from germ cell neoplasia in situ (i.e. seminoma and nonseminoma) and those which have not.

Seminoma

Seminomas have a characteristic histological appearance (Figure 17.2).[35] Macroscopically, the cut surface of seminomas is grayish-white, bulging, and glistening. Microscopically, the tumor cells are large with abundant pale or amphophilic cytoplasm, depending on the glycogen content. Stains for PLAP (staining seminoma) and cytokeratin and AFP (staining nonseminomatous elements) can be performed and will help distinguish difficult cases from non-seminoma.

A recognized variation of seminoma is seen. In these cases, cells have high rates of mitosis and cellular atypia and look more pleomorphic. They may also stain for CD 30. Clinically, these tumors may present at the higher stage[36] and have been interpreted by some as showing early differentiation towards embryonal carcinoma, although this view is not uniform.

Spermatocytic seminoma is not a true germ-cell tumor and typically has a different appearance in which carcinoma in situ (CIS)

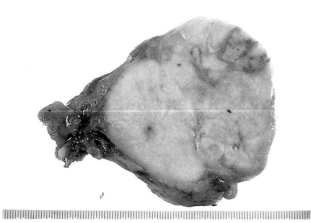

FIGURE 17.2 Orchidectomy specimen. Typical cross-section of seminoma of the testis.

is absent. Overall, these tumors are large, and the surface is yellowish, soft, and mucoid, with cystic or spongy areas. Microscopically, three cell types are seen: Large mononucleated or multinucleated cells with abundant cytoplasm, intermediate cells, and small cells with hyperchromatic nuclei. The nuclei of the large and intermediate cells have a characteristic filamentous chromatin distribution. It is usually a tumor of males over the age of 50, with a good prognosis. Metastasis from the primary site has only rarely been reported. Occasionally, spermatocytic seminomas can be associated with a sarcoma.[37] In these cases, the foci of spermatocytic seminoma will show marked cellular pleomorphism. The sarcoma is often undifferentiated and metastasizes readily.

Non-seminomatous tumors

Non-seminomatous germ-cell tumors are commonly heterogeneous tumors with different proportions of each malignant element. A discussion of these elements follows.

Teratoma

Pure teratoma is a rare entity in adult patients occurring in approximately 4% of germ-cell tumors.[38] Lesions contain a mixture of cellular elements ranging from benign (mature) features to more immature features. Benign lesions are commonly cystic in nature and may contain mesodermal, endodermal, and ectodermal cell types. In immature teratoma, a varying degree of cellular atypical is seen. Given the unstable composition of cell types, there is a recognized potential for secondary cancer to arise within deposits of mature teratoma.[39] Occasionally, this can also metastasize to sites such as the retroperitoneum.

Embryonal

This is also known as malignant teratoma undifferentiated. This relatively featureless tumor is uncommonly found in pure form (3–4% of all germ-cell tumors). It comprises of approximately 40% of mixed germ-cell tumors.[35] It is associated with a higher propensity for lymphovascular invasion and metastatic spread than the other tumor types. In the pure form, elevated serum levels of AFP are not seen. Macroscopically, tumors are often small and located close to the rete. The cut surface is grayish-white with foci of hemorrhage and necrosis. Microscopically, the cells are large and embryonic in appearance and have pale, amphophilic or eosinophilic cytoplasm. The cell borders are ill-defined, and there is frequent nuclear overlap.

Yolk-sac tumor

In its pure form, this is more common in children than in adults, although is a component of other mixed germ-cell tumors. It is associated with a high serum AFP rise. Microscopically, these tumors have ten different histological patterns including reticular/multicystic, solid, hepatoid, glandular alveolar, endodermal sinus, and polyvesicular vitalline.

Choriocarcinoma

Choriocarcinomas are known as trophoblastic tumors. They are rarely found in their pure form (less than 1%). They are aggressive tumors, associated with high hCG, and are often present with disseminated disease. Microscopically, tumors are small, hemorrhagic, and contain a mixture of syncytiotrophoblastic, cytotrophoblastic and intermediate trophoblastic cells.

Assessment and staging of disease

Once a diagnosis of testicular cancer has been confirmed, the patient should be staged. The TNM or the Royal Marsden classification (see Table 17.3) are commonly used for staging. The recent 8th edition of the TMN amends include a subdivision of the pT1 seminomas as a low risk of recurrence is seen in tumors of less than 3-cm diameter.[40] The International Germ Cell Cancer Collaborative Group (IGCCCG) prognostic score should be documented in all cases of metastatic disease. Assessment of all patients should include the following:

1. A thorough history to ascertain if any risk factors for testicular cancer are present. Particular consideration should be given to patients with a history of contralateral testicular cancer, cryptorchidism, or a family history of testicular cancer amongst first-degree relatives.
2. Clinical examination including assessment for gynecomastia and for evidence of cervical, abdominal, and inguinal masses. The remaining testis should also be examined and its size assessed.
3. Measurement of the serum markers AFP/hCG/-lactate dehydrogenase (LDH). If these are found to be elevated, measurement should be repeated weekly to determine if they are rising or falling. Fertility of patients of reproductive age should be assessed and sperm banking should be offered where applicable.
4. A chest X-ray and computed tomography (CT) scan of the chest, abdomen, and pelvis. Brain CT or magnetic

TABLE 17.3   Royal Marsden Staging Classification

Stage	Location of Disease	Maximum Size of Abdominal Nodes
I	Disease confined to testis	N/A
IM	Rising post-orchidectomy tumor marker	N/A
II A	Abdominal lymphadenopathy	<2 cm
IIB		2–5 cm
IIC		>5 cm
III	Supra-diaphragmatic disease	No abdominal nodes
IIIA		<2 cm
IIIB		2–5 cm
IIIC		>5 cm
IV	Extra-lymphatic metastases	

resonance imaging (MRI) should also be performed in patients with a significantly elevated hCG, extensive lung metastases, or if there are symptoms suggestive of intracranial metastatic involvement. Positron emission tomography (PET) scanning has, as yet, no definite role in initial staging, but may be important after chemotherapy in metastatic seminoma (see the following).

Serum markers

Alpha-fetoprotein

AFP is an oncofetal antigen produced in the liver, yolk sac, and gastrointestinal tract. Elevation of AFP is found in approximately 70% of non-seminatous germ-cell tumors pre-orchidectomy and a comparable number of cases prechemotherapy for metastatic disease. It is never elevated in patients with pure seminoma. High levels of AFP can also occur in patients with malignant hepatoma and occasional other gastrointestinal malignancies, and in patients with liver-cell damage and accompaning proliferation (e.g. cirrhosis with regeneration). It has a half-life of approximately 5–6 days.

Beta subunit of human chorionic gonadotrophin

hCG is a glycopeptide secreted by the placenta in pregnancy. In germ-cell malignancies it is produced by the trophoblastic tumor elements. It has a half-life of 24–36 hours. hCG comprises an alpha and a beta subunit. The alpha subunit is common to luteinizing hormone (LH), follicle-stimulating hormone (FSH), and thyroid-stimulating hormone (TSH); and the beta subunit is found in hCG only. Elevation of hCG can occur in both seminoma (present in 35% pre-orchidectomy), and non-seminoma (approximately 70% pre-orchidectomy). It also occurs in low levels in a variety of other cancers, including lung cancer, stomach, and bladder cancer.[41] An elevated hCG is therefore not specific to germ-cell cancer. It has also been described in hypogonadal patients with high FSH or LH levels, presumably reflecting cross-reactivity in the immunoassay. Elevation of hCG has also been described in marijuana users.

Lactate dehydrogenase

LDH is a glycolytic enzyme present in all living cells with the highest concentration in the heart, skeletal muscle, liver, kidney, and red blood cells. It is often raised at the diagnosis of germ-cell malignancies, and the precise etiology of its elevation is unknown. Minor elevations of LDH are, however, rather non-specific, and sensitivity and specificity tend to be low. As assays vary between hospitals, it is conventional to quote the degree of elevation of LDH as a ratio when compared with the upper limit of normal of each laboratory (e.g. level 900 IU, normal range 200–450 L, LDH ratio = 2). LDH is not a useful marker during or shortly after chemotherapy, as levels are increased at the time of bone-marrow recovery. It is unclear whether LDH is useful in detecting relapse.

Fertility

A baseline fertility assessment should be performed in all patients of reproductive age. This includes the determination of total testosterone level, LH, FSH, and semen analysis. Where relevant the patient must be offered counseling about cryopreservation. This should occur ideally before orchidectomy, and certainly before systemic cytotoxic therapy.

Radiological assessment

Chest X-ray

A plain chest radiograph is a useful baseline investigation for patients with testicular cancer. It is a cheap, reproducible, and readily available imaging modality. Evidence of pulmonary metastasis or a mediastinal mass may be detected, and further investigation of these may be indicated. An association between sarcoid-like granulomatous lung disease and testicular cancer has been described,[42] and therefore in patients with isolated mediastinal or hilar node enlargement without abdominal nodal involvement, consideration should be given to biopsy the nodes to confirm metastatic disease before commencing treatment.

Computed tomography scanning

CT is the imaging modality of choice for cross-sectional staging in all patients with a germ-cell tumor. CT is used to accurately stage patients, assess response to treatment and help detect relapse. It can also be useful in aiding the diagnosis of germ-cell tumors in the unknown primary setting as germ-cell tumors have a characteristic metastatic distribution; and a suitable site for obtaining a tissue biopsy can be identified and performed under CT guidance.

Staging CT includes the chest, abdomen, and pelvis. Significant lymphadenopathy is defined as nodal size of 10 mm or greater in the retroperitoneum. CT has a 70–80% sensitivity of detecting metastatic disease in the abdomen.[43] The abdominal lymphatic spread in both tumor types occurs in characteristic sites (the so-called "landing zones"); these are the para-aortic area for left-sided primary tumors and the inter-aorto-caval and para-caval area for right-sided tumors. All scans of new patients should be reviewed by the specialist center in a multidisciplinary meeting to ensure accurate staging at the outset. In cases where the nodal distribution is atypical or the size of the nodal lesions is borderline (approximately 10 mm), it is often reasonable to perform an interval scan to help clarify the staging before therapy. Thoracic CT has a higher sensitivity, but a lower specificity compared to chest radiography in detecting pulmonary nodules.[44] Lung nodules of uncertain significance can also be followed up with interval scanning.

Magnetic resonance imaging

The potential advantage of MRI is the absence of irradiation in this young patient population. However, lack of oral contrast agents and claustrophobia limit the use of this technique. It has not been validated to date in comparison with CT scanning. The results of the UK trial (TRISST) comparing the use of MRI scans and CT scans in the management of stage 1 seminoma patients on active surveillance are eagerly awaited.

MRI scanning is the diagnostic imaging investigation of choice in patients with brain metastases or spinal-cord compression. It may also be useful to differentiate between equivocal findings in the liver or bones. However, it is not as effective as CT at examining the lungs, although there may be advantages in some cases with regard to the examination of mediastinal structures.

Positron emission tomography scanning

PET images are dependent on the uptake of a radiolabeled fluorodeoxyglucose (FDG) by metabolically active tissue. A theoretical advantage of this technique when compared with CT or MRI is the possibility of detecting malignant infiltration of normal-size lymph nodes. However, lesions less than 5 mm cannot be visualized. PET scans may be difficult to obtain and may be costly.

There is no validated role for PET scans in staging of germ-cell tumors.[45,46] PET scans have been utilized in assessment of patients following chemotherapy to assess for residual disease. This is particularly true of seminomas where it may be useful to help decide if a patient should undergo surgery or surveillance following chemotherapy.[47,48] The sensitivity of detection of a lesion over 3 cm in diameter is approx. 80% with a high negative predictive uptake value (94%).[49]

The use of PET CT in metastatic non-seminoma is contentious.[50] Although active cancer will have PET uptake, necrotic tissue can contribute to a false-positive PET scan. Moreover, mature teratoma has either low or negligible uptake.

Summary of assessment and staging

If a germ cell tumor is suspected, all patients should undergo the investigations listed in Table 17.4.

The tumor markers AFP and hCG, and the LDH should be measured in the first instance. In presentations with advanced disease and if the diagnosis needs to be made urgently, the presence of urinary hCG and a suspicious testicular mass on ultrasound give a strong indication that the patient has a testicular germ-cell tumor. Where a suspicious lesion is present in the testis, testicular exploration should be performed by an inguinal incision, and a radical orchidectomy should be performed if a tumor is found.

Occasionally, patients presenting with metastatic disease are diagnosed as a result of biopsy of one of these sites or are found to have diagnostic elevation of AFP and/or hCG. In such cases, particularly if metastatic disease is widespread, orchidectomy should be delayed and urgent chemotherapy should be initiated first. It is recommended that orchidectomy be performed once systemic treatment is completed.[51]

Stage 1 disease

Prognosis and risk of relapse

Seminoma

Stage 1 disease represents around 80% of patients with seminoma at presentation. This patient group therefore represents the most common diagnosis in this tumor type.

Surveillance studies in stage I seminoma have demonstrated that in the absence of adjuvant therapy, it will recur in 15–20% of the patients.[52–54] Retrospective analyses of pooled series of patients managed by surveillance suggest that the risk factors for relapse are increasing size of the primary tumor (with those >4 cm in diameter at most increased risk) along with

tumor involvement of the rete testis.[52,55] There is evidence that patients with both of these features have a 31.5% risk of relapse, patients with either feature are at approximately 15% chance of relapse, and patients with neither feature are at a 12% risk of relapse.[52]

Non-seminoma

The presence of vascular invasion is an independent prognostic factor in stage 1 non-seminomas. On active surveillance, 48% of patients with vascular invasion will develop metastatic disease. In contrast, only 14–22% of patients without this feature go on to develop metastases.[56] Other less consistently demonstrable indicators of poor prognosis and higher risk of relapse include a high proliferation rate (over 70%), no yolk sac elements, and a larger percentage of embryonal carcinoma, although at present these are not routinely used to guide treatment.

Treatment

Stage 1 disease: Seminoma

Risk factors for recurrence are considered when deciding on the appropriate adjuvant treatment. Active surveillance and a single dose of adjuvant carboplatin (AUC 7) are the main options. Adjuvant radiotherapy is rarely used now.

Surveillance

Surveillance, with treatment of relapse, may be an attractive option for a select group of patients. It, however, requires a compliant patient and greater follow-up intensity including more CT scans. There are a number of prospective non-randomized studies of surveillance that have been conducted. Previous analysis from four studies showed a 5-year relapse-free rate of 82.3%.[54,55,57] Most of the relapses are first detected in infra-diaphragmatic lymph node. Patients without risk factors for relapse (small tumors without rete testis invasion) can have relapse rates of approximately 12% over 5 years.[55]

Adjuvant chemotherapy

Owing to concerns relating to the risk of secondary malignancies induced by radiotherapy, most oncologists currently recommend chemotherapy as the adjuvant therapy of choice after orchidectomy for stage 1 seminoma. The landmark joint trial by the MRC and the European Organisation for Research and Treatment of Cancer (EORTC) (MRC TE 19 trial), which compared one cycle of carboplatin (area under curve [AUC] 7) with adjuvant

TABLE 17.4 **Prognostic Factors for Relapsed Germ-Cell Tumors**

Parameter	0	1	2	3
Primary site	Gonadal	Extragonal		Mediastinal (NSGCT)
Prior response to treatment	CR or PR with negative markers	PR with positive markers or SD	PD	
Progression-free interval (months)	<3	>3		
AFP salvage	0	<1000	>1000	
hCG salvage	<1000	>1000		
Liver/bone/brain mets	No	Yes		

Calculating the score
1. Sum of values from 0 to 10.
2. Regroup score sum into categories: (0) = 0; (1 or 2) = 1; (3 or 4) = 2; (5 or more) = 3.
3. Add histology score points: pure seminoma = −1; non-seminoma or mixed tumors = 0.
4. Final prognostic score (−1 = very low risk; 0 = low risk; 1 = intermediate risk; 2 = high risk; 3 = high risk).

Source: Lorch et al., 2010.

radiotherapy, showed no difference with regard to recurrence rate, time to recurrence, and overall survival after a median follow-up of 4 years.[58] The trial also reported a reduction in contralateral testicular cancers from 2% to 0.5% with the use of adjuvant carboplatin in comparison to radiotherapy. The chemotherapy treatment is relatively well-tolerated in the short to medium term. Long-term toxicity data are not as yet available.

However, the site of relapse differed among patients treated with radiotherapy and chemotherapy. Most chemotherapy patients relapsed in the para-aortic nodes, whereas patients receiving para-aortic radiotherapy relapsed most commonly in the pelvis or supra-diaphragmatic nodes. Only one patient in the trial died from germ-cell cancer.

Radiotherapy for stage 1 seminoma

Seminomas are extremely radiosensitive. Adjuvant radiotherapy remains a valid, although decreasingly used, management approach. Historically, stage 1 seminoma was managed by treatment with dog-leg (DL) radiotherapy to a dose of 30 Gy. Two landmark Medical Research Council (MRC)-funded studies have helped to mold modern radiotherapy approaches. The first is the study by Fossa et al.,[59] which randomized 478 patients (T1–T3, no previous ipsilateral inguinal surgery) to either DL or para-aortic radiotherapy to a dose of 30 Gy. Three-year relapse-free survival (96.6% versus 96%) and survival were equivalent, with only one cancer-related death. Gastrointestinal toxicity and sperm-count toxicity were lower in the para-aortic arm. When relapses occurred, the para-aortic-only arm was noted to have a higher number of relapses in ipsilateral pelvic nodes. This prompted concerns about appropriate pelvic CT follow-up in this group (as this was not routine). However, in view of the reduction in acute toxicity, para-aortic irradiation was recommended.

In a second study, appropriate radiation dose was evaluated.[60] The MRC-led study compared two different radiation doses (30 Gy versus 20 Gy) in patients treated with para-aortic radiotherapy (or DL where previous ipsilateral inguinal surgery had been performed). Patients (n = 625) were randomized into the above groups and 5-year relapse-free survival (97% versus 96.4%) and survival rates were equivalent. Again, there was only one death resulting from seminoma. Therefore, most centers would now administer 20 Gy to the para-aortic field.

Summary of the management of stage 1 seminomas

Stage 1 disease is the most common presentation for seminomas. Presently, the main options post-orchidectomy are to consider active surveillance, single-agent carboplatin, or in certain circumstance para-aortic radiotherapy. The risk of relapse is 13–20% for patients on active surveillance and 3–4% for patients who have received adjuvant treatment.[52–55,59,60] Patients can be stratified according to the risk of recurrence with rete testis involvement and tumors larger than 4 cm in size defining the high-risk category. For patients who are likely to be non-compliant on follow-up, those with a higher risk of recurrence, or with whom there may be difficulties in delivering adequate doses of BEP chemotherapy in the future, adjuvant carboplatin may be an attractive option.

Stage 1 disease: Non-seminoma

Approximately 60% of patients diagnosed with a non-seminoma will be stage 1 on presentation. Stage 1 non-seminomas can be risk stratified based on the presence or absence of lymphovascular invasion. This feature is present in approximately 25% of the cases and, when present, predicts a risk of subsequent relapse of approximately 50%.[61,62] There is currently no proven scope for PET scanning in these patients to assess for occult disease.

Treatment options after orchidectomy include surveillance, adjuvant chemotherapy, or retroperitoneal lymph–node dissection (RPLND). The routine use of RPLND in stage 1 disease varies globally and will not be discussed in detail in this chapter.

Surveillance for stage 1 non-seminoma

Following orchidectomy, the overall risk of relapse is 25–30% for patients diagnosed with stage 1 non-seminoma.[56] If patients without evidence of vascular invasion are selected for surveillance, the risk of relapse is only 15% versus 40–50% for those with this feature.[56] The overall cure rate for relapsed stage 1 non-seminoma managed with surveillance should approach 98–99% as deferred chemotherapy is highly effective.

Relapses usually occur within a few months following orchidectomy and are rare after 24 months. In an MRC trial (TE-08), the frequency of CT scanning was evaluated for patients going onto surveillance for stage 1 testis non-seminoma. This compared a total of three whole-body scans (0, 3, and 12 months after orchidectomy) with six whole-body scans (0, 3, 6, 9, 12, and 24 months). No difference in relapses was found. In addition, this study supported the results of an earlier series suggesting that CT scanning of the thorax post-staging could be replaced by a chest X-ray without being detrimental to the patient.[63] This CT surveillance program—initial whole-body staging CT scan followed by abdominal scanning only at 3 months and 1 year—is now the standard approach in many centers.[21]

Adjuvant chemotherapy for stage 1 non-seminoma

Adjuvant chemotherapy has been evaluated in patients with stage I non-seminoma with a high risk of subsequent spread (identified by the presence of vascular invasion).[64,65] Two cycles of modified BEP chemotherapy, given with a total dose of etoposide of 360 mg/m^2 in each cycle (BE(360)P), has been shown to reduce the relapse rate to approximately 2%.[66]

However, three randomized trials have since evaluated the impact of one cycle of BEP. Albers et al. compared one cycle of BEP to RPLND.[67] The 2-year recurrence-free survival was 99.6% in the chemotherapy group and 91.87% in the RPLND arm. However, this trial included patients with both low and high risk of recurrence (i.e. the presence or not of vascular invasion) and therefore does not represent standard practice in the United Kingdom. Secondly, the Swedish–Norwegian testicular cancer group reported study of 157 stage 1 non-seminomatous germ-cell tumor patients with vascular invasion treated with 1 cycle of adjuvant BEP.[68] After a median follow-up of 4.8 years, the number of relapses was 3.2%. There were no recurrences seen after 2 years.

Finally, the BEP111 trial (n = 246), the largest prospective trial of single-dose adjuvant chemotherapy in NSGCT, was a single-arm study in which one cycle of bleomycin (30,000 IU day 1, 8, and 15), etoposide (165 mg/m^2 day 1, 2, and 3), and cisplatin (50 mg/m^2 day 1 and 2) was administered to patients at a high risk of recurrence from stage 1 NSGCT. The 2-year recurrence rate was 1.3% (95% CI: 0.4 to 4.0%).[69] This is comparable to the rate seen with two doses of BE(360)P. The standard adjuvant therapy for stage 1 non-seminoma should therefore be considered to be BE(500)P.

Metastatic disease

Prognostic classification

Historically, a number of different prognostic classifications were used to aid treatments. It was known that, unlike other malignancies, disease bulk may have little relevance to prognosis, as many of the more bulky non-seminomatous metastatic masses largely comprise teratoma differentiated. More importantly, it was suspected that the degree of elevation of tumor markers (hCG, AFP, LDH) may show a closer relationship to prognosis in this case. The large number of classifications contained few similarities, and it became increasingly difficult to cross-interpret and translate their use into clinical practice. The situation was resolved through worldwide collaboration and development of the IGCCC published in 1997.[70] Retrospective clinical data were collected on more than 5000 patients with metastatic testicular non-seminoma/extra-gonadal primary non-seminoma and 660 patients with metastatic seminoma who had been treated with cisplatin-containing chemotherapy. The median duration of follow-up was 5 years.

Through analysis of this extensive dataset, it soon became apparent that the main determinant of prognosis in metastatic non-seminomas was the degree of elevation of all the serum markers. Two additional adverse features were the presence of a mediastinal primary and spread to extra-thoracic visceral sites (e.g. liver, bone, and brain). Three prognostic groups for metastatic non-seminomas were identified: Good prognosis, intermediate prognosis, and poor prognosis (Table 17.5).

For seminomas the presence of non-pulmonary visceral metastases was the main adverse feature. In contrast to non-seminoma,

TABLE 17.5 Prognosis Factors in Metastatic Non-Seminoma, IGCCC

- Good prognosis
  - 56% of cases
  - 5-year progression-free survival, 89%; survival, 92%
  - Testis/retroperitoneal primary
  - No non-pulmonary visceral metastases
- Good markers—all of:
  - AFP <1000 KU/L and
  - hCG <5000 IU/L and
  - LDH <1.5 × upper limit of normal
- Intermediate prognosis
  - 28% of cases
  - 5-year progression-free survival, 75%; survival, 80%
  - Testis/retroperitoneal primary
  - No non-pulmonary visceral metastases
- Intermediate markers—any of:
  - AFP ≥1000 and ≤10,000 KU/L or
  - hCG ≥5000 IU/L and ≤50,000 IU/L or
  - LDH ≥1.5 × N and ≤10 × N upper limit of normal
- Poor prognosis
  - 16% of cases
  - 5-year progression-free survival, 41%; survival, 48%
  - Mediastinal primary
  - Non-pulmonary visceral metastases
  - Poor markers—any of:
  - AFP >10,000 KU/L or
  - hCG >50,000 IU/L (10,000 IU/L) or
  - LDH >10 × upper limit of normal

AFP, alpha-fetoprotein; hCG, human chorionic gonadotrophin; LDH, lactate dehydrogenase

TABLE 17.6 Prognosis Factors in Metastatic Seminoma, IGCCC

- Good prognosis
  - 90% of patients
  - 5-year progression-free survival, 82%; survival, 86%
  - Any primary site
  - No non-pulmonary visceral metastases
  - Normal AFP, any hCG and LDH
- Poor prognosis
  - 10% of patients
  - 5-year progressive-free survival 67%; survival 72%
  - Seminoma
  - Any primary site
  - Non-pulmonary visceral metastases
  - Normal AFP, any hCG any LDH

AFP, alpha-fetoprotein, hCG, human chorionic gonadotrophin; LDH, lactate dehydrogenase.

no poor prognosis group is identified (Table 17.6). Of particular note, seminoma arising from extra-gonadal sites (including the mediastinum) seemed to confer similar prognosis, compared to other types of metastatic testicular seminoma. Patients with metastatic seminoma are divided into a good-prognosis or intermediate-prognosis group based on the presence of non-pulmonary metastases. Marker elevation does not influence outcome.

This easy-to-use classification has been used in clinical practice (to standardize the number of cycles of treatments patients receive) and in the design and reporting of clinical trials to aid international collaboration and understanding.

Overview of chemotherapy

Metastatic testicular germ-cell cancers are a highly chemosensitive disease. However, 40 years ago, deaths following a diagnosis of metastatic disease were common. Some patients with metastatic disease were cured by radiotherapy, but outcomes were poor with only 5–10% of patients cured. In the 1970s there were significant advances in therapies. First, a 35% complete response rate was seen in patients treated with vinblastine and bleomycin. Subsequently, the introduction of cisplatin, vinblastine, and bleomycin (PVB) by the Indiana group in the late 1970s ranks as one of the single most important advances in oncology. Etoposide was used in the study by Peckham et al. in 1983[71] and its efficacy confirmed by a subsequent study by Williams et al. which showed BEP to be less toxic and to have improved survival outcomes compared to PVB.[72] Compared to BEP, the regimen VIP (etoposide, ifosfamide, and cisplatin) has shown a tendency to better outcomes (complete response [CR] of 79% versus 74%), although there were more deaths secondary to toxicity in the VIP treatment arms.[73]

Optimal delivery of chemotherapy is key to its success. Each cycle of chemotherapy should be delivered at full dose, and on time (every 3 weeks). Table 17.7 outlines the current dosing regimes. Dose reduction or treatment delays should be avoided. Cisplatin, given as part of BEP, is generally administered in divided doses. Bleomycin can be delivered virtually regardless of blood counts as it is minimally myelosuppressive. Care should be taken in older patients (>40 years) or if the serum creatinine is elevated or the creatinine clearance reduced below 60 mL/min as this may exacerbate toxicities.[74]

The number of cycles of BEP has been investigated in the context of good-prognosis disease. There are two studies that have

TABLE 17.7   **BEP (3-Day) Treatment Schedule (Cycle Length 21 Days)**

Name of Drug	Dose	Day Given	Notes
a) 7BEP (3 day) treatment schedule (cycle length 21 days)			
Bleomycin	30,000 IU	1, 8, 15	Respiratory assessment prior to each dose
Etoposide	165 mg/ m²	1–3	
Cisplatin	50 mg/m²	1–2	Given with iv fluids
b) BEP (5-day) treatment schedule (cycle length 21 days)			
Bleomycin	30,000 IU	1, 8, 15	Respiratory assessment prior to each dose
Etoposide	100 mg/m²	1–5	
Cisplatin	20 mg/m²	1–5	Given with iv fluids

compared four cycles of BEP to three cycles. The first study performed by the South Eastern Cancer Study Group (SECSG)[75] randomized 184 patients between receiving 3 or 4 cycles of BEP. The outcomes for both arms were equivalent with reduction in toxicity for patients receiving three cycles of chemotherapy. Concerns were initially raised about the statistical power of the study, and therefore this trial was repeated by the MRC/European Organisation for Research into Treatment of Cancer (EORTC) group. The results of this study were in agreement with the SECSG. In the latter study, 812 patients were randomized between the 2 groups. Free from relapse and overall survival were 0.4% and 89.4% and 97.0% and 97.1%, respectively.[76]

This MRC/EORTC study also examined whether cisplatin and etoposide should be administered over a 3-day versus 5-day period. Equivalence in cure rates was found between both groups. However, toxicity did vary with increased gastrointestinal toxicity, ototoxicity, peripheral neuropathy, and Raynaud's phenomenon in patients treated over 3 days rather than 5 days, particularly if treated for 4 cycles.

Bleomycin is a generally well-tolerated and established treatment for advanced GCTs. A rare, though significant, complication is pulmonary toxicity (see "Complications of Treatment"). Owing to this complication, attempts have been made to omit bleomycin from curative chemotherapy regimens. Increased risk of bleomycin toxicity occurs with increasing dose (recommended maximum lifetime dose of 400,000 IU), but also occurs when renal clearance is impaired (bleomycin should be given with caution to any patient with an elevated creatinine or creatinine clearance <60 mL/min) or in older (>40 years) patients.[74,77] In several large trials, the inclusion of bleomycin in BEP (three or four cycles) for treatment of metastatic non-seminoma shows a slight increase in toxicity but improved overall failure-free survival rates.[78–80] One study compared three cycles of BEP with four cycles of EP (etoposide and cisplatin). The complete response rate was greater for patients receiving BEP. Although overall survival in this study was not statistically different (92% in the EP arm and 96% in the BEP arm), more recurrences occurred in the group of patients receiving EP.[81]

To further minimize chemotherapy-related toxicity, carboplatin has been investigated as an alternative to cisplatin. However, although preliminary phase II data suggested equivalence when carboplatin was substituted for cisplatin in BEP, two randomized trials[82,83] demonstrated inferiority of carboplatin compared to cisplatin. Therefore at present, the use of carboplatin in the initial therapy of metastatic GCTs is not routinely recommended. It can, however, be considered in cases where delivery of cisplatin is not possible (e.g. significant renal impairment).

As germ-cell tumors are uncommon and their treatment complex, there is clear evidence that referral to specialist high-volume treatment centers improves survival. This particularly is true for patients with intermediate- and poor-prognosis disease.[84] All patients with metastatic disease should be discussed in a multidisciplinary team meeting. Treatment should be based on IGCCCG prognostic classification and protocols should be strictly adhered to. Following cytotoxic treatment, surgery should be considered for the primary lesion (if still in situ at the start of chemotherapy) and any residual masses. Patients without imminently life-threatening metastatic disease should be offered sperm banking before chemotherapy.

Complications of treatment

Short-term complications of chemotherapy

The treatment of germ-cell tumors with cisplatin-containing chemotherapy is associated with a wide range of toxicities, particularly for patients receiving salvage treatment for relapsed disease. Nausea and vomiting can usually be adequately controlled with 5HT3 antagonists used with dexamethasone. Addition of the neurokinin modulator aprepitant has been shown to improve control of emesis in patients given such doses of cisplatin as administered with BEP.[85] Alopecia occurs universally. Myelosuppression occurs routinely within 10 days of treatment and many centers now routinely using growth factor support. There is a risk of neutropenic fever, which may necessitate admission and treatment with intravenous antibiotics.

Specific side effects of cisplatin include tinnitus or high-tone hearing loss, which may become apparent during or after treatment. In 20% of patients this may be permanent. In addition, impaired renal function, with an overall loss of 10–20%, commonly occurs when BEP is given as full dose.[86] Assessment of hearing (via audiogram) and creatinine clearance (via EDTA clearance test) can be tested before commencing chemotherapy. Cisplatin may also cause a peripheral neuropathy and Raynaud's phenomenon.

One of the most concerning toxicities of BEP chemotherapy is the development of bleomycin lung changes. Bleomycin is a sulfur-containing chemotherapeutic, which is excreted in the urine. It is inactivated by most tissues in the body by an enzyme, bleomycin hydrolase. The sites of the body that do not contain this enzyme are the skin and the lungs and therefore these are commonly the sites of bleomycin toxicity. In the lungs, bleomycin causes pneumonitis with progressive pulmonary fibrosis occurring with an overall incidence of 6.8% in patients receiving BEP chemotherapy at full dose (360,000 units), with a mortality of 1–2%.[74] Pulmonary toxicity is dose-related, and it rarely occurs after small quantities have been administered. Patients are at an increased risk of developing this with increasing age (>40 years) and deteriorating renal function. In its early stages, bleomycin lung changes may be hard to detect—the findings of bilateral basal crepitations on chest auscultation, bilateral basal changes on chest X-ray, or persistent cough or dyspnea may all indicate early toxicity. Concerns of bleomycin toxicity warrant further investigation with thoracic CT scanning and, if confirmed, bleomycin should be discontinued.

Infertility is likely to be universal during chemotherapy, but sperm counts usually recover to their previous levels. In a study of spermatogenesis and cisplatin-containing chemotherapy, 64% of patients whose spermatogenesis was normal before receiving chemotherapy had normal counts at 1 year post-treatment. At this stage, 16% were oligospermic and 20% azospermic.[87] Recovery may take years if sperm counts are low at the initiation of chemotherapy or if more than four courses of cisplatin are given. All patients wishing to retain fertility should therefore undergo sperm banking before treatment commences. There have been no reports of an increase in teratogenicity in the children of survivors of testicular cancer though it is routine to advise patients to use contraception for at least 6 months after the completion of chemotherapy.

Long-term complications of chemotherapy

The long-term side effects of BEP chemotherapy have been investigated in epidemiological studies. There is an increased risk of both systolic and diastolic hypertension. In addition, patients who have received BEP chemotherapy have an increased tendency for raised body mass index and an increased risk of hyperlipidemia and coronary artery disease.[3,88] Routine monitoring of late effects (blood pressure/lipids) should be incorporated into follow-up protocol and patients, and their general practitioners, should also be informed of the increased risks and the ways to prevent them.

Secondary cancers have been reported occurring with an increased relative risk of 1.7.[89,90] These are often hematological and develop after a latent period of at least 10 years from treatment. Other types of long-term toxicity including hypogonadism, nephrotoxicity, Raynaud phenomenon, and ototoxicity may occur in approximately 25% of long-term survivors.[91]

Complications of radiotherapy treatment

Post-abdominal radiotherapy gastrointestinal symptoms are common. These may persist in a small number of cases. The use of modern radiotherapy techniques has reduced incidence of these effects. Infertility due to scatter radiation dose can be prevented with shielding of the residual testicle.[26]

Seminoma: Stage IIA/B

In approximately 10% of patients with seminoma, evidence of low-volume para-aortic adenopathy (≤5 cm) will be found at presentation. Such patients can be treated with chemotherapy or radiation.

Traditionally, radiation fields encompassed the para-aortic, ipsilateral iliac, and obturator nodes in a DL field to a dose of 30 Gy. A number of small studies have described a 5-year recurrence-free survival of 93–100%.[92,93] However, patients with more bulky para-aortic nodes on presentation are more likely to relapse. Studies have been published regarding the use of neoadjuvant carboplatin before radiotherapy treatment. The largest study described by Horwich et al. is a single-arm study of 51 patients with stage IIA/B disease.[94] With a median follow-up of 55 months, no relapses were described. In this study the radiation field was reduced from an extended abdominopelvic field to just the para-aortic region, and the radiation dose from 35 Gy to 30 Gy in 39 patients to help reduce late-term toxicities. Late toxicities when treated with radiotherapy (in isolation or combination) include a risk of secondary malignancy (commonly leukemia) and a marginal increase of cardiovascular disease.

Regarding chemotherapy, three cycles of BEP are considered treatment for stage IIA/B seminoma. A Spanish multicenter prospective observational study (*n* = 78) of cisplatin-based chemotherapy in low-volume stage II seminoma has been reported.[95] These data revealed a high disease-free survival (DFS) with

cisplatin-based chemotherapy using four cycles of E400P (400 mg per cycle of etoposide plus cisplatin) or three cycles of BEP. It should be noted that the dose intensity of the etoposide in this regime was lower than considered standard. Five-year DFS for the whole group was 90% (100% IIA, 87% IIB), and overall survival was 95%. Grade 3 or 4 hematological toxicities were reported in 10–15%, including 11% febrile neutropenia. Eight percent had Grade 3 or 4 emesis. No significant late toxicity had been reported at 6 years, although the risk of late secondary malignancies from etoposide typically occurs 10–15 years post-treatment. There is evidence that single-agent carboplatin given over multiple cycles at AUC 10 may be effective with favorable disease-free survival demonstrated.

Patients with IIA and IIB seminoma require post-treatment CT scanning. Residual masses are almost always sterile and can be watched. There is no indication for prophylactic treatment of the mediastinum with irradiation, a common practice in the past that was of doubtful benefit and resulted in cardiac toxicity. Relapse, when it occurs following radiotherapy, is almost always sited in the mediastinum or cervical region. However, relapse can occur to other sites (lung, pleura, or bone) but is relatively rare.

Stage IIC and higher: Seminoma—good prognosis

Patients with bulky (more than 5 cm) stage II as well as stage III and stage IV seminoma should undergo primary treatment with combination chemotherapy. The majority of these patients present with nodal disease in the retroperitoneum, posterior mediastinum, or left cervical area.

Metastatic seminoma is extremely chemosensitive, and the treatment of choice is three to four cycles of BEP chemotherapy depending on whether the disease is good or intermediate prognosis. To reduce toxicity, alternative regimens have been studied, in particular single-agent carboplatin regimens. Previously, data from two studies have not shown single-agent carboplatin to be effective. The MRC led a study of 130 patients randomized to either single-agent carboplatin (400 mg/m² intravenously) or combination chemotherapy with etoposide and cisplatin which was terminated early because of inferior outcomes seen in patients treated for metastatic seminoma.[96] At the same time, a German study randomized patients between single-agent carboplatin (400 mg/ m² intravenously) and combination chemotherapy with cisplatin, etoposide, and ifosfamide.[97] Combined data clearly indicated that carboplatin alone produced inferior outcomes for both progression-free survival (72% versus 92%) and overall survival (89% versus 94%). More recently, increased doses of single-agent carboplatin ([AUC] 10) have been used in select groups of metastatic seminoma patients with promising results.[98] However, randomized data versus BEP are lacking and long-term data outcomes are not yet available. Therefore, the treatment of choice for patients with metastatic seminoma of good prognosis should continue to be three cycles of BEP chemotherapy, though there is scope for future prospective randomized trials within this area.

Almost all patients with seminoma will respond to chemotherapy. In patients with bulky disease at presentation, there may be residual masses following treatment. Although surgery can be considered for these patients it can be challenging. This is due to the desmoplastic nature of seminomas and the proximity to a number of important retroperitoneal structures (e.g. aorta, inferior vena cava [IVC], vertebra). Often masses less than 3 cm do not progress on, and approximately 90% of masses resected do not reveal any active cancer. PET-CT may be useful in differentiating between necrosis and viable tumor in such cases.[99]

Metastatic non-seminoma—good prognosis

Patients should be treated according to their IGCCCG-defined prognostic group. BEP chemotherapy remains the first-line treatment of choice for patients with good prognosis metastatic non-seminoma. The standard management is to administer BEP as either a 3- or 5-day regimen for a total of 3 cycles. Patients considered to be at high risk of bleomycin lung toxicity can be treated with four cycles of etoposide and cisplatin (EP) although outcomes may be inferior, or three cycles of VIP. Post-chemotherapy RPLND should be considered in patients with radiologically enlarged residual masses.

Metastatic GCT: Intermediate/poor prognosis

Standard first-line treatment for patients with intermediate or poor prognosis disease is with 4 cycles of 5-day BEP. Bleomycin is delivered weekly (30,000 units per week to a maximum dose of 360,000 units).

Approximately 30% of the patients presenting with non-seminomatous and 10% with seminomatous GCTs have IGCCCG intermediate- to poor-prognosis disease at presentation. Assessment should be made to the extent of the metastatic disease. Bulky pulmonary metastases may present with intrathoracic hemorrhage and dyspnea. Bulky abdominal disease may cause occlusion to the inferior vena cava (either direct compression or thrombus formation) and ureters. The latter may require the insertion of a nephrostomy or ureteric stent. Patients with extensive lung or abdominal disease should be assessed for the possibility of CNS metastases. Patients who present in extremis or with extensive liver, pulmonary, or central nervous system (CNS) metastases may be initially stabilized with a low-dose induction treatment (e.g. low-dose EP) before full-dose chemotherapy commences.[26]

As this group of patients may not respond to first-line chemotherapy, there are a number of ongoing clinical trials investigating the best treatment schedule. Some centers in the UK have adopted the regimen from the randomized phase II trial, TE23, which showed improved tumor shrinkage, although increased toxicity, compared to BEP, in poor-prognosis patients treated with carboplatin, vincristine, bleomycin, etoposide, and cisplatin (CBOP/BEP).[100] An international phase III trial would be needed to confirm these findings. The P3BEP study is currently recruiting patients with intermediate- or poor-prognostic disease to see whether dose intensification of BEP ("accelerated" BEP with the EP component given 2-weekly) leads to better patient outcomes. At present there is no evidence for high-dose chemotherapy with stem cell support. Studies have indicated a trend towards improved DFS, but no improvement in overall survival with high-dose chemotherapy,[101,102] and therefore, it cannot currently be recommended.

Treatment of central nervous system metastases

CNS metastases are uncommon, occurring in only 1–2% of germ-cell tumors. CNS disease is most commonly seen in patients with a high presenting hCG (e.g. >10,000 IU/L) or with multiple (>20) lung metastases. A CT or MRI brain scan is indicated for initial evaluation in such cases. Metastatic CNS disease is associated with an increase in morbidity and presents a clinical challenge. Metastases may be single or multiple. As well as being present at initial diagnosis, CNS disease can occur at relapse or during systemic treatment. The long-term survival of a patient who presents with CNS disease is 30–40%.[103] In comparison, CNS disease at relapse has a 5-year survival of only 2–5%.[104] Meningeal involvement is rare and spinal cord compression may occur secondary to contiguous tumor spread.

The optimal management of CNS disease remains controversial. Although chemotherapy, radiotherapy, and surgery have been used, the optimal sequence of therapy is unclear.[104–106] Most patients undergo primary combination chemotherapy treatment, normally with BEP. A multivariate analysis has shown that the addition of whole-brain radiotherapy may improve outcomes. Doses of up to 40–45 Gy have been used. Treatment can be delivered synchronously or sequentially to chemotherapy. If a single metastasis is present and is potentially surgically resectable, and the systemic disease is clinically non-threatening, craniotomy and resection should be considered as an initial measure. In practice, such cases are extremely rare.

Some centers have developed CNS-specific regimens, and there is a suggestion that CNS-specific protocols or dose dense regimes may improve outcomes in patients, although the data supporting this are sparse.

Monitoring response to first-line treatment

While receiving chemotherapy and following its completion, patients should have their tumor markers (AFP and hCG) monitored sequentially. All patients with known chest disease can have the extent of their pulmonary metastases monitored by serial chest radiographs. Patients with a high tumor burden may exhibit an initial tumor flare (elevation of markers for 7–10 days after commencing chemotherapy probably secondary to tumor cell necrosis). Tumor marker should then fall. Occasionally patients with very high markers on presentation or with a pure choriocarcinoma may develop a marker plateau. Patients may undergo resection of their residual masses which can show no evidence of residual cancer. However, in 50% of cases markers fall to normal after surgery. The remaining cases may experience a rapid relapse, and monitoring of markers following surgery should be very regular to enable relapse to be detected early.

Radiologically, post-chemotherapy imaging will usually show a complete or partial response in involved tissue. Occasionally tumors can appear to grow in size as markers are falling. This can represent "growing teratoma syndrome" and may not indicate a failure of chemotherapy, but an expansion of mature teratoma in the residual nodes.[107,108] Surgical resection is indicated in such cases.

Resection of residual disease

The most common site of residual disease is in the para-aortic region. A RPLND can be performed if indicated. RPLND should be performed by an experienced surgeon with a nerve-sparing technique. Despite a nerve-sparing approach, the risk of retrograde ejaculation following such surgery is still as high as 6–8%.[109,110]

In seminoma a residual mass (<3 cm) of pure seminoma should not be primarily resected especially if tumor markers have normalized. Patients should undergo close surveillance with marker monitoring and serial imaging with CT or PET-CT. PET-CT is of prognostic value in such patients.[47,99] No surgery is usually required if post-chemotherapy PET-CT is negative. On the contrary, a positive PET-scan performed 4–5 weeks after day 21 of chemotherapy may be a predictor of residual viable tumor.[47,99] Resection (or another means of obtaining histological confirmation) is often advised in this situation. On progression, salvage therapy is indicated.

In non-seminoma, residual masses are relatively common, particularly if the initial disease burden was large or where elements of teratoma differentiated were present in the primary tumor. Following BEP chemotherapy, 10–15% of residual masses contain viable cancer, 30% contain mature teratoma, and 50% contain necrotic tissue.[111–113] It is recommended that all abnormal masses visualized on abdominal CT scan be excised if they measure more than 1-cm diameter.[114] However, further shrinkage of large masses may be possible and clinical sense dictates if a large mass has resolved to 1.0–1.5 cm; it may be observed for a short while to see if it regresses further. In the United Kingdom, template RPLND is used where possible, in addition to the removal of all visibly abnormal disease sites. When residual disease is bulky, this surgery can be complex, and occasionally patients will require resection of surrounding structures opposed to the residual mass such as the kidney, the IVC, or even a length of aorta in order to achieve complete removal of tumor masses.

Residual lung masses should also be resected if this is technically feasible, and combined thoroco–laparotomy is a possibility if both abdominal and lung masses require resection. When this combined approach is not reasonable, laparotomy is generally performed first, with observation of the pulmonary masses during the time of recovery. Patients with residual liver masses should undergo biopsy at the time of laparotomy and be considered for resection if there is viable cancer or mature teratoma present.

If the primary tumor is still present, orchidectomy is recommended post-chemotherapy.[30,31]

Careful histological evaluation of all resected tissue by an experienced histopathologist is essential. Completely resected necrotic tissue or teratoma differentiated (which may appear quite dysplastic) requires no further therapy (Figure 17.3). Patients in whom viable cancer is resected should be considered for further chemotherapy. There is some evidence to suggest that patients who have undergone complete resection may have a favorable outcome without the use of adjuvant chemotherapy if the resected specimen contains <10% vital tumor cells.[113]

Relapsed disease

Unlike most malignancies, relapsed metastatic germ-cell tumors are still potentially curable. However, there is currently no

TABLE 17.8   First Salvage Regimes

Name of Regimen	Drugs/Dose	Day Given
VIP (CDCT)	Cisplatin 20 mg/m^2	1–5
4 x 3 weekly cycles	Etoposide 100 mg/m^2	1–5
	Ifosfamide 1.2 g/m^2	1–5
TIP (CDCT)—MSK	Paclitaxel 250 mg/m^2	1
protocol	Cisplatin 25 mg/m^2	2–5
4 × 3 weekly cycles	Isfosfamide 1.5g/m^2	2–5
TI-CE (HD-CT)	Paclitaxel (T) 200 mg/m^2	Day 1 (TI cycle)
2 × TI cycles (repeated	Isfosfamide (I) 2 g/m^2	Days 2–4 (TI cycle)
after 2 weeks) followed	Carboplatin (C) AUC 8	Days 1–3 (CE cycle)
by 3 × CE cycles (repeated after 3 weeks)	Etoposide (E) 400 mg/m^2	Days 1–3 (CE cycle)
VIP-CE (HD-CT)	Carboplatin 500 mg/m^2	Days 1–3
1 × VIP cycle (see above) followed by 3 × CE cycles (repeated after 3 weeks)	Etoposide 500 mg/m^2	Days 1–3
Indiana-CE (HD-CT)	Carboplatin 700 mg/m^2	Days 1–3
2 cycles to be repeated after hematopoietic recovery	Etoposide 750 mg/m^2	Days 1–3

Source: Adapted from ESMO Clinical Guidelines.

consensus as to the optimal chemotherapy regime for these patients. Both conventional-dosed regimes (CDCT) and high-dose regimes (HDCT) are employed (see Table 17.8 for examples of regimes). At present no conventional-dose salvage regimen has shown unequivocal superiority over another conventional-dose cisplatin-containing salvage regime. In addition, it is currently unresolved whether conventional-dosed chemotherapy alone is sufficient, or whether high-dose chemotherapy is also needed. For this reason these patients should be treated at experienced centers and where possible within prospective randomized trials such as the currently recruiting international TIGER study.[115] A discussion of the two treatment options can be found in the following sections.

Response to further treatment following relapse of germ-cell tumors can be difficult to predict. A recently collated international dataset collected from 1984 patients with relapsed disease has identified a number of adverse prognostic features.[116] These included non-seminomatous histology, poor response to first-line therapy, high tumor markers at relapse, short progression-free interval, and site of relapsed disease (liver and brain). This led to the development of a prognostic index where patients are classified into five risk categories: very low risk, low risk, intermediate risk, high risk, and very high risk.

Conventional-dose chemotherapy

Retrospective studies have described the outcomes from the use of CDCT (either etoposide, ifosfamide, cisplatin [VIP] or vinblastine, ifosfamide, cisplatin [VeIP]).[117,118] These show CR rates of between 36 and 56% with a long-term durable CR of 23–42%. The main toxicities were similar for both regimens, namely, myelotoxicity and nephrotoxicity. There are a small number of prospective studies evaluating CDCT. The first, a trial of 135 patients, showed a CR rate of 50% with 24% being disease-free at 6 years.[119] This trial excluded those patients who progressed within 3 weeks of receiving cisplatin-based chemotherapy (cisplatin refractory disease). All patients with extragonadal non-seminoma progressed, whereas two patients with extragonadal seminoma had a durable CR. The second is the European run trial (IT_94) that compared

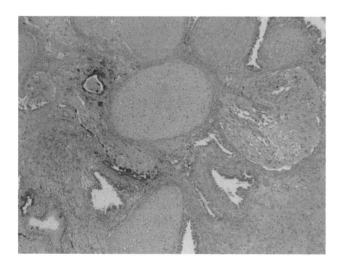

FIGURE 17.3   Mature teratoma: This figure shows a mixture of tissues islands of cartilage, neural tissue, glands and pigmented epithelium. (Courtesy of Dr. A Warren, consultant histopathologist, Addenbrooke's hospital.)

CDCT with HDCT.[120] In the CDCT arm patients received either VeIP or VIP with a CR rate of 42% and a durable CR of 26%. A summary of this is in the subsequent section.

More recently, the combination of paclitaxel, ifosfamide, cisplatin has been used in clinical practice. A number of phase II trials have reported the CR as 70–77% with a durable CR of 65–73% in selected patients (CR with first-line therapy, testicular primary, progression-free interval of over 6 months).[121,122] A multicenter MRC phase II trial attempted to replicate the results, with 43 patients including those outside the previously mentioned selection criteria.[123] This reported CR rate of 31% with a 5-year progression-free survival of 38%. The trial used a lower dose of paclitaxel (175 mg/m^2) and also different selection criteria, which may have accounted for some of this discrepancy. A subgroup analysis took place and patient with "good risk" features were shown to have a favorable response in 73% of patients compared to 41% of patients with "poor risk" factors.

High-dose chemotherapy

A number of characteristics of germ-cell tumors suggest a potential to respond well to high-dose chemotherapy: The established chemosensitivity, the lack of bone marrow involvement, and the young and relativity fit patient population. Traditionally, the most commonly used high-dose agents were carboplatin and etoposide.

To date there has been only one published randomized control trial comparing CDCT and HDCT in the relapsed setting.[120] This was European phase III trial (IT_94) of 280 patients who were randomized to receive either four cycles of VeIP or three cycles of CDCT followed by one cycle of HDCT. Rates of complete response, progression-free survival, and overall survival where similar in both arms, and therefore the primary endpoint of superiority of HDCT was not met. The study, however, had a number of shortcomings, in particular, 81% of those randomized to high-dose treatment did not receive it, and there were concerns regarding the safety of delivery of treatment at smaller hospitals. It has been suggested that in light of this trial there is no benefit with high-dose chemotherapy, especially among patients with good prognostic features.[26] However, a number of retrospective studies have been reported showing a more favorable outcome with the use of high-dose chemotherapy, especially among patients with poor prognostic features.[124–126]

In summary, the randomized studies to date, which have compared high-dose with conventional-dose chemotherapy, have not shown any unequivocal overall survival benefit with high-dose chemotherapy though the data are limited and flawed. The internationally recruiting trial, TIGER, of conventional-dose (TIP) and high-dose (TICE), hopes to address this question definitively (ClinicalTrials.gov Identifier: NCT02375204).

Surgery

Patients with residual masses following salvage chemotherapy should be considered for surgery. Viable tumor is found in half of these cases and correlates to a poorer outlook.[127] If there is radiological and marker progression after salvage treatment surgical resection may still be considered. If complete resection is feasible, then the long-term survival rate is approximately 25%.[128–130]

Management of the contralateral testicle

Patients diagnosed with a testicular germ-cell tumor have increased risk of developing a contralateral testicular primary. Rarely, patients present with synchronous bilateral tumors. More commonly the development of a second tumor is delayed by 5–10 years.[131]

Testicular intraepithelial neoplasia

The main risk factor for a second cancer is underlying TIN in the remaining testicle. In a large German series,[132] routine testicular biopsy was performed at the time of orchidectomy for cancer, and CIS was detected in the contralateral testis in 4.9% of cases, which equates approximately to the recognized risk of contralateral disease. The risk of TIN was identified in an MRC study.[133] This found patients aged less than 30 years with a small remaining testis (16 mL or less on ultrasound) have a risk of contralateral TIN of more than 30%. For the remaining patients, the risk was between 2% and 4%.

Patients should be carefully counseled on the detection of TIN. If detected, there are two main options for its management. One is surveillance with regular assessments through ultrasound. However, as there is strong clinical evidence that TIN carries a very high risk of subsequent malignancy (70% risk by 7 years),[11] treatment is often advised. This involves radiotherapy to the remaining testicle or prophylactic orchidectomy. The recommended dose for radiotherapy is 20 Gy in 10 daily fractions.[134] This will often result in infertility and occasionally testosterone insufficiency. Sperm banking should be offered before radiotherapy commences.

Contralateral testicular cancer

After detection of a contralateral testicular cancer, patient should have repeat staging investigations to ensure there is no metastatic spread. A second radical orchidectomy is the best treatment option in the majority of cases. Surgical castration necessitates hormonal replacement. Hypogonadism commonly causes flushes, sweats, swinging moods, and impotence, with a long-term complication of osteoporosis. Patients may go onto testosterone replacement (which has various forms) though it is advised that a specialist endocrinologist be involved in monitoring of the replacement therapy.

To preserve endocrine function a partial orchidectomy may be considered in a select number of cases.[135] The size and location of the tumor and the patient's current endocrine function must be assessed before any such surgery.

Mediastinal primary

Primary mediastinal germ-cell tumors are rare. Mediastinal seminomas do not confer a worse prognosis; however, these make up the minority of mediastinal primaries. Clinically, mediastinal NSGCT behave differently compared with other primary sites; they are often less chemosensitive and associated with poorer prognosis. Mediastinal tumors of seminomatous histology have a long-term chance of cure of approximately 90%, whereas only 45% of patients with mediastinal non-seminomas are alive at 5 years.[136] As a non-seminoma mediastinal primary is a poor prognostic feature it should be treated urgently with chemotherapy in the first instance. Following chemotherapy cardiothoracic surgery is often required to remove the residual masses. Viable tumor cells in the mediastinal specimen post-chemotherapy are often predictive for poor outcomes with a hazard ratio of 15 compared to necrosis alone.[137]

The most common symptoms at presentation include dyspnea (25%), chest pain (23%), cough (17%), fever (13%), weight loss (11%), superior vena cava obstruction (6%), fatigue (6%), and pain at other sites (5%).[136] Tumors are aggressive with a high tumor burden and often have significantly elevated tumor markers on presentation.

Primary mediastinal non-seminomas may in some cases be associated with Kleinfelter's syndrome.[138,139] In addition, the development of secondary malignancy within the tumor mass (e.g. sarcoma)[140,141] or the coexistence of hematological malignancy (myelodysplasia, acute myeloid leukemia, or malignant histiocytosis) is recognized.[142]

Other testicular cancers

Leydig-cell and Sertoli-cell tumors

Patients with Leydig-cell and Sertoli-cell tumors together comprise perhaps 2–3% of patients with testicular tumors.[143] These tumors can occur at any age, and at least 90% of cases are benign.

It is difficult to differentiate which sex-cord stromal tumors have metastatic potential. A large size, increased mitotic activity, vascular invasion, necrosis, increased pleomorphism, and extra capsular extension lean toward a more malignant tumor.[144–147]

Most cases of sex-cord stromal tumors present with testicular swelling. Patients may present with gynecomastia (30%) as these tumors may occasionally be hormone-secreting, with associated elevation of estrogen levels. Management is with orchidectomy/partial orchidectomy.

Post-orchidectomy CT scanning should be performed. Majority of the patients are in stage I and require no further therapy. If there is a high suspicion of malignant potential, a prophylactic RPLND may be considered.[148]

Metastatic disease may be seen in 10% of cases. When this occurs, chemotherapy and radiotherapy are generally ineffective, and control is only possible with radical surgery. The prognosis is very poor in such cases.

Conclusion

Germ-cell tumors are an interesting group of histological subtypes. The multidisciplinary approach to their management, intrinsic chemosensitivity of the tumors, and use of strict treatment and follow-up protocols have led them to be a success of modern oncology. Cure rates for early disease are approaching 100% and for metastatic disease with good prognostic features are approximately 95%.

Although cure rates are high for early-stage disease, there are a number of areas for further development including the understanding of familial risk and management of poor risk or relapsed disease. Patients with relapsed disease in particular should be encouraged to enter clinical trials where available as the mortality from these is significantly higher and there is no clear consensus on salvage therapy.

Treatment of metastatic disease and subsequent follow-up can be extensive and the long-term morbidity (both physical and psychological) should be considered in these patients.

Key learning points

- Testicular malignancies are rare with germ-cell tumors making up the majority of these malignancies.
- Germ-cell tumors commonly express tumor markers, bHCG and AFP, and these can be used for diagnosis, predicting prognosis, and monitoring of tumors.
- Stage 1 germ-cell tumors have a high cure rate with just surgery alone; however risk factors assessment is used to guide adjuvant therapy for cases with a high risk of recurrence.
- First-line treatment for metastatic germ-cell tumors is BEP chemotherapy.
- Risk stratification, using the IGCCG prognostic guidelines, is useful to predict response to first-line treatment.

- Although the cure rates from good-prognosis disease are high, the treatment of poor-prognosis disease and relapsed germ-cell tumor is still an area of ongoing research.

References

1. UK CR. *Testicular Cancer Incidence Statistics.* 2016. Available from: https://www.cancerresearchuk.org.
2. Bray F, Richiardi L, Ekbom A et al. Trends in testicular cancer incidence and mortality in 22 European countries: Continuing increases in incidence and declines in mortality. *Int J Cancer.* 2006; 118(12):3099–111.
3. Haugnes HS, Aass N, Fossa SD et al. Components of the metabolic syndrome in long-term survivors of testicular cancer. *Ann Oncol.* 2007; 18(2):241–8.
4. Bray F, Ferlay J, Soerjomataram I et al. Global cancer statistics 2018: GLOBOCAN estimates of incidence and mortality worldwide for 36 cancers in 185 countries. *CA Cancer J Clin.* 2018; 68(6):394–424.
5. Ruf CG, Isbarn H, Wagner W et al. Changes in epidemiologic features of testicular germ cell cancer: Age at diagnosis and relative frequency of seminoma are constantly and significantly increasing. *Urol Oncol.* 2014; 32(1):33 e1–6.
6. Aetiology of testicular cancer: Association with congenital abnormalities, age at puberty, infertility, and exercise. United Kingdom Testicular Cancer Study Group. *BMJ.* 1994; 308(6941):1393–9.
7. Stone JM, Cruickshank DG, Sandeman TF et al. Laterality, maldescent, trauma and other clinical factors in the epidemiology of testis cancer in Victoria, Australia. *Br J Cancer.* 1991; 64(1):132–8.
8. Forman D, Oliver RT, Brett AR et al. Familial testicular cancer: A report of the UK family register, estimation of risk and an HLA class 1 sib-pair analysis. *Br J Cancer.* 1992; 65(2):255–62.
9. Dieckmann KP, Pichlmeier U. The prevalence of familial testicular cancer: An analysis of two patient populations and a review of the literature. *Cancer.* 1997; 80(10):1954–60.
10. Dieckmann KP, Rube C, Henke RP. Association of Down's syndrome and testicular cancer. *J Urol.* 1997; 157(5):1701–4.
11. Hoei-Hansen CE, Rajpert-De Meyts E, Daugaard G et al. Carcinoma in situ testis, the progenitor of testicular germ cell tumours: A clinical review. *Ann Oncol.* 2005; 16(6):863–8.
12. von der Maase H, Rorth M, Walbom-Jorgensen S et al. Carcinoma in situ of contralateral testis in patients with testicular germ cell cancer: Study of 27 cases in 500 patients. *Br Med J.* 1986; 293(6559):1398–401.
13. Petersen PM, Giwercman A, Daugaard G et al. Effect of graded testicular doses of radiotherapy in patients treated for carcinoma-in-situ in the testis. *J Clin Oncol.* 2002; 20(6):1537–43.
14. Christensen TB, Daugaard G, Geertsen PF et al. Effect of chemotherapy on carcinoma in situ of the testis. *Ann Oncol.* 1998; 9(6):657–60.
15. van Echten J, Oosterhuis JW, Looijenga LH et al. No recurrent structural abnormalities apart from i(12p) in primary germ cell tumors of the adult testis. *Genes Chromosomes Cancer.* 1995; 14(2):133–44.
16. Looijenga LH, Zafarana G, Grygalewicz B et al. Role of gain of 12p in germ cell tumour development. *APMIS.* 2003; 111(1):161–71; discussion 172–3.
17. Reuter VE. Origins and molecular biology of testicular germ cell tumors. *Mod Pathol.* 2005; 18(Suppl 2):S51–60.
18. Kao HW, Wu CJ, Chen CY et al. Malignant tumor of testis imitating epididymo-orchitis. *Arch Androl.* 2005; 51(5):407–11.
19. Hassan HC, Cullen IM, Casey RG et al. Gynaecomastia: An endocrine manifestation of testicular cancer. *Andrologia.* 2008; 40(3):152–7.
20. McKendrick JJ, Theaker J, Mead GM. Nonseminomatous germ cell tumor with very high serum human chorionic gonadotrophin. *Cancer.* 1991; 67(3):684–9.
21. Albers P, Albrecht W, Algaba F et al. EAU guidelines on testicular cancer: 2011 update. *Eur Urol.* 2011; 60(2):304–19.

22. Bach AM, Hann LE, Hadar O et al. Testicular microlithiasis: What is its association with testicular cancer? *Radiology.* 2001; 220(1):70–5.

23. Costabile RA. How worrisome is testicular microlithiasis? *Curr Opin Urol.* 2007; 17(6):419–23.

24. Fabre E, Jira H, Izard V et al. "Burned-out" primary testicular cancer. *BJU Int.* 2004; 94(1):74–8.

25. Scholz M, Zehender M, Thalmann GN et al. Extragonadal retroperitoneal germ cell tumor: Evidence of origin in the testis. *Ann Oncol.* 2002; 13(1):121–4.

26. Krege S, Beyer J, Souchon R et al. European consensus conference on diagnosis and treatment of germ cell cancer: A report of the second meeting of the European Germ Cell Cancer Consensus Group (EGCCCG): Part II. *Eur Urol.* 2008; 53(3):497–513.

27. Harding M, Paul J, Kaye SB. Does delayed diagnosis or scrotal incision affect outcome for men with non-seminomatous germ cell tumours? *Br J Urol.* 1995; 76(4):491–4.

28. Capelouto CC, Clark PE, Ransil BJ et al. A review of scrotal violation in testicular cancer: Is adjuvant local therapy necessary? *J Urol.* 1995; 153(3 Pt 2):981–5.

29. Leibovitch I., Little JS Jr., Foster RS et al. Delayed orchiectomy after chemotherapy for metastatic nonseminomatous germ cell tumors. *J Urol.* 1996; 155(3):952–4.

30. Simmonds PD, Mead GM, Lee AH et al. Orchiectomy after chemotherapy in patients with metastatic testicular cancer. Is it indicated? *Cancer.* 1995; 75(4):1018–24.

31. Albers P, Algaba F, Bokemeyer C, et al. EAU Guidelines on Testicular Cancer. 2017; Available from: https://uroweb.org/wp-content/uploads/EAU-Guidelines-Testicular-Cancer-2016-1.pdf

32. Czaja JT, Ulbright TM. Evidence for the transformation of seminoma to yolk sac tumor, with histogenetic considerations. *Am J Clin Pathol.* 1992; 97(4):468–77.

33. Moch H, Cubilla AL, Humphrey PA et al. The 2016 WHO classification of tumours of the urinary system and male genital organspart A: Renal, penile, and testicular tumours. *Eur Urol.* 2016; 70(1):93–105.

34. Williamson SR, Delahunt B, Magi-Galluzzi C et al. The World Health Organization 2016 classification of testicular germ cell tumours: A review and update from the International Society of Urological Pathology Testis Consultation Panel. *Histopathology.* 2017; 70(3):335–346.

35. Sesterhenn IA, Davis CJ, Jr., Pathology of germ cell tumors of the testis. *Cancer Control.* 2004; 11(6):374–87.

36. Tickoo SK, Hutchinson B, Bacik J et al. Testicular seminoma: A clinicopathologic and immunohistochemical study of 105 cases with special reference to seminomas with atypical features. *Int J Surg Pathol.* 2002; 10(1):23–32.

37. Floyd C, Ayala AG, Logothetis CJ et al. Spermatocytic seminoma with associated sarcoma of the testis. *Cancer.* 1988; 61(2):409–14.

38. Simmonds PD, Lee AH, Theaker JM et al. Primary pure teratoma of the testis. *J Urol.* 1996; 155(3):939–42.

39. Garcia-Labastida L, Gomez-Macias GS, Flores-Gutierrez JP et al. Secondary malignant transformation of testicular teratomas: Case series and literature review. *Actas Urol Esp.* 2014; 38(9):622–7.

40. Chung P, Daugaard G, Tyldesley S et al. Evaluation of a prognostic model for risk of relapse in stage I seminoma surveillance. *Cancer Med.* 2015; 4(1):155–60.

41. Stenman UH, Alfthan H, Hotakainen K. Human chorionic gonadotropin in cancer. *Clin Biochem.* 2004; 37(7):549–61.

42. Kaikani W, Boyle H, Chatte G et al. Sarcoid-like granulomatosis and testicular germ cell tumor: The "Great Imitator." *Oncology.* 2011; 81(5–6):319–24.

43. Fernandez EB, Moul JW, Foley JP et al. Retroperitoneal imaging with third and fourth generation computed axial tomography in clinical stage I nonseminomatous germ cell tumors. *Urology.* 1994; 44(4):548–52.

44. See WA, Hoxie L, Chest staging in testis cancer patients: Imaging modality selection based upon risk assessment as determined by abdominal computerized tomography scan results. *J Urol.* 1993; 150(3):874–8.

45. Albers P, Bender H, Yilmaz H et al. Positron emission tomography in the clinical staging of patients with Stage I and II testicular germ cell tumors. *Urology.* 1999; 53(4):808–11.

46. Cremerius U, Wildberger JE, Borchers H et al. Does positron emission tomography using 18-fluoro-2-deoxyglucose improve clinical staging of testicular cancer? Results of a study in 50 patients. *Urology.* 1999; 54(5):900–4.

47. De Santis M, Becherer A, Bokemeyer C et al. 2–18fluoro-deoxy-D-glucose positron emission tomography is a reliable predictor for viable tumor in postchemotherapy seminoma: An update of the prospective multicentric SEMPET trial. *J Clin Oncol.* 2004; 22(6):1034–9.

48. Hinz S, Schrader M, Kempkensteffen C et al. The role of positron emission tomography in the evaluation of residual masses after chemotherapy for advanced stage seminoma. *J Urol.* 2008; 179(3):936–40; discussion 940.

49. Treglia G, Sadeghi R, Annunziata S et al. Diagnostic performance of fluorine-18-fluorodeoxyglucose positron emission tomography in the postchemotherapy management of patients with seminoma: Systematic review and meta-analysis. *Biomed Res Int.* 2014; 2014:852681.

50. Huddart RA, O'Doherty MJ, Padhani A et al. 18fluorodeoxyglucose positron emission tomography in the prediction of relapse in patients with high-risk, clinical stage I nonseminomatous germ cell tumors: Preliminary report of MRC Trial TE22--the NCRI Testis Tumour Clinical Study Group. *J Clin Oncol.* 2007; 25(21):3090–5.

51. Geldart TR, Simmonds PD, Mead GM. Orchidectomy after chemotherapy for patients with metastatic testicular germ cell cancer. *BJU Int.* 2002; 90(4):451–5.

52. Warde PR, Gospodarowicz MK, Goodman PJ et al. Results of a policy of surveillance in stage I testicular seminoma. *Int J Radiat Oncol Biol Phys.* 1993; 27(1):11–5.

53. Warde P, Gospodarowicz MK, Panzarella T et al. Stage I testicular seminoma: Results of adjuvant irradiation and surveillance. *J Clin Oncol.* 1995; 13(9):2255–62.

54. Horwich, A, Alsanjari N, A'Hern R et al. Surveillance following orchidectomy for stage I testicular seminoma. *Br J Cancer.* 1992; 65(5):775–8.

55. Warde P, Specht L, Horwich A et al. Prognostic factors for relapse in stage I seminoma managed by surveillance: A pooled analysis. *J Clin Oncol.* 2002; 20(22):4448–52.

56. Read G, Stenning SP, Cullen MH et al. Medical Research Council prospective study of surveillance for stage I testicular teratoma. Medical Research Council Testicular Tumors Working Party. *J Clin Oncol.* 1992; 10(11):1762–8.

57. von der Maase H, Specht L, Jacobsen GK et al. Surveillance following orchidectomy for stage I seminoma of the testis. *Eur J Cancer.* 1993; 29A(14):1931–4.

58. Oliver RT, Mason MD, Mead GM et al. Radiotherapy versus single-dose carboplatin in adjuvant treatment of stage I seminoma: A randomised trial. *Lancet.* 2005; 366(9482):293–300.

59. Fossa SD, Horwich A, Russell JM et al. Optimal planning target volume for stage I testicular seminoma: A Medical Research Council randomized trial. Medical Research Council Testicular Tumor Working Group. *J Clin Oncol.* 1999; 17(4):1146.

60. Jones WG, Fossa SD, Mead GM et al. Randomized trial of 30 versus 20 Gy in the adjuvant treatment of stage I Testicular Seminoma: A report on Medical Research Council Trial TE18, European Organisation for the Research and Treatment of Cancer Trial 30942 (ISRCTN18525328). *J Clin Oncol.* 2005; 23(6):1200–8.

61. Albers P, Siener R, Kliesch S et al. Risk factors for relapse in clinical stage I nonseminomatous testicular germ cell tumors: Results of the German Testicular Cancer Study Group Trial. *J Clin Oncol.* 2003; 21(8):1505–12.

62. Pont J, Holtl W, Kosak D et al. Risk-adapted treatment choice in stage I nonseminomatous testicular germ cell cancer by regarding vascular invasion in the primary tumor: A prospective trial. *J Clin Oncol.* 1990; 8(1):16–20.

63. Rustin GJ, Mead GM, Stenning SP et al. Randomized trial of two or five computed tomography scans in the surveillance of patients

with stage I nonseminomatous germ cell tumors of the testis: Medical Research Council Trial TE08, ISRCTN56475197–The National Cancer Research Institute Testis Cancer Clinical Studies Group. *J Clin Oncol.* 2007; 25(11):1310–5.

64. Madej G, Pawinski A. Risk-related adjuvant chemotherapy for stage I non-seminoma of the testis. *Clin Oncol.* 1991; 3(5):270–2.

65. Bohlen D, Borner M, Sonntag RW et al. Long-term results following adjuvant chemotherapy in patients with clinical stage I testicular nonseminomatous malignant germ cell tumors with high risk factors. *J Urol.* 1999; 161(4):1148–52.

66. Cullen MH, Stenning SP, Parkinson MC et al. Short-course adjuvant chemotherapy in high-risk stage I nonseminomatous germ cell tumors of the testis: A Medical Research Council report. *J Clin Oncol.* 1996; 14(4):1106–13.

67. Albers P, Siener R, Krege S et al. Randomized phase III trial comparing retroperitoneal lymph node dissection with one course of bleomycin and etoposide plus cisplatin chemotherapy in the adjuvant treatment of clinical stage I Nonseminomatous testicular germ cell tumors: AUO trial AH 01/94 by the German Testicular Cancer Study Group. *J Clin Oncol.* 2008; 26(18):2966–72.

68. Tandstad T, Dahl O, Cohn-Cedermark G et al. Risk-adapted treatment in clinical stage I nonseminomatous germ cell testicular cancer: The SWENOTECA management program. *J Clin Oncol.* 2009; 27(13):2122–8.

69. Huddart RA, White JD, Hutton P et al. 111: A single-arm trial evaluating one cycle of BEP as adjuvant chemotherapy in high-risk, stage 1 non-seminomatous or combined germ cell tumors of the testis (NSGCTT). 2017; 400.

70. International Germ Cell Consensus Classification: A prognostic factor-based staging system for metastatic germ cell cancers. International Germ Cell Cancer Collaborative Group. *J Clin Oncol.* 1997; 15(2):594–603.

71. Peckham MJ, Barrett A, Liew KH et al. The treatment of metastatic germ-cell testicular tumours with bleomycin, etoposide and cisplatin (BEP). *Br J Cancer.* 1983; 47(5):613–9.

72. Williams SD, Birch R, Einhorn LH et al. Treatment of disseminated germ-cell tumors with cisplatin, bleomycin, and either vinblastine or etoposide. *N Engl J Med.* 1987; 316(23):1435–40.

73. de Wit R, Stoter G, Sleijfer DT et al. Four cycles of BEP vs. four cycles of VIP in patients with intermediate-prognosis metastatic testicular non-seminoma: A randomized study of the EORTC Genitourinary Tract Cancer Cooperative Group. European Organization for Research and Treatment of Cancer. *Br J Cancer.* 1998; 78(6):828–32.

74. O'Sullivan JM, Huddart RA, Norman AR et al. Predicting the risk of bleomycin lung toxicity in patients with germ-cell tumours. *Ann Oncol.* 2003; 14(1):91–6.

75. Einhorn LH, Williams SD, Loehrer PJ et al. Evaluation of optimal duration of chemotherapy in favorable-prognosis disseminated germ cell tumors: A Southeastern Cancer Study Group protocol. *J Clin Oncol.* 1989; 7(3):387–91.

76. de Wit R, Roberts JT, Wilkinson PM et al. Equivalence of three or four cycles of bleomycin, etoposide, and cisplatin chemotherapy and of a 3- or 5-day schedule in good-prognosis germ cell cancer: A randomized study of the European Organization for Research and Treatment of Cancer Genitourinary Tract Cancer Cooperative Group and the Medical Research Council. *J Clin Oncol.* 2001; 19(6):1629–40.

77. Dalgleish AG, Woods RL, Levi JA. Bleomycin pulmonary toxicity: Its relationship to renal dysfunction. *Med Pediatr Oncol.* 1984; 12(5):313–7.

78. Loehrer PJ, Sr., Johnson D, Elson P et al. Importance of bleomycin in favorable-prognosis disseminated germ cell tumors: An Eastern Cooperative Oncology Group trial. *J Clin Oncol.* 1995; 13(2):470–6.

79. Levi JA, Raghavan D, Harvey V et al. The importance of bleomycin in combination chemotherapy for good-prognosis germ cell carcinoma. Australasian Germ Cell Trial Group. *J Clin Oncol.* 1993; 11(7):1300–5.

80. de Wit R, Stoter G, Kaye SB et al. Importance of bleomycin in combination chemotherapy for good-prognosis testicular non-seminoma: A randomized study of the European Organization for Research and Treatment of Cancer Genitourinary Tract Cancer Cooperative Group. *J Clin Oncol.* 1997; 15(5):1837–43.

81. Culine S, Kerbrat P, Kramar A et al. Refining the optimal chemotherapy regimen for good-risk metastatic nonseminomatous germ-cell tumors: A randomized trial of the Genito-Urinary Group of the French Federation of Cancer Centers (GETUG T93BP). *Ann Oncol.* 2007; 18(5):917–24.

82. Horwich A, Sleijfer DT, Fossa SD et al. Randomized trial of bleomycin, etoposide, and cisplatin compared with bleomycin, etoposide, and carboplatin in good-prognosis metastatic nonseminomatous germ cell cancer: A Multiinstitutional Medical Research Council/ European Organization for Research and Treatment of Cancer Trial. *J Clin Oncol.* 1997; 15(5):1844–52.

83. Bajorin DF, Sarosdy MF, Pfister DG et al. Randomized trial of etoposide and cisplatin versus etoposide and carboplatin in patients with good-risk germ cell tumors: A multiinstitutional study. *J Clin Oncol.* 1993; 11(4):598–606.

84. Mead GM. Who should manage germ cell tumours of the testis? *BJU Int.* 1999; 84(1):61–7.

85. Albany C, Brames MJ, Fausel C et al. Randomized, double-blind, placebo-controlled, phase III cross-over study evaluating the oral neurokinin-1 antagonist aprepitant in combination with a 5HT3 receptor antagonist and dexamethasone in patients with germ cell tumors receiving 5-day cisplatin combination chemotherapy regimens: A hoosier oncology group study. *J Clin Oncol.* 2012; 30(32):3998–4003.

86. Hartmann JT, Kollmannsberger C, Kanz L et al. Platinum organ toxicity and possible prevention in patients with testicular cancer. *Int J Cancer.* 1999; 83(6):866–9.

87. Lampe H, Horwich A, Norman A et al. Fertility after chemotherapy for testicular germ cell cancers. *J Clin Oncol.* 1997; 15(1):239–45.

88. Willemse PM, Burggraaf J, Hamdy NA et al. Prevalence of the metabolic syndrome and cardiovascular disease risk in chemotherapy-treated testicular germ cell tumour survivors. *Br J Cancer.* 2013; 109(1):60–7.

89. Travis LB, Fossa SD, Schonfeld SJ et al. Second cancers among 40,576 testicular cancer patients: Focus on long-term survivors. *J Natl Cancer Inst.* 2005; 97(18):1354–65.

90. Bokemeyer C, Schmoll HJ. Secondary neoplasms following treatment of malignant germ cell tumors. *J Clin Oncol.* 1993; 11(9):1703–9.

91. Fung C, Dinh P, Jr., Ardeshir-Rouhani-Fard S. et al. Toxicities aassociated with cisplatin-based chemotherapy and radiotherapy in long-term testicular cancer survivors. *Adv Urol.* 2018; 2018:8671832.

92. Classen J, Schmidberger H, Meisner C et al. Radiotherapy for stages IIA/B testicular seminoma: Final report of a prospective multicenter clinical trial. *J Clin Oncol.* 2003; 21(6):1101–6.

93. Chung PW, Gospodarowicz MK, Panzarella T et al. Stage II testicular seminoma: Patterns of recurrence and outcome of treatment. *Eur Urol.* 2004; 45(6):754–59; discussion 759–60.

94. Horwich A, Dearnaley DP, Sohaib A et al. Neoadjuvant carboplatin before radiotherapy in stage IIA and IIB seminoma. *Ann Oncol.* 2013; 24(8):2104–7.

95. Garcia-del-Muro X, Maroto P, Guma J et al. Chemotherapy as an alternative to radiotherapy in the treatment of stage IIA and IIB testicular seminoma: A Spanish Germ Cell Cancer Group Study. *J Clin Oncol.* 2008; 26(33):5416–21.

96. Horwich A, Oliver RT, Wilkinson PM et al. A medical research council randomized trial of single agent carboplatin versus etoposide and cisplatin for advanced metastatic seminoma. MRC Testicular Tumour Working Party. *Br J Cancer.* 2000; 83(12):1623–9.

97. Bokemeyer C, Kollmannsberger C, Stenning S et al. Metastatic seminoma treated with either single agent carboplatin or cisplatin-based combination chemotherapy: A pooled analysis of two randomised trials. *Br J Cancer.* 2004; 91(4):683–7.

98. Tookman L, Rashid S, Matakidou A et al. Carboplatin AUC 10 for IGCCCG good prognosis metastatic seminoma. *Acta Oncol.* 2013; 52(5):987–93.

99. De Santis M, Bokemeyer C, Becherer A et al. Predictive impact of 2–18fluoro-2-deoxy-D-glucose positron emission tomography for residual postchemotherapy masses in patients with bulky seminoma. *J Clin Oncol.* 2001; 19(17):3740–4.

100. Christian JA, Huddart RA, Norman A et al. Intensive induction chemotherapy with CBOP/BEP in patients with poor prognosis germ cell tumors. *J Clin Oncol.* 2003; 21(5):871–7.

101. Bokemeyer C, Kollmannsberger C, Meisner C et al. First-line high-dose chemotherapy compared with standard-dose PEB/VIP chemotherapy in patients with advanced germ cell tumors: A multivariate and matched-pair analysis. *J Clin Oncol.* 1999; 17(11):3450–6.

102. Motzer RJ, Nichols CJ, Margolin KA et al. Phase III randomized trial of conventional-dose chemotherapy with or without high-dose chemotherapy and autologous hematopoietic stem-cell rescue as first-line treatment for patients with poor-prognosis metastatic germ cell tumors. *J Clin Oncol.* 2007; 25(3):247–56.

103. Bokemeyer C, Nowak P, Haupt A et al. Treatment of brain metastases in patients with testicular cancer. *J Clin Oncol.* 1997; 15(4):1449–54.

104. Spears WT, Morphis JG, 2nd, Lester SG et al. Brain metastases and testicular tumors: Long-term survival. *Int J Radiat Oncol Biol Phys.* 1992; 22(1):17–22.

105. Kollmannsberger C, Nichols C, Bamberg M et al. First-line high-dose chemotherapy +/– radiation therapy in patients with metastatic germ-cell cancer and brain metastases. *Ann Oncol.* 2000; 11(5):553–9.

106. Fossa SD, Bokemeyer C, Gerl A et al. Treatment outcome of patients with brain metastases from malignant germ cell tumors. *Cancer.* 1999; 85(4):988–97.

107. Panicek DM, Toner GC, Heelan RT et al. Nonseminomatous germ cell tumors: Enlarging masses despite chemotherapy. *Radiology.* 1990; 175(2):499–502.

108. Jeffery GM, Theaker JM, Lee AH et al. The growing teratoma syndrome. *Br J Urol.* 1991; 67(2):195–202.

109. Baniel J, Foster RS, Rowland RG et al. Complications of primary retroperitoneal lymph node dissection. *J Urol.* 1994; 152(2 Pt 1):424–7.

110. Heidenreich A, Albers P, Hartmann M et al. Complications of primary nerve sparing retroperitoneal lymph node dissection for clinical stage I nonseminomatous germ cell tumors of the testis: Experience of the German Testicular Cancer Study Group. *J Urol.* 2003; 169(5):1710–4.

111. Fossa SD, Ous S, Lien HH et al. Post-chemotherapy lymph node histology in radiologically normal patients with metastatic nonseminomatous testicular cancer. *J Urol.* 1989; 141(3):557–9.

112. Hartmann JT, Schmoll HJ, Kuczyk MA et al. Postchemotherapy resections of residual masses from metastatic non-seminomatous testicular germ cell tumors. *Ann Oncol.* 1997; 8(6):531–8.

113. Fizazi K, Tjulandin S, Salvioni R et al. Viable malignant cells after primary chemotherapy for disseminated nonseminomatous germ cell tumors: Prognostic factors and role of postsurgery chemotherapy–Results from an international study group. *J Clin Oncol.* 2001; 19(10):2647–57.

114. Toner GC, Panicek DM, Heelan RT et al. Adjunctive surgery after chemotherapy for nonseminomatous germ cell tumors: Recommendations for patient selection. *J Clin Oncol.* 1990; 8(10):1683–94.

115. Rashid S, Lim L, Powles T. Treatment of relapsed/refractory germ cell tumours: An equipoise between conventional and high dose therapy. *Curr Treat Options Oncol.* 2012; 13(2):201–11.

116. International Prognostic Factors Study G, Lorch A, Beyer J et al. Prognostic factors in patients with metastatic germ cell tumors who experienced treatment failure with cisplatin-based first-line chemotherapy. *J Clin Oncol.* 2010; 28(33):4906–11.

117. Farhat F, Culine S, Theodore C et al. Cisplatin and ifosfamide with either vinblastine or etoposide as salvage therapy for refractory or relapsing germ cell tumor patients: The Institut Gustave Roussy experience. *Cancer.* 1996; 77(6):1193–7.

118. McCaffrey JA, Mazumdar M, Bajorin DF et al. Ifosfamide- and cisplatin-containing chemotherapy as first-line salvage therapy in germ cell tumors: Response and survival. *J Clin Oncol.* 1997; 15(7):2559–63.

119. Loehrer PJ, Sr., Gonin R, Nichols CR et al. Vinblastine plus ifosfamide plus cisplatin as initial salvage therapy in recurrent germ cell tumor. *J Clin Oncol.* 1998; 16(7):2500–4.

120. Pico JL, Rosti G, Kramar A et al. A randomised trial of high-dose chemotherapy in the salvage treatment of patients failing first-line platinum chemotherapy for advanced germ cell tumours. *Ann Oncol.* 2005; 16(7):1152–9.

121. Kondagunta GV, Bacik J, Donadio A et al. Combination of paclitaxel, ifosfamide, and cisplatin is an effective second-line therapy for patients with relapsed testicular germ cell tumors. *J Clin Oncol.* 2005; 23(27):6549–55.

122. Motzer RJ, Sheinfeld J, Mazumdar M et al. Paclitaxel, ifosfamide, and cisplatin second-line therapy for patients with relapsed testicular germ cell cancer. *J Clin Oncol.* 2000; 18(12):2413–8.

123. Mead GM, Cullen MH, Huddart R et al. A phase II trial of TIP (paclitaxel, ifosfamide and cisplatin) given as second-line (post-BEP) salvage chemotherapy for patients with metastatic germ cell cancer: A medical research council trial. *Br J Cancer.* 2005; 93(2):178–84.

124. Beyer J, Kramar A, Mandanas R et al. High-dose chemotherapy as salvage treatment in germ cell tumors: A multivariate analysis of prognostic variables. *J Clin Oncol.* 1996; 14(10):2638–45.

125. Lorch A, Bascoul-Mollevi C, Kramar A et al. Conventional-dose versus high-dose chemotherapy as first salvage treatment in male patients with metastatic germ cell tumors: Evidence from a large international database. *J Clin Oncol.* 2011; 29(16):2178–84.

126. Motzer RJ, Mazumdar M, Sheinfeld J et al. Sequential dose-intensive paclitaxel, ifosfamide, carboplatin, and etoposide salvage therapy for germ cell tumor patients. *J Clin Oncol.* 2000; 18(6):1173–80.

127. Eggener SE, Carver BS, Loeb S et al. Pathologic findings and clinical outcome of patients undergoing retroperitoneal lymph node dissection after multiple chemotherapy regimens for metastatic testicular germ cell tumors. *Cancer.* 2007; 109(3):528–35.

128. Coogan CL, Foster RS, Rowland RG et al. Postchemotherapy retroperitoneal lymph node dissection is effective therapy in selected patients with elevated tumor markers after primary chemotherapy alone. *Urology.* 1997; 50(6):957–62.

129. Eastham JA, Wilson TG, Russell C et al. Surgical resection in patients with nonseminomatous germ cell tumor who fail to normalize serum tumor markers after chemotherapy. *Urology.* 1994; 43(1):74–80.

130. Murphy BR, Breeden ES, Donohue JP et al. Surgical salvage of chemorefractory germ cell tumors. *J Clin Oncol.* 1993; 11(2):324–9.

131. Fossa SD, Chen J, Schonfeld SJ et al. Risk of contralateral testicular cancer: A population-based study of 29,515 U.S. men. *J Natl Cancer Inst.* 2005; 97(14):1056–66.

132. Dieckmann KP, Loy V. Prevalence of contralateral testicular intraepithelial neoplasia in patients with testicular germ cell neoplasms. *J Clin Oncol.* 1996; 14(12):3126–32.

133. Harland SJ, Cook PA, Fossa SD et al. Intratubular germ cell neoplasia of the contralateral testis in testicular cancer: Defining a high risk group. *J Urol.* 1998; 160(4):1353–7.

134. Dieckmann KP, Besserer A, Loy V. Low-dose radiation therapy for testicular intraepithelial neoplasia. *J Cancer Res Clin Oncol.* 1993; 119(6):355–9.

135. Lawrentschuk N, Zuniga A, Grabowksi AC et al. Partial orchiectomy for presumed malignancy in patients with a solitary testis due to a prior germ cell tumor: A large North American experience. *J Urol.* 2011; 185(2):508–13.

136. Bokemeyer C, Nichols CR, Droz JP et al. Extragonadal germ cell tumors of the mediastinum and retroperitoneum: Results from an international analysis. *J Clin Oncol.* 2002; 20(7):1864–73.

137. Kesler KA, Rieger KM, Hammoud ZT et al. A 25-year single institution experience with surgery for primary mediastinal nonseminomatous germ cell tumors. *Ann Thorac Surg.* 2008; 85(2):371–8.

138. Nichols CR, Heerema NA, Palmer C et al. Klinefelter's syndrome associated with mediastinal germ cell neoplasms. *J Clin Oncol.* 1987; 5(8):1290–4.

139. Volkl TM, Langer T, Aigner T et al. Klinefelter syndrome and mediastinal germ cell tumors. *Am J Med Genet A.* 2006; 140(5):471–81.

140. Gonzalez-Vela JL, Savage PD, Manivel JC et al. Poor prognosis of mediastinal germ cell cancers containing sarcomatous components. *Cancer.* 1990; 66(6):1114–6.

141. Malagon HD, Valdez AM, Moran CA et al. Germ cell tumors with sarcomatous components: A clinicopathologic and immunohistochemical study of 46 cases. *Am J Surg Pathol.* 2007; 31(9): 1356–62.

142. Hartmann JT, Nichols CR, J.P. Droz et al. Hematologic disorders associated with primary mediastinal nonseminomatous germ cell tumors. *J Natl Cancer Inst.* 2000; 92(1):54–61.

143. Conkey DS, Howard GC, Grigor KM et al. Testicular sex cord-stromal tumours: The Edinburgh experience 1988–2002, and a review of the literature. *Clin Oncol.* 2005; 17(5):322–7.

144. Cheville JC, Sebo TJ, Lager DJ et al. Leydig cell tumor of the testis: A clinicopathologic, DNA content, and MIB-1 comparison of non-metastasizing and metastasizing tumors. *Am J Surg Pathol.* 1998; 22(11):1361–7.

145. McCluggage WG, Shanks JH, Arthur K et al. Cellular proliferation and nuclear ploidy assessments augment established prognostic factors in predicting malignancy in testicular Leydig cell tumours. *Histopathology.* 1998; 33(4):361–8.

146. Kratzer SS, Ulbright TM, Talerman A et al. Large cell calcifying Sertoli cell tumor of the testis: Contrasting features of six malignant and six benign tumors and a review of the literature. *Am J Surg Pathol.* 1997; 21(11):1271–80.

147. Giglio M, Medica M, De Rose AF et al. Testicular sertoli cell tumours and relative sub-types. Analysis of clinical and prognostic features. *Urol Int.* 2003; 70(3):205–10.

148. Mosharafa AA, Foster RS, Bihrle R et al. Does retroperitoneal lymph node dissection have a curative role for patients with sex cord-stromal testicular tumors? *Cancer.* 2003; 98(4):753–7.

18 RENAL CELL CANCER

Sarah Ellis and Joanna Hack

Introduction and Epidemiology

Malignant renal tumors are the 14th most common cancer worldwide with varying rates dependent on region. In 2018 there were more than 400,000 cases recorded.[1] Kidney cancer affects men more commonly than women with a 1.5:1 ratio, estimated to represent 5% of all cancer cases in men and 3% in women in the United States.[2,3] More than half of renal tumors are now localized when identified likely due to the increasing use of ultrasound and cross-sectional imaging resulting in incidental pick up in the absence of symptoms.[3]

The incidence of renal cancer increases with age peaking between 60 and 70 years. The age-standardized rates are 0.5 per 100,000, increasing to 35 per 100,00 in those over 75 years of age.[2] See Figure 18.1.

Classification of renal tumors

Eighty to ninety percent of malignant renal tumors arise from the renal parenchymal tissue with the remainder being uroepithelial in origin. The vast majority of renal uroepithelial tumors are transitional cell carcinomas (TCCs) arising from the renal pelvis, and treatment principles are those of TCCs occurring at other sites such as the bladder and ureter (see Chapter 13).

Renal parenchymal tumors were originally considered to arise from ectopic adrenal nests, hence the coining of the term hypernephroma. In 1960, on the basis of electron microscopic features, Oberling et al. demonstrated a proximal renal tubular origin, and tumors were renamed renal cell adenocarcinoma or renal cell carcinoma (RCC).[4] Subsequently, RCC has been further reclassified and subdivided into a number of differing subtypes with distinct histopathological, clinical, and molecular features. The World Health Organisation introduced a number of new sub-types in the 2016 classification which are listed in Table 18.1. However clear-cell tumors are by far the most common renal carcinomas and together with papillary and chromophobe subtypes account for more than 90% of renal carcinomas.[5]

Clear-cell (conventional) renal cell carcinoma

Macroscopically clear-cell RCCs have a characteristic appearance with solid areas often interspersed with areas of cystic degeneration. These tumors are richly vascular with numerous vessels throughout the supporting stroma. Microscopically, tumor cells have a clear cytoplasm with a low nuclear to cytoplasmic ratio. The Fuhrman and WHO/ISUP grading systems can aid in the prediction of clinical tumor behavior. Both consist of four grades (I–IV) on the basis of morphologic tumor appearance. Sarcomatoid change may be seen, and represents a poor prognostic feature occurring in approximately 5% of tumors. The presence of tumor necrosis is also of prognostic significance and is associated with a worse survival.[6] For the vast majority of patients with clear-cell RCC, the key molecular driver underlying development and progression of both sporadic and hereditary disease is loss of function of the Von Hippel–Lindau (VHL)

gene through a process of deletion, mutation, or methylation.[7,8] Increasingly evident with the progress in genetic sequencing is that multiple other genes are also responsible for malignant cell proliferation. Located on chromosome 3p in addition to VHL are PBRM1, SETD2, and BAP1 epigenetic/chromatin regulators. Loss of function of these tumor suppressor genes is thought to play a key role in cancer progression. PBRM-1 is mutated in around 40% ccRCC, and subclonal mutations in BAP-1 and SETD2 identified in 10–15% of tumor samples.[8,9]

Papillary (chromophil) renal carcinoma

Papillary (chromophil) RCCs are significantly rarer, but with a prevalence of approximately 15% are the second most common variant of RCC.[5] There is a male predominance. Papillary architecture is a key finding in these tumors. Papillary tumors may be further subclassified into type I or type II. Type I (basophilic) tumors are the most common variant and typically behave in a more indolent fashion than type II tumors. They consist of small cells with scanty cytoplasm and small nuclei.[5] Mutation in the proto-oncogene *met*, which encodes for a tyrosine kinase receptor whose ligand is hepatocyte growth factor is associated with hereditary type I papillary renal carcinoma and has been demonstrated in some patients with sporadic papillary RCC.[10,11]

Type II (eosinophilic) tumors have large cells with abundant eosinophilic cytoplasm and large nuclei. Type II tumors are typically associated with a higher nuclear grade, clinical stage, and shorter survival than Type I. In patients with hereditary type II papillary RCC (hereditary leiomyomatosis RCC [HLRCC]), a mutation in the fumarate hydratase gene has been identified.[5]

Chromophobe renal carcinoma rare subtypes, benign renal tumors, and nephroblastoma

Chromophobe RCCs account for approximately 5% of renal carcinomas. In contrast to clear-cell and papillary tumors, which characteristically arise from the proximal tubule, chromophobe carcinomas are thought to arise from the cortical collecting duct.[12] Microscopically, chromophobe tumors consist of large polygonal cells forming a compact growth pattern with pale cytoplasm and prominent cell membranes. Chromophobe carcinomas are often localized and associated with a more favorable prognosis.[5]

Rare subtypes

Less than 5% of RCCs may be of a rare subtype with ten included in the WHO 2016 classification

Key features are summarized in Table 18.1.

Benign renal tumors

Benign renal tumors include papillary and metanephric adenomas, renal oncocytomas, angiomyolipomas, fibromas, and lipomas. Although occasionally symptomatic, these benign tumors are often detected incidentally. Surgical excision or thermal ablation, where appropriate, represents definitive treatment.

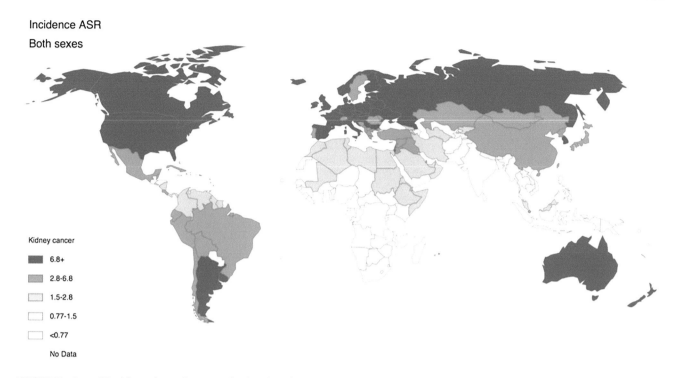

Incidence ASR

Both sexes

Kidney cancer

- 6.8+
- 2.8-6.8
- 1.5-2.8
- 0.77-1.5
- <0.77
- No Data

FIGURE 18.1 World incidence (age-standardized rate) for renal cancer for both sexes. (From Capitano et al., 2019.)

Nephroblastoma (Wilms' tumor)

Nephroblastomas are malignant mixed embryonic tumors of the kidney and one of the most common neoplasms in young children, occurring with a peak incidence in the second year of life. Their diagnosis and treatment is discussed in Chapter 32.

Inherited syndromes and the molecular biology of renal cell carcinoma

A number of hereditary syndromes are associated with the development of kidney cancer, which tends to present at a younger age with multifocal or bilateral disease. These represent around 5% of all RCC cases,[14] and investigation into the underlying genetic abnormalities continues to provide important insights into the mechanisms for the development and treatment of hereditary and sporadic cancers. With advances in genetic sequencing more than ten hereditary renal cancer syndromes have now been identified: Von Hippel–Lindau (VHL) disease, hereditary papillary renal carcinoma (HPRC), hereditary leiomyomatosis and renal cell cancer (HLRCC), Birt–Hogg–Dubé syndrome (BHD), tuberous sclerosis complex (TSC), and succinate dehydrogenase (SDH)-associated familial cancer. Hereditary paraganglioma-pheochromocytoma syndrome (HPPS), Cowden syndrome, chromosome 3p translocation-associated (Ch3pTA) kidney cancer syndrome, BAP-1 cancer susceptibility syndrome (BAP1CSS). Their key features are detailed in Table 18.2.

Risk factors

A number of risk factors have been implicated in the development of RCC, including increasing age, cigarette smoking, obesity, and hypertension. Evidence from case-control and cohort studies consistently supports a relationship between these factors and RCC. The VITAL study followed 77,260 US residents prospectively over a period of 8 years. Body mass index (BMI) >35 kg/m^2 versus < 25kg/m^2 conferred increased risk HR 1.71 (CI 1.06–2.79). A smoking history of >37.5 pack-years versus never-smokers gave HR 1.71 (CI 1.16–2.42). The presence of hypertension demonstrated HR 1.7 (CI 1.3–2.22).[15]

Other factors that have shown associations include chronic kidney disease, presumably relating to the development of acquired renal cystic disease with pre-existent renal failure and dialysis. The occurrence of RCC is around ten times higher than the general population.[2]

Viral hepatitis has been highlighted as a possible risk in a number of studies, with HR 1.8 (CI 1.03–3.14) in the VITAL study. Exposure to trichloroethylene initially administered as an anesthetic in the 20th century, and still in use as an industrial solvent, is seen to increase RCC risk.[2]

The chronic use of analgesics appears to be contributory to the development of RCC in addition with acetaminophen, and non-aspirin non-steroidal anti-inflammatory drugs suggested as the causative agents.[2]

Clinical features

Kidney cancer remains occult for much of its clinical course. More than half of all patients with kidney cancer are now diagnosed incidentally following diagnostic imaging performed for another indication, a phenomenon that has led to size and stage migration with increasing numbers of earlier, smaller tumors being detected.[1,3] The National Cancer Database in the US demonstrated under 20% of tumors were stage III or IV at presentation (2004–2015), with no evidence of further stage migration after 2007.[17]

Symptoms relating to the primary tumor tend to occur late. Macroscopic hematuria, flank pain, and a palpable mass represent the classical triad of symptoms although this presentation occurs in a minority of patients and generally indicates locally advanced disease. Disease may occasionally be locally invasive into adjacent structures including ipsilateral adrenal gland, liver,

TABLE 18.1 **Subtypes of Renal Cell Tumors**

Renal Cell Tumor Subtypes	Clinical Features	Morphological/Immunohistochemical Features	Molecular Features
CCRCC	65–70% of adult RCCs	Clear/eosinophilic cells with thin-walled, staghorn-shaped vasculature; positive for CAIX and CD10, negative for CK7 and AMACR	Loss of function of *VHL*, Chr 3p deletion, inappropriate stabilization of HIFs, genetic mutations in PI3K/AKT pathway, mutations of *SETD2*, *BAP1*, and *MTOR*, aggressive CCRCC demonstrating a metabolic shift
PRCC	15–20% of adult RCCs, type 1 shows a better prognosis than type 2	Papillary structure, foamy macrophages; type 1: Scanty cytoplasm; type 2: Abundant eosinophilic cytoplasm; positive for CD10, CK7, and AMACR, negative for CAIX	Gain of Chr 7 and/or Chr 17, loss of Chr Y; type 1: *MET* alteration; type 2: *CDKN2A* silencing, *SETD2* mutation; three subtypes according to the TCGA, including CIMP-associated aggressive subtype with an *FH* mutation
ChRCC	5–7% of adult RCCs, favorable prognosis, Birt–Hogg–Dubé syndrome with an FLCN mutation	Prominent cell membrane, irregular nuclei, perinuclear halo, pale to eosinophilic cytoplasm; positive for KIT and CK7, negative for CAIX and CD10	Loss of Chrs 1, 2, 6, 10, 13, and 17, somatic mutation in mitochondrial DNA, mutations of TP53 and PTEN, imbalanced chromosome duplication (ICD), high TERT expression by DNA rearrangement within the TERT promoter region with kataegis
Rarer Tumor Subtypes			
Collecting duct (Bellini's)	Aggressive clinical course	High grade, papillary or sarcomatoid patterns. Eosinophilic cells	Limited data, various genomic alterations detected in small studies
Medullary	Aggressive clinical course, strong association with sickle disease/trait. Resistant to VEGF TKIs	Adenocarcinoma—high grade within renal medulla. Sickled erythrocytes within tumor specimen/adjacent kidney tissue. SMARCB1 loss on IHC	Loss of protein expression of tumor suppressor gene *SMARCB1*, commonly inactivated by deletions and inactivating translocations
Mucinous tubular and spindle cell	Favorable prognosis, female predominance	Tubular and spindle cells within mucinous stroma	Limited data—a range of chromosomal losses and gains recorded in small studies
Multilocular cystic renal neoplasm of low malignant potential	Excellent prognosis	Numerous cysts lined by clear cells; positive for CAIX and CK7	VHL mutation, Chr 3p deletion
MiT family TRCC	Pediatric to young adult patients, mean age of 30 years	Papillary pattern, psammoma bodies, large epithelioid cells and small cells; positive for TFE3 or TFEB	Xp11 TRCC: TFE3 rearrangement, t(6;12) RCC: TFEB rearrangement
Tubulocystic RCC	Male predominance, mean age of 60 years, indolent	Dilated tubules with a single layer of cells	Gain of Chrs 7 and 17, loss of Chr Y
ACD-associated RCC	End-stage renal disease or ACD, indolent	Eosinophilic cytoplasm, sieve-like pattern, intratumoral oxalate crystals; positive for AMACR and CD10, negative for CK7	Gain of Chrs 3, 16, and Y
CCPRCC	3–4% of renal tumors, indolent, end-stage renal disease, VHL disease	Clear cytoplasm, papillary pattern, apical-oriented nuclei; positive for CK7 and CAIX, negative for CD10	Lack of the genomic alterations observed in CCRCC/PRCC
SDH-deficient RCC	0.05–0.2% of renal carcinomas, mean age of 37 years, good prognosis, germline mutation in one of the *SDH* genes	Cytoplasmic vacuoles and inclusion-like spaces; negative for SDHB, KIT, and CK7 a	Double-hit inactivation of one of the *SDH* genes, most commonly *SDHB*, no mutations in *VHL*, *PIK3CA*, *AKT*, *MTOR*, *MET*, or *TP53*
HLRCC-associated RCC	HLRCC syndrome, aggressive	Large nuclei with inclusion-like eosinophilic nucleoli and perinuclear clearing, abundant eosinophilic cytoplasm, papillary/tubular pattern; positive for S-(2-succino)-cysteine (2SC), negative for FH, CK19, 34betaE12, and CK7	Germline mutation in *FH*, metabolic shift to aerobic glycolysis, increased fumarate and HIF1A

Source: WHO Classification 2016, adapted from Inamura, 2017.
Abbreviations: CCRCC, clear cell RCC; Chr, chromosome; ChRCC, chromophobe RCC; CIMP, CpG island methylator phenotype; HIF, hypoxia-inducible factor; PRCC, papillary RCC; RCC, renal cell carcinoma; TCGA, The Cancer Genome Atlas; ACD, acquired cystic disease; CCPRCC, clear cell papillary RCC; Chr, chromosome; HLRCC, hereditary leiomyomatosis and RCC; MiT, microphthalmia transcription factor; SDH, succinate dehydrogenase, TRCC, translocation RCC; VHL, von Hippel–Lindau; WHO, World Health Organization.

pancreas, spleen, and abdominal wall. Local vascular invasion is a typical feature of RCC with tumor extension into the renal vein and can progress into the inferior vena cava. Vena caval extension may be longitudinally extensive with associated bland thrombus.

Metastatic spread may occur via lymphatic and hematogenous routes. Early lymphatic spread typically gives rise to loco-regional/retroperitoneal lymphadenopathy and is an adverse prognostic feature.[16] Involvement of more distant nodal groups including mediastinal and peripheral nodes can be seen. Hematogenous spread is frequently encountered resulting in lung, bone, liver, and brain metastases. Lung metastases may present as an incidental finding on a chest X-ray or computed tomography (CT)

TABLE 18.2   Hereditary Renal Cancer Syndromes

Syndrome	Gene	Chromosome	Renal cancer histology	Clinical syndrome
VHL	VHL	3p25	Clear cell	Bilateral, multifocal renal tumors
				Pheochromocytomas, hemangioblastomas, angiomas, islet cell tumors, paragangliomas, endolymphatic sac tumors
HPRC	MET	7q31	Papillary (type I)	Bilateral, multifocal renal tumors
HLRCC	FH	1q42	Papillary (type II)	Skin/uterine leiomyomas
				Solitary RCCs with early metastatic potential
BHD	FLCN	17p11	Chromophobe Oncocytomas	Bilateral, multifocal renal tumors
				Fibrofolliculomas, pulmonary cysts
TSC	TSC	9q34 (TSC1) 16p13 (TSC2)	Clear cell, Angiomyolipomas	Multiple fibromas, hamartomas, skin lesions, epilepsy, developmental delay, astrocytomas
HPPS	SDH		Renal cell	Head and neck paragangliomas, pheochromocytomas
Cowden's syndrome	PTEN		Papillary Chromophobe Clear cell	Intestinal hamartomatous polyps, benign skin tumors, macrocephaly, breast/thyroid/uterine/prostate Ca
Ch3pTA	VHL BAP1 PBRM1 SETD2	3p	Clear cell	Early onset
BAP1CSS	BAP1		Clear cell	Early onset, bilateral

Source: Adapted from Hasumi and Yao, 2018.

or with symptomatic breathlessness, cough, and occasionally hemoptysis. In patients with involvement of the inferior vena cava, pulmonary embolic disease (tumor or bland thrombus) may occur as a presenting feature. Patients with isolated pulmonary metastases are thought to comprise a better prognostic group compared to those with spread to other visceral sites, and such patients may remain asymptomatic for a considerable period of time without treatment. Bone metastases are typically lytic and commonly present with pain or pathological fracture. In contrast to other epithelial malignancies, metastatic spread to other intra-abdominal organs such as the gastrointestinal tract, pancreas, and contralateral adrenal gland is not uncommon. Metastatic involvement of the gastrointestinal tract may present acutely with bleeding, obstruction, or intussusception.

Systemic symptoms are common in patients with locally advanced or metastatic kidney cancer and include fatigue, night sweats, anorexia, weight loss, and fever. Anemia, hypercalcemia, and an elevated lactate dehydrogenase are of adverse prognostic significance.[6]

Paraneoplastic syndromes can be seen even in the absence of metastatic disease related to secreted endocrine factors leading to conditions such as hypercalcemia, polycythemia, and liver dysfunction (Stauffer's syndrome).

Clinical evaluation and staging

As with most cancers, prognosis is clearly related to stage at diagnosis. Small operable tumors are associated with an excellent 5-year survival whereas patients presenting with metastatic disease have a much poorer prognosis. Over the past 40 years, there has been a significant improvement in the 5-year survival rates.

Ultrasound and contrast-enhanced CT of abdomen, pelvis, and chest +/− head are the most commonly used diagnostic imaging modalities and staging tools for renal tumors. Clear-cell RCCs are highly vascular and are typically avidly enhancing following injection of intravenous contrast. Particular attention should be paid to the assessment of direct extension into adjacent organs, enlargement of retroperitoneal lymph nodes, adrenal involvement, invasion of the ipsilateral renal vein (with

or without extension into the inferior vena cava), and the presence or absence of distant metastatic disease. Technetium-99m bone scanning typically underestimates or under-stages bony disease but may be helpful in evaluating individuals with symptomatic bone pain or elevated alkaline phosphatase.[18] Plain films are helpful in evaluation of local bony disease. Magnetic resonance imaging (MRI) is a particularly sensitive modality for evaluating sites of bony metastatic disease in the spine and may also be used as an alternative to CT for local staging. Positron emission tomography (PET) scanning is not in routine diagnostic use.

For patients who are not managed surgically, a core biopsy of primary or metastatic disease is recommended for tissue confirmation of diagnosis and to provide important information about grade and histopathological subtype. In keeping with other solid tumors, RCCs should be staged according to Union for International Cancer Control (UICC) and American Joint Committee on Cancer (AJCC) staging system (Table 18.3).[19]

TABLE 18.3   Kidney Cancer Staging

Renal Tumor (T)

T1	Tumor ≤7 cm in greatest dimension, limited to the kidney
T2	Tumor >7 cm in greatest dimension, limited to the kidney
T3	Tumor extends into major veins or peri-nephric tissues but not into the ipsilateral adrenal gland and not beyond Gerota's fascia
T4	Tumor invades beyond Gerota's fascia (including contiguous extension into the ipsilateral adrenal gland)

Prognostic Stage Groups

Stage	Tumor Size	Regional Nodes	Distant Metastasis
I	T1	−	−
II	T2	−	−
III	T1/T2	+	−
	T3	+/−	−
IV	T4	+/−	−
	Any T	+/−	+

Source: Adapted from Amin et al., 2017.

Localized disease

Surgical management

Patients with localized RCC (T1-T4), who are medically fit, should be considered for open or laparoscopic surgery with curative intent. Radical nephrectomy (RN) involves en-bloc excision of Gerota's fascia and its contents (kidney and ipsilateral adrenal gland). Ipsilateral adrenalectomy in low-stage tumors without involvement on imaging or macroscopic changes is not routine.[20] Where technically possible, nephron-sparing surgery (partial nephrectomy, PN) should be considered for smaller, appropriately positioned tumors. PN is shown to have equivalent outcomes to RN in T1a tumors and selected, more advanced tumors may also be considered, particularly where preservation of renal function is important. Regional lymphadenectomy may be performed at the time of nephrectomy. Positivity rate increases with T stage; a survival benefit has not been conclusively demonstrated, however it may give prognostic information highlighting those at higher risk of relapse.[16,20] A variety of surgical techniques are currently practiced and include anterior transperitoneal, flank, thoracoabdominal, laparoscopic, and robot-assisted approaches with the choice of approach relating to the size and location of the tumor, presence or absence of inferior venal caval invasion, and the body habitus of the patient. Image-guided renal vessel embolization may be performed electively before operative intervention and may help to facilitate surgery by reducing tumor vascularity and minimizing surgical blood loss. In patients with symptomatic primary tumors where surgery is considered inappropriate or where the primary is felt to be inoperable, renal embolization may be used alone as effective palliation.[21] Extensive caval infiltration particularly with supradiaphragmatic extension does not preclude surgical intervention but may require intraoperative cardiopulmonary bypass. Where tumor extends into vena cava, caval removal may be required. These operations can have high morbidity and mortality and careful patient selection must be undertaken.

Thermal ablation

Thermal ablation using microwave ablation/radiofrequency or cryotherapy approaches has become an established treatment for smaller localized, early-stage renal cell cancer, particularly in patients with operable disease who are considered high risk due to significant comorbidity or advancing age or in patients with bilateral disease.[22] A treatment probe is inserted percutaneously into the lesion with imaging guidance following local/general anesthesia. Treatment is generally carried out over one or more sessions. Confirmatory, pre-ablational biopsies should be performed at the same sitting to obtain histological diagnosis, which would not otherwise be available with such an approach. Follow-up CT imaging is standard to ensure satisfactory ablation. Redo ablation in the setting of inadequate treatment or local recurrence may be undertaken.

Surveillance

Active surveillance for small primary tumors, particularly in the elderly, patients with short life expectancy, and individuals with multiple comorbidities is an option.[3]

Disease relapse

Approximately 30% of patients will relapse following radical nephrectomy performed with curative intent. The median time to relapse is between 1 and 2 years although the range may be very wide with some patients relapsing many years after initial surgery. Pulmonary metastatic disease is the most common site of spread, occurring in up to two-thirds of patients.[23]

A number of prognostic scoring systems have been developed and validated for use in assessing risk of progression for patients who have undergone definitive treatment of their primary tumors. These include the University of California, Los Angeles integrated staging system (UISS) which incorporates all pathological sub-types (ECOG Performance Status, Fuhrman grade, TNM stage) and the Mayo Clinic stage, size, grade, and necrosis (SSIGN) score validated for use in clear cell carcinoma.[3] They estimate disease-specific survival and overall survival respectively. A further, large, retrospective multivariate analysis of risk factors for relapse has also been reported by Leibovich et al.[6]

The Leibovich score uses the same five parameters as the SSIGN score, T stage, size, N stage, Fuhrman grade, and tumor necrosis, but scoring is weighted slightly differently. Patients are then placed in three prognostic groups (low, intermediate, and high) predicting risk of relapse following radical nephrectomy (see Table 18.4). Leibovich score has been used as a criterion for entry in a number of adjuvant trials such as SORCE and RAMPART.

Adjuvant treatment

Adjuvant therapy is not yet extensively used following resection of RCC performed with curative intent. To date trials in intermediate- and high-risk RCC post-nephrectomy using VEGF tyrosine kinase inhibitors have failed to show a clear overall survival benefit.

The phase III ASSURE trial included 1943 patients randomized to sunitinib, sorafenib, or placebo. No disease-free (DFS) or overall survival benefit was shown. Toxicity was a significant issue resulting in loss of patients from the active treatment arms, and the need for dose reductions.[24] Another phase III randomized controlled trial PROTECT included 1538 patients randomized to placebo, or pazopanib for 1 year. During the trial the dose of pazopanib was reduced to 600 mg due to toxicity and tolerability issues. No DFS was shown; on sub-group analysis there was DFS

TABLE 18.4   Leibovich Scoring System

Tumor Stage	Score	Risk Group	Overall Score	Estimated Metastasis Free Survival at 5 years
pT1a	0	Low	0–2	97%
pT1b	2			
pT2	3			
pT3–4	4			
Nodal Stage				
pNx/pN0	0	Intermediate	3–5	74%
pN1/pN2	2			
Dimension				
<10 cm	0			
>10 cm	1			
Fuhrman Nuclear Grade				
1–2	0	High	>=6	31%
3	1			
4	3			
Tumor Necrosis				
Absent	0			
Present	1			

Source: Data from Leibovich et al., 2003.

benefit in those started on 800 mg HR of 0.69 (95% CI 0.51–0.94), but the trial was not powered to confirm this.[25] The STRAC Trial randomized high-risk patients to sunitinib or placebo for up to 1 year. Median DFS was 6.8 years in the sunitinib arm, and 5.6 years in the placebo arm with HR 0.76 (95%CI 0.59–0.98). As in the other trials toxicity was an issue with 60% of patients in the sunitinib arm suffering grade 3 or 4 adverse events.[26] To date sunitinib has been approved for adjuvant use in the USA but not in Europe. Trials of other oral targeted agents are yet to report and include EVEREST (everolimus), and axitinib (ATLAS).

Carbonic anhydrase IX is a transmembrane protein expressed in most RCCs, and is upregulated in hypoxic conditions. Girentuximab, a carbonic anhydrase IX antibody, was given adjuvantly within the ARISER trial. No DFS or OS benefit was shown. An unplanned analysis of those with high CAIX expression demonstrated a DFS benefit.[27]

With increasing evidence for immunotherapy drugs in the advanced RCC setting there are a number of trials ongoing. Earlier adjuvant trials of IL-2 and interferon gamma did not show benefit. A 2004 study using autologous tumor cell vaccines in 379 patients showed a PFS benefit of 10% at 5 years;[28] however this has not been expanded into clinical practice. Nivolumab (PROSPER), atezolizumab (IMMoTION), pembrolizumab (KEYNOTE), ipilimumab with nivolumab (CheckMate 214), and durvalumab monotherapy/combination with tremelimumab (RAMPART) are actively recruiting or in follow-up; additional trials and more information can be seen in Table 18.5.

Metastatic disease—surgical management

Cytoreductive nephrectomy

Historically surgical removal of the involved kidney (cytoreductive nephrectomy) in patients presenting with metastatic RCC was undertaken for palliation of symptomatic primary tumors. Occasionally metastatic disease can be seen to regress spontaneously. What is not clear is whether removal of the primary tumor is beneficial to survival. Trials in the early immunotherapy era with interferon gamma did demonstrate some benefit. A combined analysis of two trials of nephrectomy prior to interferon gamma in highly selected fit patients demonstrated a weighted mean difference in median survival of 4.8 months (12.6 versus 7.8 months) in favor of the surgical arm.[29]

On the basis of these trials, cytoreductive nephrectomy became a standard of care in appropriately selected patients. With the development of active targeted agents for RCC the benefit of CN in addition to systemic therapy was questioned. CN is not without complications, and can lead to a prolonged recovery, meaning that some patients do not subsequently receive effective systemic treatments.

The CARMENA trial enrolled 450 patients of a planned 576, with intermediate- or poor-risk disease. Patients were randomized to CN followed by sunitinib, or primary sunitinib. The trial met its end point demonstrating non-inferiority of sunitinib alone, median OS 18.4 months sunitinib (95%CI 11.8–18.3) versus 13.9 months (95%CI 14.7–23) surgery.[30] It should be noted the trial group had a high median metastatic tumor burden, and the OS was relatively short compared to other trials with similar cohorts, raising the possibility that lower volume fitter patients were not placed in the trial, intimating selection bias. A second trial SURTIME was shut due to poor accrual at 99 patients who were randomized to initial versus deferred nephrectomy. There was a trend to longer OS with deferred nephrectomy but the trial was underpowered.[31]

Cytoreductive nephrectomy remains an option for selected patients with good prognostic disease, low tumor burden, and adequate fitness. Some patients may benefit from a period of systemic therapy first. For patients who do not immediately need therapy, for example in the presence of a solitary metastasis, surgery remains gold standard.

Resection of loco-regionally recurrent or metastatic disease

Patients with kidney cancer may present or relapse with macroscopically isolated, resectable loco-regional, or oligometastatic disease. Metastectomy has an established role, particularly in patients who have experienced long treatment-free intervals. Ultimately virtually all patients will relapse. Immunotherapy trials in resected stage IV disease may change the landscape in future.

Recurrent renal fossa disease can be managed by resection or ablation in appropriately selected patients but randomized evidence is lacking. Following radical nephrectomy in a large retrospective RCC cohort, local recurrence was uncommon with 54 cases in 2945 patients.[32]

Resection of pulmonary metastatic disease is also widely practiced. A 2016 meta-analysis included 16 retrospective cohort studies with 5-year OS estimated at 43%; poor prognostic factors identified included lymph node positivity of the primary RCC, lymph node involvement of the metastases, incomplete resection, larger or multiple metastases, synchronous metastases, and a short disease-free interval.[33]

Pancreatic metastases may indicate a more indolent course of disease. Surgery for isolated pancreatic lesions can be performed. Even in those with multiple disease sites those with co-existing pancreatic metastases are seen to do better.[34] Careful consideration prior to surgery is required given the risks and long-term side effects of extensive pancreatic surgery.

Isolated or threatening bone disease is a particular management problem; where appropriate and technically feasible, aggressive surgical intervention is warranted. In the presence of long bone metastases regular surveillance with plain X-ray, in addition to routine staging, is recommended with a low threshold for additional MRI scanning where appropriate. In malignant cord compression, randomized evidence suggests that early surgical intervention followed by radiotherapy is superior to radiotherapy alone, and in a less radiosensitive tumor such as renal cell cancer, this may be particularly true.[35]

Brain metastases convey a poor prognosis. Surgical resection of brain oligometastatic disease may be considered for fit patients whose disease is technically resectable and where disease elsewhere is amenable to treatment. Stereotactic radiotherapy techniques may remove the need for invasive surgery in visceral and non-visceral sites (see "Radiotherapy" section).

Careful patient selection is key to identifying appropriate cases to manage with local therapies or surgery, and should be done in conjunction with an experienced multidisciplinary team. A number of factors need to be taken in to account including synchronicity, number of sites, location, fitness, and tumor biology.

Metastatic disease—prognostic factors

Prognostic factors

RCC can behave in a biologically diverse fashion with survival for patients with metastatic disease ranging from a few weeks to many years or even decades. A number of prognostic factors have

TABLE 18.5   Clinical Trials of RCC

	NCT Number/Study Name	Agents	Comparator	Histology	Phase	Primary Endpoint	Treatment Line	Trial Status
Adjuvant/ neoadjuvant	NCT02575222	Nivolumab	-	ccRCC	I	Safety	Neo-adjuvant	Active not recruiting
	NCT01575548	Pazopanib	Placebo	ccRCC	III	DFS	Resected stage IV	Active not recruiting
	NCT03055013	Nivolumab	Observation	ccRCC	III	DFS	Adjuvant	Recruiting
	NCT03138512/CheckMate 914	Nivolumab + ipilimumab	Placebo	ccRCC	III	DFS	Adjuvant	Recruiting
	NCT03142334/Keynote-564	Pembrolizumab	Placebo	ccRCC	III	DFS	Adjuvant inc resected IV	Recruiting
	NCT03024996/IMmotion010	Atezolizumab	Placebo	ccRCC	III	DFS	Adjuvant	Active, not recruiting
	NCT03138512/RAMPART	Durvalumab/durvalumab + tremelimumab	Placebo	Cc/nccTCC	III	DFS, OS	Adjuvant	Recruiting
First line/all lines	NCT03260894	Pembrolizumab + epacadostat	Sunitinib/pazopanib	ccRCC	III	ORR	First line	Active not recruiting
	NCT02446860/ADAPTeR	Nivolumab	-	ccRCC	II	Safety	Pre- and post-operative Stage IV	Recruiting
	NCT02917772/TITAN RCC	Nivolumab +/- nivolumab + ipilimumab dependent on response		ccRCC	II	ORR	First or second line	Recruiting
	NCT03793166/PDIGREE	Nivolumab + ipilimumab	Nivolumab + cabozantinib	ccRCC	III	OS	First line	Recruiting
	NCT02960906/BIONIKK	Nivolumab/nivolumab + ipilimumab/ sunitinib	Treatment arm dependent on molecular stratification	ccRCC	II	ORR	First line	Recruiting
	NCT02811861/CLEAR	Lenvatinib + everolimus/ pembrolizumab	Sunitinib	ccRCC	III	PFS	First line	Recruiting
	NCT03141177/CheckMate 9ER	Nivolumab + cabozantinib	Sunitinib	ccRCC	III	PFS	First line	Recruiting
	NCT03172754	Nivolumab + axitinib		ccRCC	I/II	Safety/ORR	At least second line/first line	Recruiting
	NCT02348008	Pembrolizumab + bevacizumab		ccRCC	I/II	Safe dose, RR	I-at least second line/II-first line	Active not recruiting
	NCT02853344/Keynote-427	Pembrolizumab	-	cc/nccRCC	II	ORR	All lines	Active not recruiting
	NCT02964078	Pembrolizumab + interleukin-2	-	ccRCC	II	ORR	All lines	Active not recruiting
	NCT03200587	Avelumab + cabozantinib		ccRCC	Ib	Safe dose	All lines	Recruiting
	NCT02501096	Pembrolizumab + lenvatinib		ccRCC	I/II	DLT, ORR	All lines	Recruiting
Second/third line	NCT02989714	Nivolumab + interleukin-2	-	ccRCC	I/II	Safety/ORR	Up to two prior lines (VEGF/ mTOR)	Active, not recruiting
	NCT03308396	Durvalumab + guadecitabine	-	ccRCC	I/II	DLT/ORR	At least second line	Recruiting
	NCT03428217/CANTATA	Cabozantinib + CB839	Cabozantinib	ccRCC	II	PFS	At least second line	Recruiting
	NCT03066427/INMUNOSUN	Sunitinib	-	ccRCC	II	ORR	Second line post antiPD1/CTLA4 Ab's	Recruiting
	NCT02819596/Calypso	Durvalumab /tremelimumab/savolitinib combinations dependent on histology/ biomarkers	-	cc/pRCC	II	DLT, OR	At least second line	Recruiting
	NCT03024437	Atezolizumab + bevacizumab + entinostat	-	ccRCC	I/II	Safe dose, ORR	Various dependent on cohort	Recruiting

been identified that currently help to predict response to treatment, stratify patients for clinical trials, and help guide estimation of overall survival.

Clinical prognostic scoring systems

Both the Memorial Sloane–Kettering Cancer Center (MSKCC) and the International Metastatic RCC Database Consortium (IDMC) scoring can be used to help estimate median survival, and group patients into favorable-, intermediate-, and poor-risk groups with regards to prognosis. The MSKCC group identified five independent variables in advanced RCC clinical trial cohorts in 1999; these included low performance status, elevated lactate dehydrogenase, low serum hemoglobin, elevated corrected serum calcium, and absence of prior nephrectomy. This was revised with patient data from further prospective randomized trials in the advent of cytokine treatments (see "Interferon Alpha" section). In this analysis, interval from diagnosis to introduction of IFN-α therapy replaced absence of prior nephrectomy as one of the five risk factors used to create the risk model. Patients classified as favorable risk (zero risk factors) had a median survival of 30 months in comparison to an intermediate-risk group (one or two risk factors) with a survival of 14 months and a poor-risk group (three or more risk factors) whose median survival was poor at 5 months.[36]

The IDMC multivariate analysis published in 2009 involved patients treated with vascular endothelial growth factor (VEGF) targeted therapies (see "Targeted Therapies" section).[37] All pathological subtypes of RCC were included. Six independent adverse prognostic factors were identified and included hemoglobin less than lower limit of normal, raised serum corrected calcium, Karnofsky performance status less than 80%, time from diagnosis to treatment initiation of less than 1 year, raised neutrophil count, and a raised platelet count. Patients without any poor prognostic factors had median OS of 43 months. Intermediate-risk patients (1–2 risk factors) had a median OS of 22.5 months, with a 2-year OS of 53%. Patients with 3–6 risk factors were identified as particularly poor risk with a median OS 7.8 months and 2-year OS of only 7%.

Molecular biomarkers as putative prognostic markers

Increasingly molecular biomarkers are likely to play a role in how patients are stratified for prognostic risk and appropriate treatments selected. The identification of loss of multiple tumor suppressor genes from chromosome 3p and other prevalent mutations in ccRCC has had implications both for the design of new treatments but also for providing information about prognosis. Identifying the molecular profile on an individual level is likely to provide greater information as RCC shows marked interpatient and intratumoral heterogeneity. Targeted sequencing of 341 cancer genes in 258 tumor samples from the RECORD-3 Trial identified the multiple common mutations in tumor suppressor genes including VHL (75%), PBRM1 (46%), SETD2 (30%), BAP1 (19%), KDM5C (15%), PTEN (12%).[39] BAP1 mutations are seen to be associated with higher tumor grade and shorter overall survival; the prognostic role of PBRM1 is less clear but those with PBRM1 mutations are seen to do well on VEGF TKI, MTOR inhibitors, and checkpoint inhibitors. PBRM1 mutant patients had 12.8-month PFS on everolimus first line versus 5.5 months in wild type (WT) patients in RECORD3. BAP1 mutant patients did better with first-line sunitinib (4.9 months everolimus PFS versus 10.5 months). Those with KDM5C mutations demonstrated 20.6 months PFS on sunitinib first line versus 8.3 months with everolimus.[39]

The Memorial Sloane–Kettering Cancer Center and Cancer Genome Atlas Cohort provided outcome data on 609 patients with genetic mutations in these chromosome 3p chromatin regulating genes. Around one-third of patients exhibited PBRM1 mutations which were not seen to impact cancer-specific survival. Approximately 10% had mutations in SETD2, and just under 10% BAP1 mutations. Both were seen to negatively affect cancer-specific survival, BAP1 in both patient cohorts (MSKCC-HR 7.71 95%CI 2.08–28.6, TGCA-HR 2.21 95%CI 1.35–3.63), and SETD2 in the TCGA cohort (HR 1.68 95%CI 1.04–2.73).[40]

With the increasing use of immune checkpoint inhibitors there is interest in immune biomarkers of response. To date PDL1 expression, seen to predict response to anti-PD1 Ab therapies in some cancer types, does not seem to be of use in RCC. Evidence from meta-analyses indicates high expression may be a negative prognostic indicator.[41]

Location of metastases at presentation

The presence of brain metastases at presentation is a poor prognostic factor. Analysis of the SEER and National Cancer Databases in the United States estimated 1.5% of cases presented with brain lesions. Routine imaging of the CNS is not recommended in most guidelines for RCC so the prevalence is likely to have been underestimated as it would not include those with asymptomatic brain metastases. Median OS was 6.4 months in the brain metastasis cohort versus not reached in those without CNS disease at presentation.[42] With the development of new treatments, particularly immunotherapy agents which have shown activity in the melanoma population in the CNS, and the increasing uses of SRS for local control we may see improvements in OS in future.

Bone metastases are also associated with poorer prognosis, although retrospective evidence supports the case that surgical resection may increase survival in those with solitary bone metastases.[43]

Metastatic disease—non-surgical management

Observation

The prognosis and rate of progression of renal cancer can vary widely in patients with metastatic disease. For selected patients, a period of observation before starting chronic long-term therapy may be considered. Patients with low-volume, non-threatening metastatic disease (often lung only) are often considered for this approach and considerable intervals may elapse before any systemic treatment is required. A recent prospective phase II trial looked at active surveillance. Forty-eight asymptomatic patients with low tumor burden were included; all but one were good or intermediate IDMC risk, with prior nephrectomy. Median time to initiation of systemic treatment was 14.9 months (95%CI 10.6–25).[44] The trial did not include an immediate treatment arm for comparison, so whether delayed initiation affects disease outcome is unknown.

Radiotherapy

Although RCCs are classically considered to be a less radiosensitive malignancy when compared to other solid tumors, radiotherapy still plays an important part in the management of local treatment for symptomatic (often bone and brain) metastatic disease. Case series suggest that the vast majority of patients will experience symptomatic benefit from treatment although duration of response varies. Post-surgical radiotherapy is also commonly used to decrease local recurrence/progression rates following orthopedic intervention in the spine or long bones.

Individual cases and case series using stereotactic ablative radiotherapy (SABR) show this to be a promising less invasive option for oligometastatic disease at both bone, soft tissue, and visceral sites in RCC. A phase II trial of patients with oligometastatic RCC is currently recruiting to see if it is able to delay the start of systemic therapy in selected patients. Several trials incorporating SRS and systemic treatment are recruiting (see Table 18.6).

Increasingly stereotactic radiosurgery is being used for brain metastases in multiple cancer types, giving a single fraction of high-dose radiation. It is not suitable for lesions >3 cm, or multiple lesions with a high cumulative volume. It is generally well-tolerated and less invasive than surgery. A Canadian case series reported a 91% control rate for RCC brain metastases at 12 months.[45]

Chemotherapy

Historically, the use of cytotoxic chemotherapy in advanced RCC has proven to be disappointing with low response rates and little impact on survival. Collecting duct and renal medullary carcinomas may respond to platinum-based chemotherapy regimens; extensive trial data are lacking due to the rarity of these subtypes. Overall RCC is considered to be an inherently chemorefractory tumor and chemotherapy is not in routine use.

Bisphosphonates/denosumab

In patients with solid tumors and bony metastatic disease, a number of clinical trials of bisphosphonates or denosumab have been conducted.[46] Subset analysis of patients with metastatic RCC has revealed a reduction in skeletal-related events. These agents represent a treatment option for selected patients. Osteonecrosis of the jaw is a rare but important toxicity of these agents, which may be increased with concurrent use of VEGF-directed therapies.

Immunotherapy

The treatment options for RCC have expanded rapidly since the early 21st century. Up until the early 2000s recombinant cytokine therapies with interferon alpha (IFN-α) and interleukin-2 (IL-2) were in widespread use, exploiting the observation that RCC exhibits variable behavior with some having indolent disease and spontaneous regressions, supporting the theory that host immunity plays an important role. Bio-chemotherapy, adoptive immunotherapy, vaccination, and allogeneic stem cell transplantation were also attempted with limited success.

Cytokine-based treatments were largely superseded following the development of active targeted agents, but the arrival of immune checkpoint inhibitors has again focused interest back on immune modulation as the backbone of treatments for RCC. See Figure 18.2 for first-line treatment timeline.

Interferon alpha

The immunoregulatory cytokine IFN-a became the previous standard of care for the treatment of advanced RCC in the 1990s, although the benefit of treatment for most patients was modest at best.[47] A key randomized phase III study from the Medical Research Council evaluated the use of IFN-α at a dose of 10 million units subcutaneously, 3 times weekly against medroxyprogesterone acetate (MPA) 300 mg orally once daily for 12 weeks in 335 patients with metastatic RCC.[47] The primary endpoint was survival and IFN-α was associated with a 28% reduction in the risk of death (hazard ratio [HR] 0.72 [95% CI 0.55–0.94], p = 0.017). Both median survival (8.5 versus 6 months) and 1-year survival (43% versus 31%) were improved in the IFN-α arm. Response rates were low (14%; CR 2%) with 42% patients achieving stable disease. IFN-α use is associated with significant dose-related toxicity. Patients with conventional (clear-cell) histology appear more likely to respond than patients with other histological subtypes. IFNa as a single agent is now not in routine use.

Interleukin-2

IL-2 is a critical cytokine in the activation of cellular and humoral immune responses. IL-2 induces proliferation of antigen-primed CD4- and CD8-positive T-cells and enhances the cytotoxic activity of NK cells. Approval for the use of IL-2 as treatment for advanced renal cell cancer in the United States was granted following the publication of data collated from a series of seven phase II trials from the National Cancer Institute (NCI). Two hundred and fifty-five highly selected patients were treated with

TABLE 18.6   Clinical Trials of Immunotherapy Drugs in the Advanced RCC Setting

	NCT Number/ Study Name	Agents	Comparator	Histology	Phase	Primary Endpoint	Treatment Line	Trial Status
Non-clear cell histology	NCT03177239/ ANZUP1602 UNISON	Nivolumab + ipilimumab	Sequencing dependent on response	nccRCC	II	ORR	All lines	Recruiting
	NCT03075423/ SUNIFORECAST	Nivolumab + ipilimumab	Sunitinib	nccRCC	II	OS	First line	Recruiting
	NCT03091192	Savolitinib	Sunitinib	pRCC(METmt)	II	Safety and PFS	Any line (not sutent.METi)	Active, not recruiting
	NCT02724878	Atezolizumab + bevacizumab		nccRCC	II	ORR	All lines	Recruiting
	NCT03635892	Nivolumab + cabozantinib		nccRCC	II	ORR	All lines	Recruiting
	NCT03595124	Nivolumab Nivolumab + axitinib Axitininb		TFE/tRCC	II	Clinical activity	All lines	Recruiting
SRS combinations	NCT03065179/ RADVAX	Nivolumab + ipilimumab + SBRT	-	ccRCC	II	ORR	All lines	Recruiting
	NCT02019576	Sunitinib + SRS		ccRCC	II	LCR	First line	Recruiting
	NCT03469713/ NIVES	Nivolumab + SBRT	-	ccRCC	II	ORR	At least second line	Recruiting

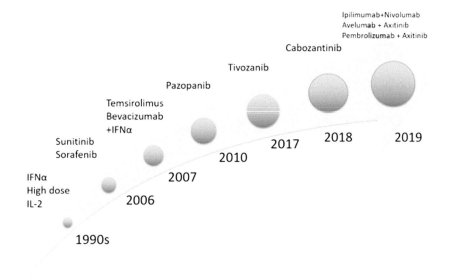

FIGURE 18.2 Treatment timeline for first-line advanced RCC.

high-dose IL-2 (600,000 or 720,000 IU/kg intravenously every 8 hours over 5 days) repeated after 5–9 days of rest. Courses were repeated every 6–12 weeks in stable or responding patients.[48]

Objective responses were seen in 15%, with 7% complete responses and 8% partial responses. Median survival time was 16.3 months. Despite the highly selected cohort of patients, treatment was associated with significant acute toxicity. Severe vascular leak syndrome predominated, leading to peripheral and pulmonary edema, hypotension, oliguria, and multiorgan failure. For many clinicians, the toxicity, potential morbidity, and mortality of high-dose IL-2 was seen as unacceptable, but for some it offers the potential of prolonged post-treatment remission.[48] Patient selection is able to increase observed responses. [49]

Immune checkpoint inhibitors

Immune checkpoint inhibitors are a form of immunotherapy that target mechanisms developed by tumor cells to evade immune destruction. Nivolumab is a human monoclonal antibody against the programmed death receptor 1 (PD1). PD1 is an immuno-regulatory receptor expressed on activated T-cells. Nivolumab acts to block T-cell inactivation seen following PD1 ligand (PDL1 and 2) binding and allows the immune system to mount an anti-tumor response. CTLA4 is another immunoregulatory receptor expressed on activated T-cells. The interaction of the CTLA4 with CD80/86 results in T-cell inactivation. Ipilimumab is a monoclo-nal antibody which acts to block this interaction.

The CheckMate 025 study was a pivotal phase III RCT compar-ing the use of nivolumab and everolimus in 821 patients with pre-viously treated (one or two lines of antiangiogenic therapy) renal cell cancer. The objective response rate was 25% for nivolumab compared to 5% for everolimus, with an odds ratio of 5.98 (95% CI 3.68–9.72); $p = < 0.001$. Median overall survival was 25 months (95% CI 21.8–not estimable) in the nivolumab group compared to 19.6 months (95% CI 17.6–23.1 months) in the everolimus group, with a hazard ratio for death of 0.73 (0.57–0.93, $p = 0.002$).[50] In 2016, following the publication of these data, NICE recom-mended the use of nivolumab in the setting of previously treated advanced RCC in the UK.

The combination of ipilimumab (1 mg/kg) and nivolumab (3 mg/kg) has shown to be effective in metastatic melanoma. The CheckMate 214 study was a large phase III RCT which com-pared the use of ipilimumab/nivolumab combination treatment to sunitinib in 1096 patients with previously untreated advanced clear-cell RCC. Median follow-up was 25.2 months in the inter-mediate-/poor-risk population. In this population median overall survival was not reached in the ipilimumab/nivolumab group and was 26 months in the sunitinib group, with a hazard for death of 0.63 (95%CI 0.44–0.89; $p < 0.001$). Progression-free survival was 11.6 months and 8.4 months for each respective group, with a haz-ard ratio for progression/death of 0.82, though this did not meet the pre-specified level of significance. The objective response rate was 42% with the combination treatment compared to 27% with sunitinib ($p < 0.001$). In the favorable-risk population sunitinib was superior to the combination treatment for both progression-free survival (HR 2.18, 99.1%CI 1.29–3.68, $p < 0.001$) and objec-tive response-rate (29% versus 52%, $p < 0.001$).[51]

Drug-related adverse events with ipilimumab and nivolumab are typically immune-related and include colitis, vitiligo, hepati-tis, hypophysitis, thyroiditis, pneumonitis, and nephritis. As use of these drugs increases, real-world data regarding toxicity are beginning to emerge. Within CheckMate 214 immune-mediate adverse events occurred in 80% of patients on the combination treatment, with 35% requiring high-dose steroids to manage these events and a discontinuation rate of 22%.[51]

Based on the results of CheckMate 214 the combination of ipi-limumab and nivolumab is now being used as first-line treatment for intermediate- and poor-risk patients with advanced clear-cell RCC. CheckMate 214 did not contain a nivolumab-only arm, and as part of its recommendation the EMA have mandated that a randomized trial is set up to evaluate whether the effectiveness of combination ipilimumab/nivolumab justifies the additional tox-icity of ipilimumab compared to nivolumab alone.

Targeted therapies

The development of targeted treatment options revolutionized the outlook and treatment approach for patients with locally advanced and metastatic renal cancer.

Therapeutic rationale

As outlined in the section "Clear Cell (Conventional) Renal Cell Carcinoma," loss of function of the *VHL* gene represents a key genetic event in both hereditary and sporadic clear-cell RCC.[7,8,9,14] This tumor suppressor gene located on chromosome 3p25 encodes a 213 amino acid protein (pVHL) that forms part of a larger ubiquitin ligase complex that is critically involved in the degradation of hypoxia-inducible factor (HIF), a protein transcription factor. HIF induces transcription of a variety of genes that allow cells to grow and survive in hypoxic conditions. In hypoxic conditions or in the presence of VHL mutation, HIF escapes degradation by VHL and remains constitutively active, leading to increased transcription of a number of genes important for angiogenesis (VEGF, platelet-derived growth factor [PDGF]), cellular growth and proliferation (transforming growth factor alpha and beta [TGF-a/-b]), glucose uptake (glut1), and acid–base balance (carbonic anhydrase IX [CAIX]), amongst others.[11,14]

Additional genes have now been implicated, both ubiquitous and sub-clonal, many of them located on chromosome 3.[8,9,14] The m-TOR pathway also drives cancer progression in some RCC cases.[10,11]

Knowledge of the underlying biology of hereditary and sporadic clear-cell RCC and the key role played by VHL and VEGF was a landmark discovery in the understanding of RCC and has resulted in a step change in the development of treatments for patients with advanced disease.

Vascular endothelial growth factor inhibition

Seven agents targeting the VEGF receptor pathway are now licensed and in routine use for the treatment of advanced kidney cancer. Six licensed agents—sunitinib, pazopanib, axitinib, sorafenib, tivozanib, and cabozantinib—are multi-targeted tyrosine kinase inhibitors targeting VEGFR function and other related receptor signaling. The seventh licensed agent, bevacizumab, is a monoclonal antibody that is able to bind and neutralize circulating VEGF ligand.

Sunitinib

Sunitinib is an orally active multi-targeted receptor tyrosine kinase inhibitor (rTKI) with activity against VEGFR, PDGFR, KIT, RET, CSF-1R, and flt3. In a landmark, randomized, phase III trial, sunitinib was compared to standard IFN-a in 750 untreated patients with metastatic clear-cell RCC.[53,54] Sunitinib 50 mg p.o. was given in 6-weekly cycles on a 4 weeks on, 2 weeks off schedule with IFN-a given subcutaneously, at a standard dose of 9 MU 3 times weekly until progression or unacceptable toxicity. Sunitinib was associated with a dramatically improved median PFS (11 months versus 5 months; $p = 0.001$) and response rate (47% versus 12%; $p = 0.001$). Following cessation of trial medication, the majority of patients in the interferon arm crossed over to second-line VEGFR-directed therapy, confounding median OS results (median OS 26.4 versus 21.8 months; HR 0.82, 95% CI 0.67–1.0; $p = 0.051$). Despite this, OS outcomes vastly exceeded previous results seen in historical IFNa studies with a doubling of median survival in the sunitinib arm.

Key sunitinib toxicities included hypertension, fatigue, diarrhea, hand–foot sensitivity, stomatitis, and skin color changes. Mild pancytopenia is common but rarely dose-limiting. Post-marketing surveillance and expanded access programs have also revealed drug-induced hypothyroidism to be common, and routine monitoring of thyroid function and supplementation when required while on treatment with sunitinib (and related agents) are recommended.

The effectiveness and chronic dosing schedule of sunitinib and other targeted therapies mean that supportive therapies and pro-active management of treatment-related toxicity are of great importance, not only in reducing side-effect severity and duration but in maintaining dose intensity and the best possible outcome for patients.[55,56] Intriguingly, a number of subsequent analyses of sunitinib and other VEGF-directed treatment toxicities suggest that the development of treatment-induced side effects such as hypertension may act as biological surrogate markers of efficacy.[57]

Pazopanib

Pazopanib (Votrient) is another orally active rTKI with activity against VEGFR, PDGFR, and C-KIT.

A phase III trial evaluating pazopanib 800 mg p.o. daily continuously against placebo was evaluated in 453 treatment-naïve (54%) and cytokine pre-treated (46%) patients with metastatic clear-cell RCC in a 2:1 randomization.[58]

Median PFS was superior in the pazopanib arm in all patient groups (overall 9.2 versus 4.2 months; HR 0.46, 95% CI 0.34–0.62; $p = 0.0001$; treatment-naïve subjects 11.1 versus 2.8 months, second line 7.4 versus 4.2 months). There was no significant difference in median OS (22.9 months versus 20.5 months, $p = 0.224$), which was again confounded by cross-over to pazopanib treatment.[58] Overall response rates were 30% versus 3%. Common adverse events were similar to that seen with sunitinib and other VEGF rTKIs, although hair color depigmentation is much more commonly seen with pazopanib. In contrast with sunitinib, elevations in liver transaminases occur more frequently and require routine liver function test monitoring, particularly within the first 3 months of therapy.

Sunitinib versus pazopanib

Two trials have compared sunitinib and pazopanib as a first-line treatment for metastatic RCC in a head-to-head randomization.

The COMPARZ trial evaluated treatment in 1110 treatment-naïve patients with advanced clear-cell RCC. The study was designed to demonstrate non-inferiority of pazopanib with PFS as a primary endpoint.[59] Pazopanib was found to be non-inferior to sunitinib (PFS 8.4 months versus 9.5 months; HR 1.047, 95% CI 0.898–1.22). Disease control rates were similar in both arms at 70% and 69%, respectively. Liver function test abnormalities, weight loss, and hair depigmentation were more commonly seen in patients on pazopanib while those on sunitinib experienced more fatigue, hand–foot syndrome, mucositis, and myelosuppression.

The PISCES trial was a double-blind, patient and clinician preference cross-over trial.[60] All patients received 22 weeks of treatment with pazopanib given continuously for 10 weeks followed by a 2-week washout followed by sunitinib on a 4-week on 2-week off schedule for a further 10 weeks or the reverse. Both patients and clinicians were then asked which drug they preferred, and continued their drug of choice. Seventy percent of patients and 61% of clinicians preferred pazopanib over sunitinib with 22% of both patients and clinicians preferring sunitinib. Overall quality of life, fatigue, and gastrointestinal toxicities were the predominant reasons given for treatment preference.

Axitinib

Axitinib (Inlyta) is a potent oral selective inhibitor of VEGFR1-3 with phase III data supporting its use as a second-line treatment option.[61] The AXIS study compared axitinib to sorafenib in a randomized open label phase III trial in 723 patients with advanced clear-cell RCC. First-line treatments included sunitinib (54%), cytokines alone (35%), bevacizumab/IFNa (8%), and temsirolimus (3%).

Median PFS was 6.7 months versus 4.7 months with sorafenib (HR 0.665, 95% CI 0.544–0.822, p = 0.0001). Objective response rates were 19% with axitinib and 9% sorafenib (p = 0.0001). Median OS was 20.1 months (95% CI 16.7–23.4) with axitinib and 19.2 months (17.5–22.3) with sorafenib (HR 0.969, 95% CI 0.800–1.174; one-sided p = 0.3744). On subgroup analysis, those treated with cytokines first line gained most benefit (median PFS 12.1 versus 6.5 months); PFS was still improved for those with prior sunitinib treatment (4.8 months versus 3.4 months; HR 0.741, 95% CI 0.573–0.958; p = 0.0107). In keeping with other VEGFR TKIs, side effects of axitinib that should be pro-actively managed include diarrhea, nausea, hypertension (a potential biological marker of efficacy), and fatigue. In contrast to other rTKIs, reversible dysphonia is not uncommon.[56]

Sorafenib

Sorafenib (Nexavar) is a multi-targeted rTKI with activity against BRAF, KIT, flt-3, RET, VEGRF-1-3, and PDGFR-ß. It was one of the earliest rTKIs to be evaluated in a phase III setting in 903 patients with advanced RCC following cytokine failure.[62] Disease control rates were high (80%), although only 2% of patients achieved a partial response. Median PFS was low in comparison to other first-line VEGF targeted agents at 5.5 months in the sorafenib arm versus 2.8 months for placebo (HR 0.44, 95% CI 0.35–0.55; p = 0.000001). On the basis of interim results, the protocol was amended to allow cross-over, confounding overall survival results (17.8 versus 15.2 months; HR 0.88; p = 0.146). A disappointing first-line phase II trial evaluating sorafenib against standard-dose IFNa coupled with higher response rates and longer PFS figures seen for other targeted treatments has meant that sorafenib is now a less commonly used first-line agent.[63]

Cabozantinib

Cabozantinib is a multi-kinase inhibitor with activity against VEGF, MET, and AXL. It is now approved for use in both untreated and previously treated advanced RCC.

METEOR was a phase III RCT that compared the use of cabozantinib with everolimus in 658 patients with previously treated advanced RCC. In an intention-to-treat population overall survival improved with cabozantinib compared with everolimus (21.4 versus 16.5 months; hazard ratio 0.66; 95% CI 0.53 to 0.83; p = 0.00026). Median progression-free survival also improved with cabozantinib (7.4 versus 3.9 months, hazard ratio 0.51, p < 0.001). The objective response rate was 17% (95% CI 13–22) for cabozantinib versus 3% (95% CI 2–6) for everolimus with p < 0.0001. The results of METEOR led to the recommendation of cabozantinib as an option for those with previously treated RCC.[64]

CABSOSUN was a phase II trial that then compared cabozantinib with sunitinib in 157 patients with treatment-naïve intermediate- or poor-risk advanced RCC. Median progression-free survival was 8.6 months for cabozantinib compared to 5.3 months with sunitinib, with a hazard ratio of 0.66 (95%CI 0.46–0.95, p = 0.012). The overall response rate was 33% (95% CI 23–44%) for cabozantinib and 12% (95% CI 5.4–21%) for sunitinib. Levels of grade 3 or 4 toxicity were 67% for cabozantinib and 68% for sunitinib. Diarrhea, fatigue, hypertension, and palmar-plantar erythrodysesthesia were some of the most commonly noted events. Hematologic adverse events were more common with sunitinib (22% versus 3%). It was noted that the benefit of cabozantinib

was larger in MET-positive patients compared to MET-negative patients (hazard ratios 0.32 versus 0.67). There was a high proportion of patients within the trial who had bone metastases, which is a known negative prognostic factor for advanced RCC. However, subgroup analyses of the results showed the improvement in PFS was similar for patients with and without bone metastases.[65] Based on the CABOSUN results cabozantinib began to be used as a first-line treatment for advanced RCC. With the advent of combination nivolumab and ipilimumab as first-line treatment in intermediate- and poor-risk patients it is likely to be used more frequently in second-line treatment.

Tivozanib

Tivozanib is a novel and highly selective VEGF1-3 receptor oral TKI. In a phase III study of 517 patients with advanced clear-cell RCC, tivozanib was compared to sorafenib. Seventy percent of patients were treatment-naïve with 30% of patients having received prior cytokine therapy. Despite better than expected results for sorafenib, median PFS and response rates were superior for tivozanib (11.9 months versus 9.1 months; HR 0.797; p = 0.042 with response rates of 33% versus 23%; p = 0.014). Long-term follow-up data failed to demonstrate any survival benefit for tivozanib over sorafenib median OS 28.8 months (95% CI 22.5–NA) versus 29.3 months (95% CI 29.3–NA; p = 0.105) with results confounded by unbalanced cross-over following failure of first-line treatment. Only 10% of patients in the tivozanib arm received subsequent anti-VEGF treatments (with only 36% receiving any further treatment lines at all), compared to 70% in the sorafenib arm.[66] The high selectivity of tivozanib for the VEGFR was characterized by lower rates of certain off-target AEs and fewer dose adjustments, so it remains a valid option for selected patients.

Bevacizumab

In contrast to the oral TKIs, bevacizumab is an intravenously delivered, recombinant, humanized monoclonal antibody that selectively targets circulating VEGF ligand. Following demonstration of single-agent activity in cytokine refractory disease, two phase III trials have evaluated its efficacy in combination with IFNa in the first-line treatment of advanced clear-cell RCC.[67–68]

Both trials evaluated IFNa given at a standard dose of 9MU s/c three times weekly plus bevacizumab 10 mg/kg every 2 weeks intravenously or placebo. The addition of bevacizumab in the AVOREN trial resulted in a marked improvement in median PFS (10.2 months versus 5.4 months; HR 0.63, 95% CI 0.55–0.75; p = 0.0001) and response rate (31% versus 12%; p = 0.0010). Median OS was not significantly different between the two arms but was again confounded by cross-over (23.3 months versus 21.3 months; HR 0.91; 95% CI 0.76–1.10; p = 0.34). In an exploratory analysis, patients who received post-protocol therapy that included a TKI had significantly longer median OS (38.6 months versus 33.6 months; HR = 0.80; 95% CI 0.56–1.13).[67]

In the CALGB study improved median PFS and response rates were seen in the combination arm of 8.5 months (95% CI 7.5–9.7) versus 5.2 months (95% CI 3.1–5.6, p = 0.0001), and 25.5% versus 13.1%, respectively (p = 0.0001).[68] Side effects from IFNa monotherapy were predictable in both studies. The addition of bevacizumab added relatively little toxicity to IFNa although hypertension and proteinuria are recognized toxicities.

Mammalian target of rapamycin (mTOR) inhibition

mTOR signaling has been identified as a potential driver of malignancy in a variety of different tumor types, including RCC.[10,11]

mTOR is an intracellular protein kinase downstream of AKT within the PI3K-AKT signaling pathway with a key role in the regulation of cell growth, proliferation, and survival. Two mTOR inhibitors, temsirolimus and everolimus, are currently licensed for use in the treatment of advanced RCC.

Temsirolimus

The mTOR inhibitor temsirolimus was evaluated against standard IFNa or combination treatment in a phase III trial in patients with advanced RCC.[70] In contrast to other phase III clinical trials that have evaluated treatment in patients with predominantly good or intermediate prognosis risk factors and exclusively clear-cell histology, the Global ARCC trial included patients with both clear and non-clear-cell histology (80%/20% of patients, respectively) and poor-risk disease: All patients had three or more poor prognostic features (elevated serum LDH, low hemoglobin, high corrected serum calcium, time from initial diagnosis to randomization of less than 1 year, Karnofsky performance score 60–70, or metastases in multiple organs).

Six hundred and twenty-six patients were randomized to receive IFNa dosed at 3–18 MU s/c three times per week, temsirolimus 25 mg weekly intravenously, or IFN and temsirolimus at reduced dose in combination. There was no significant difference in objective response rates between arms (4.8%, 8.6%, 8.1%), but PFS and OS data favored single-agent temsirolimus with a median OS of 10.9 months (95% CI: 8.6–12.7, HR 0.73 [0.58–0.92]; $p = 0.0078$) for single-agent treatment compared to 7.3 months for IFNa alone (95% CI: 6.1–8.8). Increased toxicity was seen in the combination arm with no improvement in efficacy. Side effects of temsirolimus included stomatitis, rash, peripheral edema, mild myelosuppression, hyperglycemia, and hyperlipidemia with pneumonitis being recognized as a rare but potentially important treatment-related adverse event. Single-agent temsirolimus is a first-line treatment option with phase III evidence to support its use in poor prognosis and non-clear-cell RCC.

Everolimus

Everolimus, an orally active mTOR inhibitor, was initially evaluated as a treatment option for patients failing prior VEGF-directed or cytokine treatment. There were 416 patients enrolled in the phase III RECORD-1 study comparing everolimus or placebo.[72] Median PFS was 4.9 months on everolimus versus 1.9 months for placebo (HR 0.33, $p = 0.001$) and on the basis of a pre-planned interim PFS analysis, the trial was stopped early and patients on placebo were offered active drug. OS data were confounded by cross-over at 14.8 months versus 14.4 months, respectively (HR 0.87, 95% CI 0.65–1.17). Treatment effects were predominantly disease-stabilizing with only 1% of patients achieving a partial response. Of the patients, 63% on everolimus had stable disease compared to 32% for placebo. Grade 3 and 4 toxicities were low with a pattern similar to that seen with temsirolimus. On the basis of this study, everolimus became a treatment option for patients progressing through VEGF-directed therapy.

In common with other targeted agents, proactive management of treatment-related toxicities is key. This is particularly true for patients receiving second-line treatment where previous exposure to side effects from first-line therapy may be an issue alongside greater disease burden and deteriorating fitness.

The HOPE 205 trial was a randomized phase II multicenter trial that compared the use of single-agent everolimus (10 mg), single-agent lenvatinib (24 mg, multi-receptor targeted TKI), or the combination of everolimus (5 mg) plus lenvatinib (18 mg) in 153 patients with advanced clear-cell RCC which had progressed on first-line VEGF-targeted TKI. The combination treatment significantly prolonged median PFS (14.6 months, 95% CI 5.9–20.1) compared to everolimus alone (5.5 months, 95% CI 3.5–7.1), with a HR of 0.4 (95% CI 0.24–0.68, $p = 0.0005$), but not compared to lenvatinib alone, which had a median PFS of 7.4 months (95% CI 5.6–10.2) with a HR of 0.66 (95%CI 0.39–1.1, $p = 0.12$).[73] The level of grade 3 or 4 toxicity was higher with single-agent lenvatinib (79%) than combination treatment (71%) or single-agent everolimus (50%).[73] Based on these results the combination of everolimus and lenvatinib has now been approved by both the EMA and FDA. Due to the size of the trial, the combination is generally recommended when either nivolumab or cabozantinib cannot be used.[3]

VEGF-targeted agents with checkpoint inhibitors

Recent studies have shown that anti-angiogenic VEGF-targeted agents can mediate an anti-tumor immune response and thereby work synergistically with immunotherapy. They have been shown to increase the sensitivity of tumor cells to T-cell mediated lysis, to increase the production and infiltration of T-cells into the tumor microenvironment, and to reduce the function of immune suppressor cells.[74]

Several groups published their initial results in 2019, with further to follow with trials ongoing.[69,75,76] The IMMOTION-151 trial is a phase III RCT comparing the use of bevacizumab plus atezolizumab (anti-PDL1) with sunitinib as first-line treatment in 915 patients with metastatic RCC. Forty percent of patients had PDL1-positive disease, and in this population the median PFS (median follow-up 15 months) was 11.2 months in the combination group and 7.7 months in the sunitinib group, with a HR of 0.74 (95%CI 0.57–0.96, $p = 0.0217$). With a median follow-up of 24 months, overall survival had HR of 0.93 and did not cross the significance boundary. Further follow-up is needed to determine whether a better survival advantage will develop. Levels of grade 3 or higher toxicity were 40% in the combination group and 54% in the sunitinib group.[69]

The phase III KEYNOTE-426 trial compared the use of the combination of pembrolizumab (anti-PD1) and axitinib with sunitinib in 861 patients with previously untreated advanced clear-cell RCC. The 12-month overall survival rate was 89.9% with the combination treatment compared to 78.3% with sunitinib, with a HR of 0.53 (95% CI 0.38–0.74, $p < 0.0001$). The overall response rate was 59.3% (95% CI 54.5–63.9%) versus 35.7% (95% CI 31.1–40.4%, $p < 0.001$). Median progression-free survival was 15.1 months in the combination group compared to 11.1 months in the sunitinib group with a hazard ratio of 0.69 (95% CI 0.57–0.84, $p < 0.001$). The benefit was seen across all prognostic groups. The level of grade 3 or higher toxicity was 75.8% in the combination group and 70.6% in the sunitinib group.[75] Following the KEYNOTE-426 results the pembrolizumab–axitinib combination was approved for use by the FDA in April 2019 for the first-line treatment of advanced RCC.

The JAVELIN Renal 101 is another recently published phase III RCT that compared the use of avelumab (anti-PDL1) plus axitnib with sunitinib in 886 patients with previously untreated advanced RCC. Median PFS in the overall population was 13.8 months for the combination treatment compared with 8.4 months for the sunitinib group, with a HR for disease progression or death of 0.69 (95% CI 0.56–0.84, $p < 0.001$). In those with PDL1-postive tumors median PFS was 13.8 months compared to 7.2 months with a HR of 0.61 (95% CI 0.47–0.79, $p < 0.001$). Levels of grade 3 or higher toxicity were similar to those in KEYNOTE-426, at 71.2% in the combination group and 71.5% in the sunitinib group.[76]

Results from both these trials confirm the effectiveness of anti-PD1/anti-PDL1 treatment in combination with TKIs for untreated advanced RCC. Studies are also underway looking at other immunotherapy/TKI combinations. Cabozantinib is being combined with pembrolizumab (NCT03149822), atezolizumab (NCT03170960), and nivolumab (NCT03141177), with results expected in late 2019 and 2020. Lenvatinib is also being combined with pembrolizumab in a phase III RCT (NCT02811861).

Combination immunotherapy (ipilimumab/nivolumab) has also recently been approved, and there now needs to be a comparison of the different types of combination treatments to see if either has a superior outcome.

Treatment options in non-clear-cell histology

Clear-cell RCC represents the most common variant of RCC accounting for more than 70% of histologically proven diagnoses. The majority of phase III clinical trials of newer agents have excluded non-clear-cell variants and as such robust clinical trial data to guide treatment is lacking. The clinical course of non-clear-cell RCC varies widely.

For papillary and chromophobe variants, the most common subtypes of non-clear-cell RCC, case series suggest that response rates to historic and newer treatment options are typically significantly lower than those seen with clear-cell RCC but potentially useful treatment responses may still be seen.[77]

ESPN was a phase II RCT comparing the use of sunitinib with everolimus in patients with untreated non-clear-cell RCC, or clear-cell RCC with >20% sarcomatoid features. One hundred and eight patients were needed to show an improvement in median PFS. At interim analysis data from 68 patients were analyzed. Median PFS was 6.1 months with sunitinib (95% CI 4.2–9.4) compared to 4.1 months with everolimus (95% CI 2.7–10.5), $p = 0.6$, showing that everolimus was not superior.[78] The ASPEN trial was a multicenter phase II trial also comparing the use of sunitinib with everolimus in 108 patients with untreated metastatic papillary, chromophobe, or unclassified non-clear-cell RCC. The overall median PFS was significantly increased with sunitinib at 8.3 months (80% CI 5.8–11.4), compared to 5.6 months (80% CI 5.5–6.0) for everolimus, with a hazard ratio of 1.41 (80% CI 1.03–1.92, $p = 0.16$). Results varied greatly depending on histological subtype and prognostic group. Those in the poor prognostic category and those with chromophobe histology tended to do better with everolimus. In the poor-prognosis category median PFS was 4.0 months (0.9–5.8) for sunitinib and 6.1 months (3.1–7.3) for everolimus, with a HR of 0.3 (0.1–0.7). In those with chromophobe histology median PFS with sunitinib was 5.5 months (3.2–19.7) compared to 11.4 (5.7–19.4) months with everolimus.[79]

Based on current data there is no clear recommendation for sequencing of treatment after first-line therapy in those with non-clear-cell RCC. In those with papillary histology the use of clear-cell RCC treatment algorithms is an acceptable option.[3] A better understanding of the genetic basis of sporadic non-clear-cell RCC holds promise for the development of more active systemic therapies; early-phase trials of MET inhibition in papillary non-clear-cell RCC have already demonstrated proof of principle with other clinical trials ongoing (see Table 18.5). For those with sarcomatoid tumors the combination of nivolumab and ipilimumab

immunotherapy is an option given data that suggest they are sensitive to immune checkpoint inhibitors.[3]

Sequencing of treatments: First-line, second-line, and beyond

Figure 18.3 outlines the vast number of possible treatment choices and sequencing on the basis of published evidence, MSKCC prognostic group, and regulatory approval.[3]

For the first time in over a decade the position of VEGF-targeted agents at the forefront of treatment has been challenged by combination immunotherapy, demonstrating superior results in intermediate- and poor-risk patients. An increasing body of evidence for the combination of VEGF and checkpoint inhibitors means that they are unlikely to be side-lined for long. Despite the potential for longer-term remissions with immunotherapy most patients will still require subsequent therapies for progressive disease. How these are then sequenced is being evaluated in clinical trials, but at present requires individualized decision-making with patients. Route of administration, local availability, and treatment toxicity profile remain of key importance when evaluating which treatment is best suited to be given to patients in the setting of multiple treatment options.

A working knowledge of treatment-related toxicity is the key, with pro-active management of side effects vital. Checkpoint inhibition brings with it a raft of varied autoimmune toxicities, which unless promptly treated can be life-threatening. Oral-targeted agents must also be managed with appropriate supportive therapies to maintain dose intensity where able, acknowledging that patients may remain on chronic long-term therapy until their cancer is no longer sensitive to active treatment options or treatment is no longer considered appropriate or desirable.

Conclusion

Renal cancers represent 5% of cancer cases in men, and 3% in women globally. In areas with comprehensive healthcare services they are predominantly picked up at an early stage when they may be effectively cured following open or laparoscopic surgical resection or thermal ablation. Despite this some patients will go on to relapse with subsequent metastatic disease. Adjuvant treatment is not widely used due to lack of consistent data, and significant toxicity associated with its use in trials to date. A number of trials remain open, or will shortly report their results, meaning this could imminently change.

The past 10 years have seen many important developments in both the understanding of the underlying genetics of renal cell cancers and effective treatment options. Molecular profiling of tumors has identified multiple aberrant tumor suppressor genes, many in chromosome 3p. Some are prognostic, and some have implications for treatment response. It is likely that in the near future our treatment decisions will be routinely guided by the underlying molecular profile of a patient's tumor.

The advent of checkpoint inhibitor therapies, and their incorporation into the current treatment landscape again offer further benefits for those with advanced disease. Combinations of checkpoint inhibitors and targeted agents are already showing great promise across all prognostic groups, with more trial results still to report. None yet offer a cure for a large proportion of patients, and with marked interpatient and intratumoral heterogeneity, a one-size-fits-all approach is unlikely to be effective.

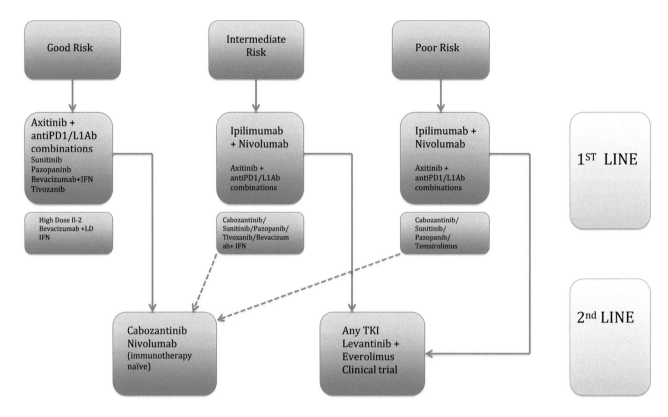

FIGURE 18.3   Suggested treatment algorithm for clear cell renal cell carcinoma (adapted from ESMO Guidelines).

With a huge number of trials still ongoing in the field what is clear is that further changes are likely to keep coming, offering promising new options for patients, and guidance around treatment selection and sequencing.

Key points/info boxes

First-line immunotherapy for RCC
- Ipilimumab (1 mg/kg) + nivolumab (3 mg/kg) OR 42% (intermediate- and poor-risk groups)
- IrAE all grades 80%
- 35% required high-dose steroids
- 22% discontinuation rate

Localized RCC
- 30% relapse following radical nephrectomy
- Median time to relapse 1–2 years
- 66% pulmonary metastases
- No clear OS benefit with adjuvant TKI therapy
- Immunotherapy trial results pending

Risk factors for RCC
- Increasing age
- Smoking
- High BMI
- Hypertension
- CKD

Toxicity of VEGF-targeted TKIs
- Diarrhea
- Sore mouth
- Sore hands and feet
- High blood pressure
- Bleeding and poor wound healing
- Venous/arterial thromboembolic events

- Thyroid dysfunction
- Depigmentation hair/skin
- Cardiomyopathy

Immune-related adverse events (IrAE)
- Rash and itching
- Hepatitis
- Endocrine disorders
- Colitis
- Nephritis
- Pneumonitis
- Neuropathy/CNS symptoms
- Any organ can be affected

References

1. World Cancer Research Fund Kidney Cancer Statistics 2018. https://www.wcrf.org/dietandcancer/cancer-trends/kidney-cancer-statistics
2. Capitano U, Bensalah K, Bex A et al. Epidemiology of renal cell cancer. *Eur Urol.* 2019; 75(1):74–84
3. Escudier B, Porta C, Scmidit M et al. Renal cell carcinoma: ESMO clinical practice guidelines for diagnosis, treatment and follow-up. *Ann Oncol.* 2019; 1–15.
4. Oberling C, Riviere M, Haguenau F. Ultrastructure of the clear cells in renal carcinomas and its importance for the demonstration of their renal origin. *Nature.* 1960; 186:402–3.
5. Inamura K. Renal Cell Tumors: Understanding the molecular pathological epidemiology and the 2016 WHO classification. *Int J Mol Sci.* 2017; 18(10):2195.
6. Leibovich BC, Blute ML, Cheville JC et al. Prediction of progression after radical nephrectomy for patients with clear cell renal cell carcinoma. *Cancer.* 2003; 7(97):1663–71.
7. Latif F, Tory K, Gnarra J et al. Identification of the von Hippel–Lindau disease tumor suppressor gene. *Science.* 1993; 260(5112):1317–20.

8. Liao L, Testa JR, Yang H. The roles of chromatin remodelers and epigenetic modifiers in kidney Cancer. *Cancer Genet.* 2015; 208(5):206–14

9. Hakimi AA1, Ostrovnaya I, Reva B. Adverse outcomes in clear cell renal cell carcinoma with mutations of 3p21 epigenetic regulators BAP1 and SETD2: A report by MSKCC and the KIRC TCGA research network. *Clin Cancer Res.* 2013; 19(12):3259–67.

10. Schmidt L, Duh FM, Chen F et al. Germline and somatic mutations in the tyrosine kinase domain of the MET proto-oncogene in papillary renal carcinomas. *Nat Genet.* 1997; 16(1):68–73.

11. Finley DS, Pantuck AJ, Belldegrun AS. Tumor biology and prognostic factors in renal cell carcinoma. *Oncologist.* 2011; 16 Supplement 2:4–13.

12. Storkel S, Steart PV, Drenckhahn D, Thoenes W. The human chromophobe cell renal carcinoma: Its probable relation to intercalated cells of the collecting duct. *Virchows Arch B Cell Pathol Incl Mol Pathol.* 1989; 56(4):237–45.

13. Msaouel P, Hong AL, Mullen EA et al. Updated recommendations on the diagnosis, management and clinical trial eligibility criteria for patients with renal modullary carcinoma. *GU Cancer.* 2019; 17(1):1–6.

14. Hasumi H, Yao M. Herditary kidney cancer syndromes: Genetic disorders driven by alterations in metabolism and epigenome regulation. *Cancer Sci.* 2018; 109(3):581–6.

15. Macleod LC, Hotaling JM, Wright JL et al. Risk factors for renal cell carcinoma in the Vitamin and Lifestyle (VITAL) Study. *J Urol.* 2013; 190(5):1657–61.

16. Schafhauser W, Ebert A, Brod J, Petsch S, Schrott KM. Lymph node involvement in renal cell carcinoma and survival chance by systematic lymphadenectomy. *Anticancer Res.* 1999; 19(2C):1573–8.

17. Patel DH, Gupta M, Joice GA. Clinical stage migration and survival for renal cell carcinoma in the United States. *Eur Urol Oncol.* 2019 Jul 1;2(4):343–8.

18. Koga S, Tsuda S, Nishikido M et al. The diagnostic value of bone scan in patients with renal cell carcinoma. *J Urol.* 2001; 166(6):2126–8.

19. Amin MB, Edge S, Greene F et al. *AJCC Cancer Staging Manual* (8th ed.). New York, NY: Springer, 2017.

20. Krabbe LM, Bagrodia A, Margulis V. Surgical management of renal cell carcinoma. *Semin Intervent Radiol.* 2014; 31(1):27–32.

21. Munro NP, Woodhams S, Nawrocki JD, Fletcher MS, Thomas PJ. The role of transarterial embolization in the treatment of renal carcinoma. *BJU Int.* 2003; 92(3):240–4.

22. Breen DJ, Rutherford EE, Stedman B et al. Management of renal tumors by image-guided radiofrequency ablation: Experience in 105 tumors. *Cardiovasc Intervent Radiol.* 2007; 30(5):936–42.

23. Stephenson AJ, Chetner MP, Rourke K et al. Guidelines for the surveillance of localized renal cell carcinoma based on the patterns of relapse after nephrectomy. *J Urol.* 2004; 172(1):58–62.

24. Haas NB, Manola J, Uzzo RG et al. Adjuvant sunitinib or sorafenib for high-risk, non-metastatic renal-cell carcinoma (ECOG-ACRIN E2805): A double-blind, placebo-controlled, randomised, phase 3 trial. *Lancet.* 2016; 387(10032):2008–16

25. Motzer RJ, Haas NB, Donskov F. Randomized phase III trial of adjuvant pazopanib versus placebo after nephrectomy in patients with localized or locally advanced renal cell carcinoma. *J Clin Oncol.* 2017; 35(35):3916–23

26. Ravaud A, Motzer RJ, Pandha HS. STRAC Adjuvant sunitinib in high-risk renal-cell carcinoma after nephrectomy. *N Engl J Med.* 2016; 375:2246–54

27. Chamie K, Donin NM, Klopfer P et al. Adjuvant weekly Girentuximab following nephrectomy for high risk renal cell carcinoma: The ARISER randomized clinical trial. *JAMA Oncology.* 2017; 3(7):913–20.

28. Jocham D, Richter A, Hoffmann L. Adjuvant autologous renal tumour cell vaccine and risk of tumour progression in patients with renal-cell carcinoma after radical nephrectomy: Phase III, randomized controlled trial. *Lancet.* 2004; 363(9409):594–9

29. Flanigan RC, Salmon SE, Blumenstein BA et al. Nephrectomy followed by interferon alfa-2b compared with interferon alfa-2b alone for metastatic renal-cell cancer. *N Engl J Med.* 2001; 345(23):1655–9.

30. Mejean A, Ravaud A, Thezenas S et al. Sunitnib alone or after nephrectomy in metastatic renal cell carcinoma. *N Engl J Med.* 2018; 379:417–27

31. Bex A, Mulders P, Jewett M et al. Comparison of immediate vs. deferred cytoreductive nephrectomy in patients with metastatic renal cell carcinoma receiving Sunitinib. *JAMA Oncol.* 2019; 5(2):164–70.

32. Margulis V, Mcdonald M, Tamboli P. Predictors of Oncological outcome after resection of locally recurrent renal cell carcinoma. *J of Urol.* 2009; 181(5):2044–51.

33. Zhao Y, Li J, Li C et al. Prognostic factors for overall survival after lung metastectomy in renal cell cancer patients: A systematic review and metanalysis. *Int J of Surg.* 2017; 41:70–77.

34. Yuasa T, Inoshota N, Saiura A et al. Clinical Outcome of patients with pancreatic metastases from RCC. *BMC Cancer.* 2015; Dec 1;15(1):46.

35. Patchell RA, Tibbs PA, Regine WF et al. Direct decompressive surgical resection in the treatment of spinal cord compression caused by metastatic cancer: A randomised trial. *Lancet.* 2005; 366(9486):643–8.

36. Motzer RJ, Bacik J, Murphy BA, Russo P, Mazumdar M. Interferon-alfa as a comparative treatment for clinical trials of new therapies against advanced renal cell carcinoma. *J Clin Oncol.* 2002; 20(1):289–96.

37. Heng DY, Xie W, Regan MM et al. Prognostic factors for overall survival in patients with metastatic renal cell carcinoma treated with vascular endothelial growth factor–targeted agents: Results from a large, multicenter study. *J Clin Oncol.* 2009; 27:5794–9.

38. Hsieh JJ, Chen D, Pi W et al. Genomic biomarkers of randomized controlled trial comparing first line Everolimus and Sunitinib in patients with metastatic renal cell carcinoma. *Cancer Eur Urol.* 2017; 71(3):405–14.

39. Adverse outcomes in clear cell renal cell carcinoma with mutations of 3p21 epigenetic regulators BAP1 and SETD2: A report by MSKCC and the KIRC TCGA research network. *Clin Cancer Res.* 2013; 19(12):3259–67.

40. Lacovelli R, Verri F. Prognostic role of PD-L1 expression in Renal Cell Carcinoma. A systematic review and meta-analysis. *Target Oncol.* 2016; 11(2):143–8.

41. Sun M, De Velasco G, Brastianos PK et al. The development of brain metastases in patients with renal cell carcinoma: Epidemiology, trends, survival and clinical risk factors using a population based cohort. *Eur Urol Focus.* 2019 May 1;5(3):474-81.

42. Fuchs B, Trousdale RT, Rock MG. Solitary bony metastasis from renal cell carcinoma: Significance of surgical treatment. *Clin Orthop Relat Res.* 2005 Feb 1;431:187-92.

43. Rini B, Dorff TB, Elson P. Active Surveillance in metastatic renal cell carcinoma:a prospective, phase 2 trial. *Lancet Oncol.* 2016; 17(9):1317–24.

44. Lwu S, Goetz P, Monsalves E et al. Stereotactic radiosurgery for the treatment of melanoma and renal cell carcinoma brain metastases. *Oncol Rep.* 2013; 29(2):407–12.

45. Lipton A, Zheng M, Seaman J. Zoledronic acid delays the onset of skeletal-related events and progression of skeletal disease in patients with advanced renal cell carcinoma. *Cancer.* 2003; 98(5):962–9.

46. Hancock B, Griffiths G, Ritchie A et al. Updated results of the MRC randomised controlled trial of alpha interferon vs. MPA in patients with metastatic renal carcinoma. *Proc Am Soc Clin Onc.* 2000; Vol. 1336.

47. Fisher RI, Rosenberg SA, Fyfe G. Long-term survival update for high-dose recombinant interleukin-2 in patients with renal cell carcinoma. *Cancer J Sci Am.* 2000; 6(1) Supplement 1:S55–7.

48. Shablak A, Sikand K, Shanks JH et al. High-dose interleukin-2 can produce a high rate of response and durable remissions in appropriately selected patients with metastatic renal cancer. *J Immunother.* 2011; 34(1):107–12.

49. Motzer J, Escudier B, McDermott DF et al. Nivolumab versus everolimus in advanced renal cell carcinoma. *NEJM.* 2015; 373:1803–13.

50. Motzer J, Tannir NM, McDermott D et al. Nivolumab plus Ipilimumab versus Sunitinib in advanced renal cell carcinoma. *NEJM.* 2018; 378:1277–90.

51. Haanen J, Carbonnel F, Robert C et al. Management of toxicities from immunotherapy: ESMO clinical practice guidelines. *Ann Oncol.* 2017; 28(suppl 4):iv119–iv142

52. Motzer RJ, Hutson TE, Tomczak P et al. Sunitinib versus interferon alfa in metastatic renal-cell carcinoma. *N Engl J Med.* 2007; 356:115–24.

53. Motzer RJ, Hutson TE, Tomczak P et al. Overall survival and updated results for sunitinib compared with interferon alfa in patients with metastatic renal cell carcinoma. *J Clin Oncol.* 2009; 27:3584–90.

54. Ravaud A. Treatment-associated adverse event management in the advanced renal cell carcinoma patient treated with targeted therapies. *Oncologist.* 2011; 16 Supplement 2:32–44.

55. Larkin J, Fishman M, Wood L et al. Axitinib for the treatment of metastatic renal cell carcinoma: Recommendations for therapy management to optimize outcomes. *Am J Clin Oncol.* 2014 Aug 1;37(4):397–403.

56. Rini BI, Cohen DP, Lu DR et al. Hypertension as a biomarker of efficacy in patients with metastatic renal cell carcinoma treated with sunitinib. *J Natl Cancer Inst.* 2011; 103(9):763–73.

57. Sternberg CN, Hawkins RE, Wagstaff J et al. A randomised, double-blind phase III study of pazopanib in patients with advanced and/or metastatic renal cell carcinoma: Final overall survival results and safety update. *Eur J Cancer.* 2013; 49(6):1287–96.

58. Motzer RJ, Hutson TE, Cella D et al. Pazopanib versus sunitinib in metastatic renal-cell carcinoma. *N Engl J Med.* 2013; 369(8):722–31.

59. Escudier B, Porta C, Bono P et al. Randomized, controlled, double-blind, cross-over trial assessing treatment preference for pazopanib versus sunitinib in patients with metastatic renal cell carcinoma: PISCES Study. *J Clin Oncol.* 2014; 32(14):1412–8.

60. Motzer RJ, Escudier B, Tomczak P et al. Axitinib versus sorafenib as second-line treatment for advanced renal cell carcinoma: Overall survival analysis and updated results from a randomised phase 3 trial. *Lancet Oncol.* 2013; 14(6):552–62.

61. Escudier B, Eisen T, Stadler WM et al. Sorafenib for treatment of renal cell carcinoma: Final efficacy and safety results of the phase III treatment approaches in renal cancer global evaluation trial. *J Clin Oncol.* 2009; 27:3312–18.

62. Escudier B, Szczylik C, Hutson TE et al. Randomized phase II trial of first-line treatment with sorafenib versus interferon alfa-2a in patients with metastatic renal cell carcinoma. *J Clin Oncol.* 2009; 27:1280–89.

63. Cabozantinib versus everolimus in advanced renal cell carcinoma(METEOR): Final results from a randomized open label phase 3 trial. *Lancet Oncol.* 2016; 17(7):917–27.

64. Choueiri TK, Halabi S, Sanford BL et al. Cabozantinib versus sunitinib as initial targeted therapy for patients with metastatic renal cell carcinoma of poor and intermediate risk: The Alliance A031203 CABOSUN Trial. *J Clin Oncol.* 2017; 25(6):591–97

65. Motzer RJ1, Nosov D, Eisen T et al. Tivozanib versus sorafenib as initial targeted therapy for patients with metastatic renal cell carcinoma: Results from a phase III trial. *J Clin Oncol.* 2013; 31(30):3791–9.

66. Escudier B, Pluzanska A, Koralewski P et al. Bevacizumab plus interferon alfa-2a for treatment of metastatic renal cell carcinoma: A randomised, double-blind phase III trial. *Lancet.* 2007; 370:2103–11

67. Rini BI, Halabi S, Rosenberg JE et al. Bevacizumab plus interferon alfa compared with interferon alfa monotherapy in patients with metastatic renal cell carcinoma: CALGB 90206. *J Clin Oncol.* 2008; 26:5422–8.

68. Rini B, Atkins MB, Escudier B et al. Atezolizumab plus bevacizumab versus sunitinib in patients with previously untreated metastatic renal cell carcinoma (IMmotion151): A multi-centre, open label, phase 3, randomized controlled trial. *Lancet.* 2019; Jun 15;393(10189):2404–15.

69. Hudes G, Carducci M, Tomczak P et al. Temsirolimus, interferon alfa,α or both for advanced renal-cell carcinoma. *N Engl J Med.* 2007; 356(22):2271–81.

70. Motzer RJ, Escudier B, Oudard S et al. Phase 3 trial of everolimus for metastatic renal cell carcinoma: Final results and analysis of prognostic factors. *Cancer.* 2010; 116:4256–65.

71. Motzer RJ, Hutson TE, Glen H et al. Lenvatinib, everolimus, and the combination in patients with metastatic renal cell carcinoma: A randomized, phase 2, open-label, multicenter trial. *Lancet Oncol.* 2015; 16(15):1473–82.

72. Kwilas AR, Donahue RN, Tsang KY et al. Immune consequences of tyrosine kinase inhibitors that synergize with cancer immunotherapy. *Cancer Cell Microenv.* 2015; 2(1)

73. Rini B, Plimack ER, Stus V et al. Pembrolizumab plus axitinib versus sunitinib for advanced renal cell carcinoma. *N Engl J Med.* 2019; 380(12):1116–27.

74. Motzer RJ, Konstantin P, Haanen J et al. Avelumab plus Axitinib for advanced renal cell carcinoma. *N Engl J Med.* 2019; 380:1103–15.

75. Choueiri TK, Plantade A, Elson P et al. Efficacy of sunitinib and sorafenib in metastatic papillary and chromophobe renal cell carcinoma. *J Clin Oncol.* 2008; 26:127–31.

76. Tannir NM, Jonasch E, Albiges L et al. Everolimus versus sunitinib prospective evaluation in metastatic non-clear cell renal cell carcinoma (ESPN): A randomized multicenter phase 2 trial. *Eur Urol.* 2016; 69(5):866–74.

77. Armstrong AJ, Halabi S, Eisen T et al. Everolimus versus sunitinib for patients with metastatic non-clear cell renal cell carcinoma (ASPEN): A multicentre, open-label, randomised phase 2 trial. *Lancet Oncol.* 2016; 17(3):378–88.

19 OVARIAN, FALLOPIAN TUBE, AND PRIMARY PERITONEAL CANCER

Robert D. Morgan, Andrew R. Clamp, and Gordon C. Jayson

Epithelial tumors of the ovary

Introduction

Cancer of the ovary is the eighth commonest cause of cancer-related death in females worldwide, accounting for 184,799 deaths each year.[1] In the United Kingdom and North America, there are greater than 7000 and 22,000 new cases diagnosed annually, respectively. Ovarian adenocarcinoma is a disease that occurs predominantly in peri- and post-menopausal women, with a peak incidence occurring between the ages of 55 and 65 years old. Fewer than 1% of epithelial ovarian cancers occur before the age of 20 years old, and two-thirds of ovarian malignancies in this latter age group are ovarian germ cell tumors. Epithelial malignancies arising from the fallopian tube, and the peritoneum in females, occur through similar etiological pathways and demonstrate similar clinical behavior; therefore, they are managed using the same treatment algorithm(s) as epithelial ovarian cancer.

Although advances over the last 40 years in surgical techniques and systemic therapies have improved the median survival rate, the overall mortality of ovarian cancer has remained largely unchanged. In the West, more women die from ovarian cancer than from any other gynecological malignancy,[2] largely because it often remains undiagnosed until a late stage, when symptoms result from invasion of other pelvic organs and/or from widespread peritoneal metastases.

Epidemiology and risk factors

The most significant risk factors for ovarian cancer are age and a family history of the disease. The odds ratio for ovarian cancer in first-degree and second-degree relatives of ovarian cancer cases, compared with controls, is 3.6 and 2.9, respectively.[3]

Epidemiological studies have suggested that the risk of ovarian cancer is associated with ovulation, in that early onset of menarche and late menopause are associated with a slightly higher risk of ovarian cancer, whereas pregnancy, the contraceptive pill,[4] and tubal ligation[5] reduce risk. Nulliparity and infertility are associated with increased risk. There is an increased risk of developing borderline ovarian tumors in women who undergo in vitro fertilization treatment.[6] There is also evidence that prolonged use of hormone replacement therapy is associated with a small increased risk of ovarian cancer.[7]

The use of perineal talc[8] is now largely discounted as a cause of ovarian cancer, whereas tobacco smoking appears to increase the risk of mucinous tumours.[9] There is an association between body mass index and ovarian cancer risk.[10] Endometriosis is associated with an increased risk of clear cell and endometrioid histotypes.[11] Dietary intake and consumption of alcohol are not associated with epithelial ovarian cancer.[12,13]

Genetic factors

Between 15% and 20% of epithelial ovarian cancer cases are associated with germline mutations.[14] The commonest genetic variants that predispose to ovarian cancer involve genes involved in DNA repair mechanisms, in particular homologous recombination (HR) repair and the mismatch repair (MMR).

The most frequently detected genetic mutations in epithelial ovarian cancer occur in BRCA1 and BRCA2; these are estimated to occur in 10–15% of all high-grade serous cases. BRCA1 and BRCA2 have a number of important cellular functions; however, it is their role in DNA repair, in particular HR repair, that is linked to carcinogenesis.[15] HR repair is an error-free DNA repair mechanism able to repair DNA double-strand breaks (DSBs).[16] It occurs during the S/G2-phase of the cell cycle, at which stage a sister chromatid, containing a homologous DNA sequence, can act as a template for homology-directed repair. In the absence of BRCA1/2 proteins, the alternative error-prone DNA repair pathway, non-homologous end joining (NHEJ), is relied upon to repair DSBs that have resulted from either exogenous or endogenous genotoxins.[17] A greater reliance upon the error-prone NHEJ pathway potentiates the risk of acquiring somatic mutations in oncogenes/tumor suppressor genes, thereby risking tumorigenesis. A deficiency in BRCA1/2 proteins in cells containing a germline mono-allelic/heterozygous BRCA1/2 mutation often occurs through somatic loss of the remaining BRCA1/2 wild-type allele, leading to a bi-allelic/homozygous mutation; in keeping with the concept of BRCA1/2 being tumor suppressor genes.

The cumulative lifetime risk of developing ovarian cancer in carriers of mutations in BRCA1 or BRCA2 is 40–60% and 10–30%, respectively.[18] This compares with a lifetime risk in the general population of approximately 1%. The pattern of inheritance of BRCA1/2 is autosomal dominant with incomplete penetrance. Women diagnosed with BRCA-mutant ovarian cancer have a better 5-year prognosis, even after adjustment for disease stage and age.[19] This is likely due to the hypersensitivity of BRCA-deficient tumor cells to DNA-damaging agents, such as carbo- and cisplatin, and pegylated liposomal doxorubicin.

Female carriers of BRCA1 or BRCA2 mutations are offered prophylactic bilateral salpingo-oophorectomy, following completion of childbearing, in order to reduce the risk of developing ovarian cancer. However, the peritoneum remains at risk, with subsequent development of primary peritoneal carcinoma in approximately 1% of women who have undergone risk-reducing oophorectomy.[20]

Other genes associated with hereditary ovarian cancer, which also have a functional role in HR repair, include RAD51C, RAD51D, and BRIP1,[21–23] although variants in these genes are much less frequently detected (<1% of all cases).

Loss-of-function mutations in genes involved in the MMR pathway lead to microsatellite instability and are associated with Lynch syndrome (hereditary nonpolyposis colorectal cancer). Germline mutations in genes involved in MMR, in particular MLH1, MSH2, MSH6, and PMS2, are associated with <3% of all ovarian cancer cases. Cases of Lynch syndrome–associated ovarian cancer more frequently include endometrioid or clear cell subtypes, well- or moderately differentiated tumors, and early-stage disease. Women with germline mutations in MLH1, MSH2, and MSH6 have a lifetime risk of ovarian cancer between 10% and 17%.[24] Other cancers related to Lynch syndrome include colorectal, gastric, pancreatic, ureteral and renal pelvis, biliary tract, and brain. It is important to note that most women diagnosed with hereditary ovarian cancer present at a younger age compared with sporadic cases.

Histopathology

Epithelial ovarian carcinomas are classified into four main histological subtypes: serous, endometrioid, clear cell, and mucinous (Figures 19.1 and 19.2).[25] Each subtype represents a morphologically and genetically distinct disease.

Serous carcinomas of the ovary are classified as either high-grade (historically Grade 2/3, moderately/poorly differentiated) or low-grade (Grade 1, well differentiated). High-grade serous (HGS) carcinomas are the commonest type of epithelial ovarian cancer, representing approximately 80% of cases. They often present late with metastatic disease and elevated serum CA 125 levels. Histologically, HGS carcinomas have high-grade nuclear atypia, WT-1 staining, and aberrant p53 expression on immunohistochemistry (IHC). Aberrant p53 patterns include either complete absence (null-type) or strong diffuse staining. HGS carcinomas frequently contain somatic mutations in *TP53* (>95%) or germline or somatic mutations in *BRCA1* or *BRCA2* (~15–20%) and are considered to have chromosomal instability.[26,27]

Low-grade serous (LGS) carcinomas are much rarer than HGS carcinomas, representing ~5% of all serous tumors. They present in patients roughly 10 years earlier than HGS tumors. LGS carcinomas are invasive tumors with low-grade malignant cytological atypia and comparatively slow growth. These tumors are therefore associated with a better prognosis than HGS carcinoma, especially if detected at an early stage. WT-1 staining is often positive in LGS carcinoma, but they rarely demonstrate aberrant p53 expression (i.e., wild-type staining). LGS carcinomas frequently contain *KRAS* or *BRAF* mutations.[28]

Endometrioid carcinomas are the second commonest subtype of epithelial ovarian tumors, accounting for approximately 10–15% of all cases. They are subdivided into Grade 1 (well differentiated), Grade 2 (moderately differentiated), or Grade 3 (poorly differentiated) tumors based on architecture ± nuclear atypia.[29] Most tumors are well differentiated and present with Federation Internationale de Gynecologie et d'Obstetrique (FIGO) Stage I disease. In addition, endometrioid carcinoma is associated with ovarian endometriosis and endometrial carcinoma.

Epithelial tumors
Serous tumors
    Benign (serous cystadenoma, serous adenofibroma, serous surface papilloma)
    Borderline (atypical proliferative serous tumor, non-invasive low-grade serous carcinoma)
    Malignant (low-grade serous carcinoma, high-grade serous carcinoma)
Mucinous tumors
    Benign (mucinous cystadenoma, mucinous adenofibroma)
    Borderline (atypical proliferative mucinous tumor)
    Malignant (mucinous carcinoma)
Endometrioid tumors
    Benign (endometriotic cyst, endometrioid cystadenoma, endometrioid adenofibroma)
    Borderline (endometrioid cystadenoma, endometrioid adenofibroma)
    Malignant (endometrioid carcinoma)
Clear cell tumors
    Benign (clear cell cystadenoma, clear cell adenofibroma)
    Borderline (atypical proliferative clear cell tumor)
    Malignant (clear cell carcinoma)
Brenner tumors
    Benign (Brenner tumor)
    Borderline (atypical proliferative Brenner tumor)
    Malignant (malignant Brenner tumor)
Seromucinous
    Benign (seromucinous cystadenoma, seromucinous adenofibroma)
    Borderline (atypical proliferative seromucinous tumor)
    Malignant (seromucinous carcinoma)
Undifferentiated carcinoma

Mixed epithelial and mesenchymal tumors   (e.g. carcinosarcoma)

Sex-cord stromal tumors
Pure stromal tumors (e.g. fibroma, Leydig cell tumor, Steroid cell tumor)
Pure sex cord tumors (e.g. granulosa cell tumor, Sertoli cell tumor)

Mixed sex cord-stromal tumors   (e.g. Sertoli-Leydig cell tumors)

Germ cell tumors   (e.g. dysgerminoma, yolk sac tumor, teratoma, non-gestational carcinoma)

Secondary tumors

FIGURE 19.1   2014 WHO Classification of tumors of the ovary. (Adapted from Kurman et al., 2014.)

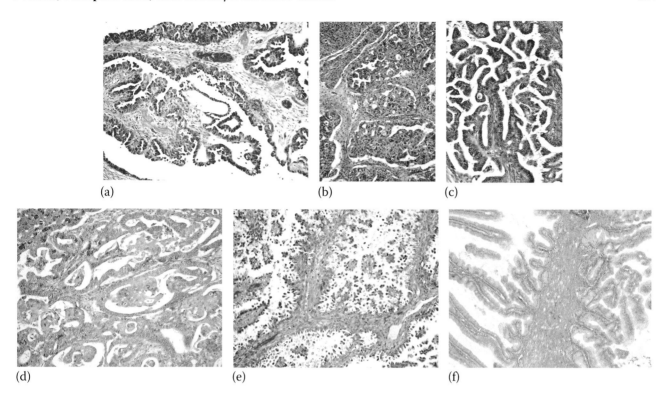

FIGURE 19.2 Five main subtypes of epithelial ovarian carcinoma. Hematoxylin and eosin stained images. (a) High-grade serous: Papillary architecture with multilayering of nuclei and tufting and budding of cells. (b) High-grade serous: Cells contain pleomorphic high-grade nuclei. (c) Low-grade serous: Papillary architecture covered by uniform cells with low-grade nuclei. (d) Endometrioid: Glandular architecture with endometrioid morphology and foci of squamous metaplasia. (e) Clear cell: Papillary architecture and papilla are covered by hobnail cells with clear cytoplasm and apical nuclei. (f) Mucinous: Complex papillary and glandular architecture with tall columnar cells containing mucin and mildly atypical nuclei. (Images courtesy of Dr. Sudha Desai, Consultant Pathologist at The Christie NHS Foundation Trust, Manchester.)

Immunohistochemistry is unlikely to show positive WT-1 staining or aberrant p53 expression. Mutations in *PIK3CA*, *PTEN*, *ARID1A*, *CTNNB1*, and MMR genes are most commonly found in endometrioid ovarian carcinoma.

The incidence of ovarian clear cell carcinoma (OCCC) is higher in Japan compared with the West. These tumors often present with Stage I disease, as a large unilateral solid/cystic mass arising from the pelvis, and are commonly associated with endometriosis. Patients with OCCC may also present with thromboembolic complications and paraneoplastic hypercalcemia. Immunohistochemistry staining is often negative for WT-1, ER and PR, and p53 wild-type but positive for HNF-1β. Clear cell carcinoma of the ovary is associated with mutations in *PIK3CA*, *PTEN*, and *ARID1A*.[30] No internationally accepted grading system exists for OCCC, so all cases are reported as "clear cell carcinoma" and assumed to be high-grade. These tumors are particularly chemotherapy-resistant, and so the prognosis of patients presenting with metastatic/relapsed disease is poor.[31]

Mucinous ovarian carcinoma accounts for ~3% of all epithelial ovarian tumours.[32] These tumors are composed of gastrointestinal-type cells containing intra-cytoplasmic mucin. They often present in relatively younger women between the ages of 40 and 50 years, with early-stage disease detected as a large (frequently >10 cm) unilateral solid/cystic mass arising from the pelvis. Tumor markers such as CEA and CA 19-9 may be elevated. Histological examination may reveal a precursor/borderline lesion, suggestive of transformation from benign to malignant tissue. IHC expression of CK7 and an absence of CK20 expression, in the context of an atypical/borderline proliferative tumor, provide supportive evidence of a primary mucinous ovarian adenocarcinoma versus metastasis to the ovary from a primary gastrointestinal cancer. Mutations in mucinous tumors include *KRAS*, *BRAF*, *CDKN2A*, and *TP53* as well as amplifications in *MYC* and *HER2*.[33]

Ovarian cancer staging

Ovarian cancer spreads via local shedding into the peritoneal cavity and local invasion of bowel and bladder. It also often metastases to the pelvic and para-aortic lymph nodes. Trans-diaphragmatic spread to the pleura is also common. Hematogenous spread to involve the parenchyma of other organs is uncommon, particularly at initial diagnosis.

The FIGO staging system (2014) reflects this metastatic pattern (Table 19.1).[34] Definitive staging of ovarian cancer requires laparotomy by a vertical midline incision. It is customary to examine and biopsy or obtain cytological brushings of the diaphragm, both paracolic gutters, the pelvic peritoneum, para-aortic and pelvic nodes, and infracolic omentum, and to obtain peritoneal washings, particularly in suspected early-stage disease. In this staging operation, about a third of patients thought to have either Stage I or II tumors will be found to have advanced-stage disease.[35] Pelvic and para-aortic lymphadenectomy has no impact on overall survival (OS) in women with complete or optimally (≤1 cm of residual tumor visible) debulked advanced-stage ovarian carcinoma.[36,37]

TABLE 19.1   2014 International Federation of Gynecology and Obstetrics (FIGO) Staging Criteria for Cancer of the Ovary, Fallopian Tube, and Peritoneum

Stage I	**Tumor confined to ovaries or fallopian tube(s)**
IA	Tumor limited to one ovary (capsule intact) or fallopian tube; no tumor on ovarian or fallopian tube surface; no malignant cells in the ascites or peritoneal washings
IB	Tumor limited to both ovaries (capsules intact) or fallopian tubes; no tumor on ovarian or fallopian tube surface; no malignant cells in the ascites or peritoneal washings

IC	Tumor limited to one or both ovaries or fallopian tubes, with any of the following:
	    IC1: surgical spill
	    C2: capsule rupture before surgery or tumor on ovarian or fallopian surface
	    IC3: malignant cells in ascites or peritoneal washings

Stage II	**Tumor involves one or both ovaries or fallopian tubes with pelvic extension (below pelvic brim) or primary peritoneal cancer**
IIA	Extension and/or implants on uterus and/or fallopian tubes and/or ovaries
IIB	Extension to other pelvic intraperitoneal tissues
Stage III	**Tumor involves one or both ovaries or fallopian tubes, or primary peritoneal cancer, with cytologically or histologically confirmed spread to the peritoneum outside the pelvis and/or metastasis to the retroperitoneal lymph nodes**

IIIA	Positive retroperitoneal lymph nodes only (cytologically or histologically proven):
	    IIIA1(i): metastasis up to 10 mm in greatest dimension
	    IIIA1(ii): metastasis more than 10 mm in greatest dimension
	    IIIA2: microscopic extrapelvic (above the pelvic brim) peritoneal involvement with or without positive retroperitoneal lymph nodes

IIIB	Macroscopic peritoneal metastasis beyond the pelvis up to 2 cm in greatest dimension, with or without metastasis to the retroperitoneal lymph node
IIIC	Macroscopic peritoneal metastasis beyond the pelvis more than 2 cm in greatest dimension, with or without metastasis to the retroperitoneal lymph nodes (includes extension of tumor to capsule of liver and spleen without parenchymal involvement of either organ)
Stage IV	**Distant metastasis excluding peritoneal metastases**
IVA	Pleural effusion with positive cytology
IVB	Parenchymal metastases and metastases to extra-abdominal organs (including inguinal lymph nodes and lymph nodes outside the abdominal cavity)

Source: Adapted from Prat, 2014.

Diagnosis

Ninety-five percent of women with ovarian cancer experience symptoms before diagnosis. Symptoms initially tend to be vague but may include abdominal distension, bloating or pain, alterations in bowel or bladder habits, and gynecological complaints such as dyspareunia. These symptoms are often initially misdiagnosed as irritable bowel syndrome (IBS), although symptoms are generally progressive in patients with underlying ovarian malignancy. In the United Kingdom, to avoid delays in diagnosis, guidance from the National Institute for Health and Clinical Excellence suggest that all women over the age of 50 with symptoms suggestive of IBS should have their serum CA 125 measured. A pelvic ultrasound examination should also be considered. A diagnosis of ovarian cancer should be considered in any pre-menopausal woman with an unexplained enlargement of the ovary or any post-menopausal woman with a palpable ovary. Ascites, pleural effusions, and an umbilical tumor mass, referred to as a Sister Mary Joseph's nodule, may also be found on physical examination.

Paraneoplastic syndromes may occasionally be present, including hypercalcemia in clear cell carcinoma of the ovary, paraneoplastic cerebellar degeneration, peripheral polyneuropathy, and dermatomyositis. Paraneoplastic syndromes can be associated with the presence of onconeural antibodies.

Tumor markers

CA 125 is a protein that is released into the plasma of approximately 80% of patients diagnosed with advanced-stage epithelial ovarian cancer. CA 125 concentrations alone are neither sufficiently sensitive nor specific enough to be diagnostic of ovarian cancer,[38] as CA 125 may be elevated in other benign gynecological conditions, including endometriosis and pelvic inflammatory disease, and pregnancy, as well as cancers of the uterus, breast, lung, and gastrointestinal tract and other illnesses such as congestive heart failure and liver disease.

However, CA 125 has most value when interpreted in the context of transvaginal ultrasound (TVUS).[39] A number of other potential tumor markers for ovarian cancer have been identified, in particular HE4, although there is little evidence that the incorporation of HE4 in a multi-modality screening panel is sufficiently superior to CA 125 to justify use in routine clinical practice.[40] In adolescent and young females, there is a greater risk of an ovarian tumor being a germ cell tumor, in which case the plasma concentration of alpha fetoprotein (AFP), beta-human chorionic gonadotropin (β-HCG), and lactate dehydrogenase (LDH) should be checked.

Imaging

The conventional initial imaging investigation of a suspected ovarian mass is TVUS. In most centers, findings from this are then scored and incorporated into the "risk of malignancy index" (RMI) with the patient's menopausal status and CA 125 concentration. A final result of greater than 250 is relatively sensitive and specific for the diagnosis of malignant ovarian cysts.[39] However, the optimum RMI threshold for further management has yet to be defined. In the United Kingdom, a RMI >250 leads to surgery by specialist gynecological cancer surgeons, as treatment by such surgeons is associated with an improved outcome, albeit in retrospective studies.[41]

Pre-operative imaging usually also includes computed tomography (CT), which provides information on the stage of cancer, and occasionally magnetic resonance imaging. These investigations may also provide information that can contraindicate surgery. For instance, massive ascites or porta hepatis, mesenteric, or extensive upper abdominal disease is often used to justify postponing surgery until cytotoxic (neoadjuvant) chemotherapy has brought the disease under control. Such a pre-operative chemotherapy approach requires histological confirmation of the diagnosis by radiologically guided percutaneous or laparoscopic biopsy before cytotoxic therapy can be initiated.

Screening

Despite considerable efforts directed at early detection, no cost-effective screening tests have been developed. The suggested screening tests for ovarian cancer include bimanual pelvic examination, TVUS, and CA 125 antigen. The Pap smear and cytological examination of peritoneal lavage obtained by culdocentesis have low sensitivities and are not recommended. Similarly, for women with no known genetic predisposition to ovarian cancer, there is no conclusive evidence to support routine screening.[42,43]

Initial studies that tested the value of TVUS and CA 125 showed that a significant proportion of women who were initially identified as having an abnormal test and who subsequently underwent laparotomy did not have ovarian cancer, and so most of these patients did not benefit from the procedure.[44] This study led to the United Kingdom Collaborative Trial of Ovarian Cancer Screening (UKCTOCS) trial, which randomized 202,638 post-menopausal women, aged between 50 and 74 years old, to undergo annual screening by TVUS, or a multimodal approach incorporating both TVUS and serial CA 125 levels, or no screening. After a median follow-up of 11.1 years, ovarian cancer had been diagnosed in 1282 (0.6%) women within the study. However, neither TVUS nor the multimodal approach led to a significant reduction in mortality over 0–14 years of screening.[42]

Treatment for Stage I and II ovarian cancer

If early-stage ovarian cancer is suspected on the basis of the physical examination and imaging, cytoreductive surgery is performed for histological confirmation, formal staging, and tumor debulking. Surgical staging provides important information that can guide post-operative decision-making in early-stage disease. Full staging surgery has been described earlier.

In selected patients with Stage I disease who wish to retain their fertility, a more conservative fertility-sparing approach consisting of a unilateral salpingo-oophorectomy with conservation of the contralateral ovary/fallopian tube and uterus is associated with a low risk of recurrence.[45] However, careful surgical staging is still required to exclude occult omental or nodal metastatic disease. The majority of patients with early-stage epithelial ovarian cancer, especially those considered as having a higher risk of relapse, will also require post-operative adjuvant chemotherapy in an attempt to eradicate residual disease.

Two large Phase 3 trials, ACTION and ICON1, randomized patients with early-stage (predominantly FIGO Stage I) epithelial ovarian carcinoma to adjuvant platinum-based chemotherapy or observation.[46,47] A combined analysis of data from both trials showed a significant improvement in 5-year recurrence-free survival (76% versus 65%; HR 0.64, 95% confidence interval [CI] 0.50–0.82) and 5-year OS (82% versus 74%; HR 0.67, 95%CI 0.50–0.90) in favor of adjuvant chemotherapy.[48] However, it is important to note that one of these trials, ACTION, showed that the benefit of adjuvant chemotherapy was limited to only those patients who were not optimally debulked and therefore at higher risk of recurrence.[47]

There is broad consensus that those women with early-stage disease who do not require adjuvant chemotherapy have been diagnosed with either Stage IA LGS, Stage IA mucinous (expansile-type), or Stage IA Grade 1–2 endometrioid ovarian cancer.[49]

Adjuvant chemotherapy is usually recommended for all other tumor histotypes, grades, and stages.

Stage III and IV ovarian cancer

The outcome of patients with Stage IV disease is less favorable than that of patients with Stage III disease. Usually, patients with Stages III and IV are treated with the same chemotherapeutic strategies; however, the role of surgery for patients with Stage IV disease is less clear. Although the efficacy of cytotoxic therapy is assessed by CT scanning, changes in CA 125 are also a reliable way of assessing response to treatment.[50]

Primary cytoreductive surgery

Considerable evidence from retrospective analyses of large patient cohorts indicates that the volume of disease left at the completion of the primary cytoreductive surgery is related to patient survival.[51–53] Complete macroscopic debulking (i.e., no residual disease) was associated with a median OS of 81.1 months in one analysis of 1779 patients diagnosed with FIGO Stage IIIC disease, treated in three separate trials, compared with 34.2 months for those with residual disease (HR 0.36, 95%CI 0.31–0.42).[51] Furthermore, for those patients with residual disease following primary cytoreductive surgery, there was an OS benefit in favor of those with 1–10 mm of residual disease ("optimal" cytoreduction) versus those with >10 mm of residual disease ("suboptimal" cytoreduction) (HR 0.80, 95%CI 0.70–0.91). However, what remains unclear is how much of this improvement reflects aggressive surgical resection and/or is related to an intrinsically more aggressive biological phenotype in unresectable disease. Indeed, it would be ethically challenging to disentangle the relative contributions of these factors in a randomized trial assessing the role of cytoreductive surgery, and so the goal of primary surgery should be to achieve complete cytoreduction, provided this is achieved with acceptable post-operative morbidity and mortality.

Neoadjuvant chemotherapy

For patients where complete macroscopic debulking is not considered possible, neoadjuvant (i.e., pre-operative) chemotherapy followed by delayed cytoreductive surgery is now an established standard of care treatment. Factors precluding successful primary surgery include, for instance, extensive upper abdominal disease, in particular that involving the porta hepatis or mesentery, and poor performance status secondary to symptoms associated with ovarian cancer and/or comorbidities. In such patients, two randomized Phase 3 trials demonstrated that administering three cycles of platinum-based chemotherapy before surgery does not negatively impact on survival and results in reduced perioperative morbidity and a shorter hospital stay for those patients undergoing surgery after chemotherapy.[54,55]

Second-look laparotomy

It is now widely accepted that second-look laparotomy performed after the completion of primary chemotherapy is not associated with a survival advantage. Similarly, a second cytoreductive procedure after primary cytoreductive surgery followed by three to four cycles of chemotherapy in patients with suboptimally (i.e., >1 cm of residual disease) resected disease at initial laparotomy is not associated with any clinical benefit, provided that the primary surgery was performed by a gynecological oncologist.[56,57]

Primary chemotherapy

The platinum analogues, carboplatin and cisplatin, are the most active agents in the treatment of ovarian cancer and have formed the backbone of standard of care chemotherapy regimens for the last 25 years. In the initial trials investigating cisplatin, a relationship between survival and dose-intensity was reported at 75 mg/m[2] administered every 3 weeks, and this was adopted as the standard.[58,59] For carboplatin, similar results were found with an improved outcome shown for an area under the curve (AUC) of 5 and 6[60] administered 3-weekly.[61] It is also well established that cisplatin and carboplatin yield equivalent clinical results.

Since the 1990s, the administration of six to eight 3-weekly cycles of intravenous platinum–taxane chemotherapy has been the international standard of care for advanced-stage ovarian cancer after a survival advantage was demonstrated in most studies adding paclitaxel to platinum.[62–65] Paclitaxel may also be substituted by docetaxel, with similar survival outcomes and lower neurotoxicity but at the expense of greater neutropenia.[66]

Up to around 90% of patients with advanced-stage disease who are treated with cytoreductive surgery and platinum–taxane chemotherapy achieve clinical remission by the end of first-line treatment. Despite this, relapse still occurs in most women, and only 10–15% of patients with advanced-stage disease are long-term survivors. The majority of responding patients develop recurrent disease within 18 months of starting their initial platinum-based chemotherapy. Many trials have attempted to improve upon the carboplatin–paclitaxel doublet therapy by incorporating a third cytotoxic agent or using maintenance cytotoxic chemotherapy, but neither strategy has demonstrated any improvement in OS.[62,67]

The utility of first-line weekly dose-dense platinum–taxane therapy remains unclear. Four randomized Phase 3 trials have reported results comparing 3-weekly and weekly carboplatin–paclitaxel regimens. The Japanese trial JGOG-3016 showed a significant improvement in survival outcomes in women treated with weekly paclitaxel (80 mg/m[2]) plus 3-weekly carboplatin versus those treated with 3-weekly carboplatin and paclitaxel (180 mg/m[2]).[68,69] In contrast, three randomized Phase 3 trials, GOG-0262, MITO7, and ICON8, have demonstrated equivalent progression-free survival (PFS) benefits between groups treated with 3-weekly or weekly paclitaxel in combination with 3-weekly carboplatin.[70,71] Furthermore, data from JGOG-3016 and GOG-0262 revealed higher rates of hematological and neurological toxicity in those groups of women treated with weekly paclitaxel, although these differences in toxicity were not replicated in MITO7 or ICON8.

Intraperitoneal chemotherapy

The delivery of chemotherapy to the peritoneal cavity is an attractive strategy, given the fact that the spread of ovarian cancer often remains limited to this space until late in the disease course. Pharmacologically, intraperitoneal (IP) therapy delivers orders of magnitude higher concentrations of cytotoxic therapy directly to the tumor by repeated "baths" that strip away cancer cells layer by layer with each cycle of therapy.[72] Although several randomized trials[73–77] suggested increased efficacy using the IP route, there were methodological weaknesses and toxicity concerns that prevented the adoption of IP. Indeed, in some studies, IP cytotoxic agents acted as a reservoir that allowed chemotherapy drugs to achieve sustained intra-vascular concentrations, leading to severe local and distant toxicity. This significantly reduced the patients' ability to complete therapy, leading to reduced levels of total drug exposure.[74]

More recently, the randomized Phase 3 trial GOG-0252 reported that six cycles of 3-weekly intravenous (IV) versus IP carboplatin (AUC6) in combination with weekly IV paclitaxel (80mg/m[2]) and 3-weekly IV bevacizumab demonstrated no difference in PFS (HR 0.925, 95%CI 0.802–1.07) between groups.[78]

Bevacizumab treatment

The adult pre-menopausal ovary demonstrates a striking reliance on angiogenesis: the formation of new blood vessels, and in particular vascular endothelial growth factor (VEGF). Many preclinical and clinical studies have also indicated the importance of angiogenesis in ovarian cancer, and it is not surprising that the addition of anti-VEGF treatment strategies to first-line regimens have proven clinical benefit.[79]

Two large randomized Phase 3 trials, ICON7 and GOG-0218, evaluated the addition of concurrent and maintenance 3-weekly bevacizumab, an anti-VEGF monoclonal antibody, to first-line standard 3-weekly carboplatin–paclitaxel chemotherapy. Both trials demonstrated a significant improvement in PFS,[80,81] with a modest increase in toxicity (predominantly hypertension) in the study arm (Table 19.2). Following data maturation in both trials,[82,83] an OS benefit for the use of bevacizumab was reported, but only in patients considered at high risk of progressive disease (Stage IV disease, inoperable Stage III disease, or suboptimally debulked disease).[83]

TABLE 19.2   Randomized Phase III Trials Investigating the Anti-Angiogenic Agent Bevacizumab

Trial	FIGO stage	Chemotherapy	Bevacizumab	Median progression-free survival
First line				
ICON7 (1, 2)*Adjuvant*	Stage I/IIA (clear cell or Grade 3 tumors) or Stage IIB–IV	Carboplatin (AUC5/6) and paclitaxel (175 mg/m[2])	7.5 mg/kg every 3 weeks for 18 cycles in total	19.0 vs. 17.3 months (HR 0.81, 95%CI 0.70–0.94)
GOG-0218 (3, 4)*Adjuvant*	Stage III–IV	Carboplatin (AUC6) and paclitaxel (175 mg/m[2])	15 mg/mg every 3 weeks for 22 cycles in total	14.2 vs. 10.3 months (HR 0.717, 95%CI 0.625–0.824)
Recurrent disease				
OCEANS*Palliative*	Relapsed, platinum-sensitive epithelial ovarian cancer	Carboplatin (AUC4) and gemcitabine (1000 mg/m[2])	15 mg/kg every 3 weeks	12.4 vs. 8.4 months (HR 0.484, 95%CI 0.388–0.605)
AURELIA (5)*Palliative*	Relapsed, platinum-resistant epithelial ovarian cancer	Investigator choice (paclitaxel, pegylated liposomal doxorubicin, or topotecan)	10 mg/kg every 2 weeks or 15 mg/kg every 3 weeks	6.7 vs. 3.4 months (HR 0.48, 95%CI 0.38–0.60)

Sources: Perren et al., 2011; Oza et al., 2015; Burger et al., 2011; Tewari et al., 2019; Pujade-Lauraine et al., 2014.

Poly(ADP-ribose) polymerase inhibitors

In the last 10 years, poly(ADP-ribose) polymerase (PARP) inhibitors have changed the treatment of HGS ovarian cancer.[84] Poly(ADP) ribose polymerase is a family of 17 different enzymes involved in a number of essential cellular mechanisms.[85] It is the role of PARP-1 and PARP-2 in the response to DNA damage that has led to the utility of PARP inhibitors as anti-cancer therapy.[86]

At sites of DNA single-strand breaks (SSBs), PARP-1/2 catalyzes the formation of polymers of ADP-ribose (PAR chains) from the coenzyme nicotinamide adenine dinucleotide (NAD+). Consequently, linear and branched PAR chains form at sites of SSBs in a process called PARylation. These PAR chains attract proteins involved in the repair of SSBs.[87] In order for the repair proteins to access sites of SSBs, PARP-1/2 must dissociate. PARP inhibitors trap PARP-1/2 at sites of SSBs, thereby delaying repair of SSBs.[88] Unrepaired SSBs may form lethal, replication-associated DNA DSBs if the approaching replication fork collapses.[89,90] Collapsed replication forks are substrates for another DNA repair mechanism, called HR repair.[91] Cancer cells with a functional HR repair pathway are able to repair DSBs; however, cancer cells with a deficiency in HR repair, such as those with a deficiency of BRCA1 or BRCA2 proteins, are unable to repair DSBs. Thus, an accumulation of lethal DSBs leads to cell death. It is this synthetically lethal mechanism that explains the cytotoxicity of PARP1/2 inhibitors.[92] Indeed, synthetic lethality states that a deficiency in one gene/gene product (i.e., either *BRCA1/2* or PARP1/2) can be tolerated by a cell, but a deficiency in two genes/gene products (both *BRCA1/2* and PARP1/2) is lethal to the cell.

The relatively high frequency of germline and somatic *BRCA1/2* mutations in HGS carcinoma means that PARP1/2 inhibitors provide a realistic therapeutic option for a substantial number of women diagnosed with ovarian cancer. Large genetic studies have shown that approximately 15–20% of HGS cancers contain a germline or somatic mutation in *BRCA1* or *BRCA2*.[93,94] These mutations are most commonly germline (10–15%) rather than somatic (5–7%). Moreover, mutations in *BRCA1* and *BRCA2* are often clonal, occurring early in carcinogenesis.[95] Seminal preclinical work established the efficacy of PARP1/2 inhibitors in *BRCA1/2* deficient cells.[89,90] Thereafter, a series of Phase 1 to 3 trials established that PARP1/2 inhibitors were highly efficacious in *BRCA*-mutant tumors.[96–103] Most recently, SOLO1, a Phase 3 randomized trial, showed that 24 months of first-line maintenance therapy with the PARP1/2 inhibitor olaparib (300 mg twice daily) improved PFS compared with placebo in FIGO Stage III/IV *BRCA*-mutant HGS or endometrioid ovarian carcinoma following a complete/partial response to primary therapy (HR 0.30, 95%CI 0.23–0.41).[99] Furthermore, there are a number of ongoing trials investigating other PARP1/2 inhibitors (e.g., talazoparib, veliparib, and niraparib) as maintenance first-line therapy. The results of these trials are eagerly anticipated.

Recurrent/relapsed ovarian cancer

Although recurrent disease is generally incurable, and palliation of symptoms remains a key management goal, longitudinal evaluation of clinical trial data from the past 20 years suggests that survival outcomes are improving for patients with recurrent ovarian cancer.

The earliest indicator of disease relapse is often a rise in the serum CA 125 level in the absence of both symptoms and signs on physical examination and/or CT scan.[104] Frequently, the development of disease-related symptoms is delayed, by a median of approximately 5 months, after a doubling of CA 125 levels, and one important decision facing the patient and the oncologist is

when to start further chemotherapy. The MRC OV05 trial,[105] which randomized women in complete remission after platinum-based first-line therapy to receive second-line treatment on the basis of CA 125 marker-defined progression or clinical/symptomatic relapse, has provided important information to guide this decision. This study showed no OS advantage to commencing chemotherapy early, and those women who received chemotherapy while they were asymptomatic had inferior quality of life. Although some centers have interpreted this study to indicate that it is not necessary to monitor CA 125 during follow-up, many institutions continue to do this to avoid missing patients who present with an isolated site of disease relapse and therefore may gain benefit from secondary cytoreduction. The value of secondary cytoreductive surgery is the subject of ongoing clinical trials.

Platinum-free interval

The choice of second-line cytotoxic agents generally depends on the platinum-free interval. Patients who have relapsed disease more than 6 months after the completion of platinum therapy are generally considered to have platinum-sensitive disease,[106] with response rates of around 40% to a second platinum-based regimen. As the median PFS from first-line chemotherapy in advanced-stage disease is approximately 18 months, most patients fall into this category at first relapse, and the greater the time-to-relapse, the higher the chances of response to platinum re-challenge.[107,108] Patients with a short remission, lasting less than 6 months after first-line chemotherapy, usually (but not always) have relatively platinum-resistant disease. It is notable that with each successive chemotherapy regimen, the treatment-free interval often becomes shorter, until ultimately chemotherapy resistance develops, and active treatment is withdrawn. Attempts to extend the platinum-free interval using non-platinum-based regimens prior to reintroducing platinum therapy for platinum-sensitive disease did not improve survival.[109] The 10% of patients with disease that progresses on first-line therapy (referred to as platinum-refractory disease) have the worst prognosis.

Platinum-sensitive recurrent disease

Several randomized trials have shown that treatment with doublet chemotherapy[110] consisting of carboplatin in combination with either paclitaxel,[111] gemcitabine,[112,113] or pegylated liposomal doxorubicin,[114] is associated with improved PFS. Single-agent chemotherapy with carboplatin is also a reasonable treatment option for frail patients, as it is often better tolerated.[115] The median OS for recurrent platinum-sensitive disease is 3 years.

It should be noted that up to 40% of patients receiving multiple lines of platinum chemotherapy develop hypersensitivity to carboplatin. Historically, this required switching to cisplatin or withdrawing platinum chemotherapy entirely; however, hypersensitivity can now often be managed successfully using desensitization regimens.

Platinum-resistant recurrent disease

When disease recurs within 6 months of previous platinum-based treatment or progresses on treatment, standard of care therapies involve single-agent non-platinum-based chemotherapy, including weekly paclitaxel,[116] pegylated liposomal doxorubicin,[117] or topotecan.[117] All these drugs have response rates in the 10–20% range in this clinical setting. As no drug has been shown to be more effective than any other in platinum-resistant disease, the choice of chemotherapy regimen should be based on comorbidities, the presence of residual toxicity, and potential adverse impact on the patient's quality of life. The median OS for recurrent platinum-resistant disease is approximately 12–13 months.

Several studies have investigated the use of dose-dense platinum-based combination regimens in patients with platinum-resistant disease[118,119] with response rates approximating 40%. However, because of a lack of proven survival advantage, these dose-dense regimens are routinely used in all centers.

The use of endocrine therapies such as tamoxifen and aromatase inhibitors (e.g., letrozole and anastrozole) is often reserved for tumors with positive estrogen receptor (ER) and/or progesterone receptor (PR) immunohistochemistry[120] and can represent an alternative treatment option in patients considered unlikely to tolerate further cytotoxic therapy[121] and/or those diagnosed with LGS carcinoma.[122,123]

Bevacizumab treatment for recurrent disease

Randomized trials have confirmed the utility of bevacizumab in both platinum-sensitive and platinum-resistant recurrent ovarian cancer. The OCEANS trial[113] showed that the addition of bevacizumab to carboplatin-gemcitabine improved PFS in platinum-sensitive disease, although no OS benefit was reported,[124] probably because of the confounding effects of cross-over and subsequent lines of therapy.

The AURELIA trial[116] randomized patients with platinum-resistant ovarian cancer to standard chemotherapy (single-agent paclitaxel, pegylated liposomal doxorubicin, or topotecan) with or without bevacizumab. This trial demonstrated an improvement in PFS associated with bevacizumab, particularly when weekly paclitaxel (80 mg/m^2) was the chosen concurrent chemotherapy, although again, no OS benefit was reported (Table 19.2).

It is clear from these trials, along with those in the first-line setting,[80,81] that anti-VEGF therapy is a key treatment option in ovarian cancer, but the optimal positioning of this in the management pathway has yet to be defined, as there is a low risk of serious gastrointestinal toxicity, in particular bowel perforation and fistula formation, which is higher in patients with extensive pre-treatment or evidence of bowel obstruction.[125]

PARP inhibitors for recurrent disease

PARP inhibitors are now a standard of care maintenance treatment in relapsed, platinum-sensitive HGS or endometrioid ovarian cancer. Data from three randomized Phase 3 trials showed that olaparib (300 mg twice daily), niraparib (300 mg once daily), and rucaparib (600 mg twice daily) maintenance monotherapy significantly improves PFS, compared with placebo, in women with relapsed, platinum-sensitive HGS or endometrioid carcinoma, following a complete/partial response to the latest line of platinum-based therapy[97,100,103] (see Table 19.3). As a result of these trials, all three PARP inhibitors have been licensed as maintenance treatment in this clinical setting. PARP inhibitors are well tolerated and have little impact on quality of life compared with placebo. The commonest side effects associated with PARP1/2 inhibitors include myelosuppression, in particular anemia and thrombocytopenia, fatigue, nausea and vomiting, and less frequently, liver transaminitis. In addition, trial data suggests an approximate 1% risk of myelodysplastic syndrome (MDS), acute myeloid leukemia (AML), or other secondary malignancies. However, it remains unclear whether the onset of secondary malignancies resulted from exposure to PARP inhibitors or prior chemotherapy use.

The use of PARP inhibitors as single-agent therapies has also been reported in both platinum-sensitive[96,98] and platinum-resistant[98,101] recurrent ovarian cancer. In these Phase 2 trials, the greatest PFS benefits were shown in *BRCA*-mutant tumors. Consequently, data from these trials led to olaparib and rucaparib being licensed for platinum-resistant *BRCA*-mutant epithelial ovarian cancer.

Combinational therapy that includes a PARP inhibitor with another targeted agent and/or immune therapy are also being investigated in patients with recurrent disease.[126,127] One of the most promising combinations includes olaparib (300 mg twice daily) and the oral anti-angiogenic agent cediranib (20 mg once daily). A randomized Phase 2 trial recently showed that this combination significantly improved PFS (HR 0.42, 95%CI 0.23–0.76), compared with olaparib alone, in relapsed, platinum-sensitive HGS or endometrioid ovarian cancer.[127]

Immune therapy

Despite the optimism surrounding immune therapy in many other tumor types, efficacy data from early phase trials in ovarian cancer have been disappointing, with response rates of around 10–20%.[126,128–132] Indeed, two randomized Phase 3 trials,

TABLE 19.3   Randomized Phase III Trials Investigating PARP Inhibitors in Ovarian Cancer

Trial	Demographics	Study arms	Subgroups	Median progression-free survival
First line				
SOLO1(1)	FIGO III/IVHGS/EOCCR/PR following first-line therapy	Olaparib 300 mg twice daily (for up to 24 months) versus placebo	g*BRCA1/2*m	60% vs. 27% freedom from progressive disease or death at 3 years (HR 0.30, 95%CI 0.23–0.41)
Recurrent disease				
SOLO2(2)	Relapsed, platinum-sensitive HGS/EOC	Olaparib 300 mg twice daily versus placebo	g*BRCA1/2*m	19.1 vs. 5.5 months (HR 0.30, 95%CI 0.22–0.41)
NOVA(3)	Relapsed, platinum-sensitive HGSC	Niraparib 300 mg once daily versus placebo	g*BRCA1/2*m	21.0 vs. 5.5 months (HR 0.27, 95%CI 0.17–0.41)
			Non-g*BRCA1/2*m/ HRD-positive	12.9 vs. 3.8 months (HR 0.38, 95%CI 0.24–0.59)
			Non-g*BRCA1/2*m	9.3 vs. 3.9 months (HR 0.45, 95%CI 0.34–0.61)
ARIEL3(4)	Relapsed, platinum-sensitive HGS/EOC	Rucaparib 600 mg twice daily versus placebo	g/s*BRCA1/2*m	16.6 vs. 5.4 months (HR 0.23, 95%CI 0.16–0.34)
			HRD carcinoma	13.6 vs. 5.4 (HR 0.32, 95%CI 0.24–0.42)
			ITT population	10.8 vs. 5.4 (HR 0.36, 95%CI 0.30–0.45)

Source: Data from Moore et al., 2018; Pujade-Lauraine et al., 2017; Mizra et al., 2016; Coleman et al., 2017.

Abbreviations: g/s*BRCA*m, germline or somatic *BRCA1/2* mutation; EOC, epithelial ovarian cancer; HGSOC, high-grade serous ovarian cancer; HGSOC, high-grade serous or endometrioid ovarian cancer; HRD, homologous recombination deficiency; ITT, intention to treat.

JAVELIN 100 and JAVELIN 200, have failed to show a survival benefit for the addition of the anti-PD-L1 therapy avelumab in either treatment-naïve or relapsed platinum-resistant/refractory epithelial ovarian cancer.

The hitherto disappointing outcomes for immune therapy in ovarian cancer have led to a determination to find predictive biomarkers, with current efforts focused on improving our understanding of the tumor microenvironment. Prospective trials are now investigating biomarkers such as PD-1/PD-L1 expression on tumor and immune cells, tumor mutational burden, and the presence/absence of tumor-infiltrating lymphocytes within tumor biopsies. However, a major drawback of investigating predictive biomarkers from single tumor-site biopsies is the paucity of data this approach provides regarding tumor heterogeneity.[133]

Follow-up

The conventional follow-up protocol for patients, following cytoreductive surgery and platinum-based therapy, is to be seen every 3 months for the first 2 years; then every 6 months until 5 years; and then, in some centers, follow-up continues on a 6–12-monthly basis until 10 years. At each visit, the patient undergoes review of symptoms, physical examination of abdomen and pelvis, and measurement of the CA 125.

The MRC OV05 trial[105] trial addressed whether it is in the patient's interests to have recurrent disease detected earlier, leading to early treatment, or whether it is better to wait for the patient to develop recurrent disease-related symptoms before initiating treatment. This trial randomly allocated patients with CA 125 evidence of recurrent disease to immediate treatment or treatment based on the development of symptoms. Of the 1442 patients recruited, 529 developed recurrence during the trial. The median survival from randomization was 25.7 (early treatment) versus 27.1 months (delayed treatment), and there was no difference in survival between the two arms (HR 0.98, 95%CI 0.80–1.20). These data are very important, as they suggest: (A) that there is no merit in early treatment of recurrent disease; (B) that the watch-and-wait surveillance process that is practiced by many oncologists for women with low-risk recurrent disease does not disadvantage them; and (C) that there may be little advantage in measuring the CA 125 during follow-up of patients. However, one caveat that has arisen since the publication of MRC OV05 is the concern that some patients may have an asymptomatic isolated site of recurrence that can be detected through serial monitoring of CA 125, and that these patients may benefit from secondary cytoreductive surgery. Routine CT scans are not advised in follow-up because of the long-term risks of ionizing radiation.

Prognostic factors and survival

The most important favorable prognostic factors in ovarian cancer patients include earlier disease stage, smaller residual tumor following primary cytoreductive surgery, good performance status, absence of ascites, a younger age, histological subtype other than mucinous and clear cell carcinoma, a well-differentiated tumor, platinum-free interval, and pathological response to neoadjuvant chemotherapy.[51,134,135]

Historically, grade was believed to be of limited significance. However, initial findings in Stage I ovarian cancer suggested that patients with high-grade ovarian cancer, including those with clear cell histology, are the ones who most benefit from adjuvant platinum chemotherapy.[136] Low-grade tumors are indolent and relatively resistant to cytotoxic therapy, whereas high-grade tumors are characterized by transient chemo-sensitivity with

reducing treatment-free intervals between recurrences, eventually leading to the patient's death through chemoresistant disease.

Retrospective data have demonstrated that the outcome from ovarian cancer is improved if surgery is performed by gynecological cancer surgeons. If all treatment is given in a cancer center, the survival of ovarian cancer now approaches 35% at 10 years' follow-up. With respect to the stage, the survival for Stage I, II, III, and IV disease is approximately 90%, 50%, 20%, and 5%, respectively.

Low–malignant potential tumors of the ovary

Introduction

Tumors of low malignant potential (borderline tumors) are not benign, because they show cytological and architectural atypia. They are also not malignant, because there is no overt stromal destruction. They account for 15% of all epithelial ovarian tumors and often develop in women of younger age than those with invasive cancer. Approximately 75–80% of these tumors are Stage I at the time of diagnosis. Their prognosis and treatment are markedly different from adenocarcinoma, in that the 20-year survival rate is approximately 90% for all cases, but disease-related mortality depends on several factors. According to the stage, mortality ranges from <1% for Stage I to approximately 30% for Stage III disease.[137] Serous histology and younger age are associated with a better prognosis.

Pathology and staging

The histopathology of borderline ovarian tumors is complex and should be reviewed by a specialist gynecological cancer histopathologist. A comprehensive review in several centers shows that two-thirds of the patients have serous tumors, and the other third have mucinous borderline ovarian tumours.[138] The staging system is the same as that applied to ovarian adenocarcinoma. Although some studies suggest that microinvasive disease or invasive implants carry a worse prognosis,[139] others simply show that stage is significant.[138] In contrast to colorectal carcinoma, where the process of transformation has been well described, transformation of borderline tumors to invasive adenocarcinoma is thought to occur in only approximately 2% of cases.[138]

Treatment

For Stages I and II, OS after resection is close to 100%. If the diagnosis is suspected or confirmed at surgery by frozen section, full staging surgery has not been prospectively demonstrated to be of benefit, and in general, total abdominal hysterectomy and bilateral salpingo-oophorectomy is appropriate therapy in patients who have completed their families. For patients desiring to maintain fertility, more conservative surgery is appropriate. However, a large retrospectively published series suggested that fertility-preserving surgery, and particularly organ preservation by ovarian cystectomy alone, is associated with a greater risk of recurrent disease. In univariate analysis, the HR of developing recurrent disease following fertility-sparing surgery was 2.98.[138] In general, once these patients have completed their families, consideration should therefore be given to removal of the remaining ovarian tissue due to the documented risk of disease recurrence.[140] No additional treatment is indicated.

Patients with newly diagnosed Stage III disease should undergo aggressive tumor debulking surgery, as observational studies have indicated that when there is no gross residual tumor, the survival rate can be as high as 100%. Patients with bulk residual disease after surgery have a better prognosis than those with Stage III epithelial ovarian cancer, but the volume of residual disease is an important prognostic factor.[138] There is no evidence to support the use of post-operative chemo- or radiotherapy for early- or advanced-stage borderline disease.

Disease recurrence is usually managed surgically, although some patients develop inexorably progressive and indolent tumors that can eventually be fatal. The role of chemotherapy is not well defined, but it may be beneficial in patients whose disease has recurred rapidly or in whom further surgery is not possible; however, response rates are low.

Non-epithelial tumors of the ovary

Germ cell tumors

Ovarian germ cell tumors are rare but aggressive malignancies and are more prevalent among girls and young women.[141] They arise from primordial germ cells of the ovary, are commonly unilateral, and are often curable. The histological subtypes of ovarian germ cell tumors are heterogenous and include dysgerminomas, yolk sac tumors, immature teratomas, and mixed germ cell tumors, as well as other rarer subtypes.[25] The tumors are staged using the FIGO staging system used for adenocarcinoma, although there is debate regarding the extent of surgical staging required, given the favorable sensitivity of these diseases to cytotoxic chemotherapy. Whether fertility-sparing surgery or more aggressive cytoreduction is performed, all tumors except for Stage IA pure dysgerminoma and Stage IA Grade 1 pure immature teratoma are treated with cytotoxic chemotherapy. Bleomycin, etoposide, and cisplatin is the standard of care regimen.[142] Evaluation of the disease and its response to treatment can be performed using radiological imaging as well as the tumor markers AFP, β-HCG, and LDH. These diseases are curable, but rare, and so there is a strong case for them to be managed by specialist teams incorporating oncologists with experience of managing male germ cell tumors. Treatment of germ cell tumors is reviewed in more detail in Chapter 17.

Sex cord-stromal tumors

Sex cord-stromal tumors of the ovary account for <5% of all ovarian tumors, and their clinical presentation is often characterized by their ability to secrete sex hormones.[143] They are classified as pure stromal tumors (e.g., fibroma, thecoma, and Leydig cell tumor), pure sex cord tumors (e.g., granulosa cell tumor [GCT] and Sertoli cell tumor), or mixed sex cord-stromal tumors (e.g., Sertoli-Leydig cell tumor). GCTs are the commonest sex cord-stromal tumors, accounting for approximately 70%. Genetic studies have revealed somatic mutations in *FOXL2* as well as the promoter region of *TERT*, which have been linked to the pathogenesis of GCTs,[144,145] as well as mutations in *DICER1*, which has been linked to Sertoli-Leydig cell tumours.[146,147]

Estrogen secretion is noted in at least 70% of GCTs, and as the median age of diagnosis is between 50 and 55 years old, patients may present with post-menopausal bleeding or irregular menses. In such patients, it is important to exclude a synchronous endometrial cancer caused by hyperestrogenism. Precocious puberty may be the presenting complaint in the case of juvenile GCTs. Patients with Sertoli-Leydig cell tumors may show clinical features of virilization or amenorrhea due to hyperandrogenism. Along with sex hormone secretion, the tumors can also release inhibins, which can be used as tumor markers to monitor the disease. These tumors may also present only when they have reached a large size, with symptoms related to tumor bulk, such as abdominal pain and distension. Due to their vascular nature, emergency presentation with an acute abdomen due to intraperitoneal bleeding is also not uncommon.

Sex cord-stromal tumors are associated with cancer predisposition syndromes including DICER syndrome (Sertoli-Leydig cell tumors), Peutz–Jeghers syndrome (Sertoli cell tumor and sex cord tumor with annular tubules), and Gorlin syndrome (fibroma). Most sex cord-stromal tumors behave in a benign fashion and present with early-stage disease. Surgical resection is generally associated with longer-term survival rates; however, due to the rarity of most subtypes other than GCTs, there is little published evidence to guide the management of cases with advanced/recurrent disease.[142]

Management of granulosa cell tumors

The majority of patients with GCTs present with Stage I disease, and these cases are associated with good long-term survival. It is reasonable to offer unilateral salpingo-oophorectomy to those patients who wish to preserve their fertility. The most important prognostic factor for GCTs is the stage of disease at clinical presentation, with around 90% of Stage I patients alive at 10 years compared with 17–33% of patients with Stage III/IV disease.[148] However, up to 40% of patients with Stage I disease have been reported to experience disease relapse at a median of 76 months after presentation, and relapses more than 20 years after the initial diagnosis have also been reported. Although some experts recommend the use of adjuvant chemotherapy for patients with advanced-stage disease, this is not supported by evidence from randomized trials.[148]

Because of the indolent nature of this condition, long-term follow-up is required. Disease relapse often occurs intra-abdominally, but distant metastases in lung, liver, and bone have also been reported. In patients with recurrent disease, surgical debulking should be considered, but in the presence of inoperable disease, platinum-based chemotherapy or endocrine therapy can be utilized.[149,150]

Key learning points

- Epithelial ovarian cancer can be classified into five main histological subtypes: high-grade serous, low-grade serous, endometrioid, clear cell and mucinous carcinoma. High-grade serous carcinoma is the commonest form of epithelial ovarian cancer, accounting for approximately 80% of all cases.
- Epithelial ovarian cancer is believed to originate from the distal fallopian tube epithelium or the ovarian surface epithelium.
- Germline and somatic *BRCA1/2* pathogenic variants occur in approximately 20% of all cases of high-grade serous carcinoma and can be targeted with poly (ADP-ribose) polymerase inhibitors (PARPi).
- First-line therapy for advanced stage ovarian cancer includes cytoreductive surgery plus platinum-based chemotherapy followed by maintenance treatment with bevacizumab or PARPi in specific clinically- and molecularly-defined groups.
- The goal of cytoreductive surgery should be complete macroscopic debulking (i.e., no residual disease).

- Relapsed, platinum-sensitive ovarian cancer can be treated with secondary cytoreductive surgery for isolated disease followed by adjuvant platinum-based chemotherapy. For relapsed metastatic ovarian cancer treatment involves either platinum or non-platinum-based chemotherapy depending upon the platinum-free interval.

References

1. Bray F, Ferlay J, Soerjomataram I et al. Global cancer statistics 2018: GLOBOCAN estimates of incidence and mortality worldwide for 36 cancers in 185 countries. *CA Cancer J Clin.* 2018; 68(6):394–424.
2. Siegel RL, Miller KD, Jemal A. Cancer statistics, 2019. *CA Cancer J Clin.* 2019; 69(1):7–34.
3. Schildkraut JM, Thompson WD. Familial ovarian cancer: A population-based case-control study. *Am J Epidemiol.* 1988; 128(3):456–66.
4. Iversen L, Fielding S, Lidegaard O et al. Association between contemporary hormonal contraception and ovarian cancer in women of reproductive age in Denmark: Prospective, nationwide cohort study. *BMJ.* 2018; 362:k3609.
5. Gaitskell K, Coffey K, Green J et al. Tubal ligation and incidence of 26 site-specific cancers in the Million Women Study. *Br J Cancer.* 2016; 114(9):1033–7.
6. Stewart LM, Holman CD, Finn JC, Preen DB, Hart R. In vitro fertilization is associated with an increased risk of borderline ovarian tumours. *Gynecol Oncol.* 2013; 129(2):372–6.
7. Pearce CL, Chung K, Pike MC, Wu AH. Increased ovarian cancer risk associated with menopausal estrogen therapy is reduced by adding a progestin. *Cancer.* 2009; 115(3):531–9.
8. Houghton SC, Reeves KW, Hankinson SE et al. Perineal powder use and risk of ovarian cancer. *J Natl Cancer Inst.* 2014; 106(9). doi: 10.1093/jnci/dju208
9. Collaborative Group on Epidemiological Studies of Ovarian C, Beral V, Gaitskell K et al. Ovarian cancer and smoking: Individual participant meta-analysis including 28,114 women with ovarian cancer from 51 epidemiological studies. *Lancet Oncol.* 2012; 13(9):946–56.
10. Collaborative Group on Epidemiological Studies of Ovarian C. Ovarian cancer and body size: Individual participant meta-analysis including 25,157 women with ovarian cancer from 47 epidemiological studies. *PLoS Med.* 2012; 9(4):e1001200.
11. Pearce CL, Templeman C, Rossing MA et al. Association between endometriosis and risk of histological subtypes of ovarian cancer: A pooled analysis of case-control studies. *Lancet Oncol.* 2012; 13(4):385–94.
12. Rota M, Scotti L, Turati F et al. Alcohol consumption and prostate cancer risk: A meta-analysis of the dose-risk relation. *Eur J Cancer Prev.* 2012; 21(4):350–9.
13. Crane TE, Khulpateea BR, Alberts DS et al. Dietary intake and ovarian cancer risk: A systematic review. *Cancer Epidemiol Biomarkers Prev.* 2014;23(2):255–73.
14. Norquist BM, Harrell MI, Brady MF et al. Inherited mutations in women with ovarian carcinoma. *JAMA Oncol.* 2016; 2(4):482–90.
15. Venkitaraman AR. Cancer susceptibility and the functions of BRCA1 and BRCA2. *Cell.* 2002; 108(2):171–82.
16. San Filippo J, Sung P, Klein H. Mechanism of eukaryotic homologous recombination. *Annu Rev Biochem.* 2008; 77:229–57.
17. Helleday T, Lo J, van Gent DC, Engelward BP. DNA double-strand break repair: From mechanistic understanding to cancer treatment. *DNA Repair.* 2007; 6(7):923–35.
18. Kuchenbaecker KB, Hopper JL, Barnes DR et al. Risks of breast, ovarian, and contralateral breast cancer for BRCA1 and BRCA2 Mutation Carriers. *JAMA.* 2017; 317(23):2402–16.
19. Yang D, Khan S, Sun Y et al. Association of BRCA1 and BRCA2 mutations with survival, chemotherapy sensitivity, and gene mutator phenotype in patients with ovarian cancer. *JAMA.* 2011; 306(14):1557–65.
20. Kauff ND, Satagopan JM, Robson ME et al. Risk-reducing salpingo-oophorectomy in women with a BRCA1 or BRCA2 mutation. *N Engl J Med.* 2002; 346(21):1609–15.
21. Loveday C, Turnbull C, Ramsay E et al. Germline mutations in RAD51D confer susceptibility to ovarian cancer. *Nat Genet.* 2011; 43(9):879–82.
22. Loveday C, Turnbull C, Ruark E et al. Germline RAD51C mutations confer susceptibility to ovarian cancer. *Nat Genet.* 2012; 44(5):475–6; author reply 6.
23. Rafnar T, Gudbjartsson DF, Sulem P et al. Mutations in BRIP1 confer high risk of ovarian cancer. *Nat Genet.* 2011; 43(11):1104–7.
24. Moller P, Seppala TT, Bernstein I et al. Cancer risk and survival in path_MMR carriers by gene and gender up to 75 years of age: A report from the Prospective Lynch Syndrome Database. *Gut.* 2018;67(7):1306–16.
25. Kurman RJ, Carcangiu ML, Herrington CS, Young RH. *WHO Classification of Tumours of the Female Reproductive Organs. WHO Classification of Tumours.* Lyon: IARC Press, 2014.
26. Cancer Genome Atlas Research N. Integrated genomic analyses of ovarian carcinoma. *Nature.* 2011; 474(7353):609–15.
27. Hoadley KA, Yau C, Wolf DM et al. Multiplatform analysis of 12 cancer types reveals molecular classification within and across tissues of origin. *Cell.* 2014;158(4):929–44.
28. Emmanuel C, Chiew YE, George J et al. Genomic classification of serous ovarian cancer with adjacent borderline differentiates RAS pathway and TP53-mutant tumors and identifies NRAS as an oncogenic driver. *Clin Cancer Res.* 2014; 20(24):6618–30.
29. Zaino RJ, Kurman RJ, Diana KL, Morrow CP. The utility of the revised International Federation of Gynecology and Obstetrics histologic grading of endometrial adenocarcinoma using a defined nuclear grading system. A Gynecologic Oncology Group study. *Cancer.* 1995; 75(1):81–6.
30. Jones S, Wang TL, Shih Ie M et al. Frequent mutations of chromatin remodeling gene ARID1A in ovarian clear cell carcinoma. *Science.* 2010; 330(6001):228–31.
31. Sugiyama T, Okamoto A, Enomoto T et al. Randomized phase III trial of irinotecan plus cisplatin compared with paclitaxel plus carboplatin as first-line chemotherapy for ovarian clear cell carcinoma: JGOG3017/GCIG Trial. *J Clin Oncol.* 2016; 34(24):2881–7.
32. Morice P, Gouy S, Leary A. Mucinous ovarian carcinoma. *N Engl J Med.* 2019; 380(13):1256–66.
33. Ryland GL, Hunter SM, Doyle MA et al. Mutational landscape of mucinous ovarian carcinoma and its neoplastic precursors. *Genome Med.* 2015; 7(1):87.
34. Prat J, Oncology FCoG. Staging classification for cancer of the ovary, fallopian tube, and peritoneum. *Int J Gynaecol Obstet.* 2014; 124(1):1–5.
35. Young RC, Decker DG, Wharton JT et al. Staging laparotomy in early ovarian cancer. *JAMA.* 1983; 250(22):3072–6.
36. Harter P, Sehouli J, Lorusso D et al. A randomized trial of lymphadenectomy in patients with advanced ovarian neoplasms. *N Engl J Med.* 2019; 380(9):822–32.
37. Panici PB, Maggioni A, Hacker N et al. Systematic aortic and pelvic lymphadenectomy versus resection of bulky nodes only in optimally debulked advanced ovarian cancer: A randomized clinical trial. *J Natl Cancer Inst.* 2005; 97(8):560–6.
38. Bast RC, Jr., Knapp RC. Use of the CA 125 antigen in diagnosis and monitoring of ovarian carcinoma. *Eur J Obstet Gynecol Reprod Biol.* 1985; 19(6):354–6.
39. Jacobs I, Oram D, Fairbanks J et al. A risk of malignancy index incorporating CA 125, ultrasound and menopausal status for the accurate preoperative diagnosis of ovarian cancer. *Br J Obstet Gynaecol.* 1990; 97(10):922–9.
40. Karlsen MA, Sandhu N, Hogdall C et al. Evaluation of HE4, CA125, risk of ovarian malignancy algorithm (ROMA) and risk of malignancy index (RMI) as diagnostic tools of epithelial ovarian cancer in patients with a pelvic mass. *Gynecol Oncol.* 2012; 127(2):379–83.
41. Vernooij F, Heintz P, Witteveen E, van der Graaf Y. The outcomes of ovarian cancer treatment are better when provided by gynecologic oncologists and in specialized hospitals: A systematic review. *Gynecol Oncol.* 2007; 105(3):801–12.

42. Jacobs IJ, Menon U, Ryan A et al. Ovarian cancer screening and mortality in the UK Collaborative Trial of Ovarian Cancer Screening (UKCTOCS): A randomised controlled trial. *Lancet.* 2016; 387(10022):945–56.

43. Buys SS, Partridge E, Black A et al. Effect of screening on ovarian cancer mortality: The Prostate, Lung, Colorectal and Ovarian (PLCO) Cancer Screening Randomized Controlled Trial. *JAMA.* 2011; 305(22):2295–303.

44. Jacobs IJ, Skates SJ, MacDonald N et al. Screening for ovarian cancer: A pilot randomised controlled trial. *Lancet.* 1999; 353(9160):1207–10.

45. Morice P, Denschlag D, Rodolakis A et al. Recommendations of the Fertility Task Force of the European Society of Gynecologic Oncology about the conservative management of ovarian malignant tumors. *Int J Gynecol Cancer.* 2011; 21(5):951–63.

46. Colombo N, Guthrie D, Chiari S et al. International Collaborative Ovarian Neoplasm trial 1: A randomized trial of adjuvant chemotherapy in women with early-stage ovarian cancer. *J Natl Cancer Inst.* 2003; 95(2):125–32.

47. Trimbos JB, Vergote I, Bolis G et al. Impact of adjuvant chemotherapy and surgical staging in early-stage ovarian carcinoma: European Organisation for Research and Treatment of Cancer-Adjuvant ChemoTherapy in Ovarian Neoplasm trial. *J Natl Cancer Inst.* 2003; 95(2):113–25.

48. Trimbos JB, Parmar M, Vergote I et al. International Collaborative Ovarian Neoplasm trial 1 and Adjuvant ChemoTherapy In Ovarian Neoplasm trial: Two parallel randomized phase III trials of adjuvant chemotherapy in patients with early-stage ovarian carcinoma. *J Natl Cancer Inst.* 2003; 95(2):105–12.

49. Colombo N, Sessa C, du Bois A et al. ESMO-ESGO consensus conference recommendations on ovarian cancer: Pathology and molecular biology, early and advanced stages, borderline tumours and recurrent disease. *Ann Oncol.* 2019; 30:672–705.

50. Rustin GJ, Vergote I, Eisenhauer E et al. Definitions for response and progression in ovarian cancer clinical trials incorporating RECIST 1.1 and CA 125 agreed by the Gynecological Cancer Intergroup (GCIG). *Int J Gynecol Cancer.* 2011; 21(2):419–23.

51. du Bois A, Reuss A, Pujade-Lauraine E et al. Role of surgical outcome as prognostic factor in advanced epithelial ovarian cancer: A combined exploratory analysis of 3 prospectively randomized phase 3 multicenter trials: By the Arbeitsgemeinschaft Gynaekologische Onkologie Studiengruppe Ovarialkarzinom (AGO-OVAR) and the Groupe d'Investigateurs Nationaux Pour les Etudes des Cancers de l'Ovaire (GINECO). *Cancer.* 2009; 115(6):1234–44.

52. Bristow RE, Tomacruz RS, Armstrong DK, Trimble EL, Montz FJ. Survival effect of maximal cytoreductive surgery for advanced ovarian carcinoma during the platinum era: A meta-analysis. *J Clin Oncol.* 2002; 20(5):1248–59.

53. Allen DG, Heintz AP, Touw FW. A meta-analysis of residual disease and survival in stage III and IV carcinoma of the ovary. *Eur J Gynaecol Oncol.* 1995; 16(5):349–56.

54. Vergote I, Trope CG, Amant F et al. Neoadjuvant chemotherapy or primary surgery in stage IIIC or IV ovarian cancer. *N Engl J Med.* 2010; 363(10):943–53.

55. Kehoe S, Hook J, Nankivell M et al. Primary chemotherapy versus primary surgery for newly diagnosed advanced ovarian cancer (CHORUS): An open-label, randomised, controlled, non-inferiority trial. *Lancet.* 2015; 386(9990):249–57.

56. van der Burg ME, van Lent M, Buyse M et al. The effect of debulking surgery after induction chemotherapy on the prognosis in advanced epithelial ovarian cancer. Gynecological Cancer Cooperative Group of the European Organization for Research and Treatment of Cancer. *N Engl J Med.* 1995; 332(10):629–34.

57. Rose PG, Nerenstone S, Brady MF et al. Secondary surgical cytoreduction for advanced ovarian carcinoma. *N Engl J Med.* 2004; 351(24):2489–97.

58. McGuire WP, Hoskins WJ, Brady MF et al. Assessment of dose-intensive therapy in suboptimally debulked ovarian cancer: A Gynecologic Oncology Group study. *J Clin Oncol.* 1995; 13(7):1589–99.

59. Kaye SB, Paul J, Cassidy J et al. Mature results of a randomized trial of two doses of cisplatin for the treatment of ovarian cancer.

60. Calvert AH, Newell DR, Gumbrell LA et al. Carboplatin dosage: Prospective evaluation of a simple formula based on renal function. *J Clin Oncol.* 1989; 7(11):1748–56.

61. Gore M, Mainwaring P, A'Hern R et al. Randomized trial of dose-intensity with single-agent carboplatin in patients with epithelial ovarian cancer. London Gynaecological Oncology Group. *J Clin Oncol.* 1998; 16(7):2426–34.

62. Piccart MJ, Bertelsen K, James K et al. Randomized intergroup trial of cisplatin-paclitaxel versus cisplatin-cyclophosphamide in women with advanced epithelial ovarian cancer: Three-year results. *J Natl Cancer Inst.* 2000; 92(9):699–708.

63. Muggia FM, Braly PS, Brady MF et al. Phase III randomized study of cisplatin versus paclitaxel versus cisplatin and paclitaxel in patients with suboptimal stage III or IV ovarian cancer: A gynecologic oncology group study. *J Clin Oncol.* 2000; 18(1):106–15.

64. McGuire WP, Hoskins WJ, Brady MF et al. Cyclophosphamide and cisplatin compared with paclitaxel and cisplatin in patients with stage III and stage IV ovarian cancer. *N Engl J Med.* 1996; 334(1):1–6.

65. International Collaborative Ovarian Neoplasm G. Paclitaxel plus carboplatin versus standard chemotherapy with either single-agent carboplatin or cyclophosphamide, doxorubicin, and cisplatin in women with ovarian cancer: The ICON3 randomised trial. *Lancet.* 2002; 360(9332):505–15.

66. Vasey PA, Jayson GC, Gordon A et al. Phase III randomized trial of docetaxel-carboplatin versus paclitaxel-carboplatin as first-line chemotherapy for ovarian carcinoma. *J Natl Cancer Inst.* 2004; 96(22):1682–91.

67. Markman M, Liu PY, Wilczynski S et al. Phase III randomized trial of 12 versus 3 months of maintenance paclitaxel in patients with advanced ovarian cancer after complete response to platinum and paclitaxel-based chemotherapy: A Southwest Oncology Group and Gynecologic Oncology Group trial. *J Clin Oncol.* 2003; 21(13):2460–5.

68. Katsumata N, Yasuda M, Isonishi S et al. Long-term results of dose-dense paclitaxel and carboplatin versus conventional paclitaxel and carboplatin for treatment of advanced epithelial ovarian, fallopian tube, or primary peritoneal cancer (JGOG 3016): A randomised, controlled, open-label trial. *Lancet Oncol.* 2013; 14(10):1020–6.

69. Katsumata N, Yasuda M, Takahashi F et al. Dose-dense paclitaxel once a week in combination with carboplatin every 3 weeks for advanced ovarian cancer: A phase 3, open-label, randomised controlled trial. *Lancet.* 2009; 374(9698):1331–8.

70. Pignata S, Scambia G, Katsaros D et al. Carboplatin plus paclitaxel once a week versus every 3 weeks in patients with advanced ovarian cancer (MITO-7): A randomised, multicentre, open-label, phase 3 trial. *Lancet Oncol.* 2014; 15(4):396–405.

71. Chan JK, Brady MF, Penson RT et al. Weekly vs. Every-3-week paclitaxel and carboplatin for ovarian cancer. *N Engl J Med.* 2016; 374(8):738–48.

72. Dedrick RL, Myers CE, Bungay PM, DeVita VT, Jr. Pharmacokinetic rationale for peritoneal drug administration in the treatment of ovarian cancer. *Cancer Treat Rep.* 1978; 62(1):1–11.

73. Alberts DS, Liu PY, Hannigan EV et al. Intraperitoneal cisplatin plus intravenous cyclophosphamide versus intravenous cisplatin plus intravenous cyclophosphamide for stage III ovarian cancer. *N Engl J Med.* 1996; 335(26):1950–5.

74. Armstrong DK, Bundy B, Wenzel L et al. Intraperitoneal cisplatin and paclitaxel in ovarian cancer. *N Engl J Med.* 2006; 354(1):34–43.

75. Markman M, Bundy BN, Alberts DS et al. Phase III trial of standard-dose intravenous cisplatin plus paclitaxel versus moderately high-dose carboplatin followed by intravenous paclitaxel and intraperitoneal cisplatin in small-volume stage III ovarian carcinoma: An intergroup study of the Gynecologic Oncology Group, Southwestern Oncology Group, and Eastern Cooperative Oncology Group. *J Clin Oncol.* 2001; 19(4):1001–7.

76. Provencher DM, Gallagher CJ, Parulekar WR et al. OV21/PETROC: A randomized Gynecologic Cancer Intergroup phase II study of intraperitoneal versus intravenous chemotherapy

Scottish Gynecology Cancer Trials Group. *J Clin Oncol.* 1996; 14(7):2113–9.

following neoadjuvant chemotherapy and optimal debulking surgery in epithelial ovarian cancer. *Ann Oncol.* 2018; 29(2):431–8.

77. Tewari D, Java JJ, Salani R et al. Long-term survival advantage and prognostic factors associated with intraperitoneal chemotherapy treatment in advanced ovarian cancer: A gynecologic oncology group study. *J Clin Oncol.* 2015; 33(13):1460–6.

78. Walker JL, Brady MF, Wenzel L et al. Randomized trial of intravenous versus intraperitoneal chemotherapy plus bevacizumab in advanced ovarian carcinoma: An NRG Oncology/Gynecologic Oncology Group Study. *J Clin Oncol.* 2019; 37:1380–90

79. Ferrara N, Kerbel RS. Angiogenesis as a therapeutic target. *Nature.* 2005; 438(7070):967–74.

80. Burger RA, Brady MF, Bookman MA et al. Incorporation of bevacizumab in the primary treatment of ovarian cancer. *N Engl J Med.* 2011; 365(26):2473–83.

81. Perren TJ, Swart AM, Pfisterer J et al. A phase 3 trial of bevacizumab in ovarian cancer. *N Engl J Med.* 2011; 365(26):2484–96.

82. Tewari KS, Burger RA, Enserro D et al. Final overall survival of a randomized trial of bevacizumab for primary treatment of ovarian cancer. *J Clin Oncol.* 2019; 37(26):2317–28.

83. Oza AM, Cook AD, Pfisterer J et al. Standard chemotherapy with or without bevacizumab for women with newly diagnosed ovarian cancer (ICON7): Overall survival results of a phase 3 randomised trial. *Lancet Oncol.* 2015; 16(8):928–36.

84. Fong PC, Boss DS, Yap TA et al. Inhibition of poly(ADP-ribose) polymerase in tumors from BRCA mutation carriers. *N Engl J Med.* 2009; 361(2):123–34.

85. Schreiber V, Dantzer F, Ame JC, de Murcia G. Poly(ADP-ribose): Novel functions for an old molecule. *Nat Rev Mol Cell Biol.* 2006; 7(7):517–28.

86. Lord CJ, Ashworth A. The DNA damage response and cancer therapy. *Nature.* 2012; 481(7381):287–94.

87. El-Khamisy SF, Masutani M, Suzuki H, Caldecott KW. A requirement for PARP-1 for the assembly or stability of XRCC1 nuclear foci at sites of oxidative DNA damage. *Nucleic Acids Res.* 2003; 31(19):5526–33.

88. Murai J, Huang SY, Das BB et al. Trapping of PARP1 and PARP2 by clinical PARP inhibitors. *Cancer Res.* 2012; 72(21):5588–99.

89. Bryant HE, Schultz N, Thomas HD et al. Specific killing of BRCA2-deficient tumours with inhibitors of poly(ADP-ribose) polymerase. *Nature.* 2005; 434(7035):913–7.

90. Farmer H, McCabe N, Lord CJ et al. Targeting the DNA repair defect in BRCA mutant cells as a therapeutic strategy. *Nature.* 2005; 434(7035):917–21.

91. Arnaudeau C, Lundin C, Helleday T. DNA double-strand breaks associated with replication forks are predominantly repaired by homologous recombination involving an exchange mechanism in mammalian cells. *J Mol Biol.* 2001; 307(5):1235–45.

92. Ashworth A. A synthetic lethal therapeutic approach: Poly(ADP) ribose polymerase inhibitors for the treatment of cancers deficient in DNA double-strand break repair. *J Clin Oncol.* 2008;26(22):3785–90.

93. Alsop K, Fereday S, Meldrum C et al. BRCA mutation frequency and patterns of treatment response in BRCA mutation-positive women with ovarian cancer: A report from the Australian Ovarian Cancer Study Group. *J Clin Oncol.* 2012; 30(21):2654–63.

94. Hennessy BT, Timms KM, Carey MS et al. Somatic mutations in BRCA1 and BRCA2 could expand the number of patients that benefit from poly (ADP ribose) polymerase inhibitors in ovarian cancer. *J Clin Oncol.* 2010; 28(22):3570–6.

95. Patch AM, Christie EL, Etemadmoghadam D et al. Whole-genome characterization of chemoresistant ovarian cancer. *Nature.* 2015; 521(7553):489–94.

96. Swisher EM, Lin KK, Oza AM et al. Rucaparib in relapsed, platinum-sensitive high-grade ovarian carcinoma (ARIEL2 Part 1): An international, multicentre, open-label, phase 2 trial. *Lancet Oncol.* 2017; 18(1):75–87.

97. Pujade-Lauraine E, Ledermann JA, Selle F et al. Olaparib tablets as maintenance therapy in patients with platinum-sensitive, relapsed ovarian cancer and a BRCA1/2 mutation (SOLO2/ENGOT-Ov21): A double-blind, randomised, placebo-controlled, phase 3 trial. *Lancet Oncol.* 2017; 18(9):1274–84.

98. Moore KN, Secord AA, Geller MA et al. Niraparib monotherapy for late-line treatment of ovarian cancer (QUADRA): A

99. multicentre, open-label, single-arm, phase 2 trial. *Lancet Oncol.* 2019; 20(5):636–48.

99. Moore K, Colombo N, Scambia G et al. Maintenance olaparib in patients with newly diagnosed advanced ovarian cancer. *N Engl J Med.* 2018; 379(26):2495–505.

100. Mirza MR, Monk BJ, Herrstedt J et al. Niraparib maintenance therapy in platinum-sensitive, recurrent ovarian cancer. *N Engl J Med.* 2016; 375(22):2154–64.

101. Kaye SB, Fehrenbacher L, Holloway R et al. A phase II, randomized, placebo-controlled study of vismodegib as maintenance therapy in patients with ovarian cancer in second or third complete remission. *Clin Cancer Res.* 2012; 18(23):6509–18.

102. Fong PC, Yap TA, Boss DS et al. Poly(ADP)-ribose polymerase inhibition: Frequent durable responses in BRCA carrier ovarian cancer correlating with platinum-free interval. *J Clin Oncol.* 2010; 28(15):2512–9.

103. Coleman RL, Oza AM, Lorusso D et al. Rucaparib maintenance treatment for recurrent ovarian carcinoma after response to platinum therapy (ARIEL3): A randomised, double-blind, placebo-controlled, phase 3 trial. *Lancet.* 2017;390(10106): 1949–61.

104. Niloff JM, Knapp RC, Lavin PT et al. The CA 125 assay as a predictor of clinical recurrence in epithelial ovarian cancer. *Am J Obstet Gynecol.* 1986; 155(1):56–60.

105. Rustin GJ, van der Burg ME, Griffin CL et al. Early versus delayed treatment of relapsed ovarian cancer (MRC OV05/EORTC 55955): A randomised trial. *Lancet.* 2010; 376(9747):1155–63.

106. Stuart GC, Kitchener H, Bacon M et al. 2010 Gynecologic Cancer InterGroup (GCIG) consensus statement on clinical trials in ovarian cancer: Report from the Fourth Ovarian Cancer Consensus Conference. *Int J Gynecol Cancer.* 2011; 21(4):750–5.

107. Gore ME, Fryatt I, Wiltshaw E, Dawson T. Treatment of relapsed carcinoma of the ovary with cisplatin or carboplatin following initial treatment with these compounds. *Gynecol Oncol.* 1990; 36(2):207–11.

108. Markman M, Rothman R, Hakes T et al. Second-line platinum therapy in patients with ovarian cancer previously treated with cisplatin. *J Clin Oncol.* 1991; 9(3):389–93.

109. Pignata S, Scambia G, Bologna A et al. Randomized Controlled Trial Testing the Efficacy of Platinum-Free Interval Prolongation in Advanced Ovarian Cancer: The MITO-8, MaNGO, BGOG-Ov1, AGO-Ovar2.16, ENGOT-Ov1, GCIG Study. *J Clin Oncol.* 2017; 35(29):3347–53.

110. Raja FA, Counsell N, Colombo N et al. Platinum versus platinum-combination chemotherapy in platinum-sensitive recurrent ovarian cancer: A meta-analysis using individual patient data. *Ann Oncol.* 2013; 24(12):3028–34.

111. Parmar MK, Ledermann JA, Colombo N et al. Paclitaxel plus platinum-based chemotherapy versus conventional platinum-based chemotherapy in women with relapsed ovarian cancer: The ICON4/AGO-OVAR-2.2 trial. *Lancet.* 2003; 361(9375):2099–106.

112. Pfisterer J, Plante M, Vergote I et al. Gemcitabine plus carboplatin compared with carboplatin in patients with platinum-sensitive recurrent ovarian cancer: An intergroup trial of the AGO-OVAR, the NCIC CTG, and the EORTC GCG. *J Clin Oncol.* 2006; 24(29):4699–707.

113. Aghajanian C, Blank SV, Goff BA et al. OCEANS: A randomized, double-blind, placebo-controlled phase III trial of chemotherapy with or without bevacizumab in patients with platinum-sensitive recurrent epithelial ovarian, primary peritoneal, or fallopian tube cancer. *J Clin Oncol.* 2012; 30(17):2039–45.

114. Pujade-Lauraine E, Wagner U, Aavall-Lundqvist E et al. Pegylated liposomal Doxorubicin and Carboplatin compared with Paclitaxel and Carboplatin for patients with platinum-sensitive ovarian cancer in late relapse. *J Clin Oncol.* 2010; 28(20):3323–9.

115. ICON2: Randomised trial of single-agent carboplatin against three-drug combination of CAP (cyclophosphamide, doxorubicin, and cisplatin) in women with ovarian cancer. ICON Collaborators. International Collaborative Ovarian Neoplasm Study. *Lancet.* 1998;352(9140):1571–6.

116. Pujade-Lauraine E, Hilpert F, Weber B et al. Bevacizumab combined with chemotherapy for platinum-resistant recurrent ovarian

cancer: The AURELIA open-label randomized phase III trial. *J Clin Oncol.* 2014; 32(13):1302–8.

117. Gordon AN, Fleagle JT, Guthrie D et al. Recurrent epithelial ovarian carcinoma: A randomized phase III study of pegylated liposomal doxorubicin versus topotecan. *J Clin Oncol.* 2001; 19(14):3312–22.

118. Sharma R, Graham J, Mitchell H et al. Extended weekly dose-dense paclitaxel/carboplatin is feasible and active in heavily pretreated platinum-resistant recurrent ovarian cancer. *Br J Cancer.* 2009; 100(5):707–12.

119. van der Burg ME, de Wit R, van Putten WL et al. Weekly cisplatin and daily oral etoposide is highly effective in platinum pretreated ovarian cancer. *Br J Cancer.* 2002; 86(1):19–25.

120. Sieh W, Kobel M, Longacre TA et al. Hormone-receptor expression and ovarian cancer survival: An Ovarian Tumor Tissue Analysis consortium study. *Lancet Oncol.* 2013; 14(9):853–62.

121. Lindemann K, Gibbs E, Avall-Lundqvist E et al. Chemotherapy vs. tamoxifen in platinum-resistant ovarian cancer: A phase III, randomised, multicentre trial (Ovaresist). *Br J Cancer.* 2017; 116(4):455–63.

122. Gershenson DM, Bodurka DC, Coleman RL et al. Hormonal maintenance therapy for women with low-grade serous cancer of the ovary or peritoneum. *J Clin Oncol.* 2017; 35(10):1103–11.

123. Paleari L, Gandini S, Provinciali N et al. Clinical benefit and risk of death with endocrine therapy in ovarian cancer: A comprehensive review and meta-analysis. *Gynecol Oncol.* 2017; 146(3):504–13.

124. Aghajanian C, Goff B, Nycum LR et al. Final overall survival and safety analysis of OCEANS, a phase 3 trial of chemotherapy with or without bevacizumab in patients with platinum-sensitive recurrent ovarian cancer. *Gynecol Oncol.* 2015; 139(1):10–6.

125. Cannistra SA, Matulonis UA, Penson RT et al. Phase II study of bevacizumab in patients with platinum-resistant ovarian cancer or peritoneal serous cancer. *J Clin Oncol.* 2007; 25(33):5180–6.

126. Konstantinopoulos PA, Waggoner S, Vidal GA et al. Single-arm phases 1 and 2 trial of niraparib in combination with pembrolizumab in patients with recurrent platinum-resistant ovarian carcinoma. *JAMA Oncol.* 2019; 5(8):1141–9.

127. Liu JF, Barry WT, Birrer M et al. Combination cediranib and olaparib versus olaparib alone for women with recurrent platinum-sensitive ovarian cancer: A randomised phase 2 study. *Lancet Oncol.* 2014; 15(11):1207–14.

128. Matulonis UA, Shapira-Frommer R, Santin AD et al. Antitumor activity and safety of pembrolizumab in patients with advanced recurrent ovarian cancer: Results from the phase 2 KEYNOTE-100 study. *Ann Oncol.* 2019; 30(7):1080–7.

129. Hamanishi J, Mandai M, Ikeda T et al. Safety and antitumor activity of anti-PD-1 antibody, nivolumab, in patients with platinum-resistant ovarian cancer. *J Clin Oncol.* 2015; 33(34):4015–22.

130. Disis ML, Taylor MH, Kelly K et al. Efficacy and safety of avelumab for patients with recurrent or refractory ovarian cancer: Phase 1b results from the JAVELIN solid tumor trial. *JAMA Oncol.* 2019; 5(3):393–401.

131. Liu JF, Gordon M, Veneris J et al. Safety, clinical activity and biomarker assessments of atezolizumab from a Phase I study in advanced/recurrent ovarian and uterine cancers. *Gynecol Oncol.* 2019; 154(2):314–22.

132. Varga A, Piha-Paul S, Ott PA et al. Pembrolizumab in patients with programmed death ligand 1-positive advanced ovarian cancer: Analysis of KEYNOTE-028. *Gynecol Oncol.* 2019; 152(2):243–50.

133. Jimenez-Sanchez A, Memon D, Pourpe S et al. Heterogeneous tumor-immune microenvironments among differentially growing metastases in an ovarian cancer patient. *Cell.* 2017; 170(5):927–38 e20.

134. Bohm S, Faruqi A, Said I et al. Chemotherapy response score: Development and validation of a system to quantify histopathologic response to neoadjuvant chemotherapy in tubo-ovarian high-grade serous carcinoma. *J Clin Oncol.* 2015; 33(22):2457–63.

135. Peres LC, Cushing-Haugen KL, Kobel M et al. Invasive epithelial ovarian cancer survival by histotype and disease stage. *J Natl Cancer Inst.* 2019; 111(1):60–8.

136. Lawrie TA, Winter-Roach BA, Heus P, Kitchener HC. Adjuvant (post-surgery) chemotherapy for early stage epithelial ovarian cancer. *Cochrane Database Syst Rev.* 2015(12):CD004706.

137. Leake JF, Currie JL, Rosenshein NB, Woodruff JD. Long-term follow-up of serous ovarian tumors of low malignant potential. *Gynecol Oncol.* 1992; 47(2):150–8.

138. du Bois A, Ewald-Riegler N, de Gregorio N et al. Borderline tumours of the ovary: A cohort study of the Arbeitsgmeinschaft Gynakologische Onkologie (AGO) Study Group. *Eur J Cancer.* 2013; 49(8):1905–14.

139. Seidman JD, Kurman RJ. Ovarian serous borderline tumors: A critical review of the literature with emphasis on prognostic indicators. *Hum Pathol.* 2000; 31(5):539–57.

140. Snider DD, Stuart GC, Nation JG, Robertson DI. Evaluation of surgical staging in stage I low malignant potential ovarian tumors. *Gynecol Oncol.* 1991;40(2):129–32.

141. Gershenson DM. Management of ovarian germ cell tumors. *J Clin Oncol.* 2007; 25(20):2938–43.

142. Ray-Coquard I, Morice P, Lorusso D et al. Non-epithelial ovarian cancer: ESMO Clinical Practice Guidelines for diagnosis, treatment and follow-up. *Ann Oncol.* 2018; 29(Supplement_4):iv1-iv18.

143. Colombo N, Parma G, Zanagnolo V, Insinga A. Management of ovarian stromal cell tumors. *J Clin Oncol.* 2007; 25(20):2944–51.

144. Shah SP, Kobel M, Senz J et al. Mutation of FOXL2 in granulosa-cell tumors of the ovary. *N Engl J Med.* 2009; 360(26):2719–29.

145. Pilsworth JA, Cochrane DR, Xia Z et al. TERT promoter mutation in adult granulosa cell tumor of the ovary. *Mod Pathol.* 2018; 31(7):1107–15.

146. Heravi-Moussavi A, Anglesio MS, Cheng SW et al. Recurrent somatic DICER1 mutations in nonepithelial ovarian cancers. *N Engl J Med.* 2012; 366(3):234–42.

147. Rio Frio T, Bahubeshi A, Kanellopoulou C et al. DICER1 mutations in familial multinodular goiter with and without ovarian Sertoli-Leydig cell tumors. *JAMA.* 2011; 305(1):68–77.

148. Schumer ST, Cannistra SA. Granulosa cell tumor of the ovary. *J Clin Oncol.* 2003; 21(6):1180–9.

149. Brown J, Shvartsman HS, Deavers MT, Burke TW, Munsell MF, Gershenson DM. The activity of taxanes in the treatment of sex cord-stromal ovarian tumors. *J Clin Oncol.* 2004; 22(17):3517–23.

150. Homesley HD, Bundy BN, Hurteau JA, Roth LM. Bleomycin, etoposide, and cisplatin combination therapy of ovarian granulosa cell tumors and other stromal malignancies: A Gynecologic Oncology Group study. *Gynecol Oncol.* 1999; 72(2):131–7.

Useful websites

www.esmo.org/Guidelines/Gynaecological-Cancers/Newly-Diagnosed-and-Relapsed-Epithelial-Ovarian-Carcinoma

www.esmo.org/Guidelines-Practice/Clinical-Practice-Guidelines/Gynaecologic-Cancers/Non-Epithelial-Ovarian-Cancer

www.esmo.org/Guidelines/Gynaecological-Cancers/ESMO-ESGO-Consensus-Conference-Recommendations-on-Ovarian-Cancer

www.esmo.org/Guidelines/Hereditary-Syndromes/Prevention-and-Screening-in-BRCA-Mutation-Carriers-and-Other-Breast-Ovarian-Hereditary-Cancer-Syndromes

www.cancer.gov/types/ovarian

https://seer.cancer.gov/statfacts/html/ovary.html

www.ncin.org.uk/cancer_type_and_topic_specific_work/cancer_type_specific_work/gynaecological_cancer/gynaecological_cancer_hub/resources/ovarian_cancer

www.nice.org.uk/guidance

www.cancerresearchuk.org

www.cancer.net/cancer-types/ovarian-fallopian-tube-and-peritoneal-cancer

www.ovacome.org.uk

www.targetovariancancer.org.uk

https://ovarian.org.uk

www.ovariancancer.net.au

www.ovariancanada.org

20 UTERINE CANCER

Claudia von Arx, Hani Gabra, and Christina Fotopoulou

Epidemiology

Cancer of the endometrium or endometrial carcinoma (EC) is the most common gynecological malignancy in developed countries and the second most common in developing countries, where cervical cancer is more common.[1,2] It occurs most frequently in the sixth and seventh decades, with an approximate median age at presentation of 60 years. The lifetime risk of developing endometrial cancer is 3%. Stromal and mesenchymal sarcoma are uncommon subtypes of uterine neoplasms, accounting for 3% of them.[3,4]

In general, EC is associated with a favorable prognosis due to relatively early diagnosis through the symptom of vaginal bleeding/discharge. The 5-year survival rate for Stage I disease is approximately 80–90%, for Stage II it is 70–80%, and for Stages III and IV it is 20–60%.[5]

Malignant uterine epithelial tumors and uterine sarcoma have different clinicopathological and molecular features that require a different management. In this chapter, we focus on epithelial tumor types, including endometrioid adenocarcinoma (80–90%), serous carcinoma, clear cell carcinoma, undifferentiated/dedifferentiated carcinoma, and carcinosarcoma.

Risk factors, etiology, and pathogenesis

Risk factors for EC are excess of estrogen, obesity, early age at menarche and late age at menopause, nulliparity, polycystic ovary syndrome, treatment with tamoxifen, insulin resistance, and the Lynch syndrome.

Hormone-related risk factors and obesity

EC is associated with hormonally driven states in the majority of cases, with 80% of endometrial cancers being associated with either an excess of estrogen or a lack of progestin. In terms of etiology, a major cause of an estrogen/progestin imbalance is obesity, particularly through an increase in the level of aromatase in adipocytes, an enzyme that converts androgens and estradiol precursors into estrogen. Importantly, obesity is a cause of compound hormonal imbalance, not just excess estrogen but also dysregulation of the insulin/insulin-like growth factor (IGF) axis through insulin resistance/metabolic syndrome effects.

In fact, obesity is associated with increased insulin levels, which reduces the synthesis and blood levels of insulin-like growth factor binding protein 1 (IGFBP1) and IGFBP2, with a consequent increase of bioavailable IGF1. IGF1 can promote cellular proliferation and inhibit apoptosis in endometrial tissue.

In addition, insulin increases the levels of bioavailable estrogens through the reduction of sex-hormone-binding globulin in the blood.[6] Indeed, two epidemiological studies demonstrate that insulin resistance is an independent risk factor for endometrial cancer.[7,8]

In conclusion, the interaction of relative estrogen excess and activation of insulin signaling through insulin resistance associated with obesity can generate endometrial hyperplasia and ultimately, endometrial carcinogenesis.

Prolonged use of tamoxifen, a selective estrogen receptor modulator, is associated with a sevenfold increase in the development of EC and also of bowel cancer[9] in those patients who have previously had a carcinoma of the breast. However, other studies, such as the national Surgical Adjuvant Breast Cancer Prevention Trial, found a 29% increase in EC after treatment with tamoxifen, but this was not statistically significant.[10] Tamoxifen can also cause gene mutations through the production of tamoxifen–DNA adducts, and this could ultimately impact on tumorigenesis.[11]

Polycystic ovarian syndrome (PCOS), associated with high estradiol levels, can predispose younger women to develop EC due to the high number of anovulatory cycles resulting in unopposed estrogen production.[12] Therefore, adequate hormonal substitution, for example, with simple contraceptives or a progestin intrauterine device (IUD), should be considered to minimize risk.[13]

Genetic risk factors

The majority of ECs are caused by sporadic mutations. However, almost 5% of patients with EC have an inherited genetic mutation.

One genetic condition of practical importance is the Lynch syndrome/hereditary non-polyposis colorectal cancer syndrome (HNPCC). In individuals with Lynch syndrome, the following lifetime risks for cancer are seen: 52–82% for colorectal cancer; 25–60% for endometrial cancer in women; 6–13% for gastric cancer; and 4–12% for ovarian cancer.[14]

For women with EC, the Society of Gynecologic Oncologists in the United States advises genetic assessment for Lynch syndrome for those who meet any of the following criteria:

- EC diagnosed before age 50
- Presence of synchronous or metachronous colorectal, or other Lynch-associated, tumors, regardless of age
- EC with tumor infiltrating lymphocytes, peritumoral lymphocytes, or undifferentiated tumor histology, lower uterine segment origin diagnosed in a patient below age 60
- One or more first-degree relatives with a Lynch-associated tumor, with one of the cancers being diagnosed below age 50
- Endometrial or colorectal cancer diagnosed in two or more first- or second-degree relatives with Lynch-associated tumors regardless of age
- Patients with a first- or second-degree relative with a known germline mutation of a mismatch repair gene

In addition, in patients with Lynch syndrome, screening for defective DNA mismatch repair proteins (MMR) and/or microsatellite instability (MSI) should be suggested for a better clinical evaluation.

Prevention

Obesity is becoming increasingly important as a risk factor for EC in the general population. Large epidemiological studies demonstrate a close correlation between body mass index (BMI) and risk of endometrial cancer.[15,16] For this reason, maintenance of a healthy BMI is the strongest measure to prevent sporadic EC. For this reason, the concept of chemoprevention with intrauterine progestins for young women and bariatric surgery for obese women is an area of active discussion.

In high-risk women, such as women with Lynch syndrome, prophylactic hysterectomy with bilateral salpingo-oophorectomy (BSO) is an effective strategy for preventing endometrial cancer.[17]

Screening

There is no evidence that screening asymptomatic women in the general population reduces the mortality from EC.

However, in women with Lynch syndrome and their first-degree relatives, an annual screening with transvaginal ultrasound scanning and endometrial biopsy, could be offered. The screening for these women should start from the age of 35 years.

Histopathology and molecular biology

Endometrial hyperplasia is regarded as the precursor of most endometrioid ECs. Endometrial hyperplasia is mainly determined by unopposed estrogen exposure status, in which estrogen's proliferative effects are not counteracted by progesterone-like hormone's effects. Complex atypical hyperplasia carries approximately a 30% risk of malignant transformation.[18]

Malignant uterine epithelial tumors have an endometrioid growth pattern. There are two main types of EC. Type I, estrogen-related, usually presents histologically as a low-grade endometrioid tumor and is associated with atypical endometrial hyperplasia. These tumors account for approximately 80% of all ECs, and usually, they have a good prognosis. Type II tumors, non-estrogen-related, include Grade 3 endometrioid tumors as well as tumors of non-endometrioid histology, namely serous, clear cell, mucinous, squamous, transitional cell, mesonephric, and undifferentiated carcinoma. These account for 10–20% of EC, and they often have a poor prognosis. A precursor lesion is rarely identified for Type II tumors. Patients presenting with Type II tumors are often older and multiparous.[18]

Type I and Type II EC have differing molecular profiles. Type I carcinomas are mainly characterized by silencing of the PTEN gene, genetic alteration in KRAS, PIK3CA, and β-catenin, and also MSI, whereas Type II serous carcinomas typically harbor TP53 mutations, inactivation of the p16 gene, low expression of E-cadherin and over-expression/amplification of Her2 in a defined subgroup.[19] Molecular features of uterine clear cell carcinomas are still not well defined; however, mutations in the ARID1A gene appear to be a frequent event in this histological subgroup.[20]

Interestingly, The Cancer Genome Atlas (TCGA) Research network has performed a large genomic characterization on 373 samples of EC and has suggested a new molecular classification.[21] This classification divides EC into four molecular subgroups:

- POLE ultra-mutated tumors, characterized by POLE (Polymerase Epsilon) exonuclease domain mutations, with a high percentage of C>A transversions, a low percentage of C>G transversions, and more than 500 single nucleotide variants. Clinically, they are characterized by a very favorable outcome.
- Microsatellite instability hypermutated tumors, characterized by defects of the DNA mismatch repair system, high mutation frequency, and PTEN and KRAS mutation. The mismatch repair deficiency is most commonly secondary to

methylation of MLH1. These types of tumors are frequently associated with inherited cancer syndromes—e.g., Lynch syndrome—and clinically, MSI is regarded as a predictive marker of response to immunotherapy; for instance, microsatellite instability-high tumor status (MSI-H) forms the basis of a tumor agnostic Food and Drug Administration (FDA) label for the PD-1 blocking antibody pembrolizumab. The outcome is relatively good.

- Copy-number high tumors, also named serous-like tumors. This type is characterized by high copy-number alterations, mutations in TP53, FBXW7, and PPP2R1A, and clinically, by a poor outcome.
- Copy-number low tumors, characterized by genomic stability, MMR-proficiency, and a moderate number of mutations, mostly within the PI3K/Akt and Wnt signaling pathways. Clinically, the outcome is relatively good.

This classification has acquired clinical relevance especially because of its prognostic role (see next section) and its predictive role for response to immunotherapy.

Pathologic and molecular features affecting prognosis

Several non-staging pathologic features may affect the treatment and management of EC.

In the case of a carcinoma involving only an endometrial polyp: Prognosis is in general more favorable. Such carcinomas have an excellent prognosis, especially when they are of endometrioid histology and carry a low risk of lymph node metastasis; thus, extensive staging (e.g., lymph node dissection [LND]) is generally not performed. Caution should be exercised here, however, in cases of polypectomy specimens or outpatient biopsies without endometrial curettings, as this may underestimate the true extent of disease in other areas of the uterus. The coincidence of EC in a polyp does not imply that endometrial polyps are premalignant. Their association is due to the fact that endometrial polyps, carcinoma, and cancer precursors (endometrial intraepithelial neoplasia) arise at higher risk in the setting of persistent estrogen exposure (anovulatory cycles or obesity).[22]

In the case of EC confined to the polyp but of serous subtype, patients will still require a full staging procedure to determine prognosis and the true stage and extent of the disease, as serous EC has been historically considered to be an aggressive neoplasm even in the absence of myometrial invasion.[23] Interestingly, some data suggest that properly staged patients with Stage IA serous carcinoma and no residual disease at hysterectomy have a good prognosis, with no recurrence at up to 170 months' follow-up (median: 38 months) even if no platinum-based adjuvant treatment is subsequently given. In cases where residual tumor was found in the hysterectomy specimen, patients treated with platinum-based chemotherapy had a significantly more favorable prognosis compared with those who merely received follow-up.[24]

Pelvic/peritoneal washing cytology: Pelvic/peritoneal washing cytology is a way of assessing microscopic peritoneal spread. The role of peritoneal cytology as a strong independent prognostic factor has failed to be established, especially after diagnostic hysteroscopy, and is therefore not included in the new Federation Internationale de Gynecologie et d'Obstetrique (FIGO) classification of uterine cancers and does not influence indication for adjuvant treatment. In only a minority of patients, positive washings are the only evidence of neoplasm outside the endometrium. However, most clinicians will not change management based on positive peritoneal washings. It has not been established that positive cytology without other evidence of extra-uterine disease or other high risk factors indicates an increased risk of recurrence.[25]

Lymphatic or blood vessel invasion (LVI): LVI is not part of the formal staging system of endometrial carcinomas and is most often seen in high-stage (node positive) disease. Thus, when lymph node sampling is not performed, LVI may prompt either additional investigations or additional therapy. LVI is less prognostically significant in well-staged, early (node-negative) disease. Although associated with deep myometrial invasion (Stage pT1c), high-grade or non-endometrioid histology, and tumor size greater than 2 cm, LVI is not an independent predictor of distant failure and death.

This probably reflects the fact that once the neoplasm has invaded (beyond its compartment, beyond the basement membrane), it has access to lymph (extracellular fluid) and may metastasize distantly whether or not it is seen in preformed spaces (lymphatics/vessels).

ProMisE molecular classifier: ProMisE (Proactive Molecular Risk Classifier for Endometrial Cancer) is a pragmatic molecular classifier recently validated as a prognostic tool for endometrial cancer.[26] Based on the TCGA subgroups and using clinically applicable methods (i.e., immunohistochemistry for MMR proteins and p53 and sequencing for POLE exonuclease domain mutations), ProMisE identifies four prognostic molecular subtypes of EC. The four groups are similar but not identical to the TCGA ones and comprise MMR-D (deficiency) type, POLE EDMs type, p53 wild type (wt), and p53 aberrant (abn) type. POLE subtype tumors have the most favorable outcomes, whereas p53abn tumors have the worst prognosis. MMR-D and p53wt are the two intermediate subtypes in terms of outcomes, with p53wt subtype having a more favorable outcome when compared with MMR-D.

This molecular classification can be applied to diagnostic specimens,[27,28] such as endometrial biopsy and curettage, providing early information to guide the decision-making.

Although not yet formally included in the guidelines risk-stratification system, ProMisE is a very promising tool to enable a more informed management of patients with EC, including identification of patients who are more likely to benefit from checkpoint inhibitors, adjuvant treatment, and surgical vs. non-surgical management.

Diagnosis

Symptoms

In 75–90% of postmenopausal patients, initial symptoms will include postmenopausal bleeding (PMB) or vaginal discharge, which are the characteristic symptoms even for early EC and should therefore be investigated via hysteroscopy and fractionated curettage despite the fact that overall, the majority of abnormal uterine bleeding is due to benign conditions. Three to twenty percent of women with PMB are found to have EC, and another 5–15% have endometrial hyperplasia. Occasionally, women with EC who have no abnormal uterine bleeding present with abnormal findings on cervical cytology. Among women with EC, 68% are diagnosed with disease confined to the uterus, and these have a 96% 5-year survival rate.[29]

In premenopausal women with any abnormal uterine bleeding, including intermenstrual bleeding, frequent (interval between the onset of bleeding episodes less than 21 days), heavy (total volume of >80 mL), or prolonged (longer than 7 days) bleeding should be investigated further to exclude malignancy.

Other symptoms due to a pelvic mass lesion may occur in higher-stage tumors, such as hydronephrosis in extensive cervical and parametrial involvement, or even ascites in cases with peritoneal metastasis associated with typically serous papillary carcinoma.

Investigation

Clinical assessment will include abdominal and pelvic examination with speculum to assess cervical and vaginal status, along with transvaginal and transabdominal ultrasound to assess endometrial thickness, uterine size, hydronephrosis, ascites, and concomitant ovarian lesions. A direct biopsy can be taken in the clinic, for example, by pipelle or other commercial aspirators, when the endometrial thickness is greater than 5 mm[30]; however, the diagnostic efficacy of a pipelle or a solitary biopsy alone can be limited and wrongly negative. In the prospective Gynaecologic Oncology Group (GOG) 167 trial evaluating almost 300 patients, an incidence of 26% of coexistent cancer together with atypical hyperplasia was described in hysterectomy specimens, whereas in 30% of the cases, an upgrading of the initial hyperplasia to cancer occurred. For that reason, fractionated curettage is the gold standard of the diagnostic algorithm of patients with PMB.[31]

In the presence of malignant histology in the curettage, a further imaging to exclude distant metastases and demonstrate potential lymph node involvement should be performed (i.e., computed tomography [CT] of the chest and abdomen and magnetic resonance imaging [MRI] of the pelvis).

Staging and tumor classification

The FIGO 2009 staging system evolves in several ways from the chronologically prior descriptions in terms of value of cytology, classification of extension of cervical (stroma) involvement, and myometrial involvement: Endocervical glandular involvement is considered as Stage I, while positive cytology is reported separately without changing the stage. Stage IC has been discontinued, with Stage IB including myometrial invasion >50% thickness. A simplified version of the FIGO 2009 staging of uterine cancer is given in Table 20.1.

TABLE 20.1   FIGO 2009 Endometrial Cancer Staging

Stage	Definition
I	**Tumor confined to the corpus uteri**
Ia	Tumor confined to the uterus or invading less than half the myometrium
Ib	Tumor confined to the uterus or invading more than half the myometrium
II	**Tumor invading cervical stroma but not extending beyond the uterus**
III	**Tumor with local or regional extension**
IIIa	Tumor invades serosa or adnexa
IIIb	Vaginal and/or parametrial involvement
IIIc1	Pelvic node involvement
IIIc2	Para-aortic involvement
IV	**Tumor with extension to bladder and/or bowel mucosa and/or distant metastases**
IVa	Tumor invading bladder and/or bowel mucosa
IVb	Distant metastases including abdominal metastases and/or inguinal lymph nodes

Source: Adapted from Colombo et al., 2016.

Treatment

The treatment plan should be decided by a multidisciplinary team, with full consideration of diagnosis, stage, grade, medical history and comorbidities of each patient. The patient should be informed of the risks and benefits associated with each method of treatment. Patients should always be considered for and offered participation in clinical trials as part of the treatment package where appropriate.

Surgery

It has been shown that staging procedures performed by a surgical gynecological oncologist and overall management performed by gynecological oncology multidisciplinary specialist teams appear to lead to better patient outcomes, especially in metastatic or advanced disease.[32] If a gynecological oncologist is not available in an incidental finding of EC, and the surgeon is not experienced in operative management of the cancer (e.g., lymphadenectomy), a two-stage procedure should be considered with a specialist available for the second procedure. Surgery including at least total abdominal hysterectomy either open or laparoscopic and BSO is the gold standard in patients with EC in the absence of distant metastases, in which case complete tumor debulking in combination with systemic and/or radiotherapy treatment or palliative symptom control is the primary aim.

The traditional approach for surgical treatment of primary EC has involved the laparotomy approach. Nevertheless, clinical practice has demonstrated excellent results with total laparoscopic approaches, especially in the common EC population, which includes older and obese patients. This has been confirmed in the large prospective randomized LAP study, which compared open versus laparoscopic hysterectomy for EC and included more than 2600 women with clinically early-stage EC. The study confirmed the clinical experience of shorter hospital stays, fewer perioperative complications, reduced blood loss, and improved body image in patients who underwent laparoscopic surgery.[33] Laparoscopic surgery took longer, and there was a 26% conversion rate to laparotomy, with obesity being the strongest risk factor; metastatic disease was identified in 17% of patients in both groups. This provided reassurance that an initial laparoscopic approach does not compromise surgical staging. Even though the recurrence and survival rates were not significantly different between both arms, the study was deemed inconclusive because laparoscopy could not be demonstrated with 95% confidence to have a hazard ratio (HR) below the predetermined threshold of 1.4 for non-inferiority.[34] However, even so, the laparoscopic approach should be considered in apparent early-stage disease, taking into consideration the size of the uterus, extent of the disease, and the comorbidity profile of the individual patient.

Robotic surgery could also be an alternative to laparoscopy.[35,36] Of note, a study conducted on 50 obese women affected by EC showed that robotic surgery appeared to be better than laparoscopic surgery in terms of operating time, estimated blood loss, mean hospital stay, and operative complications.[37] This suggests that robotic surgery has a well-defined role in the treatment of EC, especially in obese women.

In advanced stages, and in the case of tumor dissemination within the peritoneal cavity, maximal effort tumor debulking similar to peritoneally disseminated ovarian cancer can be considered to obtain complete tumor resection whenever possible and when an acceptable morbidity profile can be anticipated.

Role of lymph node dissection

The value and the surgical extent of pelvic and para-aortic LND is one of the most controversial topics in the management of EC.[38] There is a lack of standardization regarding not only the surgical technique but also the primary purpose of the procedure and indeed, for which cases LND needs to be performed at all.[38] We have no prospective evidence so far about any potential therapeutic value of LND in endometrial cancer. Its remit is probably within a prognostic value to determine and tailor the necessity and type of adjuvant treatment. The decision to perform systematic pelvic or para-aortic lymphadenectomy appears to reflect the individual surgeon's preferences based on their personal experience and surgical expertise, patients' comorbidity profile, including BMI, and age.

Two prospectively randomized trials failed to identify any survival benefit of pelvic LND in EC, despite the fact that systematic pelvic lymphadenectomy improved surgical staging, as statistically significantly more patients with lymph node metastases were found in the lymphadenectomy arm than in the no-lymphadenectomy arm (13.3% versus 3.2%, difference = 10.1%, 95% confidence interval (CI) = 5.3–14.9%, $p < 0.001$).[39]

Through numerous mapping studies, it has been demonstrated that if EC has extended to a para-aortic node, the majority of metastases are in the area between the renal veins and the inferior mesenteric artery (IMA).[40] Mariani et al. found in a prospective assessment of more than 400 EC patients that 77% of the patients with para-aortic lymphatic spread had positive lymph nodes in the area above the IMA.[41] Therefore, when para-aortic LND is indicated, it should not be limited to the space below the IMA.

Nevertheless, defining the value of systematic LND in EC will always be challenged by the level of surgical quality and skills required for dissection in the high para-aortic area, an obstacle that is widely prevalent in multicenter international surgical trials, where the surgical requirements are often lowered to facilitate the inclusiveness of investigators and enhance enrollment.[42] Three planned prospectively randomized trials initiated by the GOG, the National Cancer Research Institute (NCRI), and the Arbeitsgemeinschaft Gynaekologische Onkologie (AGO) with parallel recruitment will attempt to definitively answer this unresolved issue of the role and extent of pelvic and para-aortic LND in EC and how the LND status will be able to determine adjuvant treatment.

Clinical high-risk features that are associated with higher risk of LN metastases are high tumor grade, deep myometrial invasion, tumor size >2 cm, cervical extension, and serous or clear cell histology.[38]

Modern approaches, like laparoscopic extra-peritoneal access or robotic surgery, may decrease the operative morbidity of LND in EC, even though tailoring of surgical treatment to patients' comorbidity profile and biological age should always be very carefully taken into consideration before planning of optimal surgical treatment.[43]

Adjuvant treatment

Adjuvant treatment applies to patients who have undergone hysterectomy for early (Stage I or II) uterine adenocarcinoma and to selected patients with a completely resected Stage III disease.

Currently, there is debate worldwide regarding the optimal treatment of EC. National guidelines differ significantly in the indication for chemotherapy and radiotherapy, and all trials so far have failed to bring consistency of optimal treatment regimens for the disease.

British Gynaecological Cancer Society (BGCS) recommendations for EC treatment[44] are summarized in the treatment algorithm at the end of the chapter. The results of the trials that have led to these recommendations are discussed in the following paragraphs.

In general, the decision-making about treatment should take into account the class of risk of the patient. In 2013, European Society for Medical Oncology (ESMO) guidelines proposed a stratification of the risk based on the new FIGO 2009 staging system.[45] Recently, a refined classification has been proposed and published after the ESMO–European Society of Gynaecological Oncology (ESGO)–European Society for Radiotherapy and Oncology (ESTRO) Consensus Conference.[46] This new classification has highlighted the prognostic role of lymphovascular space invasion (LVSI) and Grade 3 (G3) differentiation, consequently dividing the pre-existing intermediate risk group into intermediate-risk and high-intermediate-risk EC. For simplicity, the two classifications are reported in Table 20.2 with the differences in bold. Molecular factors, such the ones considered in the PromMisE system (MMR, TP53, and POLE EDMs),[26] are not incorporated in these risk classifications; however, their prognostic value has been recently validated,[26] so it is likely that in the near future, new classifications incorporating clinicopathological and molecular factors will be proposed.

Adjuvant treatment for low-risk EC

Women with low-grade (G1–2) endometrioid cancers confined to the endometrium are classified as having low-risk EC. The overall probability of recurrence in these groups is very low following surgical treatment alone, with a 5-year recurrence rate of 2.6%.[47] Postoperative vaginal brachytherapy (VBT) failed to demonstrate an advantage in disease recurrence control and overall survival (OS) when compared with postoperative observation alone in low-risk EC.[48] Similarly, endocrine therapy has not shown any advantages in terms of OS compared with observation in randomized settings; instead, an increase of thromboembolic events was noticed in association with endocrine therapy.[49] In conclusion, there is no evidence to support benefit from adjuvant therapy for patients with low-risk EC.

Adjuvant treatment for intermediate-risk EC

The intermediate risk group is a highly heterogeneous group; this heterogeneity impacts on the large clinical trials (PORTEC and GOG trials) conducted to evaluate the role of adjuvant treatment for this group and ultimately, the decision-making regarding their management.

In particular, these trials identified patients with an increased risk of recurrence of EC within the intermediate-risk population. This group of patients was defined as the high-intermediate-risk (HIR) group. However, the factors used to define the HIR group were unsurprisingly similar but non-identical in the PORTEC and GOG trials, making generalization for clinical use difficult to define.

The PORTEC trials defined the HIR group as patients with two of three clinicopathologic factors present: age >60 years, outer half myometrial invasion, and G3 histology.[50]

In contrast, the GOG defined HIR based on age and any of three pathologic factors[51]: the presence of deep myometrial invasion, G2-3 histology or the presence of LVSI. Women ≥70 years are defined as having HIR with one risk factor, age 50–69 years with two risk factors, and age ≥18 years and <50 with all three risk factors.

For this reason, in 2016, the ESMO-ESGO-ESTRO panel of experts generated a standardized sub-classification within the intermediate-risk EC clearly defining the characteristics of intermediate and HIR groups. This sub-classification was based on the results of PORTEC-1, GOG99, and ASTEC/EN5 trials[50–52] and a subsequent meta-analysis.[53] Patients with intermediate-risk EC have an excellent prognosis with only low recurrence rates: maximum 6% without adjuvant therapy. On the contrary, patients with HIR EC have a recurrence risk that can be as high as 30% without adjuvant treatment and which can be lowered to 5% with adjuvant radiation.[54] However, OS can be expected to be above 80%, regardless of the radiotherapy (RT).

The indication for the optimal adjuvant treatment depends on the accuracy and quality of surgical staging, which defines the confidence in the true staging of the disease. In patients with adequately staged and hence, true intermediate-risk disease, VBT could be an option to reduce vaginal recurrence, whereas pelvic external beam radiotherapy (EBRT) is not recommended due to the high toxicity.[46] This recommendation is based on the PORTEC-2 trial and its 10-year updated follow-up results. In this trial, the majority of enrolled women had a G1–2 EC with myometrial invasion ≥50% and without LVSI; EC that following the current consensus classification, is now considered intermediate risk. In these patients, VBT has been compared with EBRT, showing a non-inferiority in terms of 10-year vaginal recurrence rate (3.4% vs. 2.4% in VBT and EBRT, respectively, $p = 0.55$) and OS (69.5% vs. 67.6%, $p = 0.42$)[55] and a better toxicity profile. However, given the overall good prognosis of intermediate-risk patients following surgical treatment, and the little benefit gained from adjuvant RT, observation can be also considered, especially in patients aged below 60.

TABLE 20.2   **Stratification of Endometrial Cancer Risk of Recurrence**

ESMO 2013		ESMO-ESGO-ESTRO	
Risk Group	**Description**	**Risk Group**	**Description**
Low	Stage Ia, G1–2	Low	Stage Ia endometrioid, G1–2, **LVSI negative**
	Stage Ib, G1		
Intermediate	Stage Ia, G3	**Intermediate**	**Stage Ib, endometrioid, G1–2, LVSI negative**
	Stage Ib, G2		
High	Stage Ib, G3	**High-intermediate**	**Stage Ia, endometrioid, G3, regardless of LVSI status**
	Non-endometrioid		**Stage I endometrioid, G1–2, LVSI unequivocally positive**
		High	Stage Ib, endometrioid, G3 regardless of LVSI status
			Stage II
			Stage III, endometrioid, no residual disease
			Non-endometrioid

For women with HIR disease, RT has been clearly shown to reduce the risk of pelvic recurrence, although it has failed to demonstrate improved OS or rate of distant metastases.

PORTEC-1, GOG99, ASTEC/EN5 trials and the subsequent meta-analysis[50–53] evaluated the role of EBRT as adjuvant treatment and have confirmed a reduction in pelvic recurrence, but not OS benefit, in patients treated with post-surgery EBRT when compared with observation. The patients presenting with HIR disease were the ones that benefited more from the EBRT treatment.

In the non-inferiority PORTEC2-trial, VBT and EBRT were equally effective in ensuring vaginal control, and there were no statistical differences in disease-free survival (DFS) and OS in patients treated with VBT versus EBRT.[55] However, fewer gastrointestinal toxic effects (13% versus 54% for BT and EBRT, respectively), but significantly higher recurrence of pelvic nodes, have been shown in the VBT arm.

The combination of EBRT and VBT has been evaluated in a Swedish trial, and the combination has been shown to significantly reduce the 5-year locoregional relapse rates (1.5% vs. 5 %, $p = 0.013$), with rates of vaginal recurrence of 1.9% vs. 2.7% in the combination and VBT alone arm, respectively; however, no statistical difference in OS or DFS has been shown. In addition, late cumulative toxicity was significantly different in favor of VBT.[56]

In conclusion, VBT should be the adjuvant treatment of choice for patients with EC of HIR risk.[46]

With respect to the role of adjuvant chemotherapy to reduce disease relapse, there are not enough data to justify toxicity from systemic chemotherapy over radiotherapy.

In a Japanese GOG trial, 425 women with EC that had at least 50% myometrial invasion were randomly assigned to treatment with whole pelvic RT versus three or more courses of cyclophosphamide, doxorubicin, and cisplatin (CAP) chemotherapy.[57] CAP was not associated with any improvement in progression-free survival (PFS) or OS in the low-intermediate-risk cohort. However, among women in the high- to intermediate-risk group, defined as G3 EC, cervical stromal invasion, or cases with positive peritoneal cytology, the CAP group had a significantly higher PFS rate (83.8% versus 66.2%, $p = 0.024$, HR = 0.44) and OS rate (89.7% versus 73.6%, $p = 0.006$, HR = 0.24).

Participation in future trials has to be encouraged to define the role of systemic treatment in this specific group of patients who appear to benefit from systemic cytotoxic chemotherapy.

The combination of systemic treatment and RT has also been recently tested and compared with radiotherapy alone in a randomized Phase III trial of the American GOG (GOG 249), the results of which were presented at the 2019 ASCO conference. This trial has shown that pelvic RT compared with vaginal cuff brachytherapy followed by paclitaxel and carboplatin (VCB/C) in patients with high-intermediate- and high-risk Stage I or Stage II EC had similar outcomes in terms of vaginal and distant recurrence, with a statistically significantly higher number of pelvic and para-aortic recurrences in the VCB/C arm. VCB/C was not superior to pelvic RT with respect to OS, with the latter regimen having a lower rate of severe acute toxicities.[58] Thus, RT alone remains an appropriate treatment for high-intermediate- and high-risk early-stage EC; however, further trials, to test different combinations and doses, are needed.

Where complete staging has not been performed at primary surgery, there has been a debate about two approaches: either performing a second staging procedure to define the lymph node status and then consequently treating accordingly (N0 versus N1) or treating all patients on the assumption that they have involved lymph nodes.

The final decision regarding the optimal treatment approach should be based on the comorbidity status of the patient and therefore, the derived surgical morbidity profile as well as patient choice after thorough discussion of the current evidence with the patient.

Adjuvant treatment for high-risk EC

Women with high-risk EC are at an increased risk of disease progression and death, even when detected at an early stage. High-risk ECs are a very heterogeneous group, which includes tumors with different histology, i.e., endometrioid cancers, serous, clear cell, and carcinosarcomas. Beyond histologic subtype, prognosis is highly dependent on both stage and tumor grade (which is by definition high for Type II cancers). The Surveillance, Epidemiology and End Results (SEER) study of more than 44,000 women identified 5-year survival as high as 97%, 80%, 60%, and 25% for Stage I, II, III, and IV disease, respectively.[59] Among women with Stage III disease, 5-year relative survival is 83%, 68%, and 48% for Grade 1, 2, and 3 adenocarcinomas, respectively.

For high-risk patients, pelvic EBRT is the standard therapy. Controversy exists over the role of the addition of chemotherapy (CT) and/or brachytherapy to EBRT, or the use of chemotherapy instead of the RT.

The role of chemotherapy has been evaluated in several clinical trials. An Italian and a Japanese trial (JGOG 2033),[57,60] both comparing postoperative pelvic EBRT with platinum-based chemotherapy (CAP) and both conducted on a very similar population of patients with high-risk EC, have shown no difference in DFS or in OS. In general, EBRT was more effective in local recurrence control, whereas the chemotherapy better controlled distant metastasis recurrence. The toxicity rate of the two treatments was similar in the Italian study, whereas in the JGOG 2033, the reported G3–G4 toxicity rate was threefold higher in the chemotherapy arm (4.7% vs. 1.6%).

With respect to the combination treatment of CT and RT, a 20-year-old GOG trial showed no benefit from the addition of adjuvant doxorubicin to surgery and postoperative pelvic EBRT.[61] Conversely, a combined analysis of the NSGO 9501/EORTC 55991 and MaNGO-ILIADE III trials, with a total of 534 patients, has reported a significant improvement in 5-year DFS (78% versus 69%, $p = 0.009$) and a trend towards improved OS (82% versus 75%, $p = 0.07$) in the association arm.[62] However, there was significant criticism of this study related to the variability in the treatment administration schedule and sequencing (CT administered before or after the RT, RT administered as pelvic EBRT ± VBT, CT with cisplatin and adriamycin or carboplatin and paclitaxel) and also the lack of definition of important clinicopathological information (disease grade and post-surgical nodal status). However, in a subsequent metanalysis, which compared no additional treatment with platinum-based chemotherapy post-surgery and RT, a significant increase in OS (HR 0.74) in DFS (HR 0.75), with a death and distant progression absolute risk reduction of 4% and 5% respectively, has been demonstrated with the addition of chemotherapy.[63]

A triplet platinum-based chemotherapy regimen (cisplatin, doxorubicin, and paclitaxel) following surgery and RT does not provide a significant increase of DFS and is characterized by a higher toxicity profile compared with a doublet chemotherapy (cisplatin and doxorubicin).[64] Thus, in the combination treatment, a triplet regimen is not suggested or pursued in practice.

In the combined treatment, chemotherapy can be also administrated concurrently with RT. Promising results were found in the RTOG 9708 Phase II study, in which patients were treated with concurrent pelvic RT and cisplatin (two cycles) followed by a further four cycles of cisplatin. The trial reported 4-year OS rates of 85% for the overall high-risk population and 77% for patients with Stage III EC, and thus concluded that concurrent CT-RT treatment is a feasible approach for high-risk EC.[65] Given these positive results, the PORTEC-3 trial was designed to compare platinum-based chemoradiation plus adjuvant chemotherapy versus RT alone, whereas GOG 258 was designed to compare cisplatin-based chemoradiation plus adjuvant chemotherapy versus chemotherapy alone.[66,67] The PORTEC-3 trial was conducted in high-risk EC Stage I, II, and III, and 5-year updated results have recently been published. A significant improvement in 5-year OS (absolute improvement 5%, HR 0.70) and failure-free survival (FFS) (absolute improvement 7%, HR 0.70) has been reported with chemoradiotherapy; in particular, the benefit was more pronounced in women with serous cancers (absolute improvement of 19% [HR 0.48] and 12% [HR 0.42] in OS and FFS, respectively) and in patients with Stage III disease (HR 0.63 for OS, HR 0.62 for FFS). Conversely, in patients with Stage I–II disease, only a small absolute improvement of 2% and 4% in OS and FFS, respectively, has been documented with chemoradiotherapy versus RT alone.[66]

The role of concurrent chemoradiotherapy in Stage III–IV R0 disease has been further evaluated in the GOG 258 trial. In this trial, the comparison was made between chemoradiotherapy and chemotherapy alone. No differences in recurrence-free survival and OS were found (HR 0.90),[67] and a significantly worse quality of life (QOL) and gastrointestinal toxicity were documented by a subsequent analysis of patient-reported outcomes in the combination arm.[68] However, a significantly higher rate of vaginal recurrences (HR 0.36) and local recurrences (HR 0.43) was reported in patients treated with chemotherapy alone.[67]

In conclusion, taking the results of these trials together, the addition of chemotherapy to RT should be considered in adjuvant treatment of high-risk Stage III–IV R0 patients. However, the pros and cons of this combination should be discussed with patients as part of a joint decision between oncologists and their patients. The evidence is neither clear nor unanimous regarding the addition of chemotherapy to RT in the treatment of high-risk Stage I–II patients.

Regarding the addition of VBT to EBRT, there is no evidence of benefit in terms of local recurrence or OS rates in high-risk Stage I and Stage II endometrial cancer,[55,65,69–72] whereas a survival benefit was reported in patients with Stage IIIC disease and direct extension to the vagina.[73] Clarity on the indication and role of VBT in addition to ERBT was not achieved except in the rare situation of vaginal extension of the disease.

Lastly, in the GOG122 trial, women with Stage III or IV EC with a residual disease limited to <2 cm were considered eligible and were randomly assigned to treatment with whole abdominal radiation therapy (WART) or doxorubicin plus cisplatin.[74] The systemic chemotherapy arm was associated with a significantly higher 5-year PFS (42% versus 38%) and 5-year OS (53% versus 42%) compared with WART, even though a higher pelvic recurrence rate was documented in the chemotherapy arm (18% versus 13% with WART). These results could suggest that chemotherapy should be considered for microscopic (<2 cm) residual disease.

Treatment of advanced and recurrent disease

In patients with initially advanced-stage disease or with recurrent disease, it has been shown that women benefit from total macroscopic tumor clearance, when possible, regardless of histologic subtype. However, these data are mainly of a retrospective nature.[75–78]

The value of local tumor resection in women with multiple distant parenchymatous metastases (i.e., lung or liver metastases) has never been established and is performed typically only for local palliative control, for example to alleviate symptoms like bleeding or bowel obstruction.

In patients with recurrences confined to the vagina or pelvis, RT (EBRT plus brachytherapy) should be considered if no prior EBRT at recurrence site was given, whereas surgery can be offered if the patient received previous EBRT treatment.[46] In a post-recurrence analysis of the PORTEC-1 trial, the combination of EBRT and brachytherapy, given after vaginal recurrence to RT naïve patients, has been shown to provide a remission rate of 89%, with 77% of patients remaining disease free at 44 months.[50]

Palliative RT should be used in metastatic disease to alleviate the symptoms secondary to metastasis, for example bleeding, painful nodes, and bone metastasis.

Chemotherapy plays an important role in advanced and recurrent EC due to the chemo-sensitive nature of this disease. The most active agents are anthracyclines, platinum-based drugs, and taxanes, with a response rate of almost 20% achieved with each of these drugs in monotherapy. However, doublet and triplet chemotherapy regimens have shown better results when compared with monotherapy. In particular, the combination of cisplatin and doxorubicin has shown a higher response rate (43–41% versus 17–25%) than doxorubicin alone, even if no benefit of OS and worse toxicity (myelotoxicity and nausea/vomiting) have been reported.[79,80]

The triplet with paclitaxel, cisplatin, and doxorubicin (TAP) was compared in many trials with the doublet paclitaxel and platinum agents (cisplatin or carboplatin) or doxorubicin and cisplatin. The results of these trials were variable in terms of PFS and OS, but the toxicity of the triplet was always higher than that of the doublet.

In particular, the GOG 177 study compared TAP+G-CSF combination therapy with AP[81]; TAP was significantly superior to AP, with a higher objective response rate (ORR) (57% versus 34%, respectively, $p < 0.01$) and PFS 8.3 versus 5.3 months, respectively, $p < 0.01$) and a small but significant improvement in OS (15.3 versus 12.3 months, respectively, $p = 0.037$). However, given the significantly higher G2–3 toxicity in the TAP arm (39% versus 5%), the conclusion that TAP could be the standard therapeutic choice was not supported. The GOG 184 trial showed that TAP did not improve PFS compared with AP and was associated again with a worsened toxicity profile.[82] The OS results are still pending. Lastly, in GOG 209, the triplet TAP has been compared with the doublet carboplatin and paclitaxel.[83] The results of this trial indicated that the combination carboplatin and paclitaxel is non-inferior to TAP, showing an equivalent overall response rate (51.2% versus 51.3%) and similar PFS (13.5 versus 13.3 months) and OS but a significantly better toxicity profile.

In conclusion, a platinum-based doublet should be considered in patients with advanced or recurrent EC. The most frequently used doublet is currently paclitaxel and carboplatin for its more favorable toxicity profile; doxorubicin/cisplatin is an alternative choice.

Regarding the use of combination chemoradiotherapy in advanced-stage disease, one has to balance the combined toxicity that is associated with such an approach with the palliative status of the patients, their comorbidity profile, and the questionable survival benefit. Multiple single-arm clinical trials have demonstrated the feasibility of combined modality treatment, but there are only limited data from retrospective studies showing that combined modality treatment improves outcomes compared with chemotherapy alone.[65,84,85]

There is more limited evidence for second-line chemotherapy to treat recurrence after platinum-based therapy, with various regimens (ifosfamide [ORR 24.3%], oxaliplatin [ORR 13.5%], pegylated liposomal doxorubicin [ORR 9.5%], topotecan [ORR 9%], or docetaxel [ORR 7.7%]) tested in this setting but not in randomized trials.[86–89] Thus, there is no a standard of care for second-line chemotherapy in EC. Currently, the NCCN guidelines suggest that pembrolizumab could be considered in recurrent MSI-H/dMMR EC, and this indication is also under evaluation for U.K. guidelines.

Endocrine therapy

The normal endometrium proliferates in response to estrogen, whereas increasing concentrations of progestogens secreted by the corpus luteum in pregnancy allow atrophy and metaplasia of the endometrium to form the decidua. Similar effects in EC follow the use of supra-physiological doses of progestogens (e.g., megestrol 160 mg daily, medroxyprogesterone acetate 200 bid or tds), with induction of apoptosis, which requires intact apoptotic pathways.[90–93] However, a clear limitation of progestogen efficacy is due to the negative feedback on the progesterone receptor (PR), and the consequent rapid downregulation of PR, induced by progestin therapy. PR is a predictive factor for progestin response, and its downregulation is not only observed in response to progestin therapy; it is also a structural feature of the endometrial cancer epigenome, with more than 70% of cases demonstrating methylation of the PR gene. These observations have led to conceptual advances such as the addition of tamoxifen to progestin, as tamoxifen upregulates PR expression, and also the exploration of epigenetic strategies for demethylation (decitabine) or histone modification (histone deacetylase [HDAC] inhibitors) to effect epigenetic re-expression of the progestin receptor to engage progestin-mediated anticancer responses. This remains an active area of thinking and clinical research.

With respect to clinical data, endocrine therapy is not indicated as adjuvant treatment for EC, whereas it could be considered a treatment option in patients with metastatic, well-differentiated, and hormone receptor–positive EC in the absence of rapidly progressive disease. Progestins have, in fact, been shown to provide a good response rate (37% for G1 tumor and 23% for G2) and a good PFS in this group of patients.[94–96] Furthermore, tamoxifen has shown a 20% response rate (RR) in ECs that are not responsive to standard progestin treatment,[97,98] and tamoxifen plus progestins has shown a good RR but with an increased toxicity profile, especially in terms of thromboembolism.[99–101]

Aromatase inhibitors such as anastrozole could be effective and used in place of progestins. There is evidence of aromatase expression in stromal cells within endometrioid-type cancers.[102–104] Lastly, gonadotrophin-releasing hormone has demonstrated a response rate of 28% irrespective of tumor grade and paradoxically, highest in previously irradiated sites.[105,106]

Young patients who wish to preserve their fertility

Although rare, EC can arise in premenopausal patients, where there are associations with polycystic ovaries, unopposed estrogen oral contraceptives, the use of estrogens in gonadal dysgenesis, and inherited tumor suppressor gene mutations. In women with well or moderately differentiated EC and minimal invasion, progestins may be used to induce regression if fertility is to be preserved.

However, if there is imaging evidence of deep myometrial invasion (i.e., >50%), hysterectomy rather than medical therapy would be the safest approach to management, because deep myometrial invasion may signify the presence of a more aggressive cancer.

A thorough screening evaluation, including transvaginal ultrasonography and a contrast enhanced MRI of the uterus, is necessary to define whether there is evidence of myometrial invasion and to evaluate the extent of tumor involvement.[107] Although the optimal surveillance method for following patients treated with progestins is unknown, repeat pelvic ultrasound with endometrial biopsy every 3 months is a reasonable approach and part of the guidelines of different countries.

Following completion of childbearing, definitive surgical treatment should be recommended.

It is very important that all women who choose to follow the conservative pathways are counseled and informed about a 15–30% risk of the presence of more "aggressive" histology than initially anticipated in endometrial biopsy. Furthermore, there is an established risk of disease progression during medical therapy.[108]

The risks and benefits of fertility preservation were illustrated in a meta-analysis of 45 studies and 391 patients, 72% with Grade 1 EC.[109]

The majority (74%) were treated with either medroxyprogesterone or megestrol acetate with the following results:

- 78%: Complete response with a median time to response of 6 months
- 36%: Spontaneous pregnancy rate
- 25%: Recurrence with a median time to recurrence of 24 months

Megestrol acetate (160 mg/day) and medroxy progesterone acetate are the two progestins used for medical treatment. Both oral and parenteral routes for progestin therapy appear to be effective, although the optimal dose and duration of therapy are unknown. The minimum duration of progestin therapy appears to be 3 months, but some women will require a longer course.[18] After induction of response, a periodic withdrawal of progestins is usually recommended. Other modalities, such as IUDs and gonadotropin releasing hormone agonists (e.g., triptorelin), should not be routinely used outside the setting of clinical trials.[110]

Non-endometrioid histology

Uterine serous carcinoma

Compared with endometrioid adenocarcinomas, uterine serous and clear cell carcinomas represent more aggressive histologic types, as clearly shown in the SEER study of cases diagnosed from 1998 to 2001.[59] The 5-year survival rate stratified by histologic type was 45%, 65%, and 91% for serous, clear cell, and endometrioid adenocarcinomas, respectively; and this directional difference was reflected across all stages of the disease.

Serous EC tends to behave clinically more like serous ovarian cancer, so there is a risk of recurrence not only locally but also as multifocal peritoneal disease. Still, the extent of tumor involvement has a significant impact on the risk of recurrence and mortality. There are no prospectively randomized controlled data that compare the various treatment modalities especially or only for patients with the serous histological subtype. Given the disparities in national and international guidelines and also the lack of robust data that support any type of treatment in terms of superior outcome, women with Stage I or II serous carcinoma should consider treatment in the setting of a clinical trial.

To cover both distant and local recurrence risk, systemic chemotherapy and VBT appear to be a reasonable approach for women with serous EC. In the very small subgroup of patients with serous EC confined only to the endometrium, the risk of recurrence is small compared with those with myometrial invasion (9% versus 29%).[111] For that reason, observation alone or VBT is reasonable in this group of patients, provided surgical staging has been complete and no occult advanced disease is identified.

One of the largest studies for serous papillary EC, the Uterine Papillary Serous Carcinoma Consortium Study, included 142 women with serous EC. This was a retrospective, multi-institution analysis of surgically staged I–II patients.[112] Following surgery, 23% received no further treatment, whereas 14% and 63% were treated with adjuvant RT alone or adjuvant chemotherapy, respectively. Of those receiving chemotherapy, mainly carboplatin and paclitaxel, 37% also received RT. Of the 206 identified patients, 21% experienced recurrence. On univariate analysis, age, increasing percentage of uterine papillary serous carcinoma (UPSC), LVSI, and tumor size were not significantly associated with recurrence or PFS. However, substage ($p = 0.005$) and treatment with platinum/taxane-based chemotherapy ($p = 0.001$) were associated with recurrence/PFS. On multivariate analysis, only chemotherapy ($p = 0.01$) was a significant factor affecting PFS, whereas age ($p = 0.05$), substage ($p = 0.05$), and chemotherapy ($p = 0.02$) were associated with OS. The authors concluded that traditional risk factors for recurrence and survival in patients with early-stage EC may not be relevant in patients with serous papillary histology and that these patients are at a significant risk for recurrence and poor survival outcomes regardless of the percentage of serous papillary component in their uterine specimens.

Fader et al. performed a further retrospective, multi-institution study of women with only Stage II serous papillary EC after comprehensive surgical staging. Treatment included observation, RT (VBT, whole pelvic, or whole abdominal therapy), or ≥3 cycles of carboplatin/paclitaxel alone or with RT. The patients treated with chemotherapy (platinum and taxane) ± radiotherapy had a lower risk of recurrence (11%) compared with patients treated by radiotherapy alone (50%) or observation (50%). No patients treated with both modalities ($n = 12$) experienced a recurrence. Treatment with chemotherapy was also associated with a decreased risk of recurrence on multivariate analysis ($p = 0.015$). Most recurrences were extra-pelvic (70%), occurred within 2 years (85%), and were not salvageable (84%). In chemotherapy-treated patients, 5-year PFS was 86% versus 41% in those not receiving chemotherapy ($p = 0.010$); OS was 88% in chemotherapy-treated patients versus 64% in those not receiving chemotherapy ($p = 0.115$).[113] These results could suggest a leading role of chemotherapy in the adjuvant treatment of serous papillary EC.

In conclusion, platinum-based chemotherapy ± VBT and/or EBRT should be considered for patients with uterine serous carcinoma in both early and advanced stages.

Uterine clear cell carcinoma

Endometrial clear cell carcinomas (ECCC) are less frequent but more aggressive, and associated with higher stage at diagnosis and poorer outcome, than the Type I EC.

Surgery including TAH, BSO, omentectomy, and peritoneal cytology is recommended. In advanced stages, optimal cytoreduction (post-surgery residual disease ≤1 or ≤2 cm) should be pursued, the amount of post-surgical residual disease being the strongest predictor of OS.[75,76,114,115] With regard to the role of LND, the same considerations as for EC Type I are valid (see "Role of lymph node dissection" section).

Due to the rarity of ECCC, there are no prospectively randomized trials that include only patients with clear cell (CC) tumors. The GOG (GOG-209, GOG-122, and GOG-258),[67,74,83] and PORTEC (2 and 3)[55,66] trials, conducted to evaluate the role of systemic therapy and RT in high-risk EC, comprise also the CC histology; therefore, the conclusions in the previous section are also valid for ECCC treatment. However, it is important to consider that for ECCC, the risk of multifocal peritoneal recurrence and distant metastasis is higher than in Type I EC; therefore, a systemic control of the disease is an important goal to achieve with adjuvant treatment.

For this reason, international guidelines suggest a post-surgery platinum-based systemic chemotherapy ± EBRT and/or VBT for Stage IB–IV ECCC.[116] Post-surgical treatment of Stage IA ECCC is a controversial topic. In fact, although a retrospective trial, including 279 patients with Stage I–II uterine papillary serous and CC carcinoma, has shown that adjuvant treatments (RT, chemotherapy, or a combination of the two) were associated with improved OS in Stages IB–II (HR 0.14; 95% CI, 0.02 to 0.78; $p = 0.026$) but not in stage IA disease,[117] international guidelines suggest platinum-based systemic chemotherapy ± VBT also for Stage IA, reflecting the uncertainty in managing these patients.[116]

Uterine carcinosarcoma

Uterine carcinosarcomas constitute 3–8% of uterine cancers, and their incidence has increased in the last 20 years.

Despite their name, the molecular features of carcinosarcomas are more similar to those of poorly differentiated endometrial cancer than those of sarcomas, as are metastases from carcinosarcomas. For this reason, they have been included in the Type II EC class.

Regarding the management of uterine carcinosarcoma, when possible, surgery is recommended. Surgery should include TAH, BSO, omentectomy, pelvic LND, and possibly para-aortic LND. Even if the therapeutic benefit of lymphadenectomy remains unclear, the high risk of pelvic lymph node metastases shown in the GOG trial[118] has justified the recommendation of pelvic lymphadenectomy in patients with uterine carcinomas.

Adjuvant therapy should be considered post-surgery. The European Organisation for Research and Treatment of Cancer (EORTC) has evaluated the role of post-surgical radiotherapy in a Phase III trial, showing only a significant reduction in local recurrence rate without any benefit in OS. On contrary, patients treated with adjuvant RT showed a worse OS than those not treated.[119] Therefore, adjuvant EBRT cannot be recommended in uterine carcinosarcomas; however, it could be discussed in the case of positive nodes after lymphadenectomy. No clear indication exists on the role of brachytherapy; however, it could be optionally selected to reduce the risk of local relapse.

The GOG 150 trial compared adjuvant chemotherapy (cisplatin and ifosfamide) with WART and showed a trend in mortality reduction in patients receiving chemotherapy ($p = 0.085$) after the analysis was adjusted for stage and age.[120] Furthermore, a cohort study showed that adjuvant chemotherapy (cisplatin and ifosfamide or carboplatin and paclitaxel) is associated with improved PFS compared with radiation or observation alone.[121]

In conclusion, adjuvant chemotherapy ± brachytherapy is recommended in the early stage of uterine carcinosarcoma, and chemotherapy ± tumor-directed radiotherapy is the preferred option in more advanced stages.

Cisplatin and ifosfamide was the recommended regimen; however, there have been criticisms regarding its high toxicity; for this reason, carboplatin and paclitaxel was often used in clinical practice. The results of the GOG 261 trial, comparing carboplatin + paclitaxel vs. cisplatin + ifosfamide, were presented in the form of an abstract at the ASCO meeting in 2019. These results showed non-inferiority of the carboplatin + paclitaxel scheme compared with cisplatin + ifosfamide in terms of OS and PFS, with no significant differences in the grade of reported toxicities.[122]

In recurrent disease, chemotherapy is the preferred option. Usually, when a recurrence occurs less than 12 months after prior chemotherapy, the disease is likely to be platinum resistant and poorly responsive to chemotherapy. However, as second-line chemotherapy, the agents that have been shown to have higher activity are doxorubicin and ifosfamide, either alone or in combination, and platinum with paclitaxel. As third line, in fit patients, a clinical trial is suggested; otherwise, weekly paclitaxel could be considered.

Future prospects

Treatment of recurrent and metastatic EC remains in its infancy and represents an unmet clinical need.

EC is a heterogeneous disease, and it comprises different tumor histologies, each of which is characterized by different molecular alterations and consequently, different potential molecular targets for intervention.

In particular, endometrial cancers show MSI and mutations in PTEN, PIK3CA, PIK3RI, KRAS, FGFR2, and β-catenin genes, whereas serous tumors have molecular alterations in C-erbB2, STK15, p16, E-cadherin, and p53.[19]

Mutations in PTEN, PIK3CA, and PIK3RI causing a consequent constitutive activation of PI3K/AKT/mTOR pathway occur in 40–60% of endometrioid cancers. Thus, mammalian target of rapamycin (mTOR) inhibitors (everolimus, temsirolimus, and ridaforolimus) have been evaluated in clinical trials with encouraging results in the recurrent disease setting. In particular, temsirolimus demonstrated a good activity in recurrent EC, especially if chemonaïve, achieving a partial response (PR) and stable disease (SD) in 14% and 69% of the chemo-naïve population, respectively.[123] Ridaforolimus also demonstrated significant activity in recurrent EC, with a clinical benefit achieved in 29% of women with recurrent or persistent endometrial cancer that had progressed after a previous treatment.[124] Interestingly, ridaforolimus showed better disease control (35% versus 17%; $p = 0.021$) and an improved PFS (3.6 vs. 1.9 months; $p = 0.008$) compared with progestin or investigator choice chemotherapy in recurrent or metastatic EC that had progressed following at least one line of chemotherapy.[125] Currently, mTOR inhibition combined with aromatase inhibition is under investigation in the GOG 3007 trial. In this trial, everolimus plus letrozole is compared with tamoxifen or medroxyprogesterone in recurrent EC, and preliminary results suggest more favorable PFS in the everolimus plus letrozole arm.[126]

High expression of vascular endothelial growth factor (VEGF) is documented in 56% of endometrioid cancers and correlates with a poor clinical outcome.[127] Targeting VEGF, with the use of bevacizumab, has shown to be a promising therapeutic approach. In particular, in patients with recurrent EC that has progressed from a prior treatment, bevacizumab has achieved a response rate of 13.5% with a median PFS and OS of 4.2 and 10.5 months, respectively.[128] Furthermore, treatment with bevacizumab in combination with other therapies has been evaluated in two Phase II randomized trials, which reported interesting results. The GOG-86P trial evaluated the addition of bevacizumab, or temsirolimus or ixabepilone, to carboplatin-paclitaxel as first line of treatment in recurrent EC.[129] The results of the three arms

were compared with the results obtained in the GOG 209 trial for the treatment with carboplatin-paclitaxel.[83] No differences in PFS were observed, but the addition of bevacizumab to carboplatin and paclitaxel resulted in an improvement of median OS compared with carboplatin and paclitaxel without bevacizumab (34.0 versus 22.7 months, $p < 0.039$). A significant improvement in median PFS (13 versus 8.7 months, $p = 0.036$) was seen in the MITO END-2 trial, in which the regimen bevacizumab-carboplatin-paclitaxel was compared with carboplatin-paclitaxel as treatment for advanced or recurrent endometrial cancer.[130] In this trial, also a non-significant improvement in OS was documented (23.5 versus 18 months, $p = 0.24$), but these OS data remain immature.

Other targetable pathways under evaluation include the RAS-RAF-MEK-ERK signaling pathway, cyclin kinase 4/6, and fibroblast growth factor-2 receptor pathways (FGFR2).

In uterine serous carcinoma, one of the most promising targets is the human epidermal growth factor receptor 2 (HER2)/neu, a receptor that is overexpressed in 30% of uterine serous tumors. In fact, the addition of trastuzumab to the standard treatment with carboplatin and paclitaxel has recently been shown to improve PFS in Stage III/IV and recurrent uterine serous carcinoma.[131]

Lastly, the genomic classification of endometrial cancer from the TCGA has highlighted that a significant subset of endometrioid cancer is characterized by high mutation load and MSI. The high genomic instability is known to correlate with a better response to immune checkpoint inhibitors, and it has been shown that EC molecular subtypes with high mutation load (MMRd and POLE) also have high TIL with multiple immunosuppressive features.[132]

In addition, pembrolizumab was tested in the Keynote 028 trial in 24 patients with EC PD-L1 positive, and an overall response rate of 26% has been shown.[133] Additionally, in the Keynote 028/016/158 trial, an ORR of 46% was observed in the 14 enrolled patients with MSI/MMRd EC.

These findings have led to further testing of immunotherapy in MMRd and POLE subtype EC. The results obtained so far are encouraging. In particular, two Phase II trials testing the activity of durvalumab alone or in combination with tremelimumab have been presented at the ASCO meeting 2019. In the first trial, durvalumab was tested as monotherapy in advanced endometrial cancer according to mismatch repair, and it has shown an ORR of 40% in patients with MMR-D tumors and 3% in patients with a proficiency MMR.[134] In the second trial, the activity of durvalumab was tested with or without tremelimumab in persistent or recurrent EC and endometrial carcinosarcoma. A modest activity was documented for both regimens; however, a second stage accrual is ongoing (NCT03015129).

A third non-randomized Phase II study evaluated avelumab in two cohorts of recurrent/persistent EC: the MSI/POLE cohort and the MSS cohort.[135] Interestingly, the MSS cohort was closed due to futility, whereas in the MSI/POLE cohort, an overall response rate of 26.7% was achieved, and the MSI vs. MSS status appears to be correlated with avelumab response even in PD-L1 negative tumors.

These results strengthen the idea that MSI status is a stronger predictor of response to immunotherapy for EC and that immunotherapy could have a future leading role in the treatment of recurrent (or indeed, first-line treatment of) EC.

Follow-up

The majority of recurrences occur within 3–5 years of treatment. Approximately 70% of patients develop symptoms at the time of recurrence (e.g., vaginal bleeding, abdominal pain, cough, and weight loss).

After standard primary treatment, follow-up should be 3-monthly for 3 years, then 6-monthly for a further 2 years, and then annually. Vault smears can be used in surveillance follow-up but can cause significant and disruptive diagnostic uncertainty after adjuvant radiotherapy and are in general not as sensitive as cervical pap smears. The follow-up should include careful history of symptoms, clinical examination, vaginal and rectal examination, and transabdominal and transvaginal ultrasound. Where careful vaginal examination reveals an apparent recurrence, a formal incisional biopsy should be taken. Patients who

have recurrent tumors should always see a gynecological oncologist with an interest in this condition. CA 125 antigen levels are unhelpful apart from in some papillary serous variants.

A systematic review of 16 studies reported that asymptomatic recurrences were detected by the following modalities[136]:

- Physical examination (5–33%)
- Vaginal vault cytology (0–4%)
- Abdominal ultrasound (4–13%)
- Abdominal/pelvic CT (5–21%)
- Chest radiography (0–14%)
- CA 125 in selected patients (15%)

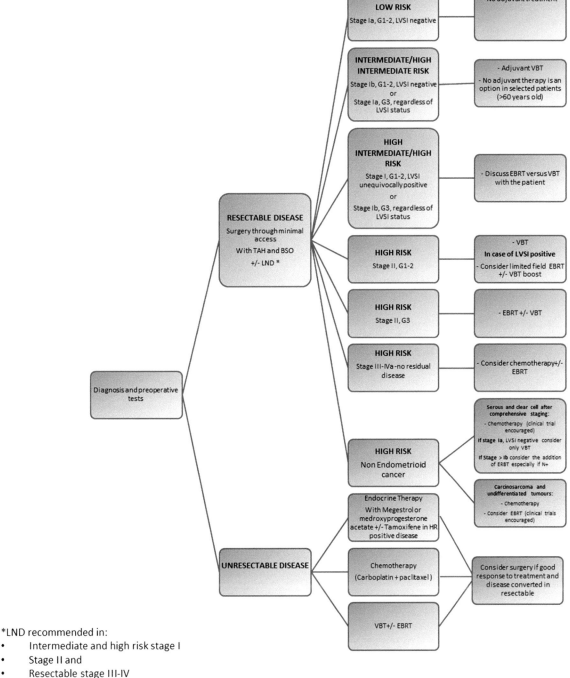

FIGURE 20.1 Endometrial cancer treatment algorithm.

Key learning points

- Uterine cancer is the most common gynaecologic malignancy in developed countries.
- There are two main types of uterine cancer: endometrial cancer and uterine sarcoma. Endometrial cancer type comprises endometrioid cancer and non-endometrioid cancer (serous carcinoma, clear cell carcinoma, undifferentiated/dedifferentiated carcinoma, and carcinosarcoma).
- Obesity is the major preventable risk factor for uterine cancer.
- 5% of all endometrial cancers arise in the context of a genetic syndrome (e.g. Lynch syndrome).
- There is no screening available in general population; however, screening with TVS and endometrial biopsy could be offered to women with Lynch Syndrome and their first-degree relatives from the age of 35 years.
- Unexpected vaginal bleeding/discharge is the most common symptom of uterine cancer at presentation.
- *ProMisE molecular classifier* has been validated as a promising prognostic and predictive tool.
- Abdominal and pelvic examination with specula and fractionated curettage is the gold standard of the diagnostic algorithm of patients with symptoms of uterine cancer.
- ESMO-ESGO-ESTRO has suggested a new risk stratification for EC that takes into account also the LVSI status.
- Surgery is the upfront treatment for EC, and optimal tumour debulking should be pursued in advanced stages. Minimal access surgery should be preferred when possible.
- There is no evidence to support routine lymphadenectomy in low risk endometrial cancers, whereas it is suggested in the other categories of risk.
- Adjuvant treatment with VBT and/or OT has not shown advantages in low risk EC, therefore should not be suggested.
- EBRT in intermediate EC has not shown an improvement of OS, therefore VBT should be preferred to EBRT in optimal staged intermediate and high-intermediate risk EC because of better toxicity profile and QOL.
- Chemoradiotherapy has been demonstrated to give an advantage in 5-years OS in high risk stage III-IV R0 EC in comparison with RT alone, while no benefit in OS has been shown in comparison with chemotherapy alone
- Doublet chemotherapy should be preferred to triplet in patient with advanced or recurrent EC not suitable for surgery and/or RT, because no-inferior in terms of PFS and OS and more tolerated.
- Endocrine therapy has shown a good response rate and a good PFS in advanced or recurrent hormone receptor-positive EC, therefore could be considered as treatment in these group of patients
- Treatment with progestins may be used to induce regression of well or moderately differentiated EC and minimal invasion if fertility is to be preserved.
- Carboplatin + paclitaxel could be used instead of cisplatin + ifosfamide as treatment in uterine carcinosarcoma having shown a no-inferiority.

References

1. Jemal A, Bray F, Center MM et al. Global cancer statistics. *Cancer J Clin.* 2011; 61(2):69–90.
2. Dickinson HO. *Cancer Survival Trends, 1971–1995.* London, UK: The Stationery Office, 1999.
3. D'Angelo E, Prat J. Uterine sarcomas: A review. *Gynecol Oncol.* 2010; 116(1):131–9.
4. Siegel RL, Miller KD, Jemal A. Cancer statistics, 2016. *CA Cancer J Clin.* 2016; 66(1):7–30.
5. Creasman WT, Odicino F, Maisonneuve P et al. Carcinoma of the corpus uteri. FIGO 26th annual report on the results of treatment in gynecological cancer. *Int J Gynaecol Obstet.* 2006; 95(1) Supplement 1:S105–43.
6. Calle EE, Kaaks R. Overweight, obesity and cancer: Epidemiological evidence and proposed mechanisms. *Nat Rev Cancer.* 2004; 4(8):579–91.
7. Soliman PT, Wu D, Tortolero-Luna G et al. Association between adiponectin, insulin resistance, and endometrial cancer. *Cancer.* 2006; 106(11):2376–81.
8. Cust AE, Kaaks R, Friedenreich C et al. Metabolic syndrome, plasma lipid, lipoprotein and glucose levels, and endometrial cancer risk in the European prospective investigation into cancer and nutrition (EPIC). *Endocr Relat Cancer.* 2007; 14(3):755–67.
9. Newcomb PA, Solomon C, White E. Tamoxifen and risk of large bowel cancer in women with breast cancer. *Breast Cancer Res Treat.* 1999; 53:271–7.
10. Fisher B, Costantino JP, Wickerham DL et al. Tamoxifen for the prevention of breast cancer: Current status of the national surgical adjuvant breast and bowel project P-1 study. *J Natl Cancer Inst.* 2005; 97:1652–62.
11. Terashima I, Suzuki N, Shibutani S. Mutagenic potential of alpha-(N2-deoxyguanosinyl) tamoxifen lesions, the major DNA adducts detected in endometrial tissues of patients treated with tamoxifen. *Cancer Res.* 1999; 59:2091–5.
12. Schmeler KM, Soliman PT, Sun CC et al. Endometrial cancer in young, normal-weight women. *Gynecol Oncol.* 2005; 99:388–92.
13. Pillay OC, Te Fong LF, Crow JC et al. The association between polycystic ovaries and endometrial cancer. *Hum Reprod.* 2006; 21(4):924–9.
14. Lu HK, Broaddus RR. Gynecologic cancers in Lynch syndrome/HNPCC. *Fam Cancer.* 2005; 4:249–54.
15. Reeves KW, Carter GC, Rodabough RJ et al. Obesity in relation to endometrial cancer risk and disease characteristics in the women's health initiative. *Gynecol Oncol.* 2011; 121(2):376–82.
16. Key TJ, Spencer EA, Reeves GK. Symposium 1: Overnutrition: Consequences and solutions. Obesity and cancer risk. *Proc Nutr Soc.* 2010; 69(1):86–90.
17. Vasen HF, Blanco I, Aktan-Collan K et al. Revised guidelines for the clinical management of Lynch syndrome (HNPCC): Recommendations by a group of European experts. *Gut.* 2013; 62(6):812–23
18. Horn LC, Schnurrbusch U, Bilek K, Hentschel B, Einenkel J. Risk of progression in complex and atypical endometrial hyperplasia: Clinicopathologic analysis in cases with and without progestogen treatment. *Int J Gynecol Cancer.* 2004; 14(2):348–53.
19. Matias-Guiu X, Prat J. Molecular pathology of endometrial carcinoma. *Histopathology.* 2013; 62:111–23.
20. Wiegand KC, Lee AF, Al-Agha OM et al. Loss of BAF250a (ARID1A) is frequent in high-grade endometrial carcinomas. *J Pathol.* 2011; 224(3):328–33.
21. Kandoth C, Schultz N, Cherniack AD et al. Integrated genomic characterization of endometrial carcinoma. *Nature.* 2013; 497:67–73.
22. Mittal K, Da Costa D. Endometrial hyperplasia and carcinoma in endometrial polyps: Clinicopathologic and follow-up findings. *Int J Gynecol Pathol.* 2008; 27(1):45–8.
23. Hui P, Kelly M, O'Malley DM, Tavassoli F, Schwartz PE. Minimal uterine serous carcinoma: A clinicopathological study of 40 cases. *Mod Pathol.* 2005; 18(1):75.
24. Kelly MG, O'malley DM, Hui P et al. Improved survival in surgical stage I patients with uterine papillary serous carcinoma (UPSC) treated with adjuvant platinum-based chemotherapy. *Gynecol Oncol.* 2005; 98(3):353.
25. Fadare O, Mariappan MR, Hileeto D et al. Upstaging based solely on positive peritoneal washing does not affect outcome in endometrial cancer. *Mod Pathol.* 2005; 18(5):673.

26. Kommoss S, McConechy MK, Kommoss F et al. Final validation of the ProMisE molecular classifier for endometrial carcinoma in a large population-based case series. *Ann Oncol*. 2018; 29(5):1180–88.

27. Stelloo E, Nout RA, Naves LC et al. High concordance of molecular tumor alterations between pre-operative curettage and hysterectomy specimens in patients with endometrial carcinoma. *Gynecol Oncol*. 2014; 133(2):197–204.

28. Talhouk A, Hoang LN, McConechy MK et al. Molecular classification of endometrial carcinoma on diagnostic specimens is highly concordant with final hysterectomy: Earlier prognostic information to guide treatment. *Gynecol Oncol*. 2016; 143(1):46–53.

29. Available from: http://seer.cancer.gov/statfacts/html/corp.html

30. Elsandabesee D, Greenwood P. The performance of Pipelle endometrial sampling in a dedicated postmenopausal bleeding clinic. *J Obstet Gynaecol*. 2005; 25:32–4.

31. Trimble CL, Kauderer J, Zaino R. Concurrent endometrial carcinoma in women with a biopsy diagnosis of atypical endometrial hyperplasia: A GOG study. *Cancer*. 2006; 106:812–9.

32. Vernooij F, Heintz P, Witteveen E, van der Graaf Y. The outcomes of ovarian cancer treatment are better when provided by gynecologic oncologists and in specialized hospitals: A systematic review. *Gynecol Oncol*. 2007; 105(3):801.

33. Walker JL, Piedmonte MR, Spirtos NM et al. Laparoscopy compared with laparotomy for comprehensive surgical staging of uterine cancer: Gynecologic oncologic group study LAP 2. *JCO*. 2009; 27:5331–6.

34. Berchuck A, Secord AA, Havrilesky LJ. Minimally invasive surgery for endometrial cancer: The horse is already out of the barn. *J Clin Oncol*. 2012; 30(7):681–2.

35. Wright JD, Burke WM, Wilde ET et al. Comparative effectiveness of robotic versus laparoscopic hysterectomy for endometrial cancer. *J Clin Oncol*. 2012; 30(8):783–91.

36. Kilgore JE, Jackson AL, Ko EM et al. Recurrence-free and 5-year survival following robotic assisted surgical staging for endometrial carcinoma. *Gynecol Oncol*. 2013; 129(1):49–53.

37. Gehrig PA, Cantrell LA, Shafer A et al. What is the optimal minimally invasive surgical procedure for endometrial cancer staging in the obese and morbidly obese woman? *Gynecol Oncol*. 2008; 111:41–5.

38. Fotopoulou C, Savvatis K, Kraetschell R et al. Systematic pelvic and aortic lymphadenectomy in intermediate and high-risk endometrial cancer: Lymph-node mapping and identification of predictive factors for lymph-node status. *Eur J Obstet Gynecol Reprod Biol*. 2010; 149(2):199–203.

39. Benedetti Panici P, Basile S, Maneschi F et al. Systematic pelvic lymphadenectomy vs. no lymphadenectomy in early-stage endometrial carcinoma: Randomized clinical trial. *J Natl Cancer Inst* 2008; 100(23):1707–16.

40. Walsh CS, Karlan BY. Lymphadenectomy's role in early endometrial cancer: Prognostic or therapeutic? *J Natl Cancer Inst*. 2008; 100(23):1660–1.

41. Mariani A, Dowdy SC, Cliby WA et al. Prospective assessment of lymphatic dissemination in endometrial cancer: A paradigm shift in surgical staging. *Gynecol Oncol*. 2008; 109(1):11–8.

42. Bakkum-Gamez JN, Mariani A, Dowdy SC et al. The impact of surgical guidelines and periodic quality assessment on the staging of endometrial cancer. *Gynecol Oncol*. 2011; 123(1):58–64.

43. Dowdy SC, Aletti G, Cliby WA, Podratz KC, Mariani A. Extraperitoneal laparoscopic paraaortic lymphadenectomy – a prospective cohort study of 293 patients with endometrial cancer. *Gynecol Oncol*. 2008; 111(3):418–24.

44. Sundar S, Balega J, Crosbie E et al. BGCS uterine cancer guidelines: Recommendations for practice. *Eur J Obstet Gynecol Reprod Biol*. 2017; 213:71–97.

45. N. Colombo E, Preti F, Landoni S et al. Endometrial cancer: ESMO Clinical Practice Guidelines for diagnosis, treatment and follow-up. *Annals of Oncology*. 2013; 24(suppl_6):vi33–vi38.

46. Colombo N, Creutzberg C, Amant F et al. ESMO-ESGO-ESTRO Consensus Conference on Endometrial Cancer: Diagnosis, treatment and follow-up. *Ann Oncol*. 2016; 27(1):16–41.

47. Sasada S, Yunokawa M, Takehara Y et al. Baseline risk of recurrence in stage I–II endometrial carcinoma. *J Gynecol Oncol*. 2018; 29(1):e9.

48. Sorbe B, Nordström B, Mäenpää J et al. Intravaginal brachytherapy in FIGO stage I low-risk endometrial cancer: A controlled randomized study. *Int J Gynecol Cancer*. 2009; 19(5):873–8.

49. Martin-Hirsch PP, Bryant A, Keep SL, Kitchener HC, Lilford R. Adjuvant progestagens for endometrial cancer. *Cochrane Database Syst Rev*. 2011.

50. Creutzberg CL, van Putten WL, Koper PC et al. Survival after relapse in patients with endometrial cancer: Results from a randomized trial. *Gynecol Oncol*. 2003; 89(2):201–9.

51. Keys HM, Roberts JA, Brunetto VL et al. A phase III trial of surgery with or without adjunctive external pelvic radiation therapy in intermediate risk endometrial adenocarcinoma: A Gynecologic Oncology Group study. *Gynecol Oncol*. 2004; 92(3):744.

52. Blake P, Swart AM, Orton J et al. Adjuvant external beam radiotherapy in the treatment of endometrial cancer (MRC ASTEC and NCIC CTG EN.5 randomised trials): Pooled trial results, systematic review, and meta-analysis. *Lancet*. 2009; 373:137–46.

53. Kong A, Johnson N, Kitchener HC, Lawrie TA. Adjuvant radiotherapy for stage I endometrial cancer: An updated Cochrane systematic review and meta-analysis. *J Natl Cancer Inst*. 2012; 104:1625–34.

54. Creutzberg CL, van Putten WL, Koper PC et al. Surgery and postoperative radiotherapy versus surgery alone for patients with stage-1 endometrial carcinoma: Multicentre randomised trial. PORTEC Study Group. Post Operative Radiation Therapy in Endometrial Carcinoma. *Lancet*. 2000; 355(9213):1404–11.

55. Sorbe B, Horvath G, Andersson H et al. External pelvic and vaginal irradiation versus vaginal irradiation alone as postoperative therapy in medium-risk endometrial carcinoma–A prospective randomized study. *Int J Radiat Oncol Biol Phys*. 2012; 82(3):1249–55.

56. Susumu N, Sagae S, Udagawa Y et al. Randomized phase III trial of pelvic radiotherapy versus cisplatin-based combined chemotherapy in patients with intermediate- and high-risk endometrial cancer: A Japanese Gynecologic Oncology Group study. *Gynecol Oncol*. 2008; 108(1):226.

57. Randall ME, Filiaci V, McMeekin DS et al. Phase III trial: Adjuvant pelvic radiation therapy versus vaginal brachytherapy plus paclitaxel/carboplatin in high-intermediate and high-risk early-stage endometrial cancer. *J Clin Oncol*. 2019; 37(21):1810–18.

58. Kosary C. Cancer of the Corpus Uteri. In *SEER Survival Monograph: Cancer Survival Among Adults: U.S. SEER Program, 1988–2001, Patient and Tumor Characteristics*. Bethesda, MD: NCI, SEER Program, National Cancer Institute, 2007.

59. Maggi R, Lissoni A, Spina F et al. Adjuvant chemotherapy vs. radiotherapy in high-risk endometrial carcinoma: Results of a randomised trial. *Br J Cancer*. 2006; 95:266–71.

60. Morrow CP, Bundy BN, Homesley HD et al. Doxorubicin as an adjuvant following surgery and radiation therapy in patients with high-risk endometrial carcinoma, stage I and occult stage II: A Gynecologic Oncology Study. *Gynecol Oncol*. 1990; 36:166–71.

61. Hogberg T, Signorelli M, de Oliveira CF et al. Sequential adjuvant chemotherapy and radiotherapy in endometrial cancer—results from two randomised studies. *Eur J Cancer*. 2010; 46:2422–31.

62. Johnson N, Bryant A, Miles T et al. Adjuvant chemotherapy for endometrial cancer after hysterectomy. *Cochrane Database Syst Rev*. 2011:CD003175.

63. Homesley HD, Filiaci V, Gibbons SK et al. A randomized phase III trial in advanced endometrial carcinoma of surgery and volume directed radiation followed by cisplatin and doxorubicin with or without paclitaxel: A Gynecologic Oncology Group study. *Gynecol Oncol*. 2009; 112:543.

64. Greven K, Winter K, Underhill K et al. Final analysis of RTOG 9708: Adjuvant postoperative irradiation combined with cisplatin/ paclitaxel chemotherapy following surgery for patients with high-risk endometrial cancer. *Gynecol Oncol*. 2006; 103:155–9.

65. de Boer SM, Powell ME, Mileshkin L et al. Adjuvant chemoradiotherapy versus radiotherapy alone in women with high-risk

endometrial cancer (PORTEC-3): Patterns of recurrence and post-hoc survival analysis of a randomised phase 3 trial. *Lancet Oncol.* 2019; 20:1273–85.

66. Matei D, Filiaci V, Randall ME et al. Adjuvant chemotherapy plus radiation for locally advanced endometrial cancer. *N Engl J Med.* 2019; 380(24):2317–26.

67. Matulonis U, Filiaci VL, Huang HQ et al. Analysis of patient-reported outcomes (PROs) for GOG-258, a randomized phase III trial of cisplatin and tumor volume directed irradiation followed by carboplatin and paclitaxel (Cis-RT+CP) vs. carboplatin and paclitaxel (CP) for optimally debulked, locally advanced endometrial carcinoma. *J Clin Oncol.* 2018; 36(15_suppl):5589.

68. Randall ME, Wilder J, Greven K, Raben M. Role of intracavitary cuff boost after adjuvant external irradiation in early endometrial carcinoma. *Int J Radiat Oncol Biol Phys.* 1990; 19:49–54.

69. Scotti V, Borghesi S, Meattini I et al. Postoperative radiotherapy in stage I/II endometrial cancer: Retrospective analysis of 883 patients treated at the University of Florence. *Int J Gynecol Cancer.* 2010; 20:1540–8.

70. Jobsen JJ, Lybeert ML, van der Steen-Banasik EM et al. Multicenter cohort study on treatment results and risk factors in stage II endometrial carcinoma. *Int J Gynecol Cancer.* 2008; 18:1071–78.

71. Crosby MA, Tward JD, Szabo A, Lee CM, Gaffney DK. Does brachytherapy improve survival in addition to external beam radiation therapy in patients with high risk stage I and II endometrial carcinoma? *Am J Clin Oncol.* 2010; 33:364–369.

72. Rossi PJ, Jani AB, Horowitz IR, Johnstone PA. Adjuvant brachytherapy removes survival disadvantage of local disease extension in stage IIIC endometrial cancer: A SEER registry analysis. *Int J Radiat Oncol Biol Phys.* 2008; 70:134–8.

73. Randall ME, Filiaci VL, Muss H et al. Randomized phase III trial of whole-abdominal irradiation versus doxorubicin and cisplatin chemotherapy in advanced endometrial carcinoma: A Gynecologic Oncology Group Study. *J Clin Oncol.* 2006; 24:36.

74. Patsavas K, Woessner J, Gielda B et al. Optimal surgical debulking in uterine papillary serous carcinoma affects survival. *Gynecol Oncol.* 2011; 121:581.

75. Rauh-Hain JA, Growdon WB, Schorge JO et al. Prognostic determinants in patients with stage IIIC and IV uterine papillary serous carcinoma. *Gynecol Oncol.* 2010; 119:299.

76. Shih KK, Yun E, Gardner GJ et al. Surgical cytoreduction in stage IV endometrioid endometrial carcinoma. *Gynecol Oncol.* 2011; 122:608.

77. Bristow RE, Zerbe MJ, Rosenshein NB et al. Stage IVB endometrial carcinoma: The role of cytoreductive surgery and determinants of survival. *Gynecol Oncol.* 2000; 78:85.

78. van Wijk FH, Aapro MS, Bolis G et al. Doxorubicin versus doxorubicin and cisplatin in endometrial carcinoma: Definitive results of a randomised study (55872) by the EORTC Gynaecological Cancer Group. *Ann Oncol.* 2003; 14:441–8.

79. Thigpen JT, Brady MF, Homesley HD et al. Phase III trial of doxorubicin with or without cisplatin in advanced endometrial carcinoma: A gynecologic oncology group study. *J Clin Oncol.* 2004; 22:3902–8.

80. Fleming GF, Brunetto VL, Cella D et al. Phase III trial of doxorubicin plus cisplatin with or without paclitaxel plus filgrastim in advanced endometrial carcinoma: A Gynecologic Oncology Group Study. *J Clin Oncol.* 2004; 22:2159–66.

81. Homesley HD, Filiaci V, Gibbons SK et al. A randomized phase III trial in advanced endometrial carcinoma of surgery and volume directed radiation followed by cisplatin and doxorubicin with or without paclitaxel: A Gynecologic Oncology study. *Gynecol Oncol.* 2009; 112:543.

82. Miller DS, Filiaci G, Mannel R et al. Randomized phase III noninferiority trial of first line chemotherapy for metastatic or recurrent endometrial carcinoma: A Gynecologic Oncology Group Study. *LBA2.* Presented at the 2012 Society of Gynecologic Oncology Annual Meeting, Austin, TX.

83. Bruzzone M, Miglietta L, Franzone P et al. Combined treatment with chemotherapy and radiotherapy in high-risk FIGO stage III–IV endometrial cancer patients. *Gynecol Oncol.* 2004; 93:345.

84. Mangili G, De Marzi P, Beatrice S et al. Paclitaxel and concomitant radiotherapy in high-risk endometrial cancer patients: Preliminary findings. *BMC Cancer.* 2006; 6:198.

85. Makker V, Hensley ML, Zhou Q et al. Treatment of advanced or recurrent endometrial carcinoma with doxorubicin in patients progressing after paclitaxel/carboplatin: Memorial Sloan-Kettering Cancer Center experience from 1995 to 2009. *Int J Gynecol Cancer.* 2013; 23:929–34.

86. Grisham RN, Adaniel C, Hyman DM et al. Gemcitabine for advanced endometrial cancer: A retrospective study of the Memorial Sloan-Kettering Cancer Center experience. *Int J Gynecol Cancer.* 2012; 22:807–11.

87. Nagao S, Nishio S, Michimae H et al. Applicability of the concept of "platinum sensitivity" to recurrent endometrial cancer: The SGSG-012/GOTIC-004/Intergroup study. *Gynecol Oncol.* 2013; 131:567–73.

88. Moore KN, Tian C, McMeekin DS et al. Does the progression-free interval after primary chemotherapy predict survival after salvage chemotherapy in advanced and recurrent endometrial cancer? A Gynecologic Oncology Group ancillary data analysis. *Cancer.* 2010; 116:5407–14.

89. Vereide AB, Kaino T, Sager G, Orbo A. Bcl-2, BAX, and apoptosis in endometrial hyperplasia after high dose gestagen therapy: A comparison of responses in patients treated with intrauterine levonorgestrel and systemic medroxyprogesterone. *Gynecol Oncol.* 2005; 97:740–50.

90. Markman M. Hormonal therapy of endometrial cancer. *Eur J Cancer.* 2005; 41:673–5.

91. Martin-Hirsch PL, Lilford RJ, Jarvis GJ. Adjuvant progestagen therapy for the treatment of endometrial cancer: Review and meta-analyses of published randomised controlled trials. *Eur J Obstet Gynecol Reprod Biol.* 1996; 65:201–7.

92. Groups C-N-UECS. Adjuvant medroxyprogesterone acetate in high-risk endometrial cancer. *Int J Gynecol Cancer.* 1998; 8:387–91.

93. Thigpen JT, Brady MF, Alvarez RD et al. Oral medroxyprogesterone acetate in the treatment of advanced or recurrent endometrial carcinoma: A dose-response study by the Gynecologic Oncology Group. *J Clin Oncol.* 1999; 17:1736–44.

94. Decruze SB, Green JA. Hormone therapy in advanced and recurrent endometrial cancer: A systematic review. *Int J Gynecol Cancer.* 2007; 17(5):964–78.

95. Dellinger TH, Monk BJ. Systemic therapy for recurrent endometrial cancer: A review of North American trials. *Expert Rev Anticancer Ther.* 2009; 9(7):905–16.

96. Quinn MA1, Campbell JJ. Tamoxifen therapy in advanced/recurrent endometrial carcinoma. *Gynecol Oncol.* 1989; 32(1):1–3.

97. Thigpen T, Brady MF, Homesley HD, Soper JT, Bell J. Tamoxifen in the treatment of advanced or recurrent endometrial carcinoma: A Gynecologic Oncology Group study. *J Clin Oncol.* 2001; 19(2):364–7.

98. Whitney CW, Brunetto VL, Zaino RJ et al. Phase II study of medroxyprogesterone acetate plus tamoxifen in advanced endometrial carcinoma: A Gynecologic Oncology Group study. *Gynecol Oncol.* 2004; 92(1):4–9.

99. Pandya KJ, Yeap BY, Weiner LM et al. Megestrol and tamoxifen in patients with advanced endometrial cancer: An Eastern Cooperative Oncology Group Study (E4882). *Am J Clin Oncol.* 2001; 24(1):43–6.

100. Barker LC, Brand IR, Crawford SM. Sustained effect of the aromatase inhibitors anastrozole and letrozole on endometrial thickness in patients with endometrial hyperplasia and endometrial carcinoma. *Curr Med Res Opin.* 2009; 25(5):1105–9.

101. Segawa T, Shozu M, Murakami K et al. Aromatase expression in stromal cells of endometrioid endometrial cancer correlates with poor survival. *Clin Cancer Res.* 2005; 11:2188–94.

102. Labrie F, Labrie C, Belanger A et al. EM-652 (SCH 57068), a third generation SERM acting as pure antiestrogen in the mammary gland and endometrium. *J Steroid Biochem Mol Biol.* 1999; 69:51–84.

103. O'Regan RM, Cisneros A, England GM et al. Effects of the antiestrogens tamoxifen, toremifene, and ICI 182,780 on endometrial cancer growth. *J Natl Cancer Inst.* 1998; 90:1552–8.

104. Jeyarajah AR, Gallagher CJ, Blake PR et al. Long-term follow-up of gonadotrophin-releasing hormone analog treatment for recurrent endometrial cancer. *Gynecol Oncol.* 1996; 63:47–52.

105. Niwa K, Tagami K, Lian Z et al. Outcome of fertility-preserving treatment in young women with endometrial carcinomas. *Br J Obst Gynecol.* 2005; 112:317–20.

106. Kinkel K, Kaji Y, Yu KK et al. Radiologic staging in patients with endometrial cancer: A meta-analysis. *Radiology.* 1999; 212(3):711.

107. Leitao MM, Jr., Kehoe S, Barakat RR et al. Comparison of D&C and office endometrial biopsy accuracy in patients with FIGO grade 1 endometrial adenocarcinoma. *Gynecol Oncol.* 2009; 113(1):105–8.

108. Gunderson CC, Fader AN, Carson KA, Bristow RE. Oncologic and reproductive outcomes with progestin therapy in women with endometrial hyperplasia and grade 1 adenocarcinoma: A systematic review. *Gynecol Oncol.* 2012; 125(2):477.

109. Jadoul P, Donnez J. Conservative treatment may be beneficial for young women with atypical endometrial hyperplasia or endometrial adenocarcinoma. *Fertil Steril.* 2003; 80(6):1315–24.

110. Havrilesky LJ, Secord AA, Bae-Jump V et al. Outcomes in surgical stage I uterine papillary serous carcinoma. *Gynecol Oncol.* 2007; 105:677.

111. Fader AN, Starks D, Gehrig PA et al. An updated clinicopathologic study of early-stage uterine papillary serous carcinoma (UPSC). *Gynecol Oncol.* 2009; 115:244.

112. Fader AN, Nagel C, Axtell AE et al. Stage II uterine papillary serous carcinoma: Carboplatin/paclitaxel chemotherapy improves recurrence and survival outcomes. *Gynecol Oncol.* 2009; 112:558.

113. Thomas M, Mariani A, Wright JD et al. Surgical management and adjuvant therapy for patients with uterine clear cell carcinoma: A multi-institutional review. *Gynecol Oncol.* 2008; 108(2):293–7.

114. Barlin JN, Puri I, Bristow RE. Cytoreductive surgery for advanced or recurrent endometrial cancer: A meta-analysis. *Gynecol Oncol.* 2010; 118:14–8.

115. National Comprehensive Cancer Network: NCCN Clinical Practice Guidelines – Endometrial Carcinoma. Version 3.2019

116. Vogel TJ, Knickerbocker A, Shah CA et al. An analysis of current treatment practice in uterine papillary serous and clear cell carcinoma at two high volume cancer centers. *J Gynecol Oncol.* 2015; 26(1):25–31.

117. Major FJ, Blessing JA, Silverberg SG et al. Prognostic factors in early-stage uterine sarcoma. A Gynecologic Oncology Group study. *Cancer.* 1993; 71(4 Suppl) Suppl: 1702–9.

118. Reed NS, Mangioni C, Malmström H et al. Phase III randomised study to evaluate the role of adjuvant pelvic radiotherapy in the treatment of uterine sarcomas stages I and II: An European Organisation for Research and Treatment of Cancer Gynaecological Cancer Group Study (protocol 55874). *Eur J Cancer.* 2008; 44(6):808–18.

119. Wolfson AH, Brady MF, Rocereto T et al. A gynecologic oncology group randomized phase III trial of whole abdominal irradiation (WAI) vs. cisplatin-ifosfamide and mesna (CIM) as post-surgical therapy in stage I–IV carcinosarcoma (CS) of the uterus. *Gynecol Oncol.* 2007; 107(2):177–85.

120. Vorgias G, Fotiou S. The role of lymphadenectomy in uterine carcinosarcomas (malignant mixed mullerian tumours): A critical literature review. *Arch Gynecol Obstet.* 2010; 282(6):659–64.

121. Powell MA, Filiaci VL, Hensley ML et al. A randomized phase 3 trial of paclitaxel (P) plus carboplatin (C) versus paclitaxel plus ifosfamide (I) in chemotherapy-naive patients with stage I-IV,

122. Oza AM, Elit L, Tsao MS et al. Phase II study of temsirolimus in women with recurrent or metastatic endometrial cancer: A trial of the NCIC Clinical Trials Group. *J Clin Oncol.* 2011; 29(24):3278–85.

123. Colombo N, McMeekin DS, Schwartz PE et al. Ridaforolimus as a single agent in advanced endometrial cancer: Results of a single-arm, phase 2 trial. *Br J Cancer.* 2013; 108(5):1021–6.

124. Oza AM, Pignata S, Poveda A et al. Randomized phase II trial of ridaforolimus in advanced endometrial carcinoma. *J Clin Oncol.* 2015; 33(31):3576–82.

125. Slomovitz, BM, Filiaci VL, Coleman RL et al. GOG 3007, a randomized phase II (RP2) trial of everolimus and letrozole (EL) or hormonal therapy (medroxyprogesterone acetate/tamoxifen, PT) in women with advanced, persistent or recurrent endometrial carcinoma (EC): A GOG Foundation study *Gynecol Oncol.* 2018; 149:2

126. Kamat AA, Merritt WM, Coffey D et al. Clinical and biological significance of vascular endothelial growth factor in endometrial cancer. *Clin Cancer Res.* 2007; 13(24):7487–95.

127. Aghajanian C1, Sill MW, Darcy KM et al. Phase II trial of bevacizumab in recurrent or persistent en-dometrial cancer: A Gynecologic Oncology Group study. *J Clin Oncol.* 2011; 29(16):2259–65.

128. Aghajanian C, Filiaci VL, Dizon DS et al. A randomized phase II study of paclitaxel/carboplatin/bevacizumab, paclitaxel/carboplatin/temsirolimus and ixabepilone/carboplatin/bevacizumab as initial therapy for measurable stage III or IVA, stage IVB or recurrent endometrial cancer, GOG86P. *J Clin Oncol.* 2015; 33(Suppl):abstract 5500.

129. Lorusso D, Ferrandina G, Colombo N et al. Randomized phase II trial of carboplatin-paclitaxel (CP) compared to carboplatin-paclitaxel-bevacizumab (CPB) in advanced (stage III–IV) or recurrent endometrial cancer: The MITO END-2 trial. *J Clin Oncol.* 2015; 33(Suppl):abstract 5502

130. Fader AN, Roque DM, Siegel E et al. Randomized Phase II trial of carboplatin-paclitaxel versus carboplatin-paclitaxel-trastuzumab in uterine serous carcinomas that overexpress human epidermal growth factor receptor 2/neu. *J Clin Oncol.* 2018; 36(20):2044–51.

131. Talhouk A, Derocher H, Schmidt P et al. Molecular subtype not immune response drives outcomes in endometrial carcinoma. *Clin Cancer Res.* 2019; 25(8):2537–48.

132. Ott PA, Bang YJ, Berton-Rigaud D et al. Safety and antitumor activity of pembrolizumab in advanced programmed death ligand 1-positive endometrial cancer: Results from the KEYNOTE-028 study. *J Clin Oncol.* 2017; 35(22):2535–41.

133. Antill YC, Kok PS, Robledo K et al. Activity of durvalumab in advanced endometrial cancer (AEC) according to mismatch repair (MMR) status: The phase II PHAEDRA trial (ANZGOG1601). *J Clin Oncol.* 2019; 37(suppl):abstr 5501

134. Konstantinopoulos PA, Liu JF, Luo W et al. Phase 2, two-group, two-stage study of avelumab in patients (pts) with microsatellite stable (MSS), microsatellite instable (MSI), and polymerase epsilon (POLE) mutated recurrent/persistent endometrial cancer (EC). *J Clin Oncol.* 2019; 37(suppl):abstr 5502.

135. Fung-Kee-Fung M, Dodge J, Elit L et al. Follow-up after primary therapy for endometrial cancer: A systematic review. *Gynecol Oncol.* 2006; 101(3):520.

136. Wortman BG, Creutzberg CL, Putter H et al. Ten-year results of the PORTEC-2 trial for high-intermediate risk endometrial carcinoma: Improving patient selection for adjuvant therapy. *Br J Cancer.* 2018; 119(9):1067–74.

21 CERVICAL CANCER

Georgios Imseeh and Alexandra Taylor

Incidence and causes

Incidence

Worldwide, cervical cancer is the fourth most common female malignancy, with 570,000 diagnosed cases and 311,000 deaths per year.[1] The incidence of cervical malignancy varies widely from one country to another and between cultures and social classes. Approximately 90% of cases occur in developing countries, where it is the most common cancer among females. Cervical cancer has the highest incidence in women aged 30–35 years, with more than 60% of cases affecting women under 50 years old.

In the United Kingdom, it is the 14th commonest cancer among women, with 3192 new cases being reported in 2016.[2] Following the introduction of the U.K. national screening program in the 1980s, a 50% reduction in invasive cervical cancer mortality was achieved.

Causes of cervical neoplasia

The major etiological factor for cervical cancer is exposure to the human papilloma virus (HPV). The great majority of tumors of the cervix arise at the squamo-columnar junction, an area known as the transformation zone, where columnar epithelium undergoes the metaplastic process of becoming squamous epithelium. The transformation zone is larger in puberty, in pregnancy, and when taking the oral contraceptive pill. This area of the cervix is the target on which a transmissible agent has its effect.

Human papilloma virus

HPV is a small deoxyribonucleic acid (DNA) virus that infects the basal cells (keratinocytes) of the skin and mucous membranes. More than 100 types of HPV have now been isolated, and at least 40 of these infect the lower female genital tract, with 12 types identified as "high risk" for developing neoplasia. More than 99% of cervical cancers are related to HPV infection. In particular, types 16 and 18 are associated with the development of invasive cancer and account for more than 70% of cervical cancer.[3]

More than 80% of the population are exposed to HPV at least once during their lifetime. For the majority of people, there are few or no symptoms, and it has no significant consequences. Within the first year, 75% of infections are cleared, and 95% by 2 years. Rarely, the infection becomes persistent, and for these women, there is a high risk of developing dysplasia and eventually, cervical cancer if untreated. This typically takes 10–20 years to occur, providing the opportunity for early detection and treatment of pre-invasive disease.[4,5]

Mechanism of action

HPV produces two proteins, E6 and E7, which play a major role in malignant transformation and immortality of infected cells by interacting with cell cycle control genes. E6 binds and deactivates the protein p53, a product of the p53 tumor suppressor gene, thus preventing cell growth arrest and apoptosis. E7 binds with pRb, a product of the retinoblastoma gene, and thereby increases levels of E2F transcription factor, which promotes cell cycle division.[5] The normal function of these genes is to prevent cells with abnormal DNA from replicating, and DNA damage may be caused by several factors, most notably age and smoking. It is likely that carcinogenesis in cervical squamous cells is a multifactorial process, with HPV clearly involved early in this process.

Sexual behavior

For many years, an etiological link between sexual intercourse and the development of cervical neoplasia has been recognized.[6] There is a higher incidence of both cervical intra-epithelial neoplasia (CIN) and invasive disease in girls who commence intercourse in their teens rather than at a later age. This suggests that the adolescent cervix is more vulnerable to potential oncogenic agents. In addition, the number of sexual partners appears to be important, and there is also an association between cervical neoplasia and the male partner having multiple other sexual partners.[7]

Smoking

The products of smoking are concentrated in cervical mucus and produce damage to the DNA of cervical squamous cells. In addition, smoking decreases the population of Langerhans cells responsible for cell-mediated immunity in the cervix. Smoking is implicated in the development of cervical neoplasia both by direct carcinogenesis and by rendering the cervix more vulnerable to infection by HPV.[8]

Immunosuppression

Systemic immunosuppression of patients who have undergone renal transplant is recognized as being a risk factor for cervical cancer. Cervical neoplasia is also more common in women with HIV, and the onset of invasive disease is an "AIDS defining illness."[9]

Pathology

Pathology of pre-invasive disease

Changes in the metaplastic process at the transformation zone may lead to dysplasia, which is known as CIN. The terms CIN1, CIN2, and CIN3 are histological terms used to describe increasing degrees of dysplasia from mild to moderate to severe. CIN1 is confined to the basal one-third of the epithelium and is usually cleared by the immune system. CIN2 is confined to the basal two-thirds, whereas CIN3 can involve the full thickness. Cervical epithelium showing severe dysplasia (CIN3) was previously known as carcinoma in situ.

It is known that a proportion of cases of CIN3 can develop into invasive carcinoma, whereas the great majority of CIN1 and most of CIN2 may revert to normal epithelium if left untreated. Most cases of CIN3 and many of CIN2 are treated. It is thought that in most women, the transformation of benign epithelium to invasive cancer takes 10–15 years.

Micro-invasive carcinoma of the cervix

Once the basement membrane beneath the epithelium is breached by the neoplastic process, the disease is referred to as being micro-invasive. In the Federation Internationale de Gynecologie et d'Obstetrique (FIGO) classification,[10] this is Stage IA, which is subdivided into Stages IA1 and IA2 (Table 21.1) according to whether the depth of invasion is up to 3 or 5 mm, respectively. When disease is more than 5 mm deep or is visible, it falls within the category of FIGO Stage IB invasive carcinoma of the cervix.

Invasive carcinoma of the cervix

Approximately 75–85% of cervical cancers are squamous cell carcinomas, the remainder being predominantly adenocarcinoma, adenosquamous carcinoma, or very rarely, small cell neuroendocrine tumors, sarcoma, lymphoma, or melanoma.

Squamous carcinoma

Most squamous cell carcinomas involve the ectocervix and are visible on a speculum examination. Some develop within the endocervical canal and remain occult until reaching quite a large size (a barrel shaped carcinoma). Visible tumors may be either exophytic or ulcerating with underlying infiltration of surrounding structures.

Histologically, tumors are graded as well-differentiated (Grade 1), moderately differentiated (Grade 2), and poorly differentiated (Grade 3). Occasionally, well-differentiated squamous carcinomas having the appearance of condylomata acuminata are seen; these are called verrucous carcinomas.

Adenocarcinoma

Adenocarcinomas arise from the glandular epithelium lining the endocervical canal and the endocervical glands. Adenocarcinoma has often been thought to carry a worse prognosis than squamous carcinoma, but this is probably due to the origin being deep in the endocervical canal, leading to a later presentation of disease on the ectocervix and an increased bulk of tumor, stage for stage, at the time of diagnosis.

As the screening campaigns have reduced the incidence of squamous neoplasia, the relative incidence of adenocarcinoma has risen. This seems not to be solely due to the selective reduction in squamous neoplasia but also due to a genuine increase in the incidence of glandular neoplasia.

Adenosquamous carcinoma

This histological type contains both malignant squamous and adenocarcinomatous elements.

Prevention and treatment of pre-invasive disease

HPV vaccination

The intention of vaccination is to inhibit HPV infection of the female genital tract and therefore prevent the formation of CIN. Three HPV vaccines—bivalent, quadrivalent, and nanovalent—have been developed, aimed primarily at HPV 16 and 18, which are responsible for 70% of invasive cancers. The vaccines comprise artificial virus-like particles (VLPs) made from recombinant HPV coat proteins that are very effective at inducing strong and durable immune responses.

TABLE 21.1   **Staging of Carcinoma of the Cervix: A Comparison of the 2009 and 2018 FIGO Staging Systems**

FIGO 2009 Staging System		FIGO 2018 Staging System	
O	Pre-invasive carcinoma (CIN)	O	Pre-invasive carcinoma (CIN)
IA1	Microinvasion <3 mm deep and <7 mm wide: diagnosed by microscopy only	IA1	Microinvasion <3 mm deep: diagnosed by microscopy only
IA2	Microinvasion <5 mm deep and <7 mm wide: diagnosed by microscopy only	IA2	Microinvasion <5 mm deep: diagnosed by microscopy only
IB1	Carcinoma more extensive than IA2 but confined to the cervix (including uterine body) <4 cm diameter	IB1	Invasive carcinoma confined to cervix (including uterine body) ≥5 mm depth of stromal invasion and <2 cm diameter
		IB2	Carcinoma confined to cervix (including uterine body) ≥2 cm and <4 cm diameter
IB2	Carcinoma confined to the cervix (including uterine body) ≥4 cm diameter	IB3	Carcinoma confined to cervix (including uterine body) ≥4 cm diameter
IIA1	Carcinoma not involving the parametria but extending beyond the cervix into the upper two-thirds of the vagina <4 cm	IIA1	Carcinoma not involving the parametria but extending beyond the cervix into the upper two-thirds of the vagina <4 cm
IIA2	Carcinoma not involving the parametria but extending beyond the cervix into upper two-thirds of the vagina ≥4 cm	IIA2	Carcinoma not involving the parametria but extending beyond the cervix into upper two-thirds of the vagina ≥4 cm
IIB	Carcinoma extending into the parametria but not reaching the pelvic sidewall	IIB	Carcinoma extending into the parametria but not reaching the pelvic sidewall
IIIA	Carcinoma involving the lower third of the vagina but not reaching the pelvic sidewall	IIIA	Carcinoma involving the lower third of the vagina but not reaching the pelvic sidewall
IIIB	Carcinoma extending to the pelvic sidewall or causing hydronephrosis or non-functioning kidney	IIIB	Carcinoma extending to the pelvic sidewall or causing hydronephrosis or non-functioning kidney
		IIIC1	Pelvic lymph node metastasis only, irrespective of tumor size and extent[a]
		IIIC2	Para-aortic lymph node metastasis[a]
IVA	Carcinoma involving the mucosa of the bladder or rectum	IVA	Carcinoma involving the mucosa of the bladder or rectum
IVB	Distant metastasis	IVB	Distant metastasis

Sources: Bray et al., 2018; Denny et al., 2012.
All stages: Imaging and pathology can be used to supplement clinical findings with respect to tumor size and extent.
[a]   Add notation of r (imaging) or p (pathology) to indicate findings that allocate case as Stage IIIC.

Vaccines offer a promising new approach to the prevention of HPV and associated conditions. The vaccine needs to be administered before exposure to the virus, as it does not affect established infection. However, it should not replace regular cervical cancer screening, because the vaccines will not prevent all HPV types, and it will be 10–20 years before the predicted reduction in invasive cancers is seen. A recent Cochrane meta-analysis demonstrated that HPV vaccination is very effective at preventing pre-invasive cervical disease, with up to 97–100% reduction in CIN2+ in the HPV-naïve population and 44–53% among the overall population, depending on the type of vaccine.[11]

Many countries have now introduced a vaccination program, which due to health economics, is usually only offered to teenage girls. In developing countries, where screening is not established or where there is poor uptake, this may be a more effective way to prevent cervical cancer. In the United Kingdom, the vaccination program commenced in 2008 with a bivalent vaccine for all girls aged 12–13 years. It now covers all 12- and 13-year-old girls and boys using the quadrivalent vaccine Gardasil®, which also prevents anogenital warts.

Cervical screening

Exfoliative cytology

CIN precedes virtually every case of invasive squamous carcinoma of the cervix. Pre-invasive disease is commonly asymptomatic but may be detected by cytological examination of exfoliated cells. The Pap smear test is named after Greek doctor Georgios Papanicolaou, who developed the technique in 1927. Cells are taken from the transformation zone of the cervix with a spatula and spread on a glass slide. Liquid-based cytology is now the preferred method, where a suspension of cells is produced by shaking the spatula or brush in a transport medium, and a thin layer of the solution is then analyzed. The cells are studied microscopically using the Papanicolaou stain and an assessment made of the size, shape, and mitotic activity of the nuclei and the nuclear–cytoplasmic ratio. On the basis of this assessment, the cells will be reported as being normal, inflammatory, or showing mild atypia, as showing low-grade or high-grade dyskaryosis, or as being characteristic of invasive disease. Those patients with moderate or severe changes require biopsy of the cervix for histological assessment.[12]

Abnormal glandular cells are much more difficult to sample and detect on exfoliative cytology due to their position higher in the endocervical canal and their situation deep within the glandular crypts of the endocervix. Criteria for the diagnosis of glandular intra-epithelial neoplasia (CGIN), now classified as adenocarcinoma-in-situ (AIS), are more complex than for the squamous counterpart because of the lack of a clearly identifiable basement membrane around endocervical glands.

Screening program

The ease and reliability of exfoliative cytology has resulted in the establishment of many screening programs. In the United Kingdom, a decrease in mortality has been seen since improved coverage of the population was achieved by the 1990s.[13] Screening in the United Kingdom commences at 25 years and is repeated 3-yearly to 50 years and then 5-yearly until 65 years. Cervical cytology can give rise to both false-positive and false-negative results, and confirmation of positive or unexpectedly negative cytological findings should be sought by biopsy. The peak incidence of CIN occurs between the ages of 25 and 30, whereas the peak incidence of invasive carcinoma occurs in a group of patients approximately 10 years older.

HPV screening and test of cure

Tests are now undertaken on cervical specimens to detect HPV subtypes using DNA or mRNA. HPV status can be used to predict patients at high risk of CIN who need more frequent assessment. It can also check whether the infection has cleared after treatment as a test of cure. Several schemes have investigated the optimal method for incorporating HPV analysis with cervical cytology. One approach was to triage patients with low-grade or borderline changes on cytology, and only those with high-risk HPV type proceed to colposcopy, whereas low-risk patients return to routine screening.[14] The preferred approach now being considered nationally in the United Kingdom is to assess HPV status as the primary screening test, and cytology is then undertaken only on samples that are HPV positive.

Colposcopy

Colposcopy is undertaken for histological confirmation when there is moderate to severe dysplasia on cytology or when there is an obvious cervical abnormality that needs further assessment. It is also recommended for women with repeated inadequate samples or borderline changes in the presence of high-risk HPV. This technique of examination involves looking at the cervix with a low-power microscope and can be carried out without the need for a general anesthetic. By staining the cervix and upper vagina with acetic acid or Lugol's iodine, areas of abnormal epithelium can be identified and directed biopsies taken. In the case of extensive abnormalities or ones that extend up to the endocervical canal and cannot be entirely visualized, cone biopsy may be necessary.

Treatment

Once diagnosed histologically, CIN may be removed under colposcopic control by surgical excision through scalpel, cutting laser, or hot wire loop (LLETZ). Excision is favored over destructive methods, as it allows more accurate histological assessment of the entire abnormality than is possible on a biopsy alone. This particularly relates to occult foci of invasion that if not recognized, may lead to under-treatment. Lesions that cannot be delineated on all sides, especially if they involve the endocervical canal, must be removed by cone biopsy (Figure 21.1).

Clinical features of invasive carcinoma of the cervix

Anatomy

Anatomy of the cervix

The female reproductive organs are represented in Figures 21.2 and 21.3. The uterus comprises the corpus and the cervix, which is the lower one-third and enters the vagina. The cervix is supported by the cardinal ligaments laterally, the uterovesical ligaments anteriorly, and the uterosacral ligaments posteriorly (Figure 21.4). The endocervical canal connects the vagina with the uterine cavity and is lined by columnar epithelium. The part of the cervix protruding into the vagina, the ectocervix, is covered by stratified squamous epithelium. The cervix and body of the uterus are small during childhood, enlarge during puberty and the reproductive years, and then atrophy after menopause. In addition to changing in size during a woman's lifetime, the

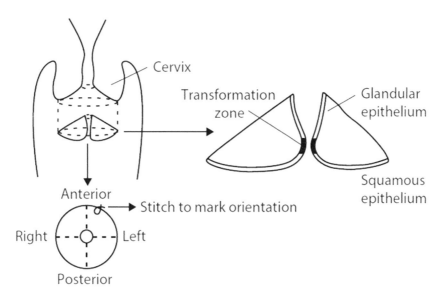

FIGURE 21.1   A cone biopsy, cut either by laser or by scalpel, must include all the transformation zone where the columnar epithelium of the endocervix meets the squamous epithelium of the ectocervix. It is marked to allow specimen orientation in the laboratory.

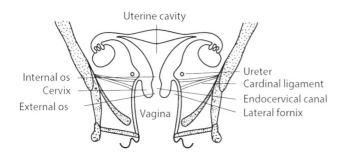

FIGURE 21.2   Diagram of the cervix, showing the relationship to the ureters and the cardinal ligaments (parametria).

transformation zone also changes in position, being usually just inside the external cervix in young women but rising up the endocervical canal after menopause.

Lymphatic drainage

There is a well-defined pattern for the lymphatic drainage of the cervix with direct drainage to the internal, external, and common iliac nodes. Other node groups that may be involved by direct lymphatic spread are the parametrial, obturator, and presacral nodes.[15,16] Spread to the para-aortic nodes is uncommon without pelvic node involvement, and the supraclavicular nodes may be involved subsequent to para-aortic node disease (Figure 21.5). Tumors involving the lower third of the vagina can drain directly to the inguinal nodes.

Spread of disease

Cervical carcinoma spreads predominantly by direct invasion and lymphatic permeation as previously described. Direct spread is superiorly into the body of the uterus and inferiorly into the vaginal mucosa. Laterally, the parametrial tissues, ligaments of the uterus, and pelvic sidewall may be involved. Rarely, the bladder anteriorly or rectum posteriorly can be invaded by advanced disease. Spread is usually contiguous, but seedlings from cervical cancer can occasionally be noted in the lower vagina.

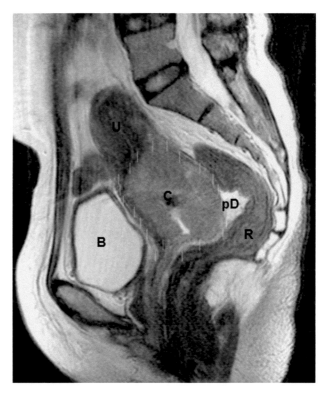

FIGURE 21.3   Sagittal T2-weighted MRI of the pelvis showing a bulky cervical tumor (C) extending into the lower aspect of the uterus (U) and the close relationship to bladder (B), rectum (R), and pouch of Douglas (pD).

Blood-borne spread is unusual, but when it does occur, it most frequently affects the lungs, bone, and liver.

Symptoms

Although an increasing number of invasive cervical carcinomas are detected in the pre-symptomatic stages by cervical screening,

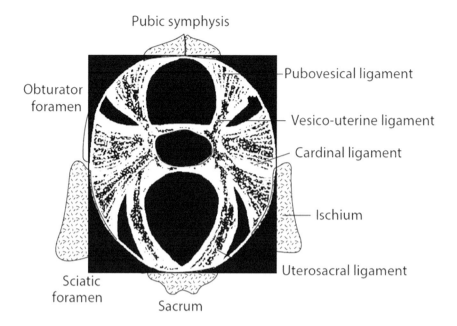

FIGURE 21.4 The ligaments supporting the uterus at the level of the cervix.

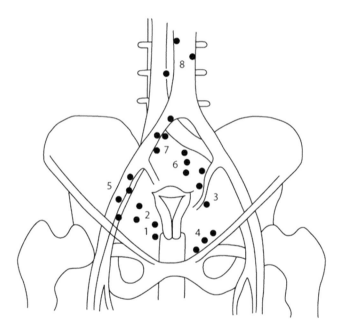

FIGURE 21.5 The lymph node drainage of the cervix: (1) para-cervical, (2) parametrial, (3) internal iliac, (4) obturator, (5) external iliac, (6) presacral, (7) common iliac, and (8) para-aortic nodes.

the majority of patients still present with symptoms. The most common symptom of invasive cervical cancer is bleeding, which may be post-coital, intermenstrual, or post-menopausal. Vaginal discharge is the second commonest symptom. These symptoms should always be investigated by clinical examination, inspection of the cervix, and exfoliative cytology and should lead to referral to a rapid referral unit according to the current referral criteria. Pain usually indicates late-stage disease. Advanced pelvic disease causes ureteric obstruction due to lateral parametrial involvement, and patients can present with confusion due to acute renal failure.

Signs

Visual inspection of the cervix may reveal it to be enlarged, have obvious growth on the surface, or be ulcerated. In addition, nodal masses may rarely be palpable in the groins or abdomen and in the left supraclavicular fossa. Patients with advanced disease may have tumors in the vagina or vulva and may have symptoms and signs of anemia, jaundice, or uremia.

Investigations for invasive disease

Clinical examination

Clinical examination of the patient should involve palpation of the abdomen to detect enlarged kidneys or liver, palpable para-aortic nodes, or an enlarged bladder. The inguinal and supraclavicular areas should be examined for metastatic lymph nodes. The vulva should be inspected and then the vagina and cervix examined using a speculum. If an abnormality is seen, a smear or punch biopsy should be taken for diagnosis.

Examination under anesthetic

Under anesthetic, both abdominal and pelvic examination will be carried out in addition to cystoscopy to rule out bladder involvement. If there is any suspicion of posterior spread, procto-sigmoidoscopy is performed. Ideally, for more advanced tumors, this should be a joint procedure with a surgeon and radiation oncologist to decide optimal management. The cervix should be examined bimanually (per vagina and per rectum) to assess the size, shape, and mobility of the uterus and any extension of tumor into surrounding tissues. Rectal examination gives additional information on posterior spread along the uterosacral ligaments, lateral parametrial invasion, and involvement of the pelvic sidewall. Biopsies should be taken from the cervix and any other abnormality in the vagina or vulva.

Hematological tests

Serum electrolytes, a full blood count, and renal and liver function tests may give an indication of ureteric involvement, liver metastases, or anemia from tumor hemorrhage.

Imaging tests

Further examination of the renal tract has traditionally been done with intravenous urography (IVU) or ultrasound scan and a chest x-ray taken to exclude lung metastases. However, cross-sectional imaging is required to determine the extent of disease.[17] Magnetic resonance imaging (MRI) has superb soft tissue contrast and is the imaging modality of choice to assess local disease extension and tumor volume.[18] Most commonly, a computed tomography (CT) scan will be used to assess the state of the chest, liver, renal tract, and para-aortic lymph nodes. Nodal disease can be imaged by CT or MRI using size criteria, measuring the nodal diameter to predict the risk of metastatic involvement. However, this method has poor sensitivity and specificity.[19] CT-positron emission tomography (CT-PET) is superior to the other imaging modalities for detecting nodal metastases (Figure 21.6).[20] In locally advanced disease, it has been shown to alter the radiation fields in approximately 20% of cases.[21]

Staging and prognostic factors

The most widely used staging system is that of FIGO.[10] Apart from micro-invasive disease, which is defined on histology, the system historically has depended largely on the examination under anesthetic. The results of cystoscopy, proctoscopy, chest x-ray, and IVU were all used in determining FIGO stage, but other imaging techniques did not alter tumor stage, because cervical carcinoma is most prevalent in developing countries where imaging resources are limited. In 2018, FIGO updated the staging system to incorporate modern imaging findings and histopathology results, particularly in relation to nodal staging.[22] A comparison of the 2009 and 2018 staging systems is shown in Table 21.1. The new staging system now includes Stage IIIC for lymph node involvement to reflect the impact of nodal status on both treatment decision-making and prognosis.

Stage

Approximately 65–75% of patients with carcinoma of the cervix can be cured of their disease (Table 21.2). Most recurrences occur within the first 2 years, and 5-year survival rates are a good measure of therapy effectiveness. More than 90% of patients with small Stage I tumors, with uninvolved lymph nodes, can be cured of their disease, but results remain disappointing for Stage III and IV tumors using the FIGO 2009 system, with 5-year survival rates of only approximately 30–50% and 10–15%, respectively.[23] Results for Stage II disease are perhaps the most variable between treatment centers. Five-year survival rates of between 40% and 75% are quoted.

Tumor volume

The FIGO system divides cervical tumors into broad prognostic groups and now takes account of tumor size in early-stage disease. Stage is the single most important factor related to prognosis (Table 21.2 and Figures 21.7 and 21.8). However, tumor volume is also an important prognostic factor, and a wide range of volumes can occur in any one FIGO stage. For example, a Stage IB

TABLE 21.2 Incidence of Lymph Node Involvement and Survival by FIGO 2009 Stage for Cervical Carcinoma

Stage	Pelvic Nodes (%)	Para-Aortic Nodes (%)	5-Year Survival (%)
IA	< 1	0	95
IB1	15	6	85
IB2	25	10	75
II	30	15	70
III	50	25	40
IVA	80	50	20
IVB	n/a	n/a	10

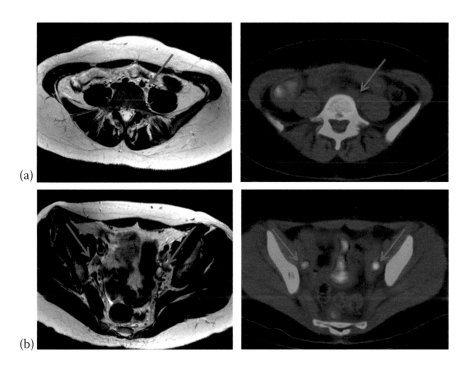

(a)

(b)

FIGURE 21.6 Comparison of MRI (left) and CT-PET (right) scans for detecting lymph node metastases. The arrows show the lymph nodes. (a) A small left common iliac lymph node is shown on both images. (b) Bilateral enlarged lymph nodes have high uptake on CT-PET.

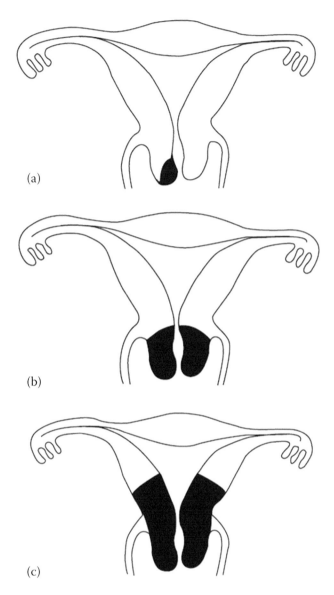

(a)

(b)

(c)

FIGURE 21.7 Stage IB carcinoma of the cervix, showing how this one stage includes a wide range of tumor volumes from (a) minimal disease of just over 0.5 cm³ to (b) involvement of the whole cervix to (c) huge tumors involving the uterine body. Although the first would now be staged as IB1 and the last as IB2, there is still a wide range of tumor volumes within each substage.

tumor can be anything from 0.25 cm³ for a tumor just exceeding the criteria for Stage IA (Figure 21.7a) to as much as 100–200 cm³ for a "barrel" tumor arising in the endocervical canal.[24] In addition to recording FIGO stage, it is also important to record tumor size or volume as measured at the time of examination under anesthetic or more accurately, on MRI scans.

Nodal status

Nodal status has a profound effect on survival. The risk of lymph node involvement increases with tumor stage and size (Table 21.2). Those patients having clinical Stage IB carcinoma of the cervix with positive pelvic nodes have a 5-year survival expectation that is half that of those with negative pelvic nodes. Patients with macroscopically involved para-aortic nodes have a much higher risk of widespread dissemination.

In addition to the distribution of nodes, the total number of nodes involved is also a powerful prognostic factor in surgically staged series.[25]

Lymphovascular permeation

Lymphovascular space involvement has a prognostic significance in being an indicator of the likelihood of pelvic nodal involvement.[26] However, it also has a prognostic effect even in the absence of pelvic nodal disease.

Depth of invasion of the cervix

Tumors invading more than 15 mm through the cervical stroma have a worse prognosis than less deeply invasive tumors.[27]

Histology

In some series, the degree of differentiation of squamous cancers has been shown to be of prognostic significance, with patients with poorly differentiated tumors faring worse than those with well- or moderately differentiated tumors. Adenocarcinomas and adenosquamous carcinomas have also been thought to have a worse prognosis, stage for stage, than squamous carcinomas, although this remains controversial.[28]

Small cell neuro-endocrine tumors of the cervix have a particularly bad prognosis because of their propensity for lymphatic and blood-borne spread, even at an early stage. As at other sites of the body, long-term survival from this type of tumor is rare.

Age

In some historical series, young age was shown to convey a survival advantage over old age, whereas in other series, no difference was found between different age groups. Furthermore, a poor prognostic effect of very young age has also been seen. The impression is that cancer of the cervix in young women is occasionally a disease of rapid onset with a high propensity for metastasis and rapid progression.

Prognostic indices and scores

The Gynecologic Oncology Group has defined a system of assigning scores to a number of prognostic factors, mostly histological, to produce an overall prognostic score. This is particularly relevant for patients treated by surgery, where the score may be used to define the need for postoperative adjuvant radiotherapy. The factors taken into consideration are lymphovascular space invasion, clinical tumor size, and depth of invasion.[27] Many oncologists use a simpler system, with absolute indicators for postoperative therapy being residual disease, positive operative margins, parametrial involvement, or lymph node involvement. Relative indicators are lymphovascular permeation, deep stromal invasion, and narrow surgical margins less than 4 mm, with the presence of any two indicating a need for adjuvant therapy.

Treatment options

The treatment of invasive cervical cancer depends on the stage of disease, tumor size, lymph node status, and the fitness of the patient.[29] It can incorporate surgery, radiotherapy, and chemotherapy. Ideally, a single definitive modality should be used, as there is no survival advantage and far greater morbidity with a combined surgical and radiotherapy approach. Although surgery

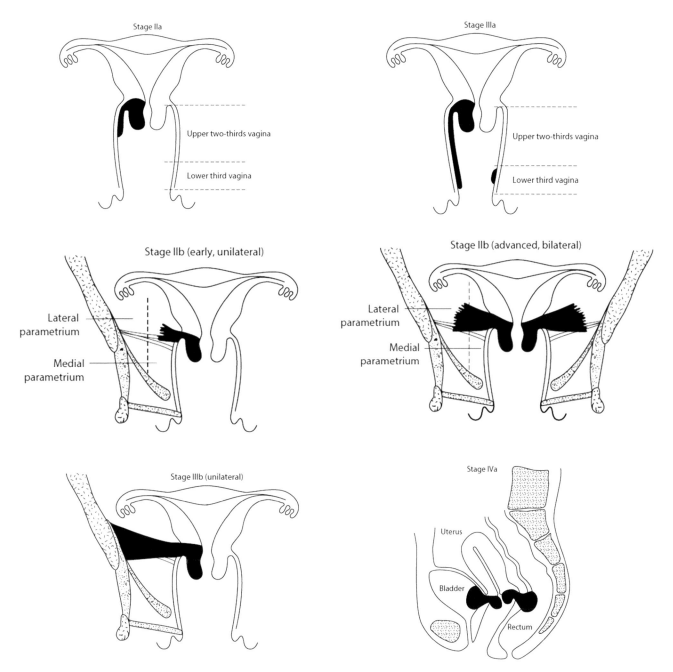

FIGURE 21.8 Stages IIA–IVA carcinoma of the cervix. Stage IIA and IIIA tumors involve the vaginal mucosa only. Stage IIB and IIIB tumors involve the parametria and pelvic sidewall, respectively. A distinction is occasionally made between medial and lateral parametrial involvement and unilateral and bilateral fixation to the pelvic sidewall. Ureteric obstruction also stages a tumor as IIIB. Stage IVA tumors involve the rectum or bladder.

is preferable for early-stage disease, radiotherapy is the treatment of choice when there is parametrial or nodal involvement, which emphasizes the need for optimal imaging to stage the disease at presentation.[30,31]

Management of micro-invasive disease

The diagnosis of Stage IA cervical cancer is made on histopathology by an expert pathologist, assessing the width and depth of tumor invasion, margin status, and whether there is any lymphovascular invasion. A cone biopsy that completely excises a IA1 lesion with clear margins should be adequate treatment provided the depth of invasion is less than 3 mm and there is no lymphovascular involvement. If a cone biopsy cannot completely encompass a lesion, then a simple hysterectomy should be undertaken in women not concerned about retaining fertility, particularly if there is a background of CIN III. For women wishing to retain the chance of further pregnancy, a trachelectomy can be performed. If the lesion invades further than 3 mm depth (Stage IA2), or if there is lymphovascular invasion, then the risk of involved lymph nodes rises and needs to be evaluated surgically.

Management of Stage IB and IIA disease

Surgery is the treatment of choice for patients with tumors less than 4 cm in diameter in whom there is a low risk of nodal metastases. Good histological differentiation, the absence of lymphatic vessel invasion, small tumor volume, and normal-sized nodes on cross-sectional imaging are indicators that lymph node metastases are unlikely. The standard surgical procedure is a radical hysterectomy with systematic pelvic lymphadenectomy. The ovaries can be conserved in pre-menopausal women.

In women who wish to preserve fertility, radical trachelectomy is also an option for treating tumors less than 2 cm in diameter. The pelvic lymph nodes must still be staged with pelvic lymphadenectomy. For tumors larger than 2 cm, neo-adjuvant chemotherapy followed by trachelectomy is being investigated as an approach for carefully selected patients provided surgical assessment of lymph nodes shows no metastases.

Radiotherapy is also an effective treatment for early-stage cervical cancer with excellent long-term tumor control. It can be used as the primary treatment if a patient is not fit for radical surgery or if there are multiple poor prognostic tumor features indicating a high risk of requiring adjuvant radiotherapy after surgery. The advantages of surgery over radiotherapy for early-stage disease include the avoidance of further shrinkage of the vagina after treatment, and the maintenance of pliability and lubrication of the vaginal mucosa. In addition, the small risk of late induction of a second malignancy is avoided.

Management of locally advanced disease

Primary radiotherapy is the treatment of choice for patients with bulky tumors or when there is extension beyond the cervix to the parametria or lymph nodes. The combination of external beam radiotherapy, concurrent chemotherapy, and intrauterine brachytherapy is used. Completion surgery with hysterectomy following radiotherapy is only required if there is any residual disease after radiotherapy. If there is a complete response following radiotherapy, the addition of surgery adds to morbidity but does not improve survival.

An alternative approach undertaken in some centers has been the use of neo-adjuvant chemotherapy followed by radical surgery for larger Stage IB tumors. In recent randomized clinical trials, there was worse progression-free survival compared with primary radiotherapy, and this method is not advised as standard of care. However, this may still be an option for selected patients, particularly if radiotherapy is contra-indicated. Rarely, primary pelvic exenterative surgery may be required for patients with very advanced local disease.

Since there can be up to 30–40% risk of future development of distant metastases in patients with lymph node involvement or with advanced local disease, there may be an advantage to the use of additional neo-adjuvant or adjuvant systemic therapy. Although previous studies did not demonstrate a significant survival advantage, there are several ongoing studies specifically for high-risk patients to investigate this strategy.

Surgery

The surgical options vary depending on the size of the primary tumor and the method for assessing the pelvic nodes. It is important to consider the potential morbidities and whether fertility preservation is an option for the patient.

Radical hysterectomy

Surgery for invasive cervical carcinoma should include a radical hysterectomy and a pelvic lymphadenectomy. This is often called a "Wertheim's" hysterectomy, which was first described in 1905, although the original operation did not include lymphadenectomy.[33] In contrast to the simple hysterectomy procedure undertaken for endometrial cancer, the parametrial and paracervical tissues and a vaginal cuff are taken. Removal of the lateral parametrium causes more morbidity with a higher risk of bladder and bowel impairment due to nerve and vascular damage. Therefore, a modified radical hysterectomy with removal of the medial half of the parametrium is usually undertaken, and nerve-sparing techniques can reduce the impact on bladder function. In a young woman with a squamous cell carcinoma, the risk of ovarian metastases in early-stage disease is low, and it is therefore possible to conserve the ovaries and avoid menopause. There is a higher risk of ovarian metastases with cervical adenocarcinoma.

Minimal access surgery with a laparoscopic or robotic approach has been reported to reduce postoperative complications and have more rapid recovery times than an open approach. Whereas retrospective studies comparing open with minimal access surgery have reported equivalent oncological outcomes, a recent randomized clinical trial and separate cohort studies have reported reduced disease-free survival in patients with cervical cancer treated with minimal access surgery. Therefore, for tumors more than 2 cm in diameter, an open surgical approach is now recommended.[34]

Fertility-preserving surgery

A less extensive radical surgical technique has been developed for women of childbearing age who want to preserve their fertility and whose tumors are smaller than 2 cm and limited to the cervix.[35] This is radical trachelectomy, in which the cervix and paracervical tissues are removed together with a cuff of vagina. The body of the uterus is left in place and anastomosed to the vagina. The new opening into the uterine cavity is narrowed with a circumferential stitch. This allows a pregnancy to be carried but requires delivery by caesarean section, and there is a higher risk of miscarriage and pre-term delivery. The procedure is usually accompanied by a pelvic lymphadenectomy, which may be carried out using minimal access surgery.

Lymph node assessment

The rich lymphatic drainage of the cervix means that lymph node metastases can occur even with very early disease. Although PET imaging has a higher sensitivity than MRI or CT for detecting nodal metastases in locally advanced disease, it has poor sensitivity in early-stage disease, and surgical assessment is recommended. Bilateral pelvic systematic lymphadenectomy is the standard staging procedure. This is usually undertaken as the first stage of the operation with frozen section of any suspicious nodes. This allows an intra-operative decision to be made to curtail the surgery if the finding of a lymph node metastasis means that radiotherapy is then going to be required.

Sentinel lymph node mapping is an alternative method for assessing lymph node status. A radioactive or fluorescent tracer is injected into the cervix and then passes via the lymphatic drainage pathways to the "first station" lymph nodes. Studies have shown equivalent sensitivity for detecting nodal metastases compared with systematic node dissection, with a low false-negative rate in early stage disease.[36] This also has the benefit that the risk of lymphoedema is significantly reduced when fewer nodes are removed. Ultrastaging of the sentinel lymph node, in which the whole lymph node is cut into very thin slices for histopathological examination, can detect micro-metastases that may not have been noted with conventional assessment. This will then help guide further management decisions based on the nodal status.

Follow-up

Following surgery, patients should have regular clinical examination, typically every 3 months for the first 2 years and then 6-monthly up to 5 years from treatment. The optimal surveillance strategy is uncertain; the use of routine MRI or CT imaging may detect more asymptomatic, and potentially curable, loco-regional recurrences than the traditional approach of imaging only in the event of new symptoms. Following fertility-preserving surgery, regular imaging and exfoliative cytology of the vaginal vault are recommended.

Radiotherapy

Radiotherapy is the recommended treatment modality for locally advanced cervical cancer. By the 1920s, the regimen of fractionated external beam radiotherapy (EBRT) followed by intracavitary brachytherapy was established as the standard of care. Advances in radiobiology, machine technologies, imaging, and systemic therapies have continued to improve outcomes over the following century. The pelvis is usually treated to a dose of 45–50 Gy over 5 weeks with concurrent chemotherapy. Intrauterine brachytherapy then delivers a very high dose directly into the cervix. When radiotherapy is required as adjuvant treatment following a hysterectomy, the brachytherapy boost following EBRT is delivered to the vaginal vault.

Radiobiological principles

There is a strong correlation between the total dose delivered to the tumor and local control rates, with overall survival similarly increasing when the dose is escalated. However, there is also a similar dose–response relationship for normal tissue toxicity that limits the dose that can be safely delivered, with dose-limiting structures including the small bowel, rectum, and bladder.

The addition of weekly cisplatin to the radiotherapy regimen has become standard practice. In 1999, the National Cancer Institute issued a clinical alert advising the use of concomitant chemoradiation for cervical cancer, resulting in an immediate worldwide change in practice. This statement was based on three published papers reporting randomized controlled trials of the addition of cisplatin-based therapies to radiotherapy, with all showing significant improvement in survival for patients in the chemoradiation arm compared with the standard radiotherapy arm.[37–39] A more recent Cochrane meta-analysis of 21 studies

concluded a 14% absolute benefit in overall survival for the addition of cisplatin chemotherapy.[40]

Studies in the late 1970s showed that women with a hemoglobin level below 10 g/dL had a lower cure rate by radiotherapy than women with a higher hemoglobin level. Women with a hemoglobin level above 12 g/dL fared better than those with a lower level, and this is independent of tumor stage and size.[41] This effect is due to a radiosensitizing effect of oxygen on the tumor, and it is recommended that the hemoglobin level be kept above 12 g/dL throughout radiotherapy.[42] Smoking decreases tumor oxygen levels and also increases normal tissue toxicity, so patients should be counseled about cessation during treatment.

Overall treatment time should not be extended beyond the planned schedule, or a decrease in effectiveness of approximately 1% per day will occur due to tumor repopulation.[43]

External beam radiotherapy

The volume encompassed by EBRT includes the loco-regional nodes as well as the primary tumor. Conventional field borders are typically from the junction of the 4th and 5th lumbar vertebrae to the bottom of the obturator foramina and laterally to 2 cm outside the bony pelvis (Figure 21.9). If it is appropriate to spare the posterior half of the rectum, in the absence of uterosacral ligament involvement, this volume can be encompassed by a four-field "box" technique; otherwise, a pair of parallel-opposed fields is used. Ideally, 10–15 MV photons are needed to ensure dose homogeneity despite the depth of the tumor volume below the surface of the lateral fields.

However, the target defined by these traditional fields has been shown to have a high risk of a geographical miss despite including a large volume of normal tissue.[44] Three-dimensional planning either with conformal radiotherapy or ideally, with intensity-modulated radiation therapy (IMRT) or volumetric arc therapy (VMAT) should be used to optimize target volume coverage and to enable individualized shielding of the normal tissues (Figure 21.10).[45] The clinical target volume includes the primary tumor, cervix, whole uterus, parametria, ovaries, and the common iliac, internal iliac, obturator, external iliac, and presacral lymph nodes.[46,47] Those patients with disease in the vaginal mucosa below the upper third have the fields extended to cover the full length of the vagina, and inguinal nodes are included when tumor involves the lower third of the vagina.

If common iliac or para-aortic nodes are involved, then the target volume should include at least the infra-renal para-aortic lymph

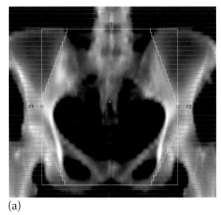
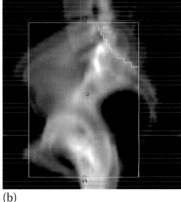

(a)   (b)

FIGURE 21.9 The conventional radiotherapy fields used to treat carcinoma of the cervix (a) anterior-posterior (b) lateral. To cover the "first station" lymph nodes, the field extends from the junction of the fourth and fifth lumbar vertebrae to the bottom of the obturator foramina.

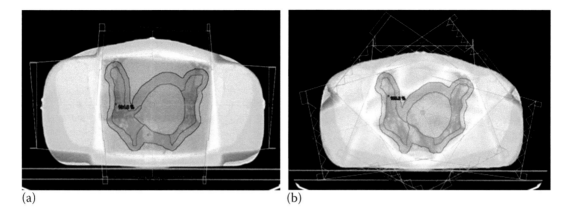

(a)   (b)

FIGURE 21.10   Radiotherapy plans designed to cover the uterus and draining lymph nodes (red outline) within the final planning target volume (blue outline). (a) Conformal plan using four fields fitted to the target volume results in a box shaped distribution of the high-dose region (shown in red on a dose color wash). (b) An IMRT plan results in the high-dose region fitting more closely to the target volume.

nodes as well as the pelvis. More bowel sparing is achieved with an IMRT technique compared with conformal or conventional radiotherapy, although care is needed to avoid the kidneys and spinal cord.

The uterus and cervix are highly mobile structures with their position dependent on bladder and rectal filling.[48] Throughout a course of radiotherapy, there is often significant tumor regression, changing the shape and location of the central disease.[49] Large margins are required around the uterus to ensure coverage throughout the 5 weeks. Reduction in these margins can only be achieved with careful image guidance involving daily scans taken immediately before treatment. Studies are ongoing to assess the application of an adaptive treatment using a "plan of the day" approach or rapid online replanning of the dose distribution.

Traditionally, the dose delivered to enlarged lymph nodes has been limited by bowel tolerance and the difficulty of matching a pelvic sidewall boost to brachytherapy dosimetry. The particular advantage of IMRT (including VMAT) is the ability to escalate the dose using a simultaneous integrated boost to involved lymph nodes without significantly impacting on the organ at risk doses (Figure 21.11).

Intracavitary brachytherapy

Brachytherapy enables a high dose of radiotherapy to be delivered directly into the cervix and uterine cavity. The rapid fall off in

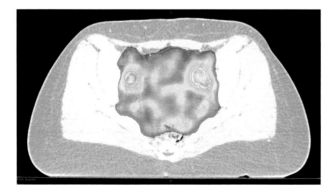

FIGURE 21.11   Simultaneous integrated boost VMAT plan delivering a higher dose of 55 Gy to the involved pelvic lymph node and 45 Gy to the rest of the target volume.

dose around the radioactive source means that there is relative sparing of the surrounding normal tissues, and the short treatment time reduces the risk of tumor repopulation. By 1903, there were published reports of women with cervical cancer who were successfully treated with radium inserted into the endocervical canal and upper vagina.[50] The radioisotope initially used for intracavitary brachytherapy was radium, which because of its gaseous daughter product radon, is hazardous. Radium was replaced by cesium-137, which decays to solid, non-radioactive products.

There is an ongoing debate about the optimal schedule for intrauterine brachytherapy.[51] Low dose rate (LDR) systems with cesium-137 were radiobiologically ideal, as they allowed ongoing repair of radiation damage to normal tissues. However, these machines are no longer manufactured and are being replaced by high dose rate (HDR) systems delivering rates in excess of 1 Gy/min, and the most common radioactive source is iridium-192. The short treatment time allows more geometrical stability of the applicator during treatment and more rapid patient throughput, but there is considerably less time for repair of radiation damage. Therefore, such treatments are fractionated over several days, and the dose is adjusted for this difference in dose rate. Pulsed dose rate brachytherapy (PDR) uses an HDR source but delivers multiple small fractions over 2 days for a single insertion to reproduce LDR radiobiology.[52] In order to be able to compare outcomes for these different dose rates and fractionation regimens, it is now standard to report 2 Gy equivalent (EQD2) total doses.

Brachytherapy procedure

Brachytherapy treatment is scheduled towards the end or immediately after completing EBRT to enable maximal tumor regression without unduly extending the total treatment time. Under general or regional anesthetic, the patient is examined to ascertain the extent of residual disease. The cervix is dilated, and applicators are placed within the uterine cavity and upper vagina. Ultrasound guidance confirms the optimal position and reduces the risk of perforation. The tubes are held in place with gauze packing, and a posterior spacer may help to reduce rectal dose. Imaging is undertaken to confirm the appropriate position and geometry of the applicators and for treatment planning. Once the patient is comfortable and in a radiation-protected environment, the radioactive source is inserted by remote control, and the individualized plan is delivered.

Conventional brachytherapy

A technique commonly used since the 1930s is the "Manchester" technique involving an intrauterine tube and two vaginal ovoids placed in the lateral vaginal fornices. The proportions of radio-isotope, initially radium and more latterly cesium, within the intrauterine tube and the vaginal ovoids were calculated to give a constant dose rate to a geometrical point "A" when using different lengths of intrauterine tube and different sizes of vaginal ovoids. Point "A" was originally defined as being 2 cm above the top of the ovoid and 2 cm lateral to the axis of the intrauterine sources. This approximates to the radiosensitive point where the uterine artery crosses the ureter, although it does vary subject to applicator type and individual anatomy.

Image-guided brachytherapy

The development of CT/MRI-compatible applicators has transformed brachytherapy treatment, enabling image-guided and individually designed treatment plans (Figure 21.12). After insertion, cross-sectional imaging confirms the applicator position, visualizes residual tumor, and allows dose distributions to be produced for the rectum, bladder, and bowel. For tumors with lateral extension, additional needles implanted into the outer cervix can increase dose to regions inadequately covered by the standard plan. This technique was pioneered at Vienna Medical University Hospital, where it demonstrated significant improvement in local control and overall survival for patients with bulky tumors.[53] An European consensus group developed the GEC-ESTRO guidelines for target volume definition, tumor doses, and organs at risk tolerances, recommending that at least 85 Gy (EQD2) is delivered to residual macroscopic disease and cervix.[54] The EMBRACE study is a large international prospective observational trial that has confirmed the benefit of image-guided brachytherapy and refined the optimal dose targets for treating the cervix and any residual disease at time of brachytherapy, as well as optimizing organ at risk doses.

Follow-up

Response to radiotherapy is assessed with clinical examination and an MRI scan after 3 months (Figure 21.13). PET imaging may be useful if there are equivocal findings, as patients with a complete metabolic response have an excellent outlook.[55] In the event of residual disease, surgery to obtain central clearance should be considered. There is no role for routine cytology in follow-up after radiotherapy.

Special situations

Neuroendocrine carcinoma of the cervix

Small cell neuroendocrine tumors of the cervix behave like small cell tumors at any other site. The most effective treatment

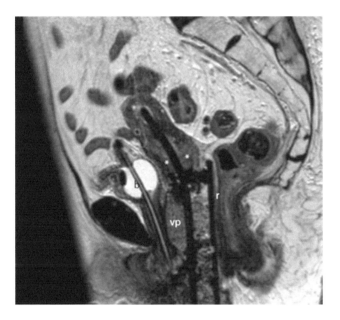

FIGURE 21.12 Sagittal T2-weighted MRI of the pelvis with a brachytherapy applicator placed in the uterus and held in place with vaginal packing (vp). Residual tumor is seen as high signal within the cervix (*). A urinary catheter is within the bladder (b), and a spacer in the vagina (r) displaces the rectum posteriorly to reduce dose.

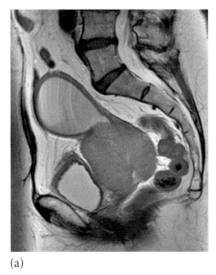
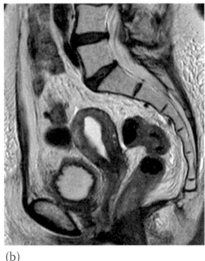

(a)   (b)

FIGURE 21.13 (a) Pre-treatment sagittal T2-weighted MRI of the pelvis showing a bulky cervical cancer causing a distended uterine cavity due to fluid collection. (b) Repeat scan 3 months after completing radiotherapy demonstrates a complete response.

is with chemotherapy (e.g., platinum and etoposide) followed by radiotherapy, surgery, or both to the sites of bulk disease. There is usually a dramatic and rapid response, but the disease metastasizes and recurs equally rapidly. Therefore, the prognosis is very poor.

Incidental finding of cervical cancer

Occasionally, invasive cervical cancer is found in the specimen following a simple hysterectomy. If the depth of invasion indicates a risk of lymphatic spread (Stage IA2 or more, or if there are other poor prognostic features), then postoperative pelvic chemoradiotherapy should be prescribed. The pelvic nodes should be imaged or undergo biopsy, as positive nodes will require surgery or a higher dose of radiotherapy than is used in the adjuvant setting. If the cuff of vagina is inadequate, then vault brachytherapy also should be delivered. With this technique, the results of treatment are no worse than with radical surgery.

Although the pelvis tolerates radiotherapy less well after surgery, it is usually possible to deliver 40–50 Gy over 5–6 weeks postoperatively, usually with concomitant cisplatin. If there is residual disease at the vaginal vault or at the margins of excision, then a second phase of treatment is needed to take the total tumor dose to at least 65 Gy with intracavitary or interstitial brachytherapy or a CT planned small volume of external beam therapy. In this circumstance, it must be accepted that there is a greater likelihood of late morbidity.

Cervical carcinoma during pregnancy

This difficult situation arises uncommonly, and treatment depends on the wishes of the parents as well as on the stage of disease. Treatment would be similar to that for non-pregnant patients in the first and second trimester of pregnancy, with treatment preceded by termination of pregnancy. Chemotherapy can be given from the second trimester if it is decided to proceed with the pregnancy. Caesarean section in the third trimester should precede definitive treatment. The commonly perceived view that carcinoma of the cervix behaves more aggressively in pregnant patients than in non-pregnant patients is not proven in long-term studies of age-matched patients.

Hemorrhage

Carcinoma of the cervix can present with severe hemorrhage that may require firm vaginal packing, bed rest, and a blood transfusion. Tranexamic acid may be helpful in stopping bleeding. Urgent EBRT may well produce hemostasis within 24–48 hours. In intractable cases, hysterectomy or embolization or ligation of the internal iliac arteries should be considered.

Management of recurrent and metastatic disease

The treatment options for recurrent or metastatic cervical cancer need to be individualized depending on the site and extent of disease, prior treatment, and patient-related factors. Localized pelvic and lymph node recurrences can potentially still be cured with surgery or radiotherapy. The most common locations for distant relapse are nodal, lung, or liver metastases, and it is less common to develop bone and brain metastases. Although it has traditionally been considered that patients with distant metastases cannot be cured, it is being increasingly recognized that when metastases are present in a limited number of sites, termed oligometastatic disease, this could also be approached with radical intent. In contrast, the development of widespread metastases necessitates a palliative approach, primarily with systemic therapies and symptomatic management.

Surgery

Surgery is usually the only potentially curative option for patients with pelvic recurrence following radiotherapy. However, in order to achieve complete resection of disease, it is necessary to undertake anterior, posterior, or total pelvic exenteration involving diversion of the urinary and gastrointestinal tracts.[56] Selection of patients for this procedure must include both physical and psychological assessment of the patient's ability to cope with the resulting stomas and potential toxicity. With good prognostic factors, including a long disease-free interval, small tumor volume, no lymph node involvement, and clear resection, up to 50% long-term survival rates are reported.[57]

Surgical resection should also be considered for resection of oligometastatic disease in the lung, liver, brain, and lymph nodes.

Radiotherapy

Pelvic recurrence occurs in approximately 10% of patients following radical hysterectomy for early-stage disease. This can still be salvaged with radical chemo-radiotherapy if a dose to the tumor in excess of 63–65 Gy can be achieved. This usually involves at least a two-phase approach to treatment, with external radiotherapy and chemotherapy followed by intracavitary brachytherapy, interstitial brachytherapy, or a CT planned small-volume external beam boost.

Pelvic and para-aortic lymph node recurrence can also be treated with radiotherapy. Whereas outcomes are poor if patients present with bulky, symptomatic disease, long-term survival rates up to 50% are reported for asymptomatic disease.[58] This may be further improved with the use of IMRT and a sequential or integrated boost to escalate the nodal dose.

Re-irradiation has historically been associated with a high risk of morbidity, although early studies did demonstrate that long-term control could be achieved. Interstitial brachytherapy can be used to deliver targeted treatment to vaginal and central pelvic recurrences for selected patients.[59] Stereotactic radiotherapy enables delivery of very targeted treatment and is increasingly being used for treatment of oligometastatic disease and for re-irradiation of small-volume disease if brachytherapy is not feasible (Figure 21.14).[60]

A short course of radiotherapy is also an effective palliative treatment for pelvic and metastatic disease, particularly when there is significant bleeding or pain.

Chemotherapy and targeted agents

Other than the role in concurrent treatment described previously, carcinoma of the cervix is not a highly chemosensitive tumor. Response rates to single agents have seldom been reported in excess of 40%, and the most effective drug is cisplatin. However, the taxanes may have a similar level of activity when combined with carboplatin 3-weekly or used alone on a weekly basis.[61] Other drugs with similar activity in combination with platinum include topotecan and gemcitabine.[62] These drugs may be used alone or in combination with others for recurrent disease, in the neo-adjuvant setting before surgery or radiotherapy, and during radiotherapy as concomitant therapy for advanced, bulky disease.

The best response rate to chemotherapy is seen in primary untreated disease (~70%). However, the response rate in metastatic disease is lower (~50%), and in recurrent disease, within an irradiated area, it is very low indeed (~15%). Therefore, with careful patient selection, chemotherapy may be used for palliation, and for a small number of patients, long-term control of disease can be achieved. Integration of a biological targeted agent,

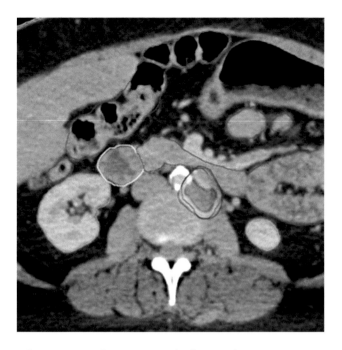

FIGURE 21.14 Stereotactic radiotherapy plan treating a para-aortic lymph node.

such as the vascular endothelial growth factor (VEGF) inhibitor bevacizumab, with chemotherapy has been shown to improve overall survival in a randomized controlled trial for patients with recurrent disease.[63] However, there is a risk of bladder and bowel fistulation and perforation, particularly in patients who have previously received radiotherapy.

Immunotherapy with pembrolizumab, a PD-1 checkpoint inhibitor, has shown promising results, which has led to approval of the drug by the U.S. Food and Drug Administration (FDA) based on early-phase trials for patients with recurrent or metastatic cervical cancer whose tumors express programmed death ligand (PD-L1). As cure of recurrent disease by chemotherapy is extremely rare, it is important to consider the toxicity of treatment when designing a palliative regimen for a patient.

Consequences of treatment

While management decisions have historically been primarily focused on oncological outcomes, it is also very important to consider the potential long-term impact of treatment. A holistic approach considering the physical, emotional, and social impact of the diagnosis and treatment of cervical cancer is required. Toxicity is typically under-reported by both patients and clinicians, and prospective assessment of morbidity and quality of life using validated clinician- and patient-reported outcomes should be incorporated into clinical studies.

Surgery

In addition to the morbidity and mortality associated with any major pelvic operation, radical hysterectomy can also cause specific problems in the pelvis. The most common of these is a degree of flaccidity of the bladder. This symptom is apparent soon after surgery and often improves with bladder drainage over a period of a few weeks. Rarely, the bladder remains flaccid, and the patient has to practice intermittent self-catheterization.

Other, more serious problems that can arise are adhesions or fistulae between the vagina, bladder, ureter, and/or rectum. Very rarely, such fistulae may also involve the small bowel. These problems are much increased in incidence if surgery is as salvage for recurrence after radical radiotherapy.

Pelvic lymphoceles may collect after a lymphadenectomy and may be asymptomatic or cause problems of pain or of obstruction to the ureters and bowel. If they become infected, then eradication of the infection may be difficult, and the risk of lower limb lymphoedema is increased. Lymphoedema affecting the lower limbs or genitalia can occur following pelvic lymphadenectomy and may progress over years after treatment. The incidence is significantly reduced if only sentinel lymph node removal is undertaken.

Radiotherapy

Treatment regimens are designed with the assumption that all patients have a similar sensitivity to radiation, although it is known that this is not the case, as a wide range of both acute and late reactions are seen at standard doses. Of particular importance is smoking, which not only reduces the chance of cure but also increases the risk of severe late effects. Patients with a history of pelvic inflammatory disease or diabetic vascular changes and those with inflammatory bowel disease, such as Crohn's disease and ulcerative colitis, may show excessive radiation reactions in the bowel. The use of IMRT reduces the risk of severe toxicity, but even low-grade long-term toxicity can significantly impact on quality of life.

Acute effects

At the dose levels necessary to treat carcinoma of the cervix with curative intent, it is common to cause some acute radiation reaction, usually in the bowel. In most patients, this results in diarrhea and urgency, which becomes apparent in the third or fourth week of a course of treatment. Diarrhea can usually be controlled by a low-roughage diet and with an anti-motility drug such as codeine phosphate or loperamide. Nausea is uncommon unless treating the para-aortic nodes, when the use of an anti-emetic such as domperidone taken 1 hour before treatment can prevent symptoms.

Radiation cystitis occurs less commonly than bowel disturbance and must be distinguished from infection by culture of a specimen of urine. With modern megavoltage radiotherapy, it is unusual to cause skin reactions that are sufficient to warrant a delay in treatment. However, moist desquamation of the skin may develop in the natal cleft or over the perineum if the whole vagina is treated.

Late effects

Late radiation effects usually become apparent months or years after treatment. Severe late effects should not occur in more than 5% of the patients treated with radical radiotherapy.

However, in up to 50% of patients, bowel habit may be permanently altered towards looseness and increased frequency of evacuation. This may be due to decreased absorption of water in the large bowel, malabsorption of bile acids from the bowel contents, bacterial overgrowth, or a number of other factors; specialist investigation is required to determine the cause.[64]

Rectal bleeding may result either from ulceration of the bowel mucosa or from telangiectasia. Recurrent cervical cancer and primary neoplasms of the bowel should be excluded by colonoscopy. Radiation fibrosis may also rarely cause stenosis or obstruction of the intestine, most commonly of the small bowel or sigmoid colon, and may occur at more than one level.

Late damage to the bladder may result in only a small volume of urine being tolerated. This can be due not only to fibrosis in the bladder restricting expansion but also to a neurological disturbance resulting in lower pressures within the bladder triggering the desire to micturate.

Fine pelvic insufficiency fractures in the sacral-iliac region can lead to pelvic pain and may be misdiagnosed as either bony metastatic disease or direct invasion.

Lower limb edema is seldom due to radiotherapy alone and is often a symptom of recurrent tumors in the pelvis or of a deep vein thrombosis. However, this symptom is much more commonly seen when there has been a combination of radiotherapy and radical surgery, especially if the latter was associated with infection or with pelvic lymphocele.

Systemic therapies

The toxic effects of cytotoxic drugs in the treatment of cancer of the cervix are similar to those caused in the treatment of other malignancies. To avoid damage to the renal system, cisplatin and carboplatin should only be given if a measure of the glomerular filtration rate, by creatinine clearance or ethylenediaminetetraacetic acid (EDTA) clearance, shows there to be adequate function. Carboplatin, cisplatin, taxanes, and topotecan can all cause myelosuppression. When scheduling intrauterine brachytherapy after chemoradiation, granulocyte-colony stimulating factor (G-CSF) may be necessary if the neutrophil count is low, whereas thrombocytopenia may prevent the use of spinal anesthesia.

Cisplatin and taxane toxicities include peripheral neuropathy, tinnitus, and damage to high-tone hearing. Unfortunately, the peripheral neuropathy and hearing changes can sometimes not be evident until after finishing chemotherapy and are often irreversible.

VEGF inhibitors cause an increased risk of bowel and bladder fistulation and perforation, particularly in patients with prior radiotherapy. Immunotherapy with checkpoint inhibitors has a very different toxicity profile, with potential auto-immune complications including colitis, pneumonitis, nephropathy, cardiotoxicity, and endocrinopathies.

Hormonal changes

Surgical removal of the ovaries at the time of radical hysterectomy can usually be avoided for pre-menopausal women unless there is involvement of the body of the uterus by tumor. However, should removal be necessary or should the ovaries lie within a radiation field, then an early menopause will occur. There is no evidence that hormone replacement therapy (HRT) has an adverse effect on survival, and it should be used to relieve menopausal symptoms and maintain bone density.

Although unopposed estrogens may be used safely in patients who have undergone a hysterectomy, those who have not should be prescribed a preparation with both estrogenic and progestogenic activity.

Fertility

As many patients with cervical cancer are less than 40 years old, fertility is an important consideration. With surgery, cone biopsy or radical trachelectomy can preserve fertility for early-stage disease. However, following radiotherapy, the uterus cannot carry a pregnancy, and any fertility options require future surrogacy. Embryo or oocyte cryopreservation requires ovarian stimulation,

and it may delay the start of treatment. It is important to refer young women to a fertility specialist to discuss options before commencing pelvic radiotherapy.

Sexuality

Both the diagnosis and the treatment of carcinoma of the cervix can have a devastating effect on a patient's sexuality and sexual functioning. Many patients fear that the cancer has been caused by sexual intercourse and may return if they re-commence intercourse. Most of these fears may be alleviated by discussion and explanation.

Radical hysterectomy should not alter sexual function markedly, although patients do report altered sensation. However, radiotherapy can lead to shortening and drying of the vagina with loss of lubrication and pliability. Shortening due to the formation of adhesions in the vagina can be avoided by using a vaginal dilator starting a few weeks after treatment. This will maintain patency of the vagina, enabling resumption of sexual activity at a later date and also examination in the follow-up clinic. Dryness of the vagina may be helped by a lubricant gel and also by HRT, which in addition, can help increase libido, which is often low in this group of patients.

New developments

There are several exciting advances in the management of cervical cancer. Sentinel lymph node mapping has the potential to detect lymph node metastases with greater sensitivity than systematic lymphadenectomy while also reducing morbidity following treatment for early-stage disease. Despite the improvement in local control observed with modern radiotherapy methods, there is still a high rate of subsequent distant metastases, particularly in patients with lymph node involvement. Ongoing randomized trials are assessing whether the addition of neo-adjuvant or adjuvant chemotherapy can improve survival. IMRT has great potential for increasing dose to lymph nodes and for recurrent disease, and adaptive image guidance will reduce normal tissue toxicity. Stereotactic radiotherapy or proton therapy have potential to improve outcomes for recurrent disease or to boost areas inaccessible for brachytherapy. Functional imaging with PET and MRI can predict and monitor response to further guide treatment decisions, while the measurement of circulating tumor cells may change follow-up and treatment strategies. An exciting area of research is the role of immunotherapy in treating early and advanced disease, which has shown promising results in initial clinical trials. Meanwhile, the HPV vaccination is redefining cancer prevention, with modeling data predicting elimination of the disease in countries with high uptake within the next two decades.

Conclusions

Cytological screening programs and rapid referral for colposcopy should continue to reduce the incidence of invasive carcinoma of the cervix. The human papilloma virus is involved in the etiology of cervical cancer. Anti-HPV vaccines have been shown to prevent the formation of CIN, the forerunner to invasive disease.

Treatment of early disease is usually with surgery, but for more advanced tumors, radiotherapy is preferable. Radiotherapy should consist of both an external beam phase and an intracavitary brachytherapy phase if curative doses are to be delivered without major normal tissue toxicity. Concomitant chemotherapy may benefit patients. Brachytherapy should be image guided to ensure optimal dose delivery to tumor.

Neo-adjuvant and adjuvant chemotherapy still do not have a proven place in the treatment of cancer of the cervix. There is a role for salvage radical surgery or radiotherapy for selected patients with recurrent disease, and this potentially still can be curative. Palliation of metastatic and recurrent disease may be achieved with carefully chosen chemotherapy regimens.

Key learning points

- The main predisposing factor for cervical cancer is chronic HPV infection (particularly types 16 and 18); other factors including early sexual intercourse, multiple partners, and smoking are associated with increased risk.
- Cervical neoplasia usually starts in the transformation zone, and pre-invasive disease may be detected by exfoliative cytology of the cervix. Invasive disease is usually preceded by CIN for several years and spreads predominantly by direct invasion and lymphatic spread to pelvic nodes.
- The FIGO staging system is the most commonly used system, traditionally based on clinical examination, chest x-ray, and imaging of the renal tract. A recent update to the FIGO staging now incorporates nodal status, cross-sectional imaging findings, and pathology results. MRI is the best imaging modality for assessing tumor volume and extent of local spread, whereas FDG-PET imaging has the highest sensitivity for nodal assessment.
- Stage is the most significant prognostic factor, as it probably represents tumor bulk. Pelvic node metastasis halves the prognosis of patients with early-stage disease, whereas para-aortic disease is often a marker of more widespread dissemination. Lymphovascular permeation increases the likelihood of nodal metastases and is a prognostic factor in itself.
- Excision of pre-invasive disease is preferable to ablation if occult invasive disease is not to be missed. Stage I disease may be treated by cone biopsy, total hysterectomy, radical trachelectomy with laparoscopic pelvic lymphadenectomy, or radical hysterectomy and lymphadenectomy, depending on the size of tumor, depth of invasion, the presence of lymphovascular permeation, and the patient's wishes to preserve fertility.
- Apart from a few patients with Stage IIA1 disease with minimal involvement of the fornices of the vagina, all patients with more advanced tumors and those unfit for surgery should be treated with primary radiotherapy. Chemoradiotherapy using concomitant cisplatin and radiotherapy offers a benefit in survival over radiotherapy alone.
- External radiotherapy should be individually planned for each patient to take account of the size and distribution of disease and the nodal groups at risk of metastasis. Ideally, it should be planned with an IMRT technique with an integrated boost to involved lymph nodes. Intracavitary therapy is vital if the primary tumor is to be cured. Image-guided brachytherapy allows individualization of the dose distribution.
- Chemotherapy can play a useful role in palliation of advanced and recurrent disease. Response rates up to 70% can be seen in previously untreated disease when using cisplatin-based combination therapy. The addition of bevacizumab can improve survival but with a risk of fistulation and perforation. The role of immunotherapy is being investigated for advanced disease.

Acknowledgments

With many thanks to Dr. Peter Blake, the original author, whose chapter we have adapted and modified.

References

1. Bray F, Ferlay J, Soerjomataram I et al. Global cancer statistics 2018: GLOBOCAN estimates of incidence and mortality worldwide for 36 cancers in 185 countries. *CA Cancer J Clin.* 2018; 68(6):394–424.
2. UK Cervical Cancer incidence statistics. Cancer Research UK. Available at: www.cancerresearchuk.org
3. Walboomers JM, Jacobs MV, Manos MM et al. Human papillomavirus is a necessary cause of invasive cervical cancer worldwide. *J Pathol.* 1999; 189:12–9.
4. Schiffman M, Castle PE, Jeronimo J et al. Human papillomavirus and cervical cancer. *Lancet.* 2007; 370:890–907.
5. Snijders PJ, Steenbergen RD, Heideman DA et al. HPV-mediated cervical carcinogenesis: Concepts and clinical implications. *J Pathol.* 2006; 208:152–64.
6. Beral V. Cancer of the cervix: A sexually transmitted infection? *Lancet.* 1974; 1:1037–40.
7. Zunzunegui MV, King MC, Coria CF et al. Male influences on cervical cancer risk. *Am J Epidemiol.* 1986; 123:302–7.
8. Barton SE, Maddox PH, Jenkins D et al. Effect of cigarette smoking on cervical epithelial immunity: A mechanism for neoplastic change? *Lancet.* 1988; 2:652–4.
9. Maiman M, Fruchter RG, Sedlis A et al. Prevalence, risk factors, and accuracy of cytologic screening for cervical intraepithelial neoplasia in women with the human immunodeficiency virus. *Gynecol Oncol.* 1998; 68:233–9.
10. Pecorelli S, Zigliani L, Odicino F. Revised FIGO staging for carcinoma of the cervix. *Int J Gynaecol Obstet.* 2009; 105:107–8.
11. Arbyn M, Xu L, Simoens C, Martin-Hirsch PP. Prophylactic vaccination against human papillomaviruses to prevent cervical cancer and its precursors. *Cochrane Database Syst Rev.* 2018; 5: CD009069.
12. Anderson MC. The pathology of cervical cancer. *Clin Obstet Gynaecol.* 1985; 12:87–119.
13. Quinn M, Babb P, Jones J et al. Effect of screening on incidence of and mortality from cancer of cervix in England: Evaluation based on routinely collected statistics. *BMJ.* 1999; 318:904–8.
14. Rebolj M, Rimmer J, Denton K et al. 2019. Primary cervical screening with high-risk human papillomavirus testing: Observational study. *BMJ.* 2019; 364:l240.
15. Henriksen E. The lymphatic spread of carcinoma of the cervix and of the body of the uterus: A study of 420 necropsies. *Am J Obstet Gynecol.* 1949; 58:924–42.
16. Benedetti-Panici P, Maneschi F, Scambia G et al. Lymphatic spread of cervical cancer: An anatomical and pathological study based on 225 radical hysterectomies with systematic pelvic and aortic lymphadenectomy. *Gynecol Oncol.* 1996; 62:19–24.
17. Bipat S, Glas AS, van der Velden J et al. Computed tomography and magnetic resonance imaging in staging of uterine cervical carcinoma: A systematic review. *Gynecol Oncol.* 2003; 91:59–66.
18. Greco A, Mason P, Leung AW et al. Staging of carcinoma of the uterine cervix: MRI-surgical correlation. *Clin Radiol.* 1989; 40:401–5.
19. Scheidler J, Hricak H, Yu KK et al. Radiological evaluation of lymph node metastases in patients with cervical cancer. A meta-analysis. *JAMA.* 1997; 278:1096–101.
20. Rose PG, Adler LP, Rodriguez M et al. Positron emission tomography for evaluating para-aortic nodal metastasis in locally advanced cervical cancer before surgical staging: A surgicopathologic study. *J Clin Oncol.* 1999; 17:41–5.
21. Salem A, Salem AF, Al-Ibraheem A et al. Evidence for the use PET for radiation therapy planning in patients with cervical cancer: A systematic review. *Hematol Oncol Stem Cell Ther.* 2011; 4:173–81.

22. Bhatla N, Berek JS, Cuello Fredes M et al. Revised FIGO staging for carcinoma of the cervix uteri. *Int J Gynaecol Obstet.* 2019; 145(1):129–35.

23. Denny L, Quinn M, Hacker N. FIGO cancer report 2012. *Int J Gynaecol Obstet.* 2012; 119 suppl 2:89.

24. Eifel PJ, Morris M, Wharton JT et al. The influence of tumor size and morphology on the outcome of patients with FIGO stage IB squamous cell carcinoma of the uterine cervix. *Int J Radiat Oncol Biol Phys.* 1994; 29:9–16.

25. Inoue T, Morita K. The prognostic significance of number of positive nodes in cervical carcinoma stages IB, IIA, and IIB. *Cancer.* 1990; 65:1923–7.

26. Kamura T, Tsukamoto N, Tsuruchi N et al. Multivariate analysis of the histopathologic prognostic factors of cervical cancer in patients undergoing radical hysterectomy. *Cancer.* 1992; 69:181–6.

27. Delgado G, Bundy B, Zaino R et al. Prospective surgical-pathological study of disease-free interval in patients with stage IB squamous cell carcinoma of the cervix: A Gynecologic Oncology Group study. *Gynecol Oncol.* 1990; 38:352–7.

28. Eifel PJ, Burke TW, Morris M et al. Adenocarcinoma as an independent risk factor for disease recurrence in patients with stage IB cervical carcinoma. *Gynecol Oncol.* 1995; 59:38–44.

29. Cibula D, Potter R, Planchamp F et al. The European Society of Gynaecological Oncology/European Society for Radiotherapy and Oncology/European Society of Pathology guidelines for the management of patients with cervical cancer. *Radiother Oncol.* 2018; 127(3):404–16.

30. Stock RG, Chen AS, Flickinger JC et al. Node-positive cervical cancer: Impact of pelvic irradiation and patterns of failure. *Int J Radiat Oncol Biol Phys.* 1995; 31:31–6.

31. Sedlis A, Bundy BN, Rotman MZ et al. A randomized trial of pelvic radiation therapy versus no further therapy in selected patients with stage IB carcinoma of the cervix after radical hysterectomy and pelvic lymphadenectomy: A Gynecologic Oncology Group Study. *Gynecol Oncol.* 1999; 73:177–83.

32. Gupta S, Maheshwari A, Parab P et al. Neoadjuvant chemotherapy followed by radical surgery versus concomitant chemotherapy and radiotherapy in patients with stage IB2, IIA, or IIB squamous cervical cancer: A randomized controlled trial. *J Clin Oncol.* 2018; 36(16): 1548–55.

33. Wertheim E. A discussion on the diagnosis and treatment of cancer of the uterus. *BMJ.* 1905; 2:689–95.

34. Ramirez PT, Frumovitz M, Pareja R et al. Minimally Invasive versus Abdominal Radical Hysterectomy for Cervical Cancer. *N Engl J Med.* 2018; 379(20):1895–904.

35. Shepherd JH, Crawford RA, Oram DH. Radical trachelectomy: A way to preserve fertility in the treatment of early cervical cancer. *Br J Obstet Gynaecol.* 1998; 105:912–6.

36. Salvo G, Ramirez PT, Levenback CF et al. Sensitivity and negative predictive value for sentinel lymph node biopsy in women with early-stage cervical cancer. *Gynecol Oncol.* 2017; 145(1):96–101.

37. Keys HM, Bundy BN, Stehman FB et al. Cisplatin, radiation, and adjuvant hysterectomy compared with radiation and adjuvant hysterectomy for bulky stage IB cervical carcinoma. *N Engl J Med.* 1999; 340:1154–61.

38. Morris M, Eifel PJ, Lu J et al. Pelvic radiation with concurrent chemotherapy compared with pelvic and para-aortic radiation for high-risk cervical cancer. *N Engl J Med.* 1999; 340:1137–43.

39. Rose PG, Bundy BN, Watkins EB et al. Concurrent cisplatin-based radiotherapy and chemotherapy for locally advanced cervical cancer. *N Engl J Med.* 1999; 340:1144–53.

40. Green JA, Kirwan JM, Tierney JF et al. Survival and recurrence after concomitant chemotherapy and radiotherapy for cancer of the uterine cervix: A systematic review and meta-analysis. *Lancet.* 2001; 358:781–6.

41. Grogan M, Thomas GM, Melamed I et al. The importance of hemoglobin levels during radiotherapy for carcinoma of the cervix. *Cancer.* 1999; 86:1528–36.

42. Fyles AW, Milosevic M, Pintilie M et al. Anemia, hypoxia and transfusion in patients with cervix cancer: A review. *Radiother Oncol.* 2000; 57:13–9.

43. Petereit DG, Sarkaria JN, Chappell R et al. The adverse effect of treatment prolongation in cervical carcinoma. *Int J Radiat Oncol Biol Phys.* 1995; 32:1301–7.

44. Russell AH, Walter JP, Anderson MW et al. Sagittal magnetic resonance imaging in the design of lateral radiation treatment portals for patients with locally advanced squamous cancer of the cervix. *Int J Radiat Oncol Biol Phys.* 1992; 23:449–55.

45. Roeske JC, Lujan A, Rotmensch J et al. Intensity-modulated whole pelvic radiation therapy in patients with gynecologic malignancies. *Int J Radiat Oncol Biol Phys.* 2000; 48:1613–21.

46. Lim K, Small W, Jr., Portelance L et al. Consensus guidelines for delineation of clinical target volume for intensity-modulated pelvic radiotherapy for the definitive treatment of cervix cancer. *Int J Radiat Oncol Biol Phys.* 2011; 79:348–55.

47. Taylor A, Rockall AG, Reznek RH et al. Mapping pelvic lymph nodes: Guidelines for delineation in intensity-modulated radiotherapy. *Int J Radiat Oncol Biol Phys.* 2005; 63:1604–12.

48. Taylor A, Powell ME. An assessment of interfractional uterine and cervical motion: Implications for radiotherapy target volume definition in gynaecological cancer. *Radiother Oncol.* 2008; 88:250–7.

49. Huh SJ, Park W, Han Y. Interfractional variation in position of the uterus during radical radiotherapy for cervical cancer. *Radiother Oncol.* 2004; 71:73–9.

50. Cleaves MA. Radium: With preliminary note on radium rays in the treatment of cancer. *Med Record.* 1903; 64:501–606.

51. Viani GA, Manta GB, Stefano EJ et al. Brachytherapy for cervix cancer: Low-dose rate or high-dose rate brachytherapy—A meta-analysis of clinical trials. *J Exp Clin Cancer Res.* 2009; 28:47.

52. Lee LJ, Das IJ, Higgins SA et al. American Brachytherapy Society consensus guidelines for locally advanced carcinoma of the cervix. Part III: Low-dose-rate and pulsed-dose-rate brachytherapy. *Brachytherapy.* 2012; 11:53–7.

53. Potter R, Dimopoulos J, Georg P et al. Clinical impact of MRI assisted dose volume adaptation and dose escalation in brachytherapy of locally advanced cervix cancer. *Radiother Oncol.* 2007; 83:148–55.

54. Potter R, Haie-Meder C, Van Limbergen E et al. Recommendations from gynaecological (GYN) GEC ESTRO working group (II): Concepts and terms in 3D image-based treatment planning in cervix cancer brachytherapy-3D dose volume parameters and aspects of 3D image-based anatomy, radiation physics, radiobiology. *Radiother Oncol.* 2006; 78:67–77.

55. Schwarz JK, Siegel BA, Dehdashti F et al. Association of post-therapy positron emission tomography with tumor response and survival in cervical carcinoma. *JAMA.* 2007; 298:2289–95.

56. Schmidt AM, Imesch P, Fink D et al. Indications and long-term clinical outcomes in 282 patients with pelvic exenteration for advanced or recurrent cervical cancer. *Gynecol Oncol.* 2012; 125:604–9.

57. Graves S, Seagle BL, Strohl AE et al. Survival after pelvic exenteration for cervical cancer: A National Cancer Database Study. *Int J Gynecol Cancer.* 2017; 27(2): 390–5.

58. Niibe Y, Kenjo M, Kazumoto T et al. Multi-institutional study of radiation therapy for isolated para-aortic lymph node recurrence in uterine cervical carcinoma: 84 subjects of a population of more than 5,000. *Int J Radiat Oncol Biol Phys.* 2006; 66(5):1366–9.

59. Martinez-Monge R, Cambeiro M, Rodriguez-Ruiz ME et al. 2014. Phase II trial of image-based high-dose-rate interstitial brachytherapy for previously irradiated gynecologic cancer. *Brachytherapy.* 2014; 13(3):219–24.

60. Mendez LC, Leung E, Cheung P, Barbera L. The role of stereotactic ablative body radiotherapy in gynaecological cancers: A systematic review. *Clin Oncol.* 2017; 29(6):378–84.

61. Moore DH, Blessing JA, McQuellon RP et al. Phase III study of cisplatin with or without paclitaxel in stage IVB, recurrent, or persistent squamous cell carcinoma of the cervix: A gynecologic oncology group study. *J Clin Oncol.* 2004; 22:3113–9.

62. Monk BJ, Sill MW, McMeekin DS et al. Phase III trial of four cisplatin-containing doublet combinations in stage IVB, recurrent, or persistent cervical carcinoma: A Gynecologic Oncology Group study. *J Clin Oncol.* 2009; 27:4649–55.

63. Tewari KS, Sill MW, Long HJ et al. Improved survival with bevacizumab in advanced cervical cancer. *N Engl J Med.* 2014; 370(8): 734–43.

64. Andreyev HJ, Vlavianos P, Blake P et al. Gastrointestinal symptoms after pelvic radiotherapy: Role for the gastroenterologist? *Int J Radiat Oncol Biol Phys.* 2005; 62:1464–71.

65. Hall MT, Simms KT, Lew JB et al. The projected timeframe until cervical cancer elimination in Australia: A modelling study. *Lancet Public Health.* 2019; 4(1): e19–27.

Useful websites

www.esmo.org/Guidelines-Practice/Clinical-Practice-Guidelines/Gynaecologic-Cancers/Cervical-Cancer

www.cancer.gov/cancertopics/types/cervical

http://seer.cancer.gov/statfacts/html/cervix.html

www.ncin.org.uk/cancer_type_and_topic_specific_work/cancer_type_specific_work/gynaecological_cancer/gynaecological_cancer_hub/resources/cervical_cancer

http://pathways.nice.org.uk/pathways/cervical-cancer?fno=1

www.cancerresearchuk.org/cancer-help/type/cervical-cancer/

www.cancer.net/cancer-types/cervical-cancer

www.jostrust.org.uk

22 CARCINOMA OF THE VAGINA AND VULVA

Sadaf Ghaem-Maghami and Kostas Lathouras

Carcinoma of vagina

Invasive vaginal cancer is rare. In 2008, the overall rate for invasive squamous tumors of the vagina was approximately 0.6 per 100,000 women; the rate rises with age to 2.5 per 100,000 for women aged 75–79 and to more than 4 per 100,000 women aged 85 and above. Since the early 1990s, vaginal cancer incidence rates have remained stable, and vaginal cancer accounts for fewer than 1% of all new cancer cases in females in the United Kingdom (2016). Between 2014 and 2016, there were approximately 250 new vaginal cancer cases in the United Kingdom every year; that's around five every week. Vaginal cancer in England is more common in females living in the most deprived areas. There are around 100 vaginal cancer deaths in the United Kingdom every year (2014–2016), accounting for fewer than 1% of all cancer deaths in females in the United Kingdom (2016). Mortality rates for vaginal cancer in the United Kingdom are highest in females aged 90+ (2014–2016), and since the early 1970s, vaginal cancer mortality rates have decreased by almost half (48%) in females in the United Kingdom.[1] However, like the cervix, the vagina has a range of pre-malignant lesions, many of which may be previously unrecognized extensions of cervical abnormalities. Coincident with the rise in prevalence of cervical intraepithelial neoplasia (CIN) is an increase in the frequency with which vaginal intraepithelial neoplasia (VAIN) is seen.

Etiology

Human papilloma virus (HPV) is found in association with vaginal carcinoma, indicating a role in its etiology.[2] Also, seropositivity to HPV 16 increases the risk of developing vaginal carcinoma by a factor of 4.5, and seropositivity for HPV 18 increases the risk of developing VAIN by a factor of 12.[3] A field effect, in the lower genital tract, has been suggested by the observation of multicentric neoplasia involving cervix, vagina, and vulva[4]; however, Sugase and Matsukura found high copy numbers of HPV virus in vaginal biopsies of patients with VAIN, a large proportion of whom had no associated CIN or vulvar intraepithelial neoplasia (VIN).[5]

Irritation caused by procidentia and vaginal pessaries has been suggested as an etiological factor, but this is an infrequent association.

Previous radiotherapy for cervical cancer in young women has been suggested as a cause of cancer of the vagina. However, a large international collaborative study of 25,995 women followed for more than 10 years after treatment with radiotherapy for cervical cancer recorded only 48 cancers of the vulva or vagina. This was not significantly different from the seven such women out of 5125 treated with surgery. These data suggest that if vaginal cancer is induced by radiotherapy, it is a very rare event.

For some time, the prevalence of clear cell adenocarcinoma of the vagina was thought to be increased by intrauterine exposure to diethylstilbestrol (DES), but with the accrual of more information, the risks now seem to be very low and lie between 0.1 and 1.0 per 1000.[6–8]

Anatomy

The upper two-thirds of the vagina are derived from the Mullerian duct and the lower third from the ectoderm of the cloaca. The vagina is related anteriorly to the bladder and the urethra. Posteriorly, the vault of the vagina is covered with the peritoneum of the Pouch of Douglas. It thus becomes closely related to loops of small or large bowel. Below this, it is closely related to the anterior wall of the rectum until the perineal body separates it from the anal canal. The ureters run close to the cervix over each side of the vaginal vault to the bladder. Laterally, the lower portion of the cardinal ligaments supports the vagina until it reaches the pelvic floor, where it is invested by the medial part of the levator ani muscles (pubococcygeus).

The vagina is lined by stratified squamous epithelium. When the transformation zone of the cervix has extended onto the vagina, clefts or glands partly lined by columnar epithelium will be seen deep within the squamous epithelium.

Pathology

VAIN is characterized by loss of stratification and polarity of the cells and by nuclear atypia. The great majority (85%–95%) of primary vaginal cancers are squamous. Of these, 60% occur in the upper one-third of the vagina, particularly in the posterior fornix. Grossly, they present as ulcerative tumors, exophytic masses, or infiltrating stenosing lesions. Histologically, squamous cell carcinomas of the vagina range from well-differentiated lesions with abundant keratin formation to poorly differentiated tumors with little squamous differentiation. The majority of lesions are moderately differentiated, non-keratinizing lesions. There appears to be little correlation between histological grade and prognosis.

Clear cell adenocarcinomas, malignant melanomas, embryonal rhabdomyosarcomas, and endodermal sinus tumors are the most common of the small number of other tumors seen very rarely in the vagina. These are discussed separately.

Natural history

Like invasive vaginal carcinoma, VAIN is also seen most commonly in the upper vagina; only 25%–30% of cases are confined to the lower vagina, usually the anterior wall. The incidence of VAIN has been reported as 0.2 per 100,000 women, and it accounts for 0.4% of intraepithelial diseases of the lower genital tract.[9] The incidence of VAIN after hysterectomy for women with CIN 3 who completed 10 years of follow-up is 0.91%.[10]

The malignant potential for VAIN is not as well-documented as for CIN, but it is clearly not a completely benign disease. Progression to invasive carcinoma probably occurs in 9%–10% of cases[11]; it would therefore seem sensible to treat it with the same respect accorded to CIN.

Squamous vaginal cancer spreads by local invasion initially. Lymphatic spread occurs by tumor embolization to the pelvic nodes from the upper vagina and to both pelvic and inguinal nodes from the lower vagina. Hematogenous spread is unusual.

Clinical presentation

Vaginal bleeding is the most common clinical presentation of vaginal cancer and is typically postmenopausal, unprovoked or postcoital. Any unscheduled vaginal bleeding should be investigated to determine whether the source is vaginal. A watery, blood-tinged, or malodorous vaginal discharge might be present. A vaginal mass might be noted. Other potential symptoms are related to local extension of disease, urinary symptoms (e.g., frequency, dysuria, or hematuria), or gastrointestinal complaints (e.g., tenesmus, constipation, or melena).[12–14] Pelvic pain from extension of disease beyond the vagina is present in 5% of patients.

Vaginal cancers may be detected as a result of cytologic screening for cervical cancer or may be an incidental finding of a vaginal mass on pelvic examination, as approximately 20% of women are asymptomatic at the time of diagnosis.[15–17]

Clinical staging

The modified clinical staging suggested by Perez and colleagues[18] has been widely adopted and updated (Table 22.1).

Diagnosis and assessment

VAIN is usually a cytological or colposcopic diagnosis. Dyskaryosis in cervical or vaginal cytology is an indication for colposcopy to determine the location and nature of the abnormality that is giving rise to the abnormal cells. As a substantial proportion of these women have undergone hysterectomy (usually for CIN) before the detection of VAIN, and as the majority of the lesions are in the vaginal vault, straddling the suture line, or in the angles of the vault, assessment and biopsy can be difficult.[19] General anesthesia is required for most cases. It should also be remembered that abnormal epithelium or invasive cancer could lie buried behind the sutures closing the vault.

Before making a diagnosis of primary vaginal cancer, the following criteria must be satisfied: the primary site of growth must be in the vagina, the uterine cervix must not be involved, and there must be no clinical evidence that the vaginal tumor is metastatic disease (International Federation of Obstetrics and Gynaecology, 1963).

The most common presenting symptom is vaginal bleeding (53%–65%), with vaginal discharge (11%–16%) and pelvic pain (4%–11%) being less common.[20]

The most important part of the pre-treatment assessment of invasive cancer of the vagina is a careful examination under anesthesia. A combined vaginal and rectal examination will help to detect extra-vaginal spread. Cystoscopy, proctosigmoidoscopy,

TABLE 22.1   **Modified FIGO Staging of Vaginal Cancer (2009)**

Stage	Definition
Stage I	Invasive carcinoma confined to the vaginal wall
Stage II	Subvaginal infiltration not extending to the pelvic side-wall
Stage III	Extends to pelvic side-wall
Stage IV	Tumor has extended beyond the true pelvis or involves the mucosa of bladder or rectum
Stage IVa	Involves mucosa of bladder or rectum or direct extension beyond the true pelvis
Stage IVb	Spread beyond the pelvis

Source: Perez, 1973. With permission.

and colposcopy may be indicated, the last to identify coexisting VAIN. A generous, full-thickness biopsy is essential for adequate histological evaluation. Other investigations include a computed tomography (CT) scan of chest abdomen and pelvis and a magnetic resonance imaging (MRI) scan to evaluate local disease and spread outside the vagina and lymph node involvement.

Treatment and complications: VAIN

The treatment of VAIN includes local ablation with the carbon dioxide laser, local excision, partial and total vaginectomy, and radiotherapy. Treatment with 5FU appears to be associated with a high recurrence rate[21] and cannot be recommended. Imiquimod 5% applied locally stimulates cellular immunity and has been used in the treatment of VIN and VAIN; it appears to be effective in the treatment of low-grade VAIN. Randomized trials are required to assess this treatment more thoroughly.[22,23] Occasionally, in a postmenopausal woman, the abnormality resolves with estrogen therapy.

Local ablation with the carbon dioxide laser is used for small lesions where there is no suspicion of invasion. Local excision is sufficient for small lesions; otherwise, partial or total colpectomy (vaginectomy) is necessary. Surgery is the only effective option available to patients previously treated with radiotherapy and is the treatment of choice for women who are post-hysterectomy. The reported recurrence rate is 0%–5%.[21]

Intracavitary radiotherapy is an option for lesions in the vaginal vault following a hysterectomy, but this will have the disadvantage that radiotherapy can cause vaginal stenosis or ovarian failure in a premenopausal woman.

Treatment of invasive cancer

Radiotherapy

Invasive vaginal cancer is usually treated with radiotherapy, which is given either as a combination of external radiation and brachytherapy (interstitial or intracavitary) or by brachytherapy alone.

Early cases of vaginal cancer occurring in the lower vagina may be treated entirely with interstitial brachytherapy, usually with [192]iridium. The objective is to achieve a tumor dose of 70–80 Gy in two fractions, 2 weeks apart. The radiation is given at a rate of 10 Gy per day.

Tumors of the upper two-thirds of the vagina are treated in an identical fashion to cancer of the cervix, either by radiotherapy or by chemo-radiotherapy, usually with cisplatin given concurrently. External radiotherapy to the pelvis includes the parametria and the pelvic nodes and is followed by brachytherapy. The lower end of the radiation field must cover the lesion in the vagina plus a 2-cm margin. If the lesion extends into the lower third of the vagina, the inguino-femoral nodes must also be included in the treatment volume. A total dose of 45–50 Gy in 25–28 fractions in 5–6 weeks is given to the pelvis. External radiotherapy is followed by intra-cavitary therapy. For lesions below the vault, the treatment boost is given with interstitial brachytherapy, which has been found to be more effective than intracavitary brachytherapy.[24] The total dose from both external radiotherapy and low–dose rate brachytherapy is 70–75 Gy to the vaginal mucosa or its equivalent using a high–dose rate system. High–dose rate radiotherapy has been reported as being as effective and as well tolerated as low–dose rate radiotherapy.[25] Recent experience suggests that treatment with intensity modulated radiation therapy (IMRT) may allow dose escalation with reduced toxicity.[26]

Complications of radiotherapy

Vaginal stenosis may occur and is more likely when advanced tumors are treated. The overall prevalence of vaginal stenosis is approximately 30% and is an undoubted problem for sexually active patients. Mucosal ulceration, either immediate or delayed, can be a distressing complication, but conservative therapy is usually effective. Vesicovaginal and rectovaginal fistulas and small bowel complications can occur but are rare. The risk of fistula formation is higher in advanced disease.

Surgery

A Stage I lesion in the upper vagina can be adequately treated by radical hysterectomy (if the uterus is still present), radical vaginectomy, and pelvic lymphadenectomy.[27] A split-thickness skin graft may be used to reconstruct a new vagina. Exenteration is required for more advanced lesions and carries the problems of stomata. However, exenterative surgery may be the treatment of choice for women who have had prior pelvic radiotherapy.

Results

Due to the rarity of vaginal cancer, there is a wide range of reported results. Probably the most reliable figures are from Kucera and Vavra,[28] who reported on 460 women with cancer of the vagina. They found that 77% of the women with Stage I disease were alive at 5 years compared with 45% with Stage II, 31% with Stage III, and 18% with Stage IV.

Although survival is predominantly stage related, the site and size of the lesion may be important, with smaller lesions and those in the upper vagina having a better prognosis. Also, the ulcerating and deeply invasive cancers have a poorer prognosis than the exophytic lesions.

Uncommon vaginal tumors

Clear cell adenocarcinoma

The histology is characterized by vacuolated or clear areas in the cytoplasm and a hob-nail appearance of the nuclei of cells lining the lumen of glands. Radical surgery or radical radiotherapy is required for invasive lesions. As most are situated in the upper vagina, they may be treated as cervical lesions. Lymph node metastases and 5-year survival figures are equivalent to cervical cancer.

Malignant melanoma

Vaginal melanoma has a 5-year survival rate of less than 10%. Vaginal bleeding and discharge are the most common presenting symptoms. The prognosis depends upon the depth of epithelial invasion. Radical surgery and radiotherapy are of little value if the lesion is deeply invasive because of its propensity to metastasize early by the blood stream. There is at present no effective chemotherapy. New immunotherapeutic agents, such as ipilimumab and small molecule inhibitors of receptor tyrosine kinase c-kit (such as imatinib), have shown promise in the treatment of melanomas.

Rhabdomyosarcoma (sarcoma botryoides)

Ninety per cent of these rare tumors occur in children younger than 5 years old. They present with vaginal bleeding and a grape-like mass in the vagina. The appearance of cross striations in the rhabdomyoblasts is characteristic of this tumor. Treatment is with combination chemotherapy, which is carried out in specialist centers. When chemotherapy produces only a partial response, local surgery is carried out. Radiotherapy is restricted to patients with unresectable tumors in view of the deleterious effects on bone growth. The overall survival rate is more than 80%.

Endodermal sinus tumors

These very rare tumors may resemble rhabdomyosarcomata, but histology shows a primitive adenocarcinoma. Most occur in infants below the age of 2. Treatment with chemotherapy is as for germ-cell tumors of the testis or ovary.

Recurrent vaginal cancer

Patients with a recurrence may be candidates for surgery. However, for those who are not candidates for surgery for whatever reason, treatment options are more limited due to the lack of prospective trials in this disease.

In patients with a central recurrence and no other sites of disease, pelvic exenteration with or without vaginal reconstruction may be curative.[29–31] Exenteration may also be considered in patients with Stage IVa disease, especially if a rectovaginal or vesicovaginal fistula is present. The role of chemotherapy in patients with recurrent or advanced vaginal cancer is unclear.

Key points

1. Invasive vaginal cancer is rare. In 2008, the overall rate for invasive squamous tumors of the vagina was approximately 0.6 per 100,000 women, and mortality rate is highest in women aged 90+.
2. HPV is found in association with vaginal carcinoma, indicating a role in its etiology.
3. Invasive vaginal cancer is a rare tumor more often seen in association with an antecedent cervical malignancy.
4. Radiotherapy is the main treatment method.
5. Interstitial therapy alone offers good cure rates in early stages I–IIa occurring in the lower vagina. External radiotherapy is required for more advanced stages.
6. Tumors of the upper two-thirds of the vagina are treated in an identical fashion to cancer of the cervix, either by radiotherapy or by chemo-radiotherapy, usually with cisplatin given concurrently.
7. A Stage I lesion in the upper vagina can be adequately treated by radical hysterectomy (if the uterus is still present), radical vaginectomy, and pelvic lymphadenectomy.
8. Exenterative surgery may be the treatment of choice for women who have had prior pelvic radiotherapy.

Carcinoma of the vulva

Invasive vulvar cancer is an uncommon cancer. It represents approximately 4% of all female gynecological cancers. There are around 1300 new vulvar cancer cases in the United Kingdom every year, that is, more than three every day (2014–2016), accounting for fewer than 1% of all new cancer cases in females in the United Kingdom (2016).

Incidence rates for vulvar and vaginal cancer in the United Kingdom are highest in females over 90 years old (2014–2016).

Since the early 1990s, vulvar cancer incidence rates have increased by around a seventh (15%) in females in the United Kingdom.

Vulvar cancer accounts for fewer than 1% of all cancer deaths in females in the United Kingdom. There are around 440 vulvar cancer deaths every year, that is, around one every day (2014–2016).

Since the early 1970s, vulvar cancer mortality rates have decreased by two-fifths (40%) in females in the United Kingdom.

More than half (53%) of women diagnosed with vaginal or vulvar cancer in England survive their disease for 10 years or more (2009–2013). More than 8 in 10 women in England diagnosed with vaginal or vulvar cancer aged 15–49 survive their disease for 5 years or more, compared with almost 6 in 10 women diagnosed aged 70–89 (2009–2013). Five-year relative survival for vaginal and vulvar cancer in women is above the European average in England but similar to the European average in Wales, Scotland, and Northern Ireland.[32] The majority of these women are elderly; fewer than 10% are below 55 years of age, and 80% are above 65 years.

Cancer of the vulva is unpleasant but potentially curable even in elderly, unfit patients if referred early and managed correctly from the outset. Surgery for this condition needs special expertise and should only be undertaken by gynecological oncologists. Initial, inappropriate surgery leads to a poor outcome.

Etiology

Little is known of the etiology of vulvar cancer. A viral factor has been suggested, as DNA from HPV types 16 and 18 has been detected in VIN. There are also recognized risks of developing cancer with lichen sclerosus (47%),[33] Paget's disease,[34] and melanoma *in situ*.[35]

Other risk factors are CIN, a prior history of cervical cancer, cigarette smoking, immunodeficiency syndromes, and northern European ancestry.[36,37]

Two independent pathways are proposed for the development of vulvar squamous cell carcinoma. The first is related to mucosal HPV infection, and the second is related to chronic inflammatory (vulvar dystrophy) or autoimmune processes.[38–40] A review of over 2000 specimens showed that HPV DNA was detected in 86.7% of VIN and 28.6% of invasive vulvar cancer cases; HPV 16 was the most common subtype (72.5%), followed by HPV 33 (6.5%) and HPV 18 (4.6%).[41]

Anatomy

The vulva includes the mons pubis, the labia majora and minora, the clitoris, the vestibule of the vagina, the bulb of the vestibule, and the greater vestibular glands (Bartholin's).

The mons pubis is a pad of fat anterior to the pubic symphysis and covered by hair-bearing skin. The labia majora extend posteriorly from the mons on either side of the pudendal cleft into which the urethra and vagina open. They merge with one another and the perineal skin anterior to the anus. They consist largely of areolar tissue and fat. On their lateral aspects, the skin is pigmented and covered with crisp hairs. On the medial side, the skin is smooth and has many sebaceous glands. The labia minora are small folds of skin that lie between the labia majora and divide anteriorly to envelop the clitoris. The clitoris is an erectile structure analogous to the male penis. Partly hidden by the anterior folds of the labia minora, the clitoris consists of a body of two corpora cavernosa, lying side-by-side and connected to the pubic and ischial rami, and a glans of sensitive, spongy erectile tissue. The vestibule is that area between the labia minora into which the urethra and vagina open. The bulbs of the vestibule are elongated masses of erectile tissue lying on either side of the vaginal opening.

Lymphatic drainage

The lymph drains from the vulva to the inguinal and femoral glands in the groin and then to the external iliac glands. Drainage from the perineum and the clitoris is to both groins, but some contra-lateral spread occurs from other sites on the vulva. Direct spread to the pelvic nodes along the internal pudendal vessels occurs only very rarely, and no direct pathway from the clitoris to the pelvic nodes has been consistently demonstrated.

Pathology

Both squamous VIN and Paget's disease occur on the vulva. The histological features of VIN are analogous to those seen in CIN and VAIN. In the same way, the histological appearance of Paget's disease is similar to the lesion seen in the breast. In a third of cases of Paget's disease, there is an adenocarcinoma in underlying apocrine glands, and these carry an especially poor prognosis. Most invasive cancers (85%) are squamous. Some 5% are melanomas, and the remainder is made up of carcinomas of Bartholin's gland, other adenocarcinomas, basal cell carcinomas, and the very rare verrucous carcinomas, rhabdomyosarcomas, and leiomyosarcomas.

In squamous cell carcinomas, the presence of infiltrative growth patterns, compared with a pushing pattern, and the presence of lymphatic vascular space invasion (LVSI) are associated with a higher local recurrence rate and poorer prognosis. However, these factors do not necessarily indicate the need for adjuvant treatment.

Natural history

A large proportion (40%) of women with VIN are below 40 years of age. VIN is histologically very similar to CIN and often occurs in association with it. It used to be said that its malignant potential is less than 5%. However, this opinion is based largely on studies of women who have been treated by excision biopsy or vulvectomy. This may not be true of untreated or inadequately treated patients, as progression to invasive cancer in 2–8 years has been reported.[42]

The definition of "microinvasion" of the vulva has proved extremely problematical. The purpose is to identify a group of women with invasive carcinoma who could safely be treated with a less mutilating procedure than radical vulvectomy. Although it was initially suggested that up to 5-mm invasion into the stroma might be acceptable,[43,44] subsequent reports have suggested lower limits. Some have suggested 2 mm,[45] others preferred 1 mm,[46] whereas further reports emphasize the importance of lymphatic or vascular invasion and the degree of differentiation[47] or confluence.[48] It seems that the safest course to follow is to perform groin node dissection in all cases with more than 1-mm stromal invasion without attempting to differentiate between superficial and deep inguinal nodes.[49,50]

Invasive disease involves the labia majora in about two-thirds of cases and the clitoris, labia minora, or posterior fourchette and perineum in the remainder. The tumor usually spreads slowly, infiltrating local tissue before metastasizing by embolization to the inguinal and femoral nodes. Overall, approximately 30% of women with operable disease have nodal spread. Spread to the contra-lateral groin can occur in up to 25% of cases with positive groin nodes. Pelvic node involvement is not common and is usually secondary to groin node involvement, but rarely, there is direct spread to the pelvic nodes via the internal pudendal vessels. Blood spread to bone or lung is rare.

Death can be a long, unpleasant process and is often due to sepsis and inanition or hemorrhage. Uremia from bilateral ureteric obstruction may supervene first. Such is the abject misery of this demise that all patients with resectable vulvar lesions should be offered surgery regardless of their age and general condition.

Clinical presentation

Many patients are asymptomatic at the time of the diagnosis. Most patients present with a vulvar lesion and/or symptoms of vulvar pruritus and/or vulvar bleeding. Most of the times, the vulvar lesion is unifocal in a form of a plaque, ulcer, or wart mass at the labia majora, labia minora, clitoris, perineum, and less commonly, the mons pubis. In 10% of cases, the lesion is too extensive to determine the site of origin, and in 5%, lesions are multifocal.[51,52]

Clinical staging

The Federation Internationale de Gynecologie et d'Obstetrique (FIGO) classification is shown in Table 22.2. In spite of the apparent limitations of this classification, it does give a reasonable guide to the prognosis. As the surgical findings are incorporated in the staging evaluation, the prognostic value is greatly improved.

Diagnosis and assessment

Intraepithelial disease of the vulva often presents as pruritus vulvae, but 20%–45% are asymptomatic. These lesions are often raised above the surrounding skin, have a rough surface, and are variable in color: white, due to hyperkeratinization; red, due to immaturity of the epithelium; or dark brown, due to increased melanin deposition in the epithelial cells. However, the full extent of the abnormality is often not apparent until 5% acetic acid is applied. After 2 minutes, VIN turns white, and mosaic or punctation may be visible. All these changes are best examined colposcopically. Biopsies must be taken from abnormal areas. This can usually be done under local anesthesia in the outpatient.

Although vulvar cancer can be asymptomatic, more than 70% patients with invasive disease complain of irritation, pruritus, pain, or soreness, and over half note a mass in the vulva or an ulcer. It is usually not until the mass appears that medical advice is sought. Bleeding and discharge are less common presentations.

Because of the multicentric nature of female lower genital tract cancer, the investigation should include inspection of the cervix and cervical cytology. The groin nodes must be palpated carefully, and any suspicious nodes may be sampled by fine needle aspiration. A CT scan is usually required; an MRI scan is also sometimes carried out. Thorough examination under anesthesia

and a full-thickness biopsy are the most important investigations. The examination under anesthesia should note particularly the size and distribution of the primary lesion, especially the involvement of the urethra or rectum, and secondary lesions in the vulvar or perineal skin must be sought.

Treatment of vulvar intraepithelial neoplasia

The treatment of VIN is difficult. Uncertainty about the malignant potential, the multifocal nature of the disorder, and the discomfort and mutilation resulting from therapy suggest that recommendations should be cautious and conservative in order to avoid making the treatment worse than the disease. The youth of many of these patients is a further, important consideration. Nonetheless, the documented progression of untreated cases to invasive cancer underlines the potential importance of these lesions. If the patient has presented with symptoms, therapy is required. Asymptomatic patients, particularly below the age of 50 years, are probably best observed closely, with biopsies repeated if there are any suspicious changes.[53]

If the lesion is small, an excision biopsy may be both diagnostic and therapeutic.[54] Larger, higher-grade, and symptomatic lesions may require simple skinning vulvectomy.

An alternative approach is to vaporize the abnormal epithelium with the carbon dioxide laser.[55] Given the very irregular surface of the vulva, it is very difficult to achieve a uniform depth of destruction. Moreover, the depth of treatment required for VIN is still unclear.[56] Even with carefully controlled depth of treatment, re-epithelialization of large areas treated with the laser will take several weeks. The other main disadvantage is not having histopathological assessment.

The use of 5-fluorouracil (5FU) cream is not widely recommended;[57] however, imiquimod has been used with some success. A recent study of more than 300 patients with high-grade VIN showed that there was a lower rate of recurrence of VIN with imiquimod and surgical excision compared with laser therapy.[58]

Treatment of invasive disease

Surgery is the mainstay of treatment. The introduction of radical vulvectomy (complete removal of the vulva and bilateral inguino-femoral lymphadenectomy) reduced the mortality from 80% to

TABLE 22.2 **FIGO Staging of Vulvar Cancer**

Stage	Definition
Stage I	Tumor confined to the vulva
IA	Lesions ≤2 cm in size, confined to the vulva or perineum and with stromal invasion ≤1.0 mm,* no nodal metastasis
IB	Lesions >2 cm in size or with stromal invasion >1.0 mm,* confined to the vulva or perineum, with negative nodes
Stage II	Tumor of any size with extension to adjacent perineal structures (1/3 lower urethra, 1/3 lower vagina, anus) with negative nodes
Stage III	Tumor of any size with or without extension to adjacent perineal structures (1/3 lower urethra, 1/3 lower vagina, anus) with positive inguino-femoral lymph nodes
IIIA	(1) With 1 lymph node metastasis (≥ 5 mm), or (2) 1–2 lymph node metastasis(es) (< 5 mm)
IIIB	(1) With 2 or more lymph node metastases (≥ 5 mm), or (2) 3 or more lymph node metastases (< 5 mm)
IIIC	With positive nodes with extra-capsular spread
Stage IV	Tumor invades other regional (2/3 upper urethra, 2/3 upper vagina), or distant structures
IVA	Tumor invades any of the following: (1) upper urethral or vaginal mucosa, bladder mucosa, rectal mucosa, or fixed to pelvic bone, or (2) fixed or ulcerated inguino-femoral lymph nodes
IVB	Any distant metastasis including pelvic lymph nodes

Source: FIGO Committee on Gynecologic Oncology, 2014. With permission.

* The depth of invasion is defined as the measurement of the tumor from the epithelial–stromal junction of the adjacent most superficial dermal papilla to the deepest point of invasion.

40%.[59] However, to control lymphatic spread, these techniques removed large areas of normal skin from the groins, and primary wound closure was rarely achieved. By using a modified incision, the same objectives could be accomplished without the removal of large areas of normal skin and with the enormous benefit that primary closure could be achieved in nearly all cases.[60] A further refinement aimed at reducing still further the problems of wound healing was the use of separate groin incisions for Stage I–II cases.[61] Studies comparing triple incision with *en bloc* dissection have not shown any significant difference in either survival or recurrence.[62,63] The corrected survival for women in Stage I disease was 95%.

More recently, there has been a move to an even more conservative approach. In early-stage disease, in the absence of clinically suspicious or involved groin nodes, the surgery to the primary tumor should be radical to remove the tumor, yet "the impetus for more conservative approaches stems from the well-recognized psychosexual sequelae."[64] The psychological morbidity of radical treatment has been reported by Andersen.[65] The management of the vulvar lesion and treatment of the groins should be considered separately.

Excision of the vulvar lesion

If the lesion is less than 2 cm in diameter and unifocal and if the rest of the vulva is healthy, then radical local excision is the treatment of choice.[66] In all other cases, a radical removal of the whole vulva is required. The deep and lateral surgical margins should be no less following radical local excision than after radical vulvectomy. The depth of resection should be to the fascia lata, and lateral margins should be at least 10 mm to minimize the risk of local recurrence.[64] The distal 1 cm of the urethra can be excised safely to achieve an adequate margin without risking incontinence. If radical surgery is likely to cause sphincter damage, leading to urinary or fecal incontinence, pre-operative radiotherapy or chemoradiotherapy should be considered to shrink the tumor.

Currently, the recommended surgical tumor-free margin distance varies between different guidelines, ranging between 1 and 2 cm.[67–69]

A recent study showed a high local recurrence rate in patients treated surgically for vulvar cancer. There was no relation found with pathologic tumor-free margin distances. Based on this study, the recommendation for a safe pathological tumor-free margin is at 3 mm. The local rate of recurrence was related to the presence of differentiated VIN (with or without lichen sclerosus (LS)). There is a lifelong increased risk after surgical treatment of vulvar cancer, especially when patients have differentiated VIN in the margin.[70]

Groin node dissection

Dissection of the groin nodes is carried out for all cases greater than Stage Ia. The groin node dissection includes both the superficial inguinal and the deep femoral nodes, as superficial groin node dissection alone is associated with a higher risk of groin node recurrence.[71] If the nodes are not obviously clinically involved, separate incisions in the groin can be used.[65] In advanced disease, the triple incision technique may be inappropriate, and a radical vulvectomy with an *en bloc* groin node dissection may be required. Because of the extensive crossover of lymphatic channels from the vulva, bilateral groin node dissection is usually performed, although in lateral tumors where the medial margin of the tumor is at least 2 cm from the mid-line, an ipsilateral groin node dissection is sufficient.[71] However, if the nodes are found to be positive, the contra-lateral groin will need to be dissected at a

second operation. Preservation of the long saphenous vein may reduce both groin wound and subsequent lower limb problems.

There is little value in performing a pelvic node dissection, as post-operative radiation therapy to the groins and pelvis gives superior results when more than two groin nodes are involved.[72]

Sentinel node detection using dye studies and lymphoscintigraphy looks promising in identifying the involved lymph nodes and requiring only limited dissection. Sentinel node identification is an accurate method for inguinal node staging in vulvar cancer. Combining radiotracer and blue dye methods and excluding patients with palpable inguinal nodes result in the highest sensitivity.[73]

Complications

The most common complication is wound breakdown and infection. With the modified surgical techniques referred to in the foregoing text, this is seldom more than a minor problem. Conservative therapy with Eusol and liquid honey packs is all that is required. Lymphocyst formation can be very troublesome. Resolution usually occurs spontaneously. Osteitis pubis is a rare but very serious complication that requires intensive and prolonged antibiotic therapy. Secondary hemorrhage occurs from time to time. Leg edema may be expected in approximately 30% of patients. Numbness and paresthesia over the anterior thigh are common due to the division of small cutaneous branches of the femoral nerve. Loss of body image and impaired sexual function undoubtedly occur, but the patients' responses to surgery are enormously variable.

Chemotherapy

Chemotherapy has not played a large role in the management of vulvar carcinoma because of the advanced age of most of the patients and the frequency of concurrent medical conditions. It may be used as an adjuvant or neo-adjuvant treatment or for recurrent disease. Single agents that have been shown to be active include cisplatin, doxorubicin, bleomycin, and methotrexate. Concomitant chemo-radiotherapy regimens have been investigated, but there are no randomized studies to show whether chemo-radiotherapy is superior to radiotherapy alone.[74,75]

Radiotherapy

Although surgery is the mainstay of treatment for vulvar carcinoma, adjuvant radiotherapy has a role in preventing recurrence. In the presence of advanced disease with bowel or bladder involvement, surgery alone can result in poor function and cosmesis, and this has led to renewed interest in the use of non-surgical treatment modalities for this situation.[76]

Radiotherapy technique

External beam radiotherapy has historically been considered too toxic a treatment to be tolerated by the epithelium of the vulva, leading to severe acute moist desquamation and severe late normal tissue damage (vulvar fibrosis, atrophy, and necrosis; vaginal and urethral stenosis; and fistula formation). However, these complications of radiotherapy are avoidable by using doses per fraction of no more than 1.8 Gy and by limiting the overall total dose.

There is general agreement on a threshold dose for improved local control at approximately 50 Gy. Fraction size is important, with 1.7 Gy being close to tolerance. The doses that have been recommended by Royal College of Obstetricians and Gynaecologists (RCOG),[67] based on the recommendations of Thomas et al.,[75] are

55 Gy as a maximum pre-operatively (with or without concurrent 5FU); 45–50 Gy as adjuvant post-operative treatment; and 65 Gy as radical therapy. Higher doses can lead to severe morbidity. Hoffman et al.[76] reported radio-necrosis in 6 of 10 patients treated with more than 70 Gy.

Limitation of the size of the radiation field is also important. When radiotherapy is given with radical intent, it is given in two phases. The first phase treats the primary and nodal sites, using external irradiation, to a dose of 45–50 Gy. For the second phase, the tumor is boosted using as small a field as possible. This is achieved by selecting the most appropriate technique, such as a direct field to the perineum using electron portals, interstitial radiotherapy, or conformal radiotherapy. The total dose from both phases of treatment, as previously stated, is 65 Gy.

Post-operative radiotherapy

Approximately 15%–33% of patients with advanced, operable vulvar carcinoma recur after radical surgery: the majority (80%–95%) at loco-regional sites in the first instance.[77]

A number of clinico-pathological variables have been defined that predict local recurrence and overall survival.[78] The clinically important features are FIGO stage, presence of clinically involved lymph nodes, tumor size independent of stage, tumor location (mid-line versus lateral, with mid-line tumors having a greater tendency to metastasize to bilateral inguinal nodes), age, and performance status.

The most significant prognostic features are size of tumor, inguinal node involvement, and the width of the vulvar tumor-free margin. Approximately one in five patients found to have metastatic involvement of groin nodes removed at surgery will also have disease in the iliac nodes. With regard to tumor margin, there is no risk of recurrence if the tumor-free margin is 8 mm or more, but the risk of recurrence is 8% if the margin is 4.8–8 mm, rising to 54% if the margin is less than 4.8 mm.[79,80]

The criteria for post-operative radiotherapy to the inguinal and pelvic nodes are the presence of a single clinically involved node, more than two histologically involved inguinal nodes, or extra-capsular spread.[81] The dose for post-operative radiotherapy to the groins and pelvic nodes is 45–50 Gy at 1.8–2.0 Gy per fraction. The recommended depth is up to 8 cm, as the depth of the deep nodes will vary from patient to patient.

Adjuvant radiotherapy to the vulva should be considered where the disease-free margin is less than 8 mm. This should be given to as small a field as possible to reduce morbidity. The recommended dose is again 45–50 Gy.

The role of chemotherapy as a post-operative adjuvant is unclear. The recent Gynaecological Oncology Group (GOG) 185 study, which closed prematurely, had tried to examine the role of radiation versus chemo/radiation but failed to achieve the recruitment target. A new international study is under development and is proposing the use of chemo/radiation. If chemotherapy is to be used in the post-operative adjuvant fashion with radiation, it is recommended that cisplatin is used as a single agent, probably at a dose of 40 mg/m^2 weekly.[67]

Radiotherapy as an alternative to surgery for occult nodal disease

Because 20%–25% of women with clinically Stage I cancer of the vulva have occult nodal metastases, some form of local treatment is required to eradicate this potential source of recurrent (and metastatic) disease. The results of adjuvant nodal irradiation[51] suggested the hypothesis that nodal irradiation could obviate the need for bilateral inguinal lymph node dissection in low-risk

groups. However, a randomized GOG study[81] did not confirm this. Fifty-two patients with clinically non-suspicious inguinal nodes undergoing radical vulvectomy were randomized to receive either node dissection or inguino-femoral nodal irradiation to a dose of 50 Gy at 2 Gy per fraction dosed at 3-cm depth. The study was closed prematurely when interim analysis revealed a significant advantage in favor of the surgical arm in terms of progression-free interval and survival. A criticism of this study is that treatment to the groins was only given to a depth of 3 cm. However, radiotherapy cannot be recommended at present as an alternative to surgery for occult nodal disease.

Pre-operative radiotherapy

The use of pre-operative neo-adjuvant therapies has been investigated in an attempt to downstage tumors and facilitate "viscera-preserving" surgery. Small studies using pre-operative radiotherapy have reported encouraging results in patients with advanced Stage III and IV disease.[82,83] The largest study consisted of 48 cases, 11 of which had recurrent disease.[84] Some of these cases had radiotherapy after surgery, but most were treated pre-operatively. The projected 5-year survival for the 37 primary cases was 75.6%, and for the recurrent cases, it was 62.6%. Only two patients subsequently underwent an exenterative procedure or stoma formation. The value of pre-operative radiotherapy for involved inguinal nodes has also been demonstrated.

In recent years, attention has been focused on the use of neo-adjuvant chemo-radiotherapy with the chemotherapy being used as a radiosensitizer rather than as a cytotoxic agent. Most of these studies have been carried out on only small numbers of patients. Koh et al.[85] treated 20 patients with bulky cancers of the vulva with radiation doses to a maximum of 70.4 Gy to bulk disease and 54 Gy to areas at risk of microscopic spread combined with 5-FU (six patients also received either cisplatin or mitomycin C). A response rate of 90% was reported, with 10 pathological complete responses and eight pathological partial responses at viscera-preserving surgery. Gerszten[86] has reported treating 18 patients with a twice-daily regime of radiotherapy, cisplatin, and 5FU followed by surgery with a complete response rate of 13 patients. Similarly, Geisler et al.[87] treated 10 patients with advanced vulvar carcinoma involving the anal sphincter or urethra with cisplatin and 5-FU followed by radical surgery. They have reported conservation of the anus and the urethra in all the patients with a 100% response rate. It would therefore appear that pre-operative radiotherapy, either alone or in combination with chemotherapy, may be useful for advanced tumors to try to downsize the tumor in order to preserve urinary and anal sphincter control.

Primary radical non-surgical therapy

The place of radiotherapy alone in the treatment of vulvar carcinoma has not been studied systematically. Data accruing from reports of non-surgical management of squamous carcinoma of the anus have led to an evaluation of the possible role of primary radical non-surgical treatment of carcinoma of the vulva based on the treatment strategy for anal carcinoma.[88,89]

Based on the success of treating anal carcinoma, definitive radical radiotherapy to the vulva and inguinal nodes is usually given with concurrent 5FU, the latter as a 4-day infusion in the first and fourth or fifth weeks of radiotherapy. The maximum radiation dose is 65 Gy.

Recent studies of locally advanced vulvar cancer showed that chemo-radiotherapy is an effective alternative to radical surgery[90,91]; these findings were also confirmed in a recent Cochrane meta-analysis.[92]

Conclusions

Radiotherapy can be delivered safely to the vulva and regional lymph nodes with or without concomitant chemotherapy. The role of chemotherapy in the treatment of carcinoma of the vulva has not yet been clearly established.

The use of radiotherapy for early-stage carcinoma of the vulva should be restricted to adjuvant therapy to the vulva and nodes in patients at high risk of local recurrence after surgery. There is no evidence to support the use of inguinal nodal irradiation as a replacement for bilateral inguinal lymph node dissection.

In advanced FIGO Stage III or IV disease, the use of pre-operative radiotherapy and chemo-radiotherapy in an attempt to facilitate viscera-preserving surgery appears promising.

Results

Published 5-year survival rates for invasive cancer vary widely due to the low incidence of this tumor and the advanced age of the majority of these patients. Probably, the most reliable information comes from a GOG study[93] that defined risk groups for 377 women with cancer of the vulva depending on size of tumor and groin node status, which on multifactorial analysis, were the only variables associated with prognosis.

The risk was minimal in lesions measuring 2 cm or less and with no groin node involvement. Nearly all these patients were alive at 5 years. Women at low risk were those with lesions larger than 2 cm but smaller than 8.1 cm with no nodal involvement. They had a survival rate at 5 years of 87%, as did lesions less than or equal to 2 cm in size but with a single node involved. The 5-year survival rate dropped to 70% for those at intermediate risk, which included lesions larger than 8 cm but with no groin node involvement and those with smaller lesions but with one or two nodes positive for metastatic disease. At high risk was any woman whose lesion was greater than 8 cm with two positive nodes or who had any size lesion with three or more ipsilateral nodes involved or with bilateral node involvement. The survival in this group at high risk was 29%.

The effect on 5-year survival rate of lymph node involvement taken as a single prognostic variable showed that a negative node status conferred a survival rate of 92%, falling to 75% with ipsilateral node involvement and 30% with bilateral node involvement. If more than two nodes were involved, the survival rate was 25%, falling to zero if more than six nodes were positive.

Uncommon tumors of the vulva

Melanoma of the vulva

Approximately 5% of melanomas in women occur on the vulva, and it is the second most common carcinoma of the vulva. Melanin production is variable, and the lesions range from black to completely amelanotic. The most usual presenting complaint is of a lump or an enlarging mole. Pruritus and bleeding are less common.

The prognosis is strongly related to the depth of invasion.[93–95] In the vulva, measurement of the thickness of the lesion as suggested by Breslow[94] is more commonly used. Breslow has five levels of invasion, from the surface epithelium to the point of deepest penetration. Level 1 is <0.76 mm in thickness, Level 2 is 1.5 mm, Level 3 is 3 mm, Level 4 is 4 mm, and Level 5 is deeper than 4 mm.

Local invasion occurs in an outward direction as well as downward, so excision margins must be very wide, 3–5 cm being suggested for all but the most superficial lesions. This usually requires a radical vulvectomy without lymphadenectomy unless there is clinical evidence of groin disease. If the groin nodes are removed, the operation should be performed *en bloc*.

Other forms of treatment, such as radiotherapy, chemotherapy, and immunotherapy, have had very little impact on this disease, although newer immunotherapeutic agents have shown some promise in modifying the disease progress (see "Uncommon Vaginal Tumors" section).

The prognosis for Level 1 melanoma of the vulva is very good, as nodal involvement is unlikely. However, approximately one-third of patients have groin lymph node metastases at presentation, and 2.6% have distant spread. Although 5-year survival is approximately 56% if the nodes are negative, the survival rate falls to 14% when the nodes are positive.[96] Involvement of the urethra or vagina, or the presence of satellite lesions, all worsen the prognosis.

Paget's disease and apocrine adenocarcinoma of the vulva

This is an uncommon condition, similar to that found in the breast. Pruritus is the presenting complaint. The lesion is indistinguishable clinically from squamous intraepithelial neoplasia, and the diagnosis must be made by biopsy. In approximately one-third of patients, there is an adenocarcinoma in the apocrine glands. This has a poor prognosis if the groin lymph nodes are involved, with no survivors at 5 years.

The treatment of Paget's disease is wide local excision, usually involving total vulvectomy, because of the propensity of this condition to involve apparently normal skin. The specimen must be examined histologically with great care to exclude an apocrine adenocarcinoma. Excluding underlying adnexal carcinomas, concomitant genital malignancies are found in 15%–25% of women with Paget's disease of the vulva.[97] These are most commonly vulvar or cervical, but transitional cell carcinoma of the bladder (or kidney) and ovarian, endometrial, vaginal, and urethral carcinomas have all been reported.

Verrucous carcinoma of the vulva

This slowly growing neoplasm is rarely seen on the vulva. Both macroscopically and histologically, it resembles condyloma acuminata, and the diagnosis can be difficult. Generous biopsies are required to provide sufficient material for the pathologist. The treatment is surgery, usually a radical vulvectomy but very occasionally wide local excision. The place of lymphadenectomy is debatable, as lymph node metastases are uncommon.

Basal cell carcinoma

This tumor is rarely found on the vulva. Wide local excision gives excellent results in most cases.

Bartholin's gland carcinoma

Usually an adenocarcinoma, this tumor may be squamous, transitional cell type, or even mixed squamous and adenocarcinoma. It has often spread widely to pelvic and groin nodes before the diagnosis is made. It must be distinguished from adenoid cystic carcinoma, which is similar to the tumor found in salivary glands and which seldom gives rise to metastatic disease. The treatment is surgery, but because of its deep origin, part of the vagina, levatores ani, and the ischio-rectal fat must be removed.

Sarcomas

These rare tumors of the vulva include leiomyosarcomas, which tend to grow slowly and metastasize late, and rhabdomyosarcomas, which are rapidly growing, aggressive tumors. A radical vulvectomy and groin node dissection is the usual treatment, but local recurrence and blood-borne metastases are common. Like sarcomas in other parts of the body, the prognosis for sarcomas of the vulva is poor.

Key points

1. Invasive vulvar cancer is an uncommon cancer. It represents approximately 4% of all female gynecological cancers.
2. The lymph drains from the vulva to the inguinal and femoral glands in the groin and then to the external iliac glands. Drainage from the perineum and the clitoris is to both groins, but some contra-lateral spread occurs from other sites on the vulva.
3. The histological features of VIN are analogous to those seen in CIN and VAIN. Most invasive cancers (85%) are squamous. Approximately 5% of melanomas in women occur on the vulva, and it is the second most common carcinoma of the vulva.
4. Two independent pathways are proposed for the development of vulvar squamous cell carcinoma. The first is related to mucosal HPV infection, and the second is related to chronic inflammatory or autoimmune processes.
5. Surgery is the mainstay of treatment.
6. In treating vulvar cancer, the groin node dissection includes both the superficial inguinal and the deep femoral nodes, as superficial groin node dissection alone is associated with a higher risk of groin node recurrence.
7. Sentinel node identification is now an accepted method for inguinal node staging in vulvar cancer. Combining radiotracer and blue dye methods and excluding patients with palpable inguinal nodes results in the highest sensitivity.
8. The most significant prognostic features of vulvar cancer are size of tumor, inguinal node involvement, and the width of the vulvar tumor-free margin.
9. Nearly all patients are alive at 5 years when the risk is minimal in lesions measuring 2 cm or less and with no groin node involvement. Women at a slightly higher risk are those with lesions larger than 2 cm but smaller than 8.1 cm with no nodal involvement. They have an 87% 5-year survival rate.
10. The effect on 5-year survival rate of lymph node involvement taken as a single prognostic variable showed that a negative node status conferred a survival rate of 92%, falling to 75% with ipsilateral node involvement and 30% with bilateral node involvement. If more than two nodes were involved, the survival rate was 25%, falling to zero if more than six nodes were positive.

References

1. Cancer Research UK. Vaginal cancer incidence. 2019. Available at: http://www.cancerresearchuk.org/cancer-info/cancerstats/types/vagina/incidence/uk-vaginal-cancer-incidence-statistics
2. Daling J, Sherman KJ. Relationship between human papillomavirus infection and tumours of anogenital sites other than the cervix. *IARC Sci Publ.* 1992; 119:223–41.
3. Bjorge T, Dillner J, Anttila T et al. Prospective seroepidemiological study of role of human papillomavirus in non-cervical anogenital cancers. *BMJ.* 1997; 315(7109):646–9.
4. Hopkins MP and Morley GW. Squamous cell carcinoma of the neovagina. *Obstet Gynecol.* 1987; 69(Pt 2):525–7.
5. Sugase M, Matsukura T. Distinct manifestations of human papillomaviruses in the vagina. *Int J Cancer.* 1997; 72(3):412–5.
6. Coppleson M. The DES story. *Med J Aust.* 1984; 141(8):487–9.
7. Herbst AL, Ulfelder H, Poskanzer DC. Adenocarcinoma of the vagina. Association of maternal stilbestrol therapy with tumor appearance in young women. *N Engl J Med.* 1971; 284(15):878–81.
8. McFarlane MJ, Feinstein AR, Horwitz RI. Diethylstilbestrol and clear cell vaginal carcinoma. Reappraisal of the epidemiologic evidence. *Am J Med.* 1986; 81(5):855–63.
9. Cramer DW, Cutler SJ. Incidence and histopathology of malignancies of the female genital organs in the United States. *Am J Obstet Gynecol.* 1974; 118(4):443–60.
10. 1Gemmell J, Holmes DM, Duncan ID. How frequently need vaginal smears be taken after hysterectomy for cervical intraepithelial neoplasia? *Br J Obstet Gynaecol.* 1990; 97(1):58–61.
11. Aho M, Vesterinen E, Meyer B et al. Natural history of vaginal intraepithelial neoplasia. *Cancer.* 1991; 68(1):195–7.
12. Choo YC, Anderson DG. Neoplasms of the vagina following cervical carcinoma. *Gynecol Oncol* 1982; 14:125.
13. Herbst AL, Ulfelder H, Poskanzer DC. Adenocarcinoma of the vagina. Association of maternal stilbestrol therapy with tumor appearance in young women. *N Engl J Med.* 1971; 284:878.
14. Livingston RC. Primary carcinoma of the vagina. In Thomas CC (Ed), Springfield, IL, 1950.
15. Underwood PB Jr., Smith RT. Carcinoma of the vagina. *JAMA.* 1971; 217:46.
16. Pride GL, Schultz AE, Chuprevich TW, Buchler DA. Primary invasive squamous carcinoma of the vagina. *Obstet Gynecol.* 1979; 53:218.
17. Gallup DG, Talledo OE, Shah KJ, Hayes C. Invasive squamous cell carcinoma of the vagina: A 14-year study. *Obstet Gynecol.* 1987; 69:782.
18. Perez CA, Arneson AN, Galakatos A, Samanth HK. Malignant tumors of the vagina. *Cancer.* 1973; 31(1):36–44.
19. Soutter WP. *Vaginal Intraepithelial Neoplasia and Colposcopy of the Vagina. A Practical Guide to Colposcopy* (pp. 144–60). Oxford, UK: Oxford Medical Publications, 1993.
20. Gallup DG, Talledo OE, Shah KJ, Hayes C. Invasive squamous cell carcinoma of the vagina: A 14-year study. *Obstet Gynecol.* 1987; 69(5):782–5.
21. Dodge JA, Eltabbakh GH, Mount SL et al. Clinical features and risk of recurrence among patients with vaginal intraepithelial neoplasia. *Gynecol Oncol.* 2001; 83(2):363–9.
22. Buck HW, Guth KJ. Treatment of vaginal intraepithelial neoplasia (primarily low grade) with imiquimod 5% cream. *J Lower Genital Tract Dis.* 2003; 7(4):290–3.
23. Iavazzo C, Pitsouni E, Athanasiou S, Falagas ME. Imiquimod for treatment of vulvar and vaginal intraepithelial neoplasia. *Int J Gynaecol Obstet.* 2008; 101(1):3–10.
24. Stock RG, Mychalczak B, Armstrong JG et al. The importance of brachytherapy technique in the management of primary carcinoma of the vagina. *Int J Radiat Oncol Biol Phys.* 1992; 24(4):747–53.
25. Mock U, Kucera H, Fellner C et al. High-dose-rate (HDR) brachytherapy with or without external beam radiotherapy in the treatment of primary vaginal carcinoma: Long-term results and side effects. *Int J Radiat Oncol Biol Phys.* 2003; 56(4):950–7.
26. Hiniker SM, Roux A, Murphy JD et al. Primary squamous cell carcinoma of the vagina: Prognostic factors, treatment patterns, and outcomes. *Gynecol Oncol.* 2013; 131(2):380–385.
27. Al-Kurdi M, Monaghan JM. Thirty-two years experience in management of primary tumours of the vagina. *Br J Obstet Gynaecol.* 1981; 88(11):1145–50.
28. Kucera H, Vavra N. Radiation management of primary carcinoma of the vagina: Clinical and histopathological variables associated with survival. *Gynecol Oncol.* 1991; 40(1):12–16.
29. Al-Kurdi M, Monaghan JM. Thirty-two years experience in management of primary tumours of the vagina. *Br J Obstet Gynaecol.* 1981; 88:1145.
30. Berek JS, Hacker NF, Lagasse LD. Vaginal reconstruction performed simultaneously with pelvic exenteration. *Obstet Gynecol.* 1984; 63:318.
31. Benson C, Soisson AP, Carlson J et al. Neovaginal reconstruction with a rectus abdominis myocutaneous flap. *Obstet Gynecol.* 1993; 81:871.

32. Cancer Research UK. Vulvar cancer incidence. 2019; Available at http://www.cancerresearchuk.org/cancer-info/cancerstats/types / vulva/incidence/uk-vulva-cancer-incidence-statistics.

33. Meffert JJ, Davis BM, Grimwood RE. Lichen sclerosus. *J Am Acad Dermatol.* 1995; 32(3):393–416.

34. Fishman DA, Chambers SK, Schwartz PE et al. Extramammary Paget's disease of the vulva. *Gynecol Oncol.* 1995; 56(2):266–70.

35. Ragnarsson-Olding B, Johansson H, Rutqvist LE, Ringborg U. Malignant melanoma of the vulva and vagina. Trends in incidence, age distribution, and long-term survival among 245 consecutive cases in Sweden 1960–1984. *Cancer.* 1993; 71(5):1893–7.

36. Madsen BS, Jensen HL, van den Brule AJ et al. Risk factors for invasive squamous cell carcinoma of the vulva and vagina—population-based case-control study in Denmark. *Int J Cancer.* 2008; 122:2827.

37. Brinton LA, Thistle JE, Liao LM, Trabert B. Epidemiology of vulvar neoplasia in the NIH-AARP Study. *Gynecol Oncol.* 2017; 145:298.

38. Jones RW, McLean MR. Carcinoma in situ of the vulva: a review of 31 treated and five untreated cases. *Obstet Gynecol.* 1986; 68(4):499–503.

39. Rutledge F, Smith JP and Franklin EW. Carcinoma of the vulva. *Am J Obstet Gynecol.* 1970; 106(8):1117–30.

40. de Koning MN, Quint WG, Pirog EC. Prevalence of mucosal and cutaneous human papillomaviruses in different histologic subtypes of vulvar carcinoma. *Mod Pathol.* 2008; 21:334.

41. Halec G, Alemany L, Quiros B et al. Biological relevance of human papillomaviruses in vulvar cancer. *Mod Pathol.* 2017; 30:549.

42. Weberpals JI, Lo B, Duciaume MM et al. Vulvar Squamous Cell Carcinoma (VSCC) as two diseases: HPV status identifies ddistinct mutational profiles including oncogenic fibroblast growth factor receptor 3. *Clin Cancer Res.* 2017; 23:4501.

43. de Sanjosé S, Alemany L, Ordi J et al. Worldwide human papillomavirus genotype attribution in over 20 cases of intraepithelial and invasive lesions of the vulva. *Eur J Cancer.* 2013; 49:3450.

44. Wharton JT, Gallager S, Rutledge FN. Microinvasive carcinoma of the vulva. *Am J Obstet Gynecol.* 1974; 118(2):159–62.

45. Wilkinson EJ, Rico MJ, Pierson KK. Microinvasive carcinoma of the vulva. *Int J Gynecol Pathol.* 1982; 1(1):29–39.

46. Iversen T, Abeler V, Kolstad P. Squamous cell carcinoma in situ of the vulva. A clinical and histopathological study. *Gynecol Oncol.* 1981; 11(2):224–9.

47. Parker RT, Duncan I, Rampone J, Creasman W. Operative management of early invasive epidermoid carcinoma of the vulva. *Am J Obstet Gynecol.* 1975; 123(4):349–55.

48. Hoffman JS, Kumar NB, Morley GW. Microinvasive squamous carcinoma of the vulva: Search for a definition. *Obstet Gynecol.* 1983; 61(5):615–8.

49. Hacker NF, Berek JS, Lagasse LD et al. Individualization of treatment for stage I squamous cell vulvar carcinoma. *Obstet Gynecol.* 1984; 63(2):155–62.

50. Monoghan JM. Management of vulval carcinoma. In Shepherd JH, MJM (Eds.), *Clinical Gynaecological Oncology.* London, UK: Blackwell, 1985, 133–53.

51. Soutter WP. *Colposcopy of the Vulva. A Practical Guide to Colposcopy* (pp. 161–86). Oxford, UK: Oxford Medical Publications, 1993.

52. Andreasson B, Bock JE. Intraepithelial neoplasia in the vulvar region. *Gynecol Oncol.* 1985; 21(3):300–5.

53. Zacur H, Genadry R, Woodruff JD. The patient-at-risk for development of vulvar cancer. *Gynecol Oncol.* 1980; 9:199.

54. Collins CG, Lee FY, Roman-Lopez JJ. Invasive carcinoma of the vulva with lymph node metastasis. *Am J Obstet Gynecol.* 1971; 109:446.

55. Townsend DE, Levine RU, Richart RM et al. Management of vulvar intraepithelial neoplasia by carbon dioxide laser. *Obstet Gynecol.* 1982; 60(1):49–52.

56. Dorsey J. Skin appendage involvement and vulvar intraepithelial neoplasia. In Sharp FJJA (Ed.), *Laser Surgery* (pp. 193–5). New York, NY: Perinatology Press, 1986.

57. Cavanagh DREH, Marsden DE. Cancer of the vulva. In Cavanagh DREH, Marsden DE (Ed.), *Gynaecological Cancer—A Clinico-Pathological Approach* (pp. 1–40). Norwalk, CT: Appleton-Century-Crofts, 1985.

58. Wallbillich JJ, Rhodes HE, Milbourne AM et al. Vulvar intraepithelial neoplasia (VIN 2/3): Comparing clinical outcomes and evaluating risk factors for recurrence. *Gynecol Oncol.* 2012; 127(2):312–5.

59. Way S. Carcinoma of the vulva. *Am J Obstet Gynecol.* 1960; 79:692–7.

60. Monaghan JM. Radical surgery for carcinoma of the vulva. In Monaghan JM (Ed.), *Bonney's Gynaecological Surgery* (9th ed., pp. 121–8). Eastbourne, UK: Balliere Tindall, 1986.

61. Hacker NF, Leuchter RS, Berek JS et al. Radical vulvectomy and bilateral inguinal lymphadenectomy through separate groin incisions. *Obstet Gynecol.* 1981; 58(5):574–9.

62. Helm CW, Hatch K, Austin JM et al. A matched comparison of single and triple incision techniques for the surgical treatment of carcinoma of the vulva. *Gynecol Oncol.* 1992; 46(2):150–6.

63. Siller BS, Alvarez RD, Conner WD et al. T2/3 vulva cancer: A case-control study of triple incision versus en bloc radical vulvectomy and inguinal lymphadenectomy. *Gynecol Oncol.* 1995; 57(3):335–9.

64. RCOG. Clinical Recommendations for Management of Vulvar Cancer. London, UK: Royal College of Obstetricians and Gynaecologists, 2006.

65. Anderson BL. Predicting sexual and psychological morbidity and improving quality of life for women with gynaecological cancer. *Cancer.* 1993; 15(71[4 Suppl]):1678–90.

66. Hacker NF. Current management of early vulvar cancer. *Ann Acad Med Singapore.* 1998; 27(5):688–92.

67. Stehman FB, Bundy BN, Dvoretsky PM, Creasman WT. Early stage I carcinoma of the vulva treated with ipsilateral superficial inguinal lymphadenectomy and modified radical hemivulvectomy: A prospective study of the Gynecologic Oncology Group. *Obstet Gynecol.* 1992; 79(4):490–7.

68. Homesley HD, Bundy BN, Sedlis A, Adcock L. Radiation therapy versus pelvic node resection for carcinoma of the vulva with positive groin nodes. *Obstet Gynecol.* 1986; 68(6):733–40.

69. The Royal College of Obstetricians & Gynaecologistas, Guidelines for the Diagnosis and Managament of Vulvar Carcinoma, 2014.

70. National Comprehensive Cancer Network (NCCN Guidelines) Vulvar Cancer (Squamous Cell Carcinoma).

71. European Society of Gynaecological Oncology, Vulvar Cancer Management Guidlines.

72. Te Grootenhuis NC, Pouwer AW, de Bock GH et al. Margin status revisited in vulvar squamous cellcarcinoma. *Gynecol Oncol.* 2019; 154(2):266–75.

73. Hassanzade M, Attaran M, Treglia G et al. Lymphatic mapping and sentinel node biopsy in squamous cell carcinoma of the vulva: Systematic review and meta-analysis of the literature. *Gynecol Oncol.* 2013; 130(1):237–45.

74. Sebag-Montefiore DJ, McLean C, Arnott SJ et al. Treatment of advanced carcinoma of the vulva with chemoradiotherapy—Can exenterative surgery be avoided? *Int J Gynecol Cancer.* 1994; 4(3):150–5.

75. Thomas G, Dembo A, DePetrillo A et al. Concurrent radiation and chemotherapy in vulvar carcinoma. *Gynecol Oncol.* 1989; 34(3):263–7.

76. Harrington KJ, Lambert HE. Current issues in the non-surgical management of primary vulvar squamous cell carcinoma. *Clin Oncol.* 1994; 6(5):331–6.

77. Thomas GM, Dembo AJ, Bryson SC et al. Changing concepts in the management of vulvar cancer. *Gynecol Oncol* 1991; 42(1):9–21.

78. Hoffman M, Greenberg S, Greenberg H et al. Interstitial radiotherapy for the treatment of advanced or recurrent vulvar and distal vaginal malignancy. *Am J Obstet Gynecol.* 1990; 162(5):1278–82.

79. Bryson SC, Dembo AJ, Colgan TJ, Iavazzo C. Invasive squamous cell carcinoma of the vulva defining low and high risk groups for recurrence. *Int J Gynecol Cancer.* 1991; 1:25–31.

80. Heaps JM, Fu YS, Montz FJ et al. Surgical-pathologic variables predictive of local recurrence in squamous cell carcinoma of the vulva. *Gynecol Oncol.* 1990; 38(3):309–14.

81. Hacker NF, Van der Velden J. Conservative management of early vulvar cancer. *Cancer.* 1993; 71(4) Supplement: 1673–7.
82. Woelber L, Eulenburg C, Choschzick M et al. Prognostic role of lymph node metastases in vulvar cancer and implications for adjuvant treatment. *Int J Gynecol Cancer.* 2012; 22(3):503–8.
83. Stehman FB, Bundy BN, Thomas G et al. Groin dissection versus groin radiation in carcinoma of the vulva: Gynecologic Oncology Group study. *Int J Radiat Oncol Biol Phys.* 1992; 24(2):389–96.
84. Hacker NF, Berek JS, Juillard GJ, Lagasse LD. Preoperative radiation therapy for locally advanced vulvar cancer. *Cancer.* 1984; 54(10):2056–61.
85. Rotmensch J, Rubin SJ, Sutton HG et al. Preoperative radiotherapy followed by radical vulvectomy with inguinal lymphadenectomy for advanced vulvar carcinomas. *Gynecol Oncol.* 1990; 36(2):181–4.
86. Boronow RC, Hickman BT, Reagan MT et al. Combined therapy as an alternative to exenteration for locally advanced vulvovaginal cancer. II. Results, complications, and dosimetric and surgical considerations. *Am J Clin Oncol.* 1987; 10(2):171–81.
87. Koh WJ, Wallace HJ, 3rd, Greer BE et al. Combined radiotherapy and chemotherapy in the management of local-regionally advanced vulvar cancer. *Int J Radiat Oncol Biol Phys.* 1993; 26(5): 809–16.
88. Gerszten K, Selvaraj RN, Kelley J, Faul C. Preoperative chemoradiation for locally advanced carcinoma of the vulva. *Gynecol Oncol.* 2005; 99(3):640–4.
89. Geisler JP, Manahan KJ, Buller RE. Neoadjuvant chemotherapy in vulvar cancer: avoiding primary exenteration. *Gynecol Oncol.* 2006; 100(1):53–7.
90. Nigro ND, Vaitkevicius VK, Considine B, Jr. Combined therapy for cancer of the anal canal: A preliminary report. *Dis. Colon Rectum.* 1974; 17(3):354–6.
91. Nigro ND, Vaitkevicius VK, Considine B, Jr. Combined therapy for cancer of the anal canal: A preliminary report. 1974. *Dis Colon Rectum.* 1993; 36(7):709–11.
92. Rogers LJ, Howard B, Van Wijk L et al. Chemoradiation in advanced vulvar carcinoma. *Int J Gynecol Cancer.* 2009; 19(4):745–51.
93. Tans L, Ansink AC, van Rooij PH et al. The role of chemo-radiotherapy in the management of locally advanced carcinoma of the vulva: Single institutional experience and review of literature. *Am J Clin Oncol.* 2011; 34(1):22–6.
94. Shylasree TS, Bryant A, Howells RE. Chemoradiation for advanced primary vulvar cancer. *Cochrane Database Sys Rev.* 2011; 4:CD003752.
95. Homesley HD, Bundy BN, Sedlis A et al. Assessment of current International Federation of Gynecology and Obstetrics staging of vulvar carcinoma relative to prognostic factors for survival (a Gynecologic Oncology Group study). *Am J Obstet Gynecol.* 1991; 164(4):997–1003; discussion -4.
96. Breslow A. Thickness, cross-sectional areas and depth of invasion in the prognosis of cutaneous melanoma. *Ann Surg.* 1970; 172(5):902
97. Clark WH, Jr., From L, Bernardino EA, Mihm MC. The histogenesis and biologic behavior of primary human malignant melanomas of the skin. *Cancer Res.* 1969; 29(3):705–27.

Useful websites

www.cancer.gov/cancertopics/types/vaginal
www.cancer.gov/cancertopics/types/vulvar
http://seer.cancer.gov/statfacts/html/vulva.html
www.ncin.org.uk/cancer_type_and_topic_specific_work/cancer_type_s
	pecific_work/gynaecological_cancer/gynaecological_cancer_hub/
	resources/vulvar_and_vagina_cancer
http://emedicine.medscape.com/article/2156990-overview
www.guideline.gov/content.aspx?id=43888
www.cancerresearchuk.org/cancer-info/cancerstats/keyfacts/vagina-
	and-vulva-cancer/
www.cancer.net/cancer-types/vaginal-cancer
www.cancer.net/cancer-types/vulvar-cancer

23 GESTATIONAL TROPHOBLASTIC NEOPLASIA

Michael J. Seckl

Introduction

Gestational trophoblastic disease (GTD) was probably first described as "dropsy of the uterus" around 400 BC by Hippocrates and his student, Diocles.[1] Marie Boivin (1773–1841), a Parisian midwife, was the first to document the chorionic origin of the hydatids.[1] However, it was not until 1895 that Marchand described a malignant uterine disease of syncytial and cytotrophoblastic origin and made the link between hydatidiform mole and other forms of pregnancy.[1]

Normal gestational trophoblast arises from the peripheral cells of the blastocyst in the first few days after conception. Trophoblastic tissue initially grows rapidly into two layers:

1. An inner cytotrophoblast of mononucleated cells, which migrate out and fuse, forming
2. An outer syncytiotrophoblast of large multinucleated cells (Figure 23.1).

The latter subsequently aggressively invades the endometrium and uterine vasculature, generating an intimate connection between the fetus and the mother, known as the placenta. Invasion is, of course, one of the features of malignancy, and indeed, normal trophoblast can even be detected in the maternal circulation.[2] Fortunately, complex biological and immunological mechanisms prevent such circulating normal trophoblast from producing metastases.

When GTD arises, such regulatory mechanisms controlling trophoblastic tissue are lost. Thus, the excessively proliferating trophoblast may invade through the myometrium, developing a rich maternal blood supply, with tumor emboli and hematogenous spread occurring frequently. GTD comprises two pre-malignant diseases, termed complete and partial hydatidiform mole (CHM and PHM), and the four malignant disorders, or gestational trophoblastic tumors (GTT): invasive mole, gestational choriocarcinoma, placental-site trophoblastic tumor, and epithelioid trophoblastic tumor.[3] The malignant conditions are also collectively known as gestational trophoblastic neoplasia (GTN). The origins, pathology, and clinical behavior of these various forms of GTD are different and will be discussed later. These tumors are important to recognize, because they are nearly always curable, and in most cases, fertility can be preserved. This is mainly because:

1. GTNs are exquisitely chemosensitive.
2. They all produce human chorionic gonadotrophin (hCG), a serum tumor marker with a sensitivity and accuracy in screening, monitoring, management, and follow-up of patients that are unparalleled in cancer medicine.
3. Detailed prognostic scoring has permitted "fine-tuning" of treatment intensity so that each patient only receives the minimum therapy required to eliminate her disease.

Genetics and pathology

Complete hydatidiform mole

CHMs nearly always only contain paternal DNA and are therefore androgenetic.[4] This occurs mostly because a single sperm bearing a 23X set of chromosomes fertilizes an ovum lacking maternal genes and then duplicates to form the homozygote, 46XX[4–10] (Figure 23.2a). However, in up to 25% of CHMs, fertilization can take place with two spermatozoa, resulting in the heterozygous 46XY or 46XX configuration[11,12] (Figure 23.2b). A 46YY conceptus has not yet been described and is presumably non-viable. Interestingly, CHMs retain some maternal elements, including the mitochondrial DNA.[13] Rarely, a CHM can arise from a fertilized ovum that has retained its maternal nuclear DNA and is therefore biparental in origin (BiCHM).[14,15] Women with BiCHM suffer repetitive molar pregnancies and rarely achieve a normal pregnancy. The condition is autosomal recessive and is also known as familial recurrent HM syndrome (FRHM). Most are due to mutations in NLRP7[16] and much less frequently in KHD3CL (C6orf221)[17] and other as yet un-identified genes. Recently, two triploid cases of FRHM have been described, which morphologically are also CHM.[18]

Macroscopically, CHM classically resembles a bunch of grapes due to generalized (complete) swelling of chorionic villi. However, this only occurs in the second trimester, and the diagnosis these days is usually made in the first trimester, when the villi microscopically contain little fluid, are branching, and consist of hyperplastic syncytio- and cytotrophoblast with many vessels. Although it was previously thought that CHM produced no fetal tissue, histology from first-trimester abortions reveals evidence of embryonic elements, including fetal red cells.[19–21] This has resulted in many CHMs being incorrectly labeled as PHMs. Consequently, the reported rate of persistent GTD after PHMs has been artificially elevated and is probably less than 0.5–1%.[3,22] The presence of embryonic tissue from a twin pregnancy comprising a fetus and a CHM is a further source of error, which can lead to the incorrect diagnosis of PHM. Sometimes, there may be diagnostic confusion between CHM and a hydropic abortion. This is resolved by using p57 immunostaining, an imprinted marker expressed only by the maternal genome. Since CHMs are androgenetic, the CHM intervillous trophoblast is negative, while the surrounding maternal tissue or villi from a hydropic abortion are positively stained for p57.[23]

Partial hydatidiform mole

Partial hydatidiform moles are genetically nearly all triploid or rarely, tetraploid, with at least two paternal chromosome sets but also some maternal contribution (Figure 23.2c). Although triploidy occurs in 1–3% of all recognized conceptions and in about 20% of spontaneous abortions with abnormal karyotype, triploids due to two sets of maternal chromosomes do not become PHMs.[24,25] Flow cytometry, in situ ploidy, or genotyping done from formalin-fixed, paraffin-embedded tissues[15] can all therefore help in differentiating CHM from PHM, and PHM from diploid non-molar hydropic abortions.[26] Although a variety of reports indicated that diploid PHM exists, genetic analysis of lesions suspected to be such has not supported this suggestion. In general, a diploid molar gestation is believed to be a complete hydatidiform mole.[27] In PHMs, swelling tends to be less intense than in CHM and affects only some villi (partial). Thus, two populations of villi

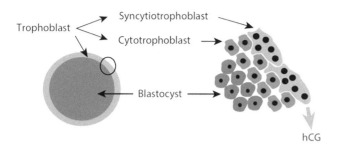

FIGURE 23.1 Schematic diagram of an embryo at the blasto-cyst stage, demonstrating trophoblast development.

usually exist in a partial mole. Both swollen and non-swollen villi can have trophoblastic hyperplasia, which is mild and focal.[28–30] Nuclear atypia is infrequent. The villi have characteristic indented or scalloped outlines and round inclusions.[31]

An embryo is usually present and can be recognized macro-scopically or inferred from the presence of nucleated red cells in villous vasculature. It may survive into the second trimester, but in most cases, it dies at about 8–9 weeks' gestation, and this is fol-lowed by loss of vessels and stromal fibrosis. In PHMs evacuated early, villus swelling and trophoblastic excess can be so mild and focal that the diagnosis of PHM may be missed.[31] Indeed, at uter-ine evacuation for a "miscarriage," it is likely that many PHMs are misclassified as products of conception. Fortunately, we only see about one patient per year with persistent GTD related to a pre-viously unrecognized PHM. Of the increasing number of PHMs that are correctly diagnosed, very few go on to develop persis-tent GTD, probably better referred to as post-mole GTN. Indeed,

studies from our center suggest just a 0.5–1.1% risk of GTN fol-lowing a PHM.[22,32] Consequently, it would be useful to have some way of identifying immediately post evacuation which patients will subsequently require chemotherapy. This would avoid many thousands of patients with a PHM undergoing unnecessary hCG follow-up. The potential for new omics technologies, such as next generation sequencing, epigenomics, expression arrays, and metabonomics, is now being actively investigated in this arena.

Other pregnancies mistaken for partial hydatidiform mole

Over half of first-trimester non-molar abortions are due to tri-somy, monosomy, maternally derived triploidy, and transloca-tions. These often develop hydrops, but this is small (<3 mm), and PHM can be excluded if they are diploid on flow cytom-etry. Syndromes such as Turner's, Edwards', and Beckwith–Wiedemann can also cause histological confusion with PHMs.[33]

Invasive hydatidiform mole

This term is applied when a CHM or rarely, a PHM invades into the myometrium. Invasive mole is common and is clinically iden-tified by the combination of an abnormal uterine ultrasound and a persistent or rising hCG level following uterine evacuation. Except under unusual circumstances when a curettage specimen contains myometrium with invasive molar villi, the diagnosis of an invasive mole can only be made on a hysterectomy speci-men. The pathological confirmation of this condition is, however, rarely required. Moreover, repeat dilatation and curettage (D&C) is often contraindicated because of the risks of uterine perfora-tion, infection, life-threatening hemorrhage, and subsequent

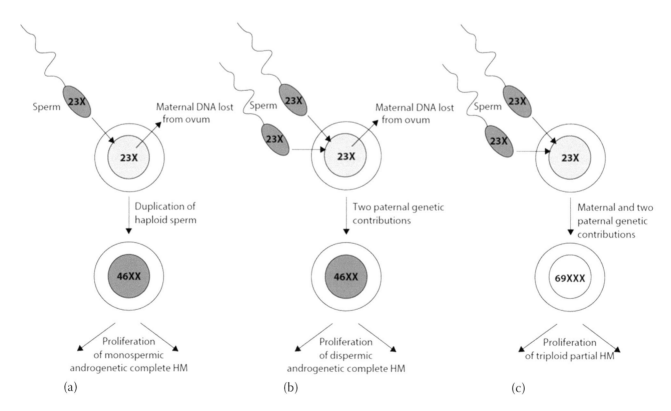

(a)　　　　　　　　　　　　　(b)　　　　　　　　　　　　　(c)

FIGURE 23.2 Schematic diagram showing that the androgenetic diploid complete HM is formed either by duplication of the chro-mosomes from a single sperm (a) or by two sperm fertilizing the ovum (b), which, in both cases, has lost its own genetic component. The triploid genetic origin of a partial HM is demonstrated in (c).

hysterectomy. In occasional cases where histology is available, invasive mole can be distinguished from choriocarcinoma by the presence of chorionic villi.

Choriocarcinoma

Gestational choriocarcinoma is the most aggressive form of GTD. Most choriocarcinomas have been shown to have grossly abnormal karyotypes with diverse ploidies and several chromosome rearrangements, none of which is specific for the disease.[34] Studies of the origin of GTN have confirmed that choriocarcinoma may arise from any type of pregnancy, including a normal term pregnancy,[35–38] a homozygous or heterozygous CHM,[36,39] or PHM.[22] Consequently, all types of hydatidiform mole (HM) need careful follow-up.

Interestingly, choriocarcinoma may not always be due to the antecedent pregnancy.[22] A patient with a history of a CHM 4 years previously developed a choriocarcinoma following the delivery of a twin pregnancy. Using PCR to amplify short tandem repeat polymorphisms in DNA, this tumor was shown to be genetically identical to the previous CHM.[15,40] As with invasive HM, obtaining tissue to make a formal histological diagnosis of choriocarcinoma is often not appropriate, and so doubt frequently exists over whether patients have one or the other form of GTN.

Choriocarcinoma is highly malignant in behavior, appearing as a soft, purple, largely hemorrhagic mass. However, in its earliest form, it may remain intraplacental in nature.[41] Detailed whole genome and epigenomic studies of one intraplacental choriocarcinoma case suggests that these tumors are a consequence of epigenomic changes matching an early stage of placental development when aggressive invasion of the uterine wall is required.[42] Microscopically, it mimics an early implanting blastocyst, with central cores of mononuclear cytotrophoblast surrounded by a rim of multinucleated syncytiotrophoblast and a distinct absence of chorionic villi. Significant cytological atypia is in place, and diffuse hCG immunostaining of the syncytiotrophoblastic cells is characteristic. There are extensive areas of necrosis and hemorrhage and frequent evidence of tumor within venous sinuses. Interestingly, the disease fails to stimulate the connective tissue support normally associated with tumors and induces hypervascularity of the surrounding maternal tissues. This probably accounts for its highly metastatic and hemorrhagic behavior.

Placental-site trophoblastic (PSTT) and epithelioid trophoblastic tumors (ETT)

PSTT accounts for 0.2% of all GTD[43,44] and is thought to derive from the intermediate trophoblasts at the implantation site.[45] PSTT, like choriocarcinoma, can arise after any type of pregnancy, including term delivery, ectopic, miscarriage, CHM, or PHM.[46] The causative pregnancy may not be the immediate antecedent pregnancy. Genetic analysis of some PSTTs has demonstrated that they are mostly diploid, either originating from a normal conceptus, and therefore biparental, or androgenetic, from a CHM.[34,43,47–50] A tetraploid PSTT has been described.[49] Interestingly, for reasons that are unclear, most PSTTs and ETTs that arise after a non-molar pregnancy are female in origin.[51] PSTTs display a pattern of vascular invasion, characterized by neoplastic cells migrating through, and replacing, vessel walls while maintaining the overall vascular architecture. PSTTs are slow-growing malignant tumors of intermediate trophoblast and so produce little hCG. However, they often stain strongly for human placental lactogen (hPL) and β1-glycoprotein. Elevated Ki-67 levels may help in distinguishing PSTT from a regressing placental nodule or exaggerated placental-site reaction.[52]

Whereas a low level of Ki-67 labelling (<1%) is seen in an exaggerated placental site, PSTTs generally show a higher index (>10%). In contrast to other forms of GTN, spread tends to occur late by local infiltration, hematogenously, and unlike other forms of GTN, also sometimes via the lymphatics.[53]

ETT is a recently described neoplastic proliferation of intermediate trophoblast that is thought by some investigators to be distinct from PSTT and choriocarcinoma,[53] but clinically, it appears to behave in the same way.[54] It has been proposed that ETT arises from the intermediate trophoblasts of the chorionic leaves.[45] Histologically, ETT displays a relatively uniform, nodular proliferation of intermediate-sized epithelioid trophoblasts, forming nests and cords. Islands of trophoblast are typically surrounded by areas of hyalinization or eosinophilic debris simulating tumor cell necrosis, resembling keratinous material in a squamous cell carcinoma. ETT can furthermore be associated with focal replacement of the cervical glandular epithelium with stratified neoplastic cells, simulating squamous cervical intra-epithelial neoplasia. The cells are positive for cytokeratin, epithelial membrane antigen, and inhibin-α, whereas the trophoblastic markers hPL, hCG, and melanoma cell adhesion molecule are only focally expressed.[55] Whether ETT is really a clinically distinct disease entity from PSTT in the GTD spectrum remains unclear.[54,56]

Atypical placental-site nodules

Recent work has revealed that placental-site nodules (PSN) can have atypical features. Importantly, these atypical placental-site nodules (APSN) may be associated with co-existing PSTT/ETT.[57] The histological criteria for distinguishing APSN from PSN are not well defined but include the presence of a hyalinized endometrial lesion containing extravillous trophoblast cells that demonstrate at least mild cytological atypia with a proliferation index above 5% but without features of invasion or other indicators of PSTT/ETT.[57] The frequency of PSN and APSN in the population is unknown. However, in our recently updated series of 77 APSN, eight have now developed or had a co-existing PSTT or ETT. Consequently, patients with a histological diagnosis of APSN should be carefully imaged and monitored for the presence or subsequent development of PSTT/ETT (Kaur et al.[57] and Naveed Sarwar et al. abstract presented at ISSTD Toronto meeting October 2019). Moreover, while the risks of PSN progressing to APSN and/or PSTT/ETT are as yet unclear, it would appear that this also merits close investigation.[58,59]

Epidemiology and etiological factors

Hydatidiform mole

Incidence and ethnic origin

From population-based studies, the incidence of CHM in countries of the Western world is approximately 0.5–1/1000 pregnancies. The previously reported increased risk in the Far East,[60] has fallen towards the stable levels found in Europe and North America,[61,62] possibly due to environmental factors, such as dietary change and better data collection.[3]

The incidence of PHM has been under-estimated in the past, and it is probably 1.5 to 2 times more frequent than CHM.[32,33]

Age

A positive relationship has been found between the risk of molar pregnancy and both upper and lower extremes of maternal age (≥45 years and ≤15 years, respectively). This association, although present for both CHM and PHM, is much greater for CHM at all maternal ages, and the degree of risk is much greater with older (≥45 years) rather than younger (≤15 years) maternal age.[63,64] Interestingly, the risk of subsequently needing chemotherapy for GTN following evacuation of a molar pregnancy also increases with age.[32]

Previous pregnancies

Risk for CHM does not rise with increasing gravidity. However, the risk of a subsequent pregnancy being a CHM rises from 1 in 1000 to about 1 in 70–100 with one previous CHM and to 1 in 4–6.5 with two previous CHMs.[32,65,66] Interestingly, the risk of a further molar pregnancy after a PHM is only very slightly increased, so most of the risk for repeat moles resides with CHM rather than PHM.[66] Tiny nests of residual molar disease may persist and can rarely reactivate in or after subsequent pregnancies. We therefore used to recommend that a serum hCG was assessed at 6 and 10 weeks after the end of any subsequent pregnancy following a previous CHM or PHM. However, a recent analysis has shown that these risks are so small that hCG testing in this situation is no longer required.[67]

Choriocarcinoma

The incidence of choriocarcinoma following term delivery without a history of CHM is approximately 1 in 50,000. However, CHM is probably the most common antecedent to choriocarcinoma, so the overall incidence of choriocarcinoma is probably much higher.[3] Proof of this is frequently difficult or inadvisable to obtain, but when histology has been available, these tumors were identified as choriocarcinoma in 3% and invasive mole in 16% of previous CHMs. Rarely, PHMs can give rise to choriocarcinoma or PSTT.[3]

Unlike HM, choriocarcinoma does not exhibit any clear geographical trends in incidence, but the effect of age remains important. Curiously, choriocarcinoma following a full-term pregnancy is more likely to be associated with a very aggressive disease course than after a CHM. This may reflect the fact that some of the choriocarcinomas after a CHM included cases of invasive mole.

Placental-site trophoblastic tumors

Data are still very limited, but using the entire U.K. experience of PSTT, it has been shown that this represents 0.23% of all GTD,[44] and no firm data currently exist for ETT.[54]

Other factors with uncertain role

Several other factors have been examined for a possible etiological role in the development of GTD. These include parity, smoking, contraceptive practice, dietary influences, and herbicide and radiation exposure. None of these has been shown conclusively to play a role in this group of diseases.[3] For example, one report has suggested that oral contraceptive use prior to conception slightly increases the risk of subsequently developing a GTN.[68] In contrast, a meta-analysis[69] and several more recent studies[70,71] have failed to show clear evidence for an association between oral contraceptive use during the post-molar follow-up period and the incidence of GTN. Consequently, it is considered safe to use oral contraception to prevent a further pregnancy following an evacuation of a CHM or PHM.

Genetic factors

All autosomal genes consist of two alleles (paternal and maternal). Some alleles are expressed from only one parent and not the other—a phenomenon called genomic imprinting. Interestingly, three closely related genes that are imprinted and located on chromosome 11p15 may be involved in GTN development and in other overgrowth syndromes.[72] These are *H19*, a putative tumor suppressor gene,[73] and *p57kip2*, a cyclin-dependent kinase inhibitor,[74] which are both normally expressed by the maternal allele, and the paternally expressed insulin-like growth factor II (*IGF-II*), a growth factor commonly implicated in tumor proliferation.[75] While *p57kip2* showed the expected pattern of expression in CHM and choriocarcinoma,[76] CHM and post-mole tumors were unexpectedly found to express *H19*,[77–79] and some post-term tumors showed bi-allelic expression of both *H19* and *IGF-II*.[80,81] This suggests that loss of the normal imprinting patterns of these genes may be an important factor in the development of GTN. Recent whole genome sequencing and methylation analysis has shown that at least for one intraplacental choriocarcinoma, there were no significant genetic mutations. However, the methylation pattern closely matched that seen in early placentation, when there is aggressive invasion of the uterine wall.[42] Further work on more cases is on-going and might provide new information about how to enable choriocarcinomas to progress past this possible block in their developmental pathway and reverse their malignant behavior.

The identification of rare families in which several sisters have repeat CHMs that are biparental in origin[14] has helped to shed further light on the genes involved in CHM formation. Classical linkage studies identified a region on chromosome 19q, and subsequent work identified NLRP7 as the causative gene in most families.[16] Recently, another causative gene was discovered (KHD3CL [C6orf221])[17] in a small number of unexplained cases, but there are additional women with FRHM that is still unexplained, presumably due to mutations in as yet un-identified genes.[18]

Risk of GTN following CHM or PHM

The risk of malignant sequelae following evacuation of a PHM is estimated be around 0.5–1%, compared with around 16% for a CHM.[22,32] Other researchers have reported somewhat higher rates of GTN developing after a PHM, with values from 2% to 6%.[82,83] The differences in these studies may have arisen because the diagnosis was made using morphological criteria without the added benefit of cytogenetics to help discriminate between CHM and PHM. Since it is not yet possible to predict in advance which patients with a CHM or PHM will develop persistent GTD, all of them must be registered for hCG monitoring. Following this strict protocol enables the identification of individuals with persistent trophoblastic growth who could benefit from lifesaving chemotherapy.

Human chorionic gonadotrophin

Molecular background and function

The family of pituitary/placental glycoprotein hormones includes hCG, follicle-stimulating hormone (FSH), luteinizing hormone (LH), and thyroid-stimulating hormone (TSH). Each hormone comprises an α-subunit, which is common between the family members, and a distinct β-subunit, which helps to confer receptor specificity. Consequently, assays to measure hCG are directed against the β-subunit. The crystal structures for both the α- and β-subunits of hCG have been solved.[84,85] The genes for βhCG and βLH have been mapped to a complex cluster of inverted and tandem genes on chromosome 19, of which six are for βhCG and the terminal seventh for βLH.[86,87] However, the precise role of each of the genes, which can all be transcribed, remains unclear.[88] Interestingly, the gene is highly conserved in nature, being found in prokaryotes.[89] So far, only one receptor for βhCG has been identified in mammals, which also serves as the main receptor for LH.[90,91] This, of course, raises the question of how hCG might exert specific effects distinct from LH. Furthermore, βhCG is now known to circulate in a variety of forms as a result of post-translational modifications of its structure, such as hyperglycosylated hCG (hCG-H), nicked hCG, nicked hyperglycosylated hCG, hCG missing the beta-subunit C-terminal extension, free alpha-subunit, free beta-subunit, free beta-subunit missing the C-terminal extension, hyperglycosylated-free beta-subunit (βhCG-H), and nicked-free beta-subunit.[92] It is therefore possible that additional βhCG receptors exist. The function(s) of the intact and the modified forms of βhCG remain obscure. During a normal pregnancy, the only forms of hCG found are intact and hCG-H, the latter being present solely during the first trimester. In contrast, in malignancy, multiple forms of hCG can be found. Whatever the functions of these different forms of hCG, the fact that hCG production clinically indicates trophoblastic proliferation suggests that this molecule may be a growth factor for normal placenta, GTD, and other hCG-producing tumors. Indeed, hCG-H produced during the first trimester of normal pregnancy promotes trophoblast proliferation and invasion into the myometrium and exerts similar effects on choriocarcinoma cells, possibly through an hCG/LH receptor–independent mechanism.[93]

hCG assays

The measurement of hCG during pregnancy is relatively straightforward, since the molecule is either intact and/or hyperglycosylated, so the antibodies used only need to detect these two forms. In contrast, the assays used to detect hCG produced by cancer should ideally be able to recognize intact and all fragments of βhCG and βhCG-H. Moreover, the assay should not produce either false negative or false positive results.[94,95] Currently, commercial assays used to measure βhCG are mostly designed to recognize intact hCG or βhCG, so they are good for pregnancy monitoring and indeed, are licensed for this purpose. However, none of these assays are approved for use in cancer, and most fail to recognize all known forms of βhCG.[95,96] This means that the assays are prone to false negatives. The commercial assays are all based on the sandwich or two-site principle using a capture antibody recognizing one site on hCG and another antibody binding to a second site on the hormone for detection. The mechanism of detection used in these assays is also variable (e.g., complement fixation, enzyme- and fluorescence-based), and this, combined with differences in antibody specificity and sensitivity, results in considerable differences in assay results,[97] particularly when the assays are used in cancer patients.[96] Added to this is a lack of agreed international standards for some of the hCG isoforms, with, for example, no standards for hCG-H. So, what does all this mean? Essentially, it is difficult to ensure direct comparability between different hCG assays in anything other than pregnancy. In addition, it means that there is a clear need for an hCG assay that can be safely used to detect this hormone in cancer patients.

At Charing Cross, we have for many years been using a non-commercial competitive one-site radio-immunoassay (RIA). Quite fortuitously, the antibody used in this assay detects a site on βhCG that is common to all the known forms of this hormone and so does not have a false negative problem. However, single-site RIA and the commercial two-site sandwich assays share a problem of false positive detection. This usually occurs as a consequence of heterophile antibodies, for example anti-mouse or anti-rabbit antibodies, produced by the patient. Fortunately, these do not cross into the urine, so simple measurement of the urine hCG can confirm whether an elevated serum result is a true positive. In addition, heterophile antibodies, in contrast to true hCG, do not produce results that diminish appropriately when the serum is serially diluted. At Charing Cross, all hCG assays are automatically set up with serial dilutions, and all patients have their hCG measured in serum and urine. Consequently, we do not see problems with false positives. This contrasts with many other centers, which depend on commercial assays that are frequently not set up in dilution and where urine is not routinely assessed in parallel with serum. Nevertheless, the Charing Cross RIA is slower to generate results, taking 24 hours rather than the commercial assays, which generally take just a few hours. Moreover, the RIA requires radioactivity. While speed of results is not usually clinically important, the use of radioactivity is becoming increasingly unacceptable. Therefore, there remains a clear need to develop a new hCG assay specifically for use in cancer, and we are currently actively exploring this area.

Use as a tumor marker

Human chorionic gonadotrophin, which has a half-life of 24–36 hours, remains the most sensitive and specific marker for trophoblastic tissue. However, hCG production is not confined to pregnancy and GTD. Indeed, hCG is produced by any trophoblastic tissue found, for example, in germ cell tumors and in up to 15% of epithelial malignancies.[98] The hCG levels in such cases can be just as high as those seen in GTD. Furthermore, the levels of hCG produced by GTD are frequently identical to those found in normal pregnancy, although very high levels outside the range for a twin pregnancy may lead to suspicion of a trophoblastic tumor. Consequently, hCG measurements per se do not reliably discriminate between pregnancy, GTD, and non-gestational trophoblastic tumors. Nevertheless, serial hCG measurements have revolutionized the management of GTD for several reasons. Thus, the amount of hCG produced correlates with tumor volume, so that a serum hCG of 5 IU/L corresponds to approximately 10^4–10^5 viable tumor cells. Consequently, these assays are several orders of magnitude more sensitive than the best imaging modalities available today. In addition, hCG levels can be used to determine prognosis.[99] Serial measurements allow progress of the disease or response to therapy to be monitored (Figure 23.3). The development of drug resistance can be detected at an early stage, which facilitates appropriate management changes. Estimates may be made of the time for which chemotherapy should be continued after hCG levels are undetectable in serum in order to reduce the tumor volume to zero. For these reasons, hCG is the best tumor marker known and is of wider interest as a model for the way in which tumor markers may be used in other cancers.

Clinical features

Complete and partial moles

CHM or PHM most commonly presents in the first trimester as a threatened abortion with vaginal bleeding. Patients with CHM may rarely notice the passing of grape-like structures (vesicles), and occasionally, the entire mole may be spontaneously delivered. The uterus may be of any size but is commonly large for gestational age. Other symptoms related to high hCG and more advanced disease, such as hyperemesis, toxemia, convulsions, theca lutein cysts, and hyperthyroidism, previously seen at a comparatively high frequency, are rarely seen today[100] because of

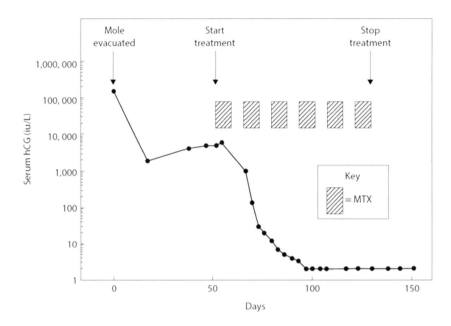

FIGURE 23.3   The use of monitoring the serum hCG concentration following evacuation of a hydatidiform mole (HM). In this case, after an initial fall, the hCG started to rise, indicating the development of invasive HM or choriocarcinoma, and so the patient was called up for staging. The prognostic score was low risk (see Table 23.5), and the patient was successfully treated with methotrexate (MTX) and folinic acid (see Table 23.6).

early ultrasound diagnosis.[3] Although pulmonary, vaginal, and cervical metastases can occur, they may spontaneously disappear following removal of the mole. Thus, the presence of metastases does not necessarily imply that invasive mole or choriocarcinoma has developed. Patients may present with acute respiratory distress not only because of pulmonary metastases and/or anemia but occasionally, as a result of tumor embolization. The risk of embolization is reduced by avoiding agents that induce uterine contraction before the cervix has been dilated to enable evacuation of the CHM.

Patients with PHM usually do not exhibit the dramatic clinical features characteristic of CHM. The uterus is often not enlarged for gestational age, and vaginal bleeding tends to occur later, so that patients most often present in the late first trimester or early second trimester with a missed or incomplete abortion. In fact, the diagnosis is rarely suspected until the histology of curettings is available. Clues to the diagnosis can occasionally be obtained by ultrasound.[101,102] The pre-evacuation hCG is >100,000 IU/L at diagnosis in over 90% of cases.

At present, a proportion of CHMs and PHMs still go undiagnosed either because of miscarriage at home or because termination centers do not carry out histopathological examination of all abortions.[103] This can result in late presentation of disease, sometimes with life-threatening complications. Clearly, there is little that can be done about miscarriages at home. However, for women attending termination centers, a pre-termination ultrasound may provide clues, and if this is abnormal, then histology should be requested. Another alternative is to measure the urine hCG 3-4 weeks post termination; this should be normal in most women but if elevated, should prompt a repeat test, which if rising, is highly suggestive of GTD.[103]

Twin pregnancies

Twin pregnancies comprising a normal fetus and a hydatidiform mole are estimated to occur in between 1 in 20,000 and 1 in 100,000 pregnancies. Some probably abort in the first trimester and so go undiagnosed. However, some are discovered on ultrasound examination, either routinely or because of complications such as bleeding, excessive uterine size, or problems related to a high hCG.[104]

Invasive moles

These are usually diagnosed because serial urine or serum hCG measurements reveal a plateaued or rising hCG level in the weeks after evacuation of the mole. Patients may complain of persistent vaginal bleeding or lower abdominal pains and/or swelling. This may occur as a result of hemorrhage from leaking tumor-induced vasculature as the trophoblast invades through the myometrium or because of vulval, vaginal, or intra-abdominal metastases. The tumor may also involve other pelvic structures, including the bladder or rectum, producing hematuria or rectal bleeding, respectively. Enlarging pulmonary metastases or tumor emboli growing in the pulmonary arteries can contribute to life-threatening respiratory complications.[105,106] The risk of these complications is clearly higher in patients in whom the initial diagnosis of a molar pregnancy was missed and who are therefore not on hCG follow-up.

Choriocarcinoma

Choriocarcinoma can present after any form of pregnancy but most commonly occurs after CHM. In the latter situation, it is often not practical to obtain histological proof of choriocarcinoma, and so it is impossible to distinguish it from invasive mole. Choriocarcinoma following an apparently normal pregnancy or non-molar abortion usually presents within a year of delivery, but in the Charing Cross series, the longest interval to date was 35 years (unpublished data). The presenting features may be similar to those of HM, with vaginal bleeding, abdominal pain, and a pelvic mass. However, one-third of all patients with choriocarcinoma present without gynecological features and instead have symptoms of distant metastases.[107,108] In these cases, lives can be saved by remembering to include choriocarcinoma in the differential diagnosis of metastatic malignancy (particularly in lungs, brain, or liver) presenting in a woman of childbearing age. Any site may be involved, including skin, producing a purple lesion, cauda equina, and heart. Pulmonary disease may be parenchymal or pleural or may result from tumor embolism and subsequent growth in the pulmonary arteries.[105,106] Thus, respiratory symptoms and signs can include dyspnea, hemoptysis, and pulmonary artery hypertension. Cerebral metastases may produce focal neurological signs, convulsions, evidence of raised intracranial pressure, and intracerebral or subarachnoid hemorrhage. Hepatic metastases may cause local pain or referred pain in the right shoulder. Although none of these presentations is specific to choriocarcinoma, performing a simple pregnancy test or quantitative hCG assay can provide a vital clue to the diagnosis. Other clues may come from features associated with a high circulating hCG level, including occasional thyrotoxicosis and ovarian theca lutein cysts.[3]

Infantile choriocarcinoma

Choriocarcinoma in the fetus or newborn is exceptionally rare, with no more than 31 reported cases.[107–111] While a primary choriocarcinoma within the infant is possible, in 18 out of 31 cases, the mother also had the tumor. This suggests that the disease can cross the placenta to flourish in both mother and child. Interestingly, the diagnosis was often made in the neonate before the mother. In all cases, the infant was anemic and had a raised hCG, but the site of metastasis was variable, including liver and lung in the majority and brain in 27% of patients. Only a few patients have been treated successfully with platinum-based chemotherapy and surgery, the rest dying within weeks of initial diagnosis, which may have been delayed.[112] Consequently, serum or urine hCG levels should be measured in all babies of mothers with choriocarcinoma. As the disease can present up to 6 months after delivery, an argument could be made for serial monitoring of hCG in these infants. However, to cause the least distress, we currently just measure it once in the infant's urine of mothers with choriocarcinomas and instruct the parents to bring the baby back for an urgent test if it is failing to thrive. The mothers of infants with infantile choriocarcinoma should be placed on regular hCG monitoring for at least a year.

PSTT/ETT and APSN

The slow growth rate of PSTT means that it can present years after term delivery, non-molar abortion, or complete HM.[53] Unlike choriocarcinoma, it tends to metastasize late in its natural history, and so patients frequently present with gynecological symptoms alone.[43] In addition to vaginal bleeding, the production of hPL by the cytotrophoblastic cells may cause hyperprolactinemia, which can result in amenorrhea and/or galactorrhea. In some instances, presumably also as a result of tumor-secreted products, patients can develop nephrotic syndrome or hematuria with deposition of fibrinogen in the glomeruli. Disseminated intra-vascular coagulation has been reported in association with these features.[113,114] Metastases may occur anywhere, including the vagina, extra-uterine pelvic tissues, retroperitoneum, lymph nodes, lungs, and brain.[43,44]

ETT, from the limited available literature, appears to behave clinically like PSTT, frequently presenting with vaginal bleeding

and low and occasionally normal levels of serum β-hCG (<2500 mIU/mL).[54] In half of the reported cases, the tumors arise in the lower uterine segment or cervix, and the distinction from a keratinizing squamous cell carcinoma can sometimes be difficult. Extra-uterine locations such as broad ligament as the primary site have also been observed.[115] Similarly to PSTT, ETT may not respond quite so well to conventional chemotherapy, and hysterectomy with close follow-up is appropriate until more experience of this rare lesion becomes available.

PSN and APSN are usually diagnosed following diagnostic curettage for vaginal bleeding that develops after a prior pregnancy. Currently, only APSN should be further investigated, but this may change with time.[57]

Management and investigations

CHM and PHM

Early bleeding in pregnancy has many causes but usually leads to a request for a pelvic ultrasound. The classical and highly suggestive, but not diagnostic, snow-storm features of a CHM are now rarely seen, as most scans are performed in the first trimester, when hydropic changes are either absent or minimal. Consequently, the scans frequently just show evidence of an abnormal or failing pregnancy. Nevertheless, although non-diagnostic, some appearances may raise suspicions of a molar pregnancy, and since the pregnancy is non-viable, termination is arranged.[116,117] The presence of a very high hCG for dates is also suspicious but not diagnostic. If there are chest symptoms, a chest x-ray (CXR) should be performed, as the disease rarely may already be metastatic to the lungs. In the event that lung metastases are already present, the case should be discussed urgently with a trophoblastic disease center. Suction D&C gives the lowest incidence of sequelae.[3] When the molar trophoblast invades the myometrium, it is relatively easy to perforate the uterus if a metal curette is used. Medical induction involving repeated contraction of the uterus induced by oxytocin or prostaglandin, or other surgical approaches including hysterectomy or hysterotomy, increases the risk of requiring chemotherapy by two- to threefold compared with suction evacuation. This is thought to be because tumor is more likely to be disseminated by uterine contraction and manipulation. For similar reasons, the prolonged use of prostanoids is not recommended, but a short use of prostanoids to ripen the cervix may be safe. If bleeding is severe immediately after suction evacuation, a single dose of ergometrine to produce one uterine contraction may stem the hemorrhage and does not appear to increase the chance of requiring chemotherapy. In the past, it has been common practice for gynecologists to perform a second and sometimes a third evacuation of the uterine cavity in patients with a molar pregnancy. However, analysis of our data has shown that the chance of requiring chemotherapy after one evacuation is only 2.4% but rises markedly to 18% after two evacuations and 81% after four evacuations (Table 23.1). Patients with an hCG plateau or with rising hCGs are at particularly high risk, and 74% of patients require chemotherapy despite undergoing a second evacuation (Table 23.2). Furthermore, high hCG values have been shown to be an indicator for low rates of benefit of a second evacuation, with 80% of patients with a pre-interventional hCG of >5000 subsequently requiring chemotherapy.[118] Consequently, repeated evacuations are not generally recommended because of the risk of complications and the high chance that the patient will require chemotherapy anyway. However, a second evacuation may be reasonable if there is a clinical indication such as bleeding

TABLE 23.1 Correlation between the Number of Evacuations Performed Following an HM and the Subsequent Requirement for Chemotherapy at Charing Cross Hospital (1973–1986)

Number of Evacuations	Patients Not Treated	Patients Treated	% Patients Treated
1	4481	109	2.4
2	1495	267	18
3	106	106	50
4	5	22	81

TABLE 23.2 hCG Levels at Second Evacuation and Subsequent Requirement for Chemotherapy

hCG at Second Evacuation	Patients Requiring Chemotherapy (%)
<1,500	50
1,500–5,000	38
5,000–10,000	83
10,000–20,000	75
20,000–50,000	68
>50,000	94
Total	74

or if repeat ultrasound shows persisting molar trophoblast within the uterine cavity and the hCG is <5000 IU/L. The use of ultrasound control during this procedure may help to reduce the risk of uterine perforation. Rarely, in more mature women who have completed their families, hysterectomy is an alternative approach to removing the hydatidiform mole.[119]

Twin pregnancies

At Charing Cross Hospital in London, we have previously reported our findings on 77 confirmed cases of CHM with a separate normal conceptus.[104] Fifty-three of these women elected to continue their pregnancy, while the remainder had a termination. Just over a third of women who continued their pregnancy achieved a live birth, while the remainder had non-viable pregnancies, which ended mostly in spontaneous abortions. Interestingly, there was no difference in the risk of developing persistent GTD/malignant change (GTN) between women who underwent an early termination and those who elected to continue their pregnancy. Moreover, no woman in this series died either from a pregnancy-related complication such as toxemia or from GTT. A recent analysis of multiple small case series suggested that there might be a more serious risks to continuing such pregnancies.[120] However, we have now seen a further 153 women across the United Kingdom with twin pregnancies, and the current healthy live birth rate is running at 51% without any maternal deaths and again, with no increased risk of developing GTN (presented at the ISSTD Toronto meeting 2019). Thus, it appears reasonably safe to allow patients with twin pregnancies in which one of the conceptions is a CHM to continue to term provided there are no other complications. This is in line with observations on singleton CHM, which suggest that later gestational age at termination does not increase the risk of subsequently requiring chemotherapy.[121,122] These results also suggest that the malignant potential of each CHM is likely determined at or very soon after conception.

Registration and follow-up after uterine evacuation

The majority of patients require no more treatment after evacuation, but 16% of patients with CHM and <0.5–1% with PHM develop malignant change (GTN) that requires chemotherapy, also known as persistent GTD. This can be invasive mole, choriocarcinoma, or very rarely, PSTT/ETT. It is vital that patients with GTN following a mole are identified as soon as possible to maximize the chances of cure with appropriate therapy. In 1973, a national follow-up service was instituted in the United Kingdom, whereby patients with GTD are registered with one of three centers, located in Dundee, Sheffield, and London, covering women living in Scotland, the north of England, and the rest of the country, respectively. Approximately 1800 U.K. women are registered per annum, and of these, about 160 need chemotherapy. After registration, the patient's details and pathology, together with two weekly blood and urine samples, are sent through the post to one of the three reference laboratories for confirmation of diagnosis and serial hCG estimations. Following the success of this scheme, other countries have now established, or are attempting to establish, a similar registration program to reduce their GTN mortality rates.

Since a molar pregnancy is a pre-malignant condition, in the majority of cases, the molar tissue dies out spontaneously. Consequently, the hCG concentration returns to normal. Once the hCG is within the normal range (<4 IU/L), a key question is how long to continue monitoring prior to attempting a further pregnancy. Having recently reviewed the outcomes on over 20,000 moles at Charing Cross, we know that most malignant change is discovered before the hCG normalizes but that there is still a small risk of malignant change after the first normal hCG value. This risk is greatest in patients with CHM and threefold higher in women whose hCG takes longer than 56 days to normalize. Consequently, for CHM, if the hCG normalizes within 56 days, monitoring continues with monthly urine samples to 6 months from the date of uterine evacuation. However, in those patients in whom the hCG is first normal >56 days post evacuation, hCG surveillance continues for 6 months of normal values. Doing this reduces the risk of missing subsequent GTN in CHM to about 1 in 1500. For women with PHM, simply one confirmatory normal hCG is sufficient to reduce the GTN risk to 1 in 3000.[123]

Indications for chemotherapy

Factors associated with an increased risk of requiring chemotherapy are summarized in Table 23.3. We previously advised women to avoid using hormone contraceptives before the hCG was normal.[124] However, more recent publications have produced discrepant results,[69] and an analysis of our own population using current-generation lower-dose contraceptives no longer shows an increased risk of developing GTN if these hormones are used while the hCG is still elevated.[70]

TABLE 23.3 Factors Increasing the Risk of Requiring Chemotherapy Following Evacuation of a Hydatidiform Mole

Factor	Reference
CHM > PHM	Seckl et al. (106)
Uterine size > gestational age	Curry et al. (131)
Pre-evacuation serum hCG level >100,000 IU/L	Berkowitz and Goldstein (100)
Bilateral cystic ovarian enlargement	Berkowitz and Goldstein (100)
Increasing maternal age	Savage et al. (2013)

The indications for intervention with chemotherapy in patients who have had a CHM or PHM are shown in Table 23.4. Human chorionic gonadotrophin values >20,000 IU/L 4 weeks after evacuation of a mole indicate that the patient is at increased risk of severe hemorrhage or uterine perforation with intra-peritoneal bleeding, and this can be reduced by starting chemotherapy. Metastases in the lung, vulva, and vagina can only be observed if the hCG levels are falling. However, if the hCG levels are not dropping, or the patient has metastases at another site, which can indicate the development of choriocarcinoma, chemotherapy is required. We and Federation of Gynaecology and Obstetrics (FIGO) previously advised commencing chemotherapy in any woman with a falling hCG at 6 months after molar evacuation. Such patients were considered to have an increased risk of acquiring further mutations in their tumors, which might make them more difficult to treat. However, recent work has shown that continued observation appears to be safe and effective, with all 66 cases normalizing their hCG without additional treatment.[125] FIGO has recently now also dropped this as an automatic indication for treatment.[126]

Prognostic factors/scoring versus FIGO staging

The principal prognostic variables for GTNs, which were originally identified by Bagshawe[99] and since modified by the World Health Organization and our own experience, are summarized in Table 23.5. Each variable carries a score, and the sum of these for an individual patient, correlates with the risk of the tumor becoming resistant to single-agent therapy. Thus, the most important prognostic variables carry the highest score and include:

1. The duration of the disease, because drug resistance of GTN varies inversely with time from the original antecedent pregnancy
2. The serum hCG concentration, which correlates with viable tumor volume in the body
3. The presence of liver and/or brain metastases

Since liver metastases correlate with a worse prognosis than brain metastases,[127,128] patients with liver involvement now score

TABLE 23.4 Indications for Chemotherapy

1. Histological evidence of choriocarcinoma
2. Evidence of metastases in brain, liver, or gastrointestinal tract, or radiological opacities >2 CHM on chest x-ray
3. Pulmonary, vulval, or vaginal metastases unless hCG falling
4. Heavy vaginal bleeding or evidence of gastrointestinal or intra-peritoneal hemorrhage
5. HCG levels that are plateaued over three consecutive or rising over two consecutive samples after evacuation
6. Serum hCG >20,000 IU/L more than 4 weeks after evacuation, because of the risk of uterine perforation
7. Raised hCG 6 months after evacuation even if still falling (no longer an automatic indication for therapy)
Any of the above are indications to treat following the diagnosis of GTD apart from 7.

TABLE 23.5a Charing Cross Scoring System for GTN

Prognostic Factor	Score			
	0	1	2	6
Age (years)	<39	>39	–	–
Antecedent pregnancy (AP)	Mole	Abortion or unknown	Term	–
Interval (end of AP to chemotherapy in months)	<4	4–7	7–12	>12
hCG (IU/L)	10^3–10^4	<10^3	10^4–10^5	>10^5
Number of metastases	0	1–3	4–8	>8
Site of metastases	None, lung, vagina	Spleen, kidney	GI tract	Brain, liver
Largest tumor mass	–	3–5 CHM	>5 CHM	–
Prior chemotherapy	–	–	Single drug	≥2 drugs

Notes: The total score for a patient is obtained by adding the individual scores for each prognostic factor. Low risk, 0–8; high risk, >9. Patients scoring 0–8 currently receive single-agent therapy with methotrexate and folinic acid, while patients scoring ≥9 receive combination drug therapy with EMA/CO (see Table 23.7).
Abbreviations: CXH, Charing Cross Hospital; hCG, human chorionic gonadotrophin; GI, gastrointestinal.

TABLE 23.5b FIGO Scoring System for GTN

Prognostic Factor	Score			
	0	1	2	4
Age (years)	<40	≥40	–	–
Antecedent pregnancy (AP)	Mole	Abortion	Term	–
Interval (end of AP to chemotherapy in months)	<4	4–6	7–13	>13
hCG (IU/L)	<10^3	10^3–10^4	10^4–10^5	>10^5
Number of metastases	0	1–4	5–8	>8
Site of metastases	Lung	Spleen, kidney	GI tract	Brain, liver
Largest tumor mass	–	3–5 CHM	>5 CHM	
Prior chemotherapy	–	–	Single drug	≥2 drugs

Notes: The total score for a patient is obtained by adding the individual scores for each prognostic factor. Low risk, 0–6; high risk, ≥7.

six points rather than four. Anatomical staging systems such as that of the International FIGO have been used by several centers managing GTN. However, surgery is virtually never indicated in the initial management of this disease, and the FIGO staging system does not appear to add anything in treatment planning to the existing scoring system. Consequently, an international committee in 2000 recommended a new combined FIGO/scoring system, which was accepted in 2002, so that all centers managing this rare group of diseases can more easily compare their results.[129] We have been using the new FIGO scoring system ever since to make our treatment decisions, as outlined in Table 23.5b, but continue to keep data for our old Charing Cross scoring system (Table 23.5a). Patients with a FIGO score of 0–6 have disease at low risk of becoming resistant to single-agent chemotherapy, and those scoring >6 have high-risk disease and so require combination-agent chemotherapy. Over time, it has become clear that the new FIGO scoring system is probably not quite as good as the old Charing Cross scoring system for predicting those low-risk patients who will develop resistance to single-agent therapy.[130,131] The problem is particularly bad for patients who have a FIGO score of 5–6, where it would be helpful to better identify the 70% who will clearly fail single-agent therapy.[56,130,131] Some clues as to how to achieve this are already available. For example, women whose hCG is in excess of 400,000 IU/L[132] but score 5 or 6 are not cured with just one drug and should be treated as high risk. In addition, those whose tumors are very vascular on Doppler ultrasound are also more likely to have disease resistant to single-agent methotrexate (MTX) chemotherapy.[133–135] However, exactly how to include these data into a revised FIGO scoring system is unclear, and work is on-going within the international community to refine and potentially simplify the FIGO scoring system.[136] This work will need to take into account the new ultra-high-risk group defined as a FIGO score >12.[137,138]

Investigation and treatment of low-risk patients

Most patients with low-risk disease have had a CHM or PHM as the antecedent pregnancy and require a history and physical examination followed by routine blood tests, including a serum hCG sample. In addition, these patients should have a Doppler ultrasound and assuming this does not identify a new pregnancy, then a CXR.[139] The latter is often normal but may reveal lung metastases. If these are visible on CXR, then a CT chest to confirm is helpful, but lesions <1 cm or not visible on CXR are not counted in the scoring system, as they do not influence the outcome.[140,141] Patients with CXR-defined lung metastases are at increased risk of central nervous system (CNS) involvement [142,143] and should have magnetic resonance imaging (MRI) of the brain.[56] If the latter is normal, then a lumbar puncture to assess the cerebrospinal fluid (CSF): serum hCG ratio can be helpful, as a ratio more than 1:60 is suggestive of occult disease. The ultrasound usually reveals a vascular mass of mixed signal intensity within the cavity and/or wall of the uterus but may appear surprisingly normal if the hCG levels are low. The degree of vascularity, assessed by measuring the pulsatility index either in the uterine arteries or even in feeding vessels to the tumor, has been shown to be an independent predictor of resistance to single-agent therapy with MTX in both a retrospective and a prospective study at Charing Cross Hospital.[133,134] Interestingly, although 1 in 50 of our patients will suffer heavy vaginal bleeding upon starting chemotherapy, this cannot be reliably predicted by the degree of endometrial vascularization seen on ultrasound.

Low-risk patients can be managed by either MTX or actinomycin D (ActD)-based regimens. There is no agreement as to

TABLE 23.6 Chemotherapy Regimen for Low-Risk and Intermediate-Risk Patients

Methotrexate/Folinic Acid

Methotrexate (MTX)	50 mg by intramuscular injection repeated every 48 h for a total of four doses
Calcium folinate (folinic acid)	15 mg orally 30 h after each injection of MTX

Note: Courses repeated every 2 weeks, i.e. days 1, 15, 29, etc.

which drug or regimen (there are at least two ActD and even more MTX regimens) is superior.[144] A trial comparing ActD 1.25 mg/m² intravenous (IV) once every 2 weeks with two different MTX regimens (one intramuscular [IM], described in Table 23.6, and the other IV) lumped into one arm was attempted but sadly closed early because of poor recruitment with insufficient numbers to draw any firm conclusions. The MTX and folinic acid (FA) regimen used since 1964 at Charing Cross Hospital and widely followed in other centers is shown in Table 23.6. Figure 23.3 illustrates a typical course of a patient responding to this therapy. The schedule is in general well tolerated and unlike ActD, does not induce alopecia. Some patients develop sore eyes and mouth ulcers. This can be prevented partly by a high fluid intake of 3 L/day while on treatment and by increasing the FA rescue from 7.5 to 15 mg. Indeed, routinely doing this from the outset has reduced the incidence of these side-effects to less than 3% without obviously decreasing efficacy.[130,131] If this approach fails, then giving the FA earlier, at 24 hours after MTX, can be helpful. Methotrexate can also induce serositis, resulting in pleuritic chest pain or abdominal pain. Myelosuppression is rare, but a full blood count should be obtained before each course of treatment. Liver and renal function should also be monitored regularly. All patients are advised to avoid sun exposure or use complete sun block for 1 year after chemotherapy, because the drugs can induce photosensitivity.

Between 30% and 40% of low-risk patients need to change treatment: 2–3% because of toxicity (usually mucositis, occasionally severe pleuritic pain or drug-induced hepatitis) and the remainder as a result of drug resistance, which occurs despite the patients being correctly scored as low risk.[130,131] Thus, careful monitoring for disease response and treatment-induced toxicity is required to ensure that these women achieve complete remission. It is also important that once the hCG is normal, sufficient consolidation therapy is given to prevent relapse. We have recently shown in a collaborative study with the Dutch that the risk of relapse is doubled in their population, where they only give two compared with our three consolidation courses.[145] Finally, in low-risk patients with post-molar GTN who have completed their families, do not have evidence of metastatic disease, and wish to avoid chemotherapy, hysterectomy is an alternative choice with acceptable outcomes.[146]

Survival in low-risk patients is excellent, currently running over the last 25 years at around 100% even though they may need to change treatment.[130,131] The only deaths in patients treated with this MTX/FA schedule following the introduction of the prognostic scoring system were one from concurrent but not therapy-induced non-Hodgkin's lymphoma, one from hepatitis,[147] and one from a subsequent lung cancer in a patient who failed to quit smoking.[137] Indeed, we found no evidence that single-agent therapy with MTX increases the risk of developing a second cancer[148,149] (Figures 23.4, 23.5, and 23.6).

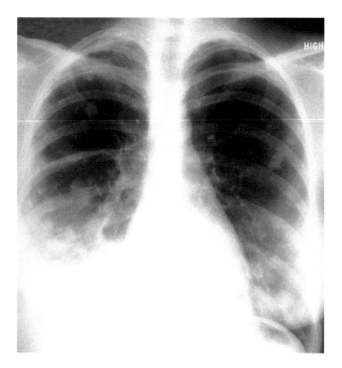

FIGURE 23.4 Chest radiograph showing multiple lung metastases and a small right pleural effusion in a patient with choriocarcinoma.

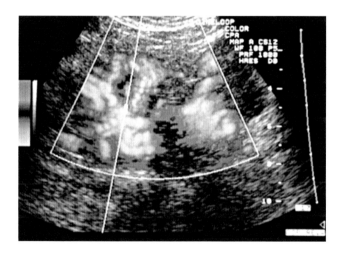

FIGURE 23.5 Ultrasonography with color Doppler showing persistent gestational trophoblastic disease following a CHM within the body and wall of the uterus. A typical vesicular or "snow storm" appearance of residual molar tissue can be seen within the uterus, together with a rich blood supply through the endometrium and myometrium. There is no evidence of a fetus.

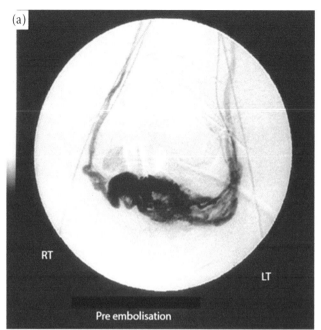

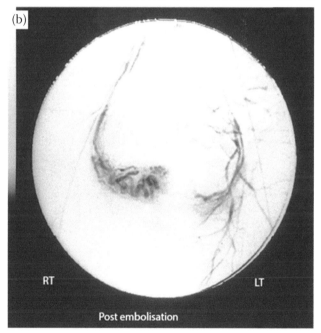

FIGURE 23.6 Arteriographic appearance of a uterine arteriovenous malformation before (a) and after selective embolization (b) in a patient with repeated vaginal hemorrhages following previous curative treatment for invasive HM. The patient's bleeding subsequently stopped, and she had a normal pregnancy.

Investigation and treatment of high-risk patients

These patients usually present without a history of molar pregnancy and may or may not have had histology showing either choriocarcinoma or PSTT/ETT. Such individuals may have widespread disease involvement and need extensive investigation beyond just simple blood tests, hCG, pelvic Doppler ultrasound, and CXR. Additional tests should include contrast-enhanced computed tomography (CT) of chest/abdomen (Figure 23.7), MRI of pelvis and brain (Figure 23.8), and biopsy if this can be obtained without precipitating life-threatening hemorrhage. Genetic analysis may be required to determine whether the disease is gestational and if so, from which previous pregnancy it has arisen, as this can guide management. Fluorodeoxyglucose positron emission tomography (FDG)-PET-CT scanning is usually not required but may be helpful later in the disease course for identifying active disease sites suitable for resection. All high-risk patients with a negative MRI of brain should have a CSF:serum hCG ratio measured to look for occult disease (see later section on CNS disease).

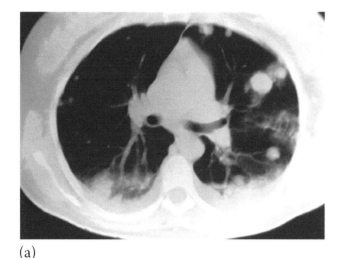

(a)

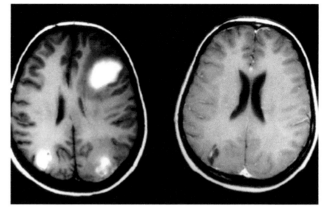

FIGURE 23.8 The MRI appearances of the brain before (a) and after (b) EMA/CO chemotherapy (see Table 23.7) for metastatic choriocarcinoma.

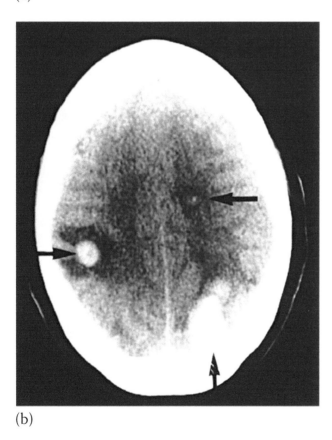

(b)

FIGURE 23.7 CT scan demonstrating (a) lung and (b) brain metastases in a patient with choriocarcinoma.

Since 1979, we have treated high-risk patients with an intensive regimen consisting of etoposide, MTX, and ActD (EMA), alternating weekly with cyclophosphamide and vincristine, otherwise known as Oncovin (CO). Table 23.7 gives details of this therapy, which can be given to most patients with only one overnight stay in hospital every 2 weeks. A patient's response to this therapy is shown in Figure 23.9. Consolidation therapy should be for 6 weeks for those with regular high-risk disease scoring 7–12 once the hCG is normal. However, for ultra-high-risk patients with a FIGO score of >12, who will likely have poor risk factors such as brain and/or liver disease, extending consolidation chemotherapy to 8 weeks with a normal hCG is

TABLE 23.7   Chemotherapy Regimen for High-Risk Patients

EMA		
Day 1	Etoposide	100 mg/m^2 by IV infusion over 30 min
	Actinomycin D	0.5 mg IV bolus
	Methotrexate	300 mg/m^2 by IV infusion over 12 h
Day 2	Etoposide	100 mg/m^2 by IV infusion over 30 min
	Actinomycin D	0.5 mg IV bolus
	Folinic acid rescue (starting 24 h after commencing the methotrexate infusion)	15 mg IM or orally every 12 h for four doses
CO		
Day 8	Vincristine	1 mg/m^2 IV bolus 1 (max. 2 mg)
	Cyclophosphamide	600 mg/m^2 IV infusion over 30 min

Note: EMA alternates with CO every week. To avoid extended intervals between courses caused by myelosuppression, it may occasionally be necessary to reduce the EMA by omitting the Day 2 doses of etoposide and actinomycin D.

probably desirable and is our standard practice. EMA/CO is myelosuppressive, but prolonged gaps in therapy, which may permit tumor regrowth, can usually be avoided by the following measures: continuing to treat unless the neutrophils are less than 0.9×10^9/L and/or platelets fall below 60×10^9/L and/or mucosal ulceration develops. Most patients require granulocyte-colony stimulating factor (G-CSF) support for 3–5 days each week to maintain treatment intensity and avoid neutropenic febrile episodes. Vincristine-induced neuropathy can be avoided by reducing the dose and if this is insufficient, stopping the drug altogether before Grade 2 symptoms are present. Nausea and vomiting are largely avoided with modern antiemetics, including 5HT3 and NK1 receptor antagonists combined with domperidone or cyclizine. This means that dexamethasone is usually not required, an advantage in young women with curable cancer, as this drug can rarely cause avascular necrosis of the femoral / humeral heads.

The cumulative 5-year survival of patients treated with EMA/CO between 1979 and 1995 was 86%, with no deaths from GTN beyond 2 years after the initiation of chemotherapy.[128] While these results were good, we noticed that deaths occurred either early, within 4 weeks of admission, due to hemorrhage and organ failure (respiratory and hepatic) associated with overwhelming

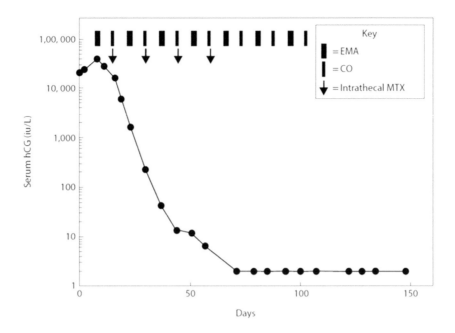

FIGURE 23.9 The fall in hCG and by inference, the tumor response to EMA/CO chemotherapy in a patient with choriocarcinoma who scored within the high-risk group. The patient had pulmonary metastases and received intrathecal methotrexate with each course of CO (cyclophosphamide and vincristine) until the hCG levels were within the normal range.

disease burden or later from drug resistant disease. The latter group appeared to include patients who in fact might have had non-gestational tumors such as lung and gastric cancers as well as those with truly drug resistant GTN. Analysis of the pre-treatment FIGO scores showed that patients at risk of early or late deaths all had a FIGO score >12, and so this could be used to define an ultra-high-risk patient group.[137,138]

To reduce early deaths in patients presenting with very advanced disease involving the chest or poorer-prognosis sites such as the brain and liver, we introduced a gentle induction chemotherapy comprising low-dose cisplatin 20 mg/m² and etoposide 100 mg/m² (EP) given on Days 1 and 2 and repeated weekly for 1–3 weeks according to the patient's response. Strikingly, the use of low-dose EP before commencing EMA/CO has almost completely eliminated early deaths.[127,137,138,150] We also introduced more regular genetic testing for tumors which we suspected might be non-gestational in origin. Doing these two things has improved overall survival for women receiving EMA/CO to nearly 95%.[137,151] The remaining 5% of deaths are nearly all due to metastatic non-resectable multidrug resistant disease, a problem discussed in the following section. However, it is important to remember that any woman of childbearing age presenting with widespread malignancy should have an hCG measurement, as very high levels of this hormone are highly suggestive of choriocarcinoma. A biopsy is not essential to make the clinical diagnosis and indeed, can be life threatening given the highly vascular nature of these tumors. Earlier recognition of choriocarcinoma will continue to help reduce disease extent and consequent early or late mortality.

The long-term risk of chemotherapy-induced second tumors in patients treated for GTNs in our center is discussed later.

Management of drug resistant disease: An emerging role for immunotherapies

Frequent measurement of the serum hCG is a simple way to detect drug resistance at an early stage, as the hormone levels will stop falling and may start to rise long before there are other clinical changes. However, it is important that decisions to alter treatment are not made on the basis of a single hCG result but on a progressive trend over two to three values. To do this in a timely fashion, the hCG should be measured at least once per week. Moreover, recent work using either normograms or kinetic analyses suggest that these approaches can identify resistance to single-agent chemotherapy earlier than by simply assessing the raw data graphically.[152,153] In patients receiving MTX for low-risk disease, if the hCG is <1000 IU/L when drug resistance occurs, the disease can often be cured simply by substituting ActD 1.25 mg/m² IV repeated every two weeks (Sita-Lumsden et al. and Taylor et al.[131,154] and Cortez Charry et al. ISSTD Amsterdam meeting 2017). This drug is slightly more toxic than MTX, inducing some hair thinning (occasionally complete alopecia), myelosuppression, nausea and vomiting, and more oral ulceration, but much less toxic than EMA/CO. To spare more women the need for EMA/CO, the United Kingdom has currently raised the hCG cut-off to <3000 IU/L to select patients for ActD. Moreover, rather than treating patients with an hCG >3000 IU/L with EMA/CO, we are trying carboplatin AUC 4 2-weekly if the hCG is between 3000 and 30,000 IU/L and reserving EMA/CO only for those women whose hCG exceeds 30,000 IU/L. This is based on limited data showing some activity for single-agent carboplatin in GTN[155,156] and the fact that this agent causes no hair loss. We hope to be able to report preliminary data on this in the next 3–4 years. The key here is to maintain a 100% cure rate while sparing more women the toxicity of EMA/CO.

While EMA/CO has saved virtually all low-risk patients failing other therapies, some high-risk patients develop disease that is resistant to this therapy. Fortunately, most of the patients who have failed EMA/CO in our center have still been salvaged by further chemotherapy and/or surgery.[128,137] Indeed, the combination of surgical removal of the main site of drug resistance (usually in the uterus, lung, or brain), together with chemotherapy, is particularly effective. Preoperative investigations include transvaginal or abdominal Doppler ultrasound of the pelvis, plain chest radiography, whole-body CT scan and MRI of the brain, lumbar puncture to measure hCG levels in the CSF, and experimental imaging techniques such as anti-hCG or ^{18}F-FDG-PET scanning. If all these investigations are negative, hysterectomy should be considered. When multiple possible sites of resistant disease are found, ^{18}F-FDG-PET imaging can potentially distinguish biologically active from dead/necrotic lesions and so guide appropriate surgery. Following surgery, or when surgery is not appropriate, we use the *cis*-platinum-containing regimen, EP (etoposide 150 mg/m^2 and *cis*-platinum 75 mg/m^2 with hydration) alternating weekly with EMA (omitting Day 2 except the FA).[157] This is not an easy schedule to administer clinically due to both myelosuppression and complications associated with even minor renal impairment. Consequently, a less toxic salvage regimen is required.

Several other anti-cancer agents have been shown to have activity in GTN, including taxanes, gemcitabine, capecitabine. and pemetrexed either alone or in combination with platinum.[56] We developed a regimen comprising paclitaxel and etoposide alternating every 2 weeks with paclitaxel and cisplatin (TE/TP; see Table 23.8), which has activity in patients with germ cell tumors and GTN that have failed prior treatment.[158–160] This regimen is much less toxic than EP/EMA and in limited data, appears to have similar efficacy in salvaging EMA/CO failures.[157,160] In China, where floxuridine is well tolerated, this is used in combination with ActD, etoposide, and vincristine (FAEV) to salvage EMA/CO failures with similarly good effect.[161] The FAEV regimen is now also being used as initial therapy for high-risk patients in China.[162]

Another approach in patients with refractory disease involves high-dose chemotherapy with autologous bone marrow or peripheral stem-cell transplantation. Patient selection here is probably important in determining outcome, as has been shown for refractory germ cell tumors, where patients with drug-sensitive disease are the ones who stay in remission.[163,164] In GTN, a previous report in just 11 patients suggested that high-dose chemotherapy may have little activity.[165] However, more recent data in 32 cases show that high-dose chemotherapy can save about

20% of multidrug resistant GTN patients, with a further 20% being salvaged by additional treatment such as surgical resection following high dose.[166] Tandem rather than high-dose procedures may offer a better chance of cure. An hCG of >12 IU/L before high-dose chemotherapy was an independent adverse prognostic factor for survival.[166] However, the experience is still small, and high-dose chemotherapy is a highly toxic procedure, so alternative therapies with fewer adverse events are needed.

Recent work has revealed a completely new approach to managing GTN using a checkpoint immunotherapy with an antibody called pembrolizumab (Keytruda) that targets the programmed cell death receptor (PD-1) on T-cells. Pregnancy is a natural allograft where half of the antigens are paternally derived and therefore foreign to the mother. Fortunately, multiple mechanisms exist to prevent maternal immunological rejection of pregnancies. Among these is strong placental expression of the ligand for PD-1, PD-L1.[167] Immunohistochemical staining also reveals very strong expression of PD-L1 in all forms of GTD, whether pre-malignant or malignant.[168,169] This raised the possibility that checkpoint immunotherapies such as pembrolizumab might be a useful strategy to treat drug resistant GTN. We therefore piloted, using pembrolizumab 2 mg/kg every three weeks, and demonstrated that three out of four patients with GTN otherwise expected to die were successfully salvaged. Another GTN patient was also successfully treated on our advice with pembrolizumab,[170] and in our cases, just five consolidation doses were given after normalization of hCG levels.[171] This meant that most patients had completed treatment within 6–7 months, which is far less time than in, for example, either lung cancer[172] or melanoma.[173] Moreover, the toxicity of pembrolizumab is significantly lower than that seen with combination-agent chemotherapy in, for example, lung cancer[172] and clearly far lower than the high-dose chemotherapy we have been using in GTN.[166] Interestingly, 6–7 months of pembrolizumab is less than half the price of a tandem high-dose procedure, so, perhaps unsurprisingly, pembrolizumab treatment was approved in January 2018 for use in the NHS in GTN patients who would otherwise require or who have failed previous high-dose chemotherapy.[174] We have now treated a total of 12 patients with drug resistant GTN, of whom nine (75%) have achieved a complete response (Ghorani et al., ISSTD Toronto 2019).

It is too early to determine how to select patients for immunotherapy, but PD-L1 staining and mutational burden are not helpful, as all tumors are PD-L1 positive and are mutational deserts, respectively ([42,168,169,171], and our unpublished observations). However, as immunotherapies can be a little slow to start working, patients with very rapidly growing tumors are unlikely to respond fast enough before they are overwhelmed by disease. These individuals might best be treated with chemotherapy first or combined chemotherapy plus immunotherapy to allow time for the latter to work. Others are now exploring using immunotherapies earlier in the disease course. In France, the Trophimmun study is assessing the efficacy of the anti-PD-L1 agent avelumab in patients failing either first-line single-agent therapy with MTX or first-line multiagent EMA-CO or EP-EMA chemotherapy. Results of the study are expected to be presented at ASCO 2020. It may be unreasonable to use immunotherapies in low-risk GTN, as these treatments are probably more toxic than other single agents such as ActD and are vastly more expensive. Moreover, it is unclear what the effect of immunotherapies might be on the success of subsequent pregnancies, while there are ample data on the safety of older chemotherapy drugs such as MTX, ActD, and EMA/CO.

TABLE 23.8   TP/TE Schedule for Relapsed GTN

Regimen	Schedule
Day 1	
Dexamethasone	20 mg oral (12 hours pre paclitaxel)
Dexamethasone	20 mg oral (6 hours pre paclitaxel)
Cimetidine	30 mg in 100 mL NS over 30 minutes IV
Chlorphenamine	10 mg bolus IV
Paclitaxel	135 mg/m^2 in 250 mL NS over 3 hours IV
Mannitol	10% in 500 mL over 1 hour IV
Cisplatin	60 mg/m^2 in 1 liter NS over 3 hours IV
Post-hydration	1 liter NS + KCl 20 mmol + 1 g MgSO$_4$ over 2 hours IV
Day 15	
Dexamethasone	20 mg oral (12 hours pre paclitaxel)
Dexamethasone	20 mg oral (6 hours pre paclitaxel)
Cimetidine	30 mg in 100 mL NS over 30 minutes IV
Chlorphenamine	10 mg bolus IV
Paclitaxel	135 mg/m^2 in 250 mL NS over 3 hours IV
Etoposide	150 mg/m^2 in 1 liter NS over 1 hour IV

Abbreviations: NS, normal saline. IV, intravenous.

Management of acute disease-induced complications

Hemorrhage

Heavy vaginal or intra-peritoneal bleeding is the most frequent immediate threat to life in patients with trophoblastic tumors.[3] The bleeding mostly settles with bed rest and after starting chemotherapy appropriate to the risk group. However, occasionally the bleeding can be torrential, requiring massive transfusion. In this situation, if the bleeding is coming from the uterus, it may be necessary to consider a uterine pack or emergency embolization of the tumor vasculature.[175] Fortunately, hysterectomy is rarely required. If the bleeding is intra-peritoneal and does not settle with transfusion and chemotherapy with or without embolization via interventional radiology, laparotomy may be required. Indeed, patients occasionally present this way.

Respiratory failure

Occasionally, patients present with respiratory failure due to multiple pulmonary metastases or more rarely, as a result of massive tumor embolism to the pulmonary circulation.[105,106] Fever with or without purulent sputum may be present, and in these cases, blood and sputum cultures should be obtained and antibiotics started to treat potential infection. If tumor embolus is suspected, a ventilation/perfusion scan, MRI, or dynamic CT of the chest (Figure 23.10) and an electrocardiogram should be obtained and a heparin infusion started.[105,106] The latter is preferable to low–molecular weight heparins as it is easily reversible by

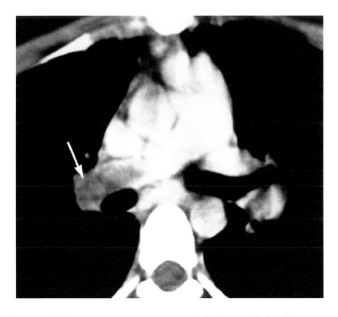

FIGURE 23.10 Contrast-enhanced CT scan of the thorax at the level of the main pulmonary arteries, showing a filling defect in the right main pulmonary artery (arrow). The patient presented with a brief history of increasing shortness of breath, which had suddenly worsened. During the previous 18 months, she had suffered from irregular heavy bleeding per vagina and had four separate positive pregnancy tests and two normal pelvic ultrasound investigations. She was successfully treated with EMA/CO chemotherapy, with some resolution of the changes seen on CT and ventilation perfusion scanning. Post-mortem examinations of similar cases have revealed that the filling defect in the main pulmonary artery is tumor embolus and not clot. (Reprinted from Seckl et al., 1991. With permission from Elsevier.)

stopping the infusion in the event of life-threatening hemorrhage into other metastases. Pulse oximetry and/or arterial blood gas should be regularly measured to allow appropriate adjustment of oxygen therapy and to monitor any deterioration in pulmonary function that may occur following the start of chemotherapy. The latter occurs probably because of edema and inflammation around tumor deposits that are becoming necrotic. To prevent this, we usually commence therapy with low-dose induction EP as described earlier[137] and introduce other drugs once pulmonary function is stable. Occasionally, patients require masked continuous positive airway pressure ventilation, but mechanical ventilation has in our experience only saved one patient. The others have died from intra-pulmonary hemorrhage, probably as a result of trauma to the tumor vasculature induced by high positive airway pressures generated on mechanical ventilation. For this reason, extra-corporeal oxygenation has been proposed.[176]

Management of cerebral metastases

Involvement of the CNS by GTN may either be overt and require intensive therapy or occult and need prophylaxis. Any patient with lung metastases is at risk of either having or developing CNS disease. Furthermore, the second most common site of metastases in high-risk patients is the CNS, and nearly all these individuals had lung deposits.[142] The presence of neurological symptoms and signs may alert the clinician to the presence of brain metastases. However, some high-risk patients do not have either overt pulmonary or CNS disease at presentation but subsequently develop cerebral metastases, which are then drug resistant. Consequently, careful investigation of patients at risk of developing brain metastases is warranted so that appropriate CNS-penetrating chemotherapy is given rather than the standard low- or high-risk treatments. Investigations include contrast-enhanced MRI of the brain and, in patients who do not have raised intracranial pressure, measurement of the hCG levels in CSF. A CSF:serum ratio greater than 1:60 suggests the presence of CNS disease.

Prophylaxis against possible CNS disease (MRI brain normal) is given to patients from all risk categories with lung metastases and all high-risk patients regardless of the absence or presence of lung deposits. The prophylaxis consists of 12.5 mg MTX administered intrathecally, followed 24 hours later by 15 mg of FA orally. This is given with every course of low-risk therapy or with each CO in the high-risk therapy for three doses. Since the introduction of this policy, the development of brain metastases without evidence of drug resistance elsewhere has been much less frequent.[143,177]

Overt CNS disease requires careful management, as therapy can induce hemorrhage into the tumor, leading to a rise in intracranial pressure and subsequent loss of life. We previously advocated early resection of solitary brain lesions, but our recent experience suggests that this is not necessary unless there are hemorrhagic complications causing acute clinical deterioration.[177] Instead, commencing therapy with low-dose induction EP seems effective in managing the acute presentation before commencing normal doses of treatment.[137,143] Cerebral edema can be reduced with high-dose corticosteroids, and so patients are given 24 mg of dexamethasone in divided doses before starting chemotherapy. Once the patient has clinically improved on the low-dose EP chemotherapy, the EMA/CO regimen is commenced but modified by increasing the dose of MTX to 1 g/m² given as a 24-h infusion on Day 1. The FA rescue is increased to 30 mg given 8-hourly intravenously for 3 days, commencing 32 hours after the start of the MTX infusion. Provided there is no evidence of raised intracranial pressure, 12.5 mg of methotrexate is given intrathecally with each CO until the hCG in serum is normal. Modified EMA/CO is then continued for a further 6–8 weeks. Overall, in approximately 85% of patients with cerebral metastases, long-term remission can be achieved.[143,177] Patients who survive the first 3 weeks of such treatment have a good prognosis, with approximately 90% chance of cure.[143,177]

Patients who develop cerebral tumor during chemotherapy have a poor prognosis, because their disease is almost certainly drug resistant. Nevertheless, a combination of immediate surgery to remove the deposit(s) and modified chemotherapy designed to provide better CNS penetration can be curative in this situation.[142,178] We have also been able to cure patients with salvage chemotherapy regimens such as EP/EMA[157] in which the MTX has been increased to 1 g/m^2 and iT MTX has been given with the EP and even with pembrolizumab.[171] Radiotherapy has been advocated as an alternative therapeutic approach. However, it has not been shown to eradicate tumor in its own right, and in combination with chemotherapy has produced either less effective or no better results than chemotherapy alone.[143,177,179] Moreover, whole brain radiotherapy adds significant short- and long-term toxicity risks for these young women. Nevertheless, stereotactic or gamma knife radiotherapy probably has a role in the treatment of isolated deep lesions that cannot be removed surgically, especially if they are still present at the end of chemotherapy.[3,177]

Management of PSTT, ETT, and APSN

The largest population-based series of PSTT, ETT or mixed PSTT/ETT comprised just 125 cases over 41 years and represented 0.23% of U.K. GTD cases.[44] Our earlier series in just 62 cases identified that these tumors were associated with a 70% long-term overall survival (OS) at 5 and 10 years.[43] Management of these cases was typically focused around surgical removal of all disease sites, with chemotherapy given to patients who had metastatic disease either upfront or following surgery and optional chemotherapy for those with Stage I disease following hysterectomy. While univariate analysis revealed several factors predictive of poor survival outcome, multivariate analysis showed that only an interval since the last known or causative pregnancy of ≥48 months was significant. Indeed, this predictor identified all 13 patients who were destined to die regardless of whether they had Stage I or more advanced stages at diagnosis. In contrast, only one out of the remaining 49 patients with an interval <48 months died, again regardless of stage. In this early series, Stage I patients were all treated with hysterectomy, and some had additional chemotherapy, mostly with EMA/CO and some with EP/EMA and/or TE/TP, and those who relapsed were considered for high-dose chemotherapy.

In view of these findings, management was changed so that all patients regardless of stage presenting ≥48 months from their causative or last known pregnancy were offered more intensive chemotherapy, preferably platinum based with EP/EMA and/or TE/TP for at least 12 weeks. These patients were then provided with the opportunity to undergo high-dose chemotherapy as a tandem procedure. Comparison of this new cohort of 63 patients with the prior cohort revealed a significantly improved median OS of 8.3 years (95% confidence interval [CI] 1.53–15.1) versus 2.6 years (95% CI 0.73–4.44, $p = 0.005$) in patients with an interval ≥48 months.[44] This correlated with significantly more cisplatin-based and high-dose chemotherapy. While the new cohort of patients were not prognostically in a better position at presentation compared with the old cohort, we cannot, of course, exclude the possibility that

the improvement seen in OS is simply due to chance. The new study obviously allowed us to combine both old and new cohorts to look for new prognostic variables. Multivariable analysis of the combined 125 patients revealed that in addition to interval, Stage IV disease was now also an independent poor prognostic factor.[44] In view of this, patients with Stage IV disease are now also offered intense platinum-based chemotherapy followed by experimental therapies such as high-dose chemotherapy.[44] The latter, though, is now superseded by the introduction of pembrolizumab, and an argument could be made to even use this immunotherapy to replace EP/EMA or TE/TP chemotherapy, particularly in those patients following a hysterectomy for Stage I disease with an interval ≥48 months.[171] However, until further data are available, we cannot yet recommend this latter suggestion.

It follows from this that hysterectomy still remains a central part of management of patients with ETT/PSTT. Nevertheless, in younger nulliparous women, there is often a strong desire to preserve fertility, particularly when there appears to be a focal abnormality in the uterus. While uterine-sparing surgery is possible,[3] multifocal microscopic uterine disease can occur,[180] which could compromise survival, and careful counseling is required. Another alternative might be to give chemotherapy and/or immunotherapy up front to try to effectively treat these cancers. Such approaches should be regarded as experimental, as there are insufficient data to be certain of efficacy and in the case of immunotherapy, the risk of interfering with subsequent fertility due to immunological rejection of new pregnancies.

Currently, it is thought that ETT behaves very similarly to PSTT and is managed in the same way.[44,53,56] Is this really justified? PSTT and ETT are so rare that it is unlikely that their treatment will ever be fully optimized, so the International Society for the Study of Trophoblastic Diseases (ISSTD) established an international PSTT/ETT database to pool cases in 2011. The first report using this database has looked at 56 patients with ETT to determine whether this has similar or distinct prognostic factors for survival compared with PSTT. As with PSTT, multivariate analysis shows that patients with ETT also do badly if the interval from the causative pregnancy to presentation is greater than 48 months or if patients present with advanced-stage disease. Thus, at the present time, ETT should be managed like PSTT until further data are available.[54]

Finally, we have recently become aware that APSN is associated with a risk of either already having or subsequently developing PSTT/ETT.[57] An update of our experience with this was presented at the 2019 ISSTD in Toronto, where 8 out of 77 patients with APSN were shown to either already have or go on to develop a PSTT/ETT. Consequently, we currently recommend that any patient with APSN should be imaged to assess the extent of the abnormality in the pelvis and elsewhere. At Charing Cross, this imaging includes an MRI of the head and pelvis and CT of the chest and abdomen, all with contrast. If all tests are negative, including the serum hCG, affected women are counseled regarding the 10% risk of an associated malignancy, and if they have completed their families, they might choose a hysterectomy, while those still wanting children might reasonably choose surveillance. The latter includes monthly monitoring of the serum hCG, gradually decreasing to 6 monthly samples out to 10 years. In addition, we offer 6-monthly MRI of the abdomen and pelvis for 2 years, then dropping to annual imaging. There are clearly no completely right answers here as we gather more data for this unusual situation. A key question as we move forwards is whether PSNs without atypical features can safely be ignored. At present, we suggest that such patients have local rather than central follow-up until more data are available.

Patient follow-up after chemotherapy

On completion of their chemotherapy, patients need to be followed up regularly, with hCG estimations to confirm that their disease is in remission. Initially, the follow-up is with serum and urine samples (Table 23.9), but in due course, the follow-up is only on urine samples. A recent analysis in over 4000 treated U.K. patients examining the rates and timings of relapse for both low-risk and high-risk patients shows that about 75% of relapses occur within the first year. Most of the rest occur in the subsequent 2 years with no further relapses beyond 7 years.[181] Consequently, we now recommend stopping hCG surveillance for low- and high-risk GTN after 10 years. The only exceptions to this are patients who were treated for ultra-high-risk GTN, those receiving high-dose chemotherapy, and any patients with PSTT/ETT, for which follow-up remains life-long until there are sufficient data to know when it is safe to stop. In the United Kingdom, our hCG surveillance is computerized, and automatic reminders are sent to patients so that they do not get lost to follow-up. Patients are advised not to become pregnant until 12 months after completing their chemotherapy. This minimizes the potential teratogenicity of treatment and avoids confusion between a new pregnancy or relapsed disease as the cause of a rising hCG. Any form of contraception can be employed as long as there are no other contraindications to its use. Despite this advice, 230 women on follow-up at our center between 1969 and 1998 became pregnant during the first year. Fortunately, this did not appear to be associated with an increased risk of relapse or fetal morbidity, and there were no maternal deaths.[182] Indeed, 71% of women continued their pregnancy to term. An update of this work in a further 242 patients has again confirmed the safety of getting pregnant within 12 months.[183] Consequently, although we continue to advise women to avoid pregnancy for 1 year after completing chemotherapy, those who do become pregnant can be reassured of a likely favorable outcome. When a patient becomes pregnant, it is important to confirm by ultrasound and other appropriate means that the pregnancy is normal. Follow-up is then discontinued until 3 weeks after the end of pregnancy, when the hCG due to the pregnancy should have returned to normal. Patients who do not require chemotherapy following evacuation of their first mole no longer need to have their hCG levels measured after the end of any subsequent pregnancy, as the risk of developing GTN is so low.[67]

TABLE 23.9 Follow-Up of Patients with GTN Who Have Been Treated with Chemotherapy

	Low-/High-Risk Post-Chemotherapy Patients, hCG Concentration Sampling	
	Urine	Blood
Year 1		
Week 1–6 after chemotherapy	Weekly	Weekly
Months, 2–6	2-weekly	2-weekly
Months, 7–12	2-weekly	–
Year 2	4-weekly	–
Year 3	8-weekly	–
Year 4	3-monthly	–
Year 5	4-monthly	–
After Year 5	6-monthly	–

Stop at 10 years unless ultra-high risk, PSTT/ETT, or treated with high dose or immunotherapy.

The follow-up of PSTT/ETT differs from that of other GTD variants, since serum hCG is a less reliable tumor marker, and late recurrences are probably more common.[43,44] Indeed, there are some reports suggesting that these tumors may fail to secrete hCG at relapse despite an extensive tumor burden.[184] One explanation for this surprising failure to detect hCG may be that some PSTTs secrete a form of the hormone that is not detected by the particular hCG assay being used by a given treatment center. Nevertheless, patients in remission from PSTT/ETT should probably be followed up serologically for life and at regular intervals in the clinic for between 5 and 10 years. It also seems sensible to organize MRI imaging of the pelvis and abdomen every 6–12 months in those with adverse prognostic features, such as an interval >4 years from the previous pregnancy. The international database of PSTT/ETTs should help to refine this guidance over time.

Long-term complications of therapy

Most patients, including those who have received intensive chemotherapy, return to normal activity within a few months, and the majority of the side-effects are reversible. Complete hair regrowth is seen in all patients with chemotherapy-induced alopecia, although sometimes it may be initially curly rather than straight. Late sequelae from chemotherapy have been remarkably rare. We previously analyzed data in 15,279 patient years of follow-up for the late sequelae from chemotherapy. This showed that patients treated with MTX and FA in the low-risk category have no significant increase in the incidence of second tumors.[148] In contrast, 26 patients receiving intensive combination chemotherapy for their GTN developed another cancer, when the expected rate was only 16.5; a significant difference.[148] Acute myeloid leukemia (AML) (relative risk 16.6) accounted for the early tumors up to 5 years, possibly reflecting the rising use of etoposide, which is now well recognized to induce this form of leukemia.[148] However, in a more recent analysis with over 30,000 patient years of follow-up, although there was still a slight increased risk of leukemia, there was no overall increased risk of second cancers induced by EMA/CO chemotherapy. Indeed, there was a modest reduction in the risk of several tumors, including breast and lung cancers.[149] Moreover, this analysis confirmed no increased risk with single-agent MTX/FA therapy. These results should be very reassuring for the young women who have to undergo chemotherapy treatment for GTN.

Fertility is an important issue in the management of patients with GTN. Although multiagent chemotherapy appears to induce a menopause 3 years earlier than would normally be expected,[185] fertility does not otherwise appear to be affected.[186] In 392 patients receiving single-agent methotrexate, 327 (83.4%) had successful live births. Interestingly, in the 336 patients receiving multiagent chemotherapy, including EMA/CO, 280 (83.3%) also succeeded in having normal pregnancies. Importantly, in this and a previous analysis there was no increase in the incidence of congenital malformations compared with the general population.[186,187]

Summary

In the past, many women have died from GTN. However, during the past 55 years, we have learnt much about the biology, pathology, and natural history of this group of disorders. Furthermore, accurate diagnostic and monitoring methods have been developed, together with effective treatment regimens. This has largely been achieved through centralized care and has enabled the

United Kingdom to lead in a complete transformation of outcomes so that overall cure rates are in excess of 99% (low-risk disease 100%, high-risk disease in excess of 95%, and PSTT/ETT >80%). The challenge now is to help others to achieve the same results elsewhere.

Key learning points

- While it is well known that CHMs can transform into choriocarcinomas and PSTTs, it had previously been thought that PHMs do not do this. However, PHMs have conclusively been shown to also transform into choriocarcinoma and PSTT/ETT, so all patients with PHMs require hCG follow-up.
- All patients with suspected GTN should be discussed with a gestational trophoblastic disease center and have their histology centrally reviewed.
- The use of serum and urine hCG measurements to follow the disease course has been a key feature in the successful management of women with GTN. However, recent work has shown that care is required in the interpretation of hCG values obtained from commercial sandwich assays. This is because (a) the epitopes of hCG detected in sandwich assays may be lost in some GTN, causing false negative results, and (b) some patients have interfering molecules such as heterophile antibodies, which bind both monoclonal antibodies used in sandwich assays, generating a false positive hCG.
- Currently, the most reliable hCG assays should detect all forms of hCG produced in cancer equally well. Fortunately, the in-house assay used at Charing Cross Hospital, which uses a polyclonal rabbit antiserum in a competitive radio-immunoassay, appears to perform exceedingly well.
- Low-risk patients with GTN are initially treated with MTX/FA, as this regimen has no long-term sequelae.
- Patients relapsing on MTX/FA are switched to actinomycin D if their hCG level is <3000 IU/L or EMA/CO combination chemotherapy if the hCG is >3000 IU/L.
- EMA/CO, like MTX/FA, does not appear to impair fertility or induce an overall increased risk of second tumors. However, EMA/CO does bring forward the date of the menopause by 3 years.
- The long-term outcome for patients with GTN is excellent, with all low-risk patients and approximately 95% of high-risk patients being cured.
- The use of low-dose induction etoposide and cisplatin chemotherapy appears to have largely eliminated early deaths.
- The management of PSTT/ETT differs from that of other GTN, reflecting a distinct biological behavior. The two key prognostic factors for adverse outcome in PSTT/ETT are a duration from the last known pregnancy to the date of presentation of >4 years and Stage IV disease.
- The discovery that checkpoint immunotherapies such as pembrolizumab are highly active in salvaging all types of GTN failing other therapies will replace most use of high-dose chemotherapy and may also impact on the use of other multiagent chemotherapy.

References

1. Ober WB, Fass, RO. The early history of choriocarcinoma. *Ann NY Acad Sci.* 1961; 172:299–426.
2. Mueller UW, Hawes CS, Wright AE et al. Isolation of fetal trophoblast cells from peripheral blood of pregnant women. *Lancet.* 1990; 336:197–200.
3. Seckl MJ, Sebire NJ, Berkowitz RS. Gestational trophoblastic disease. *Lancet.* 2010; 376(9742):717–29.
4. Davis JR, Surwit EA, Garay JP, Fortier KJ. Sex assignment in gestational trophoblastic neoplasia. *Am J Obstet Gynaecol.* 1984. 148:722–25.
5. Fisher RA, Sheppard DM, Lawler DW. Twin pregnancy with complete hydatidiform mole (46,XX) and fetus (46,XY): Genetic origin proved by analysis of chromosome polymorphisms. *Br Med J.* 1982; 1:1218–20.
6. Jacobs PA, Wilson CM, Sprenkle JA et al. Mechanism of origin of complete hydatidiform mole. *Nature.* 1980; 286:714–6.
7. Kajii T, Ohama K. Androgenetic origin of hydatidiform mole. *Nature.* 1977; 268:633–4.
8. Lawler SD, Pickthall V, Fisher R et al. Genetic studies of complete and partial hydatidiform mole (letter). *Lancet.* 1979; ii:580.
9. Lawler SD, Povey S, Fisher RA, Pickthall VJ. Genetic studies on hydatidiform moles II: The origin of complete moles. *Ann Human Gen.* 1982; 46:209–22.
10. Vassilakos P, Riotton G, Kajii T. Hydatidiform mole: Two entities. A morphologic and cytogenic study with some clinical considerations. *Am J Obstet Gynaecol.* 1977; 127:167–70.
11. Fisher RA, Povey S, Jeffreys AJ et al. Frequency of heterozygous complete hydatidiform moles, estimated by locus-specific minisatellite and Y chromosome-specific probes. *Hum Genet.* 1989; 82:259–63.
12. Ohama K, Kajii T, Okamoto E. Dispermic origin of XY hydatidiform mole. *Nature.* 1981. 292:551–52.
13. Edwards YH, Jeremiah SJ, McMillan SL et al. Complete hydatidiform moles combine maternal mitochondria with paternal nuclear genome. *Annals Human Genet.* 1984. 48:119–27.
14. Fisher RA, Khatoon R, Paradinas FJ et al. Repetitive complete hydatidiform mole can be biparental in origin and either male or female. *Hum Reprod.* 2000; 15:594–8.
15. Fisher RA, Savage PM, MacDermott C et al. The impact of molecular genetic diagnosis on the management of women with hCG-producing malignancies. *Gynecol Oncol.* 2007; 107(3):413–9.
16. Murdoch S, Djuric U, Mazhar B et al. Mutations in NALP7 cause recurrent hydatidiform moles and reproductive wastage in humans. *Nat Genet.* 2006; 38(3):300–2.
17. Parry DA, Logan CV, Hayward BE et al. Mutations causing familial biparental hydatidiform mole implicate c6orf221 as a possible regulator of genomic imprinting in the human oocyte. *Am J Hum Genet.* 2011; 89(3):451–8.
18. Fallahian M, Sebire NJ, Savage PM et al. Mutations in NLRP7 and KHDC3L confer a complete hydatidiform mole phenotype on digynic triploid conceptions. *Hum Mutat.* 2013; 34(2):301–8.
19. Paradinas F. The histological diagnosis of hydatidiform moles. *Curr Diag Pathol.* 1994; 1:24–31.
20. Paradinas FJ, Browne P, Fisher RA et al. A clinical, histopathological and flow cytometric study of 149 complete moles, 146 partial moles and 107 non-molar hydropic abortions. *Histopathology.* 1996; 28:101–10.
21. Paradinas FJ, Fisher RA, Browne P, Newlands ES. Diploid hydatidiform moles with fetal red blood cells in molar villi: I. Pathology, incidence and prognosis. *J Pathol.* 1997; 181:183–8.
22. Seckl MJ, Fisher RA, Salerno G et al. Choriocarcinoma and partial hydatidiform moles. *Lancet.* 2000; 356:36–9.
23. Sebire NJ, Seckl MJ. Immunohistochemical staining for diagnosis and prognostic assessment of hydatidiform moles: Current evidence and future directions. *J Reprod Med.* 2010; 55(5–6):236–46.
24. Jacobs PA, Hunt PA, Matsuura JS, et al. Complete and partial hydatidiform mole in Hawaii: Cytogenetics, morphology and epidemiology. *Br J Obstet Gynaecol.* 1982; 89:258–66.
25. Lawler SD, Fisher RA, Pickthall VJ et al. Genetic studies on hydatidiform moles I: The origin of partial moles. *Cancer Gen Cytogen.* 1982; 4:309–20.
26. Fukunaga M, Katabuchi H, Nagasaka T et al. Interobserver and intraobserver variability in the diagnosis of hydatidiform mole. *Am J Surg Pathol.* 2005; 29(7):942–7.

27. Genest DR, Ruiz RE, Weremowicz S et al. Do nontriploid partial hydatidiform moles exist? A histologic and flow cytometric reevaluation of nontriploid specimens. *J Reprod Med.* 2002; 47(5):363–8.

28. Samlowski WE, Abbott TM, Kepas DE et al. Placental-site trophoblastic tumor (trophoblastic pseudotumor): Case report demonstrating failure of chemotherapy, surgery, and radiotherapy to control metastatic disease. *Gynaecol Oncol.* 1985; 21:111–7.

29. Szulman A, Surti, U. The syndromes of hydatidiform mole. I. Cytogenetic and morphological correlations. *Am J Obstet Gynaecol.* 1978; 13:665–71.

30. Szulman A, Surti U. The syndromes of hydatidiform mole. II. Morphological evidence of the complete and partial mole. *Am J Obstet Gynaecol.* 1978; 132:20–7.

31. Sebire NJ, Seckl MJ. Gestational trophoblastic disease: Current management of hydatidiform mole. *BMJ.* 2008; 337:a1193.

32. Savage PM, Sita-Lumsden A, Dickson S et al. The relationship of maternal age to molar pregnancy incidence, risks for chemotherapy and subsequent pregnancy outcome. *J Obstet Gynaecol.* 2013; 33(4):406–11.

33. Paradinas FJ. The diagnosis and prognosis of molar pregnancy. The experience of the National Referral Centre in London. *Int J Gynaecol Obstet.* 1998; 60:S57–64.

34. Arima T, Imamura T, Amada S et al. Genetic origin of malignant trophoblastic neoplasms. *Cancer Genet Cytogenet.* 1994; 73:95–102.

35. Chaganti RSK, Koduru PR, Chakraborty R, Jones WB. Genetic origin of trophoblastic choriocarcinoma. *Cancer Res.* 1990; 50:6330–33.

36. Fisher RA, Newlands ES, Jeffreys AJ et al. Gestational and non-gestational trophoblastic tumours distinguished by DNA analysis. *Cancer.* 1992. 69:839–45.

37. Osada H, Newlands ES, Jeffreys AJ et al. Genetic identification of pregnancies responsible for choriocarcinomas after multiple pregnancies by restriction fragment length polymorphism analysis. *Am J Obstet Gynaecol.* 1991; 165:682–88.

38. Wake N, Tanaka KI, Chapman V et al. Chromosomes and cellular origin of choriocarcinoma. *Cancer Res.* 1981; 41:3137–43.

39. Fisher RA, Lawler SD, Povey S, Bagshawe KD et al. Genetically homozygous choriocarcinoma following pregnancy with hydatidiform mole. *Br J Cancer.* 1988; 58:788–92.

40. Fisher RA, Soteriou BA, Meredith L et al. Previous hydatidiform mole identified as the causative pregnancy of choriocarcinoma following birth of normal twins. *Int J Cancer.* 1995; 5:64–70.

41. Jiao L, Ghorani E, Sebire NJ, Seckl MJ. Intraplacental choriocarcinoma: Systematic review and management guidance. *Gynecol Oncol.* 2016; 141(3):624–31.

42. Savage P, Monk D, Mora JR et al. A case of intraplacental gestational choriocarcinoma; characterised by the methylation pattern of the early placenta and an absence of driver mutations. *BMC Cancer.* 2019; 19(1):744.

43. Schmid P, Nagai Y, Agarwal R et al. Prognostic markers and long-term outcome of placental-site trophoblastic tumours: A retrospective observational study. *Lancet.* 2009; 374(9683):48–55.

44. Froeling FEM, Ramaswami R, Papanastasopoulos P et al. Intensified therapies improve survival and identification of novel prognostic factors for placental-site and epithelioid trophoblastic tumours. *Br J Cancer.* 2019; 120(6):587–94.

45. Shih IM, Kurman RJ. The pathology of intermediate trophoblastic tumors and tumor-like lesions. *Int J Gynecol Pathol.* 2001; 20(1):31–47.

46. Palmieri C, Fisher RA, Sebire NJ et al. Placental site trophoblastic tumour arising from a partial hydatidiform mole. *Lancet.* 2005; 366(9486):688.

47. Fisher RA, Paradinas FJ, Newlands ES, Boxer GM. Genetic evidence that placental site trophoblastic tumours can originate from a hydatidiform mole or a normal conceptus. *Br J Cancer.* 1992; 65:355–58.

48. Fukunaga M, Ushigome S. Malignant trophoblastic tumours: Immunohistochemical and flow cytometric comparison of choriocarcinoma and placental-site trophoblastic tumours. *Hum Pathol.* 1993; 24:1098–106.

49. Kotylo PK, Michael H, Davis TE et al. Flow cytometric DNA analysis of placental-site trophoblastic tumours. *Int J Gynaecol Pathol.* 1992; 11:245–52.

50. Lathrop J, Lauchlan S, Nayak R, Ambler M. Clinical characteristics of placental site trophoblastic tumour (PSTT). *Gynaecol Oncol.* 1988; 31:32–42.

51. Zhao S, Sebire NJ, Kaur B et al. Molecular genotyping of placental site and epithelioid trophoblastic tumours; female predominance. *Gynecol Oncol.* 2016; 142(3):501–7.

52. Shih IM, Kurman RJ. Ki-67 labelling index in the differential diagnosis of exaggerated placental site, placental site trophoblastic tumour, and choriocarcinoma: A double staining technique using Ki-67 and Mel-CAM antibodies. *Human Pathol.* 1998; 29:27–33.

53. Horowitz NS, Goldstein DP, Berkowitz RS. Placental site trophoblastic tumors and epithelioid trophoblastic tumors: Biology, natural history, and treatment modalities. *Gynecol Oncol.* 2017; 144(1):208–14.

54. Frijstein MM, Lok CA, van Trommel NE et al. Management and prognostic factors of epithelioid trophoblastic tumors: Results from the International Society for the Study of Trophoblastic Diseases database. *Gynecol Oncol.* 2019; 152(2):361–67.

55. Hui P, Martel M, Parkash V. Gestational trophoblastic diseases: Recent advances in histopathologic diagnosis and related genetic aspects. *Adv Anat Pathol.* 2005; 12(3):116–25.

56. Seckl MJ, Sebire NJ, Fisher RA et al. Gestational trophoblastic disease: ESMO Clinical Practice Guidelines for diagnosis, treatment and follow-up. *Ann Oncol.* 2013; 24(Suppl 6):vi39–vi50.

57. Kaur B, Short D, Fisher RA et al. Atypical placental site nodule (APSN) and association with malignant gestational trophoblastic disease; a clinicopathologic study of 21 cases. *Int J Gynecol Pathol.* 2015; 34(2):152–8.

58. Chen BJ, Cheng CJ, Chen WY. Transformation of a post-cesarean section placental site nodule into a coexisting epithelioid trophoblastic tumor and placental site trophoblastic tumor: A case report. *Diagn Pathol.* 2013; 8(1):85.

59. Tsai HW, Lin CP, Chou CY et al. Placental site nodule transformed into a malignant epithelioid trophoblastic tumour with pelvic lymph node and lung metastasis. *Histopathology.* 2008; 53(5):601–4.

60. Matsuura J, Chiu D, Jacobs PA et al. Complete hydatidiform mole in Hawaii: An epidemiological study. *Genet Epidemiol.* 1984; 1:271–84.

61. Hando T, Masaguki O, Kurose T. Recent aspects of gestational trophoblastic disease in Japan. *Int J Gynaecol Oncol.* 1998; 60:S71–76.

62. Martin BH, Kim JH. Changing face of gestational trophoblastic disease. *Int J Gynaecol Oncol.* 1998; 60:S111–20.

63. Savage P, Williams J, Wong SL et al. The demographics of molar pregnancies in England and Wales from 2000–2009. *J Reprod Med.* 2010; 55(7–8):341–5.

64. Sebire NJ, Foskett M, Fisher RA et al. Risk of partial and complete hydatidiform molar pregnancy in relation to maternal age. *BJOG.* 2002; 109(1):99–102.

65. Bagshawe KD, Dent J, Webb J. Hydatidiform mole in the United Kingdom 1973–1983. *Lancet.* 1986; ii:673.

66. Eagles N, Sebire NJ, Short D et al. Risk of recurrent molar pregnancies following complete and partial hydatidiform moles. *Hum Reprod.* 2015; 30(9):2055–63.

67. Earp KE, Hancock BW, Short D et al. Do we need post-pregnancy screening with human chorionic gonadotrophin after previous hydatidiform mole to identify patients with recurrent gestational trophoblastic disease? *Eur J Obstet Gynecol Reprod Biol.* 2019; 234:117–19.

68. Palmer JR, Driscoll SG, Rosenberg L et al. Oral contraceptive use and risk of gestational trophoblastic tumors. *J. Natl. Cancer Inst.* 1999; 91:635–40.

69. Costa HL, Doyle P. Influence of oral contraceptives in the development of post-molar trophoblastic neoplasia—a systematic review. *Gynecol Oncol.* 2006; 100(3):579–85.

70. Braga A, Maestá I, Short D et al. Hormonal contraceptive use before hCG remission does not increase the risk of gestational trophoblastic neoplasia following complete hydatidiform mole: A historical database review. *BJOG.* 2016; 123(8):1330–5.

71. Dantas PRS, Maestá I, Rezende Filho J et al. Does hormonal contraception during molar pregnancy follow-up influence the risk and clinical aggressiveness of gestational trophoblastic neoplasia after controlling for risk factors? *Gynecol Oncol.* 2017; 147(2):364–70.

72. Li M, Squire JA, Weksberg R. Overgrowth syndromes and genomic imprinting: From mouse to man. *Clin. Genet.* 1998; 53:165–70.

73. Hao Y, Crenshaw T, Moulton T et al. Tumor suppressor activity of H19 RNA. *Nature.* 1993; 365:764–67.

74. Matsuoka S, Thompson JS, Edwards MC et al. Imprinting of the gene encoding a human cyclin-dependent kinase inhibitor, p57kip2, on chromosome 11p15. *Proc. Natl. Acad. Sci. USA,* 1996; 93:3026–30.

75. Ogawa O, Eccles MR, Szeto J et al. Relaxation in insulin-like growth factor II gene imprinting implicated in Wilm's tumour. *Nature.* 1993; 362:749–51.

76. Chilosi M, Piazzola E, Lestani M et al. Differential expression of p57kip2, a maternally imprinted cdk inhibitor, in normal human placenta and gestational trophoblastic disease. *Lab Invest.* 1998; 78(3):269–76.

77. Ariel I, Lustig O, Oyer CE et al. Relaxation of genomic imprinting in trophoblastic disease. *Gynaecol Oncol.* 1994; 53:212–19.

78. Mutter GL, Stewart CL, Chaponot ML et al. Oppositely imprinted genes H-19 and insulin-like growth factor 2 are co-expressed in human androgenetic trophoblast. *Am J Human Genet.* 1993; 53:1096–102.

79. Walsh C, Miller SJ, Flam F et al. Paternally derived H19 is differentially expressed in malignant and non-malignant trophoblast. *Cancer Res.* 1995; 55:1111–6.

80. Arima T, Matsuda T, Takagi N et al. Association of IGF2 And H19 imprinting with choriocarcinoma development. *Cancer Genet Cytogenet.* 1997; 93:39–47.

81. Hashimoto K, Azuma C, Koyama M, et al. Loss of imprinting in choriocarcinoma. *Nat Genet.* 1995; 9:109–10.

82. Goto S, Yamada A, Ishizuka T et al. Development of postmolar trophoblastic disease after partial molar pregnancy. *Gynaecol Oncol.* 1993; 48:165–70.

83. Rice LW, Berkowitz RS, Lage JM et al. Persistent gestational trophoblastic tumour after partial hydatidiform mole. *Gynaecol Oncol.* 1990; 36:358–62.

84. Lapthorn AJ, Harris DC, Littlejohn A et al. Crystal structure of human chorionic gonadotropin. *Nature.* 1994; 369:455–61.

85. Tegoni M, Spinelli S, Verhoeyen M, et al. Crystal structure of a ternary complex between human chorionic gonadotropin (hCG) and two Fv fragment specific for the alpha and beta-subunits. *J Mol Biol.* 1999; 289:1375–85.

86. Boorstein WR, Vamkakopoulos NC, Fiddes JC. Human chorionic gonadotropin beta subunit is encoded by at least eight genes arranged in tandem and inverted pairs. *Nature.* 1982; 300:419–22.

87. Policastro PF, Daniels-McQueen S, Carle G, et al. A map of the hCG beta-LH beta gene cluster. *J Biol Chem.* 1986; 261:5907–16.

88. Bo M, Boime I. Identification of the transcriptionally active genes of the chorionic gonadotropin beta gene cluster in vivo. *J Biol Chem.* 1992; 267:3179–84.

89. Grover S, Woodward SR, Odell WD. Complete sequence of the gene encoding a chorionic gonadotrophin-like protein from Xanthomonas maltophilia. *Gene.* 1995; 156:75–8.

90. Dufau ML, The luteinizing hormone receptor. *Annu Rev Physiol.* 1998; 60:461–96.

91. Tsai-Morris CH, Buczko E, Wang W et al. Structural organization of the rat luteinizing hormone (LH) receptor gene. *J Biol Chem.* 1991; 266:11355–59.

92. Cole LA, Sutton JM. Selecting an appropriate hCG test for managing gestational trophoblastic disease and cancer. *J Reprod Med.* 2004; 49(7):545–53.

93. Lee CL, Hautala L, Salo T et al. Human chorionic gonadotropin and its free beta-subunit stimulate trophoblast invasion independent of LH/hCG receptor. *Mol Cell Endocrinol.* 2013; 375(1–2):43–52.

94. Cole LA. Human chorionic gonadotropin tests. *Expert Rev Mol Diagn.* 2009; 9(7):721–47.

95. Mitchell H, Seckl MJ. Discrepancies between commercially available immunoassays in the detection of tumour-derived hCG. *Mol Cell Endocrinol.* 2007; 260–262:310–3.

96. Harvey RA, Mitchell HD, Stenman UH et al. Differences in total human chorionic gonadotropin immunoassay analytical specificity and ability to measure human chorionic gonadotropin in gestational trophoblastic disease and germ cell tumors. *J Reprod Med.* 2010; 55(7–8):285–95.

97. Sturgeon CM, Berger P, Bidart JM et al. Differences in recognition of the 1st WHO international reference reagents for hCG-related isoforms by diagnostic immunoassays for human chorionic gonadotropin. *Clin Chem.* 2009; 55(8):1484–91.

98. Vaitukaitis JL. Human chorionic gonadotrophin-a hormone secreted for many reasons. *New Engl J Med.* 1979; 301:324–326.

99. Bagshawe KD. Risk and prognostic factors in trophoblastic neoplasia. *Cancer.* 1976 38:1373–85.

100. Hou JL, Wan XR, Xiang Y et al. Changes of clinical features in hydatidiform mole: Analysis of 113 cases. *J Reprod Med.* 2008; 53(8):629–33.

101. Fine C, Bundy AL, Berkowitz RS et al. Sonographic diagnosis of partial hydatidiform mole. *Obstet Gynaecol.* 1989; 73:414–18.

102. Cavoretto P, Cioffi R, Mangili G et al. A pictorial ultrasound essay of gestational trophoblastic disease. *J Ultrasound Med.* 2020; 39:597–613.

103. Seckl MJ, Gillmore R, Foskett M et al. Routine terminations of pregnancy-should we screen for gestational trophoblastic neoplasia? *Lancet.* 2004; 364:705–7.

104. Sebire NJ, Foskett M, Paradinas FJ et al. Outcome of twin pregnancies with complete hydatidiform mole and healthy co-twin. *Lancet.* 2002; 359:2165–66.

105. Savage P, Roddie M, Seckl MJ. A 28 years-old woman with a pulmonary embolus. *Lancet.* 1998; 352:30.

106. Seckl MJ, Rustin GJ, Newlands ES et al. Pulmonary embolism, pulmonary hypertension, and choriocarcinoma. *Lancet.* 1991; 338:1313–15.

107. Blohm ME, Gobel U. Unexplained anaemia and failure to thrive as initial symptoms of infantile choriocarcinoma: A review. *Eur J Pediatr.* 2004; 163(1):1–6.

108. Bolze PA, Weber B, Fisher RA et al. First confirmation by genotyping of transplacental choriocarcinoma transmission. *Am J Obstet Gynecol.* 2013; 209(1):e4–6.

109. Sebire NJ, Lindsay I, Fisher RA, Seckl MJ. Intraplacental choriocarcinoma: Experience from a tertiary referral center and relationship with infantile choriocarcinoma. *Fetal Pediatr Pathol.* 2005; 24(1):21–9.

110. Kartal I, Dagdemir A, Elli M, Bilgici MC. Pulmonary metastasis in infantile choriocarcinoma: Successful outcome. *Indian Pediatr.* 2018; 55(8):699–700.

111. Taylor S, Eisenstein K, Gildenstern V et al. Metastatic choriocarcinoma masquerading as a congenital glabellar hemangioma. *Pediatr Dev Pathol.* 2019; 22(1):59–64.

112. Johnson EJ, Crofton PM, O'Neill JM et al. Infantile choriocarcinoma treated with chemotherapy alone. *Med Pediatr Oncol.* 2003; 41(6):550–7.

113. Eckstein, R, Paradinas F, and Bagshawe KD. Placental site trophoblastic tumour (trophoblastic pseudotumour): A study of four cases requiring hysterectomy including one fatal case. *Histopathology.* 1982; 6:211–226.

114. Young RH, Scully RE. Placental-site trophoblastic tumor: Current status. *Clin Obstet Gynecol.* 1984; 27(1):248–58.

115. Kuo KT, Chen MJ, Lin MC. Epithelioid trophoblastic tumor of the broad ligament: A case report and review of the literature. *Am J Surg Pathol.* 2004; 28(3):405–9.

116. Sebire NJ, Rees H, Paradinas F et al. The diagnostic implications of routine ultrasound examination in histologically confirmed early molar pregnancies. *Ultrasound Obstet Gynecol.* 2001; 18(6):662–5.

117. Fowler DJ, Lindsay I, Seckl MJ, Sebire NJ. Histomorphometric features of hydatidiform moles in early pregnancy: Relationship to detectability by ultrasound examination. *Ultrasound Obstet Gynecol.* 2007; 29(1):76–80.

118. Savage P, Seckl MJ. The role of repeat uterine evacuation in trophoblast disease. *Gynecol Oncol.* 2005; 99(1):251–2; author reply 252–3.

119. Giorgione V, Bergamini A, Cioffi R et al. Role of surgery in the management of hydatidiform mole in elderly patients: A

single-center clinical experience. *Int J Gynecol Cancer*. 2017; 27(3):550–3.

120. Lin LH, Maestá I, Braga A et al. Multiple pregnancies with complete mole and coexisting normal fetus in North and South America: A retrospective multicenter cohort and literature review. *Gynecol Oncol*. 2017; 145(1):88–95.

121. Seckl MJ, Dhillon T, Dancey G et al. Increased gestational age at evacuation of a complete hydatidiform mole: Does it correlate with increased risk of requiring chemotherapy? *J Reprod Med*. 2004; 49(7):527–30.

122. Sun SY, Melamed A, Goldstein DP et al. Changing presentation of complete hydatidiform mole at the New England Trophoblastic Disease Center over the past three decades: Does early diagnosis alter risk for gestational trophoblastic neoplasia? *Gynecol Oncol*. 2015; 138(1):46–9.

123. Coyle C, Short D, Jackson L et al. What is the optimal duration of human chorionic gonadotrophin surveillance following evacuation of a molar pregnancy? A retrospective analysis on over 20,000 consecutive patients. *Gynecol Oncol*. 2018; 148(2):254–7.

124. Stone M, Dent J, Kardana A et al. Relationship of oral contraceptive to development of trophoblastic tumour after evacuation of hydatidiform mole. *Brit J Obstet Gynaecol*. 1976; 86:913–6.

125. Agarwal R, Teoh S, Short D et al. Chemotherapy and human chorionic gonadotropin concentrations 6 months after uterine evacuation of molar pregnancy: A retrospective cohort study. *Lancet*. 2012; 379(9811):130–5.

126. Ngan HYS, Seckl MJ, Berkowitz RS et al. Update on the diagnosis and management of gestational trophoblastic disease. *Int J Gynaecol Obstet*. 2018; 143(Suppl 2):79–85.

127. Ahamed E, Short D, North B et al. Survival of women with gestational trophoblastic neoplasia and liver metastases: Is it improving? *J Reprod Med*. 2012; 57(5–6):262–9.

128. Bower M, Newlands ES, Holden L et al. EMA/CO for high-risk gestational trophoblastic tumours: Results from a cohort of 272 patients. *J Clin Oncol*. 1997; 15:2636–43.

129. Kohorn EI. Negotiating a staging and risk factor scoring system for gestational trophoblastic neoplasia. A progress report. *J Reprod Med*. 2002; 47(6):445–50.

130. McNeish IA, Strickland S, Holden L et al. Low risk persistent gestational trophoblastic disease: Outcome following initial treatment with low-dose methotrexate and folinic acid, 1992–2000. *J Clin Oncol*. 2002; 20(7):1838–44.

131. Sita-Lumsden A, Short D, Lindsay I et al. Treatment outcomes for 618 women with gestational trophoblastic tumours following a molar pregnancy at the Charing Cross Hospital, 2000–2009. *Br J Cancer*. 2012; 107(11):1810–4.

132. McGrath S, Short D, Harvey R et al. The management and outcome of women with post-hydatidiform mole "low-risk" gestational trophoblastic neoplasia, but hCG levels in excess of 100 000 IU l(−1). *Br J Cancer*. 2010; 102(5):810–4.

133. Agarwal R, Strickland S, McNeish IA et al. Doppler ultrasonography of the uterine artery and the response to chemotherapy in patients with gestational trophoblastic tumors. *Clin Cancer Res*. 2002; 8(5):1142–7.

134. Agarwal R, Harding V, Short D et al. Uterine artery pulsatility index: A predictor of methotrexate resistance in gestational trophoblastic neoplasia. *Br J Cancer*. 2012; 106(6):1089–94.

135. Sita-Lumsden A, Medani H, Fisher R et al. Uterine artery pulsatility index improves prediction of methotrexate resistance in women with gestational trophoblastic neoplasia with FIGO score 5–6. *BJOG*. 2013; 120(8):1012–5.

136. Eysbouts YK, Ottevanger PB, Massuger LF et al. Can the FIGO 2000 scoring system for gestational trophoblastic neoplasia be simplified? A new retrospective analysis from a nationwide dataset. *Ann Oncol*. 2017; 28(8):1856–61.

137. Alifrangis C, Agarwal R, Short D et al. EMA/CO for high-risk gestational trophoblastic neoplasia: Good outcomes with induction low-dose etoposide-cisplatin and genetic analysis. *J Clin Oncol*. 2013; 31(2):280–6.

138. Bolze PA, Riedl C, Massardier J et al. Mortality of gestational trophoblastic neoplasia with a FIGO score of 13 and higher. *Am J Obstet Gynecol*. 2016 Mar 1;214(3):390-e1.

139. Berkowitz RS, Goldstein, DP. Current management of gestational trophoblastic diseases. *Gynecol Oncol*. 2009; 112(3):654–62.

140. Darby S, Jolley I, Pennington S, Hancock BW. Does chest CT matter in the staging of GTN? *Gynecol Oncol*. 2009; 112(1):155–60.

141. Ngan HY, Chan FL, Au VW et al. Clinical outcome of micrometastasis in the lung in stage IA persistent gestational trophoblastic disease. *Gynecol Oncol*. 1998; 70(2):192–4.

142. Athanassiou A, Begent RH, Newlands ES et al. Central nervous system metastases of choriocarcinoma: 23 years' experience at Charing Cross Hospital. *Cancer*. 1983; 52:1728–35.

143. Newlands ES, Holden L, Seckl MJ et al. Management of brain metastases in patients with high-risk gestational trophoblastic tumors. *J Reprod Med*. 2002; 47(6):465–71.

144. Alazzam M, Hancock BW, Osborne R, Lawrie TA. First line chemotherapy in low risk gestational trophoblastic neoplasia. *Cochrane Database Syst Rev*. 2009(1):CD007102.

145. Lybol C, Sweep FC, Harvey R et al. Relapse rates after two versus three consolidation courses of methotrexate in the treatment of low-risk gestational trophoblastic neoplasia. *Gynecol Oncol*, 2012; 125(3):576–9.

146. Bolze PA, Mathe M, Hajri T et al. First-line hysterectomy for women with low-risk non-metastatic gestational trophoblastic neoplasia no longer wishing to conceive. *Gynecol Oncol*. 2018; 150(2):282–7.

147. Bagshawe KD, Dent J, Newlands ES et al. The role of low dose methotrexate and folinic acid in gestational trophoblastic tumours (GTT). *Br J Obstet Gynaecol*. 1989; 96:795–802.

148. Rustin GJS, Newlands ES, Lutz JM et al. Combination but not single-agent methotrexate chemotherapy for gestational trophoblastic tumours (GTT) increases the incidence of second tumours. *J Clin Oncol*. 1996; 14:2769–73.

149. Savage P, Cooke R, O'Nions J et al. Effects of single-agent and combination chemotherapy for gestational trophoblastic tumors on risks of second malignancy and early menopause. *J Clin Oncol*. 2015; 33(5):472–8.

150. Hak CC, Coyle C, Kocache A et al. Emergency Etoposide-Cisplatin (Em-EP) for patients with germ cell tumours (GCT) and trophoblastic neoplasia (TN). *BMC Cancer*. 2019; 19(1):770.

151. Agarwal R, Alifrangis C, Everard J et al. Management and survival of patients with FIGO high-risk gestational trophoblastic neoplasia: The U.K. experience, 1995–2010. *J Reprod Med*. 2014; 59(1–2):7–12.

152. van Trommel NE, Massuger LF, Schijf CP et al. Early identification of resistance to first-line single-agent methotrexate in patients with persistent trophoblastic disease. *J Clin Oncol*. 2006; 24(1):52–8.

153. You B, Harvey R, Henin E et al. Early prediction of treatment resistance in low-risk gestational trophoblastic neoplasia using population kinetic modelling of hCG measurements. *Br J Cancer*. 2013; 108(9):1810–6.

154. Taylor F, Grew T, Everard J et al. The outcome of patients with low risk gestational trophoblastic neoplasia treated with single agent intramuscular methotrexate and oral folinic acid. *Eur J Cancer*. 2013; 49(15):3184–90.

155. Winter MC, Tidy JA, Hills A et al. Risk adapted single-agent dactinomycin or carboplatin for second-line treatment of methotrexate resistant low-risk gestational trophoblastic neoplasia. *Gynecol Oncol*. 2016; 143(3):565–70.

156. Mora PAR, Sun SY, Velarde GC et al. Can carboplatin or etoposide replace actinomycin-d for second-line treatment of methotrexate resistant low-risk gestational trophoblastic neoplasia? *Gynecol Oncol*, 2019; 153(2):277–85.

157. Newlands ES, Mulholland PJ, Holden L et al. Etoposide and cisplatin/etoposide, methotrexate, and actinomycin D (EMA) chemotherapy for patients with high-risk gestational trophoblastic tumors refractory to EMA/cyclophosphamide and vincristine chemotherapy and patients presenting with metastatic placental site trophoblastic tumors. *J Clin Oncol*. 2000; 18:854–9.

158. McNeish IA, Kanfer EJ, Haynes R et al. Paclitaxel-containing high-dose chemotherapy for relapsed or refractory testicular germ cell tumours. *Br J Cancer*. 2004; 90(6):1169–75.

159. Osborne R, Covens A, Mirchandani D, et al. Successful salvage of relapsed high-risk gestational trophoblastic neoplasia patients

using a novel paclitaxel-containing doublet. *J Reprod Med.* 2004; 49(8):655–61.

160. Wang J, Short D, Sebire NJ et al. Salvage chemotherapy of relapsed or high-risk gestational trophoblastic neoplasia (GTN) with paclitaxel/cisplatin alternating with paclitaxel/etoposide (TP/TE). *Ann Oncol.* 2008; 19:1578–83.

161. Feng F, Xiang Y, Wan X et al. Salvage combination chemotherapy with floxuridine, dactinomycin, etoposide, and vincristine (FAEV) for patients with relapsed/chemoresistant gestational trophoblastic neoplasia. *Ann Oncol.* 2011; 22(7):1588–94.

162. Yang J, Xiang Y, Wan X et al. Primary treatment of stage IV gestational trophoblastic neoplasia with floxuridine, dactinomycin, etoposide and vincristine (FAEV): A report based on our 10-year clinical experiences. *Gynecol Oncol.* 2016; 143(1):68–72.

163. Beyer J, Kramar A, Mandanas R et al. High-dose chemotherapy as salvage treatment in germ cell tumors: A multivariate analysis of prognostic variables. *J Clin Oncol.* 1996; 14:2638–45.

164. Lyttelton MP, Newlands ES, Giles C et al. High-dose therapy including carboplatin adjusted for renal function in patients with relapsed germ cell tumor: Outcome and prognostic factors. *Br J Cancer.* 1998; 77:1672–76.

165. El-Helw LM, Seckl MJ, Haynes R et al. High-dose chemotherapy and peripheral blood stem cell support in refractory gestational trophoblastic neoplasia. *Br J Cancer.* 2005; 93(6):620–1.

166. Frijstein MM, Lok CA, Short D et al. The results of treatment with high-dose chemotherapy and peripheral blood stem cell support for gestational trophoblastic neoplasia. *Eur J Cancer.* 2019; 109:162–71.

167. Guleria I, Khosroshahi A, Ansari MJ et al. A critical role for the programmed death ligand 1 in fetomaternal tolerance. *J Exp Med.* 2005; 202(2):231–7.

168. Bolze PA, Patrier S, Massardier J et al. PD-L1 Expression in premalignant and malignant trophoblasts from gestational trophoblastic diseases is ubiquitous and independent of clinical outcomes. *Int J Gynecol Cancer.* 2017; 27(3):554–61.

169. Veras E, Kurman RJ, Wang TL et al. PD-L1 Expression in human placentas and gestational trophoblastic diseases. *Int J Gynecol Pathol.* 2017; 36(2):146–53.

170. Huang M, Pinto A, Castillo RP et al. Complete serologic response to pembrolizumab in a woman with chemoresistant metastatic choriocarcinoma. *J Clin Oncol.* 2017; 35(27):3172–74.

171. Ghorani E, Kaur B, Fisher RA et al. Pembrolizumab is effective for drug-resistant gestational trophoblastic neoplasia. *Lancet.* 2017; 390(10110):2343–45.

172. Reck M, Rodríguez-Abreu D, Robinson AG et al. Pembrolizumab versus chemotherapy for PD-L1-positive non-small-cell lung cancer. *N Engl J Med.* 2016; 375(19):1823–33.

173. Robert C, Schachter J, Long GV et al. Pembrolizumab versus Ipilimumab in advanced melanoma. *N Engl J Med.* 2015; 372(26):2521–32.

174. Jessop E. Urgent Clinical Commissioning Policy Statement: Pembrolizumab for drug-resistant gestational trophoblastic neoplasia 2018 Jan 2018 [cited 2019]; Available from: https://www.england.nhs.uk/wp-content/uploads/2018/12/Pembrolizumab-for-drug-resistant-gestational-trophoblastic-neoplasia.pdf

175. Lim AKP, Agarwal R, Seckl MJ et al. Embolization of residual uterine vascular malformations in patients with gestational trophoblastic tumours. *Radiology.* 2002; 222(3):640–4.

176. Kelly MP, Rustin GJ, Ivory C et al. Respiratory failure due to choriocarcinoma: A study of 103 dyspneic patients. *Gynaecol Oncol.* 1990; 38:149–54.

177. Savage P, Kelpanides I, Tuthill M et al. Brain metastases in gestational trophoblast neoplasia: An update on incidence, management and outcome. *Gynecol Oncol.* 2015; 137(1):73–6.

178. Rustin GJS, Newlands ES, Bergent HJ et al. Weekly alternating chemotherapy (EMA/CO) for treatment of central nervous systems of choriocarcinoma. *J Clin Oncol.* 1989; 7:900–3.

179. Neubauer NL, Latif N, Kalakota K et al. Brain metastasis in gestational trophoblastic neoplasia: An update. *J Reprod Med.* 2012; 57(7–8):288–92.

180. Pfeffer PE, Sebire N, Lindsay I et al. Fertility-sparing partial hysterectomy for placental-site trophoblastic tumour. *Lancet Oncol.* 2007; 8(8):744–6.

181. Balachandran K, Salawu A, Ghorani E et al. When to stop human chorionic gonadotrophin (hCG) surveillance after treatment with chemotherapy for gestational trophoblastic neoplasia (GTN): A national analysis on over 4,000 patients. *Gynecol Oncol.* 2019. 155(1):8–12.

182. Blagden SP, Foskett MA, Fisher RA et al. The effect of early pregnancy following chemotherapy on disease relapse and foetal outcome in women treated for gestational trophoblastic tumours. *Brit J Cancer.* 2002; 86:26–30.

183. Williams J, Short D, Dayal L et al. Effect of early pregnancy following chemotherapy on disease relapse and fetal outcome in women treated for gestational trophoblastic neoplasia. *J Reprod Med.* 2014; 59(5–6):248–54.

184. Hopkins MP, Nunez CA, Murphy JR et al. Malignant placental site trophoblastic tumour associated with placental abruption, fetal distress, and elevated CA-125. *Gynecol Oncol.* 1992; 47:267–71.

185. Bower M, Rustin GJ, Newlands ES et al. Chemotherapy for gestational trophoblastic tumours hastens menapause by 3 years. *European J Cancer.* 1998; 34:1204–7.

186. Woolas RP, Bower M, Newlands ES et al. Influence of chemotherapy for gestational trophoblastic disease on subsequent pregnancy outcome. *Br J Obstet Gynaecol.* 1998; 105:1032–5.

187. Rustin GJS, Booth M, Dent J et al. Pregnancy after cytotoxic chemotherapy for gestational trophoblastic tumours. *Brit Med J.* 1984; 288:103–6.

24 NON-MELANOMA SKIN CANCER

Irene De Francesco, Sean Whittaker, and Stephen L. Morris

Introduction

Skin cancer is the most common form of cancer in the United Kingdom. Although each cell type in the skin can give rise to a different type of cancer, it is convenient to classify skin cancer broadly into non-melanoma skin cancers (NMSC) and malignant melanoma (MM). Secondary deposits from other cancers can also be present in the skin.

Over the last decade, non-melanoma skin cancer incidence rates have increased by around two-thirds (65%) in the United Kingdom.

There are around 147,000 new non-melanoma skin cancer cases in the United Kingdom every year (more than 400 every day between 2014 and 2016). There were around 67,000 new cases in females and 88,700 new cases in males in 2016.

Every year, non-melanoma skin cancer is responsible for 950 cancer deaths in the United Kingdom, accounting for fewer than 1% of all cancer deaths (2016).[1]

This chapter will discuss the common NMSCs, basal cell carcinoma (BCC) and squamous cell carcinoma (SCC), and also cover some of the rarer tumors, including primary cutaneous lymphoma; Merkel cell carcinoma (MCC), extra-mammary Paget's disease (EMPD), and Langerhans cell histiocytosis (LCH). Melanoma is covered in another chapter. There are many other skin tumors, including superficial soft-tissue tumors that can predominantly involve the skin, such as dermatofibrosarcoma protuberans, vascular tumors such as Kaposi's sarcoma and angiosarcoma, smooth and skeletal muscle tumors such as leiomyosarcoma, and neural tumors, which are covered in other chapters.[2] There is also a wide range of rare adnexal malignant skin tumors, which often have benign counterparts. These malignant tumors may derive from different adnexal structures within normal skin such as sebaceous, eccrine, apocrine, and follicular epithelium. They may clinically simulate common forms of NMSC such as BCC and SCC but are distinguished by distinct and classical histological and immunophenotypical features. Recognition of these different malignant adnexal tumors is critical, as the prognosis and treatment may be different from common forms of NMSC. In addition, the role of sentinel lymph node biopsy for staging the more aggressive malignant adnexal tumors is unclear but currently under investigation. These tumors are referred to in the discussion of differential diagnosis where appropriate.

Etiology

In common with other cancers in the body, carcinogenesis of the skin is thought to be a multi-step process. It is generally agreed that a tumor results from the progeny of a single cell having acquired one or more somatic mutations.[3] The likelihood of acquiring these mutant clones depends on a complex interplay between the genetic susceptibility of the individual and a wide range of environmental factors, on the one hand, and the normal function of an intact immune system to rectify them, on the other. In the hereditary skin cancers discussed in this chapter, individuals are predestined to develop skin cancer because of their genetic constitutions, whereas the greatly increased incidence of skin cancers in the older population is seen as a culmination of oncogenic events and a diminished ability of the body to destroy the transformed cells with age.

The most potent environmental agent capable of inducing skin cancer is ultraviolet (UV) light exposure. The incidence of NMSC increases with decline in latitude, being highest in Australia, with an annual incidence rate per million population of 1372 for men and 702 for women.[4,5] Ozone depletion in the atmosphere, allowing more harmful radiation to reach human skin, is probably partly responsible for the alarming increase in incidence. This is compounded by the popularity of sunny holidays abroad, outdoor recreational activities, and the culture of the bronzed body beautiful. Soldiers during World War II who had high UV light exposure while serving in North Africa have a very high incidence of NMSC and are entitled to compensation from the Ministry of Defence (MOD), which many have successfully claimed.

Melanin affords some protection against UV skin damage and explains the high incidence of skin tumors in Caucasian populations. The skin sensitivity to UV damage is related to the Fitzpatrick skin phenotype,[6] and the risk of skin cancer is particularly high in those with Celtic and Caledonian ancestry (skin type I), while the incidence is lower in the more pigmented ethnic groups (skin types III–IV). Most SCCs occur in sun-exposed areas of the skin and where the skin is more sensitive to UV damage (e.g., albinism) or where the skin is unable to repair UV-induced damage to deoxyribonucleic acid (DNA), such as xeroderma pigmentosum, described later.

Most actinic keratoses and SCCs contain UV signature mutations of the *p53* tumor suppressor gene. *P53* controls the G_1 cell cycle checkpoint allowing either time for cellular DNA repair or promotion of apoptosis, and therefore, it contributes to the malignant phenotype if mutated.[7]

Other environmental factors known to induce skin cancer include arsenic, ionizing radiation, human papilloma virus (HPV), and polycyclic aromatic hydrocarbons. There are still patients alive presenting with NMSC on the head and neck who had low-dose radiation to the scalp for ringworm as a child, and multiple BCCs on the trunk are seen in patients after radiotherapy (RT) for ankylosing spondylitis. Chronic wound healing can be associated with the later development of NMSC, especially SCC (Marjolin's ulcer), as seen in patients with severe dystrophic epidermolysis bullosa in the third and fourth decades.

Patients on immunosuppressive therapy regimens for kidney and heart transplants have an increased risk of developing SCC, BCC, MM, and Kaposi sarcoma. The risk of post-transplant skin SCC is related to the degree of immunosuppression.[8] Such tumors in immunocompromised patients are invariably more aggressive, with greater local invasion and earlier metastases than in immunocompetent patients. HPV has been advocated as a possible etiological factor in these patients.[9,10] HPVs (especially types 16 and 18) have been identified in SCC cells by in situ hybridization and polymerase chain reaction (PCR) techniques, commonly in lesions affecting the genital, oral, and peri-ungual areas. However, no role for HPV has been found in those patients infected with the human immunodeficiency virus (HIV).[11] A naturally occurring model for the association of HPV and SCC is seen in epidermodysplasia verruciformis. In this autosomal recessive (AR) condition, patients develop widespread and extensive warty lesions, identical to those of the common wart, and ultimately develop intra-epithelial neoplasia and SCC following UV exposure. HPVs have been identified in these lesions, with types 5 and 8 most commonly associated with malignancy; occasionally, types 14, 17, 20, and 47 are implicated.[11–14]

A study of 252 cases of SCC and 525 of BCC found HPV antibodies more frequently in SCC patients than in controls, but no difference in patients with BCC. Seropositivity to HPV types in genus beta, particularly HPV5, was associated with SCC risk. Individuals with SCCs on chronically sun-exposed areas were more likely to be seropositive for beta-HPV than individuals with SCCs at other sites.[15]

Familial skin cancer syndromes

Nevoid basal cell carcinoma syndrome (Gorlin syndrome)

Nevoid basal cell carcinoma syndrome (NBCCS) or Gorlin syndrome is a rare autosomal dominant disorder with linkage to chromosome 9q22.[16] It is characterized by multiple BCCs and developmental defects.[17] The sexes are equally affected. Most patients are Caucasian, but cases have been reported in Afro-Caribbeans and Asians.[18] The syndrome is caused by mutations in *Patched* (*PTCH*), a tumor suppressor gene (see Figure 24.4). A single-point mutation in one *PTCH1* allele may be responsible for the malformations found in the syndrome. Inactivation of both *PTCH1* alleles results in the formation of tumors and cysts.[18] However, there is poor correlation between identifiable genetic mutations and the resulting clinical phenotype, suggesting phenotypical variability in NBCCS.[16] The skin lesions are indistinguishable from BCC, but a broader spectrum of histological subtypes is found. Multiple keratinizing odontogenic and epidermal cysts are often seen in NBCCS, and multiple keratinizing cysts within BCCs have been recorded.[19]

Clinical features

There are more than 100 recognized features of Gorlin syndrome. The diagnostic criteria are shown in Box 24.1.

BOX 24.1   DIAGNOSTIC CRITERIA FOR GORLIN SYNDROME

Major criteria

- Multiple (>2) BCCs or one under the age of 30 years or >10 basal cell nevi
- Odontogenic keratocyst (proved on histology) or polyostotic bone cyst
- Palmar or plantar pits (three or more)
- Ectopic calcification: lamellar or early (<20 years) falx calcification
- First-degree relative with Gorlin syndrome

Minor criteria

- Congenital skeletal abnormality: bifid, fused, splayed, or missing rib or fused vertebrae
- Occipitofrontal circumference (OFC) >97th percentile

- Cardiac or ovarian fibroma
- Medulloblastoma
- Lymphomesenteric cysts
- Congenital malformation: cleft lip/palate, polydactyly, eye anomaly (cataract, coloboma, microphthalmia)

A diagnosis can be made when two major or one major and two minor criteria are present.[17]

Skin tumors

Eighty percent of Caucasian patients have at least one BCC, with the first tumor occurring at a mean age of 23 years. The number of BCCs can range from 1 to more than 1000.

Jaw cysts

These are odontogenic keratocysts (OKCs) and occur in 74% of patients, with the first cysts occurring in 80% by the age of 20 years. The number of total jaw cysts can range from 1 to 28. Most sporadically occurring OKCs behave in a benign manner; however, those associated with NBCCS are clinically more aggressive in their behavior.[20] OKCs are often the first signs of NBCCS and can occasionally be detected in patients younger than 10 years of age. It is suggested that early onset of an OKC should prompt investigation for NBCCS.[19] Cutaneous cysts may be found with an identical histology to those found in the jaw.[21]

Palmar and plantar pits

These are seen in 87% of patients; they have vertical sides, are up to several millimeters in diameter, and have an erythematous

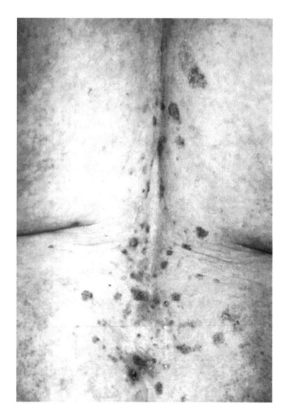

FIGURE 24.1   Nevoid BCC syndrome. Multiple basal cell carcinomas on the back of a 45-year-old woman.

base. They are said to result from impaired maturation of basal keratinocytes resulting in defective keratin.

Central nervous system

Patients with NBCCS have a predisposition to develop medulloblastoma and primitive-neuro-ectodermal tumors of the central nervous system.[22] The mean age at presentation is 2 years old, earlier than sporadic medulloblastoma. They are predominantly of the desmoplastic subtype and are often the first manifestation of the syndrome.[23]

Ovarian fibromas

These may appear in adolescent girls and women. The ovarian function may be compromised with consequent hormone imbalance.

Cardiac tumors

There now appears to be an established association between cardiac tumors and NBCCS, and evaluation of cardiac status is recommended in all patients with NBCCS.[21]

Patients with NBCCS may exhibit coarse facies, cleft lip or palate, relative macrocephaly, hypertelorism, frontal bossing, pectus deformity, or Sprengel deformity.

Radiologically, calcification may be observed in various sites, including the falx cerebri and tentorium cerebelli. Other abnormalities include bridged sella, hemivertebrae, fusion of the vertebral bodies, and flame-shaped lucencies of the phalanges and the metacarpal and carpal bones of the hands.[24]

There are no routine abnormal laboratory tests apart from, rarely, a raised alkaline phosphatase, possibly due to the presence of growing OKCs.[25]

Treatment

The first aim of treatment is to educate patients and parents as to the importance of avoiding known carcinogenic factors, with sun avoidance being of paramount importance. The BCCs may be more aggressive than their sporadic counterparts and are best treated early by one of the many options for BCCs discussed later.

Clinical experience suggests that a proportion of patients with Gorlin syndrome are extremely sensitive to ionizing radiation.[26] However, there is little in vitro evidence that the cells of individuals with Gorlin syndrome systematically demonstrate increased sensitivity to ionizing radiation. Reports are conflicting, with some studies suggesting a decrease in cultured fibroblast survival on exposure to ionizing radiation,[27,28] whereas other studies show no alteration.[29,30] These conflicting results could be explained, in part, by variable radiation sensitivity of different cell types and by the use of inappropriate methods of detecting what is likely to be a subtle difference in radiation sensitivity between tissues from normal and Gorlin syndrome patients. An alternative explanation suggests that there is genetic heterogeneity, whereby not all mutations in the *PTCH1* gene confer the same degree of radiation sensitivity.[31,32]

Vulin et al. have shown an inverse correlation between PTCH1 expression level and cellular radiosensitivity. Only cells from patients with Gorlin syndrome who presented severe deficiency in PATCHED 1 protein exhibited a significant increase in cellular radiosensitivity, affecting cell responses to both high and low radiation doses.[33]

It is sensible to limit the exposure of all patients with Gorlin syndrome to ionizing radiation. The long-term effects of radiation can be significant, with skin and soft-tissue atrophy and telangiectasia as well as induction of malignancy. The latter was demonstrated in a case of patients with Gorlin syndrome who developed a renal-cell carcinoma adjacent to a previous spinal-radiation field.[25]

Surgical excision remains the most appropriate therapy, but sun-protection advice is essential, and topical therapies such as photodynamic therapy (PDT) and imiquimod are possible alternatives. Retinoids have a therapeutic effect on existing BCCs and a prophylactic effect in inhibiting new tumor formation. However, to be of any major benefit, retinoids have to be maintained long term,[34] and in view of the need to start such therapy at an early age, the patient would be subject to long-term rheumatological complications such as diffuse idiopathic skeletal hyperostosis (DISH) and pseudo-coxarthritis.[35] Success has also been reported with a combination of topical fluorouracil (5-FU) and topical tretinoin, which may prevent the development of new tumors, inhibit the growth of existing tumors, and cause the regression of superficially invasive BCCs.[36]

Vismodegib is an oral drug that targets the hedgehog signaling pathway, and it was used in the United Kingdom until 2017 to treat patients with Gorlin syndrome. It acts as a cyclopamine-competitive antagonist of the smoothened receptor (SMO), which causes the transcription factors GLI1 and GLI2 to remain inactive, which prevents the expression of tumor mediating genes within the hedgehog pathway. A Phase II, randomized, placebo-controlled trial in Gorlin syndrome patients with BCC concluded that vismodegib was significantly better than placebo at reducing new BCC lesions ($p < 0.001$) and at decreasing the sum of the longest diameter of existing lesions ($p = 0.003$).[37] The main reported side effects are loss of taste, muscle cramps, hair loss, weight loss, and rarely, liver dysfunction. Vismodegib was initially licensed in the United Kingdom in August 2013, but it is no longer available via the cancer drug fund since 2017, when National Institute for Health and Care Excellence (NICE) guidelines concluded they could not recommend the drug because of the uncertainty in the evidence and because it was not cost effective.

Xeroderma pigmentosum

Incidence

Xeroderma pigmentosum is found worldwide in all races with an equal sex incidence. The incidence is said to be higher in Japan and Libya. Interestingly, the spectrum of disease manifestations in different countries is quite varied.[38,39] The incidence in Europe and America is 1:250,000; in Japan, 1:40,000; and in Libya, 15–20 per million.[40]

Etiology

Xeroderma pigmentosum represents a group of autosomal recessive disorders, and the genetic basis of all xeroderma pigmentosum variants has recently been elucidated. The manifestations of xeroderma pigmentosum occur as a result of a defect in excision repair of UV-induced pyrimidine dimers.[40,41] Nucleotide excision repair (NER) is one of the best-characterized DNA repair systems. The consequences of a defect in one of the NER proteins are manifested in three rare, recessive photosensitive syndromes: xeroderma pigmentosum, Cockayne's syndrome, and a photosensitive form of brittle-hair disorder, trichothiodystrophy (TTD).

Nucleotide excision repair

NER is the most flexible of all DNA repair mechanisms because of its ability to eliminate a plethora of structurally unrelated DNA lesions. Cells that are NER-deficient are sensitive to insults that cause a significant DNA helical distortion. The clinically most relevant NER substrates are *cis-syn* cyclobutane dimers (CPDs) and pyrimidine(6-4)pyrimidone photoproducts. Both are formed between adjacent pyrimidines, and they constitute the two major classes of DNA lesions induced by solar UV light.

The NER process involves the action of approximately 30 proteins, which enable damage recognition, local opening of DNA double helix around the injury, and incision of the damaged strand on either side of the lesion. After excision of the DNA lesion the resulting gap is closed by DNA repair synthesis, followed by strand ligation.[42] Using the unscheduled DNA synthesis (UDS) assay, eight complementation groups of xeroderma pigmentosum have been identified: groups A, B, C, D, E, F, G, and H.[43] The UDS measures DNA synthesis during the G_1 and G_2 phases of the cell cycle on cultured fibroblasts.

Clinical features

The clinical expression of the disease depends on the complementation group, the ethnic origin of the patient, and the geographic environment. At birth, the skin is normal. However, freckling (lentigines) and xerosis of light-exposed sites begins between 6 months and 3 years of age. This process may extend to non-sun-exposed areas. The skin becomes atrophic and telangiectatic, and superficial ulcers may develop, which can leave significant scarring (Figure 24.2).

The development of pre-malignant and malignant skin tumors will depend on the complementation group and the level of UV exposure that the patient is subjected to. Often, there are numerous actinic keratoses as well as cutaneous horns and kerato-acanthomas (KAs). Both SCCs and BCCs may appear from an early age.[38,39] Melanomas occur in up to 5% of Caucasian xeroderma pigmentosum patients, but studies of patients in Libya and South Africa have not shown a greater incidence of MM in Libyans and black South Africans.[38,39] The most common eye manifestation is photophobia with telangiectasia of the conjunctiva. There is gross hyperpigmentation of the eyelids, and severe ectropion can result

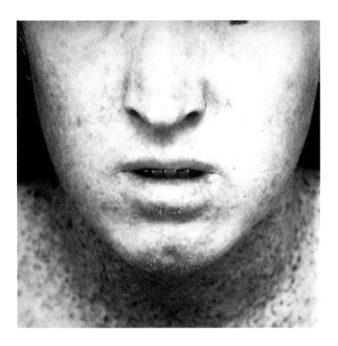

FIGURE 24.2 Xeroderma pigmentosum in a young patient with severe freckling and pigmentary skin changes.

from superficial ulceration of the skin around the eye. Scarring of the cornea and pinguecula-like growths may occur. Patients are particularly prone to SCC of the lip, and this has a particularly poor prognosis. Of xeroderma pigmentosum patients, 18% display progressive neurological abnormalities. The most severe are seen in group A patients, with mild disease seen in group D patients. This is caused by primary neuronal degeneration and loss. A mild clinical phenotype, XP variant, is recognized, which can be missed clinically but is usually associated with early onset of NMSC and marked photodamage.

Treatment

The most important single measure is UV avoidance, with the patient forbidden to go out during the peak periods of sun exposure and advised to completely cover up in the sun and to always wear a high-factor sunblock. Occasionally, patients have been treated with systemic retinoids with variable responses, but tumors tend to recur when the dose of the drug is reduced.[44,45] Patients with dysplastic and neoplastic lesions are treated as described in the sections on BCC and SCC. RT is contraindicated in these patients due to the risk of inducing further malignancy.

Pre-malignant conditions

Pre-malignant epidermal conditions include solar or actinic keratosis and Bowen's disease, which shows microscopic features of carcinoma in situ confined to the epidermis. The stage at which the lesion becomes a malignant tumor is determined by breach of the basement membrane. As well as actinic keratosis and Bowen's disease, which are discussed in the next section, skin damaged by ionizing radiation, heat, carcinogens, long-standing scars, sinuses, and ulcers may be the site of a future cancer.

Actinic keratosis and Bowen's disease

Actinic keratosis is a UV-induced pre-malignant condition with a very low malignant potential.[46,47] The etiology of Bowen's disease is unclear, as definite evidence of a pathogenic role for UV radiation is lacking, but chronic arsenic ingestion is a risk factor. Although Bowen's disease is an SCC, in situ progression to invasive SCC is very rare. It is estimated that 3–5% of Bowen's disease becomes invasive SCC and tends to be aggressive, with a metastasis rate of 30%.[48]

Actinic keratoses are small erythematous superficial keratotic lesions on sun-exposed skin. The surrounding skin shows evidence of sun exposure and damage with telangiectasia, discoloration, and non-uniform pigmentation. The scale is adherent, and attempts to remove it lead to bleeding. Bowen's disease may occur anywhere on the skin or mucous membranes and is an erythematous scaly plaque with a sharply defined margin (Figure 24.3).

When SCC in situ is found on the skin of the penis, it is called erythroplasia of Queyrat. The risk of progression of genital Bowen's disease is greater than at other sites, in the order of 10%.[49]

A biopsy or excision is required for Bowen's disease or actinic keratosis if there is suspicion of an invasive component, suggested by induration followed by development of a nodular lesion with a keratotic surface, which may break down to an ulcer with an ill-defined margin. Clinicopathological variants of actinic keratosis include hypertrophic, atrophic, acantholytic, Bowenoid, and pigmented. They all show atypical keratinocyte proliferation (dyskeratoses) within the epidermis. Initially, dysplastic changes are confined to small foci in the epidermis in which there are

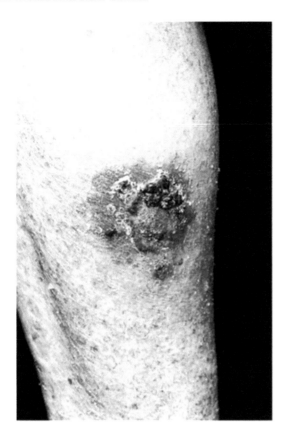

FIGURE 24.3 Bowen's disease on the lower leg of a patient with a history of arsenic ingestion.

aggregates of atypical pleomorphic keratinocytes at the basal layer. There may be hyperkeratosis and parakeratosis overlying the dysplastic keratinocytes in the epidermis. The atypical keratinocytes show loss of polarity, nuclear pleomorphism, disordered maturation, and increased numbers of mitotic figures.

There are many treatments for actinic keratosis and Bowen's disease. Cryosurgery is the most common treatment. Curettage and cautery may be used, particularly where diagnosis is in doubt to obtain histology. Topical treatment with 5-FU is a convenient and cosmetically acceptable treatment, the most common regimen being daily application of cream to the area for 4 weeks. The skin becomes inflamed, and the patient will experience pain, pruritus, and burning at the site, which sometimes extends to other subclinical areas of actinic damage.[50] There are successful reports of new topical targeted treatments, such as imiquimod, which induce an innate immune response via one of the Toll-like receptors.[51] For extensive Bowen's disease not treatable by simple topical treatment and too extensive for surgery, RT is a very successful treatment, with similar regimens to those used for SCC described later.[52] Photodynamic therapy (PDT) is a further option for extensive Bowen's disease, particularly on the lower limbs.[53]

Basal cell carcinoma

BCC (rodent ulcer or basal cell epithelioma) is the most common type of skin cancer, and it starts in the basal cell layer, the lower part of the epidermis. It derived from keratinocytes and the stroma of the pilo-sebaceous follicle,[54–56] with evidence suggesting that the tumor might be derived from follicular keratinocytes.

Incidence

BCC is the most common human cancer, affecting an estimated 750,000 Americans per year.[57] The age-standardized incidence of BCC in South Wales was estimated at 114.2 per 100,000 population in 1998.[58]

The incidence rate of BCC in the United Kingdom is 285 per 100,000 person-years and has been shown to double every 10 years, with the rapid rise attributed to the current fashion of "bronze body beautiful".[59] Widespread use of sun beds and solariums and the popularity of sunbathing holidays have resulted in more BCCs and a younger population of affected patients.[60] Estimates predict that 28% of Caucasians born after 1994 will develop a BCC in their lifetime.[57]

Etiology

There is compelling epidemiological data implicating UV radiation exposure in BCC tumorigenesis. Sixty-six per cent of BCCs occur on the head and neck. The incidence is much greater in those with fair skin and Fitzpatrick skin type I, the tumor only very rarely occurring in African-Americans.[61] The incidence of BCCs in Caucasian patients increases with decline in latitude, being highest in Australia.[62] However, the anatomical distribution of BCCs does not correspond well to the area of maximum exposure to UV. BCC is very common on the head and neck, consistently with a derivation from follicular keratinocytes, but unusual on other light-exposed areas such as the backs of the hands and forearms, unlike actinic keratoses and SCCs, which occur on all light-exposed areas. The inner canthus and eyelids, which are more shielded from sunlight than other parts of the face, are frequently involved. BCC commonly affects the trunk, and rare cases of vulval BCC also occur. The occurrence of BCCs in relatively sun-protected sites suggests that other cofactors may be important and is consistent with regional concentration of follicular sebaceous units. One series found that 7.3% of 1774 cases of BCC had a previous history of trauma to the site of the BCC.[63] BCCs may arise in congenital nevus sebaceus, skin damage by x-irradiation, burns, or vaccination scars. Arsenic salts used as tonics in the 1930s were also an important etiological factor. Arsenic-induced tumors are usually multiple, occur mainly on the trunk, and may also cause arsenical keratoses on acral sites.[64]

Although exposure to UV radiation is accepted as a critical causative factor in the pathogenesis of BCC, the magnitude of the risk associated with increased exposure seems to be insufficient to explain either why particular people get these tumors whereas others do not, or the considerable phenotypical diversity shown by patients in terms of the number and site of tumors and patterns of presentation.[65,66] Susceptibility to BCC seems to be determined by a complex interaction between duration and intensity of exposure to UV radiation and polymorphic genes. Specific and distinct clinical phenotypes include presentation with clusters of BCC (termed multiple presentation phenotype) and development of tumors on the trunk. In particular, patients with truncal BCC have more BCCs, are younger, and develop larger clusters of BCCs.[65,67] Susceptibility genes associated with multiple tumors include cytochrome P450 CYP2D6, glutathione S-transferase GSTT1, vitamin D receptor, and the tumor necrosis factor (TNF) family.[65]

The molecular basis of the basal cell nevus syndrome has been elucidated and is due to constitutive activation of the Sonic Hedgehog (SHH) signaling pathway due to germ-line inactivating mutations of the *PTCH1* gene.[2] The *PTCH1* gene is the human homologue of the *Drosophila* segment polarity gene.

PTCH1 is now known to act as a tumor suppressor gene, requiring mutations in both inherited alleles in order to be inactivated.[68] Studies on the *PTCH1* gene in patients with basal cell nevus syndrome and sporadic BCC have demonstrated abnormalities in both copies of *PTCH1* in the vast majority of tumors. *PTCH1* inhibits binding of a protein known to control growth and patterning, called SHH, which in turn binds to its transmembrane receptor, Smoothened. Inactivation of *PTCH1* results in the constitutive activation of the SHH signaling and activation of the transcription factors GLI1/2 involved in stem cell proliferation.[69,70] Activating mutations of Smoothened have been identified in some cases of sporadic BCC. Recent studies of transgenic mice overexpressing the SHH signaling pathway have demonstrated that only one mutational event is required to produce BCCs in human xenografts, which may explain why BCC is so common.[71,72] Therefore, sporadic BCCs may result from either an acquired inactivating mutation (67%) in both copies of *PTCH1* or an acquired activating mutation (10–21%) of a single copy of the Smoothened allele (Figure 24.4).

However, the correlation between the tumor biology and the clinical diversity observed in patients is currently unknown. Additional events include inactivation of the tumor suppressor gene *p53*, which controls the G_1 cell cycle checkpoint and thus regulates DNA repair or induces apoptosis of irretrievably damaged cells. Mutations of the *p53* gene have been detected in almost all human tumors, and in skin tumors, these have been shown to be UV related. The mutation of a single *p53* allele leads to the production of mutant p53 protein, which will inactivate wild-type *p53*, allowing cells that have DNA damage to proliferate. One study demonstrated that phenotypically normal UV-exposed human epidermal cells contain islands of keratinocytes that show mutant *p53* on immunostaining.[72] Such islands suggest that these cells are clonally expanded and therefore selectively out-grow those keratinocytes without mutation for *p53*.[73] Indeed, 30% of sporadic BCCs show UV-type mutations of the *p53* gene.[73] Polymorphisms in the gene for glutathione reductase, which is important in the detoxification of active oxygen species,

have been linked to BCCs, as have polymorphisms in the cytochrome P450 genes, which are important in metabolizing environmental carcinogens.[74]

Chemokines such as CXCR4 may play a critical role in the progression and angiogenesis of certain subtypes of BCC with a more aggressive nature, and functional blockade of CXCR4 has been proposed as a potential therapeutic strategy for these tumors.[75]

Clinical features

The majority of BCCs, approximately 80%, occur on the head and neck, especially the upper central portion of the face. The other 20% are mainly on the trunk and lower limbs, particularly in women. It is a common tumor on the lower eyelid, the inner canthus of the eye, and behind the ear. The palm of the hand, sole of the foot, and vermilion of the lip are never involved. Early BCCs are commonly small, translucent or pearly, with raised areas through which dilated vessels may show (telangiectasia). The classic form is the rodent ulcer, which has an indurated edge and ulcerated center.

This tumor is slow growing but if neglected, can spread deeply to cause considerable morbidity due to tissue destruction, especially around the eye, nose, or ear. It may even extend into the periorbital tissues and bone. The morphoeic type occurs almost exclusively on the face, whereas the superficial type is more common on the trunk.[76] An aggressive form may occur on the occiput. BCC has a tendency to grow along the lines of embryonic fusion, which can lead to invasive BCC migrating along the peri-chondrium, periosteum, fascia, or tarsal plate.[77] This type of spread accounts for higher recurrence rates noted in tumors involving the eyelid, nose, and scalp. The most susceptible areas include the inner canthus, philtrum, middle to lower chin, nasolabial groove, preauricular area, and retro-auricular sulcus.[77] Perineural spread is very uncommon, occurs most often in recurrent BCC,[78–82] and may present with paresthesia, pain, and weakness or in some cases, paralysis.[82–84] Involvement of the cranial nerves and in one case, thoracic spine has been reported.[79,83–85]

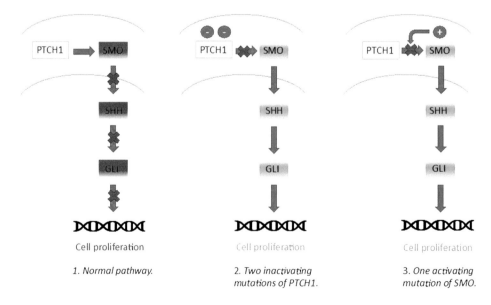

Cell proliferation

1. Normal pathway.

Cell proliferation

2. Two inactivating mutations of PTCH1.

Cell proliferation

3. One activating mutation of SMO.

FIGURE 24.4   Schematic representation of the Sonic Hedgehog Pathway. 1. Normal pathway: PTCH1 is intact and inhibits the SHH pathway and cell proliferation. 2. Two inactivating mutations of PTCH1 allow binding of SMO receptor with SHH ligand and activation of the SHH pathway. This promotes cell proliferation. 3. One activating mutation of the SMO receptor is sufficient to activate the SHH pathway, regardless of the PTCH status. This promotes cell proliferation. (By courtesy of Irene De Francesco.)

Metastatic BCC is rare, with incidence rates varying from 0.0028% to 0.1%.[85–87] Metastases, when reported, have involved lung, lymph nodes, esophagus, oral cavity, and skin.[88–93] Although long-term survival has been reported, the prognosis for metastatic BCC is generally poor, with a median survival of 8–10 months after diagnosis.[93] Platinum-based chemotherapy is the treatment of choice for metastatic BCC.[94,95]

In immunosuppressed patients, tumors may be more aggressive locally,[96] but metastasis remains extremely rare (0.1%) with spread to regional lymph nodes or lung.[97] Hematogenous spread has been only rarely reported. The interval from onset to metastasis ranged in one study from 7 to 34 years, with a median of 9 years; the 5-year survival rate was 10% for metastatic BCC in the context of immunosuppression.[98] Death may occur by local invasion of tissues such as major blood vessels and the brain.

Clinicopathological subtypes

The typical histology of BCC consists of clumps of darkly staining basaloid cells with characteristic peripheral palisading. The tumors tend to infiltrate laterally rather than deeply, and this, in conjunction with central ulceration, is responsible for the rolled border seen clinically. In addition to keratinocyte proliferation, the stroma proliferates to a varying degree according to the clinicopathological subtype of the BCC. The stroma appears as fine cellular connective tissue, which may show degenerative or metaplastic changes. There may also be an inflammatory infiltration of the stroma by lymphocytes, histiocytes, and occasionally, plasma cells.[54]

There are different clinicopathological subtypes of BCC, which are described in the following.[99,100]

Nodular basal cell carcinoma

Clinical features
This tumor starts as a small "glassy/pearly" papule, which subsequently becomes nodular and undergoes central ulceration. The margins of the tumor are well-defined and slightly raised with a rolled border and with a pearly, shiny appearance. Blood vessels traversing over the margin produce a telangiectatic appearance (Figure 24.5). In larger lesions, ulceration may be a feature, but the raised, rolled border is often prominent (Figure 24.6).

Histopathology
This tumor is composed of discrete islands of darkly staining cells with uniform nuclei and scant cytoplasm within the dermis. Typically, peripheral palisading is present. A prominent connective tissue stroma is an integral part of the tumor. If nodules measure less than 15 µm, the tumor may be called micronodular, which is an aggressive subtype. An infiltrative pattern is seen in 15–20% of BCCs and is referred to as a histologically aggressive type.

Pigmented basal cell carcinoma

Clinical features
This type of BCC is clinically similar to the nodular or superficial BCC, but the rolled margins of the tumor are irregularly pigmented. Such pigmented BCCs must be clinically distinguished from melanoma (Figure 24.7).

Histopathology
The small basaloid cells with darkly staining uniform nuclei and scant ill-defined cytoplasm may contain granules of melanin, and in such tumors, large collections of melanophages may be present in the stroma.

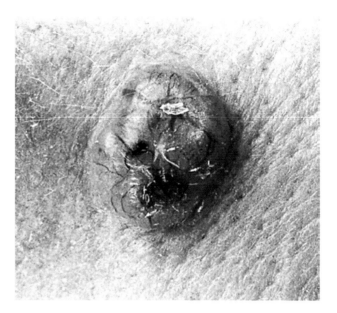

FIGURE 24.5 Typical nodular basal cell carcinoma (BCC) on a patient's face.

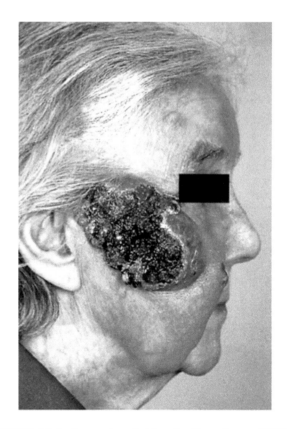

FIGURE 24.6 Large ulcerated basal cell carcinoma (BCC) in an 82-year-old woman who was terrified that she had cancer and did not leave the house for 3 years.

Cystic basal cell carcinoma

Clinical features
This is a well-defined papule that attains a pearly colored, lobulated appearance with a telangiectatic surface. The central part of the tumor may ulcerate later in its evolution. This is a relatively rare variant of nodular BCC.

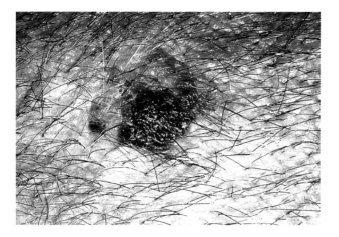

FIGURE 24.7 Pigmented basal cell carcinoma (BCC) on the chest of a 35-year-old man.

Histopathology

The hallmark of this tumor is the presence of cystic foci creating a lace-like pattern of small, darkly staining cells. It is thought that the cystic spaces may be due to the cells outgrowing their nutritional supply with the appearance of necrotic areas in the center of the epithelial strands. However, some cystic spaces may also represent sweat duct differentiation. If mucinous degeneration of the stroma occurs, as well as degeneration of the basaloid tumor, this may give rise to the appearance of the adenocystic variety of BCC, characterized by a large cystic space due to necrosis of tumor cells with a peripheral lace-like pattern caused by mucoid degeneration of the stroma.

Morphoeic (sclerosing) basal cell carcinoma

Clinical features

These tumors clinically appear as sclerotic, slightly depressed areas of skin with prominent telangiectasia (Figure 24.8). It is often difficult to clinically determine the margins of the tumor, and this type of BCC often recurs due to inadequate excision.

Histopathology

The stromal element predominates and thin epithelial cords and strands of basal cells are seen embedded in a dense, sometimes

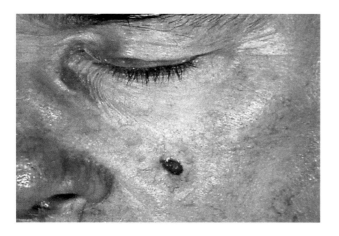

FIGURE 24.8 Morphoeic basal cell carcinoma (BCC) showing some central ulceration on the cheek of a 67-year-old man.

hyalinized connective tissue stroma. This subtype shows aggressive pattern.

Superficial basal cell carcinoma

Clinical features

This often occurs on the trunk or limbs and is characterized by a well-defined, erythematous patch that may be large (5–20 cm or more). The surface is telangiectatic and may become eroded. A thread-like margin of the tumor is present, often with a pearly appearance. Most lesions are solitary and may be pigmented. Over many years, the lesion may thicken and ulcerate. Multiple surface BCCs have been associated with arsenic ingestion.[64]

Histopathology

There are small nests of cells along the dermal/epidermal junction with an overlying atrophic epidermis. It has been demonstrated that tumor nests form direct contact with each other in three-dimensional space. This subtype usually shows non-aggressive behavior.

Linear basal cell carcinoma

Clinical features

This is an uncommon variant of BCC and was first described in 1985.[101] Clinically, it is a linear, pearly, and telangiectatic lesion and is located most often on the head and neck. This variant belongs to a more aggressive subtype and is more likely to have subclinical spread.[102] Various mechanisms have been suggested to account for this morphological variant, including a Koebner phenomenon or limited lateral spread of the BCC secondary to dermal fibrosis.[103]

Histopathology

Nodular masses of basal neoplastic cells are present in the dermis, typical of basal cell epithelioma. In the tumor and in the stroma, deposits of melanin may be found, some of which are seen in melanophages.[103]

Basosquamous carcinoma

This subtype has mixed features of basal cell carcinoma and squamous cell carcinoma. It can be more aggressive than other forms of BCC.

Diagnosis

The diagnosis of BCCs is primarily a clinical diagnosis supported by a histopathological examination. The clinical differential diagnosis of BCC includes SCC, MM (pigmented BCC), melanocytic cystic nevi (pigmented BCC), Bowen's disease (especially superficial BCC), psoriasis (superficial BCC), sebaceous hyperplasia, molluscum contagiosum, and numerous benign appendigeal tumors, especially those of follicular origin. Where clinical doubt exists, or when patients are referred for specialized forms of treatment a preoperative biopsy is recommended. Biopsy will also provide information on the histological subtype of the BCC, which influences management and prognosis. A specific adnexal tumor that needs to be distinguished histologically from BCC is microcystic adnexal carcinoma. This tumor is slow growing but is locally very aggressive and destructive, commonly affecting facial areas and specifically the lip. The treatment of choice is extensive surgical resection and preferably, micrographic surgery because of high rates of local recurrence.

There are four generally accepted methods for obtaining tissue diagnosis. These are shave biopsy, punch biopsy, cytology, or definitive surgical excision. A shave biopsy usually is adequate for raised lesions such as nodular BCC. Punch biopsy is effective for sampling superficial BCC, for which shave or excision would be technically inappropriate. An excision biopsy may be used to sample deep dermal and subcutaneous tissue. A comparison of shave biopsy versus punch biopsy was performed retrospectively in 86 cases, showing that the two techniques have equivalent diagnostic accuracy rates. Cytology provides a rapid alternative to either punch biopsy or shave biopsy, and it can yield a diagnosis during the initial outpatient appointment. The accuracy of cytology in eyelid lesions suspected clinically to be BCCs was compared retrospectively in 20 lesions from 17 consecutive patients who underwent cytology followed by excision biopsy.[104] The sensitivity of cytology for the diagnosis of BCC was 92%. This was compared with a second group of 26 clinical BCCs from 22 consecutive patients who had an incisional biopsy and histological examination followed by excision with histological confirmation, in which the sensitivity was 100% and the accuracy was 96%. Cytology is sufficiently accurate to plan excision and reconstructive surgery when the diagnosis can be confirmed histologically but may not be sufficiently sensitive for conservative regimens such as RT because of the small risk of false-negative diagnosis; however, it may be accepted clinically for subsequent diagnoses.[104]

Staging and classification

BCC rarely metastasizes, and so a staging work-up is not necessary. However, magnetic resonance imaging may delineate the extent of recurrent aggressive and neglected BCCs.

The European consensus-based multidisciplinary guidelines propose a classification including two main categories: "easy to treat BCC" (common BCC) and "difficult to treat BCC" (locally advanced or requiring complex management).[105] Ninety-five percent of BCC are "easy to treat".

The difficult-to-treat BCC are also divided into five subgroups:

1. Common BCC but difficult to treat for any reason linked to the tumor or the patient
2. BCC difficult to treat because of the number of BCCs
3. Locally advanced BCC out of critical areas
4. Locally advanced difficult-to-treat BCC in critical areas
5. Extremely advanced difficult-to-treat BCC

Management

A number of factors have a direct influence on the prognosis of BCC. Patients can be defined in terms of low- or high-risk categories by considering prognostic factors including tumor size, tumor site, tumor type and definition of margins, growth pattern/histological subtype, failure of previous treatment/recurrent tumors, and those in immunocompromised patients.[105]

Low-risk BCCs are generally small (<2 cm) and well-defined in a non-critical site with non-aggressive histology. Only 5% of well-defined BCCs <2 cm show subclinical spread beyond 5 mm.[106]

High-risk BCCs are generally large (>2 cm), indistinct or morphoeic, in a critical site such as around the eyes, ears, lips, nose, and nasolabial folds, and show aggressive histology such as morphoeic, infiltrative, micronodular or perineural spread.

The therapeutic aim is to completely eradicate the BCC with the best possible cosmetic outcome, the lowest chance of tumor recurrence, and the minimum long-term side effects.

Factors considered when determining the treatment strategy for BCC are overall health status, histological tumor type, location, size, primary versus recurrent tumor, and patient choice. Patient quality-of-life issues regarding cosmetic outcome associated with surgical procedures are also important (e.g., location of tumor leading to undesirable cosmetic outcomes or large superficial BCC). The closure of the wound needs to be considered, and larger tumors may need plastic surgical reconstruction with skin grafts and flaps, with the additional possible complications of dehiscence, necrosis, hematoma, and seroma. Not all BCCs require treatment; aggressive treatment might be inappropriate for patients of advanced age or poor general health, especially for asymptomatic low-risk lesions that are unlikely to cause significant morbidity. Furthermore, some elderly or frail patients with symptomatic or high-risk tumors might prefer less aggressive treatments designed to palliate rather than cure. Local availability of various specialized services, together with the experience and preferences of the dermatologist managing the case, are also factors that will influence the selection of therapy.

Most BCCs are adequately treated by primary excision with low risk of recurrence and no requirement for further therapy. In one study, 41 consecutive patients with 42 BCCs apparently removed surgically were treated by subsequent micrographic surgery, and blocks of tissue, sectioned consecutively until exhausted, were examined for the presence of residual tumor.[107] In 28 of 42 cases (66%), residual cancer was identified. The presence of residual cancer was not related to age, site, histological subtype, or extent of surrounding inflammation. The results indicate that patients with small BCCs that appear to be completely removed by initial biopsy may be at risk for recurrence.

Infiltrative and micronodular BCC types are the most likely to be incompletely removed by conventional excision. Rates of incomplete excision vary from 5% to 17%. Incompletely excised infiltrative and micronodular BCCs may recur at rates of 33–39%. Recurrences after RT show a tendency toward infiltrative histology and evidence of squamous transformation, and even recurrent BCC after surgical excision may become metatypical. In general, recurrences are more frequent in BCCs with infiltrative and micronodular histology, when clear margins are less than 0.38 mm, and when the histology suggests the presence of squamous differentiation.

Management options

Many series have shown that treatment by curettage and cautery, surgical excision, RT, cryotherapy, and Mohs' micrographic surgery have cure rates of well over 90%. Tumors in certain high-risk sites have a greater risk of recurrence, namely, the nasal alae, nasolabial fold, tragus, and post-auricular area. This may be due to the fusion of embryonal planes at these sites allowing covert migration of tumor cells.[108] Although most BCCs are treated by one of three methods—surgery, cryotherapy, or RT—a number of novel treatment modalities are now established. Patients with high-risk tumors are best managed by a multidisciplinary team approach to select the most appropriate treatment.[109]

Surgical treatments

Curettage and cautery (or electrodesiccation)

The tumor and 2–4 mm of adjacent normal tissue are removed by curettage under local anesthesia, and hemostasis is secured by cautery or electrosurgery (electrodesiccation or coagulation).[106,110] Typically, two or three treatment cycles are recommended to completely remove the tumor. If the dermis and fatty layer are penetrated, then surgical excision should be performed. The wound is left to heal by secondary intention. Topical antibiotics may reduce infection of the open wound. Most patients develop a white scar or occasionally a hypertrophic scar. The main indication for this treatment is for selective low-risk lesions (small, well-defined primary lesions with non-aggressive histology in non-critical sites) with 5-year cure rates up to 92.3%.[109] Recurrence rates are higher for tumors in nasal, paranasal, forehead, and mask areas and for tumors <6 mm on the cheek, forehead, scalp, and neck.[111] However, a study using micrographic surgical techniques[112] found that residual tumor was left in at least 30% of cases following curettage, which is far higher than the actual recurrence rate. It is possible that debulking of the tumor provokes an immune response that clears the residual tumor.[113]

Cryosurgery

Liquid nitrogen cryosurgery uses the effect of extreme cold (–50 to –60°C) to effect deep destruction of BCC and surrounding tissues.[109] A fine, intermittent spray is preferred, as a continuous one produces a rapid lateral extension of the ice front rather than penetration to the bottom of the tumor. A safe margin of 3–5 mm is first drawn around the tumor, as its edges are difficult to see once frozen. Satisfactory results may be obtained by spraying the center of the lesion until the ice front is maintained for 3–4 mm beyond the visible edge of the lesion for 30 seconds. After the tumor is frozen, it is allowed to thaw, and then the freeze cycle is repeated at least once, which can cause considerable transient discomfort and swelling.[114] Two freeze–thaw cycles are recommended for facial BCCs.[115] Cryosurgery is suitable for BCCs with clinically well-defined borders and non-aggressive histology but not for those tumors that are in critical facial sites.[109] Five-year cure rates up to 99% can be achieved.[116,117] Cryosurgery has also a potential role in high-risk BCC or disease recurrence, but this is limited to selected cases.[109]

The eardrum may need to be protected using dry cotton wool when the ear is being treated. Cryosurgery is not suitable for lesions bordering the lip or eyelid, as scarring leads to a contraction deformity at these sites, and should be avoided in areas of hair growth (e.g., scalp or beard). The use of cryotherapy is contraindicated in thick lesions, as the borders of these are poorly defined, and the tumor may be inadequately treated. It is also absolutely contraindicated in patients with abnormal cold tolerance, for example, cryoglobulinemia.

After treatment, there is short-term pain, tenderness, bullae or vesicle formation, erythema, sloughing of necrotic tissue, eschar formation, and often considerable edema followed by a serous discharge, which may last for 2–3 weeks. The site should be kept clean until the eschar separates. Hyper- or hypo-pigmentation can occur at the site of freezing and is more obvious the darker the skin of the patient. Scarring tends to be minimal, and this technique has rarely been associated with nerve damage. Cryosurgery has many advantages, as it is quick to perform and requires no hospitalization, and most patients require fewer than two outpatient treatment sessions.

Surgical excision

Surgical treatment of primary BCCs is highly effective and the standard of care for BCC. The major advantage is that the tumor and surgical margins can be assessed histologically.

In general, the cosmetic results are excellent, but the major problem is defining the margins of the BCC before excision. The definition of such a margin is made more difficult as 15% of BCCs show subclinical spread beyond 3 mm and 5% show subclinical spread beyond 4 mm. Morphoeic BCCs are even more difficult to define, with 18% showing subclinical spread beyond 5 mm and 5% showing subclinical spread beyond 13 mm.[118]

In a retrospective cohort analysis of 1983 BCC cases, significant risk factors for incomplete excision included lesions located on the head and neck ($p < 0.001$), surgeons performing fewer than 51 procedures during the 2-year study period ($p < 0.001$), and patients with aggressive histological BCC subtypes (e.g., morphoeic and infiltrative) ($p < 0.01$). The study further indicated that curettage before surgical excision of BCC decreased the incomplete excision rate by up to 24% ($p = 0.03$).[118]

The risk of recurrence seems highest in those lesions where both deep and lateral margins were involved.[119]

The excision of BCCs needs to take into account possible subclinical spread as well as the limitations of the tumor size and tumor site. Although histologically, a BCC may not be completely excised, its actual clinical recurrence is much lower than would be expected. Therefore, it is a matter of controversy as to whether an incompletely excised BCC needs to be re-excised. A large study of re-excisions after incomplete excision of BCCs has revealed that in most cases, re-excision will reveal residual tumor,[120] and recurrence is most likely when both lateral and deep margins are involved. Therefore, if only a lateral margin is involved in a BCC that has a non-aggressive histology and is away from a critical site, it is reasonable to take a conservative approach.[106] However, if the BCC involves a deep margin at a critical site with aggressive histology, then re-excision with micrographic surgery, or postoperative RT, would be advised.

Mohs' micrographic surgery

In this technique, the tumor is debulked with a scalpel or curette with the scalpel angled at 45 degrees to the skin. A saucer of tissue is then removed. Anatomical orientation is carefully maintained by scoring the remaining skin edge and surface of the tissue removed. The tissue is divided along the scored lines, inverted, and the edges marked with colored stains. The tissue is embedded and horizontal frozen sections cut and stained so that the whole of the under-surface of the removed tissue is examined for residual tumor. The surgeon acts as both surgeon and pathologist. The dermatological surgeon then returns to the patient and removes tissue only in areas where tumor is microscopically persistent. This process is repeated until the tumor is totally removed. This technique means that the normal surrounding tissue can be preserved while the whole of the tumor is removed. The defect can be left to heal by secondary intention, or reconstruction can commence immediately.[121] The overall risk of complications is 2%, most of which involve bleeding.[122] Mohs' micrographic surgery is regarded as a standard treatment for BCC and can give cure rates of 99% in primary and 96–98% in recurrent BCCs.[123] It is, however, expensive in both time and support facilities compared with conventional methods of treatment. The average procedure takes 5 hours. Therefore, the main indications for Mohs' micrographic surgery are for those BCCs in critical sites such as the eyelids, ears, lips, nose, and nasolabial folds, morphoeic or infiltrated histological subtype, and patients with recurrent BCC, especially after RT. It may also be used for large tumors in high-risk sites.[106,124]

Laser surgery

High-energy pulsed carbon dioxide (CO_2) lasers have been used extensively to resurface wrinkled and photo-damaged skin with a low-risk of scarring. Results of histological studies demonstrate precise ablation depths in treated skin with minimal thermal damage to underlying tissue. The ultra-pulse CO_2 laser with high energy and short pulses achieves char-free ablation of tissue, bloodless surgical field, minimal non-specific thermal damage, rapid healing, and diminished post-operative pain. Pulsed CO_2

laser treatment can also be effective in ablating superficial BCC. However, there is little published follow-up data to date. A retrospective review of 61 biopsy-proven non-recurrent nodular and superficial BCCs in 23 patients has reported only two recurrences with a mean follow-up of 41.7 months (range 15–84 months).[125] CO_2 laser surgery has also been successfully combined with a micrographic approach similar to Mohs' micrographic surgery in order to increase its cure rate in a patient with a large BCC, but as yet, there have been no trials comparing this modality with the established ones.[126,127] Because scarring is minimized with this technique, it has been particularly advocated in eyelid BCCs, although the treatment of choice for this site is micrographic surgery.

Non-surgical treatments

Radiotherapy

RT of skin cancer yields excellent results, and the cure rates for primary BCC are above 90%.[127] Review articles have reported an overall 5-year cure rate of 91.3% following RT for primary BCC and an overall 5-year cure rate of 90.2% following RT for recurrent BCC.[128,129]

In many cases, BCCs can be managed equally effectively by surgical techniques or RT. RT allows greater preservation of normal tissue than surgical excision and is useful for areas where tissue cannot be readily sacrificed because of cosmetic or functional importance.

Indications for RT include the following:

- Large superficial lesions where a better cosmetic result can be obtained with RT.
- Large lesions where surgery would cause major loss of function such as paralysis, numbness, dribbling, or ectropion.
- Extensive lesions where surgery such as nasectomy, ear amputation, or eye enucleation may be avoided.
- Older patients where possible long-term skin atrophy caused by RT is not an issue.
- Multiple superficial lesions where surgery would be onerous for the patient.
- Patients who are unfit for or refuse surgery.
- Selected tumors of the eyelids and canthi of the eyes.
- Selected tumors on the nose, ears, and lips. Larger lesions *overlying* cartilage are best treated with an electron beam rather than superficial RT.[130]
- Large lesions on the cheek, which often respond with minimum scarring.
- Recurrent lesions after surgery, incomplete excision, or perineural invasion.
- Nodal metastatic spread.

Relative contraindications include the following:

- Younger patients below 45 years: There is potential for deterioration of the cosmetic outcome over time (<5–10 years) and risk of second malignancy.
- Large lesions *involving* cartilage, bone, tendons, or joints: these may be treated with megavoltage or electron beam radiation.
- Lesions where there is uncertainty over the histology.
- Lesions that have recurred after RT.
- Hair-bearing skin such as scalp, eyebrows, and eyelashes: risk of permanent epilation.
- Lesions around the upper eyelid: Risk of lachrymal gland dryness and upper lid conjunctival keratinization.

- Medial inner canthus lesions: Risk of nasolacrimal duct stenosis.
- Lesions on the lower leg and back: Poor healing and radiation sequelae, particularly telangiectasia, pigment changes, ulceration, and atrophic scarring.

These relative contraindications need to be reviewed in each individual case, as alternative treatments may produce even more problems. The lower leg and back present particular problems for all treatment modalities. Lesions involving the mid-third of the upper lid are readily curable by RT, but mucosal changes such as keratinization and cicatricial xerosis with secondary damage to the cornea are probable.[131] If an upper lid tumor is sufficiently extensive to require complicated reconstruction, then RT may be an alternative, as there is a chance keratinization may be avoided. If it does occur, a contact lens provides a remedy. A study of 850 patients treated with RT for carcinomas of the eyelid reported a corneal complication rate of 2.3%, cataract rate of 2%, and serious ocular complication rate (including eye loss) of 1.4%.[132] The incidence of corneal complications increased from 1% for the lower lid to 6.7% for the upper lid. Damage to the lachrymal gland may cause keratoconjunctivitis sicca with a dry eye. Lesions of the outer third of the upper eyelid are therefore best avoided. If the dose to the lachrymal gland is kept below 35 Gy, then late complications (excluding asymptomatic cataracts and a mild dry eye) can be avoided.[133]

BCCs and skin cancers can be treated by a variety of RT techniques: superficial RT, electron beam RT, megavoltage external beam RT, and interstitial brachytherapy.

Most superficial lesions are treated with superficial x-rays (40–100 kV) or orthovoltage (100–300 kV). The tumor must be carefully assessed macroscopically for its lateral extent, and particular attention must be paid to the depth of the tumor in sites such as the inner canthus, nasolabial fold, ala nasi, tragus, and post-auricular area, where deep infiltration may occur. The visible tumor is drawn on the skin; typical radial margins to create the field to treat a BCC are 6 mm around the visible tumor, but this must be interpreted in the light of the clinicopathological type of BCC, the clinical site, organs at risk, and size of the lesion being treated. For example, a morphoeic BCC may require a margin of 1–1.5 cm. Percentage depth doses for different field sizes at different energies are consulted to select a beam energy that will encompass the target volume by the 90% isodose. The treatment volume needs to be larger than the target volume due to dose fall-off at the field edges. Sheets of lead cut out to surround the treatment field protect the surrounding skin and any organs at risk. The thickness of the lead depends on the energy used. A lead shield may be required to protect the eye and to protect the nasal mucosa and cartilage when the ala nasi is treated. In this case, it is inserted using local anesthetic drops.

Larger lesions more than 4 cm in diameter that are not near the eyes or complicated air spaces should be considered for electron beam therapy. Electron beam RT for periocular areas is relatively contraindicated because of lateral scatter of electron beam radiation. Where an electron beam is needed to treat the periocular skin, for example, when treating extensive cutaneous angiosarcoma, internal electron eye shields can be used. These need to be made with 3–4 mm of lead lined with 2–3 mm of silicon depending on the electron energy used. They are thicker and more uncomfortable for the patient than the thinner eye shield needed when using superficial RT. Electron beams are ideal for large flat tumors on the scalp and trunk and for treating tumors overlying cartilage, such as the nose. The depth dose characteristics of electron beams are such that bolus material is needed to increase the skin surface to 100% dose or compensate for an irregular contour, but there is a sharp fall-off in dose past the 90% isodose at a depth determined by the electron beam energy. The effective treatment depth in centimeters is approximately one-third of the beam energy in mega electron volts, depending on the field size. The RT is planned in a similar way as described earlier, but an additional margin must be added for electron beam therapy because of the shape of the isodose curves, and an electron end plate for the linear accelerator (LINAC) needs to be made. Computed tomography (CT) is useful for planning large lesions. Good results have been obtained for BCCs that are difficult to treat by other methods.[130]

The daily dose and fractionation schedule prescribed for the patient depends on the site and size of the tumor, its relationship to other structures such as the eye, ear, and nose, the age of the patient, and the ease of getting the patient to the RT center. Fractionated dose schedules are preferred to a single large dose, as these have been found to give rise to better cure rates and better cosmetic results, since tumor tissue recovers more slowly than normal tissue.[134] Many different dose schedules are in use, and all have been shown to be effective (Table 24.1).

Erythema usually develops in the first week of treatment followed by an exudative reaction. Healing is completed approximately 3 weeks after the first dose. Comedones may appear several weeks after treatment but usually resolve spontaneously. Long-term side effects include atrophy, hyper- and hypo-pigmentation, telangiectasia, and alopecia (Figure 24.9). Non-healing skin ulceration, persistent pain, and secondary skin cancers are more serious late side effects. The cosmetic acceptability of RT is high at 84%, with cosmetic acceptability being higher for smaller irradiated fields. The incidence of acute complications is normally low at 2%, and that of late complications is even lower at 0.3%.[128]

As discussed earlier, incompletely excised deep margin positive BCCs in critical sites and with aggressive histology require further treatment. The risk of recurrence is 41–58% if left untreated.[135,136] In a series of 187 incompletely excised BCCs,

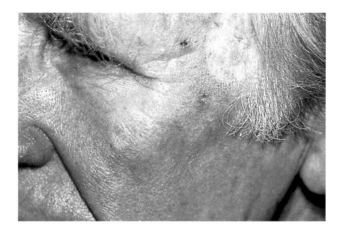

FIGURE 24.9   Two atrophic pale patches on the forehead of a 70-year-old man who had received radiotherapy for basal cell carcinomas (BCCs) 10 years earlier.

with 93% occurring on the head and neck, 119 were immediately retreated with RT, one was excised, and 67 were not treated. After a median follow-up period of 2.7 years, statistical analysis suggested a 5-year probability of cure in the RT group of 91% and in the untreated group of 61%.[137]

Photodynamic therapy

PDT involves the topical application of δ-aminolevulinic acid (ALA) to the skin, which causes an accumulation of heme precursors several hours after the initial application. These precursors act as photosensitizers, and when exposed to oxygen and an appropriate light source, a cytotoxic reaction induced by oxygen radicals occurs in cells containing these precursors.

Its use in the United Kingdom is still essentially investigational with ongoing clinical trials, and it is not widely available. A prospective study comparing PDT with cryosurgery for superficial BCC (sBCCs) and nodular BCC (nBCCs) in 88 patients reported a recurrence rate at 1 year of 25% for PDT and 15% for cryosurgery.[138] A European study in 118 patients comparing PDT with cryotherapy showed that fewer lesions recurred at 12 months with PDT, 8% versus 16%.[139] A randomized control trial on 151 patients with BCC randomized to receive two PDT illuminations with 1 hour interval or surgical excision showed a lower 5-year cumulative probability of recurrence in the surgical arm (2.3%) versus the PDT arm (30.7%). However, the cumulative probability of recurrence-free survival post-PDT was 65.0% for nBCC measuring greater than 0.7 mm in thickness and 94.4% for tumors less than or equal to 0.7 mm. Therefore, PDT might be an alternative for inoperable patients with thin (≤0.7 mm) nBCC.[140]

One advantage of PDT is that multiple BCC tumors can be treated simultaneously, but it is a relatively inconvenient treatment option. Treatment involves a two-stage process requiring several office visits. After the topical agent is applied, patients must wait several hours (e.g., 14–18 hours for ALA; 3 hours for methyl-ALA) before the light-application phase of the treatment can be initiated. This second stage of treatment must be performed within a certain time frame after agent application. Furthermore, because single PDT treatments demonstrate poor efficacy in BCC, multiple visits may be required. Increased photosensitivity during the first stage of treatment provides additional inconvenience, because patients must avoid sunlight and bright indoor lighting. Treatment with PDT is typically associated with

TABLE 24.1   **Various Radiotherapy Dose Schedules and Fractionations Currently in Use**

NMSC Features	Dose (Gy)	Fractionation	Duration
SCC <3 cm	45	9	21 days
	37.8	6	15 days
	32.4	3	15 days
	18	1	1 day
SCC >3 cm, poorly vascularized skin	45	9	21 days
	54	20	28 days
SCC >5 cm	54	20	28 days
	64	32	46 days
SCC post-op	50	20	28 days
	20	30	46 days
SCC palliative	8	1	1 day
	20	5	7 days
	36	6	Weekly
BCC <3 cm	45	9	21 days
	37.8	6	15 days
	32.4	3	15 days
	18	1	1 day
BCC >3 cm, poorly vascularized skin	45	9	21 days
	50–54	20	28 days
BCC >5 cm	50	20	28 days
	60	30	42 days

localized adverse events, including stinging or burning, erythema, and edema.[116] Treatment with PDT is contraindicated in patients with porphyria, known allergies to porphyrins, and photosensitivity to the wavelengths of the applied light sources.[116] Further development of PDT for BCC will make this a more practical and useful modality, such as, for example, the current use of methyl-ALA providing a shorter pre-exposed application phase of 3 hours.

Drug treatment

Topical fluorouracil

Topical fluorouracil (5-FU) has been used extensively for treatment of BCCs, particularly superficial BCCs. Topical formulations of 5% 5-FU can be administered once or twice daily, depending on tolerability, for 6 weeks or more. Therapy may be required for as long as 12 weeks. A study of 113 patients with sBCC treated with topical 5-FU reports 93% clearance.[116] The common type of nodular tumor is, however, too deep for 5-FU to penetrate adequately, and results in these tumors are poor. It may, however, be used to palliate tumors where a patient may be too debilitated for other treatments. In trials to improve and standardize topical 5-FU therapy, thin BCCs were treated with 25% 5-FU in petrolatum under occlusion for 3 weeks using weekly dressing changes. Of 44 thin BCCs treated, the 5-year cumulative recurrence rate was 21%.[141] In the same study, light curettage preceding the 25% 5-FU treatment in 244 BCCs yielded a better 5-year cumulative recurrence rate of 6%. Cosmetic results were good to excellent in more than 80% in both series.[142]

Side effects include local skin reactions, including pain and burning, pruritus, irritation, inflammation, swelling, tenderness, hyperpigmentation, and scarring.

Imiquimod

As BCC responds, albeit partially, to interferon therapy, treatment with imiquimod, a novel immune-response modifier that activates Toll-like receptors to stimulate the innate immune response (interferon inducer), has been investigated. It is currently licensed for the treatment of external genital and perianal warts, actinic keratoses on the face or scalp, and superficial BCCs. Randomized studies using various schedules, once daily treatments, once or twice a day three times a week, for 6 and 12 weeks to treat sBCCs have shown histological clearance rates of 70–88%.[142,143] Two randomized controlled trials comparing 5% imiquimod cream five times a week and seven times a week have shown histological clearance of 75% and 73%, respectively.[144] There is a correlation between the severity of the local reaction and the histological clearance rate. Imiquimod has also demonstrated efficacy in the treatment of nBCCs using similar schedules with histological clearance rates of 71–76%.[144,145] It has also been studied as an adjunctive therapy before excision with MMS for sBCC and nBCC and been shown to reduce the size of the target tumor and improve the resulting cosmetic defect.

A meta-analysis of 13 studies involving 4256 patients showed that imiquimod was associated with higher histological clearance rate and complete response rate compared with other treatments.[146]

Imiquimod promotes an inflammatory reaction, and treatment is associated with mild-to-moderate local skin reactions. The most common reactions are erythema, crusting, flaking, and erosion. However, these dose-related side effects are generally well-tolerated and in general, do not cause the patient to discontinue treatment. Further follow-up and long-term data are needed, but these studies suggest that imiquimod may be a useful monotherapy for BCCs, and possibly a useful adjunctive treatment.

Vismodegib

This is an oral targeted therapy used in the United Kingdom until 2017 (still approved in the United States) for patients with locally advanced or metastatic BCC that is not amenable to surgery and radiation. As discussed earlier, vismodegib is the first drug to use the Hedgehog pathway to inhibit the proliferation of tumors. A Phase II, non-randomized, multicenter, international study demonstrated a 30.3% objective response rate in metastatic BCC and a 42.9% objective response rate in locally advanced BCC. The drug was very well-tolerated, the main side effects being muscle cramps, loss of taste, hair loss, and weight loss. Rarely, it can cause liver dysfunction, and liver function tests must be monitored. There is currently uncertainty in the evidence and cost effectiveness of vismodegib.[147,148]

Follow-up

Follow-up allows detection of tumor recurrence and early treatment of new lesions. Of the patients who have a previous BCC, 36% will go on to develop a further BCC. Those especially at risk of BCCs are those with skin type I and excess sun exposure. For such high-risk patients, 20% go on to develop multiple BCCs.[149]

Recurrent BCCs tend to develop within 3 years. Although patients with multiple BCCs should be followed up at least 6-monthly on a long-term basis, it is not economically feasible to follow up every BCC patient, especially if it is a single isolated BCC in an older age group. Patient education is perhaps more important.

Squamous cell carcinoma

Primary cutaneous SCC is a malignant tumor arising from epithelial keratinocytes of the epidermis or its appendages. It can grow rapidly, invade locally, and has the rare potential to metastasize.

Incidence

Cutaneous SCC is the second most common human cancer after BCC. There are more than 60,000 cases of NMSC in the United Kingdom each year, and in the United States, there are approximately 200,000 new cases per annum of cutaneous SCC.[150] In the head and neck area, 20% of NMSC is cutaneous SCC, but this rises to 43% in sites such as the pinna.[151]

The common pre-SCC lesion is the actinic keratosis. It is estimated that 11.5% of all visits to a dermatologist in the United States are for actinic keratoses. The incidence of actinic keratoses and SCCs is dependent on cumulative sun exposure and the individual's sun sensitivity. Both are more common in individuals with skin type I. Although actinic keratoses and SCCs are more prevalent in males and tend to occur earlier in males, with advancing age, rates become more equal between the sexes.[152]

Etiology

The factors involved in the etiology and pathogenesis of cutaneous SCC are similar to those for BCC, including exposure to UV radiation, genetic mutations, immunosuppression, and HPV infections. The development of cutaneous SCC has also been associated with radiation exposure, burn scars, chronic inflammatory dermatoses, chronic ulcers, osteomyelitis, and arsenic ingestion (see the discussion earlier in the chapter).

Clinical features

Cutaneous SCC appears most frequently on sun-exposed sites but may occur anywhere. It is usually characterized by a

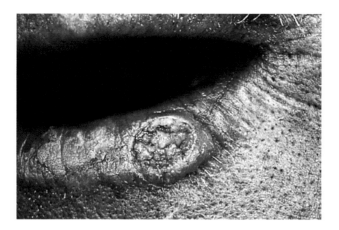

FIGURE 24.10 Squamous cell carcinoma on the lower lip of a patient.

rapidly growing indurated erythematous or skin-colored (non-pigmented) hyperkeratotic nodule or tumor that may ulcerate (Figure 24.10). An appropriate diagnostic biopsy or surgical excision should be performed on any suspicious lesion.

Natural history and risk of recurrence

Primary cutaneous SCC may grow slowly or rapidly and may metastasize, usually to the regional lymph nodes. In a review of 695 cases of cutaneous SCC of the trunk and limbs, metastases occurred in 34 cases, with a metastatic rate of 5%, an overall mortality of 3%, and a mortality in the metastatic group of 70%.[153] SCCs are more likely to spread initially to regional lymph nodes than to distant sites, but visceral metastases have been reported in as many as 5–10% of metastatic cutaneous SCCs. In addition, head and neck cutaneous SCCs can spread to the central nervous system (CNS) hematogenously or via the perineural space.

Local recurrence and regional metastasis are dependent on prior treatment, location, size, depth, cellular differentiation, histological evidence of perineural involvement, and host immune status.[154,155] Cutaneous lesions that recur after previous treatment have a higher risk of local recurrence and metastases. Overall lesions recur locally in 25%, lip lesions in 31.5%, and ear lesions in 45%.[154] Lesions found on the ears and lip are known to be at higher risk of local recurrence and metastasis. SCCs presenting on the lip have an especially high local and metastatic rate,[156] with 8% of patients presenting with clinically positive lymph node involvement and an overall 5-year mortality rate of 17%.[120] Tumors arising on non-sun-exposed sites and sites of previous radiation or thermal injury, chronic ulcers, or chronic inflammation are also reported to have higher metastatic potential.[157] SCC arising from scar tissue is rare but has a higher rate of recurrence than SCC arising in UV-damaged skin. At least 25% of such tumors may recur in 30 months. Recurrence rates double in tumors greater than 2 cm in diameter from 7.4% to 15.2%.[154] It has also been shown that local recurrence and lymph node spread is associated with a depth of invasion over 4 mm and penetration of the subcutis.[158] Local recurrence and metastatic rate increases from 6.7% to 45.7% for tumors with a depth greater than 4 mm.

Poorly differentiated and anaplastic SCCs metastasize more frequently than well-differentiated SCCs, 32.9% versus 9.2%. SCCs with perineural involvement recur in almost half of all cases (47.2%) and show a metastatic rate of 47.3%; SCCs on the mid-face and lip are especially prone to neural involvement.

Careful follow-up of patients with these high-risk features is recommended.

Pathology

Pre-malignant SCC in situ without dermal invasion, actinic keratosis and Bowen's disease, has been discussed earlier. Invasive SCC consists of irregular dermal nodules, composed of a mixture of anaplastic keratinocytes, budding from the epidermis into the dermis. Characteristically, these are relatively large cells, showing lack of maturation, nuclear atypia, and the presence of mitotic figures. In early tumors, there may be an associated lymphocytic infiltrate. They can be graded as well-, moderately-, or poorly differentiated, which has prognostic value. Perineural involvement is of prognostic significance, but lymphovascular invasion is not an independent risk factor.[157]

Special histological variants include the adenoid type (or acantholytic variant), which occurs mainly on the head in the elderly, the verrucous type, which occurs mainly in the oral mucosa, penis, or sole of the foot, and the spindle cell type. Certain types of benign skin tumor, such as KA, may mimic the appearance of SCC. KAs grow rapidly and consist of a solitary nodular lesion with a central keratin plug, which resolves spontaneously if left for up to 4–6 months; KA has a characteristic histological appearance consisting of an exophytic squamo-proliferative nodule with symmetrical buttressed edges and large tumor cells with pale eosinophilic cytoplasm. Mitoses may be seen, and there is a stromal reaction associated with blunt down-growths of squamous epithelium at the lower border of the tumor. Indeed, some authorities consider the KA to be an immunologically controlled SCC. KAs may be derived from follicular structures, and it has been proposed that their regression may be due to recapitulation of the hair cycle. They are usually treated by surgical techniques including curettage/cautery. A very rare familial autosomal dominant variant characterized by multiple self-healing KA (Ferguson Smith type) has been localized to a currently unidentified gene on chromosome 9p22 very close to the *PTCH* gene of Gorlin syndrome. As with Gorlin syndrome, RT is relatively contraindicated.

Other adnexal tumors that should be distinguished clinically and histologically from SCC include eccrine porocarcinoma (mainly located on the lower limbs in the elderly), sebaceous carcinoma (mostly located in the head and neck region, especially the ocular area, with significant risk of metastasis: 20–25%), and verrucous carcinoma (mucosal, genital, and acral sites).

Molecular pathogenesis

SCCs are associated with high rates (28%) of UV signature mutations of key tumor suppressor genes such as *p53*. In addition, inactivation of *ARF* (13%) and *P16* (13%) also contributes to loss of the G_1 cell cycle checkpoint control. Activation of the RAS pathway inducing RAF-MEK-ERK signaling has also been shown to be a critical step in SCC due to *HRAS* mutations (22%) and increased expression of RAS-GTP (75%).[159,160]

Treatment

The methods of treatment of SCC are similar to those described for BCC. However, SCC has a much greater metastatic potential, and therefore, it is important to ensure that the entire tumor is removed. High-risk tumors, especially those on the lips and ears, are treated more aggressively, as the risk of local recurrence and distant metastases is higher. As for BCCs, the treatments are highly effective and can achieve cure rates of 95%. Patients with high-risk

SCC presenting with involved lymph nodes should be reviewed by a multidisciplinary oncology team including a dermatologist, a pathologist, an appropriately trained plastic or maxillo-facial surgeon, a clinical oncologist, and a clinical nurse specialist.[157,161]

Surgical excision

Margins of 4 mm are adequate for most SCCs. However, for high-risk SCC associated with a greater risk of subclinical tumor extension, at least a 6–10 mm margin is recommended.[120,162,163]

Elective prophylactic lymph node dissection has been proposed for SCC on the lip greater than 6 mm in depth and cutaneous SCC greater than 8 mm in depth, but the evidence for this is weak.[157] It is not routinely practiced, and the risk of morbidity has to be seriously considered.

Mohs' micrographic surgery

Mohs' micrographic surgery allows precise definition and excision of the primary tumor and offers the best cure rates for high-risk tumors.[154,164] It should therefore be considered in the surgical treatment of high-risk SCC, particularly at difficult sites where wide surgical margins may be technically difficult to achieve without functional impairment.

Curettage and cautery

This technique is likely to result in inadequate clearance, and it should not be regarded as an adequate form of treatment for SCC,[157] although this is often acceptable for KAs and occasionally for palliative treatment of SCC in the elderly.

Cryotherapy

Cryotherapy may be used for actinic keratosis, but it is not recommended as treatment for SCC.

Radiotherapy

RT is generally reserved for patients above 45 years of age because of the theoretical risk of inducing further malignancies. It is not suitable for tumors invading underlying cartilage, where the risk of radiochondritis is high and cure rates are lower. There is a relative contraindication to treating SCCs in cardiac or renal transplant patients, as these patients may be particularly susceptible to further cutaneous malignancies. The 5-year cure rate for treating NMSC with RT is as high as 90%, and the cosmetic results have been evaluated as good or acceptable in 84% of treated lesions. The acute complication rate is low, and the chronic complication rate is even lower.[130] Treatment schedules are similar to those for BCC, with fractionated dose schedules. There may be a benefit to higher dose schedules, and larger lesions will require more fractionated courses. Electron beam therapy is very good for lesions in sites difficult to treat by more conventional methods.[134]

RT can be used as an adjuvant modality for high-risk SCC, for example, more than 2 cm with perineural invasion in a high-risk site. It has been shown in high-risk cutaneous SCCs of the head and neck region with lymph node spread to reduce the risk of recurrence by 50%.[165] However, the value of adjuvant RT is widely debated due to lack of prospective randomized clinical trial data.

RT may also be used palliatively for patients with lymph node metastases.

Chemotherapy

For patients with extensive SCC that has relapsed after conventional surgery or RT or for metastatic disease, a variety of drugs, including bleomycin, methotrexate, actinomycin, vincristine, vinblastine, fluorouracil (5-FU), and hydroxyurea, have been used with varying degrees of success.[166] The most commonly used are cisplatin, carboplatin, and 5-FU, either as monotherapy or in combination regimens.[167–169] Cisplatin has been used as monotherapy and in combination with other cytotoxic drugs in advanced lesions and metastatic cutaneous SCC. Eleven patients with advanced BCC or SCC of the skin were treated with cisplatin (75 mg/m^2, intravenous [IV]) plus doxyrubicin (50 mg/m^2, IV) at 3-week intervals. Responses were seen after 10–12 courses, and five of the 11 patients were in remission at the time of report.[165] A combination of cisplatin, 5-FU, and bleomycin produced partial or complete remission (CR) in 11/14 patients with advanced cutaneous SCC.[170] The search for more active combinations continues. A Phase II study of interferon-α (IFN-α), retinoic acid, and cisplatin in 39 patients with advanced SCC of the skin showed an overall response rate (ORR) of 34% with a median duration of response of 9 months.[171] In August 2019, Cemiplimab, a monoclonal antibody that binds the programmed death receptor-1 (PD-1), has become available in the UK under Cancer Drug Fund for the treatment of locally advanced or metastatic cutaneous SCC.

Follow-up

Patients with a history of SCC of skin are more likely to develop similar lesions. In a follow-up study of 101 SCC patients, 52% subsequently developed NMSC within 5 years of therapy for the first lesion,[172] and 95% of local recurrences and metastases are detected within 5 years.[157] It is recommended that patients should be followed up every 3 months for the first year and every 6 months thereafter, for a minimum of 5 years after initial treatment. Patients should be examined for local recurrence, metastatic spread, and new tumors. Recurrent lesions are treated where possible by surgical excision.[157] Mohs' surgery is particularly suitable to ensure complete clearance of recurrent tumor. Patients with recurrent lesions should be followed up indefinitely. All patients should be taught to self-examine regularly for local and regional recurrence.

Primary cutaneous lymphoma

Cutaneous lymphomas are a heterogeneous group of disorders characterized by localization of malignant lymphocytes to the skin. The term "primary cutaneous lymphoma" refers to cutaneous T-cell lymphomas (CTCL) and cutaneous B-cell lymphomas (CBCL) that present in the skin with no evidence of extracutaneous disease at the time of diagnosis. Primary cutaneous lymphomas often have a different clinical behavior, require different treatment, and have a different prognosis from histologically similar systemic lymphomas, which may involve the skin secondarily. Two-thirds of primary cutaneous lymphomas are T-cell in origin (CTCL), of which mycosis fungoides (MF) accounts for 60% of new cases. Sézary syndrome (SS) accounts for only 5% of CTCL cases, and CBCL accounts for 25% of all cutaneous lymphoma cases reported.

Incidence

The incidence of cutaneous lymphomas is 0.7 per 100,000 U.K. population with a higher incidence in men (1.6:1.0), in the elderly, and in African-Americans.[173] Most are low grade with long survival, and the overall prevalence is much higher.

Etiology

Although the fundamental etiology and molecular abnormalities that underlie the pathogenesis of different primary cutaneous lymphomas are still an enigma, there is now a wealth of data confirming a wide range of molecular changes. These are reflected in the World Health Organization–European Organization for Research and Treatment of Cancer (WHO-EORTC) classification of primary cutaneous lymphomas and are incorporated into the latest WHO Classification.[174–176] The WHO-EORTC classification provides a molecular basis for distinguishing extranodal primary cutaneous lymphomas from their nodal counterparts with a similar morphology and immunophenotype and crucially explains the different prognosis for lymphomas arising in specific extranodal sites.[174] It has been postulated that MF is a disease of antigen persistence within the skin, causing chronic lymphocyte stimulation with the eventual transformation of lymphocytes into a low-grade T-cell malignancy.[180] Studies have also demonstrated that the neoplastic cell in MF/SS is a Th2 cell. In the early stages of the disease, reactive T cells with a Th1 phenotype predominate as part of an anti-tumor response and with disease progression, the malignant Th2 cells become dominant with loss of epidermotropism.[181–183] Migration of T cells to the epidermis is mediated by various chemokines and adhesion molecules, but this is lost with the development of tumors.[184] Detailed investigation of pre-existing allergies, atopy, or biological, physical, or chemical exposure has failed to demonstrate a correlation between these factors and CTCL.[185] An association of CTCL with the human T-cell lymphoma/leukemia virus I and II (HTLV-1 and 2) has not been proven.[186,187]

In primary CBCL of marginal-zone origin, there is evidence from some geographic areas of an association with *Borrelia burgdorferi* infection. A study from Italy has shown that *B. burgdorferi*-specific sequence was detected in 15 out of 83 skin samples of patients with primary CBCL (18.1%), but in none out of 83 matched healthy controls ($p < 0.0001$).[188] A more recent study from Italy does not support a pathogenic role for *B burgdorferi* in areas nonendemic for this microorganism.[183]

Classification

Cutaneous lymphoma is classified according to the WHO 2016 classification.[176] Table 24.2 shows the classification.[176]

Primary cutaneous T-cell lymphoma

This section will discuss the features and treatment of the different types of CTCL as classified by the WHO-EORTC.

Initial assessment, staging, and diagnosis

The most common type of primary CTCL is MF. The onset of MF is often insidious, with initial manifestations difficult to distinguish from inflammatory dermatoses. The other types of primary CTCL, such as Sézary syndrome (SS), may also present insidiously or more rapidly, and their clinicopathological features are discussed in more detail later.

The clinical staging system was updated in 2007 by the International Society for Cutaneous Lymphomas (ISCL) and EORTC to incorporate advances related to tumor cell biology and new diagnostic techniques. MF and SS are staged according to the current ISCL/EORTC revision of the classification of mycosis fungoides and Sézary syndrome.[189] Early-stage disease is Stage IA and IB with just patch and plaque disease (T1 and T2). Later-stage disease is Stage IIB (T3 tumor stage), III (T4 erythroderma), IVA1 (B2 blood involvement), IVA2 (N3 effaced lymph node involvement), and IVB (M1 visceral involvement).

Recent studies in MF have shown that while prognosis is dependent on clinical stage, patients with early-stage disease can be stratified according to several factors, including the presence

TABLE 24.2 Classification of Primary Cutaneous Lymphomas

Cutaneous B-cell lymphoma
- Indolent
  - Primary cutaneous marginal zone B-cell lymphoma
  - Primary cutaneous follicle center lymphoma
- Intermediate
  - Primary cutaneous diffuse large B-cell lymphoma—leg type.
  - Primary cutaneous diffuse large B-cell lymphoma—NOS

Cutaneous T-cell lymphoma
- Indolent
  - Mycosis fungoides (Stage 1A–1B)
  - Mycosis fungoides variants (Stage 1A–1B)
    - Folliculotropic MF
    - Pagetoid reticulosis
    - Granulomatous slack disease
  - Primary cutaneous CD30+ lymphoproliferative disorders
    - Primary cutaneous anaplastic large cell lymphoma
    - Lymphomatoid papulosis
  - Subcutaneous panniculitis-like T-cell lymphoma
  - Primary cutaneous CD4+ small/medium pleomorphic T-cell lymphoproliferative disorder
  - Primary cutaneous acral CD8+ T-cell lymphoma
- Aggressive
  - Mycosis fungoides (Stage IIB–IVB)
  - Sézary syndrome
  - Primary cutaneous aggressive epidermotropic cytotoxic CD8+ T-cell lymphoma
  - Primary cutaneous γ/δ T-cell lymphoma
  - Extranodal natural killer/T-cell lymphoma, nasal type
  - Primary cutaneous peripheral T-cell lymphoma, unspecified

Source: Adapted from the WHO and EORTC classifications, Willemze et al., 2005.

of folliculotropism or plaques and age at diagnosis. This is now the subject of extensive prospective studies.[189–193]

The following are recommendations from the 2018 Joint Guidelines of the British Association of Dermatologists (BAD) and the U.K. cutaneous lymphoma group (UKCLG):[177]

- Repeated skin biopsies (ellipse rather than punch) are often required to confirm a diagnosis of CTCL.
- Histology, immunophenotypical, and preferably T-cell receptor (TCR) gene analysis should be performed on all tissue samples (ideally, molecular studies require fresh tissue).
- All patients (with the possible exception of early-stage MF [stage IA] and lymphomatoid papulosis [LyP]) should ideally be reviewed by an appropriate multidisciplinary team for confirmation of the diagnosis and to establish a management strategy.
- Initial staging CT is required in all patients with the exception of those with early stages of MF (Stage IA and IB) and LyP. The value of positron emission tomography (PET) CT in MF/SS is unclear at present but may indicate which nodal basin to sample.
- At diagnosis, peripheral blood samples should be analyzed for total white cell, lymphocyte and Sézary cell counts, serum lactate dehydrogenase (LDH), liver and renal function, lymphocyte subsets, CD4:CD8 ratios, HTLV-1 serology, and preferably, TCR gene analysis.
- Bone marrow aspirate or trephine biopsies are required for CTCL variants (with the exception of LyP) and may also be appropriate for those with late stages of MF (Stage IIB or above and SS).

Several small studies in MF and SS have shown that PET/CT is more sensitive in detecting lymph nodes and cutaneous tumors involved by lymphoma compared with CT data alone but does not adequately detect erythroderma, patches, or plaques.[194,195] Palpable lymph nodes should have histological confirmation with an excision or core biopsy, as fine needle aspirates cannot accurately establish histological lymph node involvement in MF.

A central panel, usually within the specialist cancer center, should review all histology, and it is important that the histological features are correlated with the clinical features and the patient's disease classified according to the WHO-EORTC classification.[176] In addition to morphology, immunophenotypical studies and TCR gene analysis should be performed on all tissue samples. Immunophenotypical studies should be performed on paraffin-embedded sections and include the T-cell markers CD2, CD3, CD4, CD8, B-cell marker CD20, and the activation marker CD30. Additional markers such as p53 may have prognostic significance in MF and other CTCL types such as adult T-cell leukemia/lymphoma (ATLL). Markers of cytotoxic function such as TIA-I, the monocyte macrophage marker CD68, and natural killer (NK) cell marker CD56 may be useful for specific CTCL variants.

Mycosis fungoides

Alibert, a French dermatologist, first used the term "MF" when he described a severe disorder in which large necrotic tumors presented on a patient's skin.

Clinicopathological features

MF is the classical "Alibert–Bazin" type of CTCL characterized by the slow evolution of patches, plaques, and tumors over years or sometimes decades (Figures 24.11 through 24.13).

Erythrodermic MF is characterized by more than 80% skin involvement with diffuse infiltration that can give rise to a leonine facies (Figure 24.14).

When tumors develop in MF, they commonly show ulceration, but the patient must have typical polymorphic patches and plaques of MF in other sites to confirm a diagnosis of MF. It typically affects older adults but may occur at any age. The initial skin lesions are most often on sun-protected skin around the bathing trunk distribution. In the later stages, it may involve the lymph nodes and visceral organs. If only tumors are present without the preceding evolution of patches and plaques, then another type of CTCL should be considered.

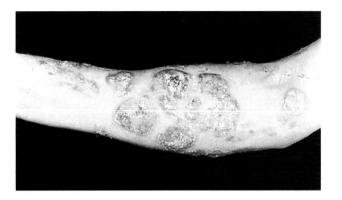

FIGURE 24.12 Plaque stage of cutaneous T-cell lymphomas (CTCL) with well-demarcated papillosquamous lesions on the forearms.

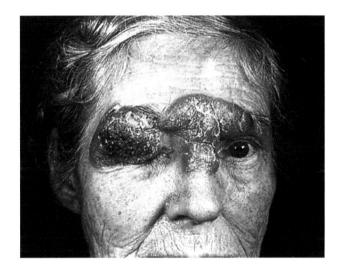

FIGURE 24.13 Tumis cutaneous T-cell lymphomas (CTCL) arising from long-standing plaque stage disease on the forehead and supraocular region.

The histopathological changes characteristic of MF are an epidermotropic proliferation of small to medium-sized T-lymphocytes with cerebriform nuclei that colonize the basal layer of the epidermis as single haloed cells or a linear configuration of cells. Epidermotropism is more pronounced in plaques than in patches. Pautrier microabscesses (intra-epidermal collections of atypical cells) are a highly characteristic feature. The dermal infiltrate becomes more diffuse and epidermotropism may be lost with progression to tumor stage. Large cell transformation may develop, and the cells may be negative or positive for CD30. Transformation is often associated with more aggressive disease and a poorer prognosis.

MF cells have a CD3+, CD4+, CD8− memory T-cell phenotype. There are rare cases of CD4−, CD8+ classical MF, which have the same clinical behavior and prognosis, although CD8+ MF is more common in childhood MF and in those patients with hypopigmented variants.

Molecular pathogenesis

In CTCL, no disease-specific balanced translocations have yet been identified, but molecular cytogenetic studies do indicate

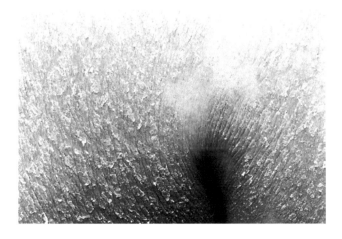

FIGURE 24.11 Patch stage of cutaneous T-cell lymphomas (CTCL) of the poikiloderma atrophicans type.

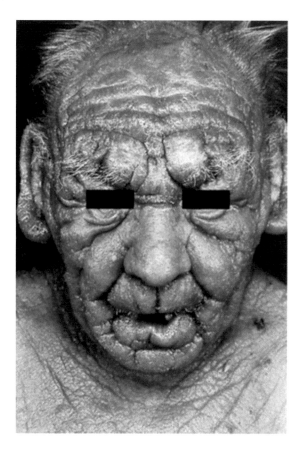

FIGURE 24.14 Erythrodermic cutaneous T-cell lymphomas (CTCL) in an elderly man with diffuse infiltration of the skin giving rise to leonine facies.

that MF and SS have a closely related pattern of chromosomal abnormalities, suggesting that the two conditions share a similar pathogenesis.[196,197] Numerical rather than structural abnormalities predominate, with losses of 1p, 10q, 13q, and 17p and gains of 4, 17q, and 18 being common.[198–200] Recent genomic studies using high throughput sequencing platforms in MF and particularly SS have shown a wide range of gene mutations specifically targeting TCR signaling, chromatin remodeling, and DNA damage response. Many of these gene variants have been shown to have functional relevance, including causing constitutive transcriptional activation of NFAT, NFkB, and AP1 as well as signal-transducers and activators of transcription, namely STAT3 and STAT5. While this complex mutational landscape has a wide variety of potential consequences, a unifying hypothesis would be that there is dysregulation of T-cell activation in MF/SS, which prevents activation-induced T-cell death.[201]

Therapy

Overview

The UKCLG guidelines for management of cutaneous lymphomas have been updated (2018).[177] The current therapeutic approach in MF consists of skin-directed therapies for early stages of the disease. The rationale for this approach is based on the randomized controlled trial by Kaye et al., which showed that intensive therapy with total skin electron beam radiotherapy (TSEB) and combination chemotherapy had a higher response rate but did not improve survival when compared with a palliative initial skin-directed approach to treatment.[202] The complete response rate

was 38% versus 18%, but the morbidity was greater on the combination treatment arm. The overall survival was the same in both groups at 75 months. There are a large number of uncontrolled trials with data showing that the disease responds to treatment but relapses, and no therapy has been shown to impact on overall survival.[203] Therapy therefore needs to be individualized to the patient and delivered by an experienced multidisciplinary team. Maintenance of quality of life is central to the therapeutic strategy. Psychological issues must be addressed, and issues such as skin pain control are important and often overlooked. The therapeutic options are discussed in detail in the following subsections. In the majority of patients with early disease and normal life expectancy, toxic and aggressive therapies should be avoided. Patients with more advanced disease should be offered entry into appropriate clinical trials, as the therapies discussed below are mostly palliative and do not have a significant impact on disease outcome. Figures 24.15 and 24.16 show the various therapeutic options by stage of disease.[177]

Topical therapy

Topical emollients can be used with aqueous cream combined with menthol, which is sometimes helpful for pruritus. Topical corticosteroids can induce complete clearance of disease, but this is usually short lived.[204] Topical mechlorethamine (nitrogen mustard, NH2) is effective for superficial disease, and there is now a European Medicines Agency (EMA)-approved gel that has shown similar efficacy to historical compounded ointment and aqueous products.[205] There is no consensus on whether it should be applied to individual lesions or to the whole skin, daily or twice daily, or the duration of treatment. Hypersensitivity reactions and irritant or allergic dermatitis occur in 10–67% but are less likely with the ointment formulation. It should not be used in pregnancy. Topical carmustine (BCNU) is a topical chemotherapeutic agent with response rates of 47–86%, dependent on stage. Alternate-day or daily treatment with 10 mg of carmustine in 60 mL of dilute alcohol (95%) or a 20–40% ointment is used. Hypersensitivity reactions are seen in 5–10% of cases. Regular blood counts should be performed to monitor for bone marrow suppression, and for this reason, maintenance therapy is not advised.[188] Bexarotene gel is a topical rexinoid that has been approved by the U.S. Food and Drug Administration (FDA) for topical therapy of early Stage I MF but is not licensed in Europe. A Phase I/II study in 67 patients reported a 63% response rate with 21% complete responses. The median time to response was 20 weeks with a median duration of 99 weeks. It is generally well-tolerated, with irritant side effects restricted to the site of application.[189]

Phototherapy

The standard for early-stage MF is psoralen ultraviolet A (PUVA), which consists of oral psoralen (8-methoxypsoralen; 8-MOP; methoxsalen) plus ultraviolet A phototherapy.[173,189] Psoralens form bifunctional and monofunctional DNA adducts when photoactivated. PUVA produces response rates of 79–88% in Stage IA and 52–59% in Stage IB. It is ideal for patients with Stage IB/IIA who are intolerant or fail to respond to topical therapy, although both therapies can be complementary. There is no significant response in Stage IIB tumor stage MF, but PUVA can occasionally be effective for erythrodermic Stage III disease, if tolerated, and combined PUVA and IFN-α has also been used for Stage III disease with some benefit. A recent EORTC Phase III trial comparing PUVA plus bexarotene with PUVA alone in early Stage IB–IIA disease showed no difference in overall response, but there was a trend to a lower cumulative UVA dose to achieve response in the combination arm.[206]

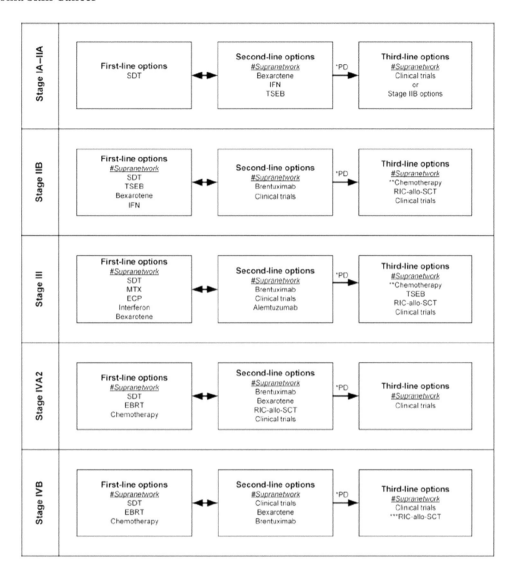

FIGURE 24.15 UKCLG recommendations for treatment of mycoidal fungoides. EBRT, external beam radiotherapy with photons or electrons for lymph node, soft tissue or visceral lymphoma; ECP, extracorporeal photopheresis; IFN, interferon; MTX, methotrexate; PD, progressive disease; RIC-allo-SCT, reduced intensity allogeneic stem cell transplantation; SDT, skin-directed therapy (topical steroids, ultraviolet B, psoralen-ultraviolet A, skin radiotherapy, topical nitrogen mustard); TSEB, total skin electron beam radiotherapy. Skin radiotherapy indicates superficial radiotherapy or EBRT to skin patches, plaques, and tumors. #Supranetwork: refers to the supranetwork multidisciplinary team (MDT) meeting for treatment decision. *PD and exhausted first- and second-line options. **Chemotherapy as recommended by the supranetwork MDT. ***Consider only if the patient has durable complete response. ↔ indicates that after treatment, patients may respond to treatments included in earlier "line" options. Patients can move between first- and second-line options. (From Gilson et al., 2018. With permission.)

Treatment schedules can vary but are usually two to three times weekly until the disease is cleared or best partial response (PR) attained. Efforts are made to restrict the total cumulative dose of PUVA to 1200 J/cm², or fewer than 200 treatment sessions, to reduce the risk of NMSC. Nausea occurs rarely but can be avoided by using 5-methoxypsoralen (5-MOP) instead of 8-MOP. PUVA is one of the most effective therapies for early-stage MF, but there is no data to establish whether it improves overall survival. Broadband and narrowband UVB and high-dose UVA1 phototherapy can also achieve good responses in early stages of MF but may not be as effective as PUVA for those with extensive plaques. UVB may have a lower risk of cutaneous carcinogenesis than PUVA, but there have been no adequate comparative studies in MF as yet.

Radiotherapy

RT is a very effective single agent for the treatment of MF. Dramatic responses to low doses of x-ray therapy were first reported in 1902.[207] RT is now widely used to treat individual thick plaques, eroded plaques, or tumors, and the whole skin can be successfully treated with TSEB.

MF is a very radiosensitive disease. Several clinical studies have evaluated the dose–response relationship in MF. There is a direct correlation between disease-free interval and dose, and split dose experiments have shown no difference in tumor regrowth at intervals of 1 or 7 days, suggesting little recovery between fractions, enabling protracted fractionation regimens.[208]

A study of fractionated RT for individual plaques and tumors has shown a response rate of 89–96%, with the likelihood of

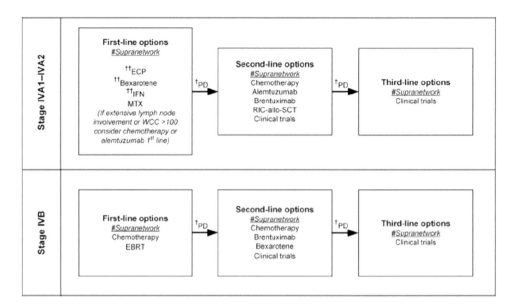

FIGURE 24.16 UKCLG recommendations for treatment of Sézary syndrome. Palliative skin-directed therapy can be used for symptom control if required. Chemotherapy is as directed by the supranetwork multidisciplinary team (MDT). EBRT, external beam radiotherapy; ECP, extracorporeal photopheresis; IFN, interferon; MTX, methotrexate; PD, progressive disease; RIC-allo-SCT, reduced-intensity allogeneic stem cell transplantation; WCC, white cell count, 9 109. #Supranetwork: refer to the supranetwork MDT meeting for treatment decision. †PD and exhausted first- and second-line options. ††May be used in combination. (From Gilson et al., 2018. With permission.)

recurrence inversely related to dose. Local recurrence occurred in 42% with doses lower than 10 Gy, 32% for doses of 10–20 Gy, 21% for doses 20–30 Gy, and no recurrences with doses over 30 Gy.[209] A study of very low-dose 4 Gy in two fractions showed that 70% of patients failed to respond. When the dose was increased to 8 Gy in two fractions, the complete response rate was 92% (60/65 lesions).[210] A similar dose–control relationship has been shown for TSEB. The Stanford data has shown the CR rate to be 18% for lower than 10 Gy, 55% for 10–20 Gy, 75% for doses of 25–30 Gy, and 94% for doses more than 30 Gy.[211]

Current standard therapy consists of low-dose superficial RT to treat individual thick or eroded plaques and tumors initially. This can be combined with other modalities such as PUVA. Large tumors may be treated with electrons depending on the tumor position, size, and thickness. Standard low fractionated schedules of 8 Gy in two fractions for patches and plaques, 12 Gy in three fractions for tumors, and 15 Gy in five fractions for large fields are used.[177,212] A single-institution center in the United States has shown that a single fraction of 7 or 8 Gy has a complete response rate of 94%, which is an excellent palliative option for some patients but limits the ability for retreatment compared with fractionated schedules.[213] Closely adjacent and overlapping fields can often be retreated successfully, and the low doses allow the safe use of TSEB later in the patient's disease. The possible exception to this is unilesional presentation of MF, which is rare, but local RT may be curative in this setting.[214] Disease-free survival following RT alone is reported as 85% at 10 years using fractionated treatment to a total dose of 20–30 Gy.[214]

Whole-body TSEB therapy has been evaluated extensively in CTCL, although it is not widely available. It was first reported for MF in 1953 by Trump et al. and informed the design of the LINAC. The most widely used technique is that reported by Stanford in 1960, and the first clinical results were published by the St John's Institute of Dermatology in 1962.[214,215] The Stanford technique involves the patient standing in six different positions

to allow maximum unfolding of the skin in areas such as the axillae. Sites such as the perineum, soles of the feet, and scalp need extra patch treatments with RT. The RT is delivered by a LINAC in high dose-rate electron mode with the beam attenuated so that the effective dose at the patient surface is approximately 4 MeV. It is a technically challenging treatment, and careful attention to dosimetry is needed. Consensus guidelines for TSEB have been published by the EORTC and make recommendations on the technique, dosimetry, patch, and boost treatments, radiation prescription dose, schedule, fractionation, and shielding.[216] The 80% isodose must be at least 4 mm deep with respect to the skin surface along the primary axis of the beam, and the dose at 20 mm should be less than 20% of the maximum skin-surface dose. Photon contamination must be reduced to less than 0.7 Gy for the full course to limit the dose to the bone marrow. Areas that are inherently shielded may be patch treated, and there are retrospective data suggesting that this may improve outcome.[216] Large tumors should be debulked with palliative short courses of RT before TSEB to improve response and to start the healing of large tumors, which helps the patient to tolerate treatment. Other techniques, such as the McGill rotating technique, are used by some centers and meet the EORTC recommendations.[217] This 2002 EORTC consensus recommends at least 26 Gy to a depth of 4 mm in the skin and 31–36 Gy to the truncal surface with similar patch treatments to inherently shielded areas such as the soles of the feet. Fractionation to 30–36 fractions over 6–10 weeks is recommended, and keeping the dose per fraction below 2–2.5 Gy reduces the long-term side effects. The availability of TSEB has now improved in the United Kingdom. There are now centers offering TSEB in London, Birmingham, Manchester, Clatterbridge, Leeds, Nottingham, Newcastle, and Belfast.

A systematic review of open uncontrolled and mostly retrospective studies of TSEB as monotherapy in 952 patients with CTCL has established that responses are stage-dependent. It has a role in every stage of the disease. In Stage IA, complete responses of 96% with 10-year recurrence-free survival (RFS) of 50% are reported.[217,218] However, this is a controversial first-line treatment for such early-stage disease, where long-term survival is similar to that of healthy controls; TSEB is, therefore, reserved for patients refractory to standard first-line skin-directed therapy.[219,220] In Stage IB/IIA disease, CR rates of 76–90% are reported but with a 10-year RFS of only 10% with TSEB alone. This indicated that TSEB is not curative, even in early disease, but significant disease control can be achieved and hopefully maintained with adjuvant therapy.[216,221–223] Retrospective data from Yale has shown that adjuvant PUVA improves the 5-year disease-free survival (DFS) from 50% to 85%, and data from Stanford shows that adjuvant use of topical mechlorethamine improves 10-year RFS from 10% to 40%.

In stage IIB disease, complete responses are less common (36–54%) with a 5-year RFS of 30% with TSEB alone.[173,217,221] Adjuvant mechlorethamine improves the 5-year RFS to 55%, and retrospective data from Yale have shown a 5-year RFS of 100% in patients treated with adjuvant photophoresis following TSEB. Other adjuvant options include IFN-α and bexarotene. The newer single-agent chemotherapy drugs can be used to debulk extensive tumors before TSEB.

The standard TSEB schedule in the United States has historically been 36 Gy in 36 fractions over 9 weeks.[211] In the United Kingdom, the standard schedule developed at St Johns has been 30 Gy in 20 fractions over 5 weeks; it has an ORR of 95% with a median duration of response of 18 months in Stage IB and 9 months in Stage IIB patients.[229] The median time to relapse in Stage IB is 18 months, and in Stage IIB it is 9 months; however, there is a small minority of patients who maintain the response to TSEB for more than 10 years.[224] The side effects of this 5-week schedule are the same as for the longer, more fractionated 9-week schedules.[224]

For erythrodermic (Stage III) disease, TSEB is very effective and can produce rapid and sustained responses. A retrospective study of erythrodermic disease has also shown 60% CR, with 26% progression free at 5 years.[223] In this study, the overall median survival was 3.4 years with a median dose of 32 Gy given as five fractions per week over 6–9 weeks. Patients with Stage III disease did best compared with those with significant nodal or hematological (IVA and IVB) disease. The duration of response was also longer for those who received more than 20 Gy using 4–9 MeV. Adjuvant photophoresis may be of benefit, and retrospective data from Yale show an improvement in 2-year cause-specific survival from 69% to 100%.[223] In Stage IVA disease, TSEB may be used palliatively with CR in the order of 70%, but this is short-lived.[216]

Acute adverse effects of TSEB are usually minor with modern techniques and attention to care of the patient's skin.[225] They include fatigue, temporary alopecia, nail loss, leg swelling and blisters, minor nose bleeds (1 in 30), reduced sweating (1 in 30), minor parotitis (1 in 30), gynecomastia (1 in 30), and skin infection, which is rare but must be treated aggressively (<1 in 100). Late effects are skin atrophy, hypothyroidism, nail and finger changes, sun sensitivity, and infertility in men. Combined with previous skin-directed therapy (SDT) and PUVA, TSEB adds to the patient's risk of other cutaneous malignancies.

Although TSEB is usually only given once in a lifetime, several reports have documented patients who have received two or three courses; however, the total doses tolerated and the duration of response have been lower with subsequent courses.[173,216] Given the high response rate of MF to low-dose RT schedules, lower-dose schedules of TSEB have been studied: A European study of very low-dose 4 Gy TSEB fractionated over 4 days showed a response rate of 88% but with a very short duration of response of only 2.7 months.[226] A small study in 21 patients treated with 10 Gy in 10 fractions of TSEB showed an ORR of 95% with a CR in 57%

of patients. The median duration of cutaneous response was 5.8 months, with very low toxicity.[227] A pooled analysis of three Phase II trials from the United States using 12 Gy reported an overall response rate of 88% with a median duration of clinical benefit of 70.7 weeks.[228] A series from the United Kingdom using 12 Gy in eight fractions over 2 weeks in 103 patients reported a median duration of response of 18 months in Stage IB and 10 months in Stage IIB with significantly less toxicity.[245] A European study of low-dose TSEB in 44 patients showed that TSEB improved disease symptoms and significantly improved emotional domains of patients' quality of life. This study showed early indications that maintenance or adjuvant therapy after TSEB may improve the progression-free survival (PFS).[230] The low-dose TSEB schedule has become the standard option, and studies are under way looking at combination and maintenance treatments.

Reduced intensity stem cell transplantation

Reduced intensity stem cell transplantation is a possible curative option for some patients with MF and Sézary syndrome. The MD Anderson reported 19 patients with advanced disease in whom TSEB was used before conditioning with fludarabine and melphalan (and anti-thymocyte globulin for mismatched donors) and an allogeneic stem cell transplant.[231] In this series, 11 patients remain in CR with a median follow-up of 19 months, and median survival has not yet been reached. A recent analysis of an EBMT cohort of 60 patients reported an OS of 46% and PFS of 32% at 5 years.[232] Relapse/progression occurred in 45% at a median of 3.8 months following hematopoietic stem cell transplantation (HSCT), but many patients were rescued with donor lymphocyte infusions. Non-relapse mortality was 22%, with the latest non-relapse death occurring 14 months following HSCT. TSEB can be considered a safe and effective debulking regimen before conditioning. Long-term results of a conditioning regimen using TSEB, total lymph node irradiation, and anti-thymocyte globulin conditioning prior to stem cell transplant are awaited; early results are encouraging, with a reduced 1-year non-relapse mortality.[233]

Immunotherapy

Immunotherapy has been used in CTCL to enhance the anti-tumor host responses by promoting the generation of cytotoxic T cells and Th1 cytokine responses.

The most commonly used immunotherapy is IFN-α, which binds to the type 1 interferon receptor expressed by CTCL. It acts via its effects on cell cycle regulation, oncogene suppression, and modulation of cell adhesion.[234] Studies have shown ORRs of 45–74% with CR rates of 10–27%.[234–237] The dosage schedule most commonly used is 3 MU three times a week, increased if tolerated to a maximum of 36 MU per week, but in practice, it is rare for patients to tolerate more than 15 MU per week. Response rates are higher with higher doses and higher in earlier compared with later stages of disease.[236,237] Side effects include dose-related "flu"-like symptoms, elevated transaminases, leukopenia, and thrombocytopenia. Recent manufacturing changes have meant that non-pegylated IFN-α is unavailable, and many centers are now using weekly pegylated IFN-α2a.[238]

IFN-α has been used in combination therapy. Adding PUVA to IFN-α has been shown to improve the CR rate from 38% to 70%, but there is no data on duration of response.[239] Uncontrolled studies of PUVA and IFN-α in MF and SS have shown an overall remission rate (RR) of 100% with a 62% CR rate, and combination therapy is useful for patients with resistant early-stage disease, such as those with thick plaques and folliculotropic disease.[240] A randomized study in early-stage disease comparing PUVA with

PUVA and IFN-α has shown a similar RR, but the cumulative dose of PUVA was lower in the combination arm. IFN-α has been used in combination with retinoids, but no improvement in RR has been shown.[241]

Small cohort studies have reported that interleukin-12 (IL-12) and IFN-α can produce clinical responses, but their role remains to be established. Cyclosporine is contraindicated, as it may cause disease progression.[242,243]

Alemtuzumab is a humanized recombinant IgG monoclonal antibody specific for the CD52 cell surface glycoprotein found on malignant B and T cells, but opportunistic infections such as cytomegalovirus (CMV) reactivation are a concern.[189] Overall, RRs of 55% with 32% CR in advanced stages of MF/SS have been reported, with a 12-month median duration of response. It is a useful agent in patients with Sézary syndrome who are CMV negative. It was withdrawn from markets in the United States and Europe in 2012 and is only available through a named patient scheme. There is some concern about its use in conditioning for reduced intensity stem cell transplantation.[244]

Denileukin difitox is a recombinant fusion protein comprising diphtheria toxin fragments and IL-2 sequences.[189] Completed studies have shown an ORR of 30% and CR rate of 10% with a median duration of 6.9 months. Steroid pre-treatment has been shown to increase the ORR to 60% and reduce adverse events. However, side effects include fever, chills, myalgia, nausea, and vomiting, and approximately one-quarter of patients developed a "vascular leak" syndrome characterized by the presence of two or more of the following: hypotension, edema, and hypoalbuminemia.[189] Denileukin difitox may be useful for advanced disease, but this drug is not currently licensed in Europe.

Chemotherapy

MF is relatively chemo-resistant, and responses are usually short-lived, as shown by the randomized controlled trial by Kaye et al.[202,203] This may reflect the low proliferative rate and a high prevalence of inactivating *p53* mutations producing a relative resistance to tumor cell apoptosis. Systematic reviews of chemotherapy have shown CR rates of 33% for single-agent chemotherapy with median duration of 2–3 months and CR rates of 38% for combination chemotherapy with median duration of 5–41 months. Patients with CTCL are prone to infection; septicemia is a common pre-terminal event and is a problem for patients receiving chemotherapy. There are now newer single-agent chemotherapy drugs with higher response rates and a safer toxicity profile, but the duration of response remains short, and patients should be offered controlled clinical trials to find more effective chemotherapeutic treatments for this disease.

Chemotherapy should only be used for patients with Stage IIB to IVB disease. Combination chemotherapy with CHOP (cyclophosphamide, doxorubicin, vincristine, and prednisolone) has a high response rate but with significant toxicity and should be reserved for patients with good performance status and Stage IIB to IVB disease as initial treatment if the patient is to be considered for a stem cell transplant, and for similarly good-performance patients with effaced lymph node disease or visceral and critical organ disease where a rapid palliative response is needed. Other patients should be considered for clinical trials or treatment with newer single-agent chemotherapy drugs to reduce the toxicity of treatment and maintain the patient's quality of life.

Single-agent chemotherapy that has been widely used includes oral chlorambucil, oral methotrexate, oral etoposide, and the intravenous use of purine analogues pentostatin (2-deoxycoformycin) and fludarabine phosphate. Open studies of pentostatin have shown RR of 35–71% with CR rates of 10–33%, and it is especially useful for erythrodermic disease and SS.[245,246] It is, however, nephrotoxic and causes T-cell depletion, increasing the risk of opportunistic infections and thus requiring prophylaxis with co-trimoxazole (Septrin), acyclovir, and antifungals. Methotrexate produces CR of 41% in patients with erythrodermic disease given as a single weekly dose ranging from 5 to 125 mg. Fludarabine in combination with cyclophosphamide has been studied in erythrodermic MF and SS, but responses are short-lived, and bone marrow toxicity is common.[247]

Other single-agent chemotherapy agents, liposomal doxorubicin hydrochloride and gemcitabine, have been shown to produce high response rates with a more favorable toxicity profile.

A Phase II study of gemcitabine monotherapy achieved an ORR of 70% (10% CR and 60% PR) in 30 previously treated patients with T3 or T4 disease. The median durations of CR and PR were 15 months (range: 6–22 months) and 10 months (range: 2–15 months), respectively. Treatment was well-tolerated; hematological toxicity was mild, and no nausea/vomiting or organ toxicity was recorded.[248] The same group previously also reported 32 untreated patients (26 MF, 5 with peripheral T-cell lymphoma not otherwise specified [PTCLnos], 1 SS) showing a CR rate of 22% and PR rate of 53% with a median duration of response of 10 months (range: 4–22 months) with only mild toxicity.[249] A U.K. multicenter trial of gemcitabine in combination with bexarotene has shown a low response rate and poor lipid control, and bexarotene did not improve the duration of response.[250]

Liposomal doxorubicin has shown good efficacy as a single agent for MF. Pegylated liposomes are stable long-circulating carriers useful for delivering doxorubicin to tumor sites with a lower toxicity profile than the free drug. A Phase II study of pegylated liposomal doxorubicin as second-line therapy in 34 patients with CTCL showed an ORR of 88.2%. Fifteen patients achieved a CR and 15 patients a PR with an overall median survival of 17.8 (±10.5) months and event free survival of 12 (±9.5) months.[251] Adverse effects were seen in 14 patients and were temporary and generally mild. Only six patients had Grade 3 or 4 adverse effects. A retrospective study of liposomal doxorubicin for patients with Stage IVB MF has shown 30% with PR and 20% with stable disease (SD) in 10 patients with limited toxicity.[252] An EORTC Phase II trial of liposomal doxorubicin for Stage IIB–IVA MF has shown an ORR of 41% with only 6% CR and an average duration of response of 6 months and time to progression of 7.4 months.[253]

Brentuximab vedotin targeting CD30+ lymphomas has been assessed in a large randomized, open-label Phase III trial (ALCANZA) designed to evaluate single-agent brentuximab vedotin compared with a control arm of investigator's choice of standard therapies, methotrexate or bexarotene, in patients with CD30-expressing CTCL, including those with primary cutaneous anaplastic large cell lymphoma (pcALCL) or MF. The primary endpoint was objective response lasting at least 4 months (ORR4) as assessed by Global Response Score. Brentuximab vedotin resulted in a statistically significant improvement in the rate of ORR4 (56.3% vs. 12.5% in the control arm). Median PFS was 16.7 months vs. 3.5 months, a significant difference favoring brentuximab ($p < 0.0001$). The FDA and EMA have since approved brentuximab vedotin for the treatment of patients with CD30-expressing MF and pcALCL who require systemic therapy and have received one prior systemic therapy.[254]

Retinoids/Rexinoids

Bexarotene is highly selective for the retinoid X receptor and was the first "rexinoid" to undergo clinical development.[255,256] The drug has received EMA approval in Europe for the treatment of skin manifestations in advanced CTCL.[257] Although the precise mechanisms are unknown, in vitro studies have shown that bexarotene can inhibit growth in tumor cell lines and cause in vivo tumor regression in animal models: the drug also stimulates apoptosis.[258] In Phase II and III studies of 152 patients with CTCL, response rates from 20% to 67% have been reported.[257,259] Bexarotene is usually administered at 300 mg/m[2]/day, and treatment is continued indefinitely in patients who respond.[173,260] Bexarotene causes severe central hypothyroidism with high frequency, associated with marked reductions in serum concentrations of thyroid-stimulating hormone and thyroxine. During treatment, patients should be monitored for thyroid function and for hyper-triglyceridemia.[172] Most patients will require concomitant treatment with a lipid-lowering agent and thyroxine.[173,260] Gemfibrozil is contraindicated in this regard because it increases plasma concentrations of bexarotene, presumably due to inhibition of cytochrome P450 3A4, which in turn, results in a paradoxical elevation of triglycerides.[173,260]

Extracorporeal photophoresis

The use of extracorporeal photophoresis (ECP) was first reported in 1987 by Edelson and colleagues, who showed a 73% RR in patients with erythrodermic CTCL.[259] Response rates were lower in earlier stages of disease (38%). In this procedure, peripheral blood leukocytes are harvested, mixed with 8-MOP, exposed to UV radiation, and then returned to the patient.[261] This is usually performed on two successive days every 4 weeks.[262] The schedule is generally continued for up to 6 months in order to assess response: maintenance therapy is tailored according to disease course. In general, ECP is well-tolerated, although patients with a history of heart disease require careful monitoring due to changing fluid volumes.[261] ECP is considered a first-line option for Stage III erythrodermic disease and SS.

Prognosis

A patient's life expectancy is not adversely affected in Stage IA disease.[177,190–192] The 5-year survival in early Stage IA and IB is 94% and 84%, respectively. In advanced disease, the 5-year survival in Stage IIB, IIIA, IVA2, and IVB is 4.7, 4.7, 2.1, and 1.4 years, respectively.[190] Studies also suggest that Stage IA and IB patients with thick plaques may have a worse prognosis, but this depends on a histological assessment of plaque thickness, which can be difficult to reproduce. Similarly, folliculotropic disease appears to have a poor prognosis compared with other patients with Stage IB disease. The presence of a peripheral blood T-cell clone may indicate which patients with early-stage disease are likely to develop disease progression.[172] SS patients, by definition, are staged as T4 N1–3 M0 B1 and have a poor prognosis, with an overall median survival of 32 months from diagnosis.[173] A multivariate analysis of 1502 patients has identified risk factors for progression and survival in a large cohort of MF/SS patients, which provides the basis for defining distinct risk groups.[190] Specifically, male gender and age (>60) are key risk factors for progression. The presence of plaques (T1b/T2b), histologic evidence of folliculotropic disease, and palpable or histologically confirmed dermatopathic peripheral nodes (N1/Nx) are also important prognostic factors in early-stage MF. For late disease, nodal involvement (N2/3) and blood and visceral disease are additional important prognostic factors. Thus, although patients with Stage IA MF are unlikely to die of their disease, patients with Stage IB disease have a variable prognosis, which is partly determined by age, gender, the presence or absence of folliculotropism, plaques, and a peripheral blood T-cell clone identical to that in skin. A cutaneous lymphoma prognostic index (CLIPi) has been proposed and defines three prognostic groups

for early and late stages of MF/SS based on modeling of these multivariate risk factors.[191] An international consortium study in 1275 patients with advanced MF/SS has shown that Stage IV, age >60, large cell transformation, and increased LDH are independent prognostic markers for worse survival.[192] The PROCLIPI study is a multinational prospective cutaneous lymphoma international prognostic index study launched in 2015 to develop a prognostic index in mycosis fungoides and Sézary syndrome.

Variants and subtypes of mycosis fungoides

There are a number of clinical variants of MF discussed here.[176] Although there have been no specific therapeutic trials in these variants, these clinical variants appear to have a good prognosis and are often responsive to skin-directed therapies such as RT. The exception is folliculotropic MF, which may have a worse prognosis. Clinical variants such as bullous and hyper- or hypopigmented MF have a clinical behavior similar to classical MF and are not considered separately.

Folliculotropic mycosis fungoides

Patients present with groups of follicular papules, indurated plaques, and sometimes tumors, often associated with alopecia. Infiltrated plaques in the eyebrows with alopecia are a common finding. Pruritus can be severe.

This variant is characterized by the presence of folliculotropic infiltrates, often sparing the epidermis, and preferential involvement of the head and neck area. Most cases show mucinous degeneration of the hair follicles (follicular mucinosis). The most relevant feature is the deep localization of the neoplastic infiltrate, which makes it less accessible to skin-directed therapies.

Folliculotropic MF is less responsive to PUVA and topical therapies. RT is an effective treatment for individual lesions, and patients with extensive disease may benefit from TSEB. In combination with retinoids or IFN-α, PUVA can also be useful. The prognosis is slightly worse, with 5-year survival of 75%.[190]

Pagetoid reticulosis

This variant of MF is characterized by the presence of localized hyperkeratotic or scaly psoriasiform patches or plaques often affecting acral sites. The histology shows a strikingly epidermotropic proliferation of atypical T cells, which may have an aberrant CD4−CD8− phenotype. This localized type is also known as Woringer–Kolopp disease, and the prognosis is excellent (Figure 24.17).

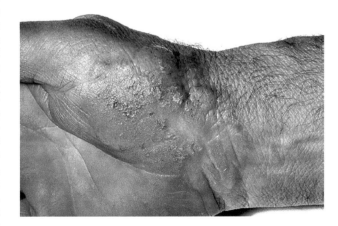

FIGURE 24.17 Woringer–Kolopp disease presenting as an isolated plaque on the hand of a 30-year-old man.

It should not be confused with the disseminated type known as Ketron–Goodman disease, which has a worse prognosis and requires aggressive treatment. Extracutaneous dissemination or disease-related deaths have not been reported. The preferred treatment is RT or surgical excision.

Granulomatous slack skin disease

This is an extremely rare subtype characterized by the slow development of folds of lax skin in flexural sites, especially the axilla. The histology is characterized by a granulomatous infiltrate with elastolysis. Discrete clonal T-cell populations are present. In most patients, it has an indolent course. Rapid recurrences after surgery are reported, and RT may be effective, but experience is limited.

Sézary syndrome

SS is defined clinically by the presence of erythroderma, generalized lymphadenopathy, and peripheral blood neoplastic T cells (Sézary cells).

It occurs exclusively in adults and in its most advanced cases, may present with a severe infiltrated erythroderma with leonine facies (see Figure 24.14) and hyperkeratosis, lichenification, edema, and fissuring of the palms and soles associated with severe pruritus. Lymphadenopathy, ectropion, alopecia, and onychodystrophy are common.

The histological features are similar to MF, but the cellular infiltrate is often more monotonous, and epidermotropism may be absent. Overall, only one-third of skin biopsies are diagnostic for lymphoma, whereas one-third are consistent with the diagnosis and one-third are not diagnostic or consistent for lymphoma. Bone marrow may be involved, but the infiltrates are often sparse and interstitial. SS is defined by the WHO by the presence of erythroderma, peripheral lymphadenopathy, and Sézary cells comprising >1000 cells μl^{-1}, or a CD4:CD8 ratio >10, or flow cytometry absolute counts of CD4+CD7− >40 or CD4+CD26 >30 with a T-cell clone for the diagnosis of B2 blood involvement.[263,264]

SS is an aggressive disease, and the 5-year survival is 26%.[190] Most patients die of opportunistic infections due to immunosuppression. The first-line treatment options include ECP, which has an ORR of 75%[265] and can be used alone or in combination with other modalities such as IFN-α or bexarotene. Chlorambucil plus prednisolone can be of benefit, but CR is uncommon. Skin-directed therapy such as RT can be used palliatively for individual tumors or lymph node regions. Second-line treatment options include single-agent chemotherapy with pentostatin or oral methotrexate and clinical trials. Combination therapy regimens are currently being evaluated. As discussed earlier for mycosis fungoides, reduced intensity allogeneic stem cell transplantation can be considered for SS patients.[232]

Adult T-cell leukemia/lymphoma

ATLL is a T-cell neoplasm etiologically associated with human T-cell leukemia virus 1 (HTLV1) infection, which can present in acute, leukemic, lymphoma, chronic, and "smoldering" forms.[266]

ATLL is endemic in regions such as southwest Japan, the Caribbean, South America, and Central Africa with a high prevalence of HTLV1. It develops in only 1–5% of seropositive individuals after more than two decades of viral persistence. The acute forms present with leukemia, lymphadenopathy, organomegaly, hypercalcemia, and skin lesions in approximately 50% of cases. The skin lesions can be nodules, tumors, generalized papules, or plaques. Chronic and smoldering variants frequently present with cutaneous involvement alone and may resemble MF, with

few, if any, circulating neoplastic T cells. The histological picture may be indistinguishable from MF, but clonally integrated HTLV1 proviral DNA can be found in all cases.

The clinical subtype is the main prognostic factor. The acute and lymphomatous types are aggressive with poor survival, and initial therapy consists of antivirals, IFN, and multi-agent chemotherapy. The chronic and smoldering forms have a less aggressive course and longer survival but may transform to an acute subtype. In the chronic and smoldering forms, skin-directed therapies such as those used in MF may be employed.[177]

Primary cutaneous CD30⁺ lymphoproliferative disorders

This is the second most common group, accounting for approximately 30% of CTCL cases. It includes primary cutaneous CD30⁺ anaplastic large cell lymphoma (C-ALCL), LyP, and borderline cases. It is a spectrum of disease, and the clinical appearance and course are used to differentiate between primary C-ALCL and LyP. Consensus treatment guidelines have been published.[267]

Primary cutaneous CD30⁺ anaplastic large cell lymphoma

Primary cutaneous C-ALCL is a primary cutaneous large cell lymphoma that presents with no previous history of MF or other CTCL variant.

It mainly affects adults and presents as a solitary tumor or localized nodules and plaques that may show ulceration. Twenty percent of patients have multifocal lesions. In some patients, C-ALCL may show partial spontaneous regression. Frequently, relapses occur in the skin, but extracutaneous dissemination is rare, and only 10% of cases develop regional lymph node disease.

The histology shows cohesive sheets of large tumor cells with a characteristic anaplastic morphology expressing CD30 in more than 75% of the tumor cells. Unlike systemic nodal CD30⁺ lymphomas, C-ALCL expresses the cutaneous lymphocyte antigen (CLA) but does not express EMA or ALK1 (anaplastic lymphoma kinase), which is due to the (2;5) translocation characteristic of systemic nodal ALCL. Unlike Hodgkin lymphoma, staining for CD15 is generally negative. Rare cases express CD56, but this does not appear to be associated with an unfavorable prognosis.

The prognosis is excellent, with 10-year disease-specific survival exceeding 90%. Aggressive loco-regional disease may indicate a poor prognosis, but this requires confirmation. The treatment of choice for localized tumors is surgical excision or RT. Multifocal skin lesions can be treated with RT if they can be encompassed by an RT field; otherwise, low-dose methotrexate is an option. The RT dose and schedule should be a fractionated course, such as 30–36 Gy in 18 fractions, to limit the long-term side effects and minimize the chance of recurrence. The rare patient who develops extracutaneous disease or rapidly progressive disease should be treated with brentuximab or combination chemotherapy such as CHOP.[177,254]

Lymphomatoid papulosis

LyP is defined as a chronic, recurrent, self-healing papulonecrotic or papulonodular skin eruption with histological features suggestive of a CD30⁺ lymphoma. It generally occurs in adults but may be seen in children. Individual lesions disappear within 3–12 weeks to leave superficial varioliform scars. Up to 20% of cases are associated with another type of cutaneous lymphoma such as MF, primary cutaneous CD30⁺ ALCL, or Hodgkin lymphoma. LyP has an excellent prognosis, and in a study of 118 patients, only five developed a systemic lymphoma, and only two died of systemic disease over 77 months' follow-up.[268] No treatment affects the course of the disease, and therefore, the short-term merits of treatment must be weighed against the potential side effects. Low-dose oral methotrexate is effective, and both PUVA and topical chemotherapy can be beneficial, but the disease recurs on discontinuation of treatment. Superficial RT is appropriate for localized or extensive regional disease.

Subcutaneous panniculitis-like T-cell lymphoma

Subcutaneous panniculitis-like T-cell lymphoma (SPTL) is a cytotoxic T-cell lymphoma that is clinically characterized by deep indurated erythematous plaques, often on the limbs, which may mimic cellulitis. There are two groups of SPTL with different histology, phenotype, and prognosis. Cases with an α/β T-cell phenotype are usually CD8⁺, restricted to subcutaneous tissue with no dermal or epidermal involvement, and run an indolent clinical course.

In contrast, in cases with a γ/δ T-cell phenotype, which are often CD4⁻ and CD8⁻ but occasionally CD56⁺, the neoplastic infiltrates may involve the epidermis and dermis, and patients invariably have a poor prognosis.

Cases of α/β SPTL have a 5-year survival of 80%.[174] Treatment of aggressive cases involves CHOP chemotherapy and RT, but recent studies suggest that patients with indolent SPTL can be controlled for long periods on systemic corticosteroids.[174]

Primary cutaneous peripheral T-cell lymphoma—unspecified

This is a heterogeneous group, which includes all CTCL variants that do not fit into any of the other well-defined categories.[174,177] Primary cutaneous aggressive CD8⁺ cytotoxic T-cell lymphoma (Berti's lymphoma) and cutaneous γ/δ T-cell lymphoma both have an aggressive course, and multi-agent systemic chemotherapy is used, but the results are disappointing. Primary cutaneous small/medium pleomorphic CD4⁺ T-cell lymphoproliferative disorder and primary cutaneous acral CD8+ lymphoma are new provisional categories with an excellent prognosis and present with solitary lesions that may be amenable to surgical excision or RT, but the optimum treatment remains to be defined. In all cases, MF must be excluded by careful clinical examination and an accurate history to identify typical subtle and polymorphic patches and plaques of MF.

Primary cutaneous B-cell lymphoma

Primary CBCL are defined as B-cell lymphomas originating in the skin without evidence of extracutaneous disease at presentation and for 6 months after diagnosis as assessed by adequate staging procedures. They represent only 25% of all cutaneous lymphomas.

There has been considerable debate over the difference between the previous EORTC and WHO classifications of primary cutaneous B-cell lymphoma.[174,177] Under the previous EORTC classification, primary cutaneous follicle center cell lymphoma (PCFCCL) defined a group of cutaneous lymphomas highly responsive to RT with an excellent prognosis. The same type of lymphoma with a diffuse growth pattern of large cells was classified under the previous WHO classification as a diffuse large B-cell lymphoma, leading to over-treatment with multi-agent chemotherapy. The other main group debated was primary cutaneous large B-cell lymphoma of the

leg (PCLBCL-leg), which was recognized under the EORTC classification as a separate subgroup, reflecting its unfavorable prognosis. Recent clinicopathological and genetic studies support the contention that PCFCCL and PCLBCL-leg are distinct groups, and a consensus was agreed in the WHO-EORTC classification with PCFCCL being defined as primary cutaneous follicle center lymphoma (PCFCL) distinct from nodal follicular lymphoma and PCLBCL-leg as primary cutaneous diffuse large B-cell lymphoma, leg type (see Table 24.2).

All patients with PCBCL should be staged with a CT scan of the neck, chest, abdomen, and pelvis and a bone marrow aspirate and trephine to exclude systemic disease. Primary cutaneous B-cell lymphoma is stage 1AE using the Ann Arbor staging system. A more useful staging system, which reflects the extent of skin involvement, is the proposed TNM classification of the ISCL and EORTC for primary cutaneous lymphomas other than MF.[269] This staging system is easy to apply but does not provide prognostic information.[270] There are no randomized controlled trials to guide management. Guidelines are published by the U.K. cutaneous lymphoma group and the EORTC.[177,178]

Primary cutaneous marginal zone B-cell lymphoma

Primary cutaneous marginal zone B-cell lymphoma (PCMZL) is considered part of the broad spectrum of extranodal marginal zone B-cell lymphomas commonly involving mucosal sites, the so-called mucosal associated lymphoid tissue (MALT). It is an indolent lymphoma composed of small cells including marginal zone cells, lymphoplasmacytoid cells, and plasma cells. It includes cases previously designated as primary cutaneous immunocytoma and exceptional cases of primary cutaneous plasmacytoma without multiple myeloma.

Most cases present with red to violaceous papules, plaques, or nodules preferentially on the trunk and extremities.[189] Multifocal lesions are frequent, ulceration is uncommon, and extracutaneous dissemination is very rare. Occasional spontaneous remission is observed, and the development of anetoderma in spontaneously resolving lesions is reported. Associated autoimmune disease is rare in PCMZL and suggests systemic lymphoma.

The prognosis is excellent, with a 5-year survival of 99%.[189] Patients with solitary lesions can be treated by surgical excision or RT. Retrospective series have shown that RT schedules delivering a total dose from 20 to 54 Gy and radiation portals with a margin of at least 2.0–3.0 cm are successful with a low risk of recurrence.[271–273] The recurrence rate is higher with smaller margins.[274] The International Lymphoma Radiation Oncology Group recommended schedule is 24 to 30 Gy in 12 to 15 fractions.[275] The St John's Institute of Dermatology schedule is 15 Gy in five fractions over 1 week.[177,210] An association with *B. burgdorferi* infection has been reported from some, but not all, geographical areas, and systemic antibiotics should be used in those patients with serological evidence of *B. burgdorferi* infection. For patients with multifocal skin lesions, chlorambucil, IFN-α, and rituximab have all produced very good results.[177] An expectant strategy similar to that used in other indolent B-cell lymphomas can be adopted.

Primary cutaneous follicle center lymphoma

PCFCL is derived from follicle center cells, with a follicular, follicular and diffuse, or diffuse growth pattern. The infiltrate consists of cleaved centrocyte-like cells with only a few large centroblasts. It must be differentiated from lymphomas with a diffuse growth pattern and monotonous proliferation, which are classified as PCLBCL-leg or other. Immunophenotype studies can help in the diagnosis. PCFCL consistently expresses Bcl6, but unlike nodal and secondary cutaneous follicular lymphomas, PCFCL rarely expresses Bcl2 and does not show the t(14:18) characteristically found in systemic follicular lymphomas.[177]

It characteristically presents as a solitary plaque or tumor or a group of plaques and tumors, usually on the scalp, forehead, or trunk and rarely on the legs. The tumors may be surrounded by erythematous papules and indurated plaques that precede the development of the tumor. Multifocal presentation is seen in a minority and not associated with a worse prognosis. If untreated, the skin lesions gradually increase in size, but dissemination is uncommon.[177]

The prognosis is excellent, with a 5-year survival of more than 95%.[177]

RT is the preferred mode of treatment and is the same as that used for PCMZL.[177,210] Cutaneous relapses occur in and out of the previous treatment fields in approximately 20% of patients and respond to treatment or retreatment with RT. Chemotherapy is occasionally needed for patients with extensive cutaneous disease or extracutaneous disease, and the regimens used are similar to that for systemic B-cell lymphoma.

Primary cutaneous diffuse large B-cell lymphoma, leg type

Primary cutaneous diffuse large B-cell lymphoma, leg type is a lymphoma characteristically presenting with skin tumors on the lower leg, but it can arise at other sites. It mainly affects elderly patients, particularly females. It presents as a rapidly growing large red or bluish tumor on the lower leg, and dissemination to extracutaneous sites is common, reflecting the more unfavorable prognosis when compared with PCFCL.[177]

The histology shows a diffuse infiltrate of large centroblasts often extending to subcutaneous tissue with a prominent stromal reaction. The neoplastic cells express CD20 and in contrast to PCFCL, show strong Bcl2 expression and express Mum1. The t(14:18) is not found, but there is evidence for chromosomal amplification of the *BCL2* gene locus. GCB.non-GCB subtype has not been found to be correlated with survival, but Bcl-2, female gender, and Bcl-6 are prognostic markers.[179]

The 5-year survival is 55%.[174] The presence of multiple skin lesions is an adverse factor. The treatment is that for systemic diffuse large B-cell lymphoma with anthracycline-containing combination chemotherapy such as CHOP plus rituximab, followed by involved field RT to the leg, but very elderly patients may require palliative RT only.[178]

Primary cutaneous diffuse large B-cell lymphoma—other

This rare group includes morphological variants of primary cutaneous diffuse large B-cell lymphoma, anaplastic or plasmablastic subtypes, or T-cell rich/histiocyte-rich large B-cell lymphomas, but prognosis and treatment are similar to that for PCLBCL.[177]

Primary cutaneous intravascular large B-cell lymphoma

This is a rare but well-defined subtype that preferentially affects the CNS, lungs, and skin and is generally associated with a poor prognosis. Cases with only skin involvement have a better survival than other presentations (3-year overall survival: 56% versus 22%). Multi-agent chemotherapy is the preferred treatment, even for disease limited to the skin.[174,177]

Other non-melanoma skin cancers

Extra-mammary Paget's disease

Sir James Paget first described the intra-epithelial carcinoma that now bears his name in the breast in 1874 and suggested that the disease might also be found in other areas.[276] The first case of EMPD was described by Crocker in 1888,[277] and peri-anal Paget's disease (PPD) was first reported in 1893.[278]

Incidence and etiology

EMPD is a rare intra-epithelial adenocarcinoma, characterized by the presence of malignant Paget cells lying within the epidermis of the skin. The etiology is unknown. It is usually a primary tumor but may be associated with an underlying adjacent or distant invasive carcinoma. Approximately 25% of cases have an underlying cutaneous adnexal carcinoma, and 10–15% have an subjacent or distant internal carcinoma.[279] In the later stages, the epidermal pagetoid cells are thought to represent metastases, and the prognosis is associated with the underlying malignancy, with a mortality rate of 50% or higher.

Clinical features

Extra-mammary Paget's disease begins as an erythematous, eczematous, slowly spreading plaque, which can bleed easily and may ulcerate. It usually affects sites with a high density of apocrine glands (e.g., vulval, perineal, and peri-anal regions). The penis, axillae, umbilicus, eyelids, and external auditory meatus are less common sites. Investigations should always include a diagnostic biopsy and exclusion of an associated underlying carcinoma.

Pathology

Within the epidermis, characteristic Paget cells are dispersed between keratinocytes. These cells have clear abundant cytoplasm and do not establish intercellular bridges with the adjacent keratinocytes. In EMPD, there is a tendency for the cells to accumulate in the basal area, especially in the interpapillary ridges. They stain positively for acid as well as neutral mucopolysaccharides and carcinoembryonic antigen.

Treatment

Evidence to guide treatment is limited to small case series. Surgery is the treatment of choice if possible.[6,279] Wide local excision is required; extensive disease requires plastic surgical reconstruction, and in the peri-anal area, abdominoperineal resection may be required. Local recurrence is a major problem because of the difficulty in accurately identifying the extent of occult disease in a multicentric process within the skin as well as accurately identifying spread into the anal canal. Local recurrence rates of 31–61% for surgery have been reported.[280] Mohs' micrographic surgery has lower recurrence rates of 23–33%.[280] Topical fluorouracil before and in addition to surgery has been advocated. Imiquimod has been used in a similar way as monotherapy and in combination with surgery to try to reduce the extent of excision.[281] Photodynamic therapy has been used, with small case series reporting responses.[282,283] RT is an effective treatment but has mainly been reserved for patients unfit for surgery and for those with recurrent disease or who decline surgery.[278] A minimum dose of >50 Gy using a single appositional field is recommended.[279,284]

Merkel cell carcinoma

MCC is a tumor of neuroendocrine cell origin. Studies have shown that MCC shares pathogenetic mechanisms with other neoplasms of neural crest derivation, such as melanoma and neuroblastoma.[285]

Incidence

It is a rare tumor, with 1515 new cases in the United Kingdom reported each year between 1999 and 2008,[286] and most often occurs in Caucasian men at a median age of 65.[287]

Etiology

Merkel cells are specialized sensory cells present in the basal or supra-basal layers of the epidermis. They are believed to be neurosensory cells that are derived from the amine precursor uptake and decarboxylation system (APUD). They function as slowly adapting type 1 mechanoreceptors, with a higher density in sun-exposed areas. Forty-seven per cent of cases occur on the head and neck, 40% on the extremities, and 8% on the trunk.[288] Risk factors include UV light and immunosuppression.[289–293] Rapid progression of MCC occurs with immunosuppressive therapy after organ transplantation.[294] A similar pattern of genomic changes has been detected in MCC and neuroendocrine tumors such as melanoma.[285] In metastatic MCC, Bcl2 is strongly expressed. In a severe combined immunodeficient (SCID) mouse xeno-transplantation model for human MCC, administration of *BCL2* antisense oligonucleotide results in either a dramatic reduction of tumor growth or CR.[295] In 2008, the Merkel cell polyoma virus was reported in MCC tumor specimens.[296] High levels of clonal integration of the virus in Merkel cell tumors has been reported, but not all cases are associated with the virus infection.[297] There may be two independent pathways for the development of MCC, one driven by the virus and the other by sun damage.

Clinical features

MCCs not only present as solitary pigmented or non-pigmented nodular tumors on the head and neck regions but may be also seen on the trunk and extremities. Multiple tumors at presentation have been reported. Lymph node areas must be examined and staged with a CT scan of the neck, chest, abdomen, and pelvis. PET has been shown to be useful in staging MCC and also for assessing response to treatment; it can, however, be negative in MCC with low proliferative rates.[298,299] Historically, five different staging systems have been used, all inconsistent with each other. The latest American Joint Committee on Cancer (AJCC) staging 2017 has been developed and should now be used for consistency.[300] Prior to the latest AJCC staging system, the favored system used in most publications was the Memorial Sloan Kettering Cancer Center (MSKCC) four-stage system: Stage I local disease <2 cm, Stage II local disease >2 cm, Stage III regional nodal disease, and Stage IV distant metastatic disease.[301]

Pathology

MCCs consist of dermal nodules with a clear Grenz zone separating the tumor from the epidermis and sheets of small, undifferentiated, and tightly packed rounded blue cells that possess only scanty cytoplasm with CK20 perinuclear dot staining. CK20 negative Merkel cell tumors and those associated with sun damage are more likely to be virus negative.[302] It may be histologically difficult to differentiate from other small cell neoplasms. A panel of immunohistochemical stains is used, and tumor cells stain positive for CK20, neurofilament, and neuron specific enolase and stain negative for CK7, TTF1 S100 protein, and leucocyte common antigen.[302] Karyotyping of neoplastic cells shows loss of chromosome Y, the significance of which is unknown.[303]

Treatment

Aggressive therapy is needed, as MCC has a high propensity for local recurrence (20–75%), regional node metastases (31–80%), and distant metastases (26–75%), and approximately one-third of patients eventually die of the disease.[288,294]

Treatment for localized disease without nodal involvement is surgical excision of the primary tumor with an adequate margin of clearance of 2 cm to investing fascia of muscle where possible.[304] Radiotherapy to the primary may be used in selected cases where complete excision is not feasible.[305] Elective lymph node dissection improves the length of the disease-free period but does not improve overall survival.[306] Sentinel lymph node biopsy (SLNB) is an important staging tool that can define subsequent treatment with observation, completion node dissection, or adjuvant radiotherapy. A review of retrospective studies showed that 93% of SLNB positive and 8% of SLNB negative patients underwent nodal basin radiotherapy, and the nodal recurrence rate was 10% for both groups.[307] The outcome of completion node dissection for SLNB positive patients is similar to that reported with nodal basin radiotherapy.[307,308]

Recurrence rates with surgery alone are reported to be between 8% and 100%. Post-excision RT to the site of the original tumor and the primary draining lymph nodes reduces recurrence rates and in some series, improves disease-free survival.[288,309] A study of 86 patients in Sydney showed that the combination of surgery and RT improved the median disease-free survival compared with surgery alone.[310] In contrast, a study from the Memorial Sloan Kettering of 251 patients showed very low recurrence rates of 8% after node-negative excision and 8%–15% after operative nodal staging but did not find a benefit for adjuvant RT.[311] However, only a minority of patients (17%) received RT in the latter study. A multivariate analysis of 5000 patients with Stage I and II disease showed a 29% and 23% reduction in the hazard of death, respectively, with the addition of adjuvant radiotherapy.[312] A prospective randomized controlled trial of adjuvant RT closed early because of the increasing use of SLNB; the study showed in 83 patients that regional recurrence was reduced from 16% to 0% with addition of radiotherapy and 3-year PFS improved from 81.2% to 85.7%, but there was no improvement in OS.279.3.

Radiotherapy to the primary site is given with a direct electron radiotherapy field except in larger tumors at difficult sites, where more complex techniques such as volumetric modulated arc therapy (VMAT) or tomotherapy are used. Radiotherapy for lymph nodal treatment is now outlined on CT scans and treated with intensity-modulated radiation therapy (IMRT) to minimize the doses to normal tissues.[313] When recommended, the RT dose to the surgical bed and draining lymph nodes for microscopic disease is 50 Gy in 2 Gy fractions.[314] When radiotherapy is used for unresected tumors or tumors with positive margins, higher doses of 60–66 Gy are recommended.[314] In the palliative setting, standard palliative schedules of 20 Gy in five fractions or 8 Gy single fractions are very effective. Chemo-radiotherapy has been investigated in a Phase II trial undertaken by the Trans Tasman Radiation Oncology Group (TROG).[315] Patients received concurrent and adjuvant combination chemotherapy (etoposide/carboplatin) and RT (50 Gy). Eligible patients needed to have one or more unfavorable features (>10 mm primary, nodal disease, residual disease post-surgery, surgical recurrence, or recurrence outside an irradiated field). The study reported an impressive 3-year overall survival, loco-regional control, and distant control rates of 76%, 75%, and 76%, respectively. Only 17% experienced loco-regional recurrence. These findings in patients with poor prognostic features, particularly the presence of nodal metastases in 33 (62% Stage III) patients, strongly suggest a benefit for the addition of combination chemotherapy in patients with unfavorable features.

MCCs are chemosensitive but rarely curable in patients with metastasis or locally advanced tumors. A high incidence of mortality directly related to chemotherapy has been reported.[316] Widely used chemotherapy regimens are those developed for other small cell cancers: cyclophosphamide, doxorubicin (or epirubicin), and vincristine (CAV or CEV), and carboplatin (or cisplatin) and etoposide (EP). Response rates around 29e75% and CR rates of between 13% and 35% have been reported.[317–320] There is current interest in immunotherapy and check point inhibitors with ongoing clinical trials. The PD-L1 inhibitor monoclonal antibody avelumab has been shown in a Phase 2 study to have a response rate of 62%, with 80% of responses ongoing at 6 months.[332] In a trial for patients who had progressed on previous chemotherapy, including 41% with more than one line of previous treatment, the overall response rate to avelumab was 33%, durable (>6 months) response rate 29%, and CR rate 9%. Three-quarters of responses lasted more than 1 year. The response was not clearly associated with tumor viral or PD-L1 status.[313] Immunotherapy trials may help to shape the optimal management of MCC in the future, but surgery and radiotherapy continue to be the prime modalities in achieving loco-regional control.

Key learning points

- The most important environmental agent capable of inducing skin cancer is exposure to ultraviolet light.
- Selection of the treatment modality for NMSC depends on a number of different factors, such as health status, site, size, histological type, and whether one is dealing with a primary or a recurrent lesion.
- Recurrent and high-risk NMSC should be managed by a multidisciplinary team to select the best treatment option for the patient.
- Primary cutaneous T-cell lymphoma treatment needs to be delivered by an experienced multidisciplinary team, with quality of life central to the therapeutic strategy.

References

1. Cancer Research UK. CancerStats: Incidence UK. 2016. Available at: www.cancerresearchuk.org/cancerstats
2. LeBoit P, Burg G, Weedon D, Sarasin A (Eds.). *WHO Classification of Tumours: Pathology and Genetics of Skin Tumours.* Lyon: IARC Press, 2006.
3. Knudson A. Hereditary cancer, oncogenes and anti oncogenes. *Cancer Res.* 1985; 45:1437–43.
4. Giles GG, Mark R, Foley P. Incidence of non-melanocytic skin cancer treated in Australia. *BMJ.* 1988; 296:13–7.
5. Scotto J, Cotton G, Urbach F et al. Biologically effective ultraviolet radiation: Surface measurements in the United States, 1974 to 1985. *Science.* 1988; 239:762–4
6. Coldiron BM, Goldsmith BA, Robinson JK. Surgical treatment of extramammary Paget's disease. A report of six cases and a re-examination of Mohs micrographic surgery compared with conventional surgical excision. *Cancer.* 1991; 67:933–8.
7. Ziegler A, Jonason AS, Leffell DJ et al. Sunburn and p53 in the onset of skin cancer. *Nature.* 1994; 372:773–6.
8. Jensen P, Hansen S, Moller B et al. Skin cancer in kidney and heart transplant recipients and different long term immunosuppressive therapy regimens. *Am Acad Dermatol.* 1999; 40:177–86.

9. Pieceall WE, Goldberg LH, Ananthaswarry HN. Presence of human papilloma virus type 16 DNA sequences in human non-melanoma skin cancers. *Invest Dermatol.* 1991; 97:880–4.
10. Shamanin V, Zur Hausen H, Lavergne D et al. Human papillomavirus infections in non-melanoma skin cancers from renal transplant recipients and non-immunosuppressed patients. *Nat Cancer Inst.* 1996; 88:802–11.
11. Maurer TA, Christian KV, Kerschmann RL et al. Cutaneous squamous cell carcinoma in human immunodeficiency virus-infected patients. A study of epidemiologic risk factors, human papillomavirus, and p53 expression. *Arch Dermatol.* 1997; 133:577–83.
12. Ostrow RR, Manias D, Mitchell AJ et al. Epidermodysplasia verruciformis. A case associated with primary lymphatic dysplasia, depressed cell-mediated immunity and Bowen's disease containing human papillomavirus 16 DNA. *Arch Dermatol.* 1987; 123:1511–6.
13. Pfister H. Human papilloma virus and impaired immunity vs. epidermodysplasia verruciform. *Arch Dermatol.* 1987; 123:1469–70.
14. Yutsudo M, Tangigaki T, Kanda R et al. Involvement of human papilloma virus type 20 in epidermodysplasia verruciformis skin carcinogenesis. *J Clin Microbiol.* 1994; 32:1076–8.
15. Karagas MR, Nelson HH, Sehr P et al. Human papillomavirus infection and incidence of squamous cell and basal cell carcinomas of the skin. *J Natl Cancer Inst.* 2006; 98:389–95.
16. Wicking C, Shanley S, Smyth I. Most germ-line mutations in the nevoid basal cell carcinoma syndrome lead to a premature termination of the PATCHED protein, and no genotype-phenotype correlations are evident. *Am J Hum Genet.* 1997; 60:21–6.
17. Levanat S, Mubrin MK, Crnic I et al. Variable expression of Gorlin syndrome may reflect complexity of the signalling pathway. *Pflugers Arch.* 2000; 439:31–3.
18. Cohen MM Jr. Nevoid basal cell carcinoma syndrome: Molecular biology and new hypotheses. *Int Oral Maxillofac Surg.* 1999; 28:216–23.
19. Lindeberg H, Jepsen FL. The nevoid basal cell carcinoma syndrome. Histopathology of the basal cell tumors. *J Cutan Pathol.* 1983; 10:68–72.
20. Lo Muzio L, Staibano S, Pannone G et al. Expression of cell cycle and apoptosis-related proteins in sporadic odontogenic keratocysts and odontogenic keratocysts associated with the nevoid basal cell carcinoma syndrome. *J Dent Res.* 1999; 78:1345–53.
21. Barr RJ, Headley JL, Jensen JL, Howell JB. Cutaneous keratocysts of nevoid basal cell carcinoma syndrome. *J Am Acad Dermatol.* 1986; 14:572–6.
22. Wolter M, Reifenberger J, Sommer C et al. Mutations in the human homologue of the Drosophila segment polarity gene patched (PTCH) in sporadic basal cell carcinomas of the skin and primitive neuroectodermal tumors of the central nervous system. *Cancer Res.* 1997; 57:2581–5.
23. Hettmer S, Teot LA, Kozakewich H et al. Mytogenic tumors in nevoid basal cell carcinoma syndrome. *J Pediatr Hematol Oncol.* 2015; 37:147–9.
24. Kimonis VE, Goldstein AM, Pastakia B et al. Clinical manifestations in 105 persons with nevoid basal cell carcinoma syndrome. *Am J Med Genet.* 1997; 31:299–308.
25. Lindeberg H, Halaburt H, Larsen PO. The naevoid basal cell carcinoma syndrome. Clinical, biochemical and radiological aspects. *J Maxillofa Surg.* 1982; 10:246–9.
26. Mitchell G, Farndon PA, Braydon P et al. Genetic predisposition to cancer: The consequences of delayed diagnosis of Gorlin syndrome. *Clinic Oncol.* 2005; 17:650–4.
27. Nagasawa H, Little FF, Burke MJ et al. Study of basal cell nevus syndrome fibroblasts after treatment with DNA-damaging agents. *Basic Life Sci.* 1984; 29:775–85.
28. Chan GL, Little JB. Cultured diploid fibroblasts from patients with the nevoid basal cell carcinoma syndrome are hypersensitive to killing by ionizing radiation. *Am J Pathol.* 1983; 111:50–5.
29. Newton JA, Black AK, Arlett CF et al. Radiobiological studies in the naevoid basal cell carcinoma syndrome. *Br J Dermatol.* 1990; 123:573–80.
30. Featherstone T, Taylor AM, Harnden DG. Studies on the radiosensitivity of cells from patients with basal cell naevus syndrome. *Am J Hum Genet.* 1983; 35:58–66.

31. Arlett CF, Priestley A. Deficient recovery from potentially lethal damage in some gamma-irradiated human fibroblast cell strains. *Br J Cancer Suppl.* 1984; 6:227–32.

32. Little JB, Nichols WW, Troilo P et al. Radiation sensitivity of cell strains from families with genetic disorders predisposing to radiation induced cancer. *Cancer Res.* 1989; 49:4705–14.

33. Vulin A, Sedkaoui M, Moratille S et al. Severe PATCHED1 deficiency in cancer-Prone Gorlin patient cells results in intrinsic radiosensitivity. *Int J Radiat Oncol Biol Phys.* 2018; 102(2):417–25.

34. Craven NM, Griffiths CEM. Retinoids in the management of non-melanoma skin cancer and melanoma. *Skin Cancer.* 1996; 26:275–6.

35. Theiler R, Hubscher E, Wagenhauser FJ et al. Diffuse idiopathic skeletal hyperostosis (DISH) and pseudo-coxarthritis following long-term etretinate therapy. *Schweiz Med Wochenschr.* 1993; 123:649–53.

36. Strange PR, Lang PG Jr. Long-term management of basal cell nevus syndrome with topical tretinoin and 5-fluorouracil. *J Am Acad Dermatol.* 1992; 27:842–5.

37. Tang JY, Mackay-Wiggan JM, Aszterbaum M et al. Inhibiting the hedgehog pathway in patients with the basal-cell nevus syndrome. *N Engl J Med.* 2012; 366(23):2180–8.

38. Jacyk WK. Xeroderma pigmentosum in black South Africans. *Int J Dermatol.* 1999; 39:511–14.

39. Khatri ML, Bemghazil M, Shafi M et al. Xeroderma pigmentosum in Libya. *Int J Dermatol.* 1999; 38:520–4.

40. Clever J. Defective repair replication of DNA in xeroderma pigmentosum. *Nature.* 1968; 218:652–6.

41. Reed W, Landing B, Sugarman G et al. Xeroderma pigmentosum: Clinical and laboratory investigations of its basic defect. *J Am Med Assoc.* 1969; 207:2073–9.

42. de Boer J, Hoeijmakers JH. Nucleotide excision repair and the human syndrome. *Carcinogenesis.* 2000; 21:453–60.

43. Lambert WC, Kuo HR, Lambert MW. Xeroderma pigmentosum. In Chu AC, Edelson RL (Eds.), *Malignant Tumours of the Skin* (pp. 119–37). London, UK: Arnold, 1999.

44. Guillot B, Favoer C, Guilhou JJ et al. Xeroderma pigmentosum. Un case traite par l'association betacarotene—canthaxanthine et retinoide aromatique. *Arch Dermatol Venereol.* 1984; 111:65–6.

45. Somos S, Farkas B, Schneider I. Cancer protection in xeroderma pigmentosum variant (XP-V). *Anticancer Res.* 1999; 3:2195–9.

46. Mittelbronn MA, Mullins DL, Ramos-Caro FA et al. Frequency of pre-existing actinic keratosis in cutaneous squamous cell carcinoma. *Int J Dermatol.* 1998; 37:677–81.

47. Montgomery H, Dorffel J. Verruca senilis und keratoma senile. *Arch Dermatol Syph.* 1932; 166:286–9.

48. Kao GF. Carcinoma arising in Bowen's disease. *Arch Dermatol.* 1986; 122:1124.

49. Mikhail GR. Cancers, precancers, and pseudo cancers on the male genitalia. *J Dermatol Surg Oncol.* 1980; 6:1027.

50. Dinehart SM. The treatment of actinic keratoses. *J Am Acad Dermatol.* 2000; 42:25–8.

51. Mackenzie-Wood A, de Kossard S, Launey J et al. Imiquimod 5% cream in the treatment of Bowen's disease. *J Am Acad Dermatol.* 2001; 44:462–70.

52. Lukas Van der Spek LA, Pond GR, Wells W, Tsang RW. Radiation therapy for Bowen's disease of the skin. *Int J Radiat Oncol Biol Phys.* 2005; 63:505–10.

53. Birnie AJ, Eedy. DJ. *Guidelines for the Management of Squamous Cell Carcinoma in situ (Bowen's Disease).* Morton, CA: British Association of Dermatologist, 2013.

54. Milne JA. *An Introduction to the Diagnostic Histopathology of the Skin.* London, UK: Edward Arnold, 1972, pp. 261–2.

55. Jih DM, Lyle S, Elenitsan R et al. Cytokine 15 expression in trichoepitheliomas and a subset of basal cell carcinomas suggests they originate from hair follicle stem cells. *J Cutan Pathol.* 1999; 26:113–8.

56. Kruger K, Blume-Peytavi U, Orfanos CE. Basal cell carcinoma possibly originates from the outer root sheath and/or the bulge region of the vellus hair follicle. *Arch Dermatol Res.* 1999; 29:253–9.

57. Miller DL, Weinstock MA. Non-melanoma skin cancer in the United States: Incidence. *J Am Acad Dermatol.* 1994; 30:774–8.

58. Holmes SA, Malinovszky K, Roberts DL. Changing trends in non-melanoma skin cancer in South Wales, 1988–1998. *Br J Dermatol.* 2000; 143:1224–9.

59. Venables ZC, Nijsten T, Wong KF, Autier P, Broggio J, Deas A. Epidemiology of basal and cutaneous squamous cell carcinoma in the UK 2013–15: A cohort study. *British J Dermatol.* 2019; https://doi.org/10.1111/bjd.17873.

60. Wallberg P, Skog E. The incidence of basal cell carcinoma in an area of Stockholm county during the period 1971–1980. *Acta Derm Venereol.* 1991; 71:134–7.

61. Aszterbaum M, Beech J, Ervin H et al. Ultraviolet radiation mutagenesis of hedgehog pathway genes in basal cell carcinomas. *J Invest Dermatol Symp Proc.* 1999; 4:41–5.

62. Staples M, Marks R, Giles G. Trends in the incidence of non-melanocytic skin cancer (NMSC) treated in Australia 1985–1995: Are primary prevention programs starting to have an effect? *Int J Cancer.* 1998; 78:144–8.

63. Noodleman FR, Pollack SV. Trauma as a possible etiologic factor in basal cell carcinoma. *J Dermatol Surg Oncol.* 1986; 12:841–6.

64. Yeh S. Skin cancer in chronic aresenicism. *Hum Pathol.* 1973; 4:469–85.

65. Ramachandran S, Fryer AA, Lovatt T et al. Susceptibility and modifier genes in cutaneous basal cell carcinomas and their associations with clinical phenotype. *J Photochem Photobiol.* 2001; 63:1–7.

66. Lear JT, Heagerty AHM, Smith A et al. Truncal site and detoxifying enzyme polymorphisms significantly reduce time to presentation of next cutaneous basal cell carcinoma. *Carcinogenesis.* 1997; 18:1499–503.

67. Ramachandran S, Fryer AA, Smith AG et al. Cutaneous basal cell carcinomas: Distinct host factors are associated with the development of tumors on the trunk and on the head and neck. *Cancer.* 2001; 92:354–8.

68. Johnson RL, Rothman AL, Xie J et al. Human homolog of patched, a candidate gene for the basal cell nevus syndrome. *Science.* 1996; 14:1668–71.

69. Riddle RO, Johnson RL, Laufer E et al. Sonic hedgehog mediates the polarising activity of the ZPA. *Cell.* 1993; 75:1401–16.

70. Roelink H, Porter JA, Chiang C et al. Floor plate and motor neuron induction by different concentrations of the amino-terminal cleavage product of sonic hedgehog autoproteolysis. *Cell.* 1995; 81:445–55.

71. Xie J, Murone M, Luoh SM et al. Activating smoothened mutations in sporadic basal-cell carcinoma. *Nature.* 1998; 391:90–2.

72. Fan H, Khavari PA. Sonic Hedgehog apposes epithelial cell cycle arrest. *J Cell Biol.* 1999; 147:71–76.

73. Johason AS, Kunala S, Price GJ et al. Frequent clones of P53-mutated keratinocytes in normal human skin. *Proc Natl Acad Sci USA.* 1996; 93:14025–9.

74. Lear JT, Smith AG, Heagerty AHM et al. Truncal site and detoxifying enzyme polymorphisms significantly reduce time to presentation of further primary cutaneous basal cell carcinoma. *Carcinogenesis.* 1997; 18:1499–503.

75. Chen GS, Yu HS, Lan CC et al. CXC chemokine receptor CXCR4 expression enhances tumorigenesis and angiogenesis of basal cell carcinoma. *Br J Dermatol.* 2006; 154:910–8.

76. MacKie R. Epidermal skin tumours. In Champion RH, Burton RH, Burns DA, Breathnach SM (Eds.), *Textbook of Dermatology* (6th ed., pp. 1651–93). Oxford, UK: Blackwell Scientific, 1998.

77. Miller SJ. Biology of basal cell carcinoma (part I). *J Am Acad Dermatol.* 1991; 24:1–13.

78. Medenhall WM, Amdur RJ, Williams LS et al. Carcinoma of the skin of the head and neck with perineural invasion. *Head Neck.* 2002; 24:78–83.

79. Di Gregorio C, Florena AM, Gebbia V et al. Mental nerve invasion by basal cell carcinoma of the chin: A case report. *Anticancer Res.* 1998; 18:4723–6.

80. Terashi H, Kurata S, Tadokoro T. Perineural and neural involvement in skin cancers. *Dermatol Surg.* 1997; 23:259–64.

81. Carlson KC, Roenigk RK. Know your anatomy: Perineural involvement of basal and squamous cell carcinoma on the face. *J Dermatol Surg Oncol.* 1990; 16:827–33.

82. Niazi ZB, Lamberty BG. Perineural infiltration in basal cell carcinomas. *Br J Plast Surg.* 1993; 46:156–7.

83. Ten Hove MW, Glaser JS, Schatz NJ. Occult perineural tumor infiltration of the trigeminal nerve. Diagnostic considerations. *J Neuroophthalmol.* 1997; 17:176–7.

84. Morselli P, Tosti A, Guerra L et al. Recurrent basal cell carcinoma of the back infiltrating the spine. *J Dermatol Surg Oncol.* 1993; 19:917–22.

85. Silbert PL, Kelsall GR, Shepherd JM et al. Enigmatic trigeminal sensory neuropathy diagnosed by facial skin biopsy. *Clin Exp Neurol.* 1992; 29:234–8.

86. Berti JJ, Sharata HH. Metastatic basal cell carcinoma to the lung. *Cutis.* 1999; 63:165.

87. Christian MM, Murphy CM, Wagner RF Jr. Metastatic basal cell carcinoma presenting as unilateral lymphedema. *Dermatol Surg.* 1998; 24:1151–3.

88. Berardi RS, Korba J, Mellow J et al. Pulmonary metastasis in nevoid basal cell carcinoma syndrome. *Int Surg.* 1991; 76:64–6.

89. Degner RA, Kerley SW, McGregor DH et al. Metastatic basal cell carcinoma: Report of a case presenting with respiratory failure. *Am J Med Sci.* 1991; 301:395–7.

90. Blinder D, Taicher S. Metastatic basal cell carcinoma presenting in the oral cavity and auditory meatus. A case report and review of literature. *Int J Oral Maxillofac Surg.* 1992; 21:31–4.

91. Cruse CW, O'Neill W, Rayhack J. Metastatic basal cell carcinoma of the upper extremity. *J Hand Surg.* 1992; 17:1093–4.

92. Mizushima J, Ohara K. Basal cell carcinoma of the vulva with lymph node and skin metastasis—Report of a case and review of 20 Japanese cases. *J Dermatol.* 1995; 22:36–42.

93. Raszewski RL, Guyuron B. Long-term survival following nodal metastases from basal cell carcinoma. *Ann Plast Surg.* 1990; 24:170–5.

94. Pfeiffer P, Hansen O, Rose C. Systemic cytotoxic therapy of basal cell carcinoma. A review of the literature. *Eur J Cancer.* 1990; 26:73–7.

95. Moeholt K, Aagaard H, Pfeiffer P et al. Platinum-based cytotoxic therapy in basal cell carcinoma—A review of the literature. *Acta Oncol.* 1996; 35:677–82.

96. Gormley DP, Hirsch P. Aggressive basal cell carcinoma of the scalp. *Arch Dermatol.* 1978; 114:782–3.

97. Cotran R. Metastasizing basal cell carcinomas. *Cancer.* 1961; 14:1036–40.

98. Wong CSM, Strange RC, Lear JT. Basal cell carcinoma. *Br Med J.* 2003; 327:794–798.

99. du Vivier A. *Atlas of Clinical Dermatology* (2nd ed., pp. 9.17–9.22). New York, NY: MosbyWolfe, 1993.

100. NICE guidelines: Improving outcomes for people with skin tumours including melanoma (update 2010). Available at: www.nice.org.uk/guidance

101. Lewis JE. Linear basal cell epithelioma. *Int J Dermatol.* 1985; 24:124–5.

102. Lim KK, Randle HW, Roenig RK et al. Linear basal cell carcinoma: Report of seventeen cases and review of the presentation and treatment. *Dermatol Surg.* 1999; 25:63–7.

103. Chopra KF, Cohen PR. Linear basal cell carcinomas: Report of multiple sequential tumors localized to a radiotherapy port and review of the literature. *Tex Med.* 1997; 93:57–9.

104. Barton K, Curling OM, Paridaens AD et al. The role of cytology in the diagnosis of periocular basal cell carcinomas. *Ophthal Plast Reconstr Surg.* 1996; 12:190–4, discussion 195.

105. Peris K, Fargnoli MC, Garbe C. Diagnosis and treatment of basal cell carcinoma: European consensus-based interdisciplinary guidelines. *Eur J Cancer.* 2019; 118:10–34.

106. Telfer NR, Colver G, Bowers PW. Guidelines for the management of basal cell carcinoma. *Br J Dermatol.* 1999; 141:415–23.

107. Holmkvist KA, Rogers GS, Dahl PR. Incidence of residual basal cell carcinoma in patients who appear tumor free after biopsy. *J Am Acad Dermatol.* 1999; 41:600–5.

108. Albright S. Treatment of skin cancer using multiple modalities. *J Am Acad Dermatol.* 1982; 7:143–71.

109. Telfer NR, Colver GB, Morton CA. Guidlines for the management of basal cell carcinoma. *Br J Dermatol.* 2008; 159:35–48.

110. Spiller WE, Spiller RE. Treatment of basal cell epithelioma by curettage and electro desiccation. *J Am Acad Dermatol.* 1984; 11:808–14.

111. Salasche SJ. Curettage and electrodessication in the treatment of primary basal cell epithelioma. *J Am Acad Dermatol.* 1984; 10:285–7.

112. Edens RL, Bartlow GA, Haghighi P et al. Effectiveness of curettage and electrodessication in the removal of basal cell carcinoma. *J Am Acad Dermatol.* 1983; 9:383.

113. Nouri K, Spencer JM, Taylor JR et al. Does wound healing contribute to the eradication of basal cell carcinoma following curettage and electrodessication? *Dermatol Surg.* 1999; 25:183–7, discussion 187–8.

114. McLean D, Haynes HA, McCarthy PI et al. Cryotherapy of basal cell carcinoma by a simple method of standardized freeze-thaw cycles. *J Dermatol Surg Oncol.* 1978; 4:175–7.

115. Ceilley RI, Del Rosso JQ. Current modalities and new advances in the treatment of basal cell carcinoma. *Int J Derm.* 2006; 45:489–98.

116. Kuflik EG, Gage AA. The five-year cure rate achieved by cryosurgery for skin cancer. *J Am Acad Dermatol.* 1991; 24:1002–4.

117. Kufic EG. Criosurgery for skin cancer: 30 year experience and cure rates. *Dermatol Surg.* 2004; 30:297–300.

118. Chiller K, Passaro D, McCalmont T et al. Efficacy of curettage before excision in clearing surgical margins of nonmelanoma skin cancer. *Arch Dermatol.* 2000; 136:1327–32.

119. Richmond JD, Davie RM. The significance of incomplete excision in patients with basal cell carcinoma. *Br J Plast Surg.* 1987; 40:63–7.

120. Griffiths RW. Audit of histologically incompletely excised basal cell carcinomas: Recommendations for management by re-excision. *Br J Plast Surg.* 1999; 52:24–8.

121. Mohs F. Chemosurgery: A microscopically controlled method of cancer excision. *Arch Surg.* 1991; 42:279–95.

122. Cook JL, Perone JB. A prospective evaluation of the incidence of complications associated with Mohs' micrographic surgery. *Arch Dermatol.* 2003; 139:143–52.

123. Cottell WI, Proper S. Mohs' surgery, fresh tissue technique: Our technique with a review. *J Dermatol Surg Oncol.* 1982; 8:576–87.

124. Smith SP, Grande DJ. Basal cell carcinoma recurring after radiotherapy: A unique, difficult treatment subclass of recurrent basal cell carcinoma. *J Dermatol Surg Oncol.* 1991; 17:26–30.

125. Iyer S, Bowes L, Kricorian G et al. Treatment of basal cell carcinoma with the pulsed carbon dioxide laser: A retrospective analysis. *Dermatol Surg.* 2004; 30:1214–8.

126. Humphreys TR, Malhotra R, Scharf MJ et al. Treatment of superficial basal cell carcinoma and squamous cell carcinoma in situ with a high-energy pulsed carbon dioxide laser. *Arch Dermatol.* 1998; 134:1247–52.

127. Krunic AL, Viehman GE, Madani S et al. Microscopically controlled surgical excision combined with ultrapulse CO_2 vaporization in the management of a patient with the nevoid basal cell carcinoma syndrome. *J Dermatol.* 1998; 25:10–12.

128. Caccialanza C Piccinno R, Beretta M. Results and side effects of dermatologic radiotherapy: A retrospective study of irradiated cutaneous epithelial neoplasms. *Am Acad Dermatol.* 1999; 41:589–94.

129. Rowe DE, Carroll RJ, Day CL Jr. Mohs' surgery is the treatment of choice for recurrent (previously treated) basal cell carcinoma. *J Dermatol Surg Oncol.* 1989; 15:424–31.

130. Miller RA, Spittle MF. Electron beam therapy for difficult cutaneous basal and squamous cell carcinomas. *Br J Dermatol.* 1982; 106:429–36.

131. Lederman M. Radiation treatment of cancer of the eyelids. *Br J Ophthal.* 1976; 60:794–805.

132. Schlienger P, Brunin F, Desjardin L et al. External radiotherapy for carcinoma of the eyelid: Report of 850 cases treated. *Int J Rad Oncol Biol Phys.* 1996; 34:277–87.

133. Stafford SL, Kozelsky TF, Garrity JA et al. Orbital lymphoma: Radiotherapy outcome and complications. *Radiother Oncol.* 2001; 59:139–44.

134. Reisner K, Haase W. Electron beam therapy of primary tumors of the skin. *Radiol Med (Torino)* 1990; 80 Supplement 1:114–15.

135. DeSilva SP, Dellon AL. Recurrence rate of positive margin basal cell carcinoma results of a five-year prospective study. *J Surg Oncol.* 1985; 28:72–4.

136. Richmond JD, Davie RM. The significance of incomplete excision in patients with basal cell carcinoma. *Br J Plast Surg.* 1987; 40:63–7.

137. Liu FF, Maki R, Warde P et al. A management approach to incompletely excised basal cell carcinomas of skin. *Int J Radiat Oncol Biol Phys.* 1991; 20:423–8.

138. Wang I, Bendsoe N, Klinteberg CA et al. Photodynamic therapy vs. cryosurgery of basal cell carcinomas: Results of a phase III clinical trial. *Br J Dermatol.* 2001; 144:832–40.

139. Basset-Seguin N, Ibbotson S, Emtestam L. Photodynamic therapy using Metvix™ is as efficacious as cryotherapy in BCC with better cosmetic results. *J Eur Acad Dermatol Venereol.* 2001; 15:226. Cited in: Foley P. Clinical efficacy of methylaminolevulinate (metvix) photodynamic therapy. *J Dermatol Treat.* 2003; 14:15–22.

140. Roozeboom MH, Aardoom MA et al. Fractionated 5-aminolevulinic acid photodynamic therapy after partial debulking versus surgical excision for nodular basal cell carcinoma: A randomized controlled trial with at least 5-year follow-up. *J Am Acad Dermatol.* 2013; 69(2):280–7.

141. Epstein E. Fluorouracil paste treatment of thin basal cell carcinomas. *Arch Dermatol.* 1985; 121:207–13.

142. Marks R, Gebauer K, Shumack S et al. Imiquimod 5% cream in the treatment of superficial basal cell carcinoma: Results of a multicenter 6-week dose–response trial. *J Am Acad Dermatol.* 2001; 44:807–13.

143. Geisse JK, Rich P, Pandya A et al. Imiquimod 5% cream for the treatment of superficial basal cell carcinoma: A doubleblind, randomized, vehicle-controlled study. *J Am Acad Dermatol.* 2002; 47:390–8.

144. Geisse J, Caro I, Lindholm J et al. Imiquimod 5% cream for the treatment of superficial basal cell carcinoma: Results from two phase III, randomized, vehicle-controlled studies. *J Am Acad Dermatol.* 2004; 50:722–33.

145. Sterry W, Ruzicka T, Herrera E et al. Imiquimod 5% cream for the treatment of superficial and nodular basal cell carcinoma: Randomized studies comparing low-frequency dosing with and without occlusion. *Br J Dermatol.* 2002; 147:1227–36.

146. Jia HX, He YL. Efficacy and safety of imiquimod 5% cream for basal cell carcinoma: A meta-analysis of randomized controlled trial. *J Dermatolog Treat.* 2019 Jul 17:1–8.

147. Sekulic A, Migden MR, Oro AE et al. Efficacy and safety of vismodegib in advanced basal-cell carcinoma. *N Engl J Med.* 2012; 366(23):2171–9.

148. Sekulic A, Migden MR, Lewis K et al. Pivotal ERIVANCE basal cell carcinoma (BCC) study: 12-month update of efficacy and safety of vismodegib in advanced BCC. 2015; 72:1021–6.

149. Robinson JK. Risk of developing another basal cell carcinoma. *Cancer.* 1987; 60:118–20.

150. Salasche SJ. Epidemiology of actinic keratoses and squamous cell carcinoma. *J Am Acad Dermatol.* 2000; 42:4–7.

151. Ahmed I, Das Gupta AR. Epidemiology of basal cell carcinoma and squamous cell carcinoma of the Pinna. *J Laryngol Otol.* 2001; 115:85–6.

152. Holman CD, Armstrong DK, Evans PR et al. Relationship of solar keratosis and history of skin cancer to objective measures of actinic skin damage. *Br J Dermatol.* 1984; 110:129–38.

153. Joseph MG, Zulueta WP, Kennedy PJ. Squamous cell carcinoma of the skin of the trunk and limbs: The incidence of metastases and their outcome. *Aust NZ J Surg.* 1992; 62:697–701.

154. Rowe DE, Carroll RJ, Day CL Jr. Prognostic factors for local recurrence, metastasis, and survival rates in squamous cell carcinoma of the skin, ear, and lip. Implications for treatment modality selection. *J Am Acad Dermatol.* 1992; 26:976–90.

155. Cherpelis BS, Marcusen C, Lang PG. Prognostic factors for metastasis in squamous cell carcinoma of the skin. *Dermatol Surg.* 2002; 28:268–73.

156. Antoniades DZ, Styanidis K, Papanayotou P et al. Squamous cell carcinoma of the lips in a northern Greek population. Evaluation of prognostic factors on 5-year survival rate. *Eur J Cancer.* 1995; 318:333–9.

157. Motley R, Kersey P, Lawrence C et al. Multiprofessional guidelines for the management of the patient with primary cutaneous squamous cell carcinoma. *Br J Dermatol.* 2002; 146:18–25.

158. Friedman HI, Cooper PH, Wanebo HJ. Prognostic and therapeutic use of microstaging of cutaneous squamous cell carcinoma of the trunk and extremities. *Cancer.* 1985; 56:1099–105.

159. Lazarov M, Kubo Y, Cai T et al. CDK4 Co-expression with Ras generates malignant human epidermal tumorigenesis. *Nat Med.* 2002; 8:1105–14.

160. Dajee M, Lazarov M, Zhang J et al. NF-kappa Beta blockade and oncogenic Ras trigger invasive human epidermal neoplasia. *Nature.* 2003; 421:639–43.

161. Motle RJ, Preston PW, Lawrence CM. Multi-professional guidelines for the management of the patient with primary cutaneous squamous cell carinoma. *BJD.* 2002; 146(1):18–25.

162. Brodland DG, Zitelli JA. Surgical margins for excision of primary cutaneous squamous cell carcinoma. *J Am Acad Dermatol.* 1992; 27:241–8.

163. Lawrence N, Cottel WI. Squamous cell carcinoma of skin with perineural invasion. *J Am Acad Dermatol.* 1994; 31:30–3.

164. Lawrence CM, Dahl MGC, Dickinson AJ, Turner RJ. Mohs micrographic surgery for cutaneous squamous cell carcinoma: Practical considerations. *Br J Dermatol.* 2001; 144:186.

165. Veness MJ, Morgan GJ, Palme CE, Gebski V. Surgery and adjuvant radiotherapy in patients with cutaneous head and neck squamous cell carcinoma metastatic to lymph nodes: Combined treatment should be considered best practice. *Laryngoscope.* 2005; 115:870–5.

166. Stephens FO, Harker GJS. The use of intra-arterial chemotherapy for treatment of malignant skin neoplasms. *Australas J Dermatol.* 1979; 20:99–107.

167. McDowell LJ, Tan TJ, Bressel M et al. Outcomes of cutaneous squamous cell carcinoma of the head and neck with parotid metastases. *J Med Imaging Radiat Oncol.* 2016; 60:668–76.

168. Sadek H, Azli N, Wendling JL et al. Treatment of advanced squamous cell carcinoma of the skin with cisplatin, 5-fluorouracil, amd bleomycin. *Cancer.* 1990; 66:1692–6.

169. Jarkowski A 3rd, Hare R, Loud P et al. Systemic therapy in advanced cutaneous squamous cell carcinoma (CSCC): The Roswell Park Experience and a Review of Literature. *Am J Clin Oncol.* 2016; 39:545–8.

170. Sadek H, Azli N, Wendling JL et al. Treatment of advanced squamous cell carcinoma of the skin with cisplatin 5-fluorouracil and bleomycin. *Cancer.* 1990; 66:1692–6.

171. Shin DM, Glisson BS, Khuri FRet al. Phase II and biologic study of interferon alfa, retinoic acid, and cisplatin in advanced squamous skin cancer. *J Clin Oncol.* 2002; 20:364–70.

172. Frankel D, Hanusa BH, Zitalli JA. New primary non-melanoma skin cancer patients with a history of squamous cell carcinoma of the skin. Implications and recommendations for follow-up. *J Am Acad Dermatol.* 1992; 26:720–6.

173. National Cancer Registration and Analysis Service. NCIN data-briefings. Available at: http://www.ncin.org.uk/publications/data_briefings (last accessed 8 October 2018).

174. Willemze R, Jaffe ES, Burg G et al. WHO-EORTC classification for cutaneous lymphomas. *Blood.* 2005; 105:3768–85.

175. Trautinger F, Eder J, Assaf C et al. European Organisation for Research and Treatment of Cancer consensus recommendations for the treatment of mycosis fungoides/Sezary syndrome—Update 2017. *Eur J Cancer.* 2017; 77:57–74.

176. Swerdlow SH, Campo E, Harris NL. *WHO Classification of Tumours of Haematopoietic and Lymphoid Tissues* (4th ed.) Lyon: IARC, 2017.

177. Gilson D Whittaker SJ, Child FJ et al. British Association of Dermatologists and UK cutaneous lymphoma guidelines for the management of primary cutaneous lymphomas 2018. *BJD.* 2019; 180:443–44.

178. Senff N, Noordijk EM, Kim YH et al. European organization for research and Treatment of Cancer and International Society for Cutaneous Lymphoma consensus recommendations for

the management of cutaneous B-cell lymphomas. *Blood.* 2008; 112(5):1600–9.

179. Felcht M, Klemke CD et al. Nicolay JP, Primary cutaneous diffuse large B-cell lymphoma, NOS and leg type: Clinical, morphologic and prognostic differences. *J Dtsch Dermatol Ges.* 2019; 17(3):275–85.

180. Tan R, Butterworth CM, Mclaughin H et al. Mycosis fungoides—A disease of antigen persistence. *Br J Dermatol.* 1974; 91:607–16.

181. Vowels BR, Cassin M, Vonderheid EC et al. Aberrant cytokine production by Sèzary syndrome patients: Cytokine secretion pattern resembles murine Th2 cells. *J Invest Dermatol.* 1992; 99:90–8.

182. Vowels BR, lessin SR, Cassin M et al. Th2 cytokine mRNA expression in skin in cutaneous T cell lymphoma. *J Invest Dermatol.* 1994; 103:29–32.

183. Saed G, Fivenson DP, Naidu T et al. Mycosis fungoides exhibits a Th1-type cell mediated cytokine profile, whereas, Sèzary syndrome expresses a Th1-type profile. *J Invest Dermatol.* 1994; 103:29–33.

184. Sugerman G, Bigby M. Preliminary function analysis of human epidermal T cells. *Arch Dermatol Res.* 2000; 292:9–15.

185. Howard K, Charif M, Martin A et al. Epidemiology and clinical manifestations of cutaneous T-cell lymphoma. *Hematol Oncol Clin North Am.* 1995; 9:5–11.

186. Lisby G, Reitz MS, Vejlsgaard GL, Reitz MS Jr. No detection of HTLV-l DNA in punch biopsies from patients with cutaneous T-cell lymphoma by the polymerase chain reaction. *J Invest Dermatol.* 1992; 98:417–20.

187. Pancake RA, Zucker-Franklin D, Coutavas EE. The cutaneous T-cell lymphoma, mycosis fungoides, is a human T-cell lymphotrophic virus-associated disease. *J Clin Invest.* 1995; 95:547–54.

188. Tothova SM, Bonin S, Trevisan G, Stanta G. Mycosis fungoides: Is it a Borrelia burgdorferi-associated disease? *Br J Cancer.* 2006; 94:879–83.

189. Trautinger F, Knobler R, Willemze R et al. EORTC consensus recommendations for the treatment of mycosis fungoides/Sèzary syndrome. *Eur J Cancer.* 2006; 42:1014–30.

190. Agar NS, Wedgeworth E, Crichton S et al. Survival outcomes and prognostic factors in mycosis fungoides/Sézary syndrome: Validation of the revised International Society for Cutaneous Lymphomas/European Organisation for Research and Treatment of Cancer staging proposal. *J Clin Oncol.* 2010; 28(31):4730–9.

191. Benton E, Crichton S, Talpur R et al. A Cutaneous Lymphoma International Prognostic Index (CLIPi) for mycosis fungoides and Sezary syndrome. *Eur J Cancer.* 2013; 49(13):2859–68.

192. Scarisbrick JJ, Prince HM, Vermeer MH et al. Cutaneous lymphoma international consortium study of outcome in advanced stages of mycosis fungoides and Sézary syndrome: Effect of specific prognostic markers on survival and development of a prognostic model. *J Clin Oncol.* 2015; 33:3766–73.

193. Olsen E, Vonderheid E, Pimpinelli N et al. Revisions to the staging and classification of mycosis fungoides and Sezary syndrome: A proposal of the International Society for Cutaneous Lymphomas (ISCL) and the cutaneous lymphoma task force of the European Organization of Research and Treatment of Cancer (EORTC). *Blood.* 2007; 110(6):1713–22.

194. Tsai EY, Taur A, Espinosa L et al. Staging accuracy in mycosis fungoides and Sèzary syndrome using integrated positron emission tomography and computed tomography. *Arch Dermatol.* 2006; 142:577–84.

195. Spaccarelli N et al. Role of 18F fluorodeoxyglucose PET imaging in the management of primary cutaneous lymphomas. *Hell J Nul Med.* 2014; 17(2):78–84.

196. Thangarelu M, Finn WG, Yelavarthi KK et al. Recurring structural chromosomal abnormalities in peripheral blood lymphocytes of patients with mycosis fungoides/Sèzary syndrome. *Blood.* 1997; 89:3371–7.

197. Mao X, Lillington DM, Czepulkowski B et al. Molecular cytogenetic characterization of Sèzary syndrome. *Genes, Chromosomes, Cancer.* 2003; 36:250–60.

198. Karenko L, Hyytinen E, Sarna S, Ranki A. Chromosomal abnormalities in cutaneous T-cell lymphoma and in its pre-malignant conditions as detected by G-banding and interphase cytogenetic methods. *J Invest Dermatol.* 1997; 108:22–9.

199. Mao X, Lillington D, Scarisbrick JJ et al. Molecular cytogenetic analysis of cutaneous T-cell lymphomas: IIentification of common genetic alterations in Sèzary syndrome and mycosis fungoides. *Br J Dermatol.* 2002; 147:464–75.

200. Fischer T, Gellrich S, Muche M et al. Genomic aberrations and survival in cutaneous T-cell lymphomas. *J Invest Dermatol.* 2004; 122:579.

201. Park J, Yang J, Wenzel AT. Genomic analysis of 220 CTCLs identifies a novel recurrent gain-of-function alteration in RLTPR (p.Q575E). *Blood.* 2017; 130(12):1430–40.

202. Kaye FJ, Bunn PA Jr, Steinberg SM et al. A randomized trial comparing combination electron beam radiation and chemotherapy with topical therapy in the initial treatment of mycosis fungoides. *N Engl J Med.* 1989; 321:1748–90.

203. Quagline P et al. Global patterns of care in advanced stage mycosis fungoides/Sezary syndrome: A multicenter retrospective follow up study from the cutaneous lymphoma international consortium. *Ann Oncol.* 2017; 28:2517–25.

204. Zackheim H, Kashani-Sabet M, Amin S. Topical corticosteroids for mycosis fungoides. *Arch Dermatol.* 1998; 134:949–54.

205. Heald P, Mehlmauer M, Martin AG et al. Topical bexarotene therapy for patients with refractory or persistent early-stage cutaneous T-cell lymphoma: Results of the phase III clinical trial. *J Am Acad Dermatol.* 2003; 49:801–15.

206. Whittaker S, Ortiz P, Dummer R et al. Efficacy and safety of bexarotene combined with psoralen ultraviolet A (PUVA) compared to PUVA treatment alone in patients with stage IB-IIA mycosis fungoides: Final results from the EORTC cutaneous lymphoma task force phase III randomised clinical trial 21011 (NCT00056056). *Br J Dermatol.* 2012; 167:678–87.

207. Scholtz W. Ueber den einfluss der rontgenstrahlen auf die haut in gesunden und krankem zustande. *Arch Dermat U Syph.* 1902; 59:421.

208. Kim JH, Nisce LZ, D'Anglo GJ. Dose-time fractionation study in patients with mycosis fungoides and lymphoma cutis. *Radiology.* 1976; 119:439–42.

209. Cotter GW, Baglan RJ, Wasserman TH, Mill W. Palliative radiation treatment of cutaneous mycosis fungoides—a dose–response. *Int J Radiat Oncol Biol Phys.* 1983; 9:1477–80.

210. Neelis KJ, Schimmel EC, Vermeer MH et al. Low-dose palliative radiotherapy for cutaneous B- and T-cell lymphomas. *Int J Radiat Oncol Biol Phys.* 2009; 74(1):154e158.

211. Morris SL. Skin lymphoma. *Clin Oncol.* 2012; 24(5):371–85.

212. Hoppe RT. Mycosis fungoides: Radiation therapy. *Dermatol Ther.* 16; 2003:347–54.

213. Thomas TO, Agrawal P, Guitart J et al. Outcome of patients treated with a single-fraction dose of palliative radiation for cutaneous T-cell lymphoma. *Int J Radiat Oncol Biol Phys.* 2013; 85(3):747–53.

214. Karzmark CJ, Loevinger R, Steele RE, Weissbluth M. A technique for large-field, superficial electron therapy. *Radiology.* 1960; 74:633–44.

215. Szur L, Silvester JA, Bewley DK. Treatment of the whole body surface with electrons. *Lancet.* 1962; 279:1373–7.

216. Jones GW, Kacinski BM, Wilson LD et al. Total skin electron radiation in the management of mycosis fungoides: Consensus of the European Organization for Research and Treatment of Cancer (EORTC) Cutaneous Lymphoma Project Group. *J Am Acad Dermatol.* 2002; 47:364–70.

217. Kim TH, Pla C, Pla M, Podgorsak EB. Clinical aspects of a rotational total skin electron beam irradiation. *Br J Radiol.* 1984; 57:501–6.

218. Jones GW, Hoppe RT, Glastein E. Electron beam treatment for CTCL. *Hematol Oncol Clin North Am.* 1995; 9:1057–76.

219. Kim YH, Jensen RA, Watanabe GL et al. Clinical stage IA mycosis fungoides. A long term outcome analysis. *Arch Dermatol.* 1996; 132:1309–13.

220. Jones G, Wilson LD, Fox-Goguen L. Total skin electron beam radiotherapy for patients who have mycosis fungoides. *Hematol Oncol Clin North Am.* 2003; 17:1421–34.

221. Kim YH, Martinez G, Varghese A et al. Topical nitrogen mustard in the management of mycosis fungoides: Update of the Stanford experience. *Arch Dermatol.* 2003; 139:165–73.

222. Chinn DM, Chow S, Kim YH et al. Total skin electron therapy with or without adjuvant topical nitrogen mustard or nitrogen mustard alone as initial treatment of T2 and T3 mycosis fungoides. *Int J Radiat Oncol Biol Phys.* 1999; 43:951–8.

223. Jones GW, Rosenthal D, Wilson LD. Total skin electron beam radiation for patients with erythrodermic cutaneous T-cell lymphoma (mycosis fungoides and the Sèzary syndrome). *Cancer.* 1999; 85:1985–95.

224. Morris SL, McGovern M, Bayne S et al. Results of a 5-week schedule of modern total skin electron beam radiation therapy. *Int J Radiat Oncol Biol Phys.* 2013; 86(5):936–41.

225. Wilson LD. Delivery and sequelae of total skin electron beam therapy. *Arch Derm.* 2003; 139:812–3.

226. Kamstrup M, Specht L, Skovgaard G et al. A prospective, open-label study of low-dose total skin electron beam therapy in mycosis fungoides. *Int J Radiat Oncol Biol Phys.* 2008; 71(4):1204–7.

227. Kamstrup MR, Lindahl LM, Gniadecki R et al. Low dose 10Gy TSEB for cutaneous t cell lymphoma: An open clinical study and pooled data analysis. *IJROBP.* 2015; 92(1):183–43.

228. Hoppe RT, Harrison C, Tavallaee M et al. Low dose TSEB as an effective modality to reduce disease burden in patients with mycosis fungoides: Results of a pooled analysis from 3 phase II clinical trials. *J Am Acad Dermatol.* 2015; 72(2):286–92.

229. Morris SL, Scarisbrick J, Frew JJ et al. The results of low dose total skin electron beam radiotherapy (TSEB), in patients with mycosis fungoides from the U.K. Cutaneous Lymphoma Group. *Int J RadiatOncol Biol Phys.* 2017; 99:627–33.

230. Elsayad K, Kroeger K, Greve B et al. Low-dose total skin electron beam therapy: Quality of life improvement and clinical impact of maintenance and adjuvant treatment in patients with mycosis fungoides or Sezary syndrome. *Strahlenther Onkol.* 2020; 196:77–84.

231. Duvic M, Donato M, Dabaja B et al. Total skin electron beam and non-myeloablative allogeneic hematopoietic stem-cell transplantation in advanced mycosis fungoides and Sezary syndrome. *J Clin Oncol.* 2010; 28(14):2365–72.

232. Duarte RF, Boumendil A, Onida F et al. Long-term outcome of allogeneic hematopoietic cell transplantation for patients with mycosis fungoides and Sezary syndrome: A European society for blood and marrow transplantation lymphoma working party extended analysis. *J Clin Oncol.* 2014; 32:3347–8.

233. Duarte R, Canals C, Onida F et al. Allogeneic hematopoietic cell transplantation for patients with mycosis fungoides and Sezary syndrome: A retrospective analysis of the Lymphoma Working Party of the European Group for Blood and Marrow Transplantation. *JCO.* 2010; 29(29):4492–9.

234. Sun WH, Pabon C, Alsayed Y et al. Interferon-alpha resistance in a cutaneous T-cell lymphoma cell line is associated with lack of STAT1 expression. *Blood.* 1998; 91:570–6.

235. Bunn PA Jr, Ihde DC, Foon KA. The role of recombinant interferon alpha-2a in the therapy of cutaneous T-cell lymphomas. *Cancer.* 1986; 57 Supplement:1689–95.

236. Olsen EA, Rosen ST, Vollmer RT et al. Interferon alfa-2a in the treatment of cutaneous T-cell lymphoma. *J Am Acad Dermatol.* 1989; 20:395–407.

237. Papa G, Tura S, Mandelli F et al. Is interferon alpha in cutaneous T-cell lymphoma a treatment of choice? *Br J Haematol.* 1991; 79 Supplement 1:48–51.

238. Spaccarelli N, Rook A. The use of interferons in the treatment of cutaneous T cell lymphoma. *Dermatol Clin.* 2015; 33:731–45

239. Stadler R, Otte HG, Luger T et al. Prospective randomized multi-centre clinical trial on the use of interferon alpha-2a plus acitretin versus interferon alpha-2a plus PUVA in patients with cutaneous T-cell lymphoma stages I and II. *Blood.* 1998; 10:3578–81.

240. Kuzel TM, Roenigk HH Jr, Samuelson E et al. Effectiveness of interferon alfa-2a combined with phototherapy for mycosis fungoides and the Sézary syndrome. *J Clin Oncol.* 1995; 13:257–63.

241. Dreno B, Claudy A, Meynadier J et al. The treatment of 45 patients with cutaneous T-cell lymphoma with low doses of interferon-alpha 2a and etretinate. *Br J Dermatol.* 1991; 125:456–9.

242. Rook AH, Wood GS, Yoo EK et al. Interleukin-12 therapy of cutaneous T-cell lymphoma induces lesion regression and cytotoxic T-cell responses. *Blood.* 1999; 94:902–8.

243. Kaplan EH, Rosen ST, Norris DB et al. Phase II study of recombinant interferon gamma for treatment of cutaneous T-cell lymphoma. *J Nat Cancer Inst.* 1990; 82:208–12.

244. Ritchie S, Qureshi I, Molloy K et al. Evaluation of haematopoietic stem cell transplantation in patients diagnosed with cutaneous T cell lymphoma at a tertiary care centre: Should we avoid chemotherapy in conditioning regimens? *Br J Dermatol.* 2020; 182(3): 807–9.

245. Kurzrock R, Pilat S, Duvic M. Pentostatin therapy of T-cell lymphomas with cutaneous manifestations. *J Clin Oncol.* 1999; 17:3117–21.

246. Dearden C, Matutes E, Catovsky D. Pentostatin treatment of cutaneous T-cell lymphoma. *Oncology.* 2000; 14 Supplement 2:37–40.

247. Scarisbrick JJ, Child FJ, Clift A et al. A trial of fludarabine and cyclophosphamide combination chemotherapy in the treatment of advanced refractory primary cutaneous T-cell lymphoma. *Br J Dermatol.* 2001; 144:1010–15.

248. Zinzani PL, Baliva G, Magagnoli M et al. Gemcitabine treatment in pretreated cutaneous T-cell lymphoma: Experience in 44 patients. *J Clin Oncol.* 2000; 18:2603–6.

249. Marchi E, Alinari L, Tani M et al. Gemcitabine as frontline treatment for cutaneous T-cell lymphoma: Phase II study of 32 patients. *Cancer.* 2005; 104:2437–41.

250. T, Chan C, Counsell N et al. Phase II study of gemcitabine and bexarotene (GEMBEX) in the treatment of cutaneous T-cell lymphoma. *Br J Cancer.* 2013; 109(10):2566–73.

251. Wollina U, Dummer R, Brockmeyer NH et al. Multicenter study of pegylated liposomal doxorubicin in patients with cutaneous T-cell lymphoma. *Cancer.* 2003; 98:993–1001.

252. Di Lorenzo G, Di Trolio R, Delfino M, De Placido S. Pegylated liposomal doxorubicin in stage IVB mycosis fungoides. *Br J Dermatol.* 2005; 153:183–5.

253. Dummer R, Quaglino P, Becker JC et al. Prospective international multicenter phase II trial of intravenous pegylated liposomal doxorubicin monochemotherapy in patients with stage IIB, IVA, or IVB advanced mycosis fungoides: Final results from EORTC 21012. *J Clin Oncol.* 2012; 30(33):4091–7.

254. Prince HM Kim YH Horwitz AM et al. Brentuximab vedotin or physicians choice in CD30 positive cutaneous T cell lymphoma (ALCANZA): An international, open label, randomized, phase 3, multicenter trial. *Lancet.* 2017; 390(10094):555–66

255. Boehm MF, Zhang L, Badea BA et al. Synthesis and structure–activity relationships of novel retinoid X receptor-selective retinoids. *J Med Chem.* 1994; 37:2930–41.

256. Duvic M, Martin AG, Kim Y et al. Phase 2 and 3 clinical trial of oral bexarotene (Targretin capsules) for the treatment of refractory or persistent early-stage cutaneous T-cell lymphoma. *Arch Dermatol.* 2001; 137:581–93.

257. Committee for proprietary medicinal products. *European Public Assessment Report (EPAR): Targretin.* London, UK: European Agency for the Evaluation of Medicinal Products, 2001.

258. Zhang C, Hazarika P, Ni X et al. Induction of apoptosis by bexarotene in cutaneous T-cell lymphoma cells: Relevance to mechanism of therapeutic action. *Clin Cancer Res.* 2002; 8:1234–40.

259. Edelson R, Berger C, Gasparro F et al. Treatment of cutaneous T-cell lymphoma by extracorporeal photochemotherapy. Preliminary results. *N Engl J Med.* 1987; 316:297–303.

260. Talpur R, Ward S, Apisarnthanarax N et al. Optimizing bexarotene therapy for cutaneous T-cell lymphoma. *J Am Acad Dermatol.* 2002; 47:672–84.

261. Knobler R, Jantschitsch C. Extracorporeal photochemoimmunotherapy in cutaneous T-cell lymphoma. *Transfus Apheresis Sci.* 2003; 28:81–9.

262. Vonderheid EC, Bernengo MG, Burg G et al. Update on erythrodermic cutaneous T-cell lymphoma: Report of the International Society for Cutaneous Lymphomas. *J Am Acad Dermatol.* 2002; 46:95–106.

263. Russell Jones RR, Whittaker S. T-cell receptor gene analysis in the diagnosis of Sézary syndrome. *J Am Acad Dermatol.* 1999; 41:254–9.

264. Scarisbrick JJ, Hodak E, Bagot M et al. Blood classification and blood response criteria in mycosis fungoides and Sézary syndrome

using flow cytometry: Recommendations from the EORTC cutaneous lymphoma task force. *Eur J Cancer.* 2018; 93:47–56.

265. Suchin KR, Cucchiara AJ, Gottleib SL et al. Treatment of cutaneous T-cell lymphoma with combined immunomodulatory therapy: A 14-year experience at a single institution. *Arch Dermatol.* 2002; 138:1054–60.

266. Bazarbachi A, Ghez D, Lepelletier Y et al. New therapeutic approaches for adult T-cell leukaemia. *Lancet Oncol.* 2004; 5:664–72.

267. Kempf W, Pfaltz K, Vermeer MH et al. EORTC, ISCL, AND USCLC Consensus recommendations for the treatment of primary cutaneous CD30-Positive lymphoproliferative disorders: Lymphomatoid papulosis and primary cutaneous anaplastic large-cell lymphoma. *Blood.* 2011; 118(15):4024–35.

268. Bekkenk M, Geelen FAMJ, van Voorst et al. Primary and secondary cutaneous CD30-positive lymphoproliferative disorders: Long term follow-up data of 219 patients and guidelines for diagnosis and treatment. A report from the Dutch Cutaneous Lymphoma Group. *Blood.* 2000; 95:3653–61.

269. Kim YH, Willemze R, Pimpinelli N et al. TNM classification system for primary cutaneous lymphomas other than mycosis fungoides and Sezary syndrome: A proposal of the International Society for Cutaneous Lymphomas (ISCL) and the Cutaneous Lymphoma Task Force of the European Organization of Research and Treatment of Cancer (EORTC). *Blood.* 2007; 110(2):479–84.

270. Senff NJ, Willemze R. The applicability and prognostic value of the new TNM classification system for primary cutaneous lymphomas other than mycosis fungoides and Sézary syndrome: Results on a large cohort of primary cutaneous B-cell lymphomas and comparison with the system used by the Dutch Cutaneous Lymphoma Group. *Br J Dermatol.* 2007; 157(6):1205–11.

271. Eich HT, Eich D, Micke O et al. Long term efficacy, curative potential and prognostic factors of radiotherapy in primary cutaneous B cell lymphoma. *Int J Radiat Oncol Biol Phys.* 2003; 55:899–906.

272. Smith BD, Glusac EJ, McNiff JM et al. Primary cutaneous B cell lymphoma treated with radiotherapy: A comparison of the EORTC and WHO classification systems. *J Clin Oncol.* 2004; 15:634–9.

273. Rijlaarsdam JU, Toomska J, Meijer OW et al. Treatment of primary cutaneous B cell lymphoma of follicle centre cell origin: A clinical follow up study of 55 patients treated with radiotherapy or polychemotherapy. *J Clin Oncol.* 1996; 14:549–55.

274. Piccinno R, Caccialanza M, Berti E et al. Radiotherapy of cutaneous B cell lymphomas: Our experience of 31 cases. *Int J Radiat Oncol Biol Phys.* 1993; 27:385–9.

275. Specht L et al. Modern radiation therapy for primary cutaneous lymphomas: Field and dose guidelines from the International Lymphoma Radiation Oncology Group. *IJROBP.* 2015; 92(1):32–9.

276. Paget J. On disease of the mammary areola preceding cancer of the mammary gland. *St Barthol Hosp Report.* 1874; 10:87–89.

277. Crocker HR. Paget's disease affecting the scrotum and penis. *Trans Path Soc.* 1888; 40:187–191.

278. Darier J, Couillaud P. Sur un cas de malade de Paget de la region perineo-anale et scrotale. *Ann Dermatol Syph.* 1893; 4:25–33.

279. Brown RSD, Lankester KJ, McCormak M et al. Radiotherapy for perianal Paget's disease. *Clin Oncol.* 2002; 14:272–84.

280. Mohs FE, Blanchard L. Microscopically controlled surgery for extramammary Paget's disease. *Arch Dermatol.* 1979; 115:706–8.

281. Mirer E, El Sayed F, Ammoury A et al. Treatment of mammary and extramammary Paget's skin disease with topical imiquimod. *J Dermatol Treat.* 2006; 17:167–71.

282. Nardelli AA, Stafinski T, Menon D. Effectiveness of photodynamic therapy for mammary and extra-mammary Paget's disease: A state of the science review. *BMC Dermatol.* 2011; 11:13.

283. Rioli DI, Samimi M, Beneton N et al. Efficacy and tolerance of photodynamic therapy for vulvar Paget's disease: A multicentric retrospective study. *Eur J Dermatol.* 2018; 28(3):351–5.

284. Besa P, Rich TA, Delclos L et al. Extramammary Paget's disease of the perineal skin: Role of radiotherapy. *Int J Radiat Oncol Biol Phys.* 1992; 24:73–78.

285. Vortmeyer AO, Merino MJ, Boni R et al. Genetic changes associated with primary Merkel cell carcinoma. *Am J Clin Pathol.* 1998; 109:565–70.

286. Rare skin cancer in England: National cancer intelligence network 2011. Available at: http://www.ncin.org.uk/publicati ons/ data_briefings/rareskincancer

287. Agelli M, Clegg LX: Epidemiology of primary Merkel cell carcinoma in the United States. *J Am Acad Dermatol.* 2003; 49(5):832–41.

288. Akhtar S, Oza KK, Wright J. Merkel cell carcinoma: Report of 10 cases and review of the literature. *J Am Acad Dermatol.* 2000; 43:755–67.

289. Simstein NL, Sduggs NK. Merkel cell tumor: Two cases. *Int Surg.* 1998; 83:60–2.

290. Barksdale SK. Advances in Merkel cell carcinoma from a pathologist's perspective. *Pathology.* 2017; 49(6):568–74.

291. Lunder EJ, Stern RS. Merkel cell carcinoma in patients treated with methoxsalen and ultraviolet radiation. *N Engl J Med.* 1998; 339:1247–8.

292. Williams RH, Morgan MB, Mathieson IM et al. Merkel cell carcinoma in a renal transplant patient: Increased incidence? *Transplantation.* 1998; 65:1396–7.

293. Ott MJ, Tanabe KK, Gadd MA et al. Multimodality management of Merkel cell carcinoma. *Arch Surg.* 1999; 134:388–92.

294. Schlagbauer-Wadl H, Klosner G, Heere-Ress E. Bcl-2 antisense oligonucleotides (G3139) inhibit Merkel cell carcinoma growth in SCID mice. *J Invest Dermatol.* 2000; 114:725–30.

295. George A, Girault S, Testard A et al. The impact of 18F-FDG-PET/CT on Merkel cell carcinoma management: A retrospective study of 66 scans from a single institution. *Nucl Med Commun.* 2014; 35(3):282–90.

296. Feng H, Shuda M, Chang Y et al. Clonal integration of a polyomavirus in human Merkel cell carcinoma. *Science.* 2008; 319(5866):1096–100.

297. Paik JY, Hall G, Clarkson A et al. Immunohistochemistry for Merkel cell polyomavirus is highly specific but not sensitive for the diagnosis of Merkel cell carcinoma in the Australian population. *Hum Pathol.* 2011; 42(10):1385–90.

298. Belhocine T, Pierard GE, Fruhling J et al. Clinical added-value of 18FDG PET in neuroendocrine-merkel cell carcinoma. *Oncol Rep.* 2006; 16:347–52.

299. Yiengpruksawan A, Coit DG, Thaler HT et al. Merkel cell carcinoma, prognosis and management. *Arch Surg.* 1991; 126:1513–9.

300. Bichakjian CK, Nghiem P, Johnson T et al. Merkel cell carcinoma. In Amin MB, Edge SB, Greene FL et al. (Eds.), *AJCC Cancer Staging Manual* (8th ed., pp 549–62). New York, NY: Springer, 2017.

301. Andea AA, Coit DG, Amin B et al. Merkel cell carcinoma: Histologic features and prognosis. *Cancer.* 2008; 113(9):2549–58.

302. Rao P, Balzer BL, Lemos BD et al. Protocol for the examination of specimens from patients with merkel cell carcinoma of the skin. *Arch Pathol Lab Med.* 2010; 134(3):341–4.

303. Tope WD, Sangueza OP. Merkel cell carcinoma. Histopathology, immunohistochemistry, and cytogenetic analysis. *J Dermatol Surg Oncol.* 1994; 20:648–54.

304. Yan L, Sun L, Guan Z et al. Analysis of cutaneous Merkel cell carcinoma outcomes after different surgical interventions. *J Am Acad Dermatol.* 2020; 82(6):1422–34.

305. Wright GP, Holtzman MP. Surgical resection improves median overall survival with marginal improvement in long-term survival when compared with definitive radiotherapy in Merkel cell carcinoma: A propensity score matched analysis of the National Cancer Database. *Am J Surg.* 2018; 215:384–7.

306. Allen PJ, Zhang ZF, Coit DG. Surgical management of Merkel cell carcinoma. *Ann Surg.* 1999; 229:97–105.

307. Gunaratne DA, Howle JR, Veness MJ. Sentinel lymph node biopsy in Merkel cell carcinoma: A 15-year institutional experience and statistical analysis of 721 reported cases. *Br J Dermatol.* 2016; 174(2):273e281.

308. Lee JS, Durham AB, Bichakjian CK et al. Completion lymph node dissection or radiation therapy for sentinel node metastasis in Merkel cell carcinoma. *Ann Surg Oncol.* 2019; 26(2):386e394.

309. Eich HT, Eich D, Staar S et al. Role of postoperative radiotherapy in the management of Merkel cell carcinoma. *Am J Clin Oncol.* 2002; 25:50–6.

310. Veness MJ, Morgan GJ, Palme CE, Gebski V. Surgery and adjuvant radiotherapy in patients with cutaneous head and neck squamous cell carcinoma metastatic to lymph nodes: Combined treatment should be considered best practice. *Laryngoscope.* 2005; 115:870–5.

311. Allen PJ, Bowne WB, Jacques DP et al. Merkel cell carcinoma: Prognosis and treatment of patients from a single institution *J Clin Oncol.* 2005; 23:2300–9.

312. Bhatia S, Storer BE, Iyer JG et al. Adjuvant radiation therapy and chemotherapy in Merkel cell carcinoma: Survival analyses of 6908 cases from the National Cancer Data Base. *J Natl Cancer Inst.* 2016; 108(9).

313. Steven N, Lawton P, Poulsen M. Merkel cell carcinoma— Current controverises and future directions. *Clin Oncol.* 2019; 31: 789–96.

314. Bichakjian CK, Olencki T, Aasi SZ et al. Merkel cell carcinoma, Version 1.2018, NCCN Clinical Practice Guidelines in Oncology. *J Natl Compr Canc Netw.* 2018; 16(6):742–74.

315. Poulsen M, Rischin D, Walpole E et al. Analysis of toxicity of Merkel cell carcinoma of the skin treated with synchronous carboplatin/ etoposide and radiation: A Trans-Tasman Radiation Oncology Group study. *Int J Radiat Oncol Biol Phys.* 2003; 51:156–63.

316. Voog E, Biron P, Martin JP et al. Chemotherapy for patients with locally advanced or metastatic Merkel cell carcinoma. *Cancer.* 1999; 85:2589–95.

317. Tai PT, Yu E, Winquist E, Hammond A et al. Chemotherapy in neuroendocrine/Merkel cell carcinoma of the skin: Case series and review of 204 cases. *J Clin Oncol.* 2000; 18(12):2493e2499.

318. Iyer JG, Blom A, Doumani R et al. Response rates and durability of chemotherapy among 62 patients with metastatic Merkel cell carcinoma. *Cancer Med.* 2016; 5(9):2294e2301.

319. Cowey CL, Mahnke L, Espirito J et al. Real-world treatment outcomes in patients with metastatic Merkel cell carcinoma treated with chemotherapy in the USA. *Future Oncol.* 2017; 13(19):1699e1710.

320. Hill ADK, Brady MS, Coit DG. Intraoperative lymphatic mapping and sentinel lymph node biopsy for Merkel cell carcinoma. *Br J Surg.* 1999; 86:518.

Useful websites

www.nice.org.uk/guidance/conditions-and-diseases/cancer/skin-cancer
www.cancer.gov/types/skin
www.ncin.org.uk/cancer_type_and_topic_specific_work/cancer_type_s
  pecific_work/skin_cancer/
www.bad.org.uk/healthcare-professionals/clinical-standards/clinical-gu
  idelines
https://lymphoma-action.org.uk/types-lymphoma/skin-lymphoma
www.clfoundation.org/

25 MALIGNANT MELANOMA

James Larkin and Lisa Pickering

Introduction

Malignant melanoma is the fifth most common cancer in the United Kingdom accounting for approximately 16,000 cases and more than 2,000 deaths a year.[1] The incidence of melanoma is rising steadily with a doubling of the number of cases every decade, a rate of increase that is more rapid than any other form of cancer. The median age of diagnosis is 57 years but increasing numbers of young people below the age of 40 are developing the disease.[1]

Malignant melanoma can be broadly divided into three main types: Cutaneous, uveal, and mucosal melanoma. Each type of melanoma is distinct in terms of its molecular genetics and clinical behavior. Cutaneous melanoma accounts for more than 90% of cases of melanoma. Uveal melanomas arise from stromal cells within the eye. Mucosal melanomas develop within mucous membranes, typically within the sinuses of the head, nasal cavity, gut, and genito-urinary tracts.

Metastatic melanoma historically had a poor prognosis, and until recently, systemic therapies have been ineffective with response rates of less than 10%. However, significant advances have been made in recent years in understanding melanoma biology and immune regulation. This knowledge has proven invaluable in the development of targeted agents and new immunotherapies that have changed practice and improved the outlook for patients.

Epidemiology

There is considerable variation in the incidence of melanoma worldwide with relatively low numbers in Afro-Caribbean, Chinese, and Japanese populations. Individuals of Hispanic origin have an intermediate risk of developing malignant melanoma with the highest rates observed in Caucasians, Australia having the highest incidence of the disease.[1] This is explained by a combination of the predominant skin type in Australia and high exposure to sunlight. Melanoma is more common among females in younger age groups, but there is a male preponderance from the age of 55.[1] Mortality rates vary according to country with Australia and New Zealand having the highest mortality rates estimated at 3.5 per 100,000 population compared to 1.5 per 100,000 population in Europe.[1]

Uveal melanoma is the most common primary intra-ocular malignancy in adults. Estimated rates of incidence within Europe and the United States are between 2 and 7.5 cases per million per year. The incidence increases to approximately 21 per million for those aged above 50 years. Males are more often affected than females. The incidence rates have remained stable over the past 35 years with no significant improvement in survival despite advances in treatment techniques for the primary tumor.

Mucosal melanoma is the rarest form of melanoma and represents less than 1.5% of all cases of malignant melanoma with an incidence of 2.6 cases per million in Europe. The incidence of mucosal melanoma has remained stable over time. The incidence of mucosal melanoma increases with age and 50% of cases are diagnosed after the age of 70. There is a female preponderance probably due to the occurrence of mucosa melanoma within the female genital tract. In terms of ethnicity, those from an Afro-Caribbean, Far Eastern, or Hispanic descent are more likely to develop mucosal melanoma than cutaneous or uveal melanomas, although the overall incidence remains higher in white non-Hispanic populations.

Etiology

Several environmental and genetic risk factors have been implicated in the development of cutaneous melanoma. Known risk factors include exposure to sunlight, particularly in childhood and adolescence, past or family history of melanoma, fair complexion, freckles, susceptibility to sunburn, and the presence of numerous dysplastic nevi.

Although there is significant evidence that ultraviolet B radiation form sunlight plays an important role in the development of melanoma, studies suggests that exposure to ultraviolet A (UVA) radiation also carries significant risks. Patients with a history of psoriasis treated with oral psoralen and UVA radiation were shown to have an increased incidence rate of all melanomas, albeit delayed up to 20 years after treatment. A significantly increased risk of melanoma has been reported in individuals following exposure to tanning beds and lamps, particularly below the age of 35.

Five to seven percent of melanoma patients have a strong family history. Many of these patients have familial atypical multiple mole melanoma syndrome previously referred to as dysplastic nevus syndrome characterized by a large number of atypical melanocytic nevi and mutations in the tumor suppressor gene CDKN2A which is critical in cell cycle regulation. Mutations in CDKN2A are associated with a 50–90% risk of melanoma by age 80 years.

The role of ultraviolet (UV) exposure in the development of uveal melanoma remains controversial. An increased risk of uveal melanoma has been found with the use of sunlamps and in individuals with lighter colored eyes and skin and in those with increased numbers of cutaneous nevi.

In contrast to cutaneous and uveal melanomas, UV radiation is not considered to play a significant role in the development of mucosal melanomas. Irritants and carcinogenic compounds such as tobacco and formaldehyde have been implicated in the development of head and neck mucosal melanomas and the human immunodeficiency virus has been associated with ano-rectal mucosal melanomas.

Prevention

Intermittent and intense sun exposure is a significant risk factor for the development of cutaneous melanoma. Therefore, minimizing exposure to sunlight is an important method of primary prevention, particularly in childhood/adolescence in those with an increased tendency to burn. Patients with a diagnosis of melanoma can reduce their risk of a second primary melanoma by reducing their sun exposure regardless of age.

The most effective way of reducing sun exposure is achieved by shade, wearing sun-protective clothing, and avoiding peak hours of sun intensity. The Anti-Cancer Council SunSmart Campaign in Australia implemented the "Slip! Slop! Slap!" program with considerable success.

The UK guidelines recommend screening, surveillance, and self-examination of high-risk individuals, for example, those with a previous primary melanoma, organ transplant, or large number of atypical nevi. Individuals with a strong family history (three or more cases of melanoma, two cases of atypical mole syndrome, or multiple primary tumors in an individual) should be referred to a cancer genetics clinic. Those with giant (>20-cm diameter) hairy pigmented nevi require lifetime follow-up because of the significant risk of malignant change.

Tumor biology

Somatic mutations in genes involved in cell proliferation and survival play a significant role in facilitating the malignant transformation of melanocytes. This knowledge forms the basis of the development of targeted therapies in melanoma. Cutaneous, uveal, and mucosal melanomas are each distinct in terms of their molecular genetics.

The mitogen-activated protein kinase (MAPK) signaling pathway is a key intracellular signaling pathway involved in cell growth, differentiation, and survival. Genetic mutations affecting key components of this pathway have been implicated in many different tumors including melanoma. Activation of the pathway occurs upon ligand-cell surface receptor tyrosine kinase binding. This causes downstream activation of Ras, a G protein with multiple isoforms, the most important in melanoma being NRAS. Phosphorylation and activation of the RAF proteins then occurs as a consequence of RAS activation. The RAF proteins, BRAF and CRAF, dimerize to activate extracellular signal-regulated kinase (ERK) which in turn activates downstream pathways to promote cell growth, differentiation, and survival.

Given the extensive "cross-talk" that occurs between intracellular signaling pathways it is difficult to identify a single cascade of signals responsible for the development of melanoma. Indeed, genetic abnormalities involving the PI3 kinase pathway have also been implicated in the development of melanoma.

The frequency of BRAF and NRAS mutations in cutaneous melanoma is 40–50% and 20%, respectively. Approximately 75% of BRAF mutations comprise a single amino acid substitution from valine to glutamic acid at codon 600 (V600E). This leads to a constitutively active BRAF protein which is responsible for the continuous downstream activation of the MAPK pathway with consequent abnormal cell growth and survival. Less frequent mutations include V600K (valine substitution to lysine), seen in approximately 10–30% of cases. The V600E mutation is more frequent in younger patients. In contrast, the V600K mutation is associated with increased age, chronic UV exposure, and cutaneous head and neck melanomas. The presence of a BRAF mutation within melanocytes is not solely responsible for the malignant transformation of a cell, rather it serves to facilitate the oncogenic process in association with other factors.

Uveal melanomas do not typically harbor BRAF or NRAS mutations, but the retinoblastoma and p53 tumor suppressor genes and the genes encoding the alpha unit of G proteins are implicated in uveal melanomas. G proteins are membrane-associated hetero-trimeric proteins, and the alpha subunits are involved in the activation of downstream effectors such as protein kinase A and C and the MAPK pathway. The genes encoding the alpha subunit of G proteins implicated in uveal melanoma are GNAQ and GNA11 and have been reported in more than 80% of cases.

Mucosal melanomas have been shown to have very different tumor biology compared to cutaneous and uveal types with mutations in the proto-oncogene c-KIT being present. This gene encodes a transmembrane tyrosine kinase receptor which activates the downstream intracellular MAPK and PI3 kinase pathways which are integral for cell proliferation, differentiation, and survival. Gain of function mutations in c-KIT, amplification, or overexpression have been reported.

Diagnosis

Early diagnosis of cutaneous melanoma allows surgery to be undertaken at a stage when cure is likely to be achieved. The "ABCD" system is widely used in public education and describes the four major clinical features of melanoma: Asymmetry, border irregularity, color variation, and diameter (>6 mm).

Cutaneous melanomas can be located anywhere on the body, and a difference between the distributions of melanomas between genders exists: In females the limbs, in males the trunk. The UK guidelines have adopted a seven-point scoring system to allow the early recognition of melanoma to prompt appropriate referral to a specialist pathway; major features include a change in size, shape, or color. Minor features include largest diameter ≥7 mm, change in sensation, and presence of inflammation or oozing. Lesions with any of the major features or three minor ones are suspicious of melanoma and should be seen by a specialist.

All patients presenting with a suspicious skin lesion should undergo a full skin examination. Any significant change in a pigmented lesion is considered to be an indication for an excision biopsy involving the entire lesion (full-thickness) with a 2–5-mm clearance margin. Punch, shave, or incision biopsies and curettage are not recommended as they can lead to misdiagnosis.

Pathology

Cutaneous melanomas can be categorized on the basis of their macroscopic appearance: Superficial spreading (70% cases), nodular (20%), acral lentiginous (5%), and lentigo maligna melanoma (5%). Superficial spreading melanoma often arises as a dark area within a pre-existing junctional nevus. Nodular melanoma typically arises from apparently normal skin and is aggressive. They are usually darker than superficial spreading melanoma, uniform in color, and often dome-shaped. Rarely, nodular melanomas are amelanotic. Acral lentiginous melanoma affects the palms, soles, and nail beds. They are more common in darker skinned individuals. Lentigo maligna melanoma tends to occur on the face or neck of older patients and has a better overall survival.

The pathology report of an excised primary lesion should include margins of excision, Breslow thickness, mitotic count, growth pattern, presence or absence of ulceration, tumor regression, lymphocytic inflammatory infiltrate, and lymphatic or vascular invasion. Immunohistochemical stains used widely in melanoma include S-100, Melan-A, and HMB45.

Staging and prognosis

Tumor stage at presentation is the most significant determinant of prognosis. The American Joint Committee on Cancer (AJCC) classification is used and was updated most recently in 2017. This is based on key histological features including Breslow thickness of the primary lesion and presence/absence of ulceration within the tumor.

Increasing tumor thickness correlates with worse prognosis; the 10-year survival for a lesion <1 mm without ulceration is 98% whereas for lesions >4 mm without ulceration it is 83%.[2] Epithelial ulceration of the primary tumor carries a worse prognosis in terms of overall survival at all stages of tumor thickness, for example 10-year survival for a lesion >4 mm with ulceration is 75%.[2]

The most common site of metastasis is the regional lymph node basin. Survival correlates with the number of nodes involved, clinically apparent (macrometastases) or clinically occult (micrometastases diagnosed at sentinel lymph node biopsy). Metastases in the sentinel lymph node are detected in <5% of patients with T1a melanomas (<0.8 mm), 5–12% of those with T1b melanomas (0.8–1 mm), and up to 35% of patients with stage IIB and IIC melanoma, i.e. with melanomas >2 mm. False-negative rates range from 4% to 9%. The presence of intra-lymphatic metastases as indicated by the presence of satellite or in-transit metastases also reflects a poorer outcome.[2]

Prognostic features in stage IV disease are the site of metastases and elevated serum lactic dehydrogenase (LDH) levels. Visceral metastases or distant metastases to any site combined with an elevated LDH carry the worst prognosis in the context of metastatic disease.

For some years there has been controversy regarding the role of sentinel lymph node biopsy and of regional completion lymph node dissection (CLND) in the management of melanoma. These were addressed by the Multicentre Selective Lymphadenectomy Trial (MSLT)-I–II trials. MSLT-I examined the impact of sentinel lymph node biopsy on survival.[3] Patients with primary melanoma were randomly assigned to wide local excision and observation or wide local excision and sentinel lymph node biopsy. Those with a positive sentinel node biopsy proceeded to lymphadenectomy. Patients with primary intermediate thickness melanomas (1.2– 3.5 mm) with a positive sentinel node biopsy had significantly higher 5-year disease-free survival rates, confirming the prognostic role of sentinel node biopsy. However, this trial failed to show an overall survival benefit. MSLT-II examined the value of CLND in 1934 patients with positive sentinel lymph node metastases.[4] Patients were randomized to have immediate CLND or nodal observation with ultrasonography but no further immediate surgery. There was no difference detected between the groups for the primary endpoint of melanoma-specific survival at 43 months median follow-up. CLND was associated with an improvement in local nodal disease control at 3 years but also with an excess of lymphedema (24.1 vs. 6.3% in the observation group). Thus current standard practice is sentinel lymph node biopsy followed by nodal surveillance but not immediate CLND.

Treatment of primary melanoma

The definitive surgical treatment for primary cutaneous melanoma is excision. Any suspected new lesion should be excised initially with a 2-mm margin and the Breslow thickness ascertained before deciding on the required wide local excision margin. The recommended surgical margin depends on the Breslow thickness of the melanoma. For cutaneous melanomas up to 1 mm in thickness, a surgical margin of 1 cm is considered safe. This is based on data obtained from the World Health Organisation (WHO) Melanoma Co-operative Group Trial 10 where patients with thin melanomas (<2 mm) were randomly assigned to 1-cm or 3-cm excision margins. In patients with melanomas <1 mm, no local

recurrence was seen and there was no significant difference in overall survival with either excision margin, supporting narrow excision as a safe procedure in such patients. In patients with melanomas between 1 mm and 2 mm, the recommendation for surgical margins is less clear; evidence from numerous randomized controlled trials supports a minimum surgical margin of 1 cm; however, 2-cm margins are also appropriate in this group of patients.[5]

In the case of melanomas between 2 mm and 4 mm, the recommended surgical margin is between 2 cm and 3 cm.[5] The Intergroup Melanoma trial compared excision margins of 2 cm and 4 cm for intermediate thickness lesions between 1 mm and 4 mm. No significant difference in recurrence rates or overall survival was demonstrated between the two groups. In contrast, the UK Melanoma Study Group/British Association of Plastic Surgeons Trial reported higher local recurrence rates but equivalent overall survival with 1 cm vs. 3 cm margins in patients with melanomas >2 mm in thickness. There has been no study directly comparing 2 cm with 3 cm margins for patients with thick primaries. The UK guidelines currently recommend a minimum surgical margin of 2 cm; however, 3 cm is also appropriate for lesions between 2-mm and 4-mm thickness.[5]

Given the significant risk of locoregional and distant metastases in patients with melanomas >4 mm in thickness, 3-cm margins are recommended in the United Kingdom. Data in patients with thick melanomas are limited with there being only one randomized trial where patients with melanomas >4 mm were included.

Special consideration is required for primary melanoma in certain sites. For example, in many head and neck primaries, the morbidity of surgery associated with achieving adequate clearance has dictated a more conservative approach.

Lymph node dissection

The presence of palpable lymph nodes, usually confirmed on fine needle aspiration biopsy, is an indication for node clearance. The aim of therapeutic lymph node dissection is local control with curative intent in many cases. Outcome is influenced by the number of lymph nodes involved and evidence of extra-capsular spread.

In patients with axillary node involvement, complete dissection to include level III nodes medial to the pectoralis minor is indicated. The main complication of lymphadenectomy is limb edema. This is more common in the lower limb, especially in patients who have had an ilio-inguinal dissection. Prospective randomized studies have failed to support a survival benefit for prophylactic elective nodal dissection.

Local treatment

There are no randomized trials showing an overall survival benefit using regional therapies such as elective lymph node dissection, isolated limb perfusion (ILP), or radiotherapy. The role of adjuvant radiotherapy following lymphadenectomy in melanoma patients identified as at high risk for further recurrence is controversial. The Tasmanian Radiation Oncology Group (ANZMTG 01.02/TROG 02.01) trial randomized patients considered at high risk of relapse following surgery (based on lymph node involvement) to receive adjuvant radiotherapy or observation.[6] The trial showed reduced recurrence in the lymph node basin area (mean follow-up of 73 months) for adjuvant radiotherapy, but there was no effect on overall survival. In the radiotherapy arm, locoregional symptoms were worse with increased limb edema and grade 2–4 long-term effects. Given the lack of survival advantage together with the significant morbidity associated with radio-therapy, adjuvant radiotherapy in high-risk patients is not practiced in all centers.

Adjuvant systemic therapy

Patients with thick primary lesions or lymph node involvement are at high risk of relapse, and there has been considerable interest in the development of adjuvant systemic therapies. Historically, no significant improvement in terms of overall survival with adjuvant cytotoxic chemotherapy was ever demonstrated. In 2011, the Food and Drug Administration (FDA) approved pegylated IFN-α-2b for stage III melanoma patients based on the results of the EORTC 18991 trial.[7] Although IFN treatment has been shown to consistently improve relapse-free survival with a relative risk reduction of approximately 20%, given the marginal effect on overall survival and significant associated toxicities, its use was limited.

More recently, given the unprecedented success of targeted agents and immunotherapies in stage IV melanoma, there has been interest in their potential use as adjuvant therapy. Randomized trials have investigated the use of immunotherapeutic agents in EORTC 18071, CheckMate-238, and KeyNote-054 and of BRAF and MEK inhibitors in BRIM8 and COMBI-AD. EORTC 18071 randomized 950 patients with resected high-risk stage III melanoma to receive the anti-CTLA-4 monoclonal antibody, Ipilimumab, or placebo.[8] This trial demonstrated that ipilimumab conferred an improvement in recurrence-free survival and overall survival compared with placebo with 5-year survival rates improved by approximately 10% with ipilimumab. As such this was practice-changing at the time but has now been superseded by trials of the anti-PD1 agents nivolumab and pembrolizumab.

CheckMate-238 randomly assigned 906 patients with resected stage IIIB, IIIC, or IV melanoma to nivolumab or ipilimumab for up to 1 year.[9] After 18 months' median follow-up, nivolumab was associated with a longer 12-month recurrence-free survival with an absolute improvement of around 10%, and a lower rate of grade III and IV adverse events. This benefit was sustained at 3 years' follow-up at which point a 32% benefit for nivolumab over ipilimumab was seen for relapse-free survival; benefit was seen regardless of BRAF status. Keynote-054 demonstrated benefit for another anti-PD1 agent, pembrolizumab, as adjuvant therapy for resected stage III melanoma;[10] 1119 patients were randomized between pembrolizumab and placebo for up to 1 year. After 15 months' follow-up there was an almost 15% improvement in recurrence-free survival from 61.0% in the placebo group to 75.4% in the pembrolizumab group. Toxicity rates are regarded as acceptable for the degree of benefit observed and similar with both nivolumab and pembrolizumab. The combination of ipilimumab with nivolumab is being compared with nivolumab alone in the CheckMate 915 study.

For patients with BRAF-mutant cutaneous melanoma, there has also been interest in the role of BRAF and MEK-directed therapies in the adjuvant setting. BRIM8 compared the BRAF inhibitor vemurafenib with placebo in resected stage IIC/III melanoma.[11] This study did show efficacy for vemurafenib but did not meet its primary endpoint for disease-free survival in the intention to treat population. The COMBI-AD trial investigated the combination of the BRAF inhibitor dabrafenib and the MEK inhibitor trametinib as adjuvant therapy in 870 patients with resected stage III melanoma that carried V600E or V600K BRAF mutations.[12] At a median of 2.8 years' follow-up the relapse-free survival rate favored dabrafenib and trametinib with an absolute

improvement of nearly 20% from 39% in the placebo group to 58% in the combination therapy group.

Thus adjuvant systemic therapy is now considered standard for patients with resected stage III and IV melanoma on the basis of consistent demonstration of improvement in relapse-free survival. Treatment should be with a PD1 inhibitor, nivolumab or pembrolizumab or, for those patients whose melanomas carry a BRAF mutation, the combination of dabrafenib and trametinib may be considered. These agents are licensed and approved by both the FDA and European Medicines Agency (EMA). Further trials are evaluating the putative role of adjuvant therapy for patients with stage IIC melanomas, i.e. thick primary melanomas without sentinel node involvement.

Loco-regional recurrent disease

Recurrent local disease is defined as occurring within 5 cm of the previous primary operative site. In-transit metastases represent lymphatic permeation towards the regional lymph nodes and are subcutaneous lesions occurring between the primary and regional lymph nodes. The majority of local recurrences occur within 5 years, and their control is an important quality of life issue.

ILP is the preferred treatment when the disease becomes beyond surgical control, that is multiple, frequent, or large recurrences in the limbs. ILP requires a general anesthetic and uses an extra-corporeal bypass circuit via the main artery and vein to the target limb and allows delivery of higher doses of antineoplastic agents than are tolerated systemically. The treatment period is approximately 90 minutes and is combined with limb hyperthermia (38–40°C). Good response rates are achievable with ILP (54–80%).

Melphalan is the most commonly used agent; however, cisplatin and dactinomycin have also been used. In a study of 114 patients with locally recurrent or metastatic limb melanoma, hyperthermic ILP with melphalan resulted in a complete and partial response in 73% and 13% of patients, respectively.[13] Complete response was durable in 37 out of 81 cases at a median follow-up of 33 months.[13]

Combinations of melphalan, TNFα, and IFNα have been investigated. A retrospective analysis of 130 patients treated with melphalan alone or melphalan and TNFα demonstrated no additional benefit with the addition of TNFα (complete response rate 45% vs. 59%, respectively; $p = 0.14$).[14] The phase III ACOSOG trial (Z0020) in which patients with locally advanced extremity melanoma were randomized to ILP with melphalan or melphalan and TNFα, demonstrated no additional benefit with TNFα.

Isolated limb infusion (ILI) is less invasive than ILP and can be easily repeated. It involves intra-arterial infusion of a cytotoxic agent into the affected limb via a percutaneous catheter. There have been suggestions, however, that ILI may be less effective than ILP. ILI is suitable for patients with low-volume disease and those with co-morbidities who may not be suitable for ILP. Laser ablation with carbon dioxide is useful for treating multiple small (<1 cm) lesions. Minimal post-operative complications are associated with laser ablation and wound healing occurs typically within 6 weeks.

Distant metastatic disease

Patients with metastatic melanoma have a poor prognosis and until recently systemic treatment was largely ineffective. This has changed dramatically with the development of targeted agents and new immune regulating monoclonal antibodies. In patients of stage IV disease, defining the mutational status of the tumor (BRAF, c-KIT, and NRAS) is key to planning management. Surgery and radiotherapy offer palliation in certain circumstances, for example, radiotherapy for bone and brain metastases and surgery for other metastases.

Cytotoxic chemotherapy

Dacarbazine, nitrosoureas, platinum compounds, vinca alkaloids, taxanes, temozolomide, and fotemustine all have some activity with response rates of 5–15% and a median progression-free survival of 2–6 months. The most commonly used of these is the alkylating agent, dacarbazine, with best response rates of approximately 10–15% and a median duration of response of up to 6 months. Dacarbazine is ineffective in cerebral metastases because it does not cross the blood–brain barrier. Temozolomide is an oral dacarbazine derivative with greater central nervous penetration. A randomized phase III trial of temozolomide and dacarbazine in 859 patients with metastatic melanoma reported response rates of 14.5% and 9.8% with temozolomide and dacarbazine, respectively.[15]

Immunotherapy: Anti-CTLA4 and anti-PD-1 antibodies

Improvements in understanding of tumor immunology have led to the development of targeted immunotherapies aimed at specific immune-checkpoints, such as cytotoxic T-lymphocyte-associated antigen 4 (CTLA-4), programmed death-1 (PD-1), and programmed death ligand-1 (PD-L1). CTLA-4 and PD-1 are inhibitory receptors with non-overlapping roles in modulating the adaptive immune response. CTLA-4 acts primarily early in the immune response to regulate T-cell proliferation and migration to the tumor, whereas PD-1 and its ligand PD-L1 regulate T-cell activation and proliferation at the tumor site.

Ipilimumab, which targets CTLA-4, was approved by the FDA and the European Medicines Agency in 2011 for the treatment of unresectable or metastatic melanoma. A survival benefit with ipilimumab was demonstrated in two randomized, controlled phase III trials (MDX010-20 and CA184-024). In study MDX010-20, previously treated melanoma patients received ipilimumab 3 mg/kg plus the melanoma peptide vaccine gp100, ipilimumab 3 mg/kg alone, or gp100 alone. The hazard ratio (HR) for death compared with gp100 alone was 0.68 ($p < 0.001$) for the ipilimumab plus gp100 group and 0.66 ($p = 0.003$) for the ipilimumab-alone group.[16] In study CA184-024, previously untreated patients received ipilimumab 10 mg/kg plus DTIC or DTIC plus placebo. There was a 28% reduction in risk of death in the ipilimumab group (HR, 0.72; $p < 0.001$).[17]

A meta-analysis of pooled OS data from ipilimumab trials, which included data from 1861 melanoma patients, reported a 3-year OS rate of 22%; furthermore, a plateau in the pooled Kaplan–Meier curve began at approximately 3 years after initiation of therapy, and extended through follow-up of as long as 10 years.[18] Ipilimumab can be associated with side effects, due to the immune system activation by CTLA-4 blockade. Collectively, the spectrum of side effects is described as immune-related adverse events (irAEs). irAEs most commonly affected the skin (rash/vitiligo/pruritis), the liver, the GI tract, and the endocrine system (hypophysitis, thyroiditis, adrenal insufficiency). More rarely, uveitis, conjunctivitis, neuropathy, myopathy, and nephritis can occur. Ipilimumab was followed by the development of additional immune-checkpoint inhibitors and the anti-PD-1 agents, nivolumab and pembrolizumab, have

demonstrated improved survival and less toxicity compared with ipilimumab.

In the phase III CheckMate 066 trial, nivolumab demonstrated superior OS in previously untreated melanoma patients without BRAF mutation[19] whilst in the CheckMate 067 trial, nivolumab demonstrated substantially improved ORR, progression-free survival (PFS), and OS compared with ipilimumab as first-line treatment.[20] In a phase III trial comparing pembrolizumab with ipilimumab (KEYNOTE-006 trial), after a median follow-up of 57.7 months, mOS was 32.7 months in the combined pembrolizumab groups and 15.9 months in the ipilimumab group. Additionally, treatment-related grade 3–5 adverse events were less frequent with pembrolizumab (13.3% and 10.1%) than with ipilimumab (19.9%).[21]

Ipilimumab in combination with nivolumab has also been studied. In the CheckMate-067 phase III trial, nivolumab alone or nivolumab plus ipilimumab were compared with ipilimumab alone in 945 previously untreated patients with metastatic melanoma. The rates of objective response were 57.6% in the nivolumab-plus-ipilimumab group, 43.7% in the nivolumab group, and 19.0% in the ipilimumab group. The mPFS was 11.5 months in the nivolumab-plus-Ipilimumab group, 6.9 months in the nivolumab group, and 2.9 months in the ipilimumab group. Treatment-related grade 3/4 adverse events were observed in 59% of patients in the nivolumab-plus-ipilimumab group, in 22% of the nivolumab group, and 28% of the ipilimumab group.[20] At the last follow-up, 5-year OS rate was 52% in the combination group and 44% in the nivolumab group, as compared with 26% in the ipilimumab group. The median overall survival was more than 60.0 months for patients treated with nivolumab plus ipilimumab, 36.9 months in the nivolumab group, and 19.9 months in the ipilimumab group.[22]

Oncolytic virotherapy is an emerging treatment modality whereby replicating viruses can be used to selectively replicate within tumors to enhance local and systemic immune responses promoting tumor regression. The phase III OPTiM trial of an oncolytic herpes simplex virus vector (talimogene laherparepvec T-VEC) encoding GM-CSF vs. GM-CSF was carried out in a total of 436 patients with stage III/IV melanoma. The T-VEC vaccine was injected intra-lesionally whereas GM-CSF was administered subcutaneously. Data from the final analysis of the trial showed that the response rate for intralesional T-VEC vaccination was 31.5% compared to 6.4% for the GM-CSF groups. Overall survival analysis favored T-VEC vaccine with a hazard ration of 0.79 and p value = 0.0494.[23]

Targeted therapies

BRAF mutant melanoma: BRAF and MEK inhibitors

The mitogen-activated protein kinase (MAPK) pathway, which includes the RAS, RAF, MEK, and ERK molecules, is a major signaling network in melanoma tumorigenesis. BRAF phosphorylates MEK and BRAF mutations are found in ~40% of melanomas, with most (70–95%) the V600E substitution. Vemurafenib, an inhibitor of mutant BRAF, was approved by the FDA in 2011 for the treatment of melanomas with the BRAF V600E mutation based on improved overall survival (OS) vs. dacarbazine (DTIC) in the BRIM-3 phase III study.[24] Another BRAF inhibitor, dabrafenib, was approved based on results from a phase III trial showing improved median progression-free survival (mPFS) vs. DTIC (5.1 months for dabrafenib vs. 2.7 months for DTIC; HR, 0.30)[25] and the MEK inhibitor trametinib was approved for melanoma harboring a BRAF V600E or V600K mutation based on results from the METRIC phase III trial showing improved mPFS vs. chemotherapy (4.8 months for trametinib vs. 1.5 months for DTIC or paclitaxel; HR, 0.45).[26] In 2014, the FDA approved dabrafenib in combination with trametinib for BRAF V600E- or V600K-mutated melanoma (the first FDA-approved targeted combination therapy for this disease) on the basis of improved overall response rate and median duration of response vs. dabrafenib monotherapy demonstrated in a phase I/II trial and then confirmed in a phase III study, Combi-D.[27] Overall, BRAF inhibitors have shown objective response rates (ORR) of approximately 50%, which increase to 70% when combined with MEK inhibitors. Additionally, mPFS increases from 7–9 months with single-agent BRAF inhibitors to around 12 months with BRAF and MEK inhibitor combination. Three BRAF–MEK combinations are now approved: Vemurafenib and cobimetinib, dabrafenib and trametinib, and encorafenib and binimetinib.[28,29] Efficacy data for these combinations are similar, taking into account the difficulties with cross-trial comparisons, whereas their pharmacokinetics and toxicity profiles differ in some regards.

NRAS mutated melanoma

Given that MEK inhibitors block the MAP kinase pathway, it was thought that they may be effective in NRAS mutation-positive melanoma. The NEMO trial randomized 402 patients with unresectable stage III or stage IV NRAS mutant melanoma to the MEK inhibitor binimetinib or standard therapy with dacarbazine.[30] Median progression-free survival was longer with binimetinib (2.8 months) than with dacarbazine (1.5 months) but still somewhat disappointing. Binimetinib is not currently approved in this setting.

KIT mutant melanoma

KIT mutations are typically seen in approximately 10–20% of acral and mucosal melanomas and multiple mutations in the KIT gene have been found. Two phase II trials of Imatinib in patients with metastatic melanoma harboring c-KIT mutations or amplifications have shown response rates of approximately 20–25%. The multi-tyrosine kinase receptor inhibitors nilotinib and dasatinib have also been of interest in advanced c-KIT mutated melanoma given their superior activity to Imatinib in other malignancies that harbor KIT mutations.

Dasatinib was investigated in the phase II E2607 trial.[31] In the cohort with KIT mutant tumors, partial response rate was 18.7% and median PFS 2.1 months which was not regarded as sufficient to recommend dasatinib over Imatinib. Nilotinib has been evaluated in several open-label phase II trials and has shown similar activity to Imatinib with objective response rates (ORR) of 17–26% including a small number of complete responses.[32–34] Disease control rates of 57% have been reported with median duration of response 35 weeks. Overall the activity of targeted therapy in KIT mutant melanoma has been relatively disappointing in comparison with the benefits seen from targeting BRAF and MEK in BRAF mutant melanoma. Ongoing trials are evaluating novel KIT inhibitors and KIT inhibition in combination with immunotherapy.

Uveal melanoma

Uveal melanoma is genetically and clinically distinct from cutaneous melanoma. As with cutaneous melanoma, historically

responses to systemic therapy have been poor. No significant improvement in overall survival with chemotherapy has ever been demonstrated.

Targeted therapies and immunotherapy have also been investigated in metastatic uveal melanoma. Responses are seen but have proven less durable than in cutaneous melanoma. Three MEK inhibitors have been evaluated either alone or in combination; selumetinib with or without dacarbazine,[35,36] trametinib,[37] and binimetinib with pan kinase C inhibitor sotrastaurin. Across these studies results were disappointing with response rates from 0 to 14% and progression-free survival 3.1 to 16 weeks. The most encouraging activity was seen with selumetinib which was compared to investigators choice of temozolomide or dacarbazine in a randomized phase II trial of 101 patients. Patients treated with selumetinib had significantly higher response rate (14% vs. 0%) and longer progression-free survival compared to temozolomide (15.9 weeks vs. 7 weeks). Overall survival was also longer with selumetinib (11.1 vs. 9.1 months) although this was not statistically significant.[35] However the phase III randomized double-blind SUMIT trial of selumetinib or placebo in combination with dacarbazine failed to show any benefit for the addition of selumetinib.[36] Other trials of MEK inhibitors are underway including in combination with paclitaxel and with AKT inhibitors.

Checkpoint inhibitors have also been investigated in metastatic uveal melanoma. Ipilimumab as a single agent has shown consistently relatively low response rates of 0–8%.[37,38] Anti PD-1 agents as monotherapy have shown similarly low activity with response rates around 5% for pembrolizumab and nivolumab and with median overall survival of less than 1 year in most of these series.[39–41] The combination of ipilimumab and nivolumab had a response rate of 17% in an open-label phase II trial although median progression-free survival was only 2.8 months.[42] This difference is thought to be related to the observation by The Cancer Genome Atlas and others that uveal melanoma has a much lower mutational load than cutaneous melanoma and thus is less immunogenic.

Despite this fact, responses have been reported to other immune-targeting approaches. A recent study of adoptive transfer of tumor-infiltrating lymphocytes in 21 patients with metastatic uveal melanoma reported response rate of 35% including one complete response ongoing 21 months after treatment.[43] Activity has also been reported to the novel bispecific immunostimulatory molecule IMCgp100 with results presented from a combined analysis of a phase I and phase II studies. The response rate was only 14.7% but prolonged disease stabilization was seen in a number of patients and 1-year survival was 73% which is considerably longer than expected in uveal melanoma.[44] Such approaches are undergoing further evaluation.

Management of brain metastases

Approximately 30–60% of patients with stage IV melanoma develop brain metastases. In a series of 686 patients with treated brain metastasis, median survival from the time of diagnosis of cerebral metastasis was 4.1 months.[46] Management of brain metastases has been difficult given the resistance to cytotoxic chemotherapy and radiotherapy. Current treatment modalities include surgery, radiotherapy (whole-brain and stereotactic irradiation), targeted therapy, and immunotherapy.

Surgery

Complete surgical resection is considered for patients with a solitary brain metastasis. Patients with multiple accessible lesions amenable to surgery may have a prognosis similar to those with a solitary metastasis, and therefore surgery is an important consideration in these patients. A retrospective study showed that the median survival for those patients undergoing surgery with or without post-operative radiotherapy (8.9 months and 8.7 months, respectively) was significantly greater than that of patients treated with radiotherapy alone or supportive care only (3.4 months and 2.1 months, respectively).[47]

Radiotherapy

There are limited data on the efficacy of whole-brain radiotherapy (WBRT) after surgical removal compared to surgery alone; the majority of data are from case series reports.[48] Case series have described improvements in survival, 18 months in irradiated group vs. 6 months in the surgery-alone group,[48] and in the time to central nervous system (CNS) recurrence from 6 to 27 months, from the addition of WBRT after surgery.

Stereotactic radiosurgery refers to radiation that is focused, and there are a number of platforms that deliver this. Surgery is often preferentially used for large superficial brain lesions (>3 cm), for infratentorial lesions, and in combination with stereotactic radiosurgery. In contrast, stereotactic surgery has minimal perioperative morbidity; however it is more effective on smaller lesions (<3 cm) with minimal mass effect or edema. It can be used in patients who have co-morbidities, thus avoiding the need for surgery, and can be used for more than one lesion. In a study of 118 melanoma brain metastases treated with stereotactic radiosurgery, freedom from progression was achieved in 90–95% of lesions with a reduction in size occurring in 55%.[49] Intracranial tumor volume and status of systemic disease are independent predictors of survival in melanoma patients undergoing radiosurgery to brain metastases. The results of RTOG 9508 demonstrated that adding stereotactic radiosurgery to WBRT for patients with 1–3 brain metastases improved survival in patients of RPA Class 1 (11.6 months vs. 9.6 months, $p < 0.0001$). A phase III trial of stereotactic radiosurgery vs. WBRT for patients with >3 brain metastases from melanoma is currently recruiting.

Systemic therapies

Vemurafenib and dabrafenib with or without trametinib have been shown to have activity within the CNS in melanoma patients.[26] The BREAK-MB trial assessed the effects of dabrafenib in 172 patients with BRAF-mutated melanoma and brain metastases. Dabrafenib showed anti-tumor activity with an overall intracranial response rate of 39% in patients without previous local treatment and 31% of those with previous local treatment. Median progression-free survival was 4 months and median overall survival approximately 8 months in both groups.[50] Vemurafenib has also shown clinical activity in a phase II clinical trial with a brain metastasis response rate of 18% but relatively short duration of response with PFS of 3.7 months.[51] Dabrafenib in combination with trametinib has shown response rates of 58% in patients with untreated melanoma brain metastases in the COMBI-MB trial, very similar to the extracranial response rates seen in that trial, although the durability of intracranial response was less than that seen for extracranial disease.[52]

Immunotherapy also has activity in melanoma patients with brain metastases with single-agent activity reported for ipilimumab, pembrolizumab, and nivolumab. A phase II trial of ipilimumab (10 mg/kg every 3 weeks) was carried out among a total of 72 patients divided into two cohorts: Neurologically asymptomatic patients (Cohort A, $n = 51$) and symptomatic patients receiving systemic corticosteroids (Cohort B, $n = 21$). Most patients had received systemic treatment or radiotherapy previously. Disease control within the brain was achieved in 24% and 10% of patients in Cohort A and B, respectively. Overall survival at 12 months and 24 months was 31% and 26% for Cohort A and 19% and 10% for Cohort B.[53] Pembrolizumab had a brain metastasis response rate of 22% in a phase II trial of 36 patients of whom 18 had melanoma brain metastases.[54] Nivolumab was evaluated alone or in combination with ipilimumab in a phase II trial which assessed patients with untreated brain metastases who had combination immunotherapy (36 patients; cohort A), nivolumab alone (27 patients; cohort B), or nivolumab alone for treatment for symptomatic and/or previously treated brain metastases (16 patients; cohort C). Brain metastases response rates were 46%, 20%, and 6% respectively.[55] The combination of ipilimumab with nivolumab was also assessed in a larger dedicated trial of 92 patients with untreated melanoma brain metastases of between 0.5 and 3 cm in size and again was striking.[56] Intracranial clinical benefit was seen in 57% of patients with partial responses in 30%, complete responses in 26%, and stable disease of at least 6 months' duration in 2%. In this cohort extracranial benefit was seen in 56% of patients.

In light of these data, it is appropriate to use systemic therapy as initial treatment of intra-cerebral metastases with surgery and radiotherapy or radiosurgery being retained for salvage.

Conclusions

The incidence of malignant melanoma continues to rise with increasing numbers of young people being affected; primary prevention strategies for malignant melanoma are of the utmost importance. For primary melanoma, surgery remains the mainstay of treatment. Our increased understanding of tumor molecular biology has led to the development of targeted therapies and newer immunotherapies. The checkpoint inhibitors and the molecularly targeted agents have revolutionized the therapeutic landscape for melanoma in both the adjuvant and metastatic settings. Adjuvant therapy is routinely recommended for Stage III melanoma with either nivolumab, pembrolizumab, or, for patients whose melanomas harbor a BRAF mutation, the combination of dabrafenib and trametinib.

Checkpoint inhibitor immunotherapies and targeted therapies also demonstrate unprecedented improvements in treatment outcomes in patients with stage IV melanoma. Ipilimumab in combination with nivolumab induces durable responses in up to 50% of patients albeit with considerable and sometimes irreversible toxicity in a proportion. Good and sometimes durable responses are also seen with nivolumab and pembrolizumab as monotherapy and to a somewhat lesser extent with Ipilimumab monotherapy. In patients with BRAF mutated melanoma the combination of a BRAF inhibitor and an MEK inhibitor is effective in inducing responses in the majority, although the responses are rarely durable. For patients whose tumors carry a BRAF mutation, in the context of symptomatic, high-volume, rapidly progressing disease it may be appropriate to use BRAF targeted therapy first whereas early commencement of immunotherapy may be better for indolent disease, reserving targeted agents for "rescue palliative therapy." Many questions remain unanswered including the optimum sequence of treatments with targeted agents and immunotherapies, and further prospective clinical trials are ongoing.

References

1. Cancer Research UK. Cancer Statistics. 2010. Available at https://www.cancerresearchuk.org/health-professional/cancer-statistics/statistics-by-cancer-type/melanoma-skin-cancer

2. Gershenwald JE, Scolyer RA, Hess KR et al. Melanoma of the skin. In Amin MB et al. (Eds.), *AJCC Cancer Staging Manual* (pp. 563–85). Basel, Switzerland: Springer, 2017.

3. Morton DL, Thompson JF, Cochrane AJ et al. Final trial report of sentinel node biopsy versus observation in melanoma. *N Engl J Med.* 2014; 370(7):599–609.

4. Faries MB, Thompson JF, Cochrane AJ et al. Completion dissection or observation for sentinel node metastasis in melanoma. *N Engl J Med.* 2017; 376(7):2211–22.

5. Marsden JR, Newton-Bishop JA, Burrows L et al. Revised U.K. guidelines for the management of cutaneous melanoma 2010. *Br J Dermatol.* 2010; 163(2):238–56.

6. Henderson MA, Burmeister BH, Ainslie J et al. Adjuvant lymph node radiotherapy versus observation only in patients with melanoma at high risk of further lymph-node field relapse after lymphadenectomy (ANZMTG 0.1.02/TROG 02.01): 6-year follow-up of a phase III randomized, controlled trial. *Lancet Oncol.* 2015; 16(9):1049–60.

7. Eggermont AM, Suciu S, Testori A et al. Long-term results of the randomized phase III trial EORTC 18991 of adjuvant therapy with pegylated interferon alfa-2b versus observation in resected stage III melanoma. *J Clin Oncol.* 2012; 30(31):3810–8.

8. Eggermont AM, Charion-Sileni V, Grob JJ et al. Adjuvant ipilimumab versus placebo after complete resection of high-risk stage III melanoma (EORTC 18071): A randomised, double-blind, phase 3 trial. *Lancet Oncol.* 2015; 16(5):522–30.

9. Weber J, Mandala M, Del Vecchio M et al. Adjuvant nivolumab versus ipilimumab in resected stage III or IV melanoma. *N Engl J Med.* 2017; 377(19):1824–35.

10. Eggermont AM, Blank CU, Mandala M. Adjuvant Pembrolizumab versus placebo in resected stage III or IV melanoma. *N Engl J Med.* 2018; 378(19):1789–801.

11. Maio M, Lewis K, Demidov L. Adjuvant vemurafenib in resected, BRAFV600 mutation-positive melanoma (BRIM8): A randomised, double-blind, placebo-controlled, multicentre, phase 3 trial. *Lancet Oncol.* 2018; 19(4):510–20.

12. Long G, Hauschild A, Santinami M. Adjuvant dabrafenib plus trametinib in stage III BRAF-mutated melanoma. *N Engl J Med.* 2017; 377(19):1813–23.

13. Thompson JF, Hunt JA, Shannon KF, Kam PC. Frequency and duration of remission after isolated limb perfusion for melanoma. *Arch Surg.* 1997; 132(8):903–7.

14. Noorda EM, Vrouenraets BC, Nieweg OE et al. Isolated limb perfusion for unresectable melanoma of the extremities. *Arch Surg.* 2004; 139(11):1237–42.

15. Patel PM, Suciu S, Mortier L et al. Extended schedule, escalated dose temozolomide versus dacarbazine in stage IV melanoma: Final results of a randomised phase III study (EORTC 18032). *Eur J Cancer.* 2011; 47(10):1476–83.

16. McDermott D, Haanen J, Chen TT et al. Efficacy and safety of ipilimumab in metastatic melanoma patients surviving more than 2 years following treatment in a phase III trial (MDX010-20). *Ann Oncol.* 2013; 24 (10):2694–8.

17. Robert C, Thomas L, Bondarenko I et al. Ipilimumab plus dacarbazine for previously untreated metastatic melanoma. *N Engl J Med.* 2011; 364(26):2517–26.

18. Schadendorf D, Hodi FS, Robert CD et al. Pooled analysis of long-term survival data from phase II and phase III trials of ipilimumab in unresectable or metastatic melanoma. *J Clin Oncol.* 2015; 33(11):1889–94.

19. Robert C, Long GV, Brady B. Nivolumab in previously untreated melanoma without BRAF mutation. *N Engl J Med.* 2015; 372(4):320–30.

20. Hodi FS, Charion-Sileni V, Gonzalez R et al. Nivolumab plus ipilimumab or nivolumab alone versus ipilimumab alone in advanced melanoma (CheckMate 067): 4-year outcomes of a multicentre, randomised, phase 3 trial. *Lancet Oncol.* 2018; 19(11):1480–92.

21. Robert C, Ribas A, Shcachter J et al. Pembrolizumab versus ipilimumab in advanced melanoma (KEYNOTE-006): Post-hoc 5-year results from an open-label, multicentre, randomised, controlled, phase 3 study. *Lancet Oncol.* 2019; 20(9):1239–51.

22. Larkin J, Charion-Sileni V, Gonzalez R et al. Five-year survival with combined nivolumab and ipilimumab in advanced melanoma. *N Engl J Med.* 2019; 381(16):1535–46.

23. Andtbacka RH, Collichio F, Harrington K et al. Final analyses of OPTiM: A randomized phase III trial of talimogene laherparepvec versus granulocyte-macrophage colony-stimulating factor in unresectable stage III–IV melanoma. *J Immunother Cancer.* 2019; 7(1):145.

24. Chapman PB, Hauschild A, Robert C et al. Improved survival with vemurafenib in melanoma with BRAF V600E mutation. *N Engl J Med.* 2011; 364(26):2507–16.

25. Hauschild A, Grob JJ, Demidov LV et al. Dabrafenib in BRAF-mutated metastatic melanoma: A multicentre, open-label, phase 3 randomised controlled trial. *Lancet.* 2012; 380(9839):358–65.

26. Flaherty KT, Infante JR, Daud A et al. Combined BRAF and MEK inhibition in melanoma with BRAF V600 mutations. *N Engl J Med.* 2012; 367(18):1694–703.

27. Long GV, Stroyakovskiy D, Gogas H et al. Combined BRAF and MEK inhibition versus BRAF inhibition alone in melanoma. *N Engl J Med.* 2014; 371(20):1877–88.

28. Larkin J, Ascierto PA, Dréno B et al. Combined vemurafenib and cobimetinib in BRAF-mutated melanoma. *N Engl J Med.* 2014; 371(20):1867–76.

29. Dummer R, Ascierto PA, Gogas HJ et al. Encorafenib plus binimetinib versus vemurafenib or encorafenib in patients with BRAF-mutant melanoma (COLUMBUS): A multicentre, open-label, randomised phase 3 trial. *Lancet Oncol.* 2018; 19(5):603–15.

30. Dummer R, Schadendorf D, Ascierto PA et al. Binimetinib versus dacarbazine in patients with advanced NRAS-mutant melanoma (NEMO): A multicentre, open-label, randomised, phase 3 trial. *Lancet Oncol.* 2017; 18(4):435–45.

31. Kalinsky K, Lee S, Rubin K et al. A phase II trial of Dasatinib in patients with locally advanced or stage IV mucosal, acral and vulvovaginal melanoma: A trial of the ECOG-ACRIN Cancer Research Group (E2607). *Cancer.* 2017; 123(14):2688–97.

32. Carvajal RD, Lawrence DP, Weber JS et al. Phase II study of nilotinib in melanoma harboring KIT alternations following progression to prior KIT inhibition. *Clin Cancer Res.* 2015; 21(10):2289–96.

33. Lee SJ, Kim TM, Kim YJ et al. Phase II trial of nilotinib in patients with metastatic malignant melanoma harboring *KIT* gene aberration: A multicenter trial of Korean Cancer Study Group (UN10-06). *Oncologist.* 2015; 20(11):1312–19.

34. Guo J, Carvajal RD, Dummer R et al. Efficacy and safety of nilotinib in patients with KIT-mutated metastatic or inoperable melanoma: Final results from the global, single-arm, phase II TEAM trial. *Ann Oncol.* 2017; 28(6):1380–87.

35. Carvajal RD, Sosman JA, Quevedo JF et al. Effect of selumetinib vs. chemotherapy on progression-free survival in uveal melanoma. *JAMA.* 2014; 311(23): 2397–405.

36. Carvajal RD, Piperno-Neuman S, Kapieijn E et al. Selumetinib in combination with dacarbazine in patients with metastatic uveal melanoma: A phase III, multicenter, randomized trial (SUMIT). *J Clin Oncol.* 2018; 36(12):1232–39.

37. Falchook GS, Lewis KD, Infante JR et al. Activity of the oral MEK inhibitor trametinib in patients with advanced melanoma: A phase 1 dose-escalation trial. *Lancet Oncol.* 2012;13(8):782–9.

38. Danielli R, Ridolfi R, Chiarion-Sileni V et al. Ipilimumab in pretreated patients with metastatic uveal melanoma: Safety and clinical efficacy. *Cancer Immunol Immunother.* 2012; 61(1):41–8.

39. Khattak MA, Fisher R, Hughes P et al. Ipilimumab activity in advanced uveal melanoma. *Melanoma Res.* 2013; 23(1):79–81.

40. Algazi PA, Tsai KK, Shoushtari AN et al. Clinical Outcomes in metastatic uveal melanoma treated with PD-1 and PD-L1 antibodies. *Cancer.* 2016; 122(21):3344–53.

41. Heppt MV, Heinzerling L, Kähler KC et al. Prognostic factors and outcomes in metastatic uveal melanoma treated with programmed cell death-1 or combined PD-1/cytotoxic T-lymphocyte antigen-4 inhibition. *Eur J Cancer.* 2017; 82:56–65.

42. Rossi R, Pagliara MM, Oreschi D et al. Pembrolizumab as first-line treatment for metastatic uveal melanoma. *Cancer Immunol Immunother.* 2019; 68(7):1179–85.

43. Shoushtari A, Navld-Azarbaljanl P, Friedman CF et al. Efficacy of nivolumab and ipilimumab (Nivo + Ipi) combination in melanoma patients (pts) treated at a single institution on an expanded-access program (EAP). *J Clin Oncol.* 2016;34:Abstr 9554.

44. Chandran SS, Somerville RPT, Yang JC et al. Treatment of metastatic uveal melanoma with adoptive transfer of tumour-infiltrating lymphocytes: A single-centre, two-stage, single-arm, phase 2 study. *Lancet Oncol.* 2017; 18(6):792–802.

45. Carvajal R, Sato T, Shoushtari AN et al. Safety, efficacy and biology of the gp100 TCR-based bispecific T cell redirector, IMCgp100 in advanced uveal melanoma in two Phase 1 trials. *J Immunother Cancer.* 2017; 5(Suppl2):P208.

46. Fife KM, Colman MH, Stevens GN et al. Determinants of outcome in melanoma patients with cerebral metastases. *J Clin Oncol.* 2004; 22(7):1293–300.

47. Fisher R, Larkin J. Treatment of brain metastases in patients with melanoma. *Lancet Oncol.* 2012; 13(5):434–5.

48. Bafaloukos D, Gogas H. The treatment of brain metastases in melanoma patients. *Cancer Treat Rev.* 2004; 30(6):515–20.

49. Mori Y, Kondziolka D, Flickinger JC et al. Stereotactic radiosurgery for cerebral metastatic melanoma: Factors affecting local disease control and survival. *Int J Radiat Oncol Biol Phys.* 1998; 42(3):581–9.

50. Long GV, Trefzer U, Davies MA et al. Dabrafenib in patients with Val600Glu or Val600Lys BRAF-mutant melanoma metastatic to the brain (BREAK-MB): A multicentre, open-label, phase 2 trial. *Lancet Oncol.* 2012; 13(11):1087–95.

51. McArthur GA, Maio M, Arance A et al. Vemurafenib in metastatic melanoma patients with brain metastases: An open-label, single-arm, phase 2, multicentre study. *Ann Oncol.* 2017; 28(3): 634–41.

52. Davies MA, Saiaq P, Robert C et al. Dabrafenib plus trametinib in patients with BRAF[V600]-mutant melanoma brain metastases (COMBI-MB): A multicentre, multicohort, open-label, phase 2 trial. *Lancet Oncol.* 2017; 18(7):863–73.

53. Margolin K, Ernstoff MS, Hamid O et al. Ipilimumab in patients with melanoma and brain metastases: An open-label, phase 2 trial. *Lancet Oncol.* 2012; 13(5):459–65.

54. Goldberg SB, Gettinger SN, Mahajan A et al. Pembrolizumab for patients with melanoma or non-small-cell lung cancer and untreated brain metastases: Early analysis of a non-randomised, open-label, phase 2 trial. *Lancet Oncol.* 2016; 17(7):976–83.

55. Long GV, Atkinson V, Lo S et al. Combination nivolumab and ipilimumab or nivolumab alone in melanoma brain metastases: A multicentre randomised phase 2 study. *Lancet Oncol.* 2018; 19(5): 672–81.

56. Tawbi HA, Forsyth PA, Algazi A et al. Combined nivolumab and ipilimumab in melanoma metastatic to the Brain. *N Engl J Med.* 2018; 379(8):722–30.

26 PRIMARY BONE TUMORS

Jeremy S. Whelan, Rob C. Pollock, Rachael E. Windsor, and Mahbubl Ahmed

Introduction

Cancers that arise in bone are exceptionally uncommon. Several discrete diseases can be identified through their differing clinico-pathological features, but for all bone tumors pain is the most common presenting symptom. As this is a feature of a vast array of musculoskeletal disorders, delay in diagnosis is a well-recognized problem. Principles of management, particularly surgical, are broadly applicable across the different histological types.[1]

Osteosarcoma and Ewing sarcoma together constitute the greatest number of cases. Occurring most often in teenagers and young adults, both diseases are now curable in a significant proportion of cases with modern multimodality treatment. Nevertheless, achieving further improvements in survival continues to prove challenging despite strong international commitment to conducting clinical trials. Chondrosarcoma, a locally aggressive tumor of adults, is often successfully cured surgically but for those with more aggressive, metastatic or recurrent disease, there are few effective treatments. Recent advances in our knowledge of the underlying biology of chondrosarcoma give encouragement for advances in treatment.

Improvements in surgical techniques have been substantial. Thus, amputation is now uncommonly performed for extremity tumors. As the use of systemic therapy has increased the number of survivors, so attention has turned to improving long-term functional outcomes.

Of critical importance in the care of these diseases is close co-operation between experienced surgeons, radiologists, pathologists, and oncologists. Appropriate supportive care facilities and experienced nursing staff are necessary for those receiving intensive chemotherapy and, as many are children and young people, a multidisciplinary approach is required to meet the additional needs which arise, including educational provision and psychosocial support for both patient and family. All those with suspected primary bone tumors should therefore be referred quickly to a recognized specialist center where management is likely to be guided by national and international consensus guidelines.[2,3]

Incidence and etiology

A classification of primary bone tumors is shown in Table 26.1.[4] These diseases do not appear to share a common etiology, although several etiological factors are apparent, particularly for osteosarcoma.

Recent publications from population-based cancer registries have provided more accurate information about the incidence of these rare diseases as well as some indication of a change in the pattern of incidence. In the UK chondrosarcoma is now the commonest bone sarcoma rather than osteosarcoma, reflecting in part an ageing population.

The patterns of incidence differ between the diseases shown in Table 26.1. Both osteosarcoma and Ewing sarcoma have a peak incidence early in adolescence. This occurs slightly earlier in girls, and the association with a pubertal growth spurt, plus the common location of tumors around the knee and in the proximal humerus, indicate an etiological association with rapid bone growth.

In contrast to Ewing sarcoma, which occur very uncommonly after the age of 40 years, there is a low incidence of osteosarcoma throughout adulthood and, indeed, a second peak of incidence in the elderly that is explained in part by an association with Paget's disease. Both osteosarcoma and Ewing sarcoma tend to have a male preponderance when occurring early in life, and Ewing sarcoma has an unexplained racial pattern, being exceptionally uncommon in Africans and African-Americans.

In the majority, the occurrence of any of the tumors shown in Table 26.1 is a sporadic event. However, there are some well-recognized etiological factors, of which the most important is radiation, including therapeutic radiation (Table 26.2).

Sarcomas are a recognized late complication of therapeutic radiation. In this setting, osteosarcoma is the most common histological subtype with a latency averaging between 8 and 20 years. Of greatest concern is the development of a radiation-associated sarcoma as a consequence of successful treatment of childhood malignancy. Although the overall incidence is low, it has become an important factor to consider in the development of new treatments which now attempt to limit use of radiation. Exposure to alkylating agents may add to this risk of sarcoma development. Radiation used in the treatment of breast and gynecological cancers in adults is also associated with the development of sarcomas. Such tumors often pose considerable management problems.

Survivors of retinoblastoma have a striking vulnerability to subsequent development of osteosarcoma. The excess risk (variously estimated as between 150- and 400-fold) is principally in those with familial retinoblastoma and is especially associated with prior treatment with radiotherapy, with most, but not all, these secondary osteosarcomas arising within a field of previous irradiation. The identification of the retinoblastoma gene as a tumor suppressor gene altered in a wide range of cancers has led to insights into osteosarcoma pathogenesis. Loss of heterozygosity for *Rb* is a frequent finding, possibly associated with an adverse prognosis.

Tumors arising in Li–Fraumeni families account for a small but significant proportion of osteosarcoma. Sporadic mutations in *p53* are thought to account for approximately 3% of osteosarcomas. Consistent chromosomal abnormalities have not been reported in osteosarcoma; thus for most, the underlying pathogenesis remains obscure.

The discovery of a chromosomal translocation specific to Ewing sarcoma (t11;22) has provided important insights, particularly in identifying primitive neuro-ectodermal tumors which share this translocation as having a common lineage. These related diseases are now usefully referred to as the Ewing sarcoma family of tumors.

Other factors associated with the development of bone tumors include Paget's disease, syndromes of aberrant DNA repair, and some rare familial skeletal dysplasias. Very occasionally bone sarcomas arise in areas of damaged bone such as a bone infarct or on a background of a previous benign lesion such as a giant cell tumor.

TABLE 26.1   Classification of Malignant Primary Bone Tumors

A Osteosarcoma
    1. Conventional
      Fibroblastic, osteoblastic, chondroblastic, osteoclast-rich, small cell, telangiectatic
    2. Low-grade central
    3. Surface
    High-grade surface, periosteal, parosteal
B Ewing sarcoma
C Chondrosarcoma
    1. Chondrosarcoma (grades 1–3)
    2. Dedifferentiated chondrosarcoma
    3. Mesenchymal chondrosarcoma
D Undifferentiated high-grade pleomorphic sarcoma of bone
E Other spindle cell tumors of bone
    Fibrosarcoma, leiomyosarcoma, liposarcoma, angiosarcoma, epithelioid hemangioendothelioma
F Primary non-Hodgkin lymphoma of bone
G Chordoma

TABLE 26.2   Etiology of Malignant Primary Bone Tumors

A	Genetic syndromes
	e.g. Familial retinoblastoma
	Li–Fraumeni syndrome
	Multiple enchondromata (diaphyseal achalasia)
	Rothmund–Thompson syndrome
B	Radiation
C	Paget's disease
D	Miscellaneous, e.g. polyostotic fibrous dysplasia

General principles of management

A broad framework of management, from initial evaluation to treatment, is appropriate for all patients with primary bone tumors. At all stages, specialist experience and liaison between disciplines are essential.

Initial evaluation

The most common presenting symptom is pain, often characterized by a gradual increase in intensity. An important distinguishing feature is night pain of sufficient severity to disturb sleep. This symptom should always be taken seriously and investigated appropriately. Swelling often accompanies pain, and again is a feature that demands rapid and careful investigation.

Most patients, even those with high-grade tumors, have no systemic symptoms. When these occur, they frequently manifest as fever, weight loss, and even episodic sweats, usually as a consequence of metastatic Ewing sarcoma. Like soft tissue sarcomas, the principal site of metastatic spread is to the lung, but this is only present in some 10–15% of patients at diagnosis, and symptoms from lung metastases are much less frequent.

Plain radiographs in two planes are the essential first investigation. Radiological features are often characteristic but occasionally radiographs may appear normal. Further evaluation of a primary tumor can then be undertaken with magnetic resonance imaging (MRI) and, particularly for lesions on the surface of the bone, computed tomography (CT). Radiological evaluation is mandatory before diagnostic biopsy is undertaken.

Biopsy

Biopsy of bone tumors is an essential but potentially hazardous investigation. Careful planning is required in the setting of a dedicated sarcoma multidisciplinary meeting. The biopsy must be sited appropriately since the biopsy tract is presumed to be contaminated and must be excised at the time of definitive surgery. Wrongly placed biopsy tracts and those that become infected or develop a hematoma may compromise future surgery.[5] An adequate volume of representative tissue must be obtained and sent fresh to the pathologist. Bone tumors are often heterogeneous, so the placement of the biopsy should take into account radiological changes that may indicate areas of higher or lower grade of malignancy which can exist within the same tumor.

Almost all bone biopsies nowadays are CT-guided core needle biopsies, and this has been shown to improve diagnostic accuracy.[6] It is unacceptable to operate on a potentially malignant bone tumor without first identifying the tissue diagnosis. There is, therefore, no role for excision biopsy in the management of primary malignant bone tumors. Incision biopsy is rarely performed on the occasions when more than two core needle biopsies are non-diagnostic. The same principles apply as far as the planning and execution of the biopsy are concerned.

Expert interpretation of the biopsy is essential as most pathologists will be unfamiliar with primary bone tumors and the appearances are often misleading, for instance when distinguishing reactive from tumor bone in bone-forming tumors such as osteosarcoma. Conventional histopathological techniques, together with immunocytochemistry, are now sufficiently advanced to provide a reliable diagnosis in most cases, but molecular diagnostics should be applied routinely for all round cell tumors and are increasingly valuable for distinguishing specific entities. The use of advanced genetic diagnostics such as whole-genome sequencing is becoming more prevalent, especially at recurrence, but the role of such approaches in routine practice is not yet well-defined.

Staging

Enneking et al. introduced the first staging system for primary malignant bone tumors in 1980, and this remains the benchmark (Table 26.3).[7] Tumors were designated low-grade, high-grade, or any grade with metastases. Tumors contained within the periosteal membrane are considered to be type A, and tumors that have extended beyond periosteum into muscle are considered type B. The majority of primary malignant bone tumors at presentation are stage IIB. Nowadays the TNM classification is also used and may be more valuable in Ewing sarcoma.

Primary malignant bone tumors most commonly metastasize to the lungs and the skeleton. The lungs are best imaged with CT whereas isotope bone scan is necessary for determining the presence of bone metastases. Whole-body MRI and PET scanning both have advantages particularly in more accurate imaging of the skeleton. MRI of the full length of the affected bone is mandatory for limb tumors to determine the presence or absence of skip lesions. Ten percent of Ewing's tumors will metastasize to the bone marrow so bone marrow biopsy is routinely performed at presentation although PET scanning may provide similar information achieved non-invasively.

Treatment

The integration of local and systemic therapies is an important feature of the management of high-grade tumors, where most will

TABLE 26.3 **Staging Notation**

Stage	Grade	Site	Treatment	Example
Ia	Low	Within pseudo-periosteum	Wide local excision	Low-grade central osteosarcoma
Ib	Low	Invading muscle	Wide local excision	Parosteal osteosarcoma, chondrosarcoma
IIa	High	Within pseudo-periosteum	Chemotherapy, local excision	Most high-grade osteosarcoma
IIb	High	Invading muscle	Chemotherapy, local excision or radiotherapy if inaccessible	Ewing tumor
IIIa	High	Oligometastatic	Chemotherapy, local excision, metastatectomy	Any sarcoma with few metastases
IIIb	High	Polymetastatic	Palliative chemotherapy and radiotherapy	Inoperable metastatic sarcoma

begin treatment with chemotherapy, local therapy being carried out anywhere between 6 and 20 weeks later. Other tumors may be managed by definitive surgery alone, after biopsy and staging as described above.

Local therapy—surgery

The guiding principles in sarcoma surgery are:

1. The aim of surgery is to achieve local control of the tumor.
2. The surgical margins must be free of tumor.
3. The safe margin of resection includes a biologically competent barrier.
4. Neoadjuvant chemotherapy may reduce or beneficially alter the local extent.
5. Preservation of function must be an additional consideration.

Margins and resection strategy

When operating on malignant bone tumors two margins need to be considered, namely the bone margin and the soft tissue margin. Good quality imaging after neoadjuvant chemotherapy is critical. The length of the tumor is determined to identify a safe bone transection point, convention being to aim for a 2-cm margin in long bones. The soft tissue margin is usually determined by the proximity of vital neurovascular structures, e.g. the popliteal vessels and the sciatic nerve in the case of distal femoral and proximal tibial tumors or the radial nerve adjacent to the proximal humerus. In order to preserve useful function, it may be necessary to perform a planned marginal excision of some part of the tumor.

For any given tumor there is always a balance between the margin of excision and the functional outcome of the limb. There is a trade-off that must be decided at the time of pre-operative planning, in discussion with the patient and also during surgery. If the surgeon aims for a really wide margin of excision and surrounding soft tissues are sacrificed in order to achieve this margin, there will be some collateral damage to the limb. Functional outcome may be compromised but the risk of local recurrence will be low. Alternatively, if a very close margin of excision is chosen and normal muscles and surrounding tissue are preserved, the functional outcome will be improved but the risk of local recurrence will be greater.

With the advent of joint-sparing surgery, the concept of the bone margin has changed in recent years. Computerized surgical navigation tools have made bone cuts much more precise and the margin of error is a lot less than using traditional techniques to decide the transection point at the time of surgery. This means that complex osteotomies can be performed in order to achieve a clear margin and also allows for pre-construction of complex, custom-made prostheses. The aim is still to achieve a clear margin, but improvements are now being seen in functional outcome

with this modern approach to limb salvage surgery with no increased risk of local recurrence.[8]

Limb salvage versus amputation

It is rare to perform amputation as the procedure of choice for primary malignant bone tumors as there is no survival advantage in amputation over limb salvage. The indications for amputation include tumors that encase vital neurovascular structures, fungating tumors, and some intra-articular tumors that are technically unresectable with a clear margin.

In the event of a primary malignant bone tumor occurring in the distal tibia, sometimes below-knee amputation is preferable to an attempt at limb salvage. Even though these tumors are often resectable, the reconstruction options are poor and have a high complication rate. Modern limb prostheses now allow extremely good function which is often superior to the function that can be achieved with limb salvage.

Reconstruction surgery

Surgical reconstruction following tumor excision varies according to size and anatomical location of the bony defect after excision, degree of soft tissue cover, age of the patient, predicted growth of the limb, functional expectations of the patient, and, finally, the resources available to the treating hospital. The relationship between the tumor, the adjacent joint, and the neurovascular structures is determined and a resection strategy is formulated. In skeletally mature patients it may be necessary to sacrifice the joint.

Broadly speaking, reconstructions may be biological or endoprosthetic. Biological reconstructions include the use of fresh frozen allograft, irradiated autograft, and free vascularized fibula grafts. These bone grafts can be used in combination with some form of joint replacement as a composite reconstruction. Endoprosthetic reconstructions, on the other hand, involve replacing the entire length of resected bone with a metal endoprosthesis. These can be modular "off the shelf" implants assembled on the operating table by the surgeon or custom-made. In most sarcoma centers reconstruction is performed with a modular endoprosthesis.

Custom-made implants use modern technology to improve the functional outcome of any given reconstruction. Examples include the use of joint-sparing prostheses around the knee and hip that allow complex fixation of the implant to very short segments of bone. Preservation of the joint means that normal function of the joint is maintained, there is less wear to the implant, and less need for revision surgery in the future. Skeletally immature patients where the physis acts as a barrier to the spread of tumor are major beneficiaries of custom implants and computer-guided navigation of bony cuts. Non-invasive growing endoprostheses are precisely manufactured to anatomically replace the section of bone removed and contain motors that can lengthen the prosthesis in an outpatient setting. This enables leg length equality to be maintained without the need for further surgery and without risk of complications associated with revision surgery.[9]

Most endoprostheses are now coated with silver as this has been shown to reduce the incidence of infection which is a devastating complication in this group of patients. Hydroxyapatite-coated collars are also routinely used in order to improve fixation of the endoprosthesis to bone by a process called osseointegration.

Axial tumors

The same principles of local control apply to axial tumors in terms of resection strategy and excision margins. Scapular tumors can usually be excised without the need for reconstruction and still leave a patient with reasonably good upper limb function.

Pelvic tumors are often large at presentation, adjacent to visceral structures, and usually closely related to iliac vessels and the sacral nerve roots. The hip joint often needs to be sacrificed, and obtaining a clear margin is challenging. Surgical navigation tools reduce the risk of positive margins and also help with the complex reconstruction required.[10] Complication rates are high in terms of wound break down and infection which can delay post-operative chemotherapy. In addition, functional outcomes are often poor. In patients with Ewing sarcoma, local control can be achieved with radiotherapy alone, and this has obvious functional advantages. In the case of chondrosarcoma and osteosarcoma, which are relatively radio-insensitive, surgery offers the only reliable option for local control and can be justified despite the morbidity involved.

Sacral tumors including chordomas provide the greatest challenge of all to orthopedic oncologists. Operations are long, wound complications are the norm, and major blood loss is expected. In order to completely excise the tumor, sacral nerve roots are sacrificed resulting in loss of bladder, bowel, and erectile function. When the S1 level is sacrificed the spine has to be reattached to the pelvis with extensive pedicle screw and rod fixation. In view of the morbidity associated with surgery, patients with a sacral Ewing sarcoma are offered radiotherapy instead.

Bone sarcomas of the spine are rare. If one of the pedicles is uninvolved with tumor it is possible to perform an *en bloc* spondylectomy with a clear margin. Often, however, patients present acutely with cord compression and undergo intralesional decompression before a diagnosis is made. The margins are then contaminated and local control is rarely achieved even with subsequent radical surgery and radiotherapy.

Local recurrence

Local recurrence is often cited as a very major cause of relapse, with the implication that inadequate surgery is a cause of death. There are no controlled data to confirm this, only the observation that the mortality rate in those centers with very aggressive surgeons is not significantly better than those with more conservative ones. In multivariate analysis, it is the size of the tumor and associated chemosensitivity that dictate this, not the type of surgery. Skip lesions may commonly be the cause of local recurrence, having developed early in the disease process as a result of a failure of cell-mediated control mechanisms. Thus, local recurrence is usually a marker of disease activity, and a failure of host tumor control mechanisms at a cellular level, rather than a cause of it.

Radiotherapy—general principles

Historically the use of radiotherapy in the treatment of primary bone tumors has been of limited value due to the radio-resistance of these tumors and also the inability of primitive radiotherapy delivery techniques safely delivering high doses of radiotherapy. Ewing sarcoma are more radio-sensitive bone tumors, and radiotherapy can be used in combination with surgery or as a definitive form of treatment after chemotherapy is complete. In a recent prospective clinical trial, surgery achieved a small but statistically significant advantage over radiotherapy alone with respect to local control of disease.[11,12] It is worth noting radiotherapy as a sole modality for definitive treatment is usually used for inoperable tumors which are likely to have poor biology and poor prognosis.

Advances in photon radiotherapy technology have allowed improved radiation dose coverage of the tumor target through improved imaging of the tumor and improvement in beam delivery techniques which can conform accurately around the tumor and reduce the dose to critical normal structures surrounding the tumor. Intensity-modulated radiotherapy (IMRT) and volumetric arc radiotherapy (VMAT) are examples of some of these advances which allow more conformal dose coverage of the tumor. Radiotherapy can also be delivered using particle therapy such as carbon ion and protons.[13,14] They have some biological advantages over photon radiotherapy such as increased relative biological dose (greater likelihood of damaging DNA in cancer cells) as well as the ability to reduce radiation dose to surrounding normal tissues. These dosimetric and biological advantages are dependent on the anatomical site of the tumor and are more likely to benefit younger patients from late radiation toxicity. The infrastructure, resources, and technologies needed to deliver particle therapy are vast and therefore are limited to nationally agreed indications for patients who are most likely to benefit the most. It is likely that as technology improves further, these treatments may be more widely available.

Even with modest dose escalation the best results are achieved with low or minimal residual volumes of tumor. The optimal local therapy for many bone tumors may require both modalities for local tumor control. Surgical techniques also evolve rapidly and previously inoperable tumors are now operable with good functional outcomes.

As some of these tumors arise in the young, the morbidity of radiotherapy is a concern, in terms of damage to adjacent organs, effects on skeletal growth, and the risk of radiation-associated malignancy. The first two may also be a concern for surgical approaches. The decision on local treatment that produces the best local control rate must be balanced against the late morbidity and, occasionally, the acute morbidity, of a selected single or planned combined approach.[15]

A third factor to be considered is the anticipated cure rate. In some individuals with a low risk of metastatic disease a local treatment plan that carries a significant adverse functional effect may be acceptable, while the same approach in a patient with a lower chance of survival may not.

Indications

Radiotherapy can be used in the definitive (inoperable) setting or pre-/post-operatively. In the pre-/post-operative setting the aim of radiotherapy is to reduce the risk of local recurrence. For osteosarcoma, pre-operative radiotherapy is not generally used. In Ewing sarcoma, pre-operative radiotherapy provides the advantages of a lower radiotherapy dose and smaller treatment volume. However, some surgeons do not favor pre-operative radiotherapy due to an increased risk of post-operative wound complications.

The indications for radiotherapy are as follows:

1. As definitive radiotherapy in in-operable tumors
2. Planned marginal excision or positive margins on resection pathology (<1 mm)
3. Residual disease in situ after surgery (R2 resection)
4. Pathological fracture with contamination of local anatomical structures
5. Poor histological response to chemotherapy (<90%) on resection pathology
6. Some anatomical sites such as spine/para/pelvis/sacrum where surgery is technically challenging

Technical factors

In most cases the radiation technique to be used is made at diagnosis to allow preparation including timing for radiotherapy. Discussion with the surgeon prior to surgery is crucial as if metal implants are required especially in the spine it is preferable to use carbon-fiber PEEK* rather than titanium. Titanium attenuates and scatters the radiotherapy beam and therefore compromises the treatment area. Protons are very difficult to deliver due to the interference of titanium or other metals.

Radiotherapy planning requires the pre-chemotherapy tumor volume imaging as well as serial chemotherapy response imaging, and pre-surgery imaging if appropriate. All imaging is reviewed including CT, MRI, and PET if available. A clinical assessment is made of the patient and using knowledge of the radiotherapy target volume and anatomical site an appropriate patient specific immobilization is created. A gross tumor volume (GTV) is delineated based on the pre-chemotherapy tumor volume.

The radiation target volume includes all tissues initially involved by tumor and is therefore based on the pre-chemotherapy extent. The clinical target volume (CTV) margin varies with the histology and anatomical site and is usually extended 1.5–3 cm from the GTV taking into account patters of microscopic spread of cancer and anatomical boundaries. For example, when a bulky tumor protrudes into a body cavity but has subsequently regressed. The planning target volume (PTV) margin depends on

---

* Polyether ether ketone.

local factors and should include results of local audit on immobilization as well as taking account of internal organ motion. If photon radiotherapy is used IMRT/VMAT is used in most cases; however if there is dosimetric advantage 3D conformal radiotherapy is still used.

In limb planning, an unirradiated "corridor" must be left along the axis of the limb to minimize late lymphedema and the full dose across the full circumference of both sides of a joint avoided if possible. In patients of childbearing age, thought must be given to fertility, with sperm storage or repositioning of gonads offered if appropriate. In tumors of the ilium, as much bowel as possible should be displaced from the radiation fields by positioning, treating with a full bladder if appropriate, or by operative placement of a retroperitoneal spacer.

In younger patients, the effects of even low-dose radiation on the growing skeleton must be considered, and fields may be extended, for at least part of the dose, to ensure an even effect on epiphyses. In many sites, IMRT may produce equivalent sparing of normal function to particle therapy, but these and VMAT techniques will almost always produce a low dose "bath" over a greater volume of tissue. In cases irradiated pre-operatively, an understanding of the planned transection plane through bone, relative to the radiation portals, may reduce adverse effects on healing.

The traditional recommendation is that the whole scar and the full length of the prosthetic material should be included in the target volume. However the length of scars often reflects the requirements of inserting the prosthesis and may be difficult to cover without compromising function. It is unclear whether scars from insertion of prosthetic stems into the receiving bone are at significant risk of microscopic contamination even when some distance from the tumor. Principles of radiotherapy for bone tumors are summarized in Table 26.4.

Adverse consequences of radiotherapy

Radiotherapy toxicity is divided into acute toxicity (toxicity during radiotherapy that resolves) and late toxicity that starts 3 months after radiotherapy and is likely to be permanent. Long-term effects relate primarily to abnormalities of growth and limb function and to induction of second malignancies. The risk of impaired function of organs such as kidney or heart from the

TABLE 26.4   **Principles of Radiotherapy for Bone Tumors**

Action	Comment
At diagnosis decide type of radiotherapy to be used, protons or photons	The type of radiotherapy to be used depends on age of patient, anatomical location of tumor, and surrounding normal tissues
At diagnosis if spinal implants are required to use carbon-fiber PEEK rather than titanium	Titanium attenuates and interferes with the radiotherapy beam
Plan with MRI and CT and after discussion with musculoskeletal radiologist and, if after surgery, the surgeon	Definition of extent difficult, especially where there is edema
GTV based on largest tumor extent (except where it originally protruded into body cavity and has regressed)	Risk of microscopic contamination after surgery or chemotherapy-induced regression
Margin along *relevant* tissue planes	Risk of spread along marrow cavity and especially in soft tissues along muscle planes. Intact fascia forms an effective barrier to spread
Include scar and all prosthetic material, but as this may considerably extend volume, consider risk of contamination in individual case	There is a risk of microscopic disease here. However the size of this risk with chemotherapy and good surgical technique is not known
Spare a "corridor" for lymphatic drainage	High doses are used for these tumors. Failure to provide for lymphatic drainage will produce very severe effects
Without compromising on target volume:	
Spare as much of joint as possible	The more spared, the less the risk of stiffness. However disability can be minimized by exercise
Spare epiphyses if possible	10 Gy will probably stop growth
Avoid gonads	Careful technique may sometimes allow this

radiotherapy must be added to the organ-specific toxic effects of chemotherapy used in multi-modality treatment.

The pattern of toxicity differs between the radiotherapy beam and technique used. In a prospective randomized trial comparing 3D-conformal radiotherapy and IMRT the rates of acute skin toxicity were 49% and 32% respectively ($p = 0.02$). Late toxicity for 3D-conformal radiotherapy versus IMRT for fracture (9.1%, 4.1%, $p = 0.18$), joint stiffness (11%, 14.5%, $p = 0.40$), lymphedema (7.9%, 14.9%, $p = 0.05$), nerve damage (1.6%, 3.5%, $p = 0.45$).[16] For patients undergoing proton radiotherapy for bone sarcoma approximately 33% develop high-grade toxicities, and the majority of these are skin toxicities.[13] Improving proton beam technology such as pencil beam scanning is likely to reduce acute and late skin toxicities.

Another serious late effect after radiotherapy is the risk of second malignancy. The risk is approximately 1 in 1000 people at 10 years; however there are many biological and environmental factors that may influence the risk.[17] With IMRT/VMAT there is an increased low-dose radiation bath to normal tissues, and it has been hypothesized that this may double the incidence of second malignancies in the future.[17] There is a theoretical increased risk of second malignancy with protons due to biological effects of the beam, however this has not been proven in follow-up data to date. In a cohort of patients having protons for Ewing sarcoma long-term follow-up data showed the cumulative incidence of second malignancy was 7% at 2 years and 15% at 3 years.[13] The second malignancies that developed were acute myeloid leukemia and myelodysplastic syndrome, more attributable to chemotherapy as it is expected that second malignancies caused by radiotherapy are more likely to be solid tumors.

Radiotherapy for palliation

Useful palliation may be achieved, where symptoms are due to pain or pressure from tumor mass even in the more resistant types such as osteosarcoma and chondrosarcoma.

Chemotherapy

Osteosarcoma and Ewing sarcoma can be fatal because of metastatic spread, principally to the lungs. Advances in chemotherapy over the past 30 years are largely responsible for the dramatic improvements in survival from these tumors. Significant proportions of patients remain incurable, generally those who have advanced disease at presentation. Furthermore, current chemotherapy regimens are associated with considerable morbidity, both in the short and long term. As many survivors of bone tumors are young, late toxic effects, particularly cardiotoxicity and infertility, are of great concern to investigators planning effective treatments.

Chemotherapy is often given after biopsy has established an appropriate diagnosis and before definitive local therapy, so-called neoadjuvant therapy. This practice began in the 1970s as orthopedic techniques to avoid amputation improved. While rates of conversion of tumors from only suitable for amputation to suitable for limb salvage surgery may be low (approximately 10%), operability is certainly facilitated in many tumors. Additionally, the prognostic information gained from histological scoring of chemotherapy response in the resected tumor remains a very valuable clinical tool. Other advantages of neoadjuvant chemotherapy are shown in Table 26.5.

The role of chemotherapy in the management of less common high-grade primary bone tumors is not clearly defined and is discussed as appropriate in specific sections below.

TABLE 26.5   Advantages of Neoadjuvant Chemotherapy for Bone Tumors

1. Rapid improvement in symptoms
2. Early treatment of micro-metastatic disease
3. Facilitation of resection in responding tumors
4. Time to manufacture customized endoprosthesis
5. Prognostic information from assessment of histological response

Osteosarcoma

This is the most common high-grade primary tumor of bone. Survival has improved dramatically since the introduction of chemotherapy. Many of the principles underpinning the treatment of osteosarcoma are applicable to other bone tumors.

Subtypes of osteosarcoma

Conventional high-grade osteosarcoma

This variant accounts for most cases. Histologically there may be areas of spindle-cell formation, malignant cartilage, fibroblastic differentiation, and variable, sometimes dense osteoblastic activity giving rise to tumor bone formation that is visible radiologically. Alkaline phosphatase produced by the malignant osteoblasts is one of the cytological stains used to confirm osteosarcoma.

Telangiectatic osteosarcoma is an uncommon and aggressive variant of osteosarcoma. Radiological appearances are of a lytic process with little new bone formation. Histologically it may be mistaken for an aneurysmal bone cyst.

Typically, high-grade tumors start at the epiphysis, expand within the bone, and break through the cortex to lift the periosteum. The tumor eventually erupts through the periosteal boundary and impinges on the adjacent soft tissues. Very large tumors behind the knee or in the axilla may incorporate the neurovascular bundle making endoprosthetic replacement extremely challenging.

Low-grade central osteosarcoma

This tumor is rare, has a slower rate of progression and is better demarcated radiologically. Histologically, it can be difficult to distinguish from fibrous dysplasia. It has a good prognosis when treated with surgery alone although recurrence with higher grade disease is recognized.

Surface steosarcomas

Some osteosarcomas arise on the surface of the bone rather than centrally. Occasionally these are high-grade tumors, but two other variants are more commonly recognized. Periosteal osteosarcoma appears to carry an intermediate course between high-grade tumors and the low-grade surface tumor, parosteal osteosarcoma. Although the prognosis is better than with classic central osteosarcoma, both parosteal and periosteal osteosarcomas may contain areas of high-grade tumor within them. They tend to arise in a more diaphyseal site than the central osteosarcomas, and the medulla of the bone is not involved until late.

Clinical presentation

The two major clinical features are pain and swelling. Typically pain precedes the swelling by weeks or months. It starts as an intermittent pain, partially relieved by ordinary analgesics but not relieved by rest. After a few weeks the pain intensifies and becomes constant. A characteristic feature, and one which would lead to earlier diagnosis if it were better appreciated, is that patients complain of intensification of pain at night-time. Often after several weeks, a second symptom appears which is swelling. At first this may not be obvious since the soft tissues of the muscle and subcutaneous fat conceal the swelling. At this point the patients or parents become alarmed and usually insist on X-rays if these have not already been arranged.

Sadly, several months often elapse before the diagnosis of a malignant bone tumor is made. This is due to the rarity of the tumors and because in the young, musculoskeletal pains, trivial injuries, and strains are common. Very often the patients will have had physiotherapy for some weeks without avail and, indeed, physiotherapy may make symptoms worse. A long period of delay in diagnosis may create great tension in the family and sometimes considerable difficulties for the relationship between the patient and the family practitioner.

Occasionally patients with osteosarcoma may have a very aggressive tumor that is accompanied by fever and constitutional malaise, anemia, and weight loss. This always implies an extremely bad prognosis and is usually associated with multiple bone or lung metastases. Osteosarcoma nearly always metastasizes to the lung in the first instance. However, bone metastases also occur and, with increasing experience of combination chemotherapy, recurrence at other sites such as skin, brain, and intra-abdominally is increasingly recognized.

In the lung, metastases are usually asymptomatic. They are typically situated subpleurally where they may give rise to pneumothorax and occasionally cavitate. If the metastasis involves the pleural space a pleural effusion develops. Centrally located metastases may compress one or other main bronchus and give rise to breathlessness, chest pain, or hemoptysis.

Investigations

Plain X-rays are essential. The characteristic features are of a permeating, lytic lesion without any clear dividing boundary. Breach of the cortex leads to elevation of the periosteum which, when accompanied by new bone formation, gives rise to a Codman's triangle (Figure 26.1). Varying degrees of tumor bone formation lead to dense sclerosis (Figure 26.2) or small areas of spiculation of bone, sometimes arranged at right angles to the long axis of the bone called "sunray spiculation." Surface osteosarcomas are associated with the typical radiological appearances shown in Figure 26.3a and b. An isotope bone scan will typically show an area of increased uptake of isotope at the site of the lesion and may show bone metastases if present. However, whole-body MRI or PET scanning provide more accurate information for skeletal staging. A CT scan of the chest is essential and may show pulmonary metastases (Figure 26.4). MRI is used to determine both the extent of the intra-medullary component of the tumor and the soft tissue extension of the mass (Figure 26.5).[18]

Accurate assessment of audiological, cardiac, renal glomerular, and tubular function should be carried out in all newly diagnosed patients with osteosarcoma. Semen cryopreservation should be offered if appropriate. Periodic re-assessment during therapy is indicated, as nephrotoxicity due to agents such as cisplatin and ifosfamide or anthracycline-induced cardiotoxicity may require adjustments in treatment to minimize the risks of permanent damage.

Surgery

General principles of surgical resection are discussed above. Osteosarcoma affects the metaphyseal region of long bones and

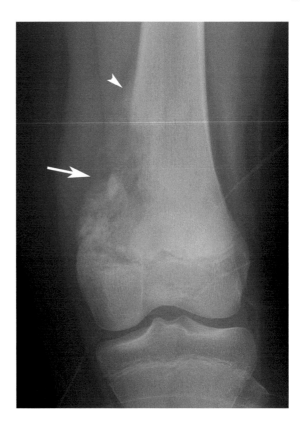

FIGURE 26.1 High-grade osteosarcoma of distal femur. A mixed lytic-sclerotic area of bone destruction is present in the metaphysis (arrows) with elevation of the periosteum at the proximal tumor margin (Codman triangle) (arrowhead).

is often closely related to the adjacent joint and neurovascular structures. Re-imaging with MRI after completion of neoadjuvant chemotherapy is a prerequisite for optimal surgical planning.

Chemotherapy

Before the 1970s osteosarcoma was a devastating disease, treatable only by amputation, with more than 80% of patients succumbing rapidly to lung metastases. This appalling outlook has been transformed by subsequent developments in chemotherapeutic and surgical treatments. First, cytotoxic agents were identified which induced responses in advanced osteosarcoma, the most important of these being very-high-dose methotrexate, doxorubicin, and cisplatin. Second was the observation that resection of pulmonary metastases was both technically possible and profitable in terms of survival. Finally, improving surgical techniques allowed limb preservation in some cases. This last development led to the concept of pre-operative chemotherapy, response to which seemed to facilitate "limb salvage" surgery and which allowed time to manufacture custom-measured metallic endoprostheses.

After 1975, evidence of a survival advantage for adjuvant chemotherapy grew, in particular through a series of uncontrolled studies conducted at the Memorial Sloan Kettering Hospital of combination chemotherapy given after surgery. These drug regimens used doxorubicin, high-dose methotrexate, and bleomycin, cyclophosphamide, and actinomycin D—a combination known as BCD. These programs evolved to produce a regimen called T10, for which impressive 2-year survival rates were claimed.[19] At the time, these studies were difficult to interpret because of the lack

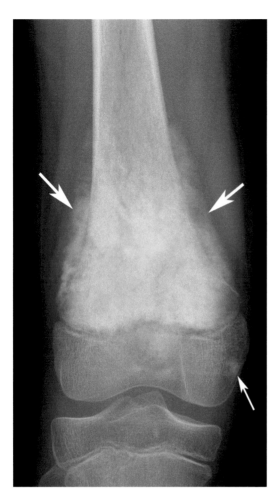

FIGURE 26.2   High-grade osteoblastic osteosarcoma of the distal femur. A densely osteoblastic lesion is present in the distal femoral metaphysis with extension into the surrounding soft tissues (arrows) and a small "skip" metastasis in the epiphysis (arrowhead).

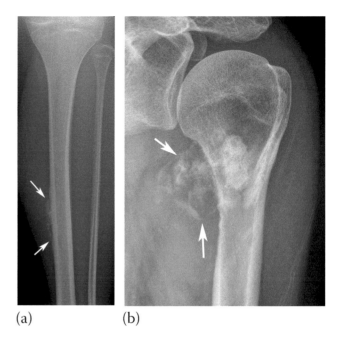

(a)   (b)

FIGURE 26.3   (a) Periosteal osteosarcoma of the tibia. AP radiograph demonstrates an area of spiculated bone formation on the surface of the tibial diaphysis (arrows). (b) Radiograph of the upper humerus, showing dense lobular ossification around the metaphysis (arrows) due to a dedifferentiated parosteal osteosarcoma.

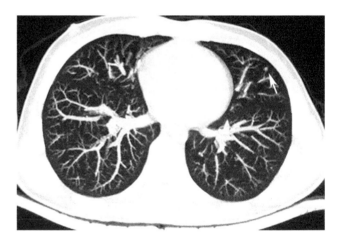

FIGURE 26.4   CT scan of the chest in a patient with osteosarcoma and a normal chest radiograph. A single sub-pleural metastasis is seen in the left lung (arrow).

of any concomitant control and the very short follow-up period. Alterations in selection criteria which had occurred during the 1970s—particularly the introduction of CT scanning—made firm assessment of the results difficult.

The doubts were allayed to a considerable extent by two randomized studies. Link and co-workers compared T10-based chemotherapy with no chemotherapy. There was a clear difference in relapse-free survival in favor of chemotherapy at diagnosis.[20] A further study from Eilber and colleagues randomized patients to receive no further chemotherapy following initial intra-arterial doxorubicin and tumor irradiation. The other arm of the randomization was to receive post-operative treatment with BCD and high-dose methotrexate. There was a significant improvement in relapse-free survival and overall survival in the small number of patients who were randomized to further chemotherapy.[21]

Subsequently, several important studies were carried out by the European Osteosarcoma Intergroup (EOI). The first aimed to define the importance of high-dose methotrexate, the second compared a prolonged multi-drug regimen, similar to T10, to a two-drug combination given for just six cycles, and the third study compared the standard two-drug regimen of cisplatin and doxorubicin with a dose-intensive schedule using granulocyte colony-stimulating factors. No advantage for dose intensity was

seen, and the overall survival in these studies falls short of that reported by groups using three or four drugs as standard.[22–24]

Adjuvant chemotherapy is now part of the accepted standard of care for high-grade osteosarcoma. Assessment of the histological response to chemotherapy has been identified as the most powerful prognostic factor in this disease; those patients who experience very extensive necrosis (in excess of 90%) have an overall survival in excess of 70% at 5 years, while those in whom the degree of necrosis falls short of this have a significantly inferior survival. There are theoretical disadvantages associated with pre-operative chemotherapy, namely that poorly or non-responsive tumors may

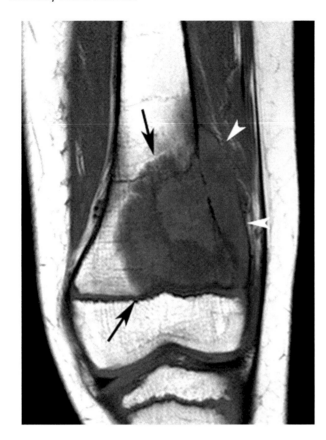

FIGURE 26.5 Coronal T1W SE MR image showing an osteosarcoma of the left distal femur extending to the open growth plate (black arrows). The tumor has extended into the soft tissues (white arrowheads).

grow during treatment, increasing the risk of amputation and of distant spread. The single randomized trial to address this issue showed that those receiving pre-operative chemotherapy enjoyed a significantly higher rate of limb salvage surgery without any survival disadvantage.[25]

Standard chemotherapy for osteosarcoma usually consists of a multi-drug regimen including methotrexate, doxorubicin, and cisplatin. Other active cytotoxic agents include ifosfamide and etoposide. There have been no important recent additions of new drugs to first-line standard of care, and clinical studies have been aimed at defining optimal treatment schedules. Intra-arterial chemotherapy has been shown to produce high rates of histological necrosis but does not improve survival and is not routinely indicated. There are relatively few randomized trials of chemotherapy for osteosarcoma that have sufficient statistical power to provide firm evidence for best practice. A large study undertaken by the Children's Oncology Group in the USA used a 2-by-2 factorial design to investigate the addition of ifosfamide to a standard arm of cisplatin, doxorubicin, and methotrexate. A second randomization compared the addition of the biological agent, MTP-PE (mifamurtide), to chemotherapy.[26,27] An unequivocal advantage for these interventions was not demonstrated although the results have attracted considerable attention. Mifamurtide has been licensed for use in patients under 30 with localized osteosarcoma in some countries but is not universally available or used. There have been no further confirmatory clinical trials.[1]

The studies described above all took many years to complete. In recognition of both the need to improve survival and the

advantages of international co-operation, individual study groups joined together to undertake EURAMOS 1, the first combined European and American randomized study in osteosarcoma.[28] This trial successfully recruited well in excess of 2000 patients. It had two primary objectives: To examine whether the addition of ifosfamide and etoposide to post-operative chemotherapy with doxorubicin, cisplatin, and methotrexate improved survival for patients with a poor histological response to pre-operative chemotherapy and to examine whether the addition of interferon-a as maintenance therapy after post-operative chemotherapy with cisplatin, doxorubicin, and methotrexate improved survival for patients with a good histological response to pre-operative chemotherapy. Neither of these interventions were demonstrated to be superior to the standard of care and indeed when additional chemotherapy was given to those with a poor histological response, there was an excess of serious toxicity and of second malignancies.[29–31] Thus, current evidence does not support changing post-operative chemotherapy based on necrosis measured in the resected tumor.

Adaptation of therapy according to risk factors remains insufficiently developed for patients with extremity osteosarcoma. This is because the most powerful indicator of outcome, histological response, is only available well into any program of systemic therapy. Furthermore, no study has clearly identified that alteration of therapy on the basis of histological response can improve survival for those with poor rates of necrosis. It is hoped that newer biological markers may provide earlier indications of outcome that can be used to plan individualized treatment. This is now an important focus for ongoing clinical studies which seek to unlock the complex biology of osteosarcoma in order to identify new targets.[32,33]

Radiotherapy

The role of radiotherapy in osteosarcoma is confined largely to the treatment of inoperable tumors, where it may extend the period of local control but is unlikely to produce local cure. This relatively radioresistant tumor does have a degree of response to radiotherapy if high doses are given. Improved control rates are reported with dose escalation approaching 70 Gy or more. Series are still small and clinically mixed but follow-up to 5 years is available and suggests local control rates at 5 years of 72%.[34] In this series the 5-year distant relapse rate was 26% indicating that attempting prolonged local control is valuable. Evidence for the use of adjuvant radiotherapy is limited but it may have a role to play where there is a high risk of residual viable microscopic disease such as R1 margins, especially with a poor histological response and where further surgery is not contemplated and in primary spinal tumors after resection. A pathological fracture occurring before resection, especially if there is significant displacement, may also prompt discussion about a role for radiotherapy, but evidence of value is slight. Doses of 60 Gy or higher, ideally 70 Gy, should be attempted but may not be achievable near sensitive normal structures such as the bowel and spinal cord.[34–36]

Treatment of metastases

Presentation with pulmonary metastasis is a grave prognostic sign, and almost no patients are cured if they present with bone metastases. Patients who present with one or two pulmonary metastases should be treated with chemotherapy. If they respond completely, a very close surveillance policy must be followed and resectable metastases should be removed if they re-appear on CT scanning. Patients presenting with multiple pulmonary metastases will almost certainly not be cured even if there is complete response to chemotherapy. Nevertheless, treatment is worthwhile and very durable responses may be obtained.

The more common situation is for metastases to appear after chemotherapy has been completed. Some patients are certainly cured by thoracotomy. Good prognostic factors for the success of thoracotomy are few metastases, unilateral rather than bilateral disease, a long period of freedom from relapse following the cessation of chemotherapy, and the peripheral location of the metastases.[37] Patients who develop pulmonary metastases while on chemotherapy have a very bad prognosis indeed. Although the introduction of new agents may produce responses, and is worthwhile, the chances of cure are very small. Similarly, relapse immediately, or a few months after, the cessation of chemotherapy is also very adverse. Pleural effusion is an extremely adverse sign and nearly always indicates intra-pleural spread of the tumor, which is incurable.

There are many questions still to be asked about optimum management of pulmonary metastases.[38] It is not clear how often repeated thoracotomies are successful. Some patients have multiple thoracotomies, each of which appears justified but which fails to produce lasting benefit. Occasionally freedom from disease may be achieved, especially when the interval between surgery is relatively long. Prophylactic pulmonary irradiation after metastatectomy has never been investigated appropriately to determine whether it might confer a lasting benefit.

Ewing sarcoma

James Ewing's original description of this disease remains pertinent today. It is a member of the group of small, round, blue cell tumors of childhood, with neuroblastoma, rhabdomyosarcoma, and some lymphomas, distinguishable only by immunocytochemistry or biological markers. Its etiology and cell of origin remain obscure despite the demonstration of characteristic chromosomal translocations, t(11;22) and, less commonly, t(21;22). These translocations have illuminated the close relationship between classical Ewing sarcoma and other related tumors, primitive neuro-ectodermal tumors of bone and soft tissue which share the same cytogenetic abnormality but may express more neural markers.[39] Recently other small round blue cell sarcomas have been identified which in the past have been loosely termed and treated as Ewing-like tumors but which have characteristic translocations and clinical behavior. These include BCOR- and CIC-DUX-associated sarcomas for which management guidelines are not yet well-defined.[40]

Clinical features and diagnosis

The presentation is as for osteosarcoma. The main symptoms are pain and swelling, and the location of the tumor is usually diaphyseal rather than epiphyseal. Unlike osteosarcoma, Ewing sarcomas are much more commonly found in the pelvis, the ribs, and the axial skeleton. The most common sites are femur, humerus, ilium, other regions of the pelvis, ribs, skull and jaw, and small bones of the hands and feet. The tumor is typically permeating, spreading widely within the medulla and the vascular spaces of the bone cortex. It causes necrosis of bone, and the tumor itself may be necrotic.

New bone is often laid down around the site of the tumor, giving rise, radiologically, to the typical "onion skin" appearance. There is often thickening and sclerosis of the cortex of the bone,

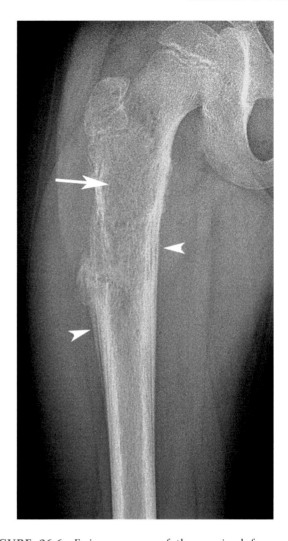

FIGURE 26.6 Ewing sarcoma of the proximal femur. AP radiograph demonstrates an area of poorly defined lytic bone destruction (arrow) with a multi-laminated periosteal response (arrowheads).

although occasionally Ewing sarcoma are purely destructive with widespread bone lysis (Figure 26.6).

Diagnosis is by biopsy, and it is important that the specimen is examined by a skilled pathologist in conjunction with the X-rays. The differential diagnosis will include non-malignant conditions such as osteomyelitis. An appropriate panel of immunocytochemical markers must be used to exclude lymphomas and carcinomas. Various degrees of neural differentiation will be indicated by markers such as S-100 and chromogranin, and expression of CD99, although not specific for Ewing sarcoma, is usually strongly positive. Access to molecular diagnostics to detect chromosomal translocations is essential and should be regarded as the gold standard for diagnostics.

Investigations

Investigations should include plain radiographs of the affected bone. A CT scan of the lungs is essential to confirm or exclude visible pulmonary metastases and an MRI of the affected bone is useful both in assessing tumor size (and thus prognosis, see below) and in planning primary treatment. An isotope bone scan will confirm the increased uptake in the presence of the primary tumor and may show other bone metastases. Staging is completed by examination of a bone marrow aspirate and trephine biopsy. As stated above, the skeleton is more effectively staged using whole-body MRI or PET scanning, the latter having the additional advantage of indicating the presence of bone marrow involvement and which can be very valuable for response assessment.[41,42] Investigations of organ function should be carried out as for osteosarcoma.

Management

When a patient with Ewing sarcoma first presents, it is essential that the treating team of medical oncologists, radiotherapists, and surgeons conducts a thorough discussion regarding local therapy options. There are no randomized studies providing clear evidence, but local control (and survival) is highest when surgery is included in local therapy and, generally, lowest when radiotherapy is the sole local therapy. The initial principle is for operation where possible, although not at the cost of profound functional defect—for example, radiotherapy would be preferred over total sacrectomy in those cases where the latter would be the necessary surgical procedure. Post-operative radiotherapy is indicated where there is a marginal (or positive) resection margin and/or a poor histological response.

More recent on-going analyses of European data indicate that even with complete resection and very good histological response there is a local relapse rate of 7–10% that may be reduced by radiotherapy.[43] Overall the best local control is achieved by using both radiotherapy and surgery, presumably because, following chemotherapy-induced regression, there is a risk of residual viable microscopic disease in tissue outside the usual operative target. There are also some indications that the outcome may be improved by pre-operative radiotherapy, for the same reason, possibly adding reduced risk of contamination at the time of operation.

The decision on local therapy taken after about 18 weeks of chemotherapy will be based on several factors to deliver the key principle of aiming to treat the entire area of tissue *initially* involved by tumor, either by surgical resection or by radiotherapy or a combination of both:

- Is the lesion likely to be resectable in its entirety with uninvolved resection margins?
- Will the functional results of surgery be acceptable?
- Is radiotherapy likely to be indicated?
- If so, would it be better delivered before or after surgery?
- Will the addition of radiotherapy significantly compromise the surgical outcome?
- If so, should a wider margin be planned to avoid the need for radiotherapy?
- What is the anticipated survival and therefore what is an acceptable morbidity for local therapy to maximize local control?
- What could be done to minimize the toxicity of radiotherapy?

Chemotherapy

Alkylating agents were among the first drugs used in Ewing sarcoma, and cyclophosphamide was the standard agent for many years. Early combination therapy comprised vincristine, actinomycin D, and cyclophosphamide (VAC). A randomized study carried out by the American co-operative group (IESS) demonstrated that the addition of doxorubicin to this combination led to a significant survival advantage, superior to that provided by pulmonary irradiation.[44] Later, ifosfamide was shown to be a highly active drug, and many current regimens use ifosfamide as the alkylating agent of choice.[45]

Combination chemotherapy regimens are based on combinations of vincristine, actinomycin, and cyclophosphamide, or vincristine, doxorubicin, and cyclophosphamide. More recently, the combinations have substituted ifosfamide for cyclophosphamide and interest increased for the use of etoposide as part of more intensive regimens.

A study between the UK and the German CESS groups compared predominantly ifosfamide-based chemotherapy with chemotherapy based on ifosfamide and cyclophosphamide in low-risk Ewing sarcomas. In another group of patients, the ifosfamide-based chemotherapy was compared with the same chemotherapy with the addition of etoposide. There appears to be no clear advantage in favor of etoposide in this schedule. Overall survival is similar to earlier studies, and there remains considerable room for improvement, particularly in patients presenting with adverse features.[46]

The European Ewing Tumor Working Initiative of National Groups Ewing Tumor Studies 1999 (EURO-E.W.I.N.G.99) completed a series of collaborative randomized studies investigating whether increased intensity of treatment leads to improved survival, particularly in patients with a poor histological response to pre-operative chemotherapy. A further aim was to reduce toxic late effects of treatment in those with good prognostic indicators. This concluded that in maintenance therapy, cyclophosphamide and ifosfamide achieved similar survival with somewhat different toxicity profiles and most significantly, that high-dose chemotherapy consolidation improved survival compared to standard chemotherapy in patients with a tightly defined poor response to chemotherapy, but this intervention was not effective in those presenting with pulmonary metastases.[47–49]

Responding to the report from The Children's Oncology Group in the USA of results of a randomized, controlled trial showing significantly improved event-free survival in patients treated with interval-compressed chemotherapy given every 14 days,[50] a wider European collaboration has rapidly conducted a further study to compare the standard chemotherapy schedule used in the EURO-E.W.I.N.G.99 studies with the American regimen.[51] Although only reported in abstract form to date, this study, EUROEWING 2012, indicated that dose-compressed chemotherapy leads to improved survival outcomes with no excess toxicity. It is likely that this will be more widely adopted as a standard of care for first-line chemotherapy. The current generation of studies is investigating whether the addition of new agents, principally tyrosine kinase inhibitors, can enhance current chemotherapy regimens.

Prognosis in this disease is multifactorial, the most important element being the presence of metastatic disease. It is evident that a proportion of patients with metastatic disease confined to the lungs will be cured by conventional chemotherapy, but there are virtually no survivors if the bone marrow or other bones are involved. Tumor volume can also be used to stratify risk, patients with tumors larger than 100–200 mL faring less well. Finally, in patients who undergo surgery, the response to pre-operative chemotherapy appears to be an important factor, as in osteosarcoma.

Surgery

Surgery for Ewing sarcoma is extremely challenging mainly because it is difficult to determine the anatomical extent of the tumor from the pre-operative MRI scan. Tumors are characterized by a large extra osseous component surrounded by edema.

Assuming that the edematous area contains tumor cells, complete surgical excision is difficult and potentially very morbid for the patient. Neoadjuvant chemotherapy is very effective in reducing the size of the extra osseous component but differentiating an infiltrative mass from one that displaces surrounding structures with a pushing edge is always difficult.

Typically, Ewing sarcoma affect the diaphysis of long bones. It is often possible to perform joint-sparing surgery using custom-made endoprostheses or biological reconstruction of some sort. Pelvic tumors present an enormous challenge. Surgery in the form of internal hemi-pelvectomy and reconstruction is extremely morbid and, whatever reconstruction is attempted, almost always ends up with a poor functional outcome. In skeletally immature patients who have resectable tumors the method of choice for reconstruction is extra-corporeal irradiation of the resected hemi-pelvis and then re-implantation.[52] This reconstructs the pelvis anatomically and usually allows preservation of the hip joint. In cases where the tumor is inoperable either because it is not possible to achieve a clear bony margin or because it infiltrates critical neurovascular structures, radiotherapy is the preferred method of local control. It is rare to have to perform a hind-quarter amputation for a Ewing sarcoma of the pelvis.

Radiotherapy

The indications for radiotherapy can be summarized as:

1. Inoperable tumors
2. Adjuvant to surgery, either pre-operatively or post-operatively

Timing of radiotherapy

Radiotherapy given as sole local therapy or as adjuvant before or after surgery is administered concurrently with chemotherapy. In current protocols it is therefore given after induction chemotherapy. Actinomycin (or doxorubicin) should be omitted during radiotherapy and, also, for the subsequent cycles as the risk of interaction can lead to significant mucosal and skin ulceration.[53] Chemotherapy dose intensity is best maintained, therefore, by starting radiotherapy with a cycle of chemotherapy.

Target definition

The principle of treatment is to treat tissues originally involved by tumor at initial diagnosis prior to chemotherapy. A shrinking volume technique may be used in some situations following surgery, with a phase I to include the tumor and involved tissues, scars, and prosthesis; and a smaller phase II to include the tumor and involved tissues only. The GTV is delineated with reference to the tumor at its maximal extent on imaging seen at diagnosis (using the MRI, CT, and PET scans). For patients who have had surgery, a GTV is reconstructed based on the tumor at its maximal extent as above. For pre-operative radiotherapy, the CTV is created by adding a margin of 1.5–2 cm to the GTV and fascial boundaries. For post-operative radiotherapy, a larger lower dose volume is created—CTV1—by adding 1.5–2 cm to the GTV. CTV2, a smaller high-dose area, is created by adding 1–2 cm to the GTV. A PTV is created by adding 0.5–1 cm to the CTV but this depends on the local institutional guidelines.

For pre-operative radiotherapy the dose is delivered in 45–50.4 Gy in 1.8 Gy per fraction. For post-operative radiotherapy a total dose of 50.4 Gy is delivered in 28 fractions with 45 Gy delivered to the larger volume and 9 Gy to the smaller volume. For definitive radiotherapy, the total dose delivered is 54 Gy in 30 fractions.

A boost of 5.4 Gy in 3 fractions can be given for large tumors (>8 cm) and those who have had <50% reduction on induction chemotherapy.

Special sites

Whole lung and hemi-thorax radiotherapy

Consolidation whole-lung radiotherapy is part of some protocols following response to chemotherapy for patients who present with pulmonary metastases. It is delivered at the end of systemic treatment and is contraindicated with high-dose chemotherapy containing busulphan. Hemi-thorax irradiation has been advocated for chest wall tumors with pleural effusion, pleural infiltration, and intraoperative contamination and may improve event-free survival.[54] For patients under 14 years of age a radiation dose of 15 Gy in 10 fractions is used and for those older than 14 years,18 Gy in 12 fractions.

Sites of metastatic disease

There is some evidence that consolidation radiotherapy to a limited number of sites of bone metastases may be associated with improved outcomes. The dose used is 40 Gy, but this strategy requires the use of whole-body MRI to select truly minimally metastatic disease.[55]

Results and prognosis

Approximately 60% of all patients with Ewing sarcoma will be cured of their disease. However, this overall figure is a simplification, since patients with small tumors have a better prognosis than those with very large lesions. The outlook for Ewing sarcoma of the small bones of the hands, feet, and jaw is already excellent. On the other hand, the prognosis in the pelvis, treated with combination chemotherapy and radiation, has remained unsatisfactory. At this site, with these very large tumors, local control with surgery or radiation is difficult to achieve.

Chondrosarcoma

Chondrosarcomas are malignant tumors of cartilage. The tumor is rare before the third decade and more common in the fourth and fifth decades. It has a predilection for the girdles and proximal long bones but may arise at any site. The tumors are usually slow-growing and, particularly in the pelvis, may reach a great size before detection. The principal presentation is with a painful lump. Grade I tumors are considered low-grade, are often incidental findings, and have low metastatic potential. Grades II and III are considered high-grade and can metastasize to the lungs and other bones. The prognosis of chondrosarcoma depends on its grade and site.[56]

Investigation

Low-grade chondral lesions have classic MRI appearances and do not need a biopsy to confirm the diagnosis.[57] If the patient is asymptomatic, they can simply be kept under surveillance. Surgery in the form of curettage is rarely indicated. High-grade lesions on the other hand, require intervention. The tissue diagnosis is confirmed with a core needle biopsy and the patient is then staged with CT scan of the chest and a whole-body bone scan.

Surgical management

The mainstay of treatment for high-grade chondrosarcomas is surgery. The resection margin depends entirely on the size and site of the lesion and the adequacy of pre-operative planning.

Although meticulous planning of approach and planes of dissection minimizes the risk of local contamination, in reality, the excision margins are frequently marginal in at least one area where the tumor is adjacent to critical neurovascular structures. This is particularly so for large pelvic tumors. Curettage of such lesions is never curative and prevents secondary surgery from ever being successful. In the elderly and debilitated, intra-lesional surgery may be contemplated for palliation where the physical cost of curative surgery is too great. In the young, however, where cure is essential, ablative surgery with reasonable margins must be undertaken to prevent a distressing prolonged illness consisting of progressive locally recurrent disease.

Radiotherapy and chemotherapy

The role of radiotherapy in this disease as an adjunct to surgery to achieve local control is evolving and in some sites such as the skull base is often used routinely, with proton beam therapy preferred. In other complex sites such as the spine or when disease is recurrent, specialist multidisciplinary discussion is essential to define whether radiotherapy may be recommended in individual cases.

Chemotherapy has traditionally only had a very limited role with responses reported occasionally in patients with recurrent high-grade disease. The identification of targetable molecular abnormalities in IDH1 and IDH2 has renewed interest in systemic disease for chondrosarcoma but this remains experimental.[58]

Other primary bone tumors

Several other histological subtypes of primary bone sarcoma occur infrequently. For clinical purposes these are often grouped as spindle cell sarcomas of bone and when high-grade, are treated as for osteosarcoma. Distinct histological subtypes include leiomyosarcoma, angiosarcoma, and fibrosarcoma.

Chordomas are rare but important tumors arising from notochordal remnants occurring at the base of skull and sacrum. Often characterized by a long clinical course, they present with pain and swelling. Due to the anatomical site and frequent presence of locally advanced disease, radical surgery is not always possible and frequently very disabling due to sacral resection. These radio-resistant tumors are showing improved control rates with higher doses of radiation and the use of proton beam therapy. The best results are seen at the base of skull and cervical spine where tumor presents with low volume. A small series using IMRT techniques to deliver dose of 65 Gy to these tumors reports local control at 5 years of over 80%. A gross tumor volume (GTV) of not more than 30 cm^3 is associated with a greater control rate than with larger tumors.[59] A series of 40 patients treated with protons to a mean dose of 72.5 RBE reports local control of 62% overall. In this group those without metal stabilization achieved 100% local control whereas in those with metal this fell to 30%. This is attributed to the adverse effect of the metal on the proton dose rather than different tumor characteristics.[60] Carbon ion therapy is reported to produce high local control rates even in the larger tumors of the sacrum and spine and without surgery, but toxicity data are limited. The largest series come from Japan where in unresectable sacral chordoma local control rates of 85% are reported with dose of 70.4 GyE delivered in 16 fractions. Fifteen percent of patients had severe sacral nerve symptoms.[61] International consensus is emerging on the best management approaches for these difficult tumors.[62,63]

Primary non-Hodgkin lymphoma of bone accounts for about 4% of primary bone tumors. The single most common type is diffuse large B-cell lymphoma with presenting symptoms similar to that of other primary bone tumors. No randomized trial has addressed optimal treatment for primary bone lymphoma, but recent series using chemotherapy and radiotherapy report 5-year survival rates of approximately 75%.[64]

Key learning points

- Primary tumors of bone are uncommon but share similar clinical features of pain and swelling. These are often misdiagnosed or ignored for a considerable time.
- Initial evaluation should be conducted in specialist centers. Appropriate imaging should be carried out before planned biopsy.
- Diagnosis can usually be made by core needle biopsy. Placement of the biopsy track should be determined after consideration of future surgery.
- Histological interpretation requires special expertise and should take account of clinical and radiological features.
- Many primary bone tumors, particularly osteosarcoma and Ewing sarcoma, may be cured by appropriate multi-modality therapy. Such treatment is intensive and complex. It requires close communication between surgical and non-surgical oncology teams and patients should be managed by experts.
- Further advances in treatment are emerging through a growing understanding of the unusual biological features of these diseases.

References

1. Whelan JS, Davis LE. Osteosarcoma, chondrosarcoma, and chordoma. *J Clin Oncol.* 2018; 36(2):188–93.
2. Biermann JS, Chow W, Reed DR et al. NCCN guidelines insights: Bone cancer, version 2.2017. *J Natl Compr Cancer Network.* 2017; 15(2):155–67.
3. Casali PG, Bielack S, Abecassis N et al. Bone sarcomas: ESMO-PaedCan-EURACAN Clinical Practice Guidelines for diagnosis, treatment and follow-up. *Ann Oncol.* 2018; 29(Suppl 4):iv79–95.
4. Fletcher CDM, Bridge JA, Hogendoorn PCW, Mertens F (Eds.). *WHO Classification of Tumours of Soft Tissue and Bone* (4th ed.). Geneva, Switzerland: WHO, 2013.
5. Mankin HJ, Mankin CJ, Simon MA. The hazards of the biopsy, revisited. Members of the Musculoskeletal Tumor Society. *J Bone Joint Surg Am.* 1996; 78(5):656–63.
6. Hau A, Kim I, Kattapuram S et al. Accuracy of CT-guided biopsies in 359 patients with musculoskeletal lesions. *Skeletal Radiol.* 2002; 31(6):349–53.
7. Enneking WF, Spanier SS, Goodman MA. A system for the surgical staging of musculoskeletal sarcoma. *Clin Orthop Relat Res.* 1980(153):106–20.
8. Wong KC, Kumta SM. Computer-assisted tumor surgery in malignant bone tumors. *Clin Orthop Relat Res.* 2013; 471(3):750–61.
9. Picardo NE, Blunn GW, Shekkeris AS et al. The medium-term results of the Stanmore non-invasive extendible endoprosthesis in the treatment of paediatric bone tumours. *J Bone Joint Surg Br.* 2012; 94(3):425–30.
10. Abraham JA, Kenneally B, Amer K, Geller DS. Can navigation-assisted surgery help achieve negative margins in resection of pelvic and sacral tumors? *Clin Orthop Relat Res.* 2018; 476(3):499–508.
11. Casey L, Meyers PA, Alektiar KM et al. Ewing sarcoma in adults treated with modern radiotherapy techniques. *Radiother Oncol.* 2014; 113(2):248–53.
12. DuBois SG, Krailo MD, Gebhardt MC et al. Comparative evaluation of local control strategies in localized Ewing sarcoma of bone: a report from the Children's Oncology Group. *Cancer.* 2015; 121(3):467–75.

13. Frisch S, Timmermann B. The evolving role of proton beam therapy for sarcomas. *Clin Oncol.* 2017; 29(8):500–6.

14. Kamada T, Tsujii H, Blakely EA et al. Carbon ion radiotherapy in Japan: An assessment of 20 years of clinical experience. *Lancet Oncol.* 2015; 16(2):e93–100.

15. Paulino AC. Late effects of radiotherapy for pediatric extremity sarcomas. *Int J Radiat Oncol Biol Phys.* 2004; 60(1):265–74.

16. Folkert MR, Singer S, Brennan MF et al. Comparison of local recurrence with conventional and intensity-modulated radiation therapy for primary soft-tissue sarcomas of the extremity. *J Clin Oncol.* 2014; 32(29):3236–41.

17. Ng J, Shuryak I. Minimizing second cancer risk following radiotherapy: Current perspectives. *Cancer Manage Res.* 2015; 7:1–11.

18. Saifuddin A, Sharif B, Gerrand C, Whelan J. The current status of MRI in the pre-operative assessment of intramedullary conventional appendicular osteosarcoma. *Skeletal Radiol.* 2019; 48(4):503–16.

19. Rosen G, Caparros B, Huvos AG et al. Preoperative chemotherapy for osteogenic sarcoma: selection of postoperative adjuvant chemotherapy based on the response of the primary tumor to preoperative chemotherapy. *Cancer.* 1982; 49(6):1221–30.

20. Link MP, Goorin AM, Miser AW et al. The effect of adjuvant chemotherapy on relapse-free survival in patients with osteosarcoma of the extremity. *N Engl J Med.* 1986; 314(25):1600–6.

21. Eilber F, Giuliano A, Eckardt J et al. Adjuvant chemotherapy for osteosarcoma: a randomized prospective trial. *J Clin Oncol.* 1987; 5(1):21–6.

22. Bramwell VH, Burgers M, Sneath R et al. A comparison of two short intensive adjuvant chemotherapy regimens in operable osteosarcoma of limbs in children and young adults: The first study of the European Osteosarcoma Intergroup. *J Clin Oncol.* 1992; 10(10):1579–91.

23. Lewis IJ, Nooij MA, Whelan J et al. Improvement in histologic response but not survival in osteosarcoma patients treated with intensified chemotherapy: A randomized phase III trial of the European Osteosarcoma Intergroup. *J Natl Cancer Inst.* 2007; 99(2):112–28.

24. Souhami RL, Craft AW, Van der Eijken JW et al. Randomised trial of two regimens of chemotherapy in operable osteosarcoma: a study of the European Osteosarcoma Intergroup. *Lancet.* 1997; 350(9082):911–7.

25. Goorin AM, Schwartzentruber DJ, Devidas M et al. Presurgical chemotherapy compared with immediate surgery and adjuvant chemotherapy for nonmetastatic osteosarcoma: Pediatric Oncology Group Study POG-8651. *J Clin Oncol.* 2003; 21(8):1574–80.

26. Meyers PA, Schwartz CL, Krailo M et al. Osteosarcoma: A randomized, prospective trial of the addition of ifosfamide and/or muramyl tripeptide to cisplatin, doxorubicin, and high-dose methotrexate. *J Clin Oncol.* 2005; 23(9):2004–11.

27. Meyers PA, Schwartz CL, Krailo MD et al. Osteosarcoma: the addition of muramyl tripeptide to chemotherapy improves overall survival—a report from the Children's Oncology Group. *J Clin Oncol.* 2008; 26(4):633–8.

28. Marina N, Bielack S, Whelan J et al. International collaboration is feasible in trials for rare conditions: the EURAMOS experience. *Cancer Treat Res.* 2009; 152:339–53.

29. Bielack SS, Smeland S, Whelan JS et al. Methotrexate, doxorubicin, and cisplatin (MAP) plus maintenance pegylated interferon Alfa-2b versus MAP alone in patients with resectable high-MAP: First results of the EURAMOS-1 good response randomized controlled trial. *J Clin Oncol.* 2015; 33(20):2279–87.

30. Marina NM, Smeland S, Bielack SS et al. Comparison of MAPIE versus MAP in patients with a poor response to preoperative chemotherapy for newly diagnosed high-grade osteosarcoma (EURAMOS-1): An open-label, international, randomised controlled trial. *Lancet Oncol.* 2016; 17(10):1396–408.

31. Whelan JS, Bielack SS, Marina N et al. EURAMOS-1, an international randomised study for osteosarcoma: results from pre-randomisation treatment. *Ann Oncol.* 2015; 26(2):407–14.

32. Behjati S, Tarpey PS, Haase K et al. Recurrent mutation of IGF signalling genes and distinct patterns of genomic rearrangement in osteosarcoma. *Nat Commun.* 2017; 8:15936.

33. Engert F, Kovac M, Baumhoer D, Nathrath M, Fulda S. Osteosarcoma cells with genetic signatures of BRCAness are susceptible to the PARP inhibitor talazoparib alone or in combination with chemotherapeutics. *Oncotarget.* 2017; 8(30):48794–806.

34. Ciernik IF, Niemierko A, Harmon DC et al. Proton-based radiotherapy for unresectable or incompletely resected osteosarcoma. *Cancer.* 2011; 117(19):4522–30.

35. DeLaney TF, Liebsch NJ, Pedlow FX et al. Phase II study of high-dose photon/proton radiotherapy in the management of spine sarcomas. *Int J Radiat Oncol Biol Phys.* 2009; 74(3):732–9.

36. DeLaney TF, Park L, Goldberg SI et al. Radiotherapy for local control of osteosarcoma. *Int J Radiat Oncol Biol Phys.* 2005; 61(2):492–8.

37. Ward WG, Mikaelian K, Dorey F et al. Pulmonary metastases of stage IIB extremity osteosarcoma and subsequent pulmonary metastases. *J Clin Oncol.* 1994; 12(9):1849–58.

38. Treasure T, Macbeth F. Doubt about effectiveness of lung metastasectomy for sarcoma. *J Thorac Cardiovasc Surg.* 2015; 149(1):93–4.

39. Gaspar N, Hawkins DS, Dirksen U et al. Ewing sarcoma: Current management and future approaches through collaboration. *J Clin Oncol.* 2015; 33(27):3036–46.

40. Machado I, Navarro S, Llombart-Bosch A. Ewing sarcoma and the new emerging Ewing-like sarcomas: (CIC and BCOR-rearranged-sarcomas). A systematic review. *Histol Histopathol.* 2016; 31(11):1169–81.

41. Kalus S, Saifuddin A. Whole-body MRI vs. bone scintigraphy in the staging of Ewing sarcoma of bone: A 12-year single-institution review. *Eur Radiol.* 2019; 29(10):5700–8.

42. Newman EN, Jones RL, Hawkins DS. An evaluation of [F-18]-fluorodeoxy-D-glucose positron emission tomography, bone scan, and bone marrow aspiration/biopsy as staging investigations in Ewing sarcoma. *Pediatr Blood Cancer.* 2013; 60(7):1113–7.

43. Foulon S, Brennan B, Gaspar N et al. Can postoperative radiotherapy be omitted in localised standard-risk Ewing sarcoma? An observational study of the Euro-E.W.I.N.G group. *Eur J Cancer.* 2016; 61:128–36.

44. Nesbit ME, Jr., Gehan EA, Burgert EO, Jr. et al. Multimodal therapy for the management of primary, nonmetastatic Ewing's sarcoma of bone: a long-term follow-up of the First Intergroup study. *J Clin Oncol.* 1990; 8(10):1664–74.

45. Grier HE, Krailo MD, Tarbell NJ et al. Addition of ifosfamide and etoposide to standard chemotherapy for Ewing's sarcoma and primitive neuroectodermal tumor of bone. *N Engl J Med.* 2003; 348(8):694–701.

46. Paulussen M, Craft AW, Lewis I et al. Results of the EICESS-92 Study: two randomized trials of Ewing's sarcoma treatment—cyclophosphamide compared with ifosfamide in standard-risk patients and assessment of benefit of etoposide added to standard treatment in high-risk patients. *J Clin Oncol.* 2008; 26(27):4385–93.

47. Dirksen U, Brennan B, Le Deley MC et al. High-dose chemotherapy compared with standard chemotherapy and lung radiation in Ewing sarcoma with pulmonary metastases: Results of the European Ewing tumour working initiative of National Groups, 99 Trial and EWING 2008. *J Clin Oncol.* 2019; 37(34):3192–202.

48. Le Deley MC, Paulussen M, Lewis I et al. Cyclophosphamide compared with ifosfamide in consolidation treatment of standard-risk Ewing sarcoma: results of the randomized noninferiority Euro-EWING99-R1 trial. *J Clin Oncol.* 2014; 32(23):2440–8.

49. Whelan J, Le Deley MC, Dirksen U et al. High-dose chemotherapy and blood autologous stem-cell rescue compared with standard chemotherapy in localized high-risk ewing sarcoma: Results of Euro-E.W.I.N.G.99 and Ewing-2008. *J Clin Oncol.* 2018:JCO2018782516.

50. Womer RB, West DC, Krailo MD et al. Randomized controlled trial of interval-compressed chemotherapy for the treatment of localized Ewing sarcoma: a report from the Children's Oncology Group. *J Clin Oncol.* 2012; 30(33):4148–54.

51. Euro Ewing 2012. Available from: http://www.isrctn.com/ISRCTN92192408

52. Krieg AH, Mani M, Speth BM, Stalley PD. Extracorporeal irradiation for pelvic reconstruction in Ewing's sarcoma. *J Bone Joint Surg Br*. 2009; 91(3):395–400.

53. Burris HA, 3rd, Hurtig J. Radiation recall with anticancer agents. *Oncologist*. 2010; 15(11):1227–37.

54. Schuck A, Ahrens S, Konarzewska A et al. Hemithorax irradiation for Ewing tumors of the chest wall. *Int J Radiat Oncol Biol Phys*. 2002; 54(3):830–8.

55. Burdach S, Thiel U, Schoniger M et al. Total body MRI-governed involved compartment irradiation combined with high-dose chemotherapy and stem cell rescue improves long-term survival in Ewing tumor patients with multiple primary bone metastases. *Bone Marrow Transplant*. 2010; 45(3):483–9.

56. Lee FY, Mankin HJ, Fondren G et al. Chondrosarcoma of bone: An assessment of outcome. *J Bone Joint Surg Am*. 1999; 81(3):326–38.

57. Douis H, Singh L, Saifuddin A. MRI differentiation of low-grade from high-grade appendicular chondrosarcoma. *Eur Radiol*. 2014; 24(1):232–40.

58. Amary MF, Bacsi K, Maggiani F et al. IDH1 and IDH2 mutations are frequent events in central chondrosarcoma and central and periosteal chondromas but not in other mesenchymal tumours. *J Pathol*. 2011; 224(3):334–43.

59. Potluri S, Jefferies SJ, Jena R et al. Residual postoperative tumour volume predicts outcome after high-dose radiotherapy for chordoma and chondrosarcoma of the skull base and spine. *Clin Oncol*. 2011; 23(3):199–208.

60. Staab A, Rutz HP, Ares C et al. Spot-scanning-based proton therapy for extracranial chordoma. *Int J Radiat Oncol Biol Phys*. 2011; 81(4):e489–96.

61. Imai R, Kamada T, Sugahara S et al. Carbon ion radiotherapy for sacral chordoma. *Br J Radiol*. 2011; 84 Spec No 1:S48–54.

62. Stacchiotti S, Gronchi A, Fossati P et al. Best practices for the management of local-regional recurrent chordoma: a position paper by the Chordoma Global Consensus Group. *Ann Oncol*. 2017; 28(6):1230–42.

63. Stacchiotti S, Sommer J, Chordoma Global Consensus G. Building a global consensus approach to chordoma: a position paper from the medical and patient community. *Lancet Oncol*. 2015; 16(2):e71–83.

64. Bruno Ventre M, Ferreri AJ, Gospodarowicz M et al. Clinical features, management, and prognosis of an international series of 161 patients with limited-stage diffuse large B-cell lymphoma of the bone (the IELSG-14 study). *Oncologist*. 2014; 19(3):291–8.

27 SOFT TISSUE SARCOMAS

Thomas F. DeLaney, David C. Harmon, Karol Sikora, and Francis J. Hornicek

Introduction

Sarcomas are malignant tumors that arise from skeletal and extra-skeletal connective tissues, including the peripheral nervous system including undifferentiated pleomorphic sarcoma (UPS; formerly called malignant fibrous histiocytoma, MFH), liposarcoma, leiomyosarcoma, synovial sarcoma, rhabdomyosarcoma, epithelioid sarcoma, angiosarcoma, fibrosarcoma, etc. In addition, malignant tumors of peripheral nerve sheaths are included despite being ectodermal in origin, as their clinical behavior is similar to that of other sarcomas. Gastrointestinal stromal tumors (GISTs) recapitulate the interstitial cells of Cajal which have neural and smooth muscle features, and thus malignant GISTs are also considered a type of soft tissue sarcoma (STS). The relative frequency of different histological subtypes of sarcomas is shown in Table 27.1.

STSs are rare with an estimated annual incidence of approximately 13,130 in the United States, representing less than 1% of all newly diagnosed malignant tumors.[1] Approximately 38% of affected patients are expected to die of their disease. In the UK there are 3,272 new patients a year of which around 45% will die of their disease.

Although the malignant tumors of soft tissue are rare, benign tumors are very common. It is estimated that the frequency of benign tumors is at least 100 times that for the malignant lesions.[2] The anatomic locations of STS in order of frequency (Table 27.2) are: Lower extremity (46%), torso (19%), upper extremity (14%), retroperitoneum (13%), head/neck (8%).[3] The small number of cases seen and the great diversity in anatomical site, histopathology, and biology complicate the understanding of these tumors and their response to diverse therapies.

A large proportion of the sarcoma patients are referred to major centers with subspecialist teams because of the following factors:

- Their relative rarity
- Appearance at all body sites
- Occurrence in all age groups
- Broad spectrum of histological types with varied biologic characteristics

When treating STSs, the major therapeutic goals are survival, local tumor control, optimal function, and minimal morbidity. Surgical resection of the primary tumor is an essential component of treatment for virtually all patients with the exception of a small percentage of selected patients with radiosensitive histologies such as extra-osseous Ewing's sarcoma or presentations in anatomical locations where resection would have unacceptable functional or cosmetic consequences. However, local control by surgery alone can be poor in selected anatomical locations if the surgical intent is also to preserve function and good cosmesis. Removal of the gross lesion by a simple excision alone with only a narrow margin is followed by local recurrence (LR) in 60%–90% of patients. Radical resections are associated with reduction in the LR rate to 10%–30% but may compromise limb function. Local control is also poor for retroperitoneal sarcomas when managed with surgery alone, where LR rates are reported to be as high as 70%, because of the difficulty in obtaining widely negative margins. Thus, the combination of surgery and radiation achieves better outcomes than either treatment alone for most patients with STSs. Chemotherapy appears to be important for selected patients with large, high-grade sarcomas and specific histologies such as extra-osseous Ewing's sarcoma, rhabdomyosarcoma, and GISTs.

The excellent results currently being obtained by more conservative treatment strategies are through a multidisciplinary approach to the overall management of these patients (diagnostic evaluation, biopsy, treatment, rehabilitation, and follow-up). The multidisciplinary team includes not only the surgeon but also the radiation, medical and pediatric oncologists, pathologists, and diagnostic radiologists. The pathologist is an extremely valuable member of the team because the staging system now employed (for other than childhood rhabdomyosarcoma) utilizes histopathological grade as the principal determinant of stage. The pathological diagnosis is now based on much more objective criteria with the introduction of immunohistochemistry and, increasingly, molecular analyses.

Meta-analyses of the phase III trials suggest an improvement in disease-free survival (DFS) and a small but not statistically significant survival gain with the use of adjuvant chemotherapy in resectable, high-grade STS in adults.[4] There are several important developments being evaluated in the laboratory and the clinic, which offer the potential of further gains.

Etiology

Genetic

Involvement of genetic factors in the genesis of STS is manifest by the strong hereditary tendency for certain sarcomas.[5] Gardner's syndrome is a hereditary disease, one feature of which is a predilection for desmoid tumors (also termed fibromatosis). Neurofibromatosis I also features tumors of the soft tissues: neurofibromas and malignant peripheral nerve sheath tumors (MPNST). A significant proportion of these patients ultimately exhibit transformation of a neurofibroma into MPNST. This disorder is associated with a mutation in the *NF1* gene. It has been proposed that malignant degeneration reflects the two-hit hypothesis in which one allele is constitutionally inactivated in the germ-line whereas the other allele undergoes somatic inactivation (the second hit). Sarcomas of soft tissue and bone, particularly osteosarcoma, have been observed later in life in surviving patients with familial or bilateral retinoblastoma. In one study of 1,604 patients with retinoblastoma, the cumulative incidence of a second cancer at 50 years after diagnosis was 51% for hereditary retinoblastoma (which is associated with mutations in the retinoblastoma tumor suppressor gene, see later), and 5% for non-hereditary (sporadic) retinoblastoma. More than 60% of the cancers were a form of sarcoma. MPNST may complicate the multiple endocrine neoplasia syndrome.

TABLE 27.1   **Frequency of Histopathological Types of STS in Large Series of Patients with Extremity and Trunk STSs**

	MGH 1994[6]	Milan 2005[7]	Lund 2004[8]	MSKCC 1996[9]
Number of patients	738	911	298	1041
UPS (%)	22	8	13	25
Liposarcoma (%)	16	31	14	29
Fibrosarcoma (%)	11	NR	13	10
Leiomyosarcoma (%)	10	14	33	8
Sarcoma, NOS (%)	9	NR	9	NR
Synovial sarcoma (%)	8	15	6	12
MPNST (%)	10	10	7	5
Rhabdomyosarcoma (%)	3	NR	NR	NR
Vascular sarcomas (%)	NR	5	1	NR
Other (%)	11	16	4	12

Abbreviations: UPS, undifferentiated pleomorphic sarcoma (formerly called MFH, malignant fibrous histiocytoma); MPNST, malignant peripheral nerve sheath tumor; NR, not reported; MGH, Massachusetts General Hospital; MSKCC, Memorial Sloan-Kettering Cancer Center.

TABLE 27.2   **Distribution (%) of Sarcoma of Soft Tissue According to Anatomical Site in Three US Surveys**

	MGH[a,10] (*n* = 788)	Russell[11] (*n* = 1215)	Lawrence[12] (*n* = 4550)
Lower extremity	44	40	46
Upper extremity	21	13	13
Head and neck	12	15	8
Torso	10	18	18
Retroperitoneum	6	13	12
Other	7	1	1

Abbreviations: MGH, Massachusetts General Hospital.
[a]   All patients seen during 1971–1993 and treated by radiation and surgery for stage M0 disease.

Patients with Li–Fraumeni syndrome often develop sarcomas. The Li–Fraumeni syndrome is inherited as an autosomal recessive trait and is primarily characterized by soft tissue and bone sarcomas and breast cancer; other features include brain tumor, leukemia, and adrenocortical cancer occurring before the age of 45. Some patients develop multiple malignancies. A germ-line mutation in the *p53* tumor suppressor gene is found in most affected families (see *p53* gene later). In addition, germ-line mutations in *hCHK2*, a protein kinase that regulates *p53* in response to deoxyribonucleic acid (DNA) damage, has also been found in a subset of families with Li–Fraumeni syndrome.[13] In one series of 151 children with STS, 5 of the families (3.3%) manifested the classic Li–Fraumeni familial cancer syndrome, another 10 (6.6%) had features consistent with the syndrome, and 16 (10.5%) had 1 parent with a possible hereditary cancer syndrome or with cancer before the age of 60. In an analysis of 754 first-degree relatives of 177 children with sarcomas of soft tissue, Birch et al. found an increased incidence of malignant tumors in relatives of patients who were male, <2 years of age, and with an embryonal rhabdomyosarcoma.

Cytogenetics

The genetics of sarcomas segregate into two major types. One type has specific genetic alterations and usually simple karyotypes, including fusion genes due to reciprocal translocations (e.g. *PAX3–FKHR* in alveolar rhabdomyosarcomas) or specific point mutations (e.g. *KIT* mutations in GISTs). A second type has non-specific genetic alterations and complex, unbalanced karyotypes, reflected by numerous genetic losses and gains (e.g. osteosarcoma, UPS [pleomorphic fibroblastic sarcoma], pleomorphic liposarcomas, angiosarcoma, leiomyosarcoma).[14]

Sarcomas with recurrent chromosome translocations account for approximately one-third of all STSs. These non-random chromosomal aberrations occur in specific types of sarcomas and are being increasingly utilized in the definitive diagnosis of these sarcomas. Furthermore, these chromosomal abnormalities have been characterized at the molecular level and many of the chimeric genes have been identified, providing clues to the molecular alterations that are fundamental for the development of STSs.

Most synovial cell sarcomas are characterized by the translocation t(x;18)(p11.2;q11.2). The breakpoint of this translocation fuses the *SYT* gene (also known as the *SS18* gene) from chromosome 18 to one of two homologous genes, *SSX1* or *SSX2*, on the X chromosome. The *SYT–SSX* gene has recently been shown to increase the transcription of genes, such as Sox2 that is necessary for synovial cell sarcoma proliferation. The nature of the chimeric gene may have prognostic and pathogenetic importance. In some studies, metastasis-free survival was higher with *SYT–SSX2* compared to *SYT–SSX1*. *SYT–SSX1* is associated with biphasic tumors (glandular epithelial differentiation on a background of spindle tumor cells), whereas *SYT–SSX2* is associated with monophasic tumors that lack glandular epithelial differentiation, although other studies have questioned these findings.

Other chromosomal changes characteristic of specific sarcoma type include the reciprocal exchange t(11:22)(q24;q12) seen in approximately 85%–90% of Ewing's sarcoma and primitive peripheral neuro-ectodermal tumor (PNET). In this translocation, the *EWS* (Ewing sarcoma breakpoint region 1) gene from chromosome 22q12 is covalently linked to the erythroblast transformation-specific (ETS) family member, *FLI-1*, to form the *EWS–FLI-1* fusion gene.[15] The chimeric proteins that result from this translocation may alter transcription of a number of genes including upregulation of the transcription factor Gli1 that promotes the oncogenic potential of the Hedgehog pathway. A less common translocation t(21;22)(q22;q12) has also been identified and links *EWS* to a different ETS family member, ETS-related gene (*ERG*). Myxoid and round cell subtypes of liposarcomas display a reciprocal translocation t(12;16) (q13;p11). In this translocation, the *CHOP* (induced by DNA damage) gene is inserted adjacent to a novel gene called *TLS*. The fusion gene, called *TLS–CHOP*, shows sequence homology to the Ewing's fusion gene. It fails to induce G_1/S arrest, which is one of the functions of the non-oncogenic form of *CHOP* (GADD153). Identification of the fusion gene has been used as a diagnostic aid for these subtypes of liposarcoma.

Alveolar rhabdomyosarcomas show a translocation at t(2;13) (q35;q14) or less often t(1;13)(p36;q14); the chimeric genes have been cloned and have been termed *PAX3–FKHR* and *PAX7–FKHR*, respectively. These translocations are associated with over-expression of the fusion product. *PAX7–FKHR* tumors more often present with extremity lesions, are more likely to be localized, and are less likely to metastasize widely than *PAX3–FKHR* tumors. A downstream target of *PAX3–FKHR* may be *MET*, which encodes a receptor involved in growth and motility signaling. Molecular determination of minimal residual disease in alveolar rhabdomyosarcoma is possible, and patients with positive peripheral blood after treatment show poorer survival than patients without micro-circulating disease.

Clear cell sarcoma has similarities to malignant melanoma, although cytogenetically the tumors are distinct. Clear cell sarcomas often exhibit a translocation at t(12;22)(q13–14;q12), which is not seen in malignant melanoma. Trisomy of chromosome 8 is also observed in clear cell sarcoma. Alveolar soft part sarcoma is another tumor that also exhibits a specific chromosomal translocation t(X;17) (p11;q25), which creates the fusion product *TFE–ASPL*.

In contrast to the sarcomas that have recurrent, non-random chromosome translocations and relatively simple karyotypes, the molecular pathogenesis of sarcomas with non-specific genetic alterations and complex karyotypes has yet to be elucidated. However, inactivation of the p53 pathway appears to be a common feature in these tumors, and it has been proposed that p53 pathway inactivation may differentiate these tumors from those with simple genetic alterations. Among the mechanisms for p53 pathway inactivation are *p53* point mutation and deletion, homozygous deletion in *CDKN2A*, and *MDM2* amplification. It should be noted, however, that inactivation of the p53 pathway has been identified in a subset of tumors with specific chromosomal translocations. For example, up to 25% of Ewing's sarcomas show *p53* mutation or loss of *CDKN2A*. Importantly, patients with Ewing's sarcomas with inactivation of the p53 pathway showed significantly worse survival.

Molecular biology

Somatic mutations in the *p53* gene are the most frequently detected molecular alteration in sporadic STS. These mutations have been detected in a variety of STSs including UPS, leiomyosarcoma, liposarcoma, and rhabdomyosarcoma.[16] Germ-line mutations of *p53* are also found in most families with the Li–Fraumeni syndrome. Germ-line mutations in this gene also may occur in other patients with STS, particularly those with other cancers that are not considered indicative of the Li–Fraumeni syndrome. Moreover, in families with Li–Fraumeni syndrome where no *p53* mutations can be identified, heterozygous mutations in *hCHK2*, which encodes a protein kinase that phosphorylates p53, may be identified.

The p53 protein is a transcriptional activator that plays a key role in the integration of signals inducing cell division, arrest of DNA synthesis following DNA damage, and programmed cell death (apoptosis). DNA damage results in increased levels of p53 protein. p53 functions to increase the expression of a number of genes including: (1) *MDM2*, which inhibits p53 function; (2) p21, a cyclin-dependent kinase inhibitor that causes cell cycle arrest; and (3) genes that initiate apoptosis. Although p53-dependent induction of apoptosis and cell cycle arrest have been proposed as key mechanisms by which p53 can suppress tumorigenesis, mice in which p53 has been mutated to lose the ability to induce apoptosis and cell cycle arrest nevertheless retain the capacity to suppress tumorigenesis. The wild-type *p53* in normal tissue has a short half-life and is not detectable by immunohistochemical methods; in comparison, mutations of the gene result in a stabilized p53 protein that accumulates in the cell and often becomes detectable by immunohistochemistry. Gross rearrangements and non-sense mutations, however, may show no immunostaining for p53, indicating that this technique fails to identify a significant proportion of tumors with *p53* alterations. Animal models are compatible with *p53* defects having a pathogenetic role in sarcoma development. Mice deficient for *p53* also develop a variety of neoplasms including bone and STSs. Similarly, irradiated transgenic mice harboring mutant *p53* show higher frequencies of sarcomas. However, transduction of wild-type *p53* genes into STSs bearing mutated *p53* genes restores enhanced cell cycle control and

suppresses sarcoma growth. In addition, restoring p53 expression in primary sarcomas in mice lacking p53 causes tumor regression. *p53* may also be activated in response to the expression of an activated oncogene. Therefore, in some settings sarcoma formation may be blocked by *p53* activation and sarcoma development may only occur when cooperating mutations occur in *p53*, *CDKN2A* that expresses *p14Arf*, or by *MDM2* over-expression. Indeed, the *MDM2* gene, located at 12q134, is over-expressed in a variety of human tumors including STSs.

In addition to p53 pathway inactivation, mutation of the retinoblastoma gene *Rb* frequently occurs in STSs. In fact, the first demonstration of a specific gene abnormality associated with malignant transformation in man was the loss of the *Rb* gene, a tumor suppressor gene, in retinoblastoma. Even before the *Rb* gene had been identified, it was recognized that some sporadic sarcomas had deletions on chromosome 13 similar to those observed in some patients with retinoblastoma. Deletions or mutations of the tumor suppressor retinoblastoma (*Rb*) gene are critical in the pathogenesis of retinoblastoma and a variety of solid tumors. Alterations in the *Rb* gene are common in STS, occurring in up to 70% of tumors.[17] It has been proposed that *Rb* alterations are primary events in human sarcomas and may be involved in tumorigenesis or the early phases of tumor progression. The *Rb* gene is critical for proper entry and transition through the cell cycle because the protein encoded by *Rb* (pRb) controls the expression of other genes necessary for G_1–S cell cycle progression. Normally, this cell cycle progression occurs when cyclin-dependent kinase 4 (cdk4) phosphorylates and inhibits pRb function. As mentioned earlier, the p53-regulated cyclin-dependent kinase inhibitor, p21, can inhibit cdk4 and prevent cell cycle progression by preventing phosphorylation of pRb. However, when *Rb* is mutated, the normal cell cycle is perturbed. This change has been shown to be associated with infrequent osteogenic or other sarcomas as second malignant neoplasms in patients with hereditary retinoblastoma.

Environmental factors

Radiation is recognized as capable of inducing sarcoma of bone and soft tissue. The frequency increases with radiation dose and with the post-radiation observation period. The most frequent histopathological type of radiation-induced sarcoma arising in soft tissues is what is now termed UPS (formerly called MFH)—approximately 70%. Although seen rarely after low doses (<40 Gy), the development of a sarcoma is predominantly a complication of high-dose treatment. The actuarial frequency at 15–20 years is approximately 0.5% for radiation of normal bone and soft tissue in the adult treated with radiation alone to full dose.

Previous studies showed that children treated for STS have increased risk for developing second cancers, and although further analysis confirms that multiple malignancies could in some cases reflect a genetic syndrome, such as neurofibromatosis type 1 or the Li–Fraumeni syndrome, the chemotherapy and radiation patients receive also contribute to their risk. Among 1,499 children reported to the Surveillance, Epidemiology, and End Results (SEER) population-based cancer registries 28 subsequent primary malignancies developed, compared with 4.5 expected malignancies based on general population rates (observed-to-expected [O/E] ratio = 6.3; 95% confidence interval [95% CI], 4.2–9.1). Initial therapy with radiation and chemotherapeutic agents was associated with a higher risk of second malignancies compared with surgery alone (O/E ratio = 15.2 versus 1.4; $p < 0.0001$). Elevated risks were observed for acute myeloid leukemia, cutaneous melanoma, breast cancer, and sarcomas of bone and soft tissue, with generally higher risks among patients who received combined modality therapy. Excess cancers of the oral cavity were prominent among long-term survivors.

This is further supported by the analysis of 1,458 patients followed after treatment for retinoblastoma for 17 years. The cumulative mortality from second primary neoplasms at 40 years was 26% and 1.5% among patients with bilateral and unilateral disease, respectively.[18] Within the bilateral population, the figures were 30% and 6.4% for irradiated and non-irradiated patients. For sarcomas (including those which arose within and without the irradiated field), the observed/expected ratios were 61% and 22% for patients with bilateral disease. The comparable figures for patients with unilateral disease were 5% and 2%. There was a difference in the use of chemotherapy in patients treated for bilateral and unilateral retinoblastoma, 48% and 13%, respectively. Chemotherapeutic agents are likewise associated with risks of sarcoma induction. For example, there are two reports describing the appearance of osteosarcoma in children treated for leukemia by drugs without radiation therapy.

Exposure to a few selected industrial chemicals including vinyl chloride, phenoxyacetic acid, arsenic, and phenoxy herbicides may be followed by the appearance of sarcomas. There are, however, a number of inherent problems in occupational epidemiology with small numbers of patients in any given series and the difficulty in isolating a single agent. For these reasons, few associations can be considered established and causal. For example, there is a clear association between vinyl chloride and hepatic angiosarcomas, oxyacetic acid and arsenic. There are reports of an increased incidence of STSs in gardeners (phenoxy herbicides), railroad workers, construction workers exposed to impregnating agents or asbestos, and unspecified chemical workers. The association between exposure to phenoxy herbicides and STS has been corroborated. The last risk may be greater with exposure to phenoxy herbicides contaminated with 2,3,7,8-tetrachlorodibenzodioxin (TCDD) or higher chlorinated dioxins. A role for dioxin per se is controversial, and most recent data question the association. A population-based case control study, however, found no increased risk for STS among Vietnam veterans, including those exposed to Agent Orange, which contains dioxin. High-intensity chlorophenol exposure in jobs involving wood preservation or machinists who use cutting fluids may increase the risk of STS, independent of phenoxy herbicides.

Chronic edema and trauma may also be contributing factors to the malignant transformation. Sarcomas of soft tissue (primarily lymphangiosarcomas) may be observed following massive and quite protracted edema. Classically, this has been seen in the post-mastectomy, lymphedematous arm (Stewart–Treves syndrome). It has also been described following chronic lymphedema due to filarial infection. Chronic irritation secondary to foreign bodies may be a factor in the induction of sarcomas. In an occasional patient, there is a history of major trauma to the affected site many months before the appearance of local symptoms of tumor. Although the trauma may merely bring the patient's attention to the presence of the mass, recent studies with *p53* mutant mice demonstrate that muscle injury can promote sarcoma development. Therefore, it is possible that trauma promotes sarcoma development in some patients.

Clinical evaluation

Clinical history

The most frequent initial complaint is that of an enlarging painless lump of a few weeks to several months' duration.

Occasionally, pain or tenderness precedes the detection of a lump. With progressive growth of tumor, symptoms appear which are secondary to infiltration of or pressure on adjacent structures (e.g. tendons, muscles, nerves) or organs. Occasionally symptoms secondary to the metabolic effects of the tumor products are seen, for example, fever, anemia, lethargy, weight loss, histamine-like reactions. To accrue clinical genetic data in sarcoma patients, the history should include details of the cause of death and history of malignant disease in siblings, parents, grandparents, and progeny.

Anatomical site, sex, and age

Sites of appearance of STS in order of frequency are listed earlier in the introduction and are shown in Table 27.2. There is a very slight preponderance of STSs in males. They are more common in older people, with 40% in persons ≥55 years of age, but the median age is 50, which is younger than that of carcinomas. It is important to emphasize that they can occur in all age groups and 15% appear in patients ≤15 years of age. Rhabdomyosarcomas almost always arise in children, synovial sarcomas develop in late adolescence and young adulthood, and liposarcoma and UPS usually occur during mid- and late adulthood.

Imaging

For the primary site, the imaging should include plain films and MRI scanning. CT scan is also the procedure of choice for evaluating intra-abdominal and retroperitoneal sarcomas.

Imaging studies alone cannot definitively distinguish malignant from benign soft tissue lesions. MRI may prove of clinical value in planning the biopsy site, using either needle or incisional techniques. Furthermore, the demonstration of necrotic regions appears to be of diagnostic importance in discrimination between benign and malignant tumors.

PET-CT scanning has been shown to be useful in discriminating between benign and high-grade lesions although it is unsuitable for distinguishing between benign and low- to intermediate-grade lesions. PET-CT may be of substantial value in defining response to pre-operative therapy. MRI studies should always include T_2-weighted sequences as these provide the optimum contrast between lesion and muscle. Contrast-enhanced T_1-weighted images (especially with fat-suppression techniques) are also helpful. Depending upon the pattern of presentation and the nature of any planned surgery, an arteriogram may be of value. For rhabdomyosarcoma, epithelioid sarcoma, high-grade synovial, clear cell sarcoma, angiosarcoma, and unclassified sarcomas, PET-CT evaluation of the regional nodes should be considered. Bone scans need not be performed unless specifically indicated by distant sites of bone pain. We do not consider a positive bone scan near or adjacent to an STS to be proof of invasion of periosteum or bone. For a diagnosis of invasion of bone there must be clear radiographic evidence of destruction of cortical bone. The single most important examination for distant metastasis is whole-lung CT; this should be obtained in all patients with intermediate- or high-grade tumors.

Imaging of the response to treatment with CT and MRI has been generally disappointing up to the present. Changes in MRI signal characteristics have been unreliable. Absence of high signal intensity on T_2-weighted images has been shown to indicate freedom from tumor. However, residual high signal may be due to tumor, edema, or fibrosis. MRI spectroscopy has been used to detect high-energy phosphate metabolism in the lesions. This has helped in the distinction between malignant and benign tumors. Several studies with phosphorus-31 magnetic resonance spectroscopy have shown changes in high-energy phosphate metabolism after effective chemotherapy, but the range of variation in sarcoma is large, and because of limitations in spatial resolution the procedure cannot be reliably done unless a large soft tissue mass is present.

Biopsy

Core needle biopsy is the preferred initial biopsy technique. For palpable lesions with a superficial component that is away from the neurovascular bundle, a Tru-Cut needle biopsy can often be obtained in the clinic without image guidance. For non-palpable, deeper lesions, and those near the neurovascular bundle, core biopsies can be obtained under CT or ultrasound guidance. There is a body of literature that supports the use of core needle biopsy for definitive diagnosis of bone and STSs.[19]

Several comments are pertinent with regard to the use of the core biopsy technique. The needle path for biopsy should allow excision of the biopsy track at the time of definitive surgery to avoid potential needle track recurrence. Image guidance with ultrasound or CT can help direct and document placement of the biopsy needle. Sufficient material for cDNA arrays can be obtained by core biopsies. It is recommended that at least three cores of tumor be retrieved for pathologic analysis. Open biopsies can be reserved for patients in whom diagnostic material cannot be obtained by needle core biopsy.

There has also been recent discussion as to whether fine needle aspiration (FNA) cytology in lieu of core biopsy can suffice for the initial diagnostic procedure. Because of the range of histological types of STSs, FNA may be insufficient to adequately characterize and subclassify the histological type of tumor. It is, however, already accepted as an important and widely used diagnostic procedure for the evaluation and documentation of LRs, as well as metastases from previously diagnosed STSs and for diagnosing benign non-neoplastic lesions and metastatic carcinomas in soft tissue. Its role as the primary modality for the initial diagnosis of STSs is not as widely accepted by all clinicians and pathologists. The core biopsies give architectural information and also provide sufficient material for ancillary studies (immunocytochemistry, electron microscopy [EM], and cytogenetic and molecular genetic analyses) permitting high degrees of diagnostic accuracy. This may be a model that is worth evaluating at other centers.

The biopsy track should go through a muscle belly rather than along fascial planes (the former tends to keep the tumor "spill" within an anatomical compartment while the latter allows transgression of two or more compartments), and careful attention should be paid to achieve hemostasis in order to avoid ecchymosis or a hematoma. The wound should be closed in layers with a narrow skin closure; as a rule, drains should not be utilized (the tract of the drain is considered to be contaminated with tumor and may greatly extend the planes of subsequent surgery or the radiation treatment volume).

For the occasional small lesion in a readily accessible site (e.g. wrist or ankle), an excisional biopsy may be the approach of choice. The surgeon should adhere to the same principles as for the definitive surgery (see below) if complications are to be avoided. The biopsy specimen needs to be of sufficient volume to be certain that it is representative. A pathological assessment of a frozen section is useful in assuring that the tissue obtained is from the lesion and is adequate for the diagnostic evaluation. Cultures should always be obtained. Specimens are processed for hematoxylin and eosin staining and various immunohisto-chemical stains considered necessary to aid in the diagnosis. A

small portion of the tissue is set aside for EM, cytogenetics, and, increasingly, for gene arrays.

Pathology

The pathologist needs to be aware of the clinical and radiographic findings and the diagnostic considerations of each case. In this way the pathologist will be best prepared to choose the appropriate methodology needed to make a complete and accurate assessment of tissue specimens.

The biopsy

Ideally, the tissue should be in the fresh state when received by the pathologist so that a portion can be used to perform a frozen section. Frozen section analysis can determine if there is adequate material for diagnosis and may even permit the rendering of a specific diagnosis. Depending on the results of the frozen section, the pathologist can then triage the tissue as necessary and submit samples for EM, DNA flow cytometry, cytogenetics, fluorescence in situ hybridization (FISH), or keep tissue frozen for other molecular studies. If a core needle biopsy is performed, then three cores of tumor-bearing tissue are usually required; if an open biopsy is performed, 0.5 cm^3 of tumor is sufficient to perform the necessary studies.

Grading

The American Joint Committee on Cancer (AJCC)[20] staging systems for sarcoma of soft tissue, shown in Table 27.3, are based on classification of the tumors into low-, intermediate-, and high-grade tumors. The designation of grade is based on a consideration and integration of each of these morphological features: Degree of cellular differentiation, extent of necrosis, number of mitoses, cellularity, pleomorphism or anaplasia, quantity of matrix, vascularity, hemorrhage, vascular invasion, and encapsulation. Among these variables, necrosis, mitoses, and degree of differentiation appear to be the best predictors of outcome.

Despite some lack of agreement on the number of grades employed and the significance of individual morphological parameters (there is inevitably a subjective component in assigning grade and only a part of the tumor is examined), grading, more than any clinical and pathological parameter available, is the most important prognosticator. The problems with current grading systems are that their criteria are not precisely defined, application and interpretation are subjective, and implementation is complex. Consistent grading requires adequate tissue and experienced pathologists.

TABLE 27.3   **2018 American Joint Committee on the Staging of Cancer (AJCC) Stage Grouping for STSs**

Stage grouping	IA	IB	II	IIIA	IIIB	IV
(histological) G(rade)	1	1	2–3	2–3	2–3	any
T(umor)*	1	2–4	1	2	3–4	any
N(ode metastases)	0	0	0	0	0	1#
(distant) M(etastases)	0	0	0	0	0	1#

Source: Adapted from Cates, 2018.
* T1, <5 cm; T2, >5 cm to <10 cm; T3, >10 cm to <15 cm; T4, >15 cm
# Either or both

Staging

The Task Force on STSs of the AJCC Staging and End Result Reporting has established a staging system for STSs that is an extension of the tumor/node/metastasis (TNM) system to include G for histological grade. Grade, size, and presence of nodal or distant metastases are the determinants of stage. This staging system is applied to all sarcomas of soft tissue except rhabdomyosarcoma (for which there is a special staging system), Kaposi's sarcoma, dermatofibrosarcoma, desmoid, and sarcoma arising from the dura mater, brain, parenchymatous organs, or hollow viscera. The current system, last updated in 2018, has separate staging categories for sarcomas of the (1) head and neck, (2) extremity and trunk, (3) retroperitoneum, (4) abdominal and thoracic viscera, (5) gastrointestinal stromal tumors, and (6) unusual histologies and sites. The system for extremity and trunk is shown in Table 27.3. Grade of sarcoma is determined on the basis of the histological features of the individual tumor. Immunohistochemistry provides additional information to classify the cell of origin, Table 27.4. T stage is determined on the basis of size. As evidence for the importance of size as a determinant of frequency of distant metastasis, Table 27.5 presents an analysis of distant metastasis versus tumor size among patients who have achieved local control. For patients with grade 1 sarcomas, distant metastases are quite uncommon. The pooled data for grade 2 and grade 3 lesions show regular increases in distant metastases with tumor size. These data make it clear that it is important to stratify patients according to grade and size in attempts to compare efficacy of different modes of treatment, defining the natural history of various histological types, or assessing the role of site, patient age, and other factors.

Management of the extremity, trunk, or head and neck primary tumor

The intent of treatment for extremity sarcomas is to eradicate tumor while optimizing limb function. For truncal and head and neck sarcomas, minimizing the functional and cosmetic defects associated with treatment is also extremely important.

TABLE 27.5 Five-Year Actuarial Distant Metastasis (DM) Probability in 501 Consecutive Patients (whose Primary Tumor was Locally Controlled) as a Function of Tumor Size for Grades 2 and 3 in Series from Massachusetts General Hospital (Treatment by Radiation and Surgery)

Size (mm)	No. of Patients	DM (%)
<25	58	3
26–50	128	22
51–100	177	34
101–150	68	43
151–200	49	58
201 plus	21	57
Total	501	35

Source: DeLaney et al., 2007.

Overview

Because sarcomas tend to infiltrate normal tissue adjacent to the evident lesion, simple excision alone is followed by LR in 60%–90% of patients. Radical resection of a wider margin of apparently normal tissue around the tumor reduces the local failure (LF) rate to approximately 25%–30%. With compartmental resections, the LF rate is only 10%–20% with surgery alone, albeit with often significant functional consequences. One study that reported a zero LF rate derives from the amputation arm of the National Cancer Institute trial comparing amputation to limb salvage treatment.

The combination of surgery and radiation achieves better outcomes than either of the treatments alone for the majority of STSs. The rationale for combining radiation with surgery is to avoid the functional and cosmetic deformity associated with radical resection, and the late consequences of high radiation doses to large volumes of normal tissue in patients treated with primary radiation alone. Radiation at moderate dose levels (60–65 Gy) is as effective as radical resection in eradicating the microscopic extensions beyond the gross lesion, resulting in similarly high rates of local control. This has allowed maximization of functional and cancer-related outcomes without the significant morbidity of radical surgery. Most centers report local control rates of

TABLE 27.4 Immunohistochemistry in STSs

Vimentin	Almost all sarcomas and some carcinomas
Keratin	Almost all carcinomas and some sarcomas (epithelioid sarcoma, synovial sarcoma)
Desmin	Leiomyosarcoma, rhabdomyosarcoma, and occasionally MFH
Glial fibrillary acidic protein	Some schwannomas
Neurofilament	Primitive neuroectodermal tumor, neuroblastoma
Leucocyte common antigen	Lymphoma
S-100 protein	Malignant schwannoma, melanoma, clear cell (melanoma of soft parts), chondrosarcoma, leiomyosarcoma, rhabdomyosarcoma, liposarcoma
Myo D1	Rhabdomyosarcoma
Myoglobin	Rhabdomyosarcoma
Factor VIII related antigen	Angiosarcoma, Kaposi's sarcoma
CD34	Angiosarcoma, epithelioid sarcoma, MFH, hemangiopericytoma, solitary fibrous tumor
Smooth muscle actin	Leiomyosarcoma
EMA	Carcinomas, synovial sarcoma, meningioma
Leu 7	Malignant schwannoma, leiomyosarcoma, synovial sarcoma, rhabdomyosarcoma
CD99 (MIC2 gene product)	Ewing's sarcoma/PNET, some rhabdomyosarcomas, some synovial sarcomas
CD117 (c-kit)	Gastrointestinal stromal tumor

Abbreviations: MFH, malignant fibrous histiocytoma; PNET, primitive peripheral neuro-ectodermal tumor.

approximately 90% for high-grade extremity STS and 90%–100% for low-grade STS depending on the size.

In addition to its benefit in improving local control rates, adjunctive radiotherapy has also had a significant impact on limb salvage for extremity sarcomas. As an example, in the 1970s, 50% of patients with extremity sarcoma underwent amputation; those patients treated by wide excision alone with limb preservation experienced a 30% rate of LR. With the subsequent application of radiotherapy and advanced reconstructive techniques, the rate of amputation at major centers has been reduced to less than 10%, and the incidence of LR with limb preservation has been reduced to 10%–15% without any measurable fall in OS. A single, prospective randomized trial showed similar rates of DFS and OS for patients treated with amputation or the combination of limb-sparing surgery and radiotherapy for extremity STS. [21]

The success of a conservative surgical approach has, as mentioned earlier, resulted in an amputation rate at major centers of only 5% in patients with extremity STS. The current indications for amputation include massive disease such that a functional limb is not achievable, severely compromised normal tissues due to age, peripheral vascular disease, and other co-morbidities. The functional and cosmetic results of conservative procedures are dependent on the size and anatomical location of the tumor, the magnitude of the surgical procedure, the extent to which muscles, tendons, or nerves must be sacrificed, the volume of tissues irradiated, and the radiation dose administered.

The role for the combined modality strategy of surgery and RT with or without chemotherapy has not been definitely established in the treatment of retroperitoneal sarcomas, for which 10-year LF rates in some series are reported to be as high as 70% with surgery alone; post-operative radiation is often difficult to administer to the required volumes and radiation doses whereas pre-operative radiation has shown promise in single-institution reports but is still being tested in randomized, phase III studies.

Surgical considerations

The technique utilized to achieve a wide or radical extirpation of the tumor will vary considerably with anatomical site and anatomical details of prior surgical procedures (especially the biopsy). The surgery, in theory at least, if it is to be successful in avoiding an LR, must include not only the complete tumor and the track of the prior biopsy, but also as wide a cuff of normal tissue as is possible without compromising function so severely as to make the procedure of limited value as limb-sparing surgery. Provided the surgical margins are *proved* to be clear, the procedure is usually successful (an LR rate of 5%). Despite the mass of muscle removed from that site, the patient demonstrates only modest disability in normal activities.

The surgical procedure as described earlier is an effective solution to the problem in sites such as the fleshy parts of the thigh or the calf, or even some parts of the arm in selected patients, but is usually unsatisfactory and more complex when the tumor lies close to vital structures or in an anatomical site where a wide margin is difficult to obtain. Tumors that lie in the popliteal or antecubital fossae are particularly problematic as are those lesions arising in the soft tissues of the volar aspects of the forearm, hands, and feet.

In general, the results of surgery alone, even with the best techniques, have an LF rate of 10%–20% when all patients on whom the surgery is performed, including those with unsatisfactory margins, are considered. The local control rate after surgery alone was 67% in a phase III trial of surgery versus surgery and brachytherapy (BRT). An LF not only enormously compounds the

management problems at the site of the original lesion but also increases the risk of distant metastases. This has been a problem especially for sarcomas of the head and neck region.

Surgical margins

The most important surgical variable that influences local control is the presence or absence of tumor cells at the surgical margins. In series that report radical resection with clear margins, such as the Scandinavian Sarcoma Group (SSG), the LF rates are quite low (8%).[22] By contrast, in a second study of 559 patients who were treated with surgery alone from the same group, an inadequate surgical margin led to a 2.9-fold greater risk of LR than did clear surgical margins. Distant metastases are extremely uncommon for low-grade lesions, but occur with high-grade lesions with a frequency that is influenced by the size of the lesion and whether local control is achieved. In the SSG experience, LR was identified as a risk factor for distant metastasis (4.4-fold higher).

The status of the surgical margins also influences the LR rate in patients treated with combined surgery and radiation. In one review of 132 consecutive patients with STS of the extremities who were treated with pre-operative RT followed by resection, the 5-year actuarial local control rates were 97% and 81% for patients with negative and positive margins, respectively. Local control was not a function of sarcoma size in patients with negative surgical margins. In a second series of 225 patients, all of whom received combined surgery and radiotherapy (either pre-operative, post-operative, or both), local control rates at 5 years were 88%, 76%, and 64% for patients with negative, uncertain, and positive margins, respectively. The policy at major sarcoma centers is to make serious efforts to achieve negative margins, although the majority of patients, even with a positive margin, will achieve local control, and conservative procedures in this setting are generally warranted, with the caveat that additional radiotherapy dose should be delivered to the area of positive margin.

The exact size of the negative margin that is optimal for local control is not known. In one study, the local control rate did not differ in patients with a negative margin ≤1 or >1 mm (local control 96% versus 97%). Most clinicians recommend that if surgery is used as the sole modality of treatment, the margin should be at least 1 cm in all directions or, if less, include a supervening fascial barrier. If surgery is combined with RT, the surgical margin can probably be safely reduced to 0.5 cm without compromising the rate of local control.

The guiding principle of surgery is total en bloc excision of the primary tumor without cutting into tumor tissue. Tissues should be cut outside of the tumor pseudo-capsule, if one exists, through normal uninvolved tissue. Violation of the tumor results in a higher LF rate. In one report, for example, the local control rate in 95 patients with extremity STS was 47% if tumor violation occurred compared to 87% without violation.[23] The majority of STS do not involve bone; as a result, it is seldom necessary to resect adjacent bone. It is also rarely necessary to resect a major nerve unless the tumor is a neurogenic sarcoma. Non-amputative surgery is now accomplished in more than 90% of patients.

In planning primary therapy for a patient who has had a suboptimal resection by a non-oncologic surgeon or insufficient imaging with pre-operative CT or MRI, it is important to consider re-resection. Approximately 37%–68% of such patients will have residual tumor in a re-resection specimen. A partial excision of the tumor before referral to a tertiary center does not appear to compromise limb preservation, local control, or survival rates in such patients, although the re-resection may entail a larger procedure than a de novo procedure and impact on the functional result. In one series of 295 patients who underwent re-resection at a single institution (final resection margins negative in 87%), local control rates at 5, 10, and 15 years were 85%, 85%, and 82%, respectively; the corresponding values for those who did not undergo re-resection were 78%, 73%, and 73%, respectively. A similar degree of benefit for re-resection was apparent for metastasis-free and disease-specific survival. Some patients, for medical, functional, or cosmetic reasons, may not be candidates for re-resection; appropriate doses of RT can help ensure local control in a substantial majority of these patients, 86% in one series.

Selection of patients for treatment with conservative surgery alone

Because of potential acute and late morbidity from RT, it is important to select patients who may be effectively treated with conservative surgery alone. Several series have evaluated wide-excision, limb-sparing surgery alone. In one report, 119 selected patients with extremity STS were grouped according to anatomical location as subcutaneous (*n* = 40), intra-muscular (*n* = 30), or extra-muscular (*n* = 49). The 70 patients with subcutaneous and intra-muscular tumors were all treated by local surgery, and a wide margin, requiring a cuff of fat tissue around the tumor and inclusion of the deep fascia beneath the tumor, was obtained in 56. These patients were followed without post-operative radiation. During a median follow-up of 5 years (range, 3.5–10 years), only four had an LR, despite the fact that 84% had high-grade tumors. The authors concluded that post-operative radiation may not be necessary in this subgroup. A prospective study at M.D. Anderson Cancer Center[24] evaluated local control for T1 tumors after excision alone with negative margins. Wide local excision was performed with the intent of including a 1- to 2-cm margin of normal tissue around the mass. Negative surgical margins were achieved in 84% of the 88 enrolled patients; the remaining 16% with microscopically positive margins received post-operative RT. In those with excision alone, the 5-year LR rate was 7.9%, and the 5-year sarcoma-specific death rate was 3.2%. In another study, 74 patients with localized STS of the extremity or trunk underwent function-sparing surgery without radiation. The overall 10-year actuarial local control rate was 93%, and was dependent on the adequacy of surgical margins (87% versus 100% for patients with margins of <1 cm and ≥1 cm, respectively). The 10-year survival rate was 73%. This approach may be appropriate for carefully selected patients with small (<5 cm), superficial tumors that can be resected with all margins ≥1 cm or a secure, intervening fascial barrier.

Combining surgery with radiation therapy

Although wide resection or amputation is often effective in achieving local control, there is usually a significant functional and cosmetic loss. Despite careful pre-operative evaluation, a portion of the resected specimen may be found to have unsatisfactory margins and mean that additional treatment is essential. The consequence is that those patients experience both radical surgery and radiation.

The available evidence indicates that the tumor control probability for an STS and an epithelial tumor of the same size and treated to the same radiation dose are similar. For example, the 5-year local control results of treatment of a patient with carcinoma of the breast or STS by resection with negative margins and radiation are essentially the same (approximately 0.9), despite the latter tumor being much the larger. There is

experience with treatment with RT alone for unresected sarcoma, discussed below, that indicates that radiation is able to effectively control a proportion of these lesions. In animal models, a significantly lower radiation dose is required to achieve local control when radiation is combined with simple excision as compared to radiation alone, which provides the laboratory basis for the combination of conservative resection and radiation in the clinic.

The rationale for utilizing radiotherapy with a conservative surgical procedure is that radiotherapy in less-than-radical doses eradicates the small number of tumor cells remaining after a less extensive excision that would be removed in the grossly normal tissue included in the radical surgical specimen, but not in that from the simple excision. Thus, moderate radiation doses can be expected to boost simple surgery, so that it provides the same gain as has been shown for radical surgery. An attractive feature of radiotherapy is the relative ease with which the treatment volume can be designed to include tissues suspected of involvement without concern for the position of nerves, vessels, and tendons. Results from several clinical studies demonstrate that this approach is clinically practical, and has achieved local control and survival results equal to those obtained by radical surgery with the important gain in cosmetic and functional results. The 5-year results of treatment of patients with STS of the extremities by radiotherapy and conservative surgery show that long-term local control is achieved in 76%–98% of patients.

Patients whose sarcomas are so extensive that even a conservative resection would result in a minimally useful limb would be best served, in most instances, by a prompt amputation. For example, the elderly patient with a large sarcoma on the ankle and who has poor vascular supply is a poor candidate for an attempted limb salvage procedure. At the opposite extreme are patients with small sarcomas (<5 cm) of the subcutaneous tissue or other anatomical sites which can be resected with wide margins and negligible functional consequences. They need only surgery as noted earlier. For the more frequent deeply sited lesions there is usually a close margin at some point on the resected specimen and a combined radiation and surgical approach is required to realize a very low likelihood of LF.

Hence, the recommended treatment for patients with extremity, truncal, and head and neck STSs who are medically and technically operable is the combination of function-preserving surgery and radiation, with the exception of that minority of patients with small, superficial lesions that can be widely excised with secure margins and good functional result. In most instances, the probability of tumor control and the late functional and cosmetic result is clearly superior following this combined modality approach.

Pre-operative (neoadjuvant) versus post-operative (adjuvant) radiotherapy

There are potential advantages to both pre-operative and post-operative administration of radiation that must be considered by the clinicians when electing the most appropriate approach for the individual patient.

Pre-operative radiation therapy

Pre-operative RT might be expected to reduce tumor burden before resection, theoretically allowing more conservative surgical therapy. At the time of surgery, the tumor is usually smaller and surrounded by a relatively dense pseudo-capsule if radiotherapy has been given pre-operatively. This means that the margins can be reduced and, hence, a more conservative approach is feasible. This should be associated with lesser disability. In addition, a lesion previously considered inoperable may regress to such an extent that it becomes operable. Radiation given pre-operatively reduces the number of viable tumor cells to such small absolute levels that the likelihood of autotransplantation in the surgical bed is virtually eliminated.

Pre-operative radiation fields can be limited to the known gross tumor and adjacent tissues at risk for microscopic infiltration. In contrast, post-operative irradiation fields must include not only the site of the tumor but also all tissues handled during the surgical procedure including the stab wound for the drain tube(s). Therefore, the treatment volume for post-operative radiotherapy will usually be larger than for pre-operative irradiation. The consequence of the smaller treatment volumes means that late radiation reactions are expected to be less severe in patients who receive radiation preoperatively. However, there is a modest increase in the acute reaction as manifest by a delay in the healing of the surgical wound. Radiation doses are lower for pre-operative RT (50 Gy pre-op versus 60–66 Gy post-op), which can reduce late effects. Pre-operative radiotherapy facilitates the development of an overall treatment plan by the surgeon, radiation therapist, and medical/pediatric oncologist before any therapeutic maneuver is implemented. Initiation of radiotherapy is not delayed when given pre-operatively. Where radiotherapy is given post-operatively, a delay of 10–14 days or even longer may occur before the treatment is started. This means that residual tumor cells are in a tumor bed flooded with growth factors and, hence, have an opportunity to increase in number. Where wound healing delays treatment further, recurrent tumor may be grossly evident at the time of initiation of irradiation (especially where surgery was not complete and the lesion was high grade).

Post-operative radiation therapy

Post-operative radiotherapy has the following advantages:

1. Histopathological diagnosis/grade is made from tissue samples taken throughout the entire tumor rather than an incisional biopsy specimen.
2. Surgery is immediate. This is important to some patients.
3. There is no delay in wound healing related to the pre-operative RT.
4. Initial surgery is the only feasible sequence for quite small lesions removed by excisional biopsy, often judged to be benign. This has rarely led to problems other than the occasionally poorly placed incision by a non-oncological surgeon.

There is one randomized controlled study comparing pre-operative and post-operative radiotherapy. This study was designed to evaluate the incidence of acute wound healing complications in patients with potentially curable extremity STS.[25] In this Canadian trial, 190 patients were randomly assigned to either pre-operative (50 Gy pre-op for all 94 patients randomized to this arm with 16–20 Gy post-op boost reserved for the 14 patients in this arm with a positive margin) or post-operative (50 Gy initial field +16–20 Gy boost field for all patients) radiotherapy. Complications were defined as secondary wound surgery, hospital admission for wound care, or the need for deep packing or prolonged wound dressings within 120 days of tumor resection.

The study was terminated when a highly significant result was obtained at the time of a planned interim analysis. With a median follow-up of 3.3 years, a significantly higher percentage of preoperatively treated patients had acute wound complications (35% versus 17%). Other factors associated with wound complications were the volume of resected tissue and lower limb location of the tumor. Late morbidity was initially not reported. Because the RT fields for the post-operative RT were larger and the dose delivered for most patients was higher, the authors indicated that more follow-up would be needed to assess whether these larger radiation volumes and higher radiation doses would lead to more late treatment effects in these patients.

In a later publication, the LR rate, regional or distant failure rate, progression-free survival, and functional outcome did not differ between the groups. When these data were updated with a median follow-up of 6.9 years, there remained no differences in local control between the patients in the two arms of the study with more than 90% local control. The regional and distant failure rates as well as the progression-free and OS rates were also no different between the two arms of the study. The post-operative patients, however, developed more grade 2–4 late toxicity (86%) when compared to the pre-operative patients (68%), $p = 0.02$. Notably, grade 3 (severe induration and loss of subcutaneous tissue or field contracture >10% linear measurement) or grade 4 (necrosis) subcutaneous fibrosis was significantly more common in the post-operative group, 36% versus 23%, $p = 0.02$.

There is thus a difference in the morbidity profile between preoperative and post-operative radiotherapy, with a higher rate of generally reversible acute wound-healing complications in the patients receiving preoperative treatment, offset by a higher rate of generally irreversible late complications, including grade 3–4 fibrosis, in those patients receiving post-operative RT. Because very few acute wound-healing complications occurred in either group when the tumor was in the upper extremity, it would seem prudent to treat these patients with pre-operative RT. We have also favored pre-operative radiation for the majority of lower extremity patients, because acute wound complications can usually be managed and will go on to heal, whereas the late treatment effects are generally irreversible. Selected patients with a high risk of acute wound-healing complications, such as those who are morbidly obese or diabetic, may be best managed with surgery followed by post-operative radiation once the wounds have healed. For patients with lower extremity lesions, this study, however, makes it clear that new strategies are needed: First, to reduce the risk of acute wound-healing problems when patients receive pre-operative RT and, second, to reduce the risk of late treatment-induced effects when higher-dose, larger-field post-operative radiation is given. Indeed, recent efforts (which will be discussed in greater detail when describing external RT treatment planning) with image-guided (IG), intensity-modulated pre-operative RT designed to reduce the radiation dose to the planned surgical flap show promise in reducing the risk of acute wound-healing delays.

Brachytherapy (BRT)

Compared to EBRT, BRT minimizes the radiation dose to surrounding normal tissues, maximizes the radiation dose delivered to the tumor, and shortens treatment times. In the usual dosage schedule, treatment is completed within 6 days and requires only one hospitalization. After loading, catheters are placed in a target area of the tumor operative bed, defined by the surgeon, and spaced at 1-cm intervals to cover the entire area of risk. BRT can also be used for delivery of a boost to the tumor bed in conjunction with EBRT.

A phase III trial of post-operative BRT versus no BRT was conducted in 126 patients who had complete resection of either extremity or superficial trunk STS.[26] The BRT dose was 45 Gy as low-dose-rate BRT. Five-year local control rates were 82% and 67% for the BRT and surgery-alone groups, respectively. The advantage of BRT was seen only in the high-grade sarcomas. It was limited to local control, as there was no difference between the groups in distant metastasis or disease-specific survival.

Although it is unclear if BRT is associated with a higher risk of wound complications the rate of wound re-operation may be higher. BRT has been combined with free flap construction as a means of enhancing primary healing in difficult anatomical situations without an increase in the incidence of wound breakdown. There have been no randomized comparisons of the relative efficacy or morbidity of EBRT compared with BRT. In a retrospective comparison of patients treated by intensity-modulated radiotherapy (IMRT) or BRT, the IMRT group appeared to have somewhat worse prognostic features, but the 5-year local control rate was significantly higher than in the BRT group (92% versus 82%).

BRT for sarcomas has traditionally been given by low-dose-rate radiation. There are increasing data available on the use of fractionated high-dose-rate schedules. High-dose-rate BRT has been used in conjunction with external beam radiotherapy for the tumor bed boost in doses of 15–24 Gy, often hyperfractionated at 2.3–4 Gy bid. One report using high-dose-rate BRT alone in doses of 40 Gy at 2.3–3 Gy bid unfortunately reported poor local control of only 20%, in contrast with 100% when BRT was combined with external beam radiation. In contrast, a more recent report showed local control of 93% with surgery and high-dose-rate BRT in patients with negative margins, whereas local control was only 48% in patients with positive margins, suggesting that for the latter group, if BRT is used, then it should be done in conjunction with external beam radiation.

External beam radiation treatment planning

The radiation treatment technique should be carefully planned so that the tissues being irradiated are only those judged to be at risk. To utilize smaller treatment volumes, the part to be irradiated must be securely and reproducibly immobilized. Most sarcoma centers have special immobilization devices prepared for the individual patient. This may require casting, especially for hand, foot, or elbow sites. For some sites the part is placed in standard plastic supports and the extremity fastened tightly in place using a Velcro fastener. Others describe their experience with casts and polyurethane foam systems.

The principal tasks involved in the development of a treatment plan are as follows:

- Design an immobilization device and a means to assure that the target is on the beam. It is important that the patient be comfortable in this position so that it can be maintained for the treatment delivery sessions.
- CT scan (or where MRI simulators are available, perform MRI scan) of the immobilized, affected extremity for radiotherapy planning. This is facilitated by the availability of a large-bore scanner that allows maximum flexibility in arranging the limb such that the contralateral extremity and the trunk will be out of the beam.
- Define the target volume(s) on the CT/MRI of the affected region. Review of these studies with the diagnostic radiologist and surgeon, as well as review of any surgical procedures performed with the surgeon, can be extremely important in defining the appropriate target volume(s).
- Image fusion of MRI scans with the treatment planning CT scan may facilitate target definition.

- Define non-target critical structures in the treatment volume and specify dose constraints for each such structure.
- Estimate the distribution of number of tumor clonogens/unit volume of tissue throughout the target volume.
- Define a series of target volumes to realize the appropriate dose distribution using "shrinking treatment volume methods."
- Design treatment techniques that achieve the closest feasible conformation of treatment to target volume. This may require complex field arrangements, treatment angles, gapped fields, wedge filters, tissue compensators, bolus, various radiation modalities (i.e. electrons, protons, IMRT, BRT, IORT).
- Avoid inclusion of an entire joint space.
- Avoid full-dose irradiation of adjacent bone to reduce the risk of pathological fracture.
- Utilize wedges and tissue compensators as needed to account for tissue heterogeneities and minimize dose inhomogeneity.
- Review the treatment plan at multiple levels along the extremity to assess dose homogeneity to the target and normal tissues.

A valuable point to keep in mind in planning treatment is that there may be a failure (recurrence or necrosis) and the plan should, if feasible, allow for potential sites for flaps, surgical incision, etc., if salvage surgery is necessary.

Radiation treatment volumes and dose

The extent of normal tissue to be irradiated adjacent to the tumor bed in the case of pre-operative RT and adjacent to the surgical bed in the case of post-operative RT is not definitively known. Nevertheless, several recent patterns of failure studies after pre-operative RT have been informative and relate the extent of the RT field to the site of local tumor recurrence.

Because sarcomas are judged to infiltrate along rather than through tissue planes, longitudinal margins proximally and distally have traditionally been considerably more generous than radial margins. Historically, fields that extended from the muscle origin to insertion or provided generous proximal–distal margins on the tumor were employed. In some centers from the 1970s through the mid-1990s, 5–10 cm proximal and distal block margins were used for large grade 1 and small grade 2 lesions and more generous fields with 10–15 cm margins were encompassed for large grade 2–3 lesions. The advent of improved MRI delineation of tumor extent and subsequent surgical experience with high rates of local control when surgical margins ≥1 cm could be obtained prompted radiation oncologists to employ ≤5-cm proximal–distal margins for small grade 1 lesions and 5–7-cm proximal–distal margins for larger, higher-grade lesions. 3-D treatment planning systems appear to allow smaller and more accurate treatment volumes in patients with extremity STS.

There are relatively few studies in the literature looking at the relationship of the treated target volume to local tumor control in patients with STS. This tends to be poorly reported. One group found a remarkable difference in 5-year local control where the proximal–distal margin was <5 cm (30%) or ≥5 cm (93%). This conflicts with the BRT data where acceptable results are achieved using ≤4-cm margins longitudinally and 2-cm laterally. A publication from the Royal Marsden Hospital has suggested that, as in other tumor sites, the great majority of LRs occur within the high-dose volume.[27] Dickie et al. recently published data on LFs with respect to irradiated volumes. The gross tumor volume

(GTV) to clinical target volume (CTV) expansion was 4 cm longitudinally and 1–1.5 cm axially. Of 768 treated extremity soft tissue sarcoma patients, LR developed in 60 patients (7.7%). All recurrences were reconstructed onto the irradiated planning target volumes (PTVs). Of the failures, 49 (82%) developed in-field, 9 were out-of-field failures (15%), and 2 were marginal failures (3%). The nine out-of-field failures (15%) were explained as "atypical" (remote from the GTV or beyond the operative bed) or "surgical" (contamination at surgery elsewhere, uninvolved flap donor site). In-field relapses could relate to surgical factors such as residual tumor cell burden after resection, the inherent radiation resistance of these cells, other biologic factors such as hypoxia or local stromal factors (i.e. proangiogenic or growth factors related to wound healing), or radiation technical factors (dose inhomogeneity, overall treatment time). The investigators concluded that only two marginal recurrences might have been prevented by larger volumes among the 768 patients treated. Similar findings were reported by Kim et al., who analyzed sites of LR with respect to the pre-operative CTV in patients treated with CT planned pre-operative radiation with 1–1.5 cm radial and 3.5 cm proximal–distal expansion of the CTV on the T1-gadolinium enhanced MRI-defined GTV (including as well any tumor-associated edema). Only 3 of 58 patients (all with positive margin) experienced LF as first relapse (2 isolated, 1 with distant failure), and 2 additional patients (all with margin <1 mm) had late LF after distant metastasis. The LFs were within the CTV in three patients and within and also extending beyond the CTV in two patients.

These data suggest that the current CTVs are adequate and may be further tailored in future clinical studies. With the advent of techniques such as IMRT and protons that allow us to selectively spare normal tissues, appropriate target volume delineation becomes particularly important. The RTOG recently completed study 0630, which assessed the use of image-guided preoperative radiation for extremity STSs in conjunction with more tailored radiation volumes. The pre-operative radiation CTV for low-grade tumors and high-grade tumors <8 cm in size included the GTV with 1.5-cm radial expansion and 2-cm proximal–distal expansion plus any tumor-associated edema; for high-grade tumors >8 cm, the proximal–distal expansion was 3 cm. This study has completed accrual and showed very good local control with these target volumes treated with image guidance.[28]

An international group of expert sarcoma radiation oncologists developed consensus guidelines for radiation treatment of extremity sarcomas that provide guidance for delineation of target volumes.[27] For the pre-operative radiation CTV, the recommended radial margin expansion on the GTV was 1.5 cm with proximal–distal margin expansion of 4.0 cm. This radial margin expansion is rationally derived from the surgical experience with high rates of local control with ≥1 cm margins. Where there is intervening bone, interosseous membrane, or major fascial planes, and these planes are intact, the CTV can be constrained at the surface of these structures. When a fascial plane has been violated, wider margins are appropriate to cover areas of potential contamination by tumor. The proximal and distal margin expansion was driven by the findings from the White study[29] showing tumor cells up to 4 cm from the gross tumor, particularly along the proximal–distal axis of the extremity because these tumors generally tend to spread along rather than through tissue planes. Because of the finding of tumor cells in tumor-associated edema, the consensus guidelines suggested including tumor-associated edema in the pre-operative CTV. Further volume expansion of 0.5–1.0 cm (institution-specific and dependent on the immobilization, image guidance, and reproducibility of daily set-up) was recommended for creating the PTV to account for any daily variability in patient set-up.

For patients receiving pre-operative radiation, 50 Gy is administered over 5 weeks, followed 3–5 weeks later by a conservative resection. With negative surgical margins and no other unfavorable prognostic features such as tumor cut-through or satellite lesions after prior surgical interventions, 50 Gy of pre-operative RT appears sufficient to provide local control in a very high proportion of patients.

For patients with positive margins following pre-operative RT, it has traditionally been recommended to use a "shrinking treatment volume technique" with delivery of either BRT or a post-operative external beam radiation boost dose of 16–18 Gy to the tumor bed once the surgical wound has healed. A boost dose to 66–68 Gy is given post-operatively or intra-operatively for microscopically positive margins, and to 75 Gy if there is gross residual disease. In patients with frozen section evidence of close or positive margins, an intra-operative boost dose can be administered by BRT or electron beam. BRT has the advantage of fractionation and one can use a low dose rate of 16 Gy for microscopically positive margins (or more recently, a high dose rate of 12–16 Gy given at 3–4 Gy bid), and 25 Gy for gross residual tumor. Although delivery of a post-operative RT boost after resection with positive margins has been the standard of care in some institutions, its efficacy in achieving local control (LC) has been called into question by the results of at least one retrospective study comparing patients with positive margins who did or did not receive a post-operative external beam boost to the tumor bed. In that study, 5-year estimated LR-free survivals were 90.4% in the no-boost group and 73.8% in the boosted group. Because most series of patients with positive surgical margins who received adjuvant radiotherapy document local control in the range of 70%–80%, this would suggest that the no-boost group was carefully selected. There is likely value in identifying patients for whom a boost is not necessary; indeed, the Princess Margaret group has identified patients with (1) a positive margin in a low-grade, well-differentiated liposarcoma or (2) planned positive margin on an anatomically fixed critical structure as low risk for local recurrence (4.2% and 3.6%, respectively).[30] Conversely, there are patients with poor histologic response, margins broadly or multifocally positive, margins positive after re-excision, and "unplanned positive margins" for whom additional treatment, if effective, is likely warranted.

For patients undergoing initial surgical resection followed by adjuvant, post-operative RT, irradiation planning usually begins 14–20 days following surgery, once the wound is healed. Following resection of large tumors, it may be necessary to wait 3–4 weeks to allow resorption of the seroma. The recommended initial radiation CTV includes all tissues handled during the surgical procedure, including the drain site, encompassing the surgical bed with 4-cm proximal–distal block margins and 1.5-cm radial margins on the surgical bed with appropriate PTV expansion of 0.5–1.0 cm as noted earlier. The dose to this initial volume is 50 Gy and then, through shrinking treatment volumes to encompass the tumor bed, the final dose is 60 Gy for negative margins, 66–68 Gy for positive margins or locally recurrent disease, and 75 Gy for gross residual sarcoma.

The available information on a dose–response relationship for the local control of sarcomas treated with surgery and post-operative RT is somewhat conflicting. Mundt et al. reported that local control was dose-dependent.[31] Although post-operative patients receiving <60 Gy had lower local control than those receiving ≥60 Gy, no difference was seen in local control between patients receiving 60–63.9 Gy (74.4%) versus those receiving 64–66 (87%)

(p = 0.5). Severe late sequelae were more frequent in patients treated with doses ≥63 Gy compared to patients treated with lower doses (23.1% versus 0%). The accepted dose for pre-operative radiotherapy is 50 Gy. Radiation doses may need to be modified for patients with diabetes or connective tissue diseases, and in those receiving chemotherapy.

For treatment of an extremity lesion, a good functional result demands that only a portion of the cross-section of the extremity be irradiated to high dose. Thus, some tissue should be spared from high dose to provide for lymphatic drainage. For very large tumors that are treated with wide resection, there may be persistent leg edema, requiring the use of a pressure-type stocking, even though the radiation treatment volume is less than circumferential. This can be a problem for patients with large (>10 cm) sarcomas of the medial thigh.

When post-operative radiation is combined with adjuvant chemotherapy, radiation daily dose has generally been reduced by 10% from 200 to 180 cGy; radiation is not given concurrently with doxorubicin. Instead, 2–3 days are allowed between the doxorubicin and radiation. Some pre-operative protocols have interdigitated chemotherapy and RT (see later); total pre-operative radiation has been reduced (i.e. 44 Gy) in this setting.

Intensity-modulated photon radiation therapy

The intent of RT is to maximize the dose delivered to the tumor while minimizing the exposure of dose-sensitive critical structures to high dose. This has been achieved traditionally by shaping the spatial distribution of the high radiation dose to conform the target volume (hence, 3-D conformal RT), thereby reducing the dose to the non-target structures. Although this approach is satisfactory in the treatment of targets that are roughly convex in shape, it is less than optimal for targets that contain complex concavities or that wrap around critical structures. Growing experience suggests that IMRT plans produce superior dose distribution in the patient as compared to 3-D conformal plans, both in terms of dose conformity in the tumor and dose reduction to the specified critical normal structures. Dosimetric studies comparing IMRT and conformal radiotherapy for STS have been reported. When evaluating sarcomas arising in the extremities, pelvis, trunk, and paranasal sinuses, IMRT plans were more conformal. In the extremities, bone and subcutaneous doses were reduced by up to 20%. A conformal-IMRT comparative planning study has been reported for a large extra-skeletal chondrosarcoma of the extremity. Not surprisingly, IMRT produced excellent conformal treatment plans for this complex target volume, with a reduction of the maximum dose to the bone as compared to the 3-D photon plan. Hong et al. performed treatment planning comparisons of IMRT and 3-D conformal radiotherapy for ten patients with STS of the thigh. They were able to document a reduction in femur dose without compromise in tumor coverage. In addition, IMRT reduced hot spots in the surrounding soft tissues and skin.

It is worth noting, however, that IMRT treatment plans often have localized areas within the high-dose volumes where dose inhomogeneities can be in the range of 10%–15% above the prescription dose. Depending on the location of these "hot spots," there can be unanticipated acute normal tissue toxicity. Because of the multiple field angles employed with IMRT, more of the extremity will see some radiation dose, albeit relatively lower levels, compared to 3-D conformal RT. The initial experience with IMRT, however, suggests that it is associated with reduced toxicity while maintaining high rates of local control. In a single-institution retrospective study, Alektiar and colleagues reported on a series of 41 adult patients with STS of the extremity treated with limb-sparing surgery and IMRT.[32] In their cohort, 51% had positive or close (<1 mm) margins, and 68% had tumors greater than 10 cm. At a median follow-up of 35 months, an encouragingly low rate of complications was observed, with 4.8% developing fractures and 32% developing edema (the majority of whom had grade 1 edema). The 5-year actuarial LC rate was 94%. Both the toxicities and LC rates reported in this study are comparable to those achieved with 3-D conformal RT techniques.

Recently, IMRT has been investigated as a tool to reduce the radiation dose to the planned surgical flap in patients receiving pre-operative RT. The Princess Margaret Group sought to determine if pre-operative IG-IMRT could reduce morbidity, including wound complications, by minimizing dose to uninvolved tissues in adults with lower extremity STS. IG-IMRT was used to conform volumes to avoid normal tissues (skin flaps for wound closure, bone, or other uninvolved soft tissues). Pre-operative IG-IMRT significantly diminished the need for tissue transfer. RT chronic morbidities and the need for subsequent secondary operations for WCs were lowered, although not significantly, whereas good limb function was maintained. There were no bone fractures and local control was good, with only a 6.8% rate of LR, none near the flaps. Hence, this appears to be a promising approach. The RTOG investigated a similar strategy in RTOG protocol 0630, the results of which confirmed a high rate of local control with image guided radiation to smaller target volumes and a reduction in late toxicities.

Proton beam radiotherapy

The rationale for the use of protons (or other charged particles) rather than photons (i.e. X-rays, which have traditionally been used for radiotherapy) is the superior dose distribution that can be achieved with protons. Protons and other charged particles deposit little energy in tissue until near the end of the proton range where the residual energy is lost over a short distance, resulting in a steep rise in the absorbed dose, known as the Bragg peak. The Bragg peak is too narrow for practical clinical applications, so for the irradiation of most tumors, the beam energy is modulated by superimposing several Bragg peaks of descending energies (ranges) and weights to create a region of uniform dose over the depth of the target; these extended regions of uniform dose are called "spread-out Bragg peaks" (SOBP). Although the beam modulation to spread out the Bragg peaks does increase the entrance dose, the proton dose distribution is still characterized by a lower-dose region in normal tissue proximal to the tumor, a uniform high-dose region in the tumor, and zero dose beyond the tumor. More recently, proton beams have been magnetically scanned to reduce entrance dose and allow intensity modulation with highly conformal doses around the tumor while maintaining low integral doses because of the absence of exit dose beyond the tumor.

Protons have been extensively employed for bony sarcomas of the skull base and spine; more recently they have been used for treatment of soft tissue tumor of the paraspinal tissues and there are clearly opportunities to employ protons with very significant sparing of normal tissues in selected patients with extremity, truncal, and retroperitoneal sarcomas. Large, medial proximal thigh lesions can be effectively treated with sparing of the femur, hip joint, genitalia, and anorectal tissue. Lesions around the shoulder can be treated without irradiating the lung apex, and avoiding the shoulder. With the recent or anticipated completion of proton beam facilities in major sarcoma centers across the world, it is anticipated that a larger proportion of these patients will be treated with protons.

Neoadjuvant doxorubicin-based chemotherapy plus radiation therapy

The UCLA group popularized pre-operative regional chemotherapy and RT followed by limb salvage surgery in patients with high-grade sarcomas.[33] They were able to achieve a high rate of primary limb salvage, low rate of LR (approximately 9%), and long-term survival in 65% of the patients. The current regimen consists of doxorubicin (30 mg per day for 3 days) followed by radiation given at 28 Gy in 8 fractions.

A number of other groups have utilized this regimen, also obtaining low rates of LR with varying degrees of toxicity. As an example, the Southeastern Cancer Study Group evaluated this protocol in 66 patients with non-metastatic high-grade extremity sarcoma who received intra-arterial doxorubicin infused directly into the vessel feeding the tumor (30 mg per 24 hours for 3 days). Concurrent RT was administered (30 Gy in 10 fractions, 35 Gy in 10 fractions, or 46 Gy in 23–25 fractions). Limb-sparing surgery was possible in 60 of 66 patients; an additional 2 patients required amputation due to wound-healing complications. Five-year survival and DFS were 59% and 44%, respectively. The LF rate was 1.5%.

It is not clear that intra-arterial administration provides added benefit to intravenous doxorubicin. One study compared these two methods of administration. The intra-arterial route was thought to be associated with a higher incidence of complications and no improvement in survival or function. Another report evaluated two separate protocols utilizing pre-operative treatment with intravenous doxorubicin and ifosfamide with or without intra-arterial cisplatin; the histological response and LF rate following surgery were better with the all-intravenous regimen.

Combination chemotherapy regimens such as mesna, doxorubicin, ifosfamide, and dacarbazine (MAID) may provide better anti-tumor activity than single-agent doxorubicin. Interesting results have been noted with neoadjuvant MAID plus RT. The experience with pre-operative MAID chemotherapy interdigitated with 44 Gy radiation, and followed by surgery, post-operative MAID, and further radiation (16 Gy) for those with positive margins was reported in a series of 48 patients with high-grade extremity sarcomas ≥8 cm.[34] Despite the low objective response rate to pre-operative therapy (partial response [PR] in 11% and stable disease in 77%), all patients were able to undergo limb-sparing surgery initially, with 15% having positive margins. Median tumor necrosis was 95%, suggesting that conventional imaging in this setting may underestimate the degree of response to therapy. At some time during treatment, 25% of the patients required hospitalization for febrile neutropenia. Wound-healing complications occurred in 14 of 48 MAID patients (29%). One MAID patient developed late fatal myelodysplasia. The 5-year rates of local control (92% versus 86%), freedom from distant metastases (75% versus 44%), DFS (70% versus 42%), and OS (87% versus 58%) all compared favorably with the outcomes of a cohort of historical control patients who were matched for tumor size, grade, patient age, and era of treatment.

Similar results were noted when this regimen was utilized in a multi-center US cooperative group trial conducted by the Radiation Therapy Oncology Group, in which 66 patients with primary high-grade extremity or truncal STSs ≥8 cm in diameter received a modified MAID regimen plus granulocyte colony-stimulating factor (G-CSF) and radiation pre-operatively, followed by resection and post-operative chemotherapy. In this report, although pre-operative chemotherapy and radiation were successfully completed by 79% and 89% of the patients, respectively, grade 4 hematological and non-hematological toxicity was experienced by 80% and 23% of the patients. Delayed wound healing was noted in 31%. With a median follow-up of 2.75 years, the estimated 3-year survival, DFS, and local control rates were 75%, 55%, and 79%, respectively. Two patients developed late myelodysplasia. It remains to be confirmed in randomized studies if these aggressive interdigitated approaches offer benefit to the subgroup of patients with large, high-grade sarcomas who are at highest risk of treatment failure.

Soft tissue sarcomas of the hand and foot

The 5-year survival rate for sarcoma of the hand and foot is approximately 80%, better than that usually given for extremity STSs.[35] This is likely related to the smaller size of these lesions at presentation. With surgical excision and the use of adjunctive radiotherapy when the minimum surgical margin is narrow (less than 2 mm), limb amputation can be avoided as primary therapy in most patients, and up to two-thirds of patients can retain a normal or fairly normal extremity.

Adjuvant chemotherapy

Although surgery and radiotherapy achieve control of the primary tumor and cure most adult patients with STSs, many patients, especially those with large grade 2 or 3 primaries, die of metastatic disease not evident at diagnosis. Several studies have shown chemotherapy to be effective against clinically evident metastases. This has suggested to many that chemotherapy used as an adjuvant therapy (in high-risk stage M0 patients) might inactivate micrometastases and increase long-term survival.

A meta-analysis of 14 randomized trials of adjuvant chemotherapy versus control in STSs demonstrated that doxorubicin-based chemotherapy yielded an absolute gain in overall recurrence-free survival of 10% from 45% to 55% ($p = 0.0001$) and a trend for improvement of OS of 4% from 50% to 54%, ($p = 0.12$). For local control the gain was 6% at 10 years, viz. 75%–81%, $p = 0.016$. The most clear evidence of a gain in survival was obtained for patients 31–60 years old, recurrent lesions, extremity, and high grade. Encouraging results with more intense adjuvant therapy were reported by investigators at MGH who evaluated doxorubicin, ifosfamide, and dacarbazine chemotherapy and radiation in adult patients with intermediate- or high-grade STSs of the extremity >8 cm.[36] A randomized trial of more intense adjuvant chemotherapy with epirubicin, ifosfamide, mesna, and G-CSF demonstrated advantage in DFS and OS. In this trial, in which two-thirds of the enrolled patients had either synovial sarcoma or liposarcoma (two particularly chemosensitive STS histologies), 144 patients with high-grade large (≥5 cm) or recurrent spindle cell sarcomas involving the extremities or girdles were randomly assigned to no post-operative therapy, or to five cycles of a dose-intensive epirubicin/ifosfamide combination (epirubicin 60 mg/m² on days 1 and 2 plus ifosfamide 1.8 g/m² on days 1 to 5) with mesna and G-CSF support. Accrual was prematurely discontinued at two years, when a significant difference in the cumulative incidence of distant metastasis was found (45% versus 28%, favoring the chemotherapy group); the OS difference (85% versus 72%), also favoring the chemotherapy group, did not reach the level of statistical significance. When the trial was reported, the 4-year OS rates were significantly higher in favor of chemotherapy (69% versus 50%, $p = 0.04$), although the distant relapse rates were by then similar in both groups (44% and 45% for the chemotherapy and control groups, respectively). It is difficult to interpret these results, since the main benefit of adjuvant systemic chemotherapy is expected to be in reducing the rate of distant relapse. There was a trend towards improved local control in the adjuvant chemotherapy group, with a 17% LF rate at 4 years in the control group compared to 6% in the adjuvantly treated group.

Two additional randomized trials have explored the benefit of doxorubicin- or ifosfamide-based chemotherapy in extremity, one of which showed a survival benefit for adjuvant chemotherapy. The second trial, also from Italy, randomly assigned 88 patients with high-risk STS to surgery with or without RT ($n = 43$), or to surgery plus chemotherapy ($n = 45$, 26 with epirubicin alone, and 19 to epirubicin plus ifosfamide) with or without RT. The 5-year survival rate of patients treated with chemotherapy was significantly higher than that of patients who did not receive chemotherapy (72% versus 47%). However, the large number of treatment variables and the small number of studied patients make interpretation of this result problematic.

The EORTC performed a randomized study of adjuvant chemotherapy in patients with macroscopically resected, Trojani grade II–III soft-tissue sarcomas at any site. Patients were randomly assigned to receive adjuvant chemotherapy or no chemotherapy. Chemotherapy consisted of five cycles of doxorubicin 75 mg/m², ifosfamide 5 g/m², and lenograstim every 3 weeks. Patients in both groups received radiotherapy if the resection was marginal or the tumor recurrent. The primary endpoint was OS and analyses were done by intention to treat. Three hundred and fifty-one patients were randomly assigned to the adjuvant chemotherapy group (175 patients) or to the control group (176 patients). Two hundred and fifty-eight (73%) of 351 patients received radiotherapy, 129 in each group. OS did not differ significantly between groups (hazard ratio [HR] 0.94 [95% CI 0.68–1.31], $p = 0.72$) nor did relapse-free survival (HR 0.91 [0.67–1.22], $p = 0.51$). In the chemotherapy group, 5-year OS rate was 66.5% (58.8–73.0) and in the control group it was 67.8% (60.3–74.2). There was a non-significant trend towards benefit in patients with high-grade tumors >10 cm.

An updated meta-analysis analyzed data from 18 randomized trials of 1953 patients reported between 1973 and 2002 but did not include data from the large EORTC trial. Five of the trials added ifosfamide to doxorubicin, whereas the others used doxorubicin alone or with other agents. The odds ratios (OR) for LR was in favor of chemotherapy. For distant and overall recurrence the OR was 0.67 (95% CI 0.56–0.82; $p = 0.0001$) in favor of chemotherapy. OR for doxorubicin combined with ifosfamide was 0.56 (95% CI, 0.36–0.85; $p = 0.01$) in favor of chemotherapy. The absolute risk reduction for doxorubicin in combination with ifosfamide was 11% (30% versus 41% risk of death). A separate update of the Sarcoma Meta-Analysis Collaboration (SMAC) included this EORTC study and had a total of 2170 patients showed a benefit of adjuvant chemotherapy for disease-free and OS after 5 years, but only a non-significant trend toward improved survival after 10 years (OR 0.87, $p = 0.12$). A pooled analysis of individual patient data from the two largest adjuvant trials conducted by EORTC using doxorubicin- and ifosfamide-based chemotherapy did not show a survival advantage for postoperative chemotherapy.

Despite many randomized trials, the role of adjuvant chemotherapy remains uncertain and cannot be adopted as the standard of practice for all extremity sarcomas. Although it has been proposed that patients be selected for adjuvant chemotherapy based upon poor prognostic tumor characteristics such as histology (i.e. synovial sarcoma), grade, or size, there is no evidence to date that this approach leads to improved outcome in any subset of patients. The absolute benefit, patient selection, and optimal regimen remain to be defined.

Functional outcome

There are increasing data available on the functional outcome of patients undergoing limb salvage procedures. The majority of patients have good or excellent functional outcome. In 1 series of 88 patients treated with surgery and either pre-operative or post-operative RT, 68 had acceptable functional results and 61 returned to work. Large tumors, neural sacrifice, proximal thigh tumors, and post-operative complications were associated with poor outcome. Subcutaneous tumors have a more favorable functional outcome. In a single institution series of 145 patients who underwent limb-sparing surgery plus post-operative RT completed over 25 years ago, long-term treatment complications included bone fracture in 6%, contracture in 20%, significant edema in 19%, moderate to severe decrease in muscle strength in 20%, requirement for a cane or crutch in 7%, and tissue induration in 57%. Three patients (2%) required amputations for treatment-related complications. The percentage of patients ambulating without assistive devices and with mild or no pain was 84%. Higher doses of RT, a long radiation portal, and irradiation of more than 75% of the extremity diameter were associated with increased complications. Another study examined issues related to quality of life in patients with STS of the lower limb. Although RT was associated with reduced muscle power and range of motion, compared to the use of surgery alone, most patients retained good to excellent limb function and quality of life.

The functional outcome is often not as good in patients requiring amputation. In a matched case-control study of patients with lower extremity sarcoma undergoing amputation ($n = 12$) or a limb-sparing approach ($n = 24$), there was a trend toward increased disability and handicap for those in the amputation group. Seven of the 12 amputees reported ongoing problems with the soft tissue overlying the stump. A few studies have assessed quality of life issues in amputees who had been treated for STS with amputation and chemotherapy compared with patients who underwent limb salvage with radiotherapy and chemotherapy. Contrary to expectations, there were no significant differences in measures of psychological outcome. Thus, a psychological advantage of limb-salvage surgery compared to amputation has yet to be demonstrated.

Treatment of local recurrence

Approximately 10%–15% of patients with extremity STS who are treated with complete resection and adjuvant radiation will develop a local tumor recurrence, the majority within the first 2 years. The approach to the patient with an isolated LR is similar to that for primary disease with some modifications. As with primary treatment, the goal is to provide limb salvage with conservative resection. However, approximately 10%–25% of patients with locally recurrent disease will require amputation. Surgery is an important component of successful salvage therapy. For patients whose primary treatment was surgery alone, re-excision combined with adjuvant radiation is the treatment of choice. If RT was used in primary treatment, further radiation may not be possible because the maximal tolerance for adjacent normal tissues would have to be exceeded, resulting in problems in wound healing and radiation fibrosis, although additional radiation given by BRT (mean dose 47.2 Gy) has been employed in these cases with a 52% local control and a 33% DFS in 1 series of 26 patients.

Optimal treatment for an LR may require both surgery and radiation. This was illustrated in one report of salvage therapy using surgery alone or surgery plus re-irradiation for 25 patients with locally recurrent extremity STS. Eighteen patients underwent surgery alone, 11 were treated by a conservative procedure, and 7 required amputation. Seven of these 18 relapsed. Of the 10 treated with surgery plus radiation, none experienced relapse with a median follow-up of 24 months. Six (60%) experienced significant wound-healing complications, but three recovered completely. Retrospective data from the M.D. Anderson Cancer Center, however, question the role for additional RT in patients previously treated by conservative surgery and radiation. They did not see a difference in local control between those who underwent surgery alone and those who underwent both surgery and radiotherapy, although selection of poorer prognosis cases for radiotherapy may have contributed to the lack of difference between the groups. In addition, 80% of those treated with excision and external beam RT required additional outpatient or surgical management of complications in contrast to only 17% of those treated with excision alone. The predominant delayed complications in the external beam RT group were soft tissue necrosis and edema. Patients resected with positive margins had worse local control. Hence, it is important to try to achieve negative margins with resections of recurrent STSs after prior surgery and radiation. Radiation would certainly be considered for patients with positive margins, but efforts should be made to use techniques to minimize the risk of radiation-associated complications.

Radiotherapy alone

It is worth also reviewing the experience with radiation alone for patients with sarcomas. Radiotherapy alone is used for those patients who, for reasons of anatomical location, medical inoperability, or refusal of any surgery, are not candidates even for a conservative surgical procedure. In 1951 Cade described 22 patients who, for a variety of reasons, were treated by radiation alone.[37] Six survived for 5–26 years. Windeyer et al. described results of radiotherapy alone in fibrosarcoma; of eight patients available for 5-year follow-up, four were free of local disease, although one had required surgery for a recurrence. McNeer et al.[38] reported their analysis of the results of treatment of 653 patients with sarcomas of soft tissue treated at the Memorial Hospital. Of the 653 patients, 25 were treated by radiotherapy alone; 15 of the 25 were surviving at 5 years, and 8 of 20 were surviving at 10 years. Local control was achieved in 14 of the 25 patients.

For small sarcomas, good local control rates can be achieved by radiation alone. However, local control probabilities of >90% for tumors of estimated volume 15–65 mL (approximately a sphere of 3–5 cm in diameter) require high radiation doses (>75 Gy).[39] For unresected sarcomas, higher rates of local control were seen in patients treated to higher dose; with the median dose of 63 Gy chosen as a cutoff, local control was significantly higher with doses above 63 Gy. Smaller tumors are significantly more likely to be controlled than larger lesions; for lesions ≤5 cm, local control of 72% was reported for doses above 63 Gy. Current recommendations for gross disease would be to deliver doses in the range of 75 Gy with shrinking field and highly conformal techniques if possible. If the volume of gross residual disease is large, the late normal tissue changes resulting from these dose levels may be significant.

Treatment of unresectable or locally advanced soft tissue sarcoma

In patients with advanced STS in whom the tumor has progressed beyond surgical resectability, treatment options depend on the site of tumor involvement. For patients with unresectable disease limited to the extremity, ILP protocols have been applied with some success. Selected patients can have their tumors, especially when small, controlled with RT with or without chemotherapy. For patients treated to a dose of 64 Gy or greater, Tepper and Suit noted control of unresected STSs in 87.5% of cases where tumors were less than 5 cm in diameter. Treatment was less effective for larger tumors, with local control falling to 53% for lesions 5–10 cm diameter (53%) and 30% for those greater than 10 cm. Kepka and colleagues updated and expanded this experience, reporting on the efficacy of radiation on 112 patients with unresected STSs. For patients receiving ≥63 Gy, local control at 5 years was 72.4% in patients with lesions ≤5 cm, 42.4% for lesions 5–10 cm in size, and 25.4% for lesions >10 cm.[39]

Management of the retroperitoneal primary lesion

Approximately 10%–15% of STSs arise in the retroperitoneum. These tumors are often asymptomatic and identified on imaging studies for unrelated complaints. In other cases, patients may present with a palpable abdominal mass or with symptoms such as abdominal pain or lower extremity neurological symptoms. Approximately 10%–20% of patients are found to have distant metastases on initial presentation.

In an analysis of 2348 patients with retroperitoneal sarcoma (RPS) in the United States SEER database, the median age of diagnosis was 64 years old and there was roughly an equal incidence among men and women.[40] Owing to the ability of the retroperitoneum to accommodate large tumors, the majority of patients with RPS remain asymptomatic until tumors are quite large. The median size in two recent, large surgical series was 17–18 cm. Patients often present with an asymptomatic abdominal mass or have an incidental retroperitoneal mass identified on radiological imaging. When symptoms do occur, they are caused by mass effect on bowel leading to abdominal discomfort, early satiety, weight loss, or bowel obstruction, compression of the inferior vena cava or iliac veins causing leg swelling, or impingement of nerves causing lower extremity pain or weakness. In 1 series of 500 patients, 80% of patients presented with an abdominal mass, 42% with lower extremity neurologic symptoms, and 37% with pain. On histological examination, approximately two-thirds of tumors are either liposarcomas or leiomyosarcomas, with the remaining tumors distributed among a large variety of histological subtypes. Retroperitoneal liposarcomas are usually classified into well-differentiated, de-differentiated, and myxoid–round cell subtypes. In a large series of retroperitoneal liposarcomas (n = 177), 56% were well-differentiated, 37% de-differentiated, and 7% myxoid–round cell. Approximately 40% of tumors are low-grade and the remaining 60% are intermediate- or high-grade. Low-grade tumors infrequently metastasize, whereas intermediate- and high-grade tumors can metastasize to the lung and liver.

Most unifocal tumors in the retroperitoneum that do not arise from adjacent organs will be either benign soft tissue tumors (e.g. schwannomas) or sarcomas. Other malignancies in the differential diagnosis include primary germ-cell tumor, metastatic testicular cancer, and lymphoma. Following a careful history and physical examination, radiological assessment of these tumors is usually performed with an abdomen and pelvic CT scan. Liposarcomas often have a characteristic appearance, with large areas of abnormal fat (well-differentiated liposarcoma) often containing higher density nodules (de-differentiated liposarcoma). In a study from the M.D. Anderson Cancer Center, CT scan features accurately identified 60 out of 60 (100%) of well-differentiated liposarcomas but was less accurate in determining areas of hypercellular well-differentiated liposarcoma from areas of de-differentiation. Leiomyosarcomas appear as heterogeneous solid tumors. MRI scans may be helpful in delineating tumors from adjacent soft tissues, nerves, or major blood vessels, particularly in the pelvis, but are usually not necessary. To evaluate for metastatic disease, the abdomen CT is adequate in evaluating the liver. Patients with intermediate- and high-grade tumors should have a chest CT to evaluate for lung metastases. A chest X-ray is obtained for low-grade tumors.

The role for image-guided (IG) biopsy of retroperitoneal tumors is somewhat controversial. The advantages of IG biopsy include the high likelihood of establishing a tissue diagnosis and the ability to give pre-operative treatment, if this is being considered. Core needle biopsy of RPS will yield a correct diagnosis of sarcoma in more than 90% of cases although there is lower accuracy in determining the correct histologic subtype and tumor grade. There are theoretical risks of needle track or intraperitoneal seeding of tumor as well as bleeding, but these risks are very low and can be minimized by avoiding a transperitoneal approach.

The primary treatment for the local control of these tumors is surgical resection. The optimal goal of surgical resection is complete gross resection with microscopically negative margins. However, even complete gross resection can be difficult to obtain, and complete gross resection rates in large series are between 54% and 67%. In about three-quarters of cases, complete gross resection requires resection of adjacent viscera. Note that for tumors abutting the kidney, the renal capsule can often be resected rather than formal nephrectomy, given that 75% of kidneys resected in one series showed no renal capsule, parenchyma, or vessel invasion.

The ability to obtain negative microscopic margins for large retroperitoneal tumors is also difficult. These tumors are surrounded by a pseudo-capsule that often contains microscopic disease, and dissection with a normal tissue margin away from the pseudo-capsule is difficult, especially along the posterior aspect of the tumor where it abuts the retroperitoneal fat and musculature. Positive or negative microscopic margin was not a prognostic factor for LR in the largest series of retroperitoneal sarcomas from MSKCC. It is likely that many large retroperitoneal tumors thought to have negative microscopic margins in fact have positive margins in areas not specifically examined under the microscope. Prognostic factors for LR in that series were incomplete gross resection, high grade, and liposarcoma histology.

Surgeons should be wary of attempting surgery if complete surgical resection cannot be performed. In some series, incomplete resection has resulted in the same OS as patients undergoing biopsy alone. However, there may be some role for debulking unresectable RPS in very select circumstances such as for very slow-growing tumors (e.g. well-differentiated liposarcomas) or for the relief of symptoms. Memorial Sloan-Kettering Cancer Center (MSKCC) studied 55 patients with unresectable liposarcomas and found increased survival (26 months versus 4 months) in patients receiving partial resection compared to biopsy alone. The majority of benefit for partial resection was seen in patients with primary disease, and patients undergoing partial resection of LR showed significantly decreased survival compared to after partial resection of primary disease (17 months versus 46 months). Several studies have shown that approximately 75% of patients report symptomatic improvement after palliative surgery. This improvement, however, can be short-lived. One study showed 71% of the patients had symptomatic improvement at 30

days but this fell to 54% by 100 days. Also in this study, palliative operations had a morbidity rate of 29% and mortality rate of 12%. Thus, selection of patients and surgical judgment is critical as these operations are often extensive and may not provide prolonged alleviation of symptoms.

Surgical resection of locally recurrent RPS is generally significantly more difficult than resection for primary disease, and the risk of another LR is even higher than that for primary disease. In studies specifically addressing resection of locally recurrent RPS, rates of complete resection ranged between 44% and 60%, and complete resection was significantly associated with increased survival. Reported 5-year OS after complete resection are between 30% and 46% compared to 27% or less in unresectable patients.

Controversy exists as to the optimal role of RT for local control of retroperitoneal sarcomas. The American College of Surgeons Oncology Group (ACOSOG) was not able to complete a phase III randomized trial of pre-operative radiation and surgery versus surgery alone for retroperitoneal sarcomas. The EORTC is currently conducting a similar trial of 50 Gy pre-operative radiation and surgery versus surgery alone; this study is reported to be accruing well and will hopefully answer the important question of whether there is a role for adjuvant radiotherapy in the management of these tumors. In the meantime, those who advocate RT usually prefer that radiation be delivered pre-operatively. With the tumor still in place, the margin around the tumor at risk of LR is more clearly defined, and the effective radiation dose to control microscopic disease is probably lower.

In a report from Massachusetts General Hospital (MGH), 29 patients were treated with pre-operative radiation to a median dose of 45 Gy and then underwent complete gross resection.[41] Intraoperative radiation 10–20 Gy was delivered to 16 patients and no IORT was delivered to 13 patients. Local control at 5 years was 83% for patients who received both pre-operative radiation and IORT and 61% for those who received only pre-operative radiation. Significant toxicity from IORT occurred in four patients and included neuropathy, ureteral stricture, and vaginal fistula. More recently, the MGH group incorporated the use of pre-operative IMRT or proton beam RT along with resection and IORT for retroperitoneal tumors and has found these techniques allow dose escalation to areas at risk while decreasing dose to adjacent organs at risk. Among 28 patients treated with these techniques, 20 patients had primary tumors and 8 had recurrent tumors. Tumors were large (median size 9.75 cm), primarily liposarcomas and leiomyosarcomas (71%), and were mostly of intermediate or high grade (81%). Proton beam RT or IMRT were delivered to all patients, preferably pre-operatively (75%), to a median dose of 50 Gy. Surgical resection included up to five adjacent organs, most commonly the colon ($n = 7$) and kidney ($n = 7$). Margins were positive for disease, usually posteriorly, in 15 patients (54%). IORT was delivered to the posterior margin in 12 patients (43%) to a median dose of 11 Gy. Surgical complications occurred in 8 patients (28.6%), and radiation-related complications in 4 patients (14%). After a median follow-up of 33 months, only 2 patients (10%) with primary disease experienced LR, while 3 patients (37.5%) with recurrent disease experienced LR.

In the extremity, the local control of sarcomas treated with RT and total gross resection with positive microscopic margins is approximately 75%. Typically, positive microscopic margins are treated with a boost of post-operative radiation to a total dose of approximately 66–68 Gy. It seems reasonable to assume that total gross resection of retroperitoneal tumors along with adequate doses of radiation could achieve local control rates similar to those seen for extremity tumors resected with positive microscopic margins. The availability of intensity-modulated RT techniques, proton beam radiation, and IORT may facilitate the efficacy and minimize morbidity of adjuvant RT for the retroperitoneal tumors and translate into improved local control.

An innovative strategy combines IMRT with a novel target volume concept for the pre-operative treatment of retroperitoneal STS. IMRT was used to deliver RT (50 Gy in 25 daily 2 Gy fractions) to a pre-operative CTV that was limited to the contact area between the tumor mass and the posterior abdominal wall.[42] All 18 patients completed the planned treatment with acceptable acute toxicity and underwent successful resection without major complications. With early follow-up (median 27 months), only two patients failed locally and one developed distant metastases. The authors concluded that this strategy was feasible, well-tolerated, and associated with better radiation sparing of critical structures, without compromising the rate of resectability. Longer follow-up is needed to assess the ultimate impact on local control and survival. Tzeng et al. were able to perform selective pre-operative radiation dose escalation to the retroperitoneal margin of a retroperitoneal sarcoma in 16 patients using IMRT to deliver 45 Gy in 25 fractions (1.8 Gy per fraction) to the entire tumor, and 57.5 Gy in 25 fractions (2.3 Gy per fraction) to the boosted retroperitoneal margin. Treatment morbidity was acceptable and the actuarial 2-year local control rate was 80%. Further dose escalation to the high-risk posterior retroperitoneal margin with either IMRT or intensity-modulated protons is currently being tested in an ongoing phase I/II clinical trial involving investigators from MGH, University of Pennsylvania, and the RTOG.

Treatment of metastatic soft tissue sarcoma

Overview

Metastatic disease rarely occurs in patients with low-grade sarcomas but occurs at an appreciable frequency in patients with high-grade sarcomas that is related to grade and size.[43] With intermediate- or high-grade sarcomas, this risk may exceed 50% when the tumor is larger than 10 cm. For extremity sarcomas, the lung is the most common site of metastatic disease. Some histologies, notably myxoid liposarcoma, which can metastasize to abdominal sites and bone, and epithelioid sarcomas, which manifest regional nodal failure, are exceptions to the more general pattern. Although most patients with metastatic sarcoma will ultimately die from their tumor, a modest proportion of patients will be long-term survivors after management with surgery or chemotherapy. Figure 27.1 outlines the current optimal care algorithm for patients with metastatic STS.

Resection of pulmonary metastases

The median survival of patients with pulmonary metastases is in the range of 15 months. Patients whose lung metastases can be resected fare better than those with unresectable metastases. In one series, patients treated with resection had a median survival after complete resection of 33 months. Their 3-year actuarial survival rate was 46%, with a 5-year actuarial survival rate of 37%. The patients who did not undergo resection had a median survival of 11 months and a 3-year actuarial survival rate of 17%.

Patients to be considered for pulmonary resection are medically fit with controlled primary tumors without pleural effusion or hilar disease. The procedure generally involves wedge resections of the nodules. Patients with a limited number of nodules fare better, but there is no consensus on the upper limit

of nodules that should be considered for resection. The role for additional adjuvant chemotherapy after resection is not settled. A subset of patients may benefit from repeat thoracotomy for recurrent disease in the chest. There are reports of resection of isolated metastatic disease in liver and other extra-pulmonic sites as well. Stereotactic body radiotherapy has been reported to successfully treat lung metastases in 86% of patients at 2 years.[44]

Chemotherapy for metastatic disease

For most patients with metastatic disease that is not resectable, treatment with chemotherapy is likely to be palliative in outcome. A small number of patients will be long-term survivors. An analysis of 1888 patients treated on studies organized by the Soft Tissue and Bone Sarcoma Group of the EORTC reported 88 5-year survivors, which translates to an 8% 5-year survival rate.[45]

Doxorubicin and ifosfamide have been demonstrated to be the most active chemotherapy agents in widely disseminated STS. For doxorubicin, objective response rates between 20% and 40% for the single agent have been reported; few are CRs and response duration averages 8 months. A steep dose–response curve for objective responses has been described. Epirubicin has similar structure and clinical features. There is also a dose–response for ifosfamide. Dacarbazine (DTIC) by itself has a modest response rate of approximately 16%. The related compound, temozolomide, has similar activity. Cyclophosphamide appears less active in adults than in children and less active than the related compound ifosfamide. Gemcitabine with or without a taxane is active in a subset of patients with sarcomas. Angiosarcoma of the scalp and face may respond to paclitaxel. A pegylated liposomal formulation of doxorubicin has activity against sarcomas. Gemcitabine has been shown to have modest single-agent activity in previously treated patients, as does vinorelbine. Studies have shown a 24% 6-month disease progression control rate using trabectidin, ecteinascidin-743, in patients with advanced pre-treated sarcoma. Other less active agents include methotrexate, topotecan, carboplatin, bendamustine, and cisplatin. Pazopanib and sunitinib are expensive and have only modest activity, but are oral agents with usually mild toxicity. Bevacizumab and sorafenib[46] are under study as are many targeted agents including mammalian target of rapamycin (MTOR) inhibitors, anti-insulin-like growth factor 1 receptor (IGF-1R) antibody, and newer agents such as brostacillin and eribulin.

Many combination chemotherapy regimens for metastatic disease have been studied in phase II trials. Most of these trials include doxorubicin (or epirubicin) and an alkylating agent. Adding dacarbazine to doxorubicin improved the response rate to 41% but the response rate has decreased over time. Randomized trials found some gain for the combination. A Southwest Oncology Group (SWOG) phase III trial compared bolus versus infusional administration of doxorubicin plus dacarbazine and reported no differences in overall response (17% in both arms) or CRs (5% in both arms). Additionally, there was no difference in the median survival, 10.5 months in both groups. Adding cyclophosphamide to the basic duo was reported to raise the response rate to 56%[47] and this was confirmed by a randomized trial. Comparisons have shown that the addition of less active drugs necessitates lower doses of doxorubicin and, accordingly, reduces overall effectiveness.

ECOG conducted a three-arm trial comparing doxorubicin alone, doxorubicin plus ifosfamide, and mitomycin plus doxorubicin plus cisplatin. Objective tumor regression occurred more frequently in the combination arms than in the single-agent arm. However, the combination regimens resulted in significantly

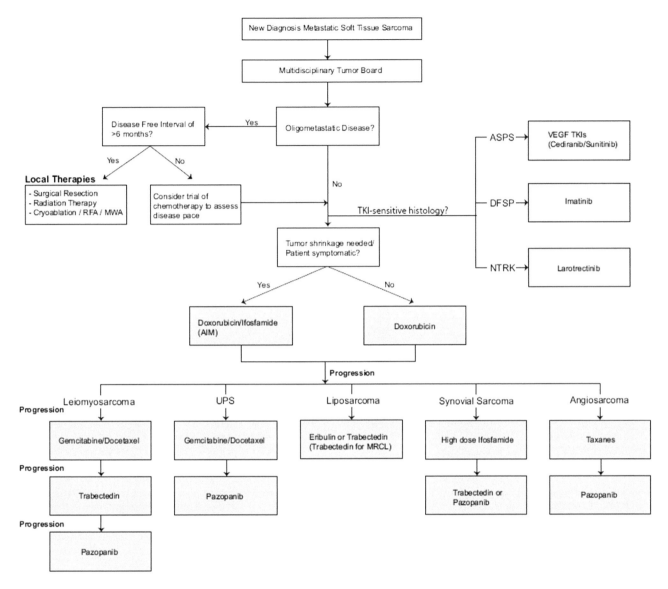

FIGURE 27.1 Treatment algorithm for metastatic soft tissue sarcomas. (From Bui et al., 2019. With permission.)

greater myelosuppression. Most notably, no significant survival differences were observed between the three treatment regimens.

A popular regimen adds ifosfamide to doxorubicin and dacarbazine and has resulted in response rates in measurable metastatic sarcomas as high as 47% with CR rates as high as 10%. The combination of just the most active agents uses doxorubicin (or epirubicin) and adds higher doses of ifosfamide. Another protocol describes activity with DTIC and cisplatin in pretreated patients. Uterine leiomyosarcoma may respond to high-dose gemcitabine with docetaxel. Gemcitabine plus vinorelbine or dacarbazine are milder combinations. Although the response rates and progression-free survival rates may be improved, in the absence of any clear benefit for the combination regimens, some clinicians favor initiation of chemotherapy with single-agent doxorubicin.

Dose intensity may be important. Very high-dose ifosfamide had been used with high response rates despite some toxicity. Higher-dose therapy with standard agents may require special supportive care such as bone marrow transplantation, but may offer a chance for higher CR rates and longer response duration. Considerable interest has been focused on maintaining dose intensity of chemotherapy using colony-stimulating factors to

alleviate myelosuppression. Granulocyte–macrophage colony-stimulating factor (GM-CSF) or G-CSF has been used with a variety of regimens to help maintain dose intensification. In a few studies this has resulted in improved response rates. Even higher-dose chemotherapy, as used at M.D. Anderson, seems to result in higher response rates (59%–69%). Attempts to intensify treatment by increasing the dose of doxorubicin in combination with ifosfamide, although promising in phase II studies, were not confirmed in a subsequent randomized trial compared with the standard doses.[48] High-dose therapy with growth factor support has been evaluated in several investigational studies but the data to date demonstrate increased toxicity without clear evidence of therapeutic gain, so this is still considered investigational treatment.

Although the foregoing generalizations apply to most STSs, different histologic subtypes of sarcomas display their own patterns of chemosensitivity. Myxoid/round cell liposarcomas appear sensitive to doxorubicin and to trabectedin. Synovial sarcoma has a strong dose response to ifosfamide. Non-uterine leiomyosarcomas appear to have lower response rates to doxorubicin and ifosfamide, but may respond to trabectedin.

Angiosarcomas are almost unique in being sensitive to paclitaxel. Rhabdomyosarcoma, desmoplastic small round cell tumors, and peripheral neuroectodermal tumors respond to combinations that include ifosfamide, etoposide, vincristine, doxorubicin, dactinomycin cyclophosphamide, and topotecan/irinotecan. Sunitinib has proven useful against solitary fibrous tumor/ hemangiopericytoma, alveolar soft part sarcoma, and clear cell sarcoma. Everolimus has activity against tumors with perivascular epithelioid cell differentiation. Imatinib can help in metastatic dermatofibroma protuberans. Cediranib is effective against alveolar soft part sarcoma. Crizotinib is active against ALK translocated inflammatory myofibroblastic tumor. Bevacizumab with temozolomide has been employed for solitary fibrous tumor.

Management of gastrointestinal stromal tumors

GISTs are the most common mesenchymal tumor of the gastrointestinal tract and are thought to differentiate along the lines of the interstitial cells of Cajal. These cells are thought to act as pacemaker cells, and have immunohistochemical and electron microscopy features of both neuronal and smooth muscle cells. Interstitial cells of Cajal and the vast majority of GISTs express KIT, which is a 145 kD trans-membrane glycoprotein that acts at the receptor for stem cell factor (SCF). Before the identification and availability of immunohistochemistry for KIT, the majority of GISTs were thought to be of smooth muscle origin and termed leiomyomas, leiomyosarcomas, and leiomyoblastomas. Ninety-five per cent of GISTs stain positive on immunohistochemistry for KIT, and approximately 80% of GISTs have a mutation in the KIT gene. A minority of GISTs have mutations in platelet-derived growth factor α (PDGFRα). Approximately 75% of the KIT gene mutations occur in exon 11, which codes for the intracellular juxtamembrane domain, and less commonly in exons 9, 13, and 17. KIT mutation results in spontaneous receptor dimerization and activation. Unlike most other solid cancers, most GISTs are highly dependent on the KIT pathway for neoplastic growth. The best guidelines are those of ESMO.[49]

GISTs can occur at nearly all ages, with the median age being approximately 60 years. The incidence is roughly equal in men and women. The tumors are located most commonly in the stomach (60%) followed by the small intestine (30%), colon/rectum (5%), and esophagus (5%). Many tumors are found on upper endoscopy, where they appear as submucosal lesions. However, even large GISTs of the stomach may not be seen on endoscopy if they are pedunculated or exophytic. Endoscopic biopsy can establish the diagnosis, especially following staining for KIT expression. For small bowel tumors, CT-guided biopsy poses the risk of inadequate tissue and spillage of tumor cells and is probably not necessary given that most isolated small bowel tumors require resection. Staging workup should include abdomen and pelvis CT scan to rule out intra-abdominal or liver metastases. GISTs are usually strongly positive on PET scans, and thus PET scans can be a valuable study for excluding metastatic disease as well as evaluating response to medical therapy such as imatinib.

Surgical resections of GISTs need to address tumors that can range from small, pedunculated lesions to large lesions with adherence or invasion of surrounding tissues and organs. Thus the surgical approach can be quite varied but certain principles should be followed. Upon surgical exploration, the liver and peritoneal cavity should be examined for possible metastatic disease. GISTs uncommonly metastasize to lymph nodes so a regional lymphadenectomy is not required. Thus, for a pedunculated

gastric tumor, wedge resection of the gastric wall along with resection of the tumor is adequate. Some gastric tumors encompass a large portion of the stomach and a formal distal, subtotal, or even total gastrectomy may be required. For small bowel and colon tumors, segmental bowel resection can be performed. Small rectal GISTs can be removed through transanal procedures whereas larger tumors may require low anterior resection or even abdominal-perineal resection. Some large GISTs with significant necrosis are susceptible to tumor rupture and spillage, which can lead to intra-peritoneal spread of disease, so tumors should be manipulated carefully.

The most common sites of GIST metastases are the liver and peritoneal cavity, and the risk of recurrence is most closely related to size and mitotic count. Before the introduction of imatinib, GIST were found to be highly resistant to chemotherapeutic agents. Imatinib inhibits both the KIT receptor and PDGFRα tyrosine kinases. Several large studies have shown imatinib to be highly effective against metastatic GIST, with a PR rate of approximately 40% and stable disease rate of approximately 30%. Given the efficacy of imatinib in treating metastatic GISTs, there has been significant interest in the use of imatinib in the adjuvant setting. The ACOSOG recently completed a phase II study of adjuvant imatinib for 1 year for patients with resected high-risk tumors (size >10 cm, tumor rupture). After a median follow-up of 4 years, the 1-, 2-, and 3-year relapse-free survivals were 94%, 73%, and 61%.[50] Another ACOSOG trial randomized patients with resected GISTs >3 cm to imatinib for 1 year or placebo. At a median follow-up of 20 months, 30 patients in the imatinib group recurred or died, versus 70 in the placebo group (8% versus 20%). The 1-year RFS rate was 98% versus 83% favoring imatinib, with a HR for RFS of 0.35, 95% CI 0.22–0.5. Given patients with relapse were subsequently allowed to take imatinib, this study found no difference in OS between groups. The Intergroup EORTC 62024 trial randomized over 900 patients with intermediate- or high-risk GIST to 2 years of imatinib or observation alone. In the first interim analysis after a median follow-up of 4.7 years, 3-year RFS was 84% versus 66% respectively and nearly all patients (99%–100%) were alive at 5 years. The SSG XVIII trial randomized 400 high-risk patients to 36 versus 12 months of adjuvant imatinib. Five-year recurrence-free survival (65.6% versus 47.9%) and 5-year OS (92.0% versus 81.7%) were both improved in the 36-month group. Thus many GIST experts recommend 3 years of adjuvant imatinib for intermediate- or high-risk patients.

Tumors with an exon 11 mutation have higher response rates to imatinib than tumors with other KIT mutations including wild-type. The median time to progression is 19–24 months. Even tumors that are sensitive to imatinib may take months to show a decrease in tumor size on CT scans, and so PET scans have been employed to assess response. GIST are usually positive on PET scans, and response to imatinib as demonstrated by decrease in PET activity can frequently be seen immediately (within days) after initiation of therapy. Two randomized trials have failed to show significantly greater efficacy for 800 mg of imatinib compared to 400 mg daily. However, in subgroup analysis, patients whose tumor has a KIT exon 9 mutation may benefit from higher doses of imatinib.

Treatment for advanced GIST that is refractory or has become resistant to imatinib includes sunitinib, regorafenib, and nilotinib. An international phase III trial of sunitinib versus placebo was performed in 312 patients with refractory disease. Patients demonstrating progression on placebo were allowed to cross over to the active treatment arm. At a median follow-up of 42 months, the primary endpoint of median time to tumor progression was 27 weeks versus 4 weeks, favoring the sunitinib group. Regorafenib was examined in a phase III trial in which 199 patients who were refractory to or intolerant of sunitinib were randomly assigned to best supportive care plus either regorafenib (160 mg once daily for 3 of every 4 weeks) or placebo. Regorafenib was associated with significantly better progression-free survival of 4.8 versus 0.9 months. In a phase III trial of 248 patients with advanced GIST who had failed imatinib and sunitinib, progression-free survival was significantly longer in the nilotinib group when the analysis was based on local investigator assessment (median 119 versus 70 days), but not when it was based on blinded central radiology review (median 109 versus 111 days).[51]

Desmoid tumors

Introduction

Desmoid tumors are deep-seated, benign, slowly growing fibro-blastic neoplasms that arise from musculo-aponeurotic stromal elements. Although they are locally aggressive, desmoids do not have the capacity to establish metastatic lesions. Nevertheless, tumor-related destruction of vital structures or organs can be fatal.

Epidemiology

Desmoid tumors are uncommon. The estimated incidence in the general population is 2–4 per million inhabitants per year, which in the United States translates into approximately 900 new tumors annually. Individuals between the ages of 15 and 60 are most often affected; desmoids are rare in the young and in the elderly. They are slightly more common in women than in men, and there is no significant racial or ethnic distribution.

The incidence of desmoids is higher in patients with familial adenomatous polyposis (FAP), affecting from 4% to 20% of patients. The simultaneous appearance of FAP and desmoid tumors was described by Gardner in 1951 and is now designated as Gardner's syndrome. Until early elective colectomy became routine in patients with FAP, the dominant cause of death in these patients was carcinoma of the colon. With the increasing use of prophylactic colectomy, desmoid tumors have become an important cause of morbidity and, in some instances, mortality.

Pathology

Desmoids tend to be large bulky tumors that lack pseudo-encapsulation and locally infiltrate adjacent tissue structures. Histologically, they are characterized by uniform spindle fibro-blasts arranged in broad sweeping fascicles in a collagenous stroma. Mitotic activity is variable, and necrosis is absent.

Etiology and pathogenesis

The etiology of desmoid tumors is unknown. However, the identification of clonal chromosomal changes in a significant fraction of cases supports the neoplastic nature of these tumors, and emerging evidence implicates dysregulated wound healing in the pathogenesis of these and other fibroblastic lesions.

Non-random clonal chromosomal changes, particularly trisomy 8 or 20, occur in one-third or more of sporadic desmoid tumors. Similar non-random genetic aberrations have been found in benign fibrous bone lesions (such as fibrous dysplasia), suggesting a similar pathogenesis. Although the clinical relevance of these genetic abnormalities is unclear, their presence appears to be associated with a higher risk of recurrence. As an example, in

one report, trisomy 8 or trisomy 20 was observed in cells cultured from 6 of 13 desmoid tumors. FISH analysis performed on the nuclei from 25 desmoid tumors from paraffin blocks or frozen tissue indicated that LR was more likely in desmoids with trisomy. Among patients followed for more than 1 year, LR was more frequent in tumors with trisomy 8 (4 of 6, as compared to 2 of 17 recurrences in trisomy 8-negative tumors). The finding of individual trisomies and their association in the same cell is rare in solid tumors, particularly mesenchymal tumors. However, these aberrations are known to occur in related benign, fibrous lesions arising in both soft tissue and bone tumors (e.g. Dupuytren's contracture, plantar fibrosis, Peyronie's disease, carpal tunnel syndrome, and infantile fibrosarcoma). Trisomy 8 is also a frequent finding in hematological malignances but is remarkably infrequent in non-fibrous solid tumors.

Gardner's syndrome

Gardner's syndrome is a variant of familial adenomatous polyposis (FAP) that is distinguished by the presence of prominent extra-intestinal lesions, such as desmoid tumors, osteomas, and cysts. When these occur in any member of an FAP family, the family has traditionally been said to have Gardner's syndrome rather than FAP, because all members of the family segregate the same mutation in the adenomatous polyposis coli (*APC*) gene. Desmoids may be the first manifestation of Gardner's syndrome. Families have also been reported that exhibit desmoids as the only manifestation of an *APC* mutation.

The estimated risk of developing a desmoid tumor in patients with FAP is between 4% and 20%. They have a particular predilection for surgical sites (e.g. the mesentery or abdominal wall following colectomy, the site of an ileal pouch–anal anastomosis). In one series, prior abdominal surgery had been performed in 68% of patients with FAP and abdominal desmoid tumors; lesions develop within 5 years after surgery in approximately one-half. One patient dramatically demonstrated this association with surgery. She had been treated, apparently successfully, with chemotherapy for an intra-abdominal desmoid tumor. To confirm the response, laparoscopy was performed. Within months, desmoid tumors began developing in each of the three trocar sites; the tumors became massive and inoperable and led to the death of the patient.

APC mutations and beta-catenin

Mutations of the *APC* gene on chromosome 5q are responsible for FAP. More than 300 mutations have been described, most of which lead to frame shifts or premature stop codons, resulting in a truncated *APC* gene product. Several studies have attempted to correlate specific *APC* mutations with the clinical phenotype. As a general rule, mutations between codons 169 and 1393 are associated with the classic form of FAP whereas mutations that are more 3′ or 5′ are associated with the attenuated form of FAP.

The site of the germ-line mutation in patients with FAP may be important for the risk of developing a desmoid tumor. Mutations between codons 1445 and 1578 have been associated with desmoid tumors in some reports, although others have not found this association.

How the abnormal gene promotes the formation of tumors such as desmoids is incompletely understood. However, increasing evidence points to involvement of germ-line *APC* mutations in the molecular pathogenesis of desmoids in patients with Gardner's syndrome. The normal APC protein prevents the accumulation of beta-catenin, a cytosolic and nuclear protein, by mediating its phosphorylation and resultant degradation. The loss of the beta-catenin regulatory domain in the truncated protein allows beta-catenin to accumulate, bind to, and activate the transcription factor Tcf-4.

In contrast, *APC* mutations are uncommon in sporadic desmoids, which usually arise from mutations in the gene for beta-catenin, *CTNNB1*. Mutations in *CTNNB1* have been found in sporadic desmoid tumors with variable prevalence (39%–87%); however, larger and more recent studies place the prevalence estimate at approximately 85%. *CTNNB1* gene mutations are therefore the most common route of Wnt pathway activation in desmoids. Phosphorylation of beta-catenin is mediated by a portion of the protein encoded by exon 3 of *CTNNB1* gene. Three specific mutations are encountered in desmoid tumors: T41A, S45F, and S45P. At least some data suggest that S45F mutations are associated with a higher rate of recurrence after surgical resection of a primary desmoid tumor.[52] It is hoped that the elucidation of the central role of beta-catenin in the pathogenesis of desmoid tumors will lead to future therapeutic advances targeting this molecule.

Trauma and pregnancy

Up to 30% of patients with desmoid tumors have a history that involves antecedent trauma, particularly surgical trauma, in patients with FAP (see earlier). A similar relationship has been observed in some sporadically occurring desmoid tumors. In one series, an antecedent history of trauma at the tumor site was elicited in 28% of 32 primary desmoid tumors.

Abdominal desmoids tend to occur in women during or following pregnancy. The classic presentation is that of an abdominal mass that is separate from the uterus. Trauma related to pregnancy and exposure to elevated hormone levels may both be contributory. As an example, one case report describes a desmoid tumor that developed at the site of a prior caesarean section scar during a subsequent pregnancy. Subsequent pregnancy is not necessarily a risk factor for recurrence or development of new disease in a woman who develops a pregnancy-related desmoid.

Clinical presentation

Most desmoid tumors present as a painless or minimally painful mass with a history of slow growth. Intra-abdominal desmoids can be associated with intestinal obstruction, mucosal ischemia, or functional deterioration in an ileo-anal anastomosis (typically in a patient who has undergone colectomy for FAP).

Desmoid tumors can develop at virtually any body site; they most commonly arise in the torso (shoulder girdle and hip–buttock region) and the extremities. The location is usually deep in the muscles or along fascial planes. Desmoid tumors may be multi-focal on an extremity, but they rarely occur in different regions in the same patient.

Diagnosis

Ultrasound is often the first method of examination of a soft tissue lesion on the torso or extremity. If the mass is solid, CT or MRI is needed to determine adherence to adjacent structures and resectability. Although desmoids can be adequately evaluated by CT, MRI is preferred for definition of the pattern and extent of involvement. There are no radiographic characteristics that can reliably distinguish desmoids from malignant soft tissue tumors. The diagnosis of a desmoid tumor can only be established by histological examination of a biopsy specimen. Core needle biopsy can establish the diagnosis in the majority of cases. There is no accepted staging system for desmoid tumors.

Natural history

Although benign, desmoid tumors are locally infiltrative and can be fatal by causing destruction of adjacent vital structures and organs. In a report of 138 patients managed at one institution between 1965 and 1984, 11 died of their disease. Factors associated with a poor outcome in this study were: Age 18–30 years, presentation with locally recurrent disease, incomplete excision, and no post-operative RT. However, this series may not be representative as many patients had advanced disease at the time of diagnosis. Other centers report an overall mortality rate <1% in patients with desmoid tumors at other than intra-abdominal sites. Indeed, spontaneous regression has been reported in patients who have initially been observed and managed expectantly following the diagnosis. Thus, even though desmoids are benign in the sense that they cannot produce distant metastases, the disease process may be devastating, and occasionally fatal. Fortunately, the pace of progression is usually relatively slow, with periods of comparative stability or even temporary regression. Re-growth is not an inevitable consequence even following grossly incomplete surgical resection.

Treatment

Because of the unpredictable nature of desmoid tumors, including the potential for spontaneous regression, the management strategy in recent years has evolved towards initial observation of patients following the diagnosis, reserving surgery or other interventions until they cause symptoms, if there is imminent risk to adjacent structures, or if they create cosmetic concerns.

Observation

Desmoids have an unpredictable clinical course, and close observation is an acceptable strategy for stable, asymptomatic primary, or recurrent desmoids, particularly if resection would entail major morbidity. In one series of 142 patients presenting with a primary (*n* = 74) or recurrent (*n* = 68), 83 were treated with observation only, whereas 59 were initially offered medical therapy (hormone therapy or chemotherapy).[53] The 5-year progression-free survival rate was 50% versus 41% for the observation and medically treated patients, respectively.

Consensus-based guidelines from the National Comprehensive Cancer Network (NCCN) suggest that patients with desmoid tumors can be followed carefully if the tumors are small and not located on the trunk, and if surgery would lead to excessive morbidity. Treatment of an extra-abdominal desmoid is indicated, as noted earlier, for symptomatic patients and patients with progressively enlarging tumors irrespective of symptoms.

Surgery

Because of their locally infiltrative nature, desmoid tumors are treated by surgical resection with a wide margin when medically and technically feasible. Because these are benign tumors, the treatment strategy should be to obtain tumor-free margins using function-preserving approaches to minimize major morbidity (functional or cosmetic). Extra-abdominal and abdominal wall desmoids are more often resectable than are intra-abdominal tumors. Surgery may be difficult and even impossible for intra-abdominal desmoids, although it may be an important option for selected patients. Medical therapy may be considered as a first-line option, particularly for tumors that involve the mesentery or encase vessels and organs.

Despite their benign character, desmoid tumors have a high rate of recurrence with surgery alone. Even patients who undergo aggressive resection with wide margins have recurrence rates of 23%–39%. When they recur, salvage therapy with RT or repeat excision is usually successful. Intra-abdominal desmoids that arise in the setting of Gardner's syndrome have a greater tendency for LR and multiple lesions. Moreover, they may be relatively refractory to RT and may be rendered more aggressive after surgical intervention. This has led some clinicians to advocate conservative management with non-cytotoxic therapy as opposed to resection or RT in these patients, although this is controversial.

Importance of resection margins

The available data are conflicting with regard to the importance of complete resection. Some authors report that the risk of recurrence is independent of margin status, whereas others demonstrate higher recurrence rates with close or positive resection margins. As an example, in one series of 203 patients undergoing surgery for either primary or recurrent desmoid tumors over a 35-year period, margins were microscopically positive in 57 and negative in 146. As expected, the DFS rate was significantly better in patients with primary disease (76% versus 59% at 10 years), but it was not significantly worse for those with microscopically positive versus negative margins at primary surgery (5-year DFS rate for those with positive and negative margins, 79% versus 82%; at 10 years, 74% versus 77%). These data have led some to conclude that aggressive attempts to achieve negative resection margins are not warranted if they result in excessive morbidity.[54] Moreover, uncertainty as to the importance of positive resection margins has led to controversy with regard to the utility of post-operative RT for patients with incompletely resected disease.

Radiation therapy

RT is an effective primary therapeutic option for patients who are not good surgical candidates, those who decline surgery, and those for whom surgical morbidity would be excessive. The time to regression after RT alone is often quite long, and several years may elapse before regression is complete. In a number of reports, RT alone (50–60 Gy) or combined with surgery in patients with positive resection margins achieves long-term control in approximately 70%–80% of desmoids. The volume of disease does not appear to affect the probability of local control. In a comparative review of published experience with treatment of desmoid tumors, local control rates after surgery alone (n = 381) were 61% overall and were 72% and 41% for those with negative or positive margins, respectively. For patients undergoing surgery plus RT (n = 297), the local control rate was 75% overall, and it was 94% and 75% for cases with negative and positive margins, respectively. The overall local control rate for RT alone (n = 102) was 78%, and was 83% and 73% for those treated for primary or recurrent tumors, respectively. Consistent with these results, the EORTC recently reported a prospective trial of RT in 44 patients with inoperable primary, recurrent, or incompletely resected desmoid tumors. Fifty-six Gy was delivered at 2 Gy per fraction, and at 3 years the local control was 81.5%.[55]

The recommended dose of RT for definitive therapy is 50–58 Gy in 6–7 weeks at 1.8–2 Gy per fraction. LR rates do not appear to be reduced by the use of higher doses. In one study, for example, 23 patients were treated with RT for unresectable disease; the relapse rate at 5 years was 31%. Radiation doses above 56 Gy did not improve outcome, and were associated with more complications (30% versus 5% with lower doses at 15 years). Positive resection margins were not an adverse prognostic factor in this report.

Post-operative radiation therapy

Post-operative RT is generally not recommended for patients with uninvolved resection margins. The benefit of post-operative RT for those with positive resection margins is controversial. As noted previously, the status of the resection margins has not been shown to significantly increase the risk of recurrence in several retrospective series. Furthermore, even in those series that did show a higher rate of recurrence in patients with positive margins in the absence of RT, successful salvage therapy at the time of recurrence has been possible in the majority of patients. From these data, many clinicians conclude that LF is not inevitable if residual tumor is left in situ. Deferring radiation is an acceptable option for patients with microscopically positive margins as long as local progression, if it occurred, would not risk significant morbidity. Post-operative irradiation is generally recommended for microscopically positive margins after resection of recurrent disease and for patients with gross or macroscopic residual disease, although some others recommend earlier use of radiation for incompletely resected disease.

Neoadjuvant therapy

An aggressive approach to reducing the rate of LR is the use of neoadjuvant (pre-operative) chemoradiotherapy. In one small series, 13 patients with potentially resectable desmoid tumors received doxorubicin 30 mg by continuous infusion daily for 3 days concurrent with RT (10 × 3 Gy), with resection performed 4–6 weeks later. With a median follow-up of 71 months, there were only two LRs (15%). Although these results are promising, this is not a standard approach and confirmation with a larger, prospective, ideally randomized trial would be needed before this approach could be more widely employed.

Systemic therapy

Patients with desmoid tumors have been treated with a variety of agents, including non-steroidal anti-inflammatory drugs (NSAIDs), hormone manipulation, IFN, cytotoxic chemotherapy, targeted agents including imatinib, and other tyrosine kinase inhibitors including sorafenib and pirfenidone (5-methyl-1-phenyl-2-[1H]-pyridone), an anti-fibroblast agent. Most of the reported data come from isolated case reports, limiting the conclusions that can be drawn as to the relative effectiveness of these agents in the treatment of desmoid tumors.

Non-cytotoxic systemic therapy

Clinical and experimental evidence suggests a hormone dependency of desmoid growth. Particularly in patients who do not have good options for surgery or radiation, treatment is often begun with a hormonal agent such as tamoxifen, the anti-estrogen toremifene, raloxifene, or progestational agents. An objective response is reported in approximately 50% of patients, mostly partial rather than complete. Response durations range from 7 months to 12 years.[56] The mechanism underlying this benefit is unclear because responses to tamoxifen have been seen in desmoids that do not express hormone receptors.

There are also documented responses as high as 70% reported with combined therapy; although regression is usually partial and may take many months after an initial period of tumor enlargement. In one report, 10 of 13 patients with FAP-associated desmoids responded to daily tamoxifen (120 mg daily) and sulindac (300 mg daily), as did 2 of 8 recurrent sporadic tumors.

The contribution of tamoxifen to these results is unclear. At least one report documents the resolution of a desmoid tumor being treated with indomethacin and ascorbic acid for 14 months.

NSAIDs alone represent a potentially attractive treatment option, particularly since they also appear to protect against colon cancer.

Several case reports describe objective response or prolonged periods of disease stabilization with IFN-alpha, in some cases following failure of sulindac and tamoxifen.

Multiple reports now suggest clinical and radiographic benefit from the tyrosine kinase inhibitor imatinib, an effect that is presumably due to tumor expression of activated receptor tyrosine kinases KIT or platelet-derived growth factor receptor (PDGFR). In a large multi-institutional phase II trial of 51 patients (45 evaluable), patients were dosed with imatinib based on body surface area (BSA), with patients ≥1.5 m² receiving 300 mg twice daily, patients 1–1.49 m² receiving 200 mg twice daily, and those <1 m² receiving 100 mg twice daily. Forty-three (84%) reached the primary endpoint defining clinical benefit (a complete or PR within 16 weeks, or stable disease lasting at least 16 weeks). Three patients had an objective PR. The progression-free survival rate at 3 years was 58%, and 5 patients remained progression-free after 4+ years of treatment.

Benefit for imatinib was also shown in a French Sarcoma Group trial in which 40 patients failing local treatment (and with documented evidence of progressive disease) received imatinib 400 mg per day (increased to 800 mg/day in the event of progression).[57] Of 35 evaluable patients at 3 months, there was 1 complete and 3 PRs, 28 had stable disease, and 3 patients progressed. The non-progression rates at 6, 9, and 12 months were 80%, 69%, and 67%, respectively. Among patients who developed progressive disease while receiving 400 mg daily, dose escalation resulted in stabilization of disease for a median time of 12 months (range 2–30 months), but eventually resulted in progression in 8 out of 10 patients. Sorafenib has become the preferred tyrosine kinase inhibitor for use in these patients.[58]

Cytotoxic chemotherapy

Chemotherapy may be effective in patients with unresectable tumors that are refractory to tamoxifen or sulindac. Low doses of methotrexate and vinblastine produce worthwhile response rates, particularly in children. In one report of 30 patients (age range 4–68 years, median 27), weekly methotrexate (30 mg/m²) and vinblastine (6 mg/m²) for between 4 months and 20 months resulted in a PR in 12 (40%), and 18 others had stable disease or a minor response with symptomatic relief.[59] The 10-year progression-free survival was 67%. The combination of methotrexate and vinorelbine may produce a similar clinical benefit with less neurotoxicity.

Liposomal doxorubicin may also be a useful agent. More aggressive doxorubicin- or ifosfamide-based regimens are not only more active, but also more toxic; thus, they are usually reserved for cases that are refractory to other therapies. In one of the largest published series, 11 patients received doxorubicin (60–90 mg/m²) plus dacarbazine (750–1000 mg/m²) for a median of five cycles.[60] Six of nine evaluable patients had an objective response (two complete, four partial). One complete responder died whereas the remainder were alive and progression-free.

Others have demonstrated activity in patients with FAP-associated desmoids using 4–5 cycles of an infusional regimen of doxorubicin (20 mg/m² daily) plus dacarbazine (150 mg/m² daily), both for 96 hours every 28 days, followed sequentially by daily administration of an NSAID (meloxicam). Three of seven patients with hormone non-responsive desmoid tumors had a CR, whereas four others had a PR. The median progression-free survival was 74 months. In a report of eight patients with desmoid

tumors and Gardner's syndrome, alternating doxorubicin/dacarbazine and carboplatin/dacarbazine resulted in two complete and four partial remissions, some durable.

A report from the French Sarcoma Group summarized the outcome of 62 patients with desmoid treated with a variety of chemotherapy regimens including methotrexate and vinblastine combination therapy as well as anthracycline-containing regimens. The response rate in this retrospective study was higher for the anthracycline-containing regimens (54% versus 12%). Median progression-free survival was 40.8 months but was significantly worse if the desmoid was located in the limb.

As randomized trials are not available, the optimal chemotherapy regimen is uncertain. In general, an approach that matches the expected toxicity of systemic therapy with the degree of symptoms caused by the tumor or the rate of tumor growth would appear to be the most reasonable.

Key learning points

- Treatment for STS requires individual tailoring of the approach because of the wide variety of clinical situations that can arise from a tumor that involves a variety of anatomical sites with a range of histologies of variable grade and size. Surgery is nearly always indicated but the use of adjuvant therapy can vary according to the site, size, and histological grade.

- In general, patients with extremity, superficial low-grade tumors that are less than 5 cm in diameter can be treated with surgical excision alone and most patients can expect excellent local control and survival rates approximating 90%.

- In patients with intermediate-grade lesions, surgical excision with negative margins in combination with radiotherapy has achieved excellent local control with OS rates approximating 80%. For larger, deep-seated tumors, pre-operative RT may facilitate resection and permits smaller fields and lower doses than post-operative radiation. Acute wound-healing complications are higher with pre-operative RT for lower extremity lesions, but generally irreversible late complications, including grade 3–4 fibrosis, are more common in those patients receiving post-operative RT.

- In patients with high-grade STS greater than 5 cm, excellent local control can be achieved with surgery and radiotherapy, but at least 50% of these patients will develop metastatic disease. In this setting, the use of adjuvant chemotherapy may benefit some and should be considered, where possible in the context of a clinical trial, to be combined with surgery and adjuvant or neoadjuvant radiotherapy.

- Complete surgical resection is the most important component of treatment for retroperitoneal sarcomas. Nevertheless, local recurrences occur in a substantial proportion of patients after surgery. Adjuvant radiotherapy is still being evaluated in an ongoing randomized study but may be of benefit; if employed, pre-operative radiotherapy is preferred.

- The management of GISTs is rapidly evolving with the development of targeted chemotherapy agents.

- Desmoid tumors are locally infiltrative, benign fibrous neoplasms that are most commonly managed initially with observation in asymptomatic patients, reserving surgery (if a function-sparing procedure can be performed) for patients with progressive or symptomatic disease. RT can be used to manage recurrent lesions, often in conjunction with additional surgery. Non-cytotoxic and cytotoxic systemic chemotherapy is available to manage recurrent desmoid tumors.

- The last 5 years have brought several new drugs licensed for metastatic STS, some heralded by great excitement. Despite a reasonable response rate and increasing personalization of therapy there has so far been little improvement in overall survival.

References

1. Siegel R, Naishadham D, Jemal A. Cancer statistics, 2013. *CA Cancer J Clin*. 2013; 63:11–30.
2. Weiss SW and Goldblum JR. *Enzinger and Weiss's Soft Tissue Tumors*. 4th ed. 2001. Philadelphia, PA: Mosby.
3. Torosian MH, Friedrich C, Godbold J et al. Soft-tissue sarcoma: Initial characteristics and prognostic factors in patients with and without metastatic disease. *Semin Surg Oncol*. 1988; 4(1):13–9.
4. Pervaiz N, Colterjohn N, Farrokhyar F et al. A systematic meta-analysis of randomized controlled trials of adjuvant chemotherapy for localized resectable soft-tissue sarcoma. *Cancer*. 2008; 113(3):573–81.
5. Rowley JD. Seminars from the University of Minnesota. Chromosome translocations: Dangerous liaisons. *J Lab Clin Med*. 1998; 132(4):244–50.
6. DeLaney TF et al. In: Price PM, Sikora K, Illidge T (eds). *Treatment of Cancer*. 5th Edition 2007. London: Hodder Arnold, 925–80.
7. Gronchi A et al. Status of surgical margins and prognosis in adult soft tissue sarcomas of the extremities: A series of patients treated at a single institution. *J Clin Oncol* 2005; 23(1):96–104.
8. Engellau J. Prognostic factors in soft tissue sarcoma Tissue micro-array for immunostaining, the importance of whole-tumor sections and time-dependence. *Acta Orthopaedica Scandinavica*. 2004; 75(314):1–52.
9. Pisters PW et al. Analysis of prognostic factors in 1041 patients with localized soft tissue sarcomas of the extremities. *J Clin Oncol* 1996; 14:1679–89.
10. Spiro IJ, Gebhardt MC, Jennings LC et al. Prognostic factors for local control of sarcomas of the soft tissues managed by radiation and surgery. *Semin Oncol*. 1997; 24(5):540–6.
11. Russell WO, Cohen J, Enzinger FM et al. A clinical and pathological staging system for soft tissue sarcomas. *Cancer* 1977; 40:1562–70.
12. Lawrence W, Jr., Donegan WL, Natarajan N et al. Adult soft tissue sarcomas. A pattern of care survey of the American College of Surgeons. *Ann Surg*. 19.
13. Bell DW, Varley JM, Szydlo TE et al. Heterozygous germ line hCHK2 mutations in Li-Fraumeni syndrome. *Science* 1999; 286(5449):2528–31.
14. Helman LJ and Meltzer P. Mechanisms of sarcoma development. *Nat Rev Cancer*. 2003; 3(9):685v94.
15. May WA, Gishizky ML, Lessnick SL et al. Ewing sarcoma 11;22 translocation produces a chimeric transcription factor that requires the DNA-binding domain encoded by FLI1 for transformation. *Proc Natl Acad Sci. USA* 1993; 90(12):5752–6.
16. Blom R, Guerrieri C, Stal O et al. Leiomyosarcoma of the uterus: A clinicopathologic, DNA flow cytometric, p53 and mdm-2 analysis of 49 cases. *Gynecol Oncol*. 1998; 68:54–61.
17. Karpeh MS, Brennan MF, Cance WG et al. Altered patterns of retinoblastoma gene product expression in adult soft-tissue sarcomas. *Br J Cancer* 1995; 72:986–91.
18. Eng C, Li FP, Abramson DH et al. Mortality from second tumors among long-term survivors of retinoblastoma. *J Natl Cancer Inst*. 1993; 85:1121–8.
19. Hau A, Kim I, Kattapuram S et al. Accuracy of CT-guided biopsies in 359 patients with usculoskeletal lesions. *Skeletal Radiol*. 2002; 31(6):349–53.
20. Cates JM. The AJCC 8th Edition staging system for soft tissue sarcoma. *JNCCN*. 2018; 16:14–152.
21. Williard WC, Hajdu SI, Casper ES and Brennan MF. Comparison of amputation with limb-sparing operations for adult soft tissue sarcoma of the extremity. *Ann Surg*. 1992; 215:389–96.
22. Alvegard TA, Sigurdsson H, Mouridsen H et al. Adjuvant chemotherapy with doxorubicin in highgrade soft tissue sarcoma: A randomized trial of the Scandinavian Sarcoma Group. *J Clin Oncol*. 1989; 7(10):1504–13.
23. Tanabe KK, Pollock RE, Ellis LM et al. Influence of surgical margins on outcome in patients with preoperatively irradiated extremity soft tissue sarcomas. *Cancer* 1994; 73:1652–9.
24. Pisters PW, Pollock RE, Lewis VO, Yasko AW, Cormier JN, Respondek PM et al. Long-term results of prospective trial of surgery alone with selective use of radiation for patients with T1 extremity and trunk soft tissue sarcomas. *Ann Surg*. 2007; 246(4):675–82.
25. O'Sullivan B, Davis AM, Turcotte R et al. Preoperative versus postoperative radiotherapy in soft-tissue sarcoma of the limbs: A randomized trial. *Lancet* 2002; 359:2235–41.
26. Harrison LB, Franzese F, Gaynor JJ et al. Long-term results of a prospective randomized trial of adjuvant brachytherapy in the management of completely resected soft tissue sarcomas of the extremity and superficial trunk. *Int J Radiat Oncol Biol Phys* 1993; 27:259–65.
27. Haas RL, Delaney TF, O'Sullivan B et al. Radiotherapy for management of extremity soft tissue sarcomas: Why, when, and where? *Int J Radiat Oncol Biol Phys*. 2012;84(3):572–80.
28. Wang D, Zhang Q, Eisenberg BL et al. Significant reduction of late toxicities in patients with extremity sarcoma treated with image-guided radiation therapy to a reduced target volume: Results of Radiation Therapy Oncology Group RTOG-0630 trial. *J Clin Oncol*. 2015; 33(20):2231–8.
29. White LM, Wunder JS, Bell RS et al. Histologic assessment of peritumoral edema in soft tissue sarcoma. *Int J Radiat Oncol Biol Phys*. 2005; 61(5):1439–45.
30. Gerrand CH, Wunder JS, Kandel RA et al. Classification of positive margins after resection of soft-tissue sarcoma of the limb predicts the risk of local recurrence. *J Bone Joint Surg Br*. 2001; 83(8):1149–55.
31. Mundt AJ, Awan A, Sibley GS et al. Conservative surgery and adjuvant radiation therapy in the management of adult soft tissue sarcoma of the extremities: clinical and radiobiological results. *Int J Radiat Oncol Biol Phys*. 1995; 32:977–85.
32. Alektiar KM, Brennan MF, Healey JH et al. Impact of intensity-modulated radiation therapy on local control in primary soft-tissue sarcoma of the extremity. *J Clin Oncol*. 2008; 26(20): 3440–4.
33. Eilber FC, Rosen G, Eckardt J et al. Treatment-induced pathologic necrosis: A predictor of local recurrence and survival in patients receiving neoadjuvant therapy for high-grade extremity soft tissue sarcomas. *J Clin Oncol*. 2001; 19(13):3203–9.
34. DeLaney TF, Spiro IJ, Suit HD et al. Neoadjuvant chemotherapy and radiotherapy for large extremity soft-tissue sarcomas. *Int J Radiat Oncol Biol Phys*. 2003; 56:1117–27.
35. Johnstone PAS, Wexler LH, Venzon DJ et al. Sarcomas of the hand and foot: Analysis of local control and functional result with combined modality therapy in extremity preservation. *Int J Radiat Oncol Biol Phys*. 1994; 29:735–45.
36. Spiro IJ, Suit H, Gebhardt M et al. Neoadjuvant chemotherapy and radiotherapy for large soft tissue sarcomas. *Proc Am Soc Clin Oncol*. 1996; 15:524.
37. Cade S. Soft tissue tumours: Their natural history and treatment. *Proc R Soc Med*. 1951; 44:19–36.
38. McNeer GP, Cantin J, Chu F et al. Effectiveness of radiation therapy in management of sarcoma of soft somatic tissues. *Cancer* 1968; 22:391–7.
39. Kepka L, DeLaney TF, Goldberg SI, Suit HD. Results of radiation therapy for unresected soft tissue sarcomas. *Int J Radiat Oncol Biol Phys*. 2005; 63:852–9.
40. Porter GA, Baxter NN, Pisters PW. Retroperitoneal sarcoma: A population-based analysis of epidemiology, surgery, and radiotherapy. *Cancer*. 2006; 106(7):1610–6.

41. Gieschen HL, Spiro IJ, Suit HD et al. Long-term results of intra-operative electron beam radiotherapy for primary and recurrent retroperitoneal soft tissue sarcoma. *Int J Radiat Oncol Biol Phys.* 2001; 50(1):127–31.

42. Bossi A, De Wever I, Van Limbergen E, Vanstraelen B. Intensity modulated radiation-therapy for preoperative posterior abdominal wall irradiation of retroperitoneal liposarcomas. *Int J Radiat Oncol Biol Phys.* 2007; 67:164–70.

43. Coindre JM, Terrier P, Bui NB et al. Prognostic factors in adult patients with locally controlled soft tissue sarcoma. A study of 546 patients from the French Federation of Cancer Centers Sarcoma Group. J Clin Oncol. 1996; **14**(3):869–77.

44. Baumann BC, De Amorim Bernstein K, DeLaney TF et al. Multi-institutional analysis of stereotactic body radiotherapy for sarcoma pulmonary metastases: High rates of local control with favorable toxicity. *J Surg Oncol.* 2020. doi:10.1002/jso.26078. PMID: 32588468.

45. Blay J-Y, van Glabbeke M, Verweij J et al. Advanced soft-tissue sarcoma: A disease that is potentially curable for a subset of patients treated with chemotherapy. *Eur J Cancer.* 2003; 39:64–9.

46. Agulnik M, Yarber JL, Okuno SH et al. An open-label, multicenter, phase II study of bevacizumab for the treatment of angiosarcoma and epithelioid hemangioendotheliomas. *Ann Oncol.* 2013; **24**(1):257–63.

47. Blum RH, Corson JM, Wilson RE et al. Successful treatment of metastatic sarcomas with cyclophosphamide, adriamycin, and DTIC (CAD). *Cancer.* 1980; 46:1722–6.

48. Le Cesne A, Judson I, Crowther D et al. Randomized phase III study comparing conventional-dose doxorubicin plus ifosfamide versus high-dose doxorubicin plus ifosfamide plus recombinant human granulocyte-macrophage colony-stimulating factor in advanced soft tissue sarcomas: A trial of the European Organization for Research and Treatment of Cancer/Soft Tissue and Bone Sarcoma Group. *J Clin Oncol.* 2000; 18:2676–84.

49. Available from: https://www.esmo.org/guidelines/sarcoma-and-gist/gastrointestinal-stromal-tumours

50. Dematteo RP, Ballman KV, Antonescu CR et al. Long-term results of adjuvant imatinib mesylate in localized, high-risk, primary gastrointestinal stromal tumor: ACOSOG Z9000 (Alliance) Intergroup Phase 2 Trial. *Ann Surg.* 2013;258(3):422–9.

51. Reichardt P, Blay JY, Gelderblom H et al. Phase III study of nilotinib versus best supportive care with or without a TKI in patients with gastrointestinal stromal tumors resistant to or intolerant of imatinib and sunitinib. *Ann Oncol.* 2012; 23(7):1680–7.

52. Lazar AJ, Tuvin D, Hajibashi S et al. Specific mutations in the beta-catenin gene (CTNNB1) correlate with local recurrence in sporadic desmoid tumors. *Am J Pathol*, 2008; **173**(5):1518–27.

53. Fiore M, Rimareix F, Mariani L et al. Desmoid-type fibromatosis: A front-line conservative approach to select patients for surgical treatment. *Ann Surg Oncol.* 2009; 16(9):2587–93.

54. Gronchi A, Casali PG, Mariani L et al. Quality of surgery and outcome in extra-abdominal aggressive fibromatosis: A series of patients surgically treated at a single institution. *J Clin Oncol.* 2003; 21:1390–7.

55. Keus RB, Nout RA, Blay JY et al. Results of a phase II pilot study of moderate dose radiotherapy for inoperable desmoid-type fibromatosis—An EORTC STBSG and ROG study (EORTC 62991-22998). *Ann Oncol.* 2013;24(10):2672–6.

56. Janinis J, Patriki M, Vini L et al. The pharmacological treatment of aggressive fibromatosis: A systematic review. *Ann Oncol.* 2003; 14:181–90.

57. Penel N, Le Cesne A, Bui BN et al. Imatinib for progressive and recurrent aggressive fibromatosis (desmoid tumors): An FNCLCC/French Sarcoma Group phase II trial with a long-term follow-up. *Ann Oncol.* 2011; 22(2):452–7.

58. Gounder MM, Mahoney MR, Van Tine BA et al. Sorafenib for advanced and refractory desmoid tumors. *N Engl J Med.* 2018; 379(25):2417–28. doi: 10.1056/NEJMoa1805052. PMID: 30575484.

59. Azzarelli A, Gronchi A, Bertulli R et al. Low-dose chemotherapy with methotrexate and vinblastine for patients with advanced aggressive fibromatosis. *Cancer.* 2001; 92:1259–64.

60. Patel S, Evans H, Benjamin R. Combination chemotherapy in adult desmoid tumors. *Cancer* 1993; **72**:3244–7

Useful websites

www.esmo.org/guidelines/sarcoma-and-gist

www.ncin.org.uk/cancer_type_and_topic_specific_work/cancer_type_specific_work/sarcomas/www.cancer.gov/cancertopics/types/soft-tissue-sarcoma

www.cancerresearchuk.org/cancer-help/type/sarcoma/

www.cancer.net/cancer-types/sarcoma

www.ctos.org/

www.sarctrials.org/

http://sarcomahelp.org/

https://liferaftgroup.org/

https://sarcoma.org.uk/

28 LEUKEMIAS

Tariq I. Mughal

Introduction

As a pedagogical device, hematological malignancies are divided into three broad categories, leukemias, lymphomas, and myelomas; however, the three categories have as many similarities as differences and can manifest at different stages of hematopoietic differentiation. Indeed, they reflect the architectural complexity of hematopoiesis, its inherent genetic heterogeneity, and the intricacies associated with the bone marrow (BM) niches.[1,2] These niches can be defined as a specialized "local" BM tissue microenvironment that directly maintains and regulates the hematopoietic stem cell (HSC), which in turn, generates all the lineages of the blood and immune system. Myeloid malignancies arise from a clonal evolution from within the HSC, and in some cases, a maturing progenitor cell from the myeloid lineage, which has turned into a cancer-initiating cell. Lymphoid malignancies are derived from the lymphoid lineage, encompassing B-, T-, and natural killer (NK)-cells; rarely, they may arise from a histiocytic cell (a macrophage). Unlike myeloid malignancies, mature lymphoid malignancies do not appear to result from transformation of normal HSCs or progenitors; rather, they evolve from mature lymphoid cells, but many still harbor cancer stem cell compartments.[3]

In this chapter, I review the *leukemias* and highlight how the astonishing pace of advances in cancer biology and the breakthroughs in gene-sequencing methods and bioinformatics have ushered in a new era in precision medicine. Powerful analytic tools help improve the way we diagnose, classify, risk stratify, and treat our patients. We are now able to identify many genetic defects and potential cancer targets in and on the cancer cells that can be exploited for treatment and the monitoring of disease regression and progression.[4] This has also helped to understand the multi-step leukemogenesis process, whereby somatic driver mutations that arise as a direct consequence of DNA-damaging insults are serially acquired in the HSCs destined to transit to leukemic stem cells (LSCs). The majority of LSCs exist in a quiescent phase and are often not amenable to being killed by conventional therapies or by many targeted therapies and immunotherapies. Recent work has also identified the presence of age-related somatic mutations (ARCH) that are associated with clonal hematopoiesis of indeterminate potential (CHIP) and in some cases, may be associated with an increased risk of leukemias.[5] And since the incidence of many leukemias increases with age, there has been speculation that associates CHIP with the increase, particularly with acute myeloid leukemia (AML), myeloproliferative neoplasms (MPN), and myelodysplastic syndromes (MDS). Interestingly, the incidence of CHIP greatly exceeds that of hematological malignancies, reported to occur in about 10–40% of individuals 60–80 years of age. Current estimates suggest that the annual risk of transformation of CHIP to myeloid malignancies is quite low, at about 0.5–1.0% per year. CHIP is also associated with an increased risk of cardiovascular mortality attributed to the genes that are involved in regulating inflammation and accelerating atherosclerosis. Furthermore, the impact of the cellular eco-system, which includes the tumor microenvironment and the immune system, remains poorly understood at present.

Classification of leukemias

Leukemias in general comprise a heterogeneous group of clonal disorders of hematopoiesis, affecting both HSC and progenitor cells within the myeloid and lymphocytic lineages. The main feature is stem cell-derived hematopoiesis with altered proliferation and differentiation leading to an excessive accumulation of abnormal leukemia cells in the bone marrow and peripheral blood. Historically, leukemias are often considered as "acute" and "chronic." Acute leukemias are typically of rapid onset, whereas chronic leukemias usually appear to have evolved slowly before diagnosis; neither term refers to the severity of the disease.

Numerous classifications of leukemias introduced since the turn of the last century have now been amalgamated into the latest revision (2016) of the *WHO Classification of Tumours,* based on cytogenetic and mutational analysis.[6] Table 28.1 depicts the 2016 revised WHO classification of myeloid neoplasms and acute leukemia. Leukemias are divided into 10 major subgroups and *one provisional entity*: (i) AML and related neoplasms that comprise precursor cells with impaired maturation; (ii) acute leukemias (AL) of ambiguous lineage, which includes undifferentiated leukemia and mixed phenotype AL; (iii) B lymphoblastic leukemia/ lymphoma (B-ALL), which is comprised of precursor B-cells with impaired maturation; (iv) T lymphoblastic leukemia/lymphoma (T-ALL), which is comprised of precursor T-cells with impaired maturation; (v) MPN, which is comprised of mature cells with effective proliferation; (vi) mastocytosis; (vii) myeloid/lymphoid neoplasms with significant eosinophilia and molecular/genetic abnormalities involving *PDGFRα* (also known as *PDGFRA*), *PDGFRβ* (also known as PDGFRB), and *FGFR*; (viii) myelodysplastic/myeloproliferative neoplasms (MDS/MPN), comprised of mature cells with both effective and ineffective proliferation of various lineages, (ix) MDS, in which immature and mature cells are observed with abnormal, dysplastic, and ineffective maturation; and (x) myeloid neoplasms with germline predisposition; the *sole provisional entity comprises NK-cell lymphoblastic leukemia/ lymphoma*. Additionally, there are rare ALs that are derived from an ambiguous lineage, which are currently classified as *five provisional entities: AML with BCR-ABL1, AML with mutated RUNX1, B lymphoblastic leukemia/lymphoma, BCR-ABL1-like, B lymphoblastic leukemia/lymphoma with iAMP21, and early T-cell precursor lymphoblastic leukemia.*

The chronic myeloid disorders include MPNs, which are divided into "classic," comprising chronic myeloid leukemia (CML), primary myelofibrosis (PMF), essential thrombocythemia (ET), and polycythemia vera (PV), and "non-classic," which include chronic neutrophilic leukemia (CNL), chronic eosinophilic leukemias (CEL), and "unclassifiable" MPN (MPN-U) (Table 28.2). They also include rare groups, such as myeloid/lymphoid neoplasms with eosinophilia and specific genetic abnormalities, and a group of disorders with proliferative/dysplastic features (MDS/MPN), which include chronic myelomonocytic (CMML) and juvenile myelomonocytic leukemia (JMML). Mastocytosis was previously classified under MPNs and is now recognized as a separate chronic myeloid neoplasm entity. Other myeloid malignancies include MDS, comprising six subtypes and *one provisional entity*:

- Myeloproliferative neoplasms (MPN)
- Mastocytosis
- Myeloid/lymphoid neoplasms with eosinophilia and abnormalities of PDGFRA, PDGFRB or FGFR1, or with PCM1-JAK2
- Myelodysplastic/myeloproliferative neoplasms (MDS/MPN)
- Myelodysplastic syndromes (MDS)
- Myeloid neoplasms with germline predisposition
- Acute myeloid leukaemia (AML) and related neoplasms
- Acute leukaemias of ambiguous lineage
- Blastic plasmacytoid dendritic cell neoplasm
- B lymphoblastic leukaemia/lymphoma
- T lymphoblastic leukaemia/lymphoma
- Provisional entity: Natural killer (NK) cell lymphoblastic leukaemia/lymphoma

Source: Swerdlow et al., 2017. With permission.

MDS with single lineage dysplasia; MDS with ring sideroblasts and either single lineage dysplasia or multilineage dysplasia; MDS with multilineage dysplasia; MDS with excess blasts; MDS with isolated del(5q); MDS, unclassifiable; and the *provisional entity of refractory cytopenia of childhood*. Additionally, a new category, inherited myeloid neoplasms associated with germline mutations, was added. The chronic lymphoid leukaemias include chronic lymphocytic leukaemia (CLL)/small lymphocytic lymphoma (SLL), monoclonal B-cell lymphocytosis (MBL), B-cell prolymphocytic leukaemias (B-PLL), and hairy cell leukaemia (HCL). In addition, there are several forms of lymphomas, such as mantle cell lymphoma (MCL), which frequently affect the blood and bone marrow and can present with a so-called "leukemic phase."

Acute leukemias

Acute myeloid leukemia

AML is a heterogeneous clonal disease characterized by recurrent genetic, epigenetic, and metabolic abnormalities. It arises from the malignant transformation of immature hematopoietic cells following the acquisition of multiple driver mutations in the HSC and committed progenitors.[7] These mutations inform on the World Health Organization (WHO) classification and the prognosis. Though there are some unique subtypes, such as acute promyelocytic leukemia (APL), characterized by a t(15;17) translocation with fusion of *PML-RARA* genes and cell-cycle arrest at the promyelocyte stage, and *RUNX1* encoding core binding factor (CBFα) AML, the prognosis of most patients is poor, with a 5-year survival of 28%, following conventional treatment. The outcome in older patients is even worse, with a median survival of less than 12 months.[8]

Epidemiology

AML accounts for nearly 80% of all adult acute leukemias with an annual incidence of approximately 3.55 per 100,000 adults; its incidence increases progressively with age to greater than 20 per 100,000 adults aged 80 years or older. In contrast, AML accounts for 10% of childhood leukemias with an annual incidence of less than 1 per 100,000 children.[9] The median age at diagnosis is about 70 years. Some subtypes, such as APL, are more common in younger adults, with a median age of 40 years, and in the United States, appear to affect Hispanics more than any other races/ethnicities. The incidence of APL is about 0.33 per 100,000 persons. Among the risk factors for AML are ARCH/CHIP, chronic myeloproliferative diseases, MDS, paroxysmal nocturnal hemoglobinuria (PNH), and therapy-related causes, such as radiotherapy and drugs. Indeed, therapy-related AML is now recognized as a subgroup of the 2016 WHO classification of AML, classified as a therapy-related myeloid neoplasm (t-MN), which also includes therapy-related MDS (t-MDS).

Clinical and diagnosis

Most patients with AML present with signs and symptoms arising from bone marrow failure and organ infiltration by leukemic cells. Pallor, lethargy, dyspnea, infections, and bleeding manifestations are all common. Patients with monocytic or myelomonocytic lineage AML might present with striking gingival hyperplasia (Figure 28.1). Occasionally, patients present as a consequence of hyperleukostasis. The diagnosis of AML is often made when more than 20% leukemic blast cells (myeloblasts) are found in the bone marrow or peripheral blood, with the exception of a

TABLE 28.2	2016 WHO Classification of Myeloproliferative Neoplasms and Other Related Myeloid Neoplasms

Myeloproliferative Neoplasms	Myeloid/Lymphoid Neoplasm with Eosinophilia and Rearrangement of *PDGFA, PDGFRB,* or with *PMC1-JAK2*	Myelodysplastic/ Myeloproliferative Neoplasm
- Chronic myeloid leukemia BCR-ABL1 positive - Chronic neutrophilic leukemia - Polycythemia vera - Primary myelofibrosis - PMF, prefibrotic/early stage - PMF, overt fibrotic stage - Essential thrombocythemia - Chronic eosinophilic leukemia, not otherwise specified - Mastocytosis - Myeloproliferative neoplasm, unclassifiable	- Myeloid/lymphoid neoplasms with *PDGFRA* rearrangement - Myeloid/lymphoid neoplasms with *PDGFRB* rearrangement - Myeloid and lymphoid neoplasms with *PGFR1* rearragement - Provisional entity: Myeloid/lmphoid neoplasm with *PMC1-JAK2*	- Chronic myelomonocytic leukemia - Atypical chronic myeloid leukemia, *BCR-ABL1* negative - Juvenile myelomonocytic leukemia - MDS/MPN with ring sideroblast and thrombocytosis - MDS/MPN, unclassifiable

Source: Swerdlow et al., 2017. With permission.

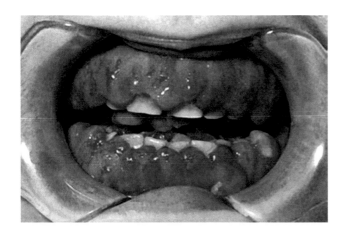

FIGURE 28.1 Gingival hypertrophy in a patient with acute monocytic leukemia.

small minority of patients with specific cytogenetic abnormalities, such as t(8;12)(q22;q22), inv(16)(p12q22), or t(15;17)(q22;q12) (Figure 28.2).

Classification

The WHO has substantially changed the French-American-British (FAB) classification introduced in 1976.[10] The 2016 WHO AML and related neoplasms classification comprises AML with recurrent genetic abnormalities, AML with myelodysplasia-related changes, t-MN, AML *not-otherwise-specified* (NOS), myeloid sarcoma, myeloid proliferations related to Down syndrome (DS),

blastic plasmacytoid dendritic cell neoplasm (BPDCN), and acute leukemias of ambiguous lineage (Table 28.3).[6] Many efforts have since validated the application of this classification in the real-world setting in the context of the 2017 European LeukemiaNet (ELN) risk stratification.

Genetics

AML is a genetically complex disease, often presenting with more than one driver mutation, which often evolves, and multiple clones often coexist. A 2016 pivotal effort provided critical insights into the pathogenesis and prognosis of AML and enabled investigators to propose 11 distinct subdivisions, each with distinguishing diagnostic and clinical outcomes; 86% of the patients had two or more driver mutations, and only 4% had no mutations.[11] In addition to the eight WHO 2016 defined subgroups, there were three heterogeneous subgroups, into which about a third of the study cohort could be grouped: AML with mutations in genes encoding chromatin, RNA splicing regulators (e.g., *SF3B1*, *U2AF1/2*), or both; AML with *TP53* mutations, chromosomal aneuploidies, or both, who had the worst prognosis; and AML with *IDH2*R172 mutations (*provisional entity*) (Table 28.4). Patients with *NPM1*-mutated AML and *FLT3*ITD or *DNMT3A* were associated with a particularly poor prognosis; in contrast, the presence of *NRAS*G12/13 mutations in *DNMT3A-NMPM1* mutated AML was favorable.[12] Patients with chromatin-splicesome mutations tended to be >60 years of age, and many had a history of antecedent MDS and a prognosis like tAML or secondary AML (s-AML). Myeloid neoplasms associated with germline mutations in *CEBPA*, *DDX41*, *RUNX1*, *ANKRD26*, *ETV6*, *GATA2*, *SRP72*, and *ATG2B/GSK1P* include AML and MDS.[13] They can

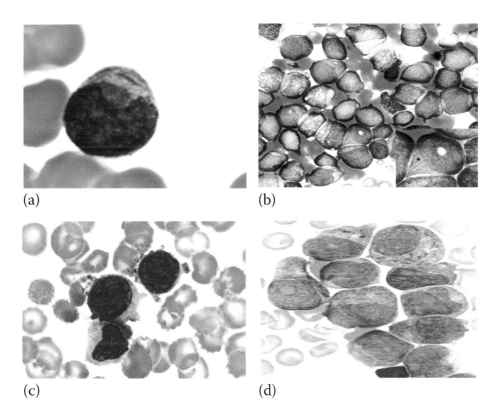

(a)

(b)

(c)

(d)

FIGURE 28.2 Photomicrographs from AML. (a) Peripheral blood smear from AML M2 showing large myeloblasts with Auer rods; (b) bone marrow aspirate from AML M5; (c) peripheral blood smear from AML M7; (d) peripheral blood smear from acute promyelocytic leukemia.

TABLE 28.3   2016 WHO Classification of AML and Related Neoplasms

AML with recurrent genetic abnormalities
 AML with t(8;21)(q22;q22.1); *RUNX1-RUNX1T1*
 AML with inv(16)(p13.1q22) or t(16;16)(p13.1;q22); *CBFB-MYH11*
 AML with *PML-RARA*
 AML with t(9;11)(p21.3;q22.3); *MLLT3-KMT2A*
 AML with inv3(3)(q21.3q26.2) or t(3;3)(q21.3;q26.2); *GATA2,MECOM*
 AML (megakaryoblastic) with t(1;22)(p13.3;q13.3); *RBM15-MKL1*
 Provisional entity: AML with mutated RUNX1
AML with myelodysplasia-related changes
Therapy-related myeloid neoplasms (t-MN)
AML, NOS
 AML with minimal differentiation
 AML without maturation
 Acute myelomonocytic leukemia
 Acute monoblastic/monocytic leukemia
 Pure erythroid leukemia
 Acute megakaryoblastic leukemia
 Acute basophilic leukemia
 Acute panmyelosis with myelofibrosis
Myeloid sarcoma
Myeloid proliferations related to DS
 Transient abnormal myelopoiesis (TAM)
 Myeloid leukaemia associated with DS
BPDCN
Acute leukemias of ambiguous lineage
 Acute undifferentiated leukemia
 Mixed phenotype acute leukemia (MPAL) with t(9;22)(q34.1;q11.2); *BCR-ABL1*
 MPAL with t(v;11q23.3); *KMT2A* rearranged
 MPAL, B/myeloid, NOS
 MPAL, T/myeloid, NOS

TABLE 28.4   A Proposed Genomic Classification of Acute Myeloid Leukemia

New Genomic Subgroup	Frequency (%)
AML with NPM1 mutation	27
AML with mutated chromatin, RNA splicing genes, or both	18
AML with TP53 mutations, chromosomal aneuploidy, or both	13
AML with MLL fusion genes	3
AML with IDH2 R172 mutations and no other class defining lesions	1
AML with driver mutations but no detected class defining lesions	11
AML with no detected driver mutations	4
AML meeting criteria for >/=2 subgroups	4

be associated with a number of well-characterized bone marrow failure syndromes, neurofibromatosis, telomere biology disorders, Noonan syndrome, and DS. Much has also been learned of the potential role of genes that encode non-coding RNA, including the microRNA (miRNA) family, though their precise importance in AML leukemogenesis and progression, and possible therapeutic implications, remain undefined. In patients with APL, research shows the presence of several gene mutations in addition to *PML-RARA*, in particular *FLT3*[ITD], *WT1*, *NRAS*, and

KRAS, but these do not appear to impact prognosis. Additionally, 12 variant *RARA* fusions have been described, of which *ZBTB16-RARA* and possibly *STAT5b-RARA* respond poorly to all-*trans*-retinoic acid and arsenic trioxide (ATRA-ATO).

Risk stratification

The revised 2017 ELN Expert Panel AML risk stratification recommendations are broadly accepted by physicians and scientists caring for adult patients with AML (Table 28.5).[14] The three-group system enables correlations of the pretreatment genomic landscape with clinical characteristics and outcome, and allows patients to be stratified into a favorable, intermediate, or adverse category. Patient-related factors, such as increasing age and comorbidities, impact treatment decisions, since outcomes of older patients, defined as >60 years, are associated with dismal outcomes following standard therapy. Another recent novel tool of interest is that based on the gene expression profile of the LSC, known as the 17-gene stemness score or LSC17 score. It has been developed for rapid determination of prognosis in AML and validated in the context of the 2017 ELN risk classification.[15]

Treatment

The principles of AML therapy have remained unchanged for almost half a century, with two sequential objectives of effective treatment.[16] The first is to restore normal hematopoiesis, and the second is to prevent relapse. The conventional treatment plan for most patients consists of a successful remission induction to achieve a complete remission (CR) and subsequent post-remission or "consolidation" therapy to prevent relapse. Currently, following standard treatment with 3 days of an anthracycline and 7 days of cytarabine, known as the "3+7" regimen, CR is achieved in 60–80% of younger adults and about 50% of older adults. Since about 70% of the patients, in particular older adults, eventually relapse, many efforts have focused on a better understanding of the biology of AML and development of individualized treatment strategies for patients who are likely to benefit.[17] Pre-transplant measurable residual disease (MRD) using a threshold of 200 copies per 10^5 *ABL* in peripheral blood (PB) and 1000 copies in BM are predictive of outcome and should be used to inform treatment decisions, including allogeneic stem cell transplantation (allo-SCT) in first CR (CR1); relapse in patients with pre-transplant MRD positivity below these thresholds appears to be solely in patients with FLT3[ITD].[18] For optimal MRD status assessment, it is important to use sensitive and well-validated assays and report the results in a non-binary manner (positive/negative).[19]

Since 2017, eight drugs, most of which are targeted agents, have been approved by the Food and Drug Administration (FDA) for diverse indications in patients with AML.[20] These include midostaurin and gilteritinib for the treatment of adults with newly diagnosed *FLT3*[ITD] AML, in combination with standard chemotherapy; venetoclax, a selective *BCL2* inhibitor, for use in combination with low-dose cytarabine in newly diagnosed older patients with AML; enasidenib, an *IDH2* inhibitor, for patients with *IDH*2R140 or *IDH*2R172 relapsed or refractory AML; vyxeos (CPX-351), a novel liposomal cytarabine-daunorubicin formulation, for patients with newly diagnosed t-MN or AML with MDS-related changes; ivosidenib, an *IDH1* inhibitor, for patients with relapsed/refractory AML; and gemtuzumab ozogamicin (mylotarg) for untreated older AML patients.

Several trials have assessed the role of "maintenance" therapy using lower doses of cytotoxic drugs for longer periods of time, hypomethylating agents (HMAs), immunotherapy, and targeted

TABLE 28.5 **European Leukemia Net Acute Myeloid Risk Stratification**

Genetic Risk Group	Survival	Subset
Favorable	65%	• t(8;21)(q22;q22); RUNX1-RUNX1T1
		• inv(16)(p13.1q22) or t(16;16)(p13.1;q22); CBFB-MYH11
		• Mutated NPM1 without FLT3-ITD (normal karyotype)
		• Mutated CEBPA (normal karyotype)
Intermediate I	50%	• Mutated NPM1 and FLT3-ITD (normal karyotype)
		• Wild-type NPM1 and FLT3-ITD (normal karyotype)
		• Wild-type NPM1 without FLT3-ITD (normal karyotype)
Intermediate II	40%	• t(9;11)(p22;q23); MLLT3-MLL
		• Any cytogenetics not classified as favorable or adverse
Adverse	20%	• inv(3)(q21q26.2) or t(3;3)(q21;q26.2); RPN1-EVI1
		• t(6;9)(p23;q34); DEK-NUP214
		• t(v;11)(v;q23); MLL rearranged
		• Monosomy 5 or del(5q); monosomy 7; abnormal 17p; complex karyotype (>/= 3 abnormalities)

Source: Adapted from data in Dohner et al., 2017.

therapies in a randomized setting. Until recently, with the sole exception of a small study including recombinant interleukin (IL)2/histamine dihydrochloride, the results were not considered robust enough for maintenance therapy to be incorporated in the general treatment algorithms.[21] In this regard, two recent prospective randomized trials that tested the use of an HMA in adult patients with high-risk AML are of interest. The HOVON97 study tested the use of intravenous or subcutaneous administration of azacytidine for a maximum of 12 months in patients >60 years of age with high-risk cytogenetics and found an improved disease-free survival (DFS) but not overall survival (OS) benefit in patients who were MRD negative compared with those who were MRD positive; the QUAZAR AML-001 study tested an oral azacytidine in patients aged 55 to 86 years and found a statistically significant improvement in OS. Further studies are ongoing and exploring the use of *FLT3* and *IDH 1/2* inhibitors in risk-adapted approaches using ELN MRD guidelines.[22]

Remission induction and consolidation therapy for patients under 60 years

Most younger patients achieve CR following treatment with the conventional 7+3 regimen, and the principal unresolved issue is how best to ensure continuing CR. The most common induction therapy consists of two courses of an anthracycline, usually daunorubicin at 60 mg/m² per day or idarubicin at 12 mg/m² for 3 days, and a continuous infusion of the cell cycle–specific drug cytarabine (cytosine arabinoside) at 100–200 mg/m² per day for 71 days. Higher dose levels of anthracyclines and cytarabine have been tested and demonstrate increased toxicity without improvement in efficacy. For patients with *FLT3*[ITD]-positive AML, midostaurin or gilteritinib should be added to the intensive chemotherapy. Post-remission therapies often comprise two to four cycles of high-dose cytarabine with or without the addition of an anthracycline. Currently, there remains a debate with regard to using an intermediate dose level of cytarabine, 1000–1500 mg/m², compared with 2000–3000 mg/m².

Stem cell transplantation

AML is the commonest indication for allo-SCT worldwide and is associated with a 50–60% chance of long-term remission and a 20% risk of relapse (Figure 28.3).[23] The relative success is due to the associated "graft-versus-leukemia" (GvL) effect and the contribution of the conditioning regimen. The transplant-related

mortality (TRM) is about 20%, largely due to immunosuppression and graft-versus-host disease (GvHD). It is therefore important to assess the risk–benefit ratio, taking into account both pre- and post-treatment factors, such as MRD status, age, comorbidities, cytogenetics, genetic features, and donor characteristics. There have been improvements in supportive care and transplant techniques resulting in a reduction in TRM. For MRD positive intermediate risk and poor risk, it is reasonable to consider an allograft using a suitable matched sibling or an alternative donor, and in some cases, using umbilical cord blood cells; *parenthetically*, patients who are MRD negative might also benefit.[19] Patients with intermediate-risk AML also obtain similar benefits from an allo-SCT, but its place is a subject of debate, in particular in those with *FLT3*[ITD] or *NPM1* AML, with some specialists considering an autologous SCT (auto-SCT) in patients who are MRD negative. Reduced intensity conditioning (RIC) compared with conventional myeloablative conditioning has, so far, not shown a substantive benefit for patients with AML, and the relapse-free survival (RFS) is significantly better with conventional allo-SCT. RIC is, however, clearly associated with less toxicity, resulting in a lower TRM, but the relapse rates are considerably higher. A recent phase randomized study confirmed the superiority of conventional conditioning compared with RIC, supporting its use as a standard of care for patients with AML who are fit and have a low SCT comorbidity index score. RIC should probably be offered only in the context of clinical trials. Patients with good-risk AML in CR1 are *not* usually offered conventional allo-SCT, since their probability of relapse is <35%. If, however, they do relapse, they may be offered transplants in second remission (CR2).

Auto-SCT has also been widely used for the past four decades, and registry data suggest a 5-year OS rate of 45–55%. Relapse is the most common reason for failure, presumably due either to residual disease in the patient or to absence of a putative GvL effect in the autograft procedure or to a combination of both causes. This is offset by the appreciably lower risk of TRM, although 5–8% of autografted patients die in CR, often because of poor engraftment. Notably, several randomized studies have failed to demonstrate the long-term benefits of auto-SCT compared with chemotherapy.

Treatment of older patients (>60 years of age)

Patients above 60 years of age account for approximately 75% of all newly diagnosed AML, and although about 60% are able to

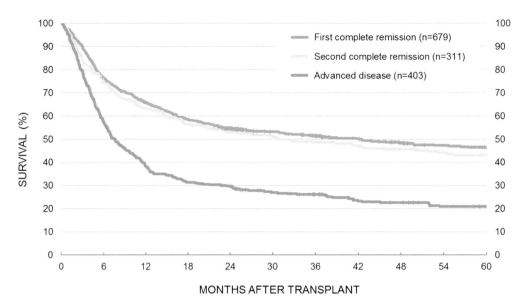

FIGURE 28.3 Acute myelogenous leukemia overall survival bone marrow transplantation for adult patients by disease status at transplant unrelated transplants facilitated by NMDP/Be The Match (2004–2013). (From CIBMTR®, the research program of NMDP/Be The Match, with permission.)

achieve a CR with standard remission induction, the relapse rates are very high, and event-free survival (EFS) is about 20% at 2 years. There has been some, but not major, improvement in these results following the use of risk scoring systems. Low-dose cytarabine has been historically used with CR rates of about 15% but dismal survival. It is possible that some of the recently approved AML drugs may improve the outcomes of older patients. As an illustration, gemtuzumab ozogamicin (GO), which has had a complicated clinical development history, was found to confer a survival benefit in older patients with favorable or intermediate-risk cytogenetics; in contrast, a large study found survival to be shorter in those aged 70 to 75 years due to early mortality. GO is approved for the treatment of adults with newly diagnosed CD33+ AML and for patients aged 2 years and older with CD33+ AML who have experienced a relapse or who have not responded to initial therapy. Vyxeos has also been found to result in a survival benefit for older patients with high-risk disease, and further studies are in progress. Venetoclax, an oral BCL-2 inhibitor, was licensed in 2018 in the United States for previously untreated older AML patients not eligible for intensive chemotherapy, in combination with low-dose cytarabine or an HMA. In randomized studies assessing therapy with HMAs, both decitabine and azacytidine have also been found to improve OS, particularly in patients with high-risk cytogenetics; patients experienced clinical benefits, such as a reduction in red cell transfusions and improved quality of life (QoL).[24] Ivosidenib is also approved for older patients with *IDH1*-mutated untreated AML.

Investigational approaches

The clinical outcomes of patients with relapsed and primary refractory disease and those with therapy-related myeloid neoplasms (t-MNs), a distinct WHO 2016 category, remain very poor with median OS of 3 to 7 months and no approved standard of care.[25] The treatment of these patients requires a carefully balanced assessment of treatment benefit versus treatment complications, and clinical trials should be considered whenever possible. The demonstration of a synergistic effect of venetoclax in combination with HMA or low-dose cytarabine led to this

combination being approved by the FDA for untreated older AML patients not suitable for intensive chemotherapy, and there have been numerous clinical single-arm studies assessing the combination in the relapsed/refractory setting. In addition, targeted immunotherapy approaches combined with a backbone of venetoclax and HMAs represent a novel approach. As an illustration, tagraxofusp, a novel, rationally designed CD123-targeted immunotherapy, is being tested in combination with venetoclax and HMAs in untreated older AML patients and relapsed/refractory patients with high CD123 expression. Tagraxofusp was licensed in 2018 for pediatric and adult patients with BPDCN.[26] The investigational therapeutic armamentarium of AML in general continues to be driven largely by targeted agents and immunotherapy. Additionally, the lessons learned from the mechanism of resistance against these agents is paving the way for the next-generation drugs. For example, following the licensing of midostaurin and gilteritinib for *FLT3*[ITD] AML, the rational development of the next generation of *FLT3* inhibitors is in progress, with drugs such as quizartinib (licensed in Japan), estaurtinib, pexidartinib, and crenolanib. Also, following the approval of the *IDH1* and *IDH2* inhibitors ivosidenib and enasidebib, respectively, new drugs are being developed to target the recurrent mutations in isocitrate dehydrogenase (IDH) enzymes. A principal challenge in assessing many of these agents is the actual design of a clinical trial, where the objective is to find treatments that make a *clinical difference* in addition to survival benefits. Moreover, in AML trials, the impact of a post-remission strategy is important and can easily negate any potential improvements achieved with a newer induction regimen.[27]

Treatment of acute promyelocytic leukemia

Though the treatment of most newly diagnosed patients with APL is remarkably successful, early deaths, mostly due to consumptive coagulopathy leading to severe hemorrhage and sometimes accompanied by thrombosis, remain a persistent problem. The risks of this coagulopathy appear to be greatest in patients presenting with a high white blood count (WBC); all newly diagnosed patients with APL should be considered as medical emergencies, and care should be supervised by APL experts. The early mortality associated with this unique coagulopathy is around 30%, which is not solely on account of diagnostic and treatment initiation delays; rather, conventional chemotherapy exacerbates it, while ATRA + ATO improves it but may require a period of 1–3 weeks for the risks to be reduced. It is possible that this unique coagulopathy is related to a novel cell death pathway (ETosis), which results in an initial increase in extracellular chromatin and affects coagulation and fibrinolysis following treatment with ATRA. The ELN APL expert panel has been providing recommendations since 2009, with the last edition in 2019.[28] These recommendations tend to be evidence-based and inform on diagnosis, including genetic tests, risk-adapted treatment, supportive measures, and specific advice on mitigating early mortality and the treatment of children and older adults.

The introduction of ATRA in 1988 and ATO in 1996 unequivocally established the principle that targeted treatment can work in this disease, with long-term remission rates exceeding 90%. The efficacy and relative safety of ATRA have been demonstrated by several well-conducted trials, first in combination with chemotherapy and then with ATO, with or without chemotherapy. The role of ATO was established by two large randomized studies, which led to the drug's approval for low-to-intermediate risk, defined as WBC <10 × 10⁹/L.[29,30] But neither ATRA nor ATO is a panacea. ATRA can be associated with a "capillary leak syndrome," often associated with leukocytosis (referred to as the "differentiation or ATRA syndrome"), QT prolongation, and acquired resistance; ATO can result in cardiac, renal, and hepatic toxicity. At present, it is reasonable to offer ATRA plus ATO to low- and intermediate-risk (WBC <10 × 10⁹/L) patients, while high-risk (WBC >10 × 10⁹/L) patients should receive ATRA plus ATO and chemotherapy, with the caveat that ATO is not currently approved for this group of patients pending the results of further studies.[31] Studies are also assessing oral formulations of ATO. Patients who are MRD negative following post-remission therapy do not require any further therapy; currently, central nervous system (CNS) prophylaxis is considered for high-risk disease in CR and for those who have had a CNS hemorrhage. Patients who have relapse (molecular/hematological) should receive further treatment based on initial therapy. For example, those who relapse after ATRA/chemotherapy should receive ATRA plus ATO plus chemotherapy, followed by an auto-SCT in CR2. Patients who fail to achieve CR1 can benefit from an allograft. Those who have a late relapse (>2 years in CR) may benefit from initial therapy. A synthetic version of ATRA, tamibarotene, is currently being tested as a monotherapy in advanced disease.

Acute lymphoblastic leukemia

Acute lymphoblastic leukemia (ALL) is a clinically aggressive, though potentially curable, and genetically complex disorder comprised of multiple subtypes of B-cell precursor (BCP) lineage (BCP-ALL) or T-cell precursor lineage (T-ALL) cells. Although the cure rates for childhood ALL have improved, with current therapies resulting in DFS >80%, the prognosis for infants and adults remains very poor, with DFS <40% dropping to <20% for those aged 60 years or more.[32] The adult ALL outcomes are worsened by the prevalence of poor-risk genetics, comorbidities, and perhaps, a lower tolerance of intensive therapy.

Epidemiology

ALL is the most common type of malignancy in children and accounts for >80% of all childhood leukemias. It is quite rare

in adults. The peak incidence in children appears to be between 2 and 5 years; in contrast, when it affects adults, the peak incidence appears to be between 30 and 50 years of age, accounting for about 20% of all adult acute leukemias. The annual worldwide incidence of ALL is about 2 per 100,000 children and about 0.7 per 100,000 adults. The disease appears to afflict more boys than girls, and there appears to be an association between genetic variants and ethnicity.[9]

Clinical and biological features

Most patients with ALL present with features of bone marrow failure and symptoms resulting from organ infiltration by leukemic lymphoblasts, in particular bone pain and arthralgias. Extramedullary involvement is not uncommon, with CNS, lymph nodes, liver, spleen, skin, and gonads affected. CNS disease appears to be twice as common in patients with T-ALL compared with B-ALL. Rarely, patients with T-ALL, and less commonly those with B-ALL, present with respiratory difficulties as a consequence of a large mediastinal mass (Figure 28.4); they also tend to have high tumor burden at diagnosis and hyperleukocytosis. The diagnosis of ALL is based on a combination of morphological features, cytochemical reactions, and genetic and immunological markers (Figure 28.5).

Classification

The 2016 WHO ALL/lymphoma classification comprises B-ALL and T-ALL (Table 28.6). The B-ALL category includes nine subtypes and *two provisional entities*, B-ALL with intrachromosomal amplification of chromosome 21 (iAMP21) and *BCR-ABL1*-like ALL, and the T-ALL category comprises *two provisional entities*, early thymic precursor (ETP)-ALL and NK-cell lymphoblastic leukemia/lymphoma.[6] The classification also highlights the unique association between low hypodiploid ALL and *TP53* mutations, which are often constitutional.

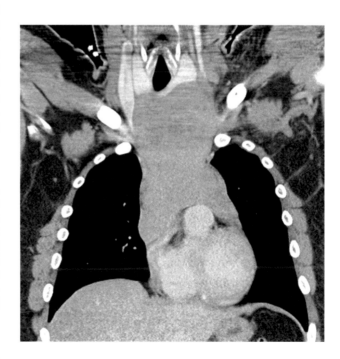

FIGURE 28.4 A patient with T-cell acute lymphoblastic leukemia presenting with a large mediastinal mass.

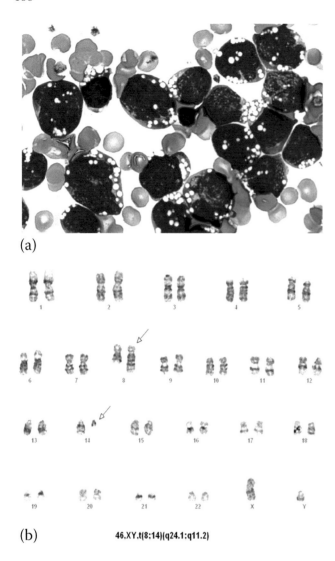

(a)

(b)   46,XY.t(8;14)(q24.1;q11.2)

FIGURE 28.5 (a) A peripheral blood smear demonstrating Burkitt's leukemia/lymphoma cells; (b) a karyotype shows the (8:14)(q24.2;q11.2) translocation (arrows).

Genetics

The recognition of structural chromosomal and genetic abnormalities in the majority of lymphoblasts has contributed enormously to understanding the molecular pathogenesis and prognosis of ALL. These abnormalities include changes in chromosome numbers (aneuploidy) and chromosomal translocations and rearrangements, which probably constitute the initiating events, followed by somatic mutations and DNA copy number alterations.[33] The ALL genome contains about 10–20 mutations at diagnosis. These mutations impact multiple cellular processes, including transcription, lymphoid development and differentiation, and cell-cycle regulation. Figure 28.6 depicts the unfolding cytogenetic and genomic landscape of ALL of both B- and T- lineages. About 10% of all ALL currently remains unclassifiable. Adolescents and adults have an usually high prevalence of poor-risk subtypes, such as BCR-ABL1 and MLL rearrangement, and a lower risk of the favorable subtypes, such as ETV6-RUNX1 and high hyperdiploidy.

In BCP-ALL, about 30% have high hyperdiploidy (>51 chromosomes) and are associated with excellent prognosis; in contrast, about 3% have hypodiploidy (<44 chromosomes), which

TABLE 28.6   2016 WHO Classification of Lymphoblastic Leukemia/Lymphoma

B lymphoblastic leukemia/lymphoma, not otherwise specified (NOS)

B lymphoblastic leukemia/lymphoma with recurrent genetic abnormalities

B lymphoblastic leukemia/lymphoma with t(9;22) (q34.1;q11.2);BCR-ABL1

B lymphoblastic leukemia/lymphoma with t(v;11q23.3);KMT2A rearranged

B lymphoblastic leukemia/lymphoma with t(12;21) (p13.2;q22.1);ETV6-RUNX1

B lymphoblastic leukemia/lymphoma with hyperdiploidy

B lymphoblastic leukemia/lymphoma with hypodiploidy

B lymphoblastic leukemia/lymphoma with t(5;14)(q31.1;q32.3); IL3-IGH

B lymphoblastic leukemia/lymphoma with t(1;19)(q23;p13.3); TCF3-PBX1

Provisional entity: B lymphoblastic leukemia/lymphoma, BCR-ABL1-like

Provisional entity: B lymphoblastic leukemia/lymphoma with iAMP21

T lymphoblastic leukemia/lymphoma

Provisional entity: Early T-cell precursor lymphoblastic leukemia

Provisional entity: Natural killer (NK) cell lymphoblastic leukemia/ lymphoma

is associated with TP53 mutations and has a poor prognosis.[34] Complex intrachromosomal amplification of chromosome 21 (iAMP21) appears to be common in older children, and it also carries a poor prognosis, which has improved following intensive treatment. Two functional classes of chromosomal translocations are recognized. The first class relocates oncogenes into regulatory regions of actively transcribed genes, such as C-MYC being moved into IGH (immunoglobulin heavy chain) or IGK or IGL (immunoglobulin light chains; K is kappa and L is lambda) in Burkitt's leukemia/lymphoma. The second class juxtaposes two genes to encode a chimeric protein, such as the ETV6 (TEL)-RUNX1, observed in about 25% of childhood ALL and <3% of adults, and is associated with a good prognosis; conversely, BCR-ABL1 is observed in 30% of adults and 3% of child ALL patients, and though it is historically associated with poor prognosis, it is often responsive to targeted therapy, and the clinical outcomes have improved substantially. Another translocation previously associated with poor prognosis, and now improved following intensive treatment, is the rare variant of the t(1;19) translocation, t(17;19)(q23;p13) translocation resulting in the TCF3-PBX1 fusion; it is also associated with a higher risk for CNS relapse.[35] Chromosomal rearrangements involving 11q23 MLL (KMT2A) appear to be observed frequently in infants under the age of 1 year and often carry a poor prognosis; about 20% of these infants also carry the FLT3-ITD mutation. Several genetic BCP-ALL subtypes with no single defining chromosomal alteration have been recognized in about 25% of children and a higher proportion of adults. These include the "BCR-ABL1-like," which have a similar gene expression profile to BCR-ABL1-positive ALL but do not have BCR-ABL1 and are recognized in the 2016 WHO classification.[36] Genome-wide approaches have also demonstrated a high frequency of IKZF1, a gene that encodes the lymphoid transcription factor IKAROS, and PAX5 deletions.[37,38] Multivariate analysis confirms the very poor prognosis conferred by any genetic alteration of IKZF1 and the unfavorable response to current standard therapy.

About half of all patients diagnosed with T-ALL demonstrate the presence of chromosomal translocations involving 14q11

Cell lineage	Cytogenetic	Genomic	Incidence: Children vs Adults	Prognosis
B	t(9;22)	BCR-ABL1	3% vs 25%	Poor
B	High hyperdiploid (51-65 chromosomes)		30% vs 7%	Good
B	Hyperdiploid (<51 chromosomes)		?	Intermediate
B	t(2;21)	TEL-AML1	22% vs 2%	Good
B	t(12;21)	ETV6-RUNX1	25% vs ?	Good
B	Hypodiploid (<44 chromosomes)		1% vs 2%	Poor
B	t(4;11), t(11;19), t(9;11)	MLL rearranged; MLL-AFF1	7% vs 10%	Poor
B	t(1;19)	TCF-PBX1	7% vs 3%	Poor
B	t(8;14),t(2;8),t(8;22)	MYC	2% vs 4%	Poor
B		BCR-ABL1-like	8% vs ?	Poor
B		DUX4 -rearranged	5% vs ?	Good
B		ETV6-RUNX1-like	3% vs ?	?Good
B		ZNF384 – rearranged	1% vs ?	Good-Intermediate
B		MEF2D - rearranged	0.5% vs ?	Poor
B	t(5;14)	IL3-IGH	<0.5% vs ?	Intermediate-Poor
T	5q35	HOX11L2	2.5% vs 1%	Poor
T	19p13	LYL1	1.5% vs 2.5%	Poor
T	1p32	TAL1	7% vs 12%	Poor
T	10q24	HOX11	0.7% vs 8%	Poor
T		MLL-ENL	0.3% vs 0.5%	Poor

FIGURE 28.6   Genetic abnormalities observed in ALL.

(T-cell receptor [TCR] α and δ genes) and 7q34 regions, juxtaposing the TCR genes to one of several transcriptional factors, such as TAL1, TAL2, TLX1 (HOX11), TLX3, NKX2-1, NKX2-5, HOXA, MYC, MYB, LYL1, OLIG2, LMO2, and others. Research has shown a pivotal role of the NOTCH1-MYC signaling and also the potential oncogenic role of RUNX1 in the early initiation of T-ALL. Some patients with T-ALL harbor rearrangements of ABL1, such as EML1-ABL1 and ETV6-ABL1, and may be candidates for ABL tyrosine kinase inhibitors (TKIs). A distinct subtype of T-ALL, ETP-ALL has also been characterized genetically. It accounts for about 15% of all T-ALL in children and about 35% in adults and involves multiple keynote cellular pathways, including RUNX1, IKZF1, ETV6, GATA3, and EP300, that are involved in hematopoiesis. Some of these patients also demonstrate involvement of JAK-STAT and PRC2 pathways and may benefit from JAK inhibitors or chromatin-modifying agents, respectively.[39]

Risk stratification

Historically, age over 55 years and total WBC >30 × 10^9/L for BCP-ALL and >100 × 10^9/L for T-ALL, at time of diagnosis, have been used to assess risk in adult patients. In pediatric ALL, the prognostic features have included age (infant or >10 years of age), WBC > 50 × 10^9/L, Hispanic or black race, male sex, and T-cell immunophenotype remain useful in the clinics for childhood ALL.[30] More recent risk stratification methods include clinical features that are present at diagnosis, cytogenetic and molecular features, and time to achieve MRD negativity following induction therapy.[40] These methods improve personalized adjustments of therapy based on prognostic markers. Poor-risk cytogenetics include t(4;11)(q21;q23), t(8;14)(q24.1;q32), complex karyotype, low hypodiploidy/near triploidy, Ph-like, and Ph chromosome; poor-risk genetics include NOTCH1, FBXW7, NRAS, KRAS, PTEN, MLL, BCR-ABL1, BCR-ABL1-like, CRLF2, iAMP21, IKZF1, MEF2D-BCL9 fusion gene, and ETP-ALL.[38] Childhood ALL with hyperdiploidy and the cryptic t(12;21) translocation encoding ETV6-RUNX1 is associated with good prognosis. MRD status is a key prognostic indicator of outcome in most subtypes of pediatric and adult ALL and as an early measure for testing new drugs.[41]

Treatment

Long-term survival of patients with ALL depends on the response to first-line therapy. The conventional approach for most patients with ALL requires prolonged therapy, comprising an intensive induction of remission followed by intensification/consolidation and maintenance treatment offered over about 2 years.[30] In general, the results are significantly better in children, in whom maintenance treatment, unlike in adults, also appears to accord some benefit. Though current results suggest that approximately 80% of all children with ALL are cured, substantial challenges remain with those with poor risk of the disease and those who fail to achieve CR following remission induction. All patients with ALL who achieve CR should receive some form of CNS prophylaxis. Unfortunately, current therapies are also associated with significant side effects, both short and long term. Although many of the drugs in use today were developed decades ago, their dosages and schedules have been modified to reduce some of these serious side effects, for example on bone development and cognitive factors. The past decade has witnessed the successful introduction and approval of targeted therapies and immunotherapies, in particular the ABL1 TKIs, monoclonal antibodies targeting CD19, CD20, and CD22 surface antigens, bispecific antibodies, and chimeric antigen receptor (CAR) T-cell therapies.[42,43] Furthermore, the importance of MRD monitoring is recognized.

Remission induction

Treatment of both children and adults involves several well-defined phases, commencing with an induction phase, with a principal objective of achieving MRD negative CR with restoration of normal hematopoiesis. Conventionally, this involves 4 to 6 weeks of combination treatment comprising vincristine, asparaginase, glucocorticoid (dexamethasone or prednisone), and sometimes an anthracycline, followed by intrathecal therapy. This accords a CR in about 98% of children and 80% of adolescents and adults. Patients with a higher risk of the disease tend to receive induction treatment with four or more drugs. It is important to tailor therapy based on an adult patient's fitness to minimize treatment-related toxicities. For patients with multiple comorbidities and those who are unable to tolerate intensive therapies, low- and moderate- intensity regimens have been developed with variable success rates. Several forms of l-asparaginase, derived from *Escherichia coli* (*E. coli*) or *Erwinia carotovora*, including a longer-acting *E. coli*–derived l-asparaginase (termed PEG-asparaginase), are now in the clinics, each with unique toxicity. The induction phase is followed by a post-remission phase, which lasts about 20 to 30 weeks and comprises intensive chemotherapy, and is followed by a maintenance phase. In general, it is difficult to assess with any precision the results of the more intensive treatments, nor is it possible to draw firm conclusions on the contribution of each individual drug. Following the achievement of a CR, all patients with ALL should receive some form of prophylaxis directed specifically at the CNS.[44]

More intensive treatment strategies, based on experiences from the treatment of children and young adults with Burkitt's lymphoma, have resulted in the inclusion of fractionated high-dose cyclophosphamide, high-dose methotrexate, and cytarabine. These modifications led to improvements in the CR rates, ascribed to the high-dose components of the protocols, although it is difficult to assess which of the high-dose combinations is more important, and the optimal doses remain debatable. The best responses have been reported with the hyper-CVAD regimen, which includes hyperfractionated cyclophosphamide, vincristine, doxorubicin, and dexamethasone alternating with high-dose methotrexate and cytarabine.[45] The treatment of *BCR-ABL1*-positive ALL has been more effective with the addition of *ABL1* TKIs to chemotherapy regimens.[46,47] The treatment of *BCR-ABL1-like* ALL has also improved with the addition of TKIs, based on the *ABL* partner gene, to chemotherapy, with durable success reported with both *ABL* TKIs and *JAK2* inhibitors, which I discuss under investigational therapy.[35] The treatment of adults has improved following the successful pediatric models.[48]

Post-remission therapy

Post-remission therapy, also known as intensification or consolidation therapy, is designed to eradicate residual leukemic cells. It comprises drugs similar to those used in remission induction or a combination of new drugs. High-dose methotrexate (8 G/m² administered continuously over 24 hours) with 6-mercaptopurine, vincristine, glucocorticoids, and asparaginase is often used for approximately 20 to 30 weeks. There is evidence that treatment results depend on the genetic characteristics. For example, patients with T-ALL, *TCF3-PBX1*, and *ETV6-RUNX1* benefit from the high doses of methotrexate, compared with those with hyperdiploid B-cell ALL, who appear to benefit more from vincristine, asparaginase, and glucocorticoids.[49] Currently, there remains some uncertainty with regard to the benefits of a second re-induction cycle in patients with high-risk ALL.

Consolidation therapy

Following the completion of consolidation therapy, the optimal duration of which remains uncertain, most patients in continuous CR, with the exception of those with mature B-cell phenotype, are offered maintenance (continuation) treatment for 2 to 3 years. It comprises daily mercaptopurine and weekly methotrexate with or without pulses of vincristine and glucocorticoid. A meta-analysis of trials assessing the value of maintenance therapy concluded that it was probably useful, particularly in children, but not for longer than 3 years. Clearly, the concept of MRD directed therapy appears attractive for all patients, and in particular those with high-risk disease.

Allogeneic stem cell transplantation

Though allo-SCT is considered to be an effective and standard post-remission induction therapy for most adults and some children with ALL who have biological features of high-risk disease, the optimal strategy for MRD negative patients remains undefined.[50] This recommendation is also being challenged in some cases, such as patients with *BCR-ABL1* positive ALL. It is also possible that with the increasing utility of pediatric remission induction and intensification regimens to treat poor-risk adult patients, the use of allo-SCT as consolidation may decrease. Allo-SCT should also be considered for patients in CR2. A principal challenge to developing a firm treatment consensus has been the lack of prospective randomized trials of allo-SCT. A 2019 Combined European Working Party for Adult Acute Lymphoblastic Leukemia (EWALL) and the Acute Leukemia Working Party of the European Society for Blood and Marrow Transplantation (EBMT) consensus panel recommended allo-SCT for all high-risk patients who have persistent MRD; TBI-based myeloablative conditioning was considered to be preferable for young adults, and for older patients, RIC based on TBI or chemotherapy was recommended; the panel felt that either PB or BM could be used as a source of stem cells, and the use of T-cell depletion to reduce chronic GvHD was recommended; and allo-SCT was not recommended for high-risk adult patients who achieve MRD negative CR following pediatric-type regimens.[51]

Autologous stem cell transplantation

The precise role of auto-SCT remains unclear despite encouraging preliminary results.[52] Most comparative studies show no major survival difference compared with chemotherapy. A small Italian study suggested a possible role for auto-SCT in patients who sustain an early CNS relapse, but in general, at present, it is probably best to offer this treatment as part of a clinical trial. *Parenthetically*, a prospective randomized study comparing allo-SCT with auto-SCT as consolidation for patients in CR1 was conducted a decade ago. Following a median follow-up of 30 months from CR1, the 3-year leukemia-free survival (LFS) was significantly better for the allo-SCT cohort compared with the auto-SCT recipients (68% versus 26%, respectively). The study was, however, criticized, since the outcome for patients who received auto-SCT was considerably poorer than that of historical studies.

Treatment of relapse and refractory disease

Despite the significant improvement in the therapy of ALL, in particular in children, about 25% of children and 50–60% of adults relapse. Second remissions (CR2) can be achieved in most of these patients, but in many cases, they are not sustained. Factors associated with a poor outcome after relapse include a shorter length of first remission, bone marrow as the initial site of relapse, older age, T-cell ALL, ETP-ALL, *BCR-ABL1*, and male sex. For patients who relapse more than 2 years after achieving CR, remission may be re-induced with the same drugs that induced the first remission. Clofarabine, a purine nucleoside, was approved over a decade ago for patients who have had two or more relapses, and the drug has had modest success.[53] Another useful licensed cytotoxic is the liposomal formulation of vincristine sulfate.

Over the past year, several new drugs, including blinatumomab, a bispecific T-cell engaging (BiTE) antibody, which binds simultaneously to CD3-positive cytotoxic T-cells and to CD19-positive B-cells, enabling the patient's T-cells to recognize and eliminate CD19-positive lymphoblasts, have been licensed in an effort to induce sustainable second and subsequent remissions for patients with relapsed/refractory ALL.[54] Inotuzumab ozagamicin, an anti-CD22 antibody conjugated to calicheamicin, was approved after it was found to accord MRD negativity with improved OS, which was improved further by allo-SCT.[55] Tisagenlecleucel, an adoptive immunotherapy using autologous T-cells genetically engineered to express a CAR, was approved in 2017 for younger patients with relapsed/refractory ALL after it was noted to confer 70–90% response rates.[56,57] As with all CAR T-cell therapy, rapid and durable responses occur but are often associated with significant acute toxicities, which can be severe and even fatal. Cytokine release syndrome is the most common side effect, affecting over 50% of patients, and ranges from low-grade constitutional symptoms to life-threatening, multi-organ failure. The second most common acute toxicity is neurotoxicity, comprising confusion, delirium, seizures, and encephalopathy (termed CAR T-cell related encephalopathy syndrome).[58]

Investigational approaches

Several promising investigational approaches involve the use of immuno-oncology products, ranging from the application of the next-generation allogenic and autologous CAR T-cell second-generation BiTE antibodies and novel combinations of currently licensed drugs, such as the combination of the monoclonal antibody rituximab with various cytotoxic chemotherapy agents. Targeted approaches, incorporating computational modeling to optimize clinical drug development, are testing the expanding list of mutations and rearrangements that characterize BCR-ABL1-like and other novel ALL subtypes, which include ABL1, JAK2, JAK-STAT, CRLF2, EPOR, and RAS, with ongoing studies assessing ABL1, JAK2, mTOR, and other rationally designed inhibitors (Table 28.7).[59]

Chronic leukemias

Myeloproliferative neoplasms

The 2016 WHO revised classification recognizes myeloproliferative neoplasms (MPNs) to comprise seven subtypes: chronic myeloid leukemia (CML), polycythemia vera (PV), essential thrombocythemia (ET), primary myelofibrosis (PMF), chronic neutrophilic leukemia (CNL), chronic eosinophilic leukemia,

not otherwise specified (CEL), and myeloproliferative neoplasm, unclassifiable (MPN-U). In addition, the WHO 2016 classification recognizes myeloid/lymphoid neoplasms with eosinophilia and rearrangements of PDGFRA, PDGFRB, FGFR1, or PCM-JAK2 (a provisional entity), and mastocytosis (see Table 28.2). CML, PV, ET, and PMF are often referred to collectively as "classic" MPNs and includes patients who transform to myelofibrosis (MF) from PV (post-PV MF) or ET (post-ET MF); in contrast, CNL, CEL, and MPN-U are referred to as "non-classic" or atypical MPNs. The classic MPNs are in turn often divided into BCR-ABL1-positive (CML) and -negative (PV, ET, and PMF).

Chronic myeloid leukemia

CML is the most common subtype of classic MPNs and is generally considered to have ushered in the current precision medicine era.[60] It is characterized by the presence of a Ph chromosome that is associated with a single hybrid fusion gene, BCR-ABL1, that encodes an onco-protein, p210$^{BCR-ABL1}$, which has dysregulated tyrosine kinase activity, considered to be the initiating event in CML.[61] The discovery that this kinase activity could be inhibited in a highly specific manner by an ABL1 TKI, imatinib, revolutionized the management of patients with CML.[62] Imatinib reduces the number of CML cells and prolongs OS very substantially. However, deep molecular responses (DMR) (also referred to as complete molecular responses [CMR] and variably defined as MR[4], MR[4,5], or MR[5]), an emerging treatment goal for patients with CML, occur only in a minority of patients. DMR informs on long-term clinical outcomes and a higher probability of successful treatment-free remission (TFR).[63]

Epidemiology

Although the incidence of CML appears to be fairly constant worldwide, with about 1 to 1.5 per 100,000 of the adult population per annum, the prevalence of the disease is increasing dramatically following the remarkable success of the ABL1 TKIs treatment.[9] It represents approximately 15% of all adult leukemias and fewer than 5% of all childhood leukemias. The median age of onset is 50 to 60 years, and there is a slight male excess. The risk of developing CML is slightly but significantly increased by exposure to high doses of ionizing radiation, such as happened to survivors of the atomic bombs exploded in Hiroshima and Nagasaki

TABLE 28.7 **Kinase Fusions in BCR-ABL1-Like Acute Lymphoblastic Leukemia and Potential Targeted Treatments**

Kinase	Tyrosine Kinase Inhibitor	Novel Partners	5' Fusion Partners
ABL1	Dasatinib	12	CENPC, ETV6, LSM14A, NUP153, NUP214, RANBP2, RCSD1, ZMIZ1
ABL2	Dasatinib	3	RCSD1, ZC3HAV1
CSF1R	Dasatinib	2	SSBP2, TBL1XR1
PDGFRB	Dasatinib	6	ATF7IP, EBF1, TNIP1, ZMYND8
CRLF2	JAK2 inhibitors	2	IGH, P2RY8
LYN	Dasatinib	2	GATAD2A
JAK2	JAK2 inhibitors	14	BCR, PAX5, PCM1, RFX3, USP25 ZNF274
EPOR	K+JAK2 inhibitors	2	IGH
NTRK3	NTRK inhibitors	1	ETV6
DGKH	?	1	ZFAND3
IL2RB	JAK1 or JAK2 inhibitors	1	MYH9
TSLP	JAK2 inhibitors	1	IQGAP2
PTK2B	FAK inhibitors	1	KDM6A, STAG2

(Japan) in 1945. There is no familial predisposition, nor any definite association with HLA genotypes. No contributory infectious agent has been incriminated.

Clinical

Patients with CML are increasingly being diagnosed following a routine blood test, and the remainder present with signs and symptoms related to anemia, hyperleukocytosis, or increasing splenomegaly; less frequently, patients may present with priapism, bone pain, gout, or skin infiltration. The diagnosis is confirmed by the presence of the *BCR-ABL1* fusion gene in all leukemic cells. Characteristically, CML is a biphasic or triphasic disease that is usually diagnosed in the initial chronic phase (CP). This CP used to last 3 to 6 years but is today very significantly longer for patients treated with TKIs. The PB smear often shows leukocytosis with basophilia, and the BM aspirate is hypercellular with an increased myeloid:erythroid ratio (Figure 28.7). Before the advent of TKIs, the disease progressed inexorably to blast transformation (BT); approximately 70% to 80% of patients entered a myeloid BT, and their survival was usually between 2 and 6 months, whereas those who entered a lymphoid BT had slightly longer survival. About half of the patients in the CP transformed directly into BT, and the remainder did so following a period of accelerated phase (AP).

Molecular pathogenesis

The Ph chromosome is formed as a result of a reciprocal translocation of genetic material of chromosomes 9 and 22 expressed as t(9;22) (q34;q11) (Figure 28.8).[64] The various genetic events are well described and result in the production of three different oncoproteins based on the breakpoints involved.[65] The CP of CML is associated with the p210$^{BCR-ABL1}$ protein and two slightly different chimeric *BCR-ABL1* genes, which in turn result in either an e13a2 or an e14a2 transcript. There appear to be no major differences in the phenotypic features of the CML associated with these two different transcripts, though recent work suggests that they might have a different impact on efforts to accord TFR. BT is characterized by the appearance of additional cytogenetic abnormalities (ACA) in Ph-positive cells and the emergence of somatic mutations, in particular *ASXL1*, *IKZF1*, and *RUNX1*.

Prognostic and predictive factors

The Sokal prognostic score, introduced in 1984, was based on the patient's age, blast cell count, spleen size, and platelet count.[65] It was modified in 1998 by the inclusion of basophils

and eosinophils and was useful in the chemotherapy and interferon-alpha (IFN-α) era for patients with CML in CP.[66] In 2011, the ELN proposed a new prognostic score specifically designed to predict the outcome of TKI treatment, EUTOS (European Treatment and Outcome Study), which required only an assessment of the spleen size and percentage of basophils in blood.[67] By 2016, it was recognized that following the success of TKI therapy, the causes of death were increasingly noted to be unrelated to CML. In order to address this, an analysis was carried out to assess long-term survival. This EUTOS effort led to a new score, which was the first effort to predict the prognosis of long-term survival considering disease-specific death in patients with CML: EUTOS Long Term Score (ELTS).[68] Older age, higher blast counts, larger splenomegaly, and low platelet count were noted to be significantly associated with a greater probability of death due to CML. The ELTS is calculated by using a mathematical formula: $0.0025 \times age/10^3 + 0.06 \times$ spleen size $+ 0.1052 \times$ PB blasts $+ 0.4104 \times$ platelet count $\times 10^9/L^{-0.5}$ and divides patients into three risk groups: low (<1.5680), intermediate (>1.5680, <2.2185), and high (>2.2185). The clinical utility of the ELTS is now incorporated in the ELN 2020 guidelines.[69] In second-line treatment, the most important risk factors are loss of hematologic response, loss of cytogenetic response, development of ACA, and kinase domain (KD) mutations.

Treatment

Clearly, TKIs have had a significant impact on the treatment of CML in CP. Until 2000, it was conventional to recommend an allo-SCT to all eligible patients with newly diagnosed CML in CP.[60] This treatment algorithm changed dramatically once the impressive success of imatinib was recognized and confirmed to be sustained. Imatinib substantially and durably reduces the number of CML cells at a daily oral dose of 400 mg, and the life expectancy of most patients now approaches that of the general population. There are now four additional licensed TKIs: dasatinib, nilotinib, bosutinib, and ponatinib. Current clinical experience suggests that patients treated with these newer TKIs achieve deeper and faster molecular responses than with imatinib, but the precise benefits of such superior responses remain an enigma.[69] Thus far, there is little evidence of a statistically significant improvement in OS, though long-term follow-up confirmed a superior rate of freedom from progression compared with patients with fewer DMRs at the same time points. It is possible that many of these patients will be able to discontinue therapy safely and effectively once they have been in DMR for about 24

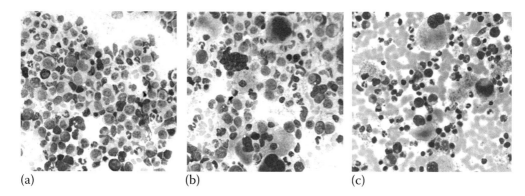

(a)   (b)   (c)

FIGURE 28.7   CML–BM aspirate. BM aspirate is hypercellular with (a) eosinophilia, (b) basophilia, and (c) clusters of megakaryocytes that have hypolobated nuclei. (From Gorczyca, 2014. With permission.)

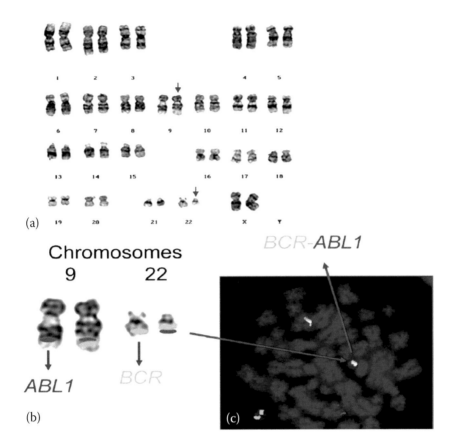

FIGURE 28.8 (a) Karyotype from a patient with chronic myeloid leukemia depicting the translocation, t(9;22)(q34;q11) (abnormal chromosomes arrowed). (b) A partial karyotype of the same chromosomes 9 and 22 with the relevant FISH probes for BCR and ABL1 is shown. The red-green fusion signals of the BCR-ABL1 and ABL1-BCR on chromosomes 22 and 9, respectively, are also shown. (c) A metaphase counterstained with DAPI (blue) indicates their appearance under the fluorescent microscope.

TABLE 28.8   2020 ELN Milestones for Treating Patients with CML in First CP

	Optimal	Warning	Failure
Baseline	NA	High-risk ACA, high-risk ELTS score	NA
3 mos	<10%	>10%	>10% if confirmed within 1–3 mos
6 mos	<1%	>1–10%	>10%
12 mos	<0.1%	>0.1–1%	>1%
Any time	<0.1%	>0.1–1%, loss of MMR	>1%, resistance mutations, high-risk ACA

Abbreviations: NA = not applicable; mos = months; ACA = additional chromosome abnormalities in Ph-positive cells; ELTS = EUTOS long-term survival score; MMR = major molecular responses (defined as BCR-ABL1 transcripts >0.1%).
Source: Adapted from Dohner et al., 2017.

months.[70] The best treatment approaches for children with CML remain unclear, and it seems reasonable to adapt dose-adjusted treatment algorithms not dissimilar to those used in adults in the first instance.[71] Table 28.8 depicts the 2020 ELN milestones for the treatment of CML in first CP.

Imatinib inhibits the enzymatic action of the activated *BCR-ABL1* tyrosine kinase by occupying the ATP-binding pocket of the kinase component of the *BCR-ABL1* oncoprotein, thereby blocking the capacity of the enzyme to phosphorylate and activate downstream effector molecules that cause the leukemic phenotype (Figure 28.9). It also binds to an adjacent part of the KD in a manner that holds the ABL–activation loop of the oncoprotein in an inactive configuration. Primary resistance to imatinib is rare and may be related to poor drug compliance, poor gastrointestinal

absorption, p450 cytochrome polymorphisms, interactions with other medications, and abnormal drug efflux and influx at the cellular level. Acquired resistance results from a variety of mechanisms, including amplification of the *BCR-ABL1* fusion gene, relative overexpression of BCR-ABL1 protein, and point mutations in the *BCR-ABL1* KD, which may impede imatinib binding. Side effects in general tend to be mild and include nausea, headache, various skin reactions, infra-orbital edema, bone pains, and sometimes, generalized fluid retention. Significant cytopenias and hepatotoxicity occur less commonly and usually in the first 6 to 12 months of therapy. The longer-term follow-up, now almost two decades, suggested no severe or late unexpected side effects but did indicate chronic low-grade debilitating fatigue, particularly in younger female patients.[72]

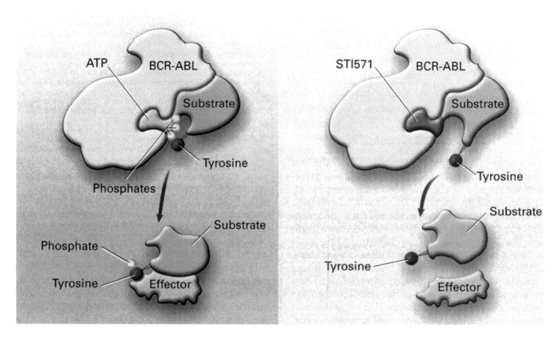

FIGURE 28.9   Mechanism of action of imatinib mesylate. (Adapted from Goldman and Mughal, 2006. With permission.)

Second-generation TKIs as first-line therapy for CML

Following the identification of resistance to imatinib, three oral second-generation TKIs, dasatinib, nilotinib, and bosutinib, entered clinical trials in 2006. Dasatinib and bosutinib are dual *SRC-ABL1* kinase inhibitors given once daily, and nilotinib was developed from imatinib by crystallographic analysis of compounds binding to imatinib-resistant *BCR-ABL1* mutants. Randomized studies showed increased benefits compared with imatinib in terms of the speed of achieving DMR in a higher proportion of patients and a reduction in the incidence of transformation to advanced phases, which was not significant; at present, there is no improvement in OS. The discontinuation rates for the drugs were about 30% at 2 years, largely due to side effects. Dasatinib was associated with myelosuppression, pleural effusions, and infrequently, pulmonary arterial hypertension and hemorrhagic colitis.[73] Bosutinib was associated with diarrhea, hepatotoxicity, and anaphylactic shock.[74] Nilotinib was associated with increased risk of peripheral arterial occlusive disease and metabolic effects, such as hyperglycemia, elevated cholesterol, and elevated lipase with frank pancreatitis.[75] It has a black box warning for QTc prolongation and cardiac death.

Second-line therapy

All the second-generation TKIs appear to be equally efficacious for the majority of imatinib-resistant/intolerant patients, but importantly, at a 5-year follow-up of the studies, only a third of patients remain on treatment. Most will then require an alternative therapy, such as ponatinib, an oral third-generation TKI, or an allo-SCT. In the imatinib-resistant patients, there are some KD mutations, such as *Y253H* and *E255K/V*, that are sensitive to dasatinib but not nilotinib, and others, such as *F317L* and *G252H*, that are sensitive to nilotinib but not dasatinib. The choice of therapy can therefore be dictated in part by the KD mutation and the side effect profile of the drug, taking into account any comorbidities present.[76,77]

Ponatinib is an oral inhibitor of *ABL1*, *SRC*, and several other kinases, which was initially developed for patients with TKIs-resistant CML as a result of a *T315I* mutation, which is resistant to imatinib, dasatinib, bosutinib, and nilotinib.[78] Subsequently, in a Phase II trial (PACE), it was found to have considerable activity in all patients with CML, irrespective of the presence or absence of the *T315I* mutation. In 2012, ponatinib was licensed for second-line use, and a Phase III randomized study (EPIC) for newly diagnosed patients with CML in CP was initiated. The study was closed in 2013 in view of an increased incidence of arterial thrombotic events, hypertension, and hepatitis in the longer-term follow-up of the PACE study, and further development of the drug for first-line use remains on hold. The considerable cardiovascular and other serious side effects appear to be dose-related, and efforts are now being made to assess lower doses. Ponatinib appears to be effective against diverse causes of TKI resistance, including *T315I* and compound mutations. Resistance to ponatinib as a consequence of new mutations, such as *T315M* and *T315L*, as well as compound mutations, has now been described.

Allogeneic stem cell transplantation

Although allo-SCT can accord long-term remission and potential cure to patients with CML in the CP under the age of 65 years, the procedure is associated with considerable morbidity and some mortality.[79,80] Clearly the outcomes can be optimized by better selection. The major factors influencing survival are patient age, disease phase at time of SCT, disease duration, degree of histocompatibility between donor and recipient, and patient/donor gender. The best results are achieved following a conventional allograft using an HLA-identical sibling donor or a suitable matched unrelated donor. The 2019 results from the Swedish CML registry assessed the role of allo-SCT in the TKI era in 118 patients allografted between 2002 and 2017 and observed that the most common indication for an allo-SCT was TKI resistance. The 5-year OS was 96.2%, 70.1%, and 36.1% when allografted in first CP, second or later CP, and AP or BT, respectively. Risk factors for relapse were EBMT score >2 and RIC, and for death, CP >2 at time of transplant. The non-relapse mortality for patients transplanted in CP was 11.6%. For patients who develop a molecular relapse following transplant, remission can be re-induced simply by withdrawal of immunosuppression or by the transfusion of donor lymphocyte infusion (DLI). DLI can induce remissions in 60–80% of patients with relapse.[81] At present, allo-SCT can be offered to patients who have failed three lines of ABL TKIs or who have *T315I* mutation, or are in AP, and have a suitable donor available; patients with BT are suitable if they can achieve a second CP using TKIs or chemotherapy.

TKI discontinuation to accord treatment-free remission

It has been generally accepted that TKI therapy should be continued indefinitely in patients who are responding optimally and tolerating the treatment well. The unresolved challenge, therefore, is really how long to continue TKI treatment in patients who have had durable deep molecular remissions and accord patients TFR.[82] The concept of TFR appears particularly attractive when the more potent second-generation TKIs are used. TFR has now been addressed in numerous single arm studies involving imatinib, dasatinib, and nilotinib and in general, is successful in about 40% of the patients. In a small minority, a second TFR is possible following the failure of the first. Nilotinib was granted a European regulatory approval in June 2017 for the inclusion of TFR. The 2020 National Comprehensive Cancer Network (NCCN) CML treatment guidelines support TFR in carefully selected persons, such as those who achieve DMRs to TKIs and can be monitored carefully; the 2020 ELN CML guidelines provide additional clarity on integrating TFR in real-world clinics (Table 28.9).

The notion of achieving TFR successfully is clearly a significant milestone, since most CML patients have a life expectancy equivalent to that of the general population following appropriate treatment with TKIs. TFR allows the safe and effective discontinuation of TKI therapy, and its inclusion should enable additional personalization of the treatment algorithm and facilitate an improved focus on daily life and improving QoL. It should reduce treatment-related risks, optimize treatment adherence and financial burdens, and better inform on the precise definition

of treatment goals and milestones, treatment choice, and monitoring. It is therefore important to identify the best validated methodology, including droplet digital polymerase chain reaction (PCR) (ddPCR), to determine DMR.[83]

Investigational approaches

There is some debate as to the effect of any of the currently licensed TKIs in affecting the progenitor/stem cells in CML. Studies have assessed alternative strategies in targeting pathways that regulate the survival and maintenance of CML stem cells.[84] Candidate pathways that appear to be activated by *BCR-ABL1* include the *JAK-STAT*, mTOR, *PI3K/AKT*, and autophagy signaling pathways and the mechanisms by which CML stem cells interact with their microenvironment. Results from clinical trials assessing the role of the allosteric inhibitor asciminib have been impressive, and the drug is now in a Phase III study, being compared with bosutinib in patients who have failed at least two TKIs.[85] Another drug of interest is radotinib, a second-generation TKI with a chemical structure similar to that of nilotinib. The drug is currently only available in South Korea, where it is licensed for both first and subsequent lines of therapy. Other interesting investigational drugs include pioglitazone, a diabetes drug, which was noted to accord MR[4,5] in about half of the newly diagnosed patients studied in a small Phase II trial. This drug, however, is associated with an increased risk of bladder cancer. Immunotherapy has, of course, been used successfully in patients with CML, not only in the allo-SCT setting but also with interferons, in particular pegylated interferon-α; anecdotal success has also been reported with vaccines developed against *BCR-ABL1* and other CML-specific peptides. Studies suggest that CML stem cells evade immune surveillance exerted by the innate immune system, which can be modulated by *JAK2* inhibitors and IFN-α.[86] Research has also shown that coordinated inhibition of nuclear export and *BCR-ABL1* selectively targets CML stem cells.[87]

Treatment of patients with CML in blast transformation

While qualified responses with TKIs have been observed in patients with CML in AP, most tend not to be durable.[69,88] The activity of TKIs in BT is even less impressive with a median survival of less than 9 months. Currently, dasatinib and bosutinib are licensed for BT; another approved drug is omacetaxine mepesuccinate, an inhibitor of protein synthesis. In younger patients, it might be reasonable to offer patients in BT intensive chemotherapy in combination with aKD mutation and prior therapy-guided TKI and consider allo-SCT if a second CP is achieved.

BCR-ABL1-negative classic myeloproliferative neoplasms

BCR-ABL1-negative MPNs are a group of clonal hematological malignancies characterized by excessive accumulation of one or more myeloid cell lineages and an inherent ability to transform to AML. An important landmark in the study of MPNs was the discovery, in 2005, of the deregulated JAK2 signaling and a recurrent somatic mutation involving *JAK2*[V617F] as a pivotal phenotypic driver, and the hyperactive JAK-STAT pathway might be considered a unifying target for therapy of all classic MPNs.[89–92] The next was the discovery of three further driver mutations, the thrombopoietin receptor (*MPL*) gene at exon 10, *JAK2* exon 12, and the calreticulin (*CALR*) gene at exon 9, between 2006 and 2013.[93–96] A third was the demonstration of safety and efficacy of INCB018424 (later named ruxolitinib), a JAK1 and JAK2 inhibitor, in myelofibrosis (MF).[97]

TABLE 28.9   2020 ELN Requirements for TKI Discontinuation

Mandatory

CML in first CP

Motivated patient with structured communication

Access to high-quality quantitative PCR using the International Scale with rapid turn-around of test results

Patient's agreement to more frequent monitoring after stopping treatment: Monthly for first 6 months, then every 2 months for 6 to 12 months, and every 3 months thereafter

Minimal (stop allowed)

First-line therapy or second-line if intolerance was the only reason for changing TKI

Typical e13a2 or e14a2 *BCR-ABL1* transcripts

Duration of TKI therapy >5 years (>4 years for second-generation TKIs)

Duration of DMR (MR[4] or better) >2 years

No prior treatment failure

Optimal (stop recommended for consideration)

Duration of TKI therapy >5 years

Duration of DMR >3 years if MR[4]

Duration of DMR >2 years if MR[4,5]

Source: Adapted from Dohner et al., 2017.

Epidemiology and etiology

ET is the most common subtype of classic *BCR-ABL1*-negative MPN, with an annual incidence rate ranging from 0.21 to 2.27 per 100,000 people and prevalence rate between 11 and 43 per 100,000 people.[9] The median age at diagnosis is around 60 years, with about 15–20% of patients <40 years and a female predominance. PV is the next most common subtype, with an annual incidence of 0.84 per 100,000 per annum, a median age of about 60–70 years, and a slight male predominance. PMF is the least frequent subtype, with an incidence of 0.22 to 1.5 per 100,000 per annum, a median age of about 65 years, and no obvious sex predominance. Fewer than 5% of patients with PMF are under the age of 40 years at the time of diagnosis, and it is a very rare condition in childhood.

Clinical features and natural history

Most patients with PV and MF present with substantial symptom burden, which includes fatigue, weight loss, pruritis, night sweats, and bone pain; in contrast, patients with ET tend to be asymptomatic, and the diagnosis is often suspected following a blood test for unrelated reasons. Patients with MPN have a significant risk of thrombotic events, which is the highest for PV. The estimated rate of thrombosis at diagnosis for PV varies from 12% to 39%, and perhaps higher for patients with "occult" disease, who do not fulfill the WHO diagnostic criteria and exhibit thrombosis in unusual anatomic sites (this led to significant lowering of the threshold for hemoglobin/hematocrit level as part of the diagnostic criteria for PV, explained later). Thrombosis resulting in myocardial ischemic strokes and venous thrombosis, which can include abdominal venous thrombosis, such as Budd–Chiari syndrome and obstruction of the portal circulation, occurs in up to a third of all patients with PV but considerably fewer with MF and ET.[98] Patients with ET may also have an increased risk of bleeding when platelet counts are $>1.5 \times 10^9$/L. Patients with MF have ineffective hematopoiesis, resulting in anemia, infection, and bleeding. Splenomegaly is found in about 10–20% of patients with PV and ET but is considerably more frequent in those with MF. Splenomegaly related symptoms are observed in about 30–50% of MF patients; hepatomegaly is found in about 40% of patients.

The estimated rate of PV and ET to transform to MF is about 12–20% and 1–10%, respectively, and is related to both disease duration and *JAK2* allelic burden, the presence of additional genetic mutations, or cytogenetic abnormalities. Progression to AML is a major complication of MF, with a 10-year risk of about 15–25%. The risk of PV and ET to progress to AML, without first transforming to MF, is considerably lower, estimated to be <2% and <0.7% at 10 years, respectively, and is associated with age >70 years and abnormal cytogenetics. The median survival of patients with PV and MF is about 14–20 years and 5–7 years, respectively; in contrast, the survival of patients with ET appears to be that of the general population.[99]

Molecular pathogenesis and genetics

Compared with CML, the *BCR-ABL1*-negative MPNs demonstrate remarkable genetic complexity, with multiple somatic mutations impacting disease biology, in particular the number of non-driver mutations present, as well as the effect of the order of acquisition of these aberrations on the phenotypic characteristics of MPN and its treatment. The phenotypic driver mutations include *JAK2*V617F, *MPL*, *CALR*, and rarely, *JAK2* exon 12. *JAK2*V617F is present in almost all patients with PV and in about 60% of those with ET or PMF; *CALR* is typically absent in PV and present in 20% ET and PMF. *MPL* mutation also tends to be

absent in PV and present in 4% of ET and 6% of PMF.[100] About 15% of all patients with ET and PMF are considered negative for all the driver mutations and labeled "triple negative" MPN. In addition to these mutations, several other somatic mutations have now been characterized, such as the epigenetic genes (*ASXL1*, *TET2*, *EZH2*, *IDH1*, *IDH2*, and *DNMT3A*), RNA splicing genes (*SRSF2*, *U2AF1*, *U2AF2*, and *SF3B1*), and transcription regulatory genes (*TP53*, *IKZF1*, *NF-E2*, and *CUX1*). Also, the order of mutation acquisition influences the biology and clinical features in MPN.[101] A novel *JAK2* insertion/deletion mutation, *JAK2*ex13InDel, associated with erythrocytosis and eosinophilia, possibly representing a variant of PV and chronic eosinophilic leukemia, was described in 2019.[102]

Diagnosis

The 2016 WHO diagnostic criteria for MPN include the presence of *JAK2*, *MPL*, or *CALR* driver mutations as a major requirement in addition to BM morphology. This has enabled MPN to be distinguished from secondary/reactive erythrocytosis or thrombocytosis. These diagnostic criteria have enabled the work-up of patients suspected to have PV by a greater reliance on the hematopathogical features; the threshold hemoglobin (Hb) has been reduced from 18.5 to 16.5 g/dL for men and from 16.5 to 16.0 g/dL for women and is now considered to be a reasonable surrogate for the historically validated increased red-cell mass measurement, which remains useful (but is often technically demanding). Tables 28.10 through 28.12 depict the 2016 WHO diagnostic criteria based on a composite assessment of clinical and laboratory characteristics for PV, ET, and PMF, respectively. A new type of PMF has also been described, in which patients present with little or no fibrosis in an otherwise hypercellular bone marrow and are considered to be in a "prefibrotic/early stage" (pre-PMF), in contrast to those with "overt fibrotic stage" (Table 28.13).[103] Both subtypes, as well as the distinction between masked PV (i.e., with high normal hemoglobin/hematocrit) and *JAK2*-mutated ET, are recognized in the 2016 WHO classification. However, since many patients with pre-PMF were previously diagnosed as ET, it is possible that the 2016 WHO ET classification will be revised.[104]

Risk stratification

Several validated risk stratification models for MPN have been developed, which allows an assessment of the risk of survival, the risk of thrombosis, and the risk of transformation. The historic prognostic scores, such as those developed by the International Working Group for MPN Research and Treatment (IWG-MRT)

TABLE 28.10 **2016 WHO Diagnostic Criteria for Polycythemia Vera**

Major criteria

1. Hb >16.5 g/dL in men, Hb >16.0 g/dL in women OR Hct >49% in men, Hct >48% in women OR Increased red-cell mass

2. Bone marrow biopsy showing hypercellularity for age with trilineage growth (panmyelosis) including prominent erythroid, granulocytic and megakaryocytic proliferation with pleomorphic megakaryocytes (differences in size)

3. Presence of *JAK2*V617F or JAK2 exon 12 mutation

Minor criterion

Subnormal serum erythropoietin level

Diagnosis of PV requires meeting either all three major criteria, or the first two major criteria and the minor criterion

Source: Adapted from Arber et al., 2016.

TABLE 28.11   2016 WHO Diagnostic Criteria for Essential Thrombocythemia

Major criteria

1. Platelet count equal to or greater than $450 \times 10^9/L$

2. Bone marrow biopsy showing proliferation of the megakaryocyte lineage with increased numbers of enlarged, mature megakaryocytes with hyperlobulated nuclei

No significant increase or left-shift of neutrophil granulopoiesis or erythropoiesis and very rarely minor increase in reticulin fibers

3. Not meeting WHO criteria for *BCR-ABL1*-positive CML, PV, PMF, myelodysplastic syndromes, or other myeloid neoplasms

4. Presence of *JAK2, CALR* or *MPL* mutation

Minor criteria

Presence of a clonal marker or absence of evidence for reactive thrombocytosis

Diagnosis of ET requires meeting all four major criteria or the first three major criteria and one of the minor criteria

Source: Adapted from Arber et al., 2016.

TABLE 28.12   2016 WHO Diagnostic Criteria for Primary Myelofibrosis (PMF)

Major criteria

1. Presence of megakaryocytic proliferation and atypia, accompanied by either reticulin and/or collagen fibrosis grade 2 or 3

2. Not meeting WHO criteria for ET, PV, BCR-ABL1-positive CML, myelodysplastic syndromes, or other myeloid neoplasms

3. Presence of *JAK2, CALR,* or *MPL* mutation or in the absence of these mutations, presence of another clonal marker or absence of reactive myelofibrosis

Minor criteria

Presence of at least one of the following, confirmed in two consecutive determinations:

a. Anemia not attributed to a co-morbid condition

b. Leukocytosis >11 x $10^4/L$

c. Palpable splenomegaly

d. LDH increased to above upper normal limit of institutional reference range

Diagnosis of PMF requires all three major criteria and one minor criterion

Source: Adapted from Arber et al., 2016.

TABLE 28.13   2016 WHO Diagnostic Criteria for Prefibrotic Primary Myelofibrosis (pre-PMF)

Major criteria

1. Presence of megakaryocytic proliferation and atypia, accompanied by either reticulin and/or collagen fibrosis grade 2 or 3

2. Not meeting WHO criteria for ET, PV, *BCR-ABL1*-positive CML, myelodysplastic syndromes, or other myeloid neoplasms

3. Presence of *JAK2, CALR,* or *MPL* mutation or in the absence of these mutations, presence of another clonal marker or absence of reactive myelofibrosis

Minor criteria

Presence of at least one of the following, confirmed in two consecutive determinations:

a. Anemia not attributed to a co-morbid condition

b. Leukocytosis >11 x $10^4/L$

c. Palpable splenomegaly

d. LDH increased to above upper normal limit of institutional reference range

Diagnosis of pre-PMF requires meeting all three major criteria and minor criteria

Source: Adapted from Arber et al., 2016.

TABLE 28.14   Molecular International Prognostic Score System (MIPSS) for PMF

	Multivariate Analysis		
Variables	**HR (95% CI)**	***p***	**Weighted Value**
Age >60 yrs	3.8 (2.60–5.51)	<.0001	1.5
Hb <100 g/L	1.4 (1.01–1.99)	.04	0.5
Constitutional symptoms	1.5 (1.13–2.16)	0.007	.5
PLT <200 × $10^9/L$	2.5 (1.77–3.42)	<.0001	1.0
Triple negativity	3.9 (2.20–6.80)	<.0001	1.5
JAK2/MPL mutation	1.8 (1.11–2.90)	.016	0.5
ASXL1 mutation	1.4 (1.06–1.99)	.02	0.5
SRSF2 mutation	1.7 (1.08–2.58)	.02	0.5

to be suppression of the inflammatory cytokine production, an important feature resulting in MPN-related symptoms, plus myelosuppression.[110]

Polycythemia vera and essential thrombocythemia

For patients with PV, phlebotomy has been the cornerstone of the treatment for over a century and improves the survival substantially. A landmark study in 1962, comparing the effects of phlebotomy alone with those of phlebotomy plus either radioactive phosphorus or chlorambucil, reported a median survival of about 14 years when aggressive phlebotomy was used alone to maintain the hematocrit below 45%. Clearly, some patients become iron deficient following frequent phlebotomy and may require iron supplementation. Following the recognition of the risk factors for thrombosis, it was established that patients with PV or ET might benefit from the addition of low-dose aspirin and/or cytoreductive therapy, such as hydroxycarbamide, for lowering the risk of thrombosis or control of symptoms, in particular those associated with microvascular episodes, such as transient ischemic attacks; in ET, they might additionally reduce the risk of bleeding. Most asymptomatic patients with ET do not require any specific therapy, and the clinical management

prognostic scoring system for PV and the revised International Prognostic Score of Thrombosis for ET (IPSET-thrombosis), were simple and served the clinics well.[105] The newer prognostic scores, such as the MIPSS70-plus, incorporate genetic information into the historical dynamic International Prognostic Scoring System (DIPSS), reflecting the progressive shift from clinical and morphological schemes to those based on genetics (Table 28.14).[106,107] Indeed, integration of the genomic data with clinical variables enabled personalized prognosis and may impact treatment choices.[108]

Treatment

In view of the long natural history, it is important to stratify the risk of all MPN patients carefully in order to avoid unnecessary treatment and treatment-related side effects.[109] At present, however, none of the licensed treatments, such as the *JAK*1/2 inhibitors, actually eliminate the malignant clone or prevent progression to AML. The drugs' major effect appears is largely based on risk stratification for vascular events, with prior vascular events and age >60 years being the strongest indications for cytoreductive treatment; a small minority might require reduction of platelet counts exceeding 1.5×10^9/L to reduce risk of bleeding due to acquire von Willebrand factor deficiency.

About 5–20% of patients with PV are either intolerant or resistant to hydroxycarbamide and may require alternative therapy, such as ruxolitinib or IFNα. IFNα has now been shown to suppress the MPN malignant clone, alleviate symptoms, and accord hematological and molecular remissions in some patients, and both therapies feature in the 2018 ELN treatment recommendations.[109] It is also of interest that the latest results of pegylated IFNα versus hydroxycarbamide as frontline therapy for patients with PV demonstrate more complete hematologic and molecular responses following IFNα treatment compared with hydroxycarbamide after prolonged therapy. For patients with high-risk ET who are refractory to hydroxycarbamide, several studies are assessing the efficacy and safety of ruxolitinib. Figure 28.10 depicts potential treatment algorithms for patients with PV and ET.

Primary and secondary myelofibrosis

Currently, the only licensed therapies for patients with MF who have disease associated symptoms or have intermediate- or high-risk disease are the JAK inhibitors ruxolitinib and fedratinib.[111–113] Ruxolitinib was approved almost a decade ago on the basis of efficacy for improving splenomegaly and MF-associated symptoms and also probably improvement in survival; ruxolitinib is being tested in the peritransplant period as a bridging strategy for allo-SCT. Though this concept appears attractive, the drug's precise impact on clinical outcome following SCT is not known, nor is the drug's long-term efficacy and safety. Fedratinib was approved in 2019 by the FDA for intermediate-2 and high-risk MF patients. In this regard, the current unmet medical need includes the optimal management of asymptomatic low-risk patients, those with thrombocytopenia with

platelets (defined as <50 × 10^9/L), and those with an associated monocytosis, which is associated with an inferior survival. For patients with higher-risk disease, it is reasonable to consider an allograft, which can accord long-term remission and may also limit clonal evolution.[114] Unfortunately, a significant proportion of candidate patients are considered ineligible, largely due to poor general condition, advanced age, or significant comorbidity. For all patients with intermediate-2 or high-risk MF, ruxolitinib should be offered in the first instance, or eligibility for a suitable clinical trial should be considered. For intermediate-1 disease, ruxolitinib should be considered for those patients who are symptomatic and require therapy; for low-risk MF patients, the drug should only be offered in the context of one of the ongoing trials. For patients who have cytopenias, in particular anemia, it is reasonable to consider erythropoietin and red blood cell transfusions. It has also been noted that patients who have low platelet counts at the beginning or end of ruxolitinib therapy, or clonal evolution while on therapy, often tend to have a poor prognosis. Figure 28.11 depicts the current ELN treatment guidelines for patients with MF.

Investigational approaches

At present, in addition to IFNα being tested as a monotherapy and in combination, many drugs including the next-generation JAK inhibitors are in clinical trials, principally for the treatment of patients with MF.[115] The clinical development of next-generation JAK2 inhibitors has been difficult, with many studies discontinued due to the emergence of serious toxicity (e.g. Wernicke's encephalopathy). Fedratinib's development in MF was discontinued in 2013, then re-evaluated in 2017, and licensed in 2019.[113] Another *JAK2* inhibitor, pacritinib, previously shown to be active in the PERSIST-1 and PERSIST-2 studies, is undergoing further development with refinement of optimal dosage. Recently, the Phase III study results show pacritinib 200 mg twice daily to be significantly better than the best available therapy, including ruxolitinib, for reducing splenomegaly and clinical symptoms in patients with MF and thrombocytopenia, both previously

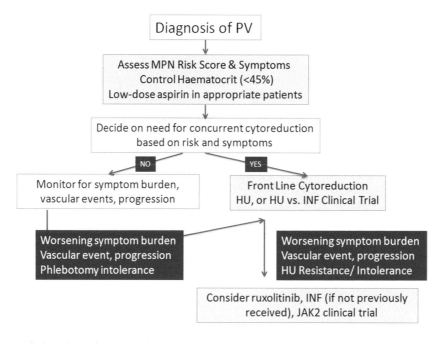

FIGURE 28.10 Proposed algorithm of therapy of PV.

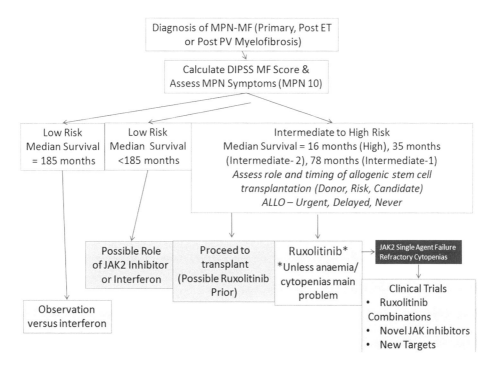

FIGURE 28.11 Proposed algorithm of therapy of MF.

untreated patients and those who had received prior ruxolitinib. Momelotinib, a *JAK2* inhibitor, was tested in the SIMPLIFY-1 and -2 studies in 2017, in first- and second-line settings, respectively, but trials failed to meet their primary endpoint. In addition to *JAK* inhibition and interferons, many other investigational agents, either alone or in combination with ruxolitinib, are being tested. These include hedgehog, aurora kinase, SMAC, HDAC, and MDM2 inhibitors, in addition to the *JAK2*-allosteric inhibitors, such as LS104 and ON044580, which have a greater specificity for *JAK2*[V617F] and are inhibitory in a non-ATP competitive manner. A novel agent, tagraxofusp, which targets CD123 and plasmacytoid dendritic cells, observed in MF patients, is currently being tested in a Phase II study.

Atypical myeloproliferative neoplasms

Chronic neutrophilic leukemia

CNL is a rare MPN subtype, which shares overlapping clinical features with an MDS/MPN subtype, aCML. It is associated with a recurrent mutation *CSF3R*), often *CSF3R*[T618I], in >80% of the patients, in addition to mutations in *SETBP1*, RNA spliceosome genes (*SRSF2*, *U2AF1*), and epigenetic modifiers (*TET2*, *ASXL2*), which may impact on the prognosis and progression to AML.[116] It is possible that at least in some cases, CNL might arise from age-related CHIP. Though *CSF3R* mutations are almost always somatic, a germline mutation involving *T618I* was reported. Since *CSF3R* is associated with a deregulated JAK/STAT pathway, it is considered a targetable lesion by a JAK inhibitor. Research has now shown the substantial morphological and genetic similarities between CNL and two related rare myelodysplastic/myeloproliferative neoplasms (MDS/MPN), aCML and MDS/MPN-U, which I discuss later.[117] The emerging evidence suggest that these diseases represent a continuum of related diseases and should, perhaps, be treated as such.

Chronic eosinophilic leukemia, not otherwise specified

Chronic eosinophilic leukemia, not otherwise specified (CEL), is distinguished from other forms of eosinophilia, in particular idiopathic hypereosinophilic syndrome, by the demonstration of clonality, increased myeloblasts, and non-specific cytogenetic abnormalities, such as trisomy 8 and i(7q). It is a rare and aggressive disorder associated with a median survival of about 20 months and a high rate of transformation to AML. It must also be carefully distinguished from other myeloid entities associated with eosinophilia by suitable cytogenetic and genetic analysis, preferably next-generation sequencing. This is critical, since the presence of specific genetic abnormalities, such as *FIP1L1-PDGFRA* or other tyrosine kinase fusions such as those involving *PDGFRA*, *PDGFRB*, *FGFR1*, or *JAK2*, is often amenable to treatment with specific targeted agents, such as imatinib. Clearly by definition, CEL is *BCR-ABL1*-negative without rearrangement of *PDGFRA*, *PDGFRB*, or *FGFR1*.[118] Recent research has also identified a mutation, *JAK2*[ex13InDel], associated with erythrocytosis and eosinophilia, possibly representing a variant of PV and CEL.[102] In general, patients with CEL, not otherwise specified, often have an aggressive clinical course, and some patients benefit from an intensive chemotherapy and allo-SCT.

Myeloid/lymphoid neoplasms with eosinophilia and rearrangements of *PDGFRA*, *PDGFRB*, *FGFR1*, or *PCM-JAK2*

The seminal discoveries of dysregulated tyrosine kinase genes in a collection of malignancies of myeloid or lymphoid lineages, sometimes, but not always, associated with eosinophilia, led to the significant revision in the 2016 WHO classification of this subtype, under the category of MPNs. It was also observed that some of these genetic lesions were amenable to being treated successfully by available TKIs. Certain genes (>70 fusion) have now been described in myeloid/lymphoid neoplasms with eosinophilia. Since many of these genetic abnormalities can be found in other malignancies, it is important to assess the morphology and clinical features carefully. *PCM1-JAK2* positive disease is classified as a *provisional entity*, since it can rarely present as T-cell or B-cell ALL and responds to ruxolitinib. Other *JAK2* rearranged neoplasms, such as *ETV6-JAK2* and *BCR-JAK2*, are best considered and treated as *BCR-ABL1*-like B-cell ALL. Patients with the *FIP1L1-PDGFRA*, *FIP1L1-PDGFRB*, *ETV6-PDGFRB*, and *ABL1-PDGFRB* rearrangements are highly sensitive to low-dose imatinib. Rarely, acquired resistance can arise, often as a consequence of the emergence of *T674I* or *D842V* mutations. Patients with *FGFR1* and *JAK2* rearrangements tend to have an aggressive TKI-resistant disease and should be treated with intensive chemotherapy and considered for an allo-SCT. Some reports suggest successful treatment of patients with clonal eosinophilia and *ETV6-FLT3* following treatment with one of the *FLT3* inhibitors, sunitinib or sorafenib.

Mastocytosis

Mastocytosis is a rare myeloid neoplasm characterized by the aberrant accumulation and infiltration of clonal mast cells in various tissues, resulting in a clinically heterogeneous disorder. The precise incidence and prevalence of mastocytosis are largely unknown, though a population-based Danish study suggests an incidence of 0.89 per 100,000 persons adults per annum for systemic mastocytosis (SM).[119] Mastocytosis is now considered as a separate entity within the myeloid malignancies rather than a subtype of MPN. In the 2016 WHO classification, the term "mastocytosis" includes cutaneous mastocytosis (CM); SM, which in turn, encompasses indolent systemic mastocytosis (ISM), smoldering systemic mastocytosis (SSM), systemic mastocytosis with associated hematological non-mast cell disease (SM-AHNMD), aggressive systemic mastocytosis (ASM), and mast cell leukemia; and mast cell sarcoma. It is caused by the accumulation of clonal mast cells in the skin and other organs and is associated with a driver mutation, KIT^{D816V}, which encodes a constitutively activated receptor tyrosine kinase, in over 90% of patients. Several other mutations, in particular *ASXL1*, *TET2*, *CBL*, and *RUNX1*, appear to contribute to the molecular pathogenesis, probably as phenotypic modifiers, and promote progression to the aggressive forms of SM. Somatic mutations in *ETNK1* have also been observed in some patients with SM and eosinophilia.[114]

The clinical features of mastocytosis result from the accumulation of neoplastic mast cells in the various organs, which results in features such as cytopenias, osteolytic bone lesions, abnormal liver function tests, and elevated serum tryptase levels.[120] The prognosis of CM is good, and most children achieve spontaneous remission. Advanced SM is associated with a poor prognosis, with a median OS of 3.5 years in ASM and 2 years for SM-AHNMD; patients with MCL fare the worst, with a median survival of <6 months. Treatment decisions are based on the presence of clinical features and symptom burden. Cladribine and IFN-α have some efficacy, which is often not sustained. Responses to imatinib tend to be transient and durable in <10% of patients, largely due to the acquired resistance conferred by several resistant mutations, including *D816V* and *T670I*. Masitinib, a TKI that selectively inhibits *KIT*, *PDGFRA*, *PDGFRB*, and *LYN* kinases, has demonstrated some efficacy in indolent, but not aggressive, disease; the drug is associated with significant diarrhea and urticaria. Another orally active multi-kinase inhibitor, midostaurin, is licensed for patients with ASM, SM-AHN, and MCL. Midostaurin may also

be effective in some patients with aggressive MCL, who are often treated with intensive chemotherapy followed by allo-SCT.

Myelodysplastic syndromes and myelodysplastic/myeloproliferative neoplasms (MDS/MPN) overlap disorders

The myelodysplastic syndromes (MDSs) are a heterogeneous group of clonal hematopoietic neoplasms characterized by morphologically abnormal progeny, an impaired ability to generate mature blood cells, manifest as cytopenias, and an inherent risk of transformation to AML. The myelodysplastic/myeloproliferative neoplasms (MDS/MPNs) are a unique group of chronic myeloid malignancies that include hematological and a biologically diverse group of disorders, all with dysplastic hematopoiesis and some with proliferative features, therefore demonstrating overlapping histological and clinical characteristics of both MDS and MPNs. These disorders exhibit considerable heterogeneity in clinical presentation, prognosis, and treatment.

Myelodysplastic syndromes

Epidemiology

Although the onset of an MDS before the age of 50 years is rare, the various subtypes of this disease are probably the most common cause of acquired bone marrow failure in older adults, among whom the annual incidence exceeds 75 per 100,000 persons.[9] The median age of occurrence is about 70 years, with males more likely to be affected than females by a ratio of 1.4:1.0, with the exception of MDS with isolated deletion 5q [del(5q) syndrome], which has a female predilection. Therapy-related MDS (t-MN) is a recognized late complication of chemotherapy or radiotherapy and to a lesser extent, occupational exposure to solvents or agricultural chemicals. The risk of MDS is increased in various genetic syndromes, such as the Diamond-Blackfan syndrome and Fanconi's anemia.

Clinical

The common presenting features relate to anemia and other cytopenias. The bone marrow cellularity is generally normal or increased, reflecting ineffective blood production, and characteristic cytological features include hypogranular and hypolobulated (pseudo-Pelger–Huët) granulocytes, small or micro-megakaryocytes with oligonuclearity or nuclear dispersion, and a variety of red-cell precursor abnormalities, ranging from ring sideroblasts to megaloblastoid changes and karyorrhexis (Figure 28.12). Dysplastic abnormalities involving >10% of a specific myeloid cell lineage are the cardinal feature of MDS. The natural history ranges from indolent, with a survival approaching that of the general population, to subtypes with clinical outcomes not dissimilar to AML. There is evidence of immune dysregulation in some patients, which may cause autoimmune myelosuppression and worsen the ineffective hematopoiesis.[121,122]

Diagnosis and classifications

The diagnosis of MDS can be difficult due to the challenges of distinguishing "true" MDS from age-related and non-malignant cytopenias.[123] Indeed, the histological differences can be taxing, in particular the accurate discrimination between aplastic anemia and hypoplastic MDS. According to the revised 2016 WHO classification system, the MDS group is comprised of six well-defined entities based upon degree of dysplasia (>10%) and blast percentage (1% in the peripheral blood with <5% bone marrow blasts) and the presence or absence of a chromosome 5q deletion or ring sideroblasts. These categories include MDS with single

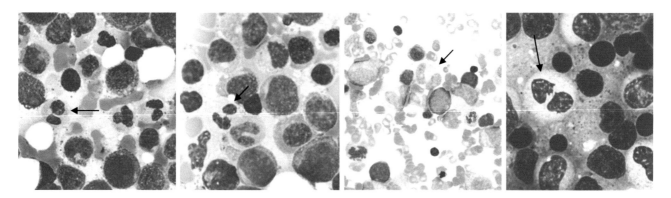

FIGURE 28.12 Bone marrow aspirate from a patient with myelodysplastic syndrome—note the dysgranulopoiesis characterized by atypical granulocytes with hypolobated nuclei, Pelgeroid features, increased size, and hypogranular cytoplasm. (From Gorczyca, 2014. With permission.)

lineage dysplasia, MDS with ring sideroblasts (with single or multilineage dysplasia), MDS with multilineage dysplasia, MDS with excess blasts, MDS with isolated del(5q) and MDS, unclassifiable, and a *provisional entity: refractory childhood cytopenia*.

Genetics

Although the precise nature of the initiating event for MDS is unknown, much has been learned about the genomic landscape, abnormalities of the bone marrow microenvironment, and how these features impact the natural history and some of the attributes of the clinical phenotype.[124] Non-specific cytogenetic abnormalities, which occur in other myeloid malignancies also, include del (5q), trisomy 8, -Y, del (20q), and monosomy 7; an isolated del(5q) is the most common cytogenetic abnormality found in MDS and is associated with specific morphological features, including a hypoplastic macrocytic anemia, small and often mononuclear megakaryocytes, normal or increased platelet count, indolent clinical course, with a female preponderance, and high probability of response to the immunomodulatory drug lenalidomide (Figure 28.13). Mutations in RNA splicing factors are the single most common class of genetic lesions in MDS,

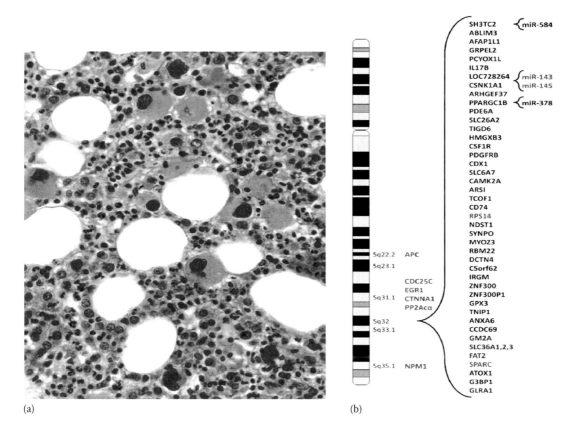

(a) (b)

FIGURE 28.13 5q-syndrome MDS Isolated Del5q ("5q-syndrome"). (a) Bone marrow trephine showing abnormal hypolobated megakaryocytes, which are increased in number; (b) schematic demonstrating the deletion between bands q31 and 33 on chromosome 5 and the associated genes.

followed by mutations in the epigenetic regulators. Mutations in the RNA splicing factor *SF3B1* are involved in 90% of patients with MDS with ring sideroblasts (MDS-RS); other mutated splicing genes include *SRSF2*, *U2AF1*, and *ZRSF2*, in order of frequency of occurrence. Importantly, these spliceosome mutations appear to be mutually exclusive, reflecting cellular intolerance and lethality of two-allele inactivation, thereby preserving a selective advantage. The epigenetic regulators are comprised of mutations of the DNA methylation genes *TET2*, *DNMT3A*, *IDH1*, and *IDH2* and the histone modifiers *ASXL1* and *EZH2*. Cohesin is a closed-loop multiprotein complex composed of *SMC1A*, *SMC3*, *RAD21*, *STAG1*, and *STAG2*, and mutations are noted in up to 17% of patients with MDS. The tumor suppressor *TP53* is involved in about 40% of patients, and those associated with deletion of the short arm of chromosome 17 have a particularly bad prognosis. Other mutations considered to play a role in the pathogenesis of MDS include transcription factors, such as *GATA*, *ETV6*, *CUX1*, and *RUNX1*, and signal transduction genes, such as *CBL*, *JAK2*, *NRAS*, *KRAS*, *MPL*, *NF1*, *PTPN11*, *KIT*, and *FLT3*. Studies also provide insights into the complex architecture and dynamics of clonal evolution in MDS. As MDS progresses, the clonal diversity, size, and order of acquisition of the individual mutations, in turn impact the phenotypic characteristics and the risk of transformation to AML.

Risk assessment

The 1997 International Prognostic Scoring System (IPSS), based on the karyotype, blast percentage, and number of cytopenias, served well until 2012, when it was revised.[125] The revised IPSS (IPSS-R) stratified patients into five prognostic groups, based on cytogenetics but not molecular characteristics (Table 28.15), and was broadly accepted.[126] It is also better able to capture fatigue severity compared with IPSS.[127] Refinements are in progress to integrate validated genetic and immunologic information to further improve prognostic discrimination and probability of response to specific therapy, including allo-SCT.[122] As an illustration, mutations in *TP53*, *RUNX1*, and *ASXL1* predict for poor prognosis, mutations involving *SF3B1* are associated with favorable prognosis, and mutations involving *PPM1D* may inform of risk of relapse from allo-SCT. Indeed, research has shown that clinical outcomes of patients with *TP53* mutated MDS are heterogenous and affected by other factors.[128]

Treatment

The remarkably heterogenous nature of MDS underscores the importance of a risk-adapted treatment strategy, informed by the R-IPSS risk score and patient-related factors, such as age, performance status, frailty, and comorbidity. At present, allo-SCT is the only treatment that can offer long-term remission, but it is not applicable for most patients in view of age and comorbidities. Allo-SCT is associated with a high TRM (about 39% at 1 year), which is significant for younger patients also. Refinements in the timing of allograft, methodology of disease risk assessment, patient selection, pre-transplant therapies, the conditioning regimens, and supportive care are being made. Recent registry data confirms that an allograft from an HLA-identical sibling offers the best outcome in younger patients with a low percentage of blasts. The 2017 ELN/EBMT risk score for allo-SCT in MDS has now been validated and recommends allo-SCT for patients with MDS who are fit and have a high-risk IPSS-R or low risk with poor genetic features, profound cytopenias, and a high transfusion burden.[129] In contrast, patients considered very high risk for allo-SCT include those with advanced age, very poor cytogenetic and genetic features, and high IPSS-R, who have a low probability of cure with allo-SCT and should be treated with an investigational approach. Long-term results for conventional allo-SCT and RIC allo-SCT show no important long-term LFS, though causes of failure differ. Iron overload related to red-cell transfusion has also been found to impact allo-SCT outcome, and appropriate iron chelating therapy should be offered pre-transplant. Figure 28.14 depicts the risk-adapted treatment approaches. The principal treatment objectives for patients with low-risk (LR) MDS are to improve cytopenias and prevent complications such as infections, reduce transfusion requirement, and improve QoL, and for patients with high-risk (HR) disease, to delay disease progression/transformation and improve survival. At present, there is a paucity of new drug approvals for MDS, in particular targeted therapies, and there is an urgent medical need for patients who fail currently licensed therapies.

A substantial proportion of patients with LR-disease are asymptomatic or have mild cytopenias at diagnosis; these may not require therapy and can be observed, which should be intensified in those with a higher-risk molecular prognostic profile, such *ASXL1*. Erythropoietin-stimulating agents (ESA) have been in global clinical use for over two decades, but clinical trials were only recently conducted. At present, erythropoietin-alpha, but not darbepoetin, is licensed for LR-MDS patients with symptomatic anemia or low red-cell transfusion burden. The drug was found to be effective in patients with a serum erythropoietin level <500 IU/L and red-cell transfusion burden <4 U within an 8-week period. For patients who remain red-cell transfusion dependent, there is an increased risk of iron overload, which may contribute to the complications of the disease. Although there remains some debate with regard to the precise benefit and survival effect, many treatment guidelines recommend a ferritin-guided (>1000 ng/ml) chelating approach for iron overload using deferasirox. For LR-disease associated with del(5q), lenalidomide can reduce the red-cell transfusion requirements in about 75% of patients and has a modest benefit on survival; the drug's success in those with a concomitant *TP53*

TABLE 28.15   Risk Stratification of Myelodysplastic Syndromes Based on the IPSS-R

Risk Group	Karyotypes	Median Survival (Months)	Proportion of Patients
Very Good	del(11q), −Y	60.8	2.9%
Good	Normal, del(20q), del(5q) +/− one other abnormality, del(12p)	48.6	65.7%
Intermediate	+8, del(7q), i(17q),+19, +21, 2 or more independent clones	26.1	19.2%
Poor	der(3q), −7, double with del(7q), complex with 3 abnormalities	15.8	5.4%
Very Poor	Complex with >3 abnormalities	5.9	6.8%

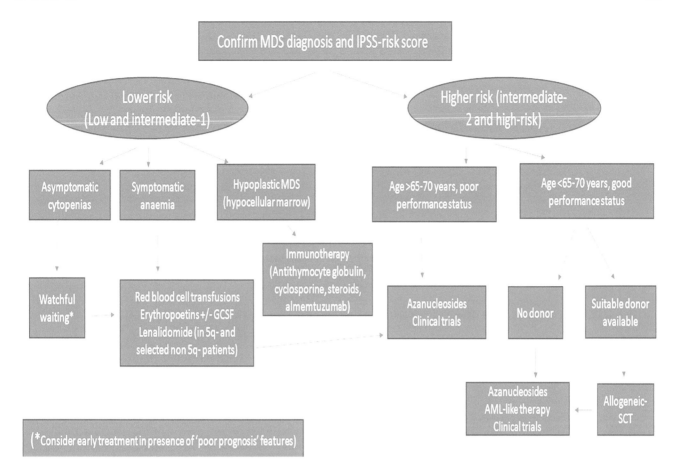

FIGURE 28.14 Potential risk-adapted, IPSS-based treatment algorithm for adult patients with MDS.

mutation and in those without del(5q) is less impressive, as is the risk of transformation. Some patients with del(5q) may have an increased risk of transformation due to the presence of additional mutations, such as *TET2* and *RUNX1*.

The hypomethylating agents (HMA), azacytidine and decitabine, are both approved by the U.S. FDA for LR- and HR-MDS, but their wider use, particularly outside the United States, is in patients with HR-disease. Clinical benefits, such as red-cell transfusion independence, were observed largely in ESA-naïve patients, but toxicity was not uncommon. Indeed, a recent Phase III placebo-controlled study in intermediate-1 risk MDS patients with red-cell transfusion dependency and thrombocytopenia was terminated prematurely due to toxicity. In patients with HR-risk disease, HMAs result in complete remission rates in 9% to 17% of patients and in some cases, delay transformation to AML. Randomized prospective studies with azacytidine, but not decitabine, show a median survival of 24.5 months as compared with 15.0 months in the conventional care group. In view of this survival benefit, azacytidine can be useful as a bridging therapy for allo-SCT. A principal current concern with HMAs in HR-disease is the relatively short-lived response duration, underscoring the need to build upon the first-line HMA outcomes.

Rare young patients who present with hypocellular MDS benefit from immunosuppressive therapy, such as antithymocyte globulin (ATG) and cyclosporine A.[130] High response rates were also observed in a study assessing the anti-CD52 antibody alemtuzumab, but the drug is no longer being developed for this indication. Clinical trials are also assessing other immune approaches through CD33 (MDSC) and Toll-like receptor signaling (TLR2).

Investigational approaches

Erythropoiesis-maturing agents (EMAs), which are specific activin fusion proteins that act as ligand traps to neutralize negative regulators of erythropoiesis, have now been tested in patients with LR-MDS. Luspartercept (ACE-536) has shown ability to increase hemoglobin levels in LR-disease and is approved for patients with beta-thalassemia. The Phase II LR-MDS study reveals 63% erythroid responses with 38% achieving red-cell transfusion independence, particularly in patients with ringed sideroblasts or *SF3B1*-defined LR-MDS. The study met its primary end-points and is anticipated to be approved in 2020.[131] Roxadustat (FG-4592) is an oral hypoxia-inducible factor inhibitor being tested in a Phase III study in LD-MDS in an effort to improve anemia.[132] Imetelstat, a telomerase inhibitor, is in a Phase II/III study in red-cell transfusion-dependent and ESA-relapsed/refractory LR-MDS patients. Drugs aimed at improving thrombocytopenia, noted in about 50% of all LR-MDS patients, are also being tested. The TPO-receptor agonists romiplostim and elthrombopag have now been tested in Phase III studies and found to have platelet responses associated with survival benefits but are not approved as yet. Several other novel approaches are being tested, including second-generation HMAs, guadecitabine and ASTX727, and combinations of azacytidine with either lenalidomide, vorinostat (a TPO-receptor agonist), or pevonedistat (an NEDD8-activating enzyme).[133] Several combination trials of venetoclax with azacytidine, including those adding tagraxofusp, a CD123-targeted drug, in the untreated and relapsed/refractory setting, and studies of immune checkpoint modulation with HMAs are also in progress. Other candidate approaches include vyxeos (CPX-351), a novel liposomal formulation of cytarabine and daunorubicin recently licensed for secondary AML or tMN, targeted *IDH1/2* or *FLT3* inhibitors, splicesome-modulator H3B-8800, CAR T-cells, and bispecific antibodies.

Myelodysplastic/myeloproliferative neoplasms (MDS/MPN) overlap disorders

MDS/MPN overlap disorders are considered distinct from MDS and MPN and classified according to the 2016 WHO classification system into chronic myelomonocytic leukemia (CMML), juvenile myelomonocytic leukemia (JMML), atypical chronic myeloid leukemia, *BCR-ABL1*-negative (aCML), MDS/MPN with ring sideroblasts and thrombocytosis (MDS/MPN-RS-T), and MDS/MPN, unclassifiable (MDS/MPN-U). The classification defines distinct biological entities with clinical and morphological features that overlap between MDS and MPN, considerable molecular heterogeneity, and the lack of specific genotypic markers. While monocytosis or eosinophilia fosters recognition of CMML/JMML or CEL, respectively, the differentiation between aCML, MDS/MPN-U, and MPN-U is often difficult. Additional diagnostic criteria have recently been proposed and require confirmation.[134]

Incidence

The precise incidence of the various subtypes of MDS/ MPN overlap disorders is unknown but considered to be low. As an illustration, CMML, the most common of the MDS/MPN overlap diseases, has a prevalence estimated to be about 10% of that for MDS and an annual incidence estimated to be 1.0 per 100,000 persons.[9] The median age of occurrence of CMML is 70 years, and there is a male predominance. Like many hematological malignancies, there is a trend towards older age for MDS/MPN, with the exception of JMML, which has a median age of occurrence of 2 years and an incidence of 0.12 per 100,000 children with a disproportionate male preponderance.

Clinical features

Most patients present with non-specific features of ineffective hematopoiesis, particularly anemia and cytopenias, and clinical heterogeneity. The respective MDS/MPN subtypes are typically identified by the type of myeloid subset that predominates in the peripheral blood.[135] For example, CMML and JMML are characterized by a unique expansion of PB monocytes that are CD14+ and CD16− and enhancement of *in vitro* sensitivity to GM-CSF; many of these monocytes also express high levels of CD123. Constitutional symptoms and splenomegaly are present in about half of patients with CMML; hepatomegaly and extramedullary involvement (skin and lymph nodes) is present less frequently. Patients with proliferative type CMML are enriched for RAS pathway mutations and may have a higher risk of transformation than other subtypes. MDS/ MPN-RS-T is hallmarked by thrombocytosis and medullary ring sideroblasts, while MDS/MPN-U has no clear association with a specific myeloid subset but instead, is identified by the presence of clinical and/or pathologic manifestations of myeloproliferation and BM failure.

Genetics

MDS/MPN overlap disorders are pathobiologically distinct from MDS and have distinct mutational profiles. Somatic mutations are significantly more common than in MDS and involve epigenetic modifiers (*TET2*, *SRSF2*, *IDH1/2*, *EZH2*, and *ASXL1*), signaling (*CSF3R*, *JAK2*, *NRAS*, *KRAS*, and *CBL*), splicing (*SF3A1* and *U2AF35*), and transcription (*RUNX1*) genes and are likely

to co-occur. Indeed, the triad of *TET2*, *ASXL1*, and *SRSF2* mutations is highly specific for CMML-0.[136] In contrast, mutations of *SF3B1* and *TP53* are observed less often than in MDS. Mutations deregulating *RAS* are found in almost all patients with JMML. Up to 80% of patients with MDS/MPN-RS-T have activated JAK-STAT signaling as a consequence of the presence of *JAK2*[V617F] or *MPL* mutations. Clonal architecture analysis in CMML has demonstrated linear acquisition of candidate mutations with limited branching through loss of heterozygosity.

Chronic myelomonocytic leukemia

The 2016 WHO classification defines CMML by the presence of monocytosis that is relative (>10% of WBC) and absolute (>1 × 10⁹/L) and must persist for >3 months, and BM findings that typically meet MDS diagnostic criteria, hypercellularity with dysplasia in >1 cell lineage and <20% blasts. Additionally, criteria diagnostic of myeloid neoplasms and alternative causes of monocytosis need to be excluded.[137] The current WHO classification divides CMML into a "proliferative type," with a total WBC >13 × 10⁹/L, and a "dysplastic type," with a WBC below this threshold, to reflect clinical and genetic distinctions, and sub-classified into three groups based on PB and BM blast proportions and not on total WBC counts: CMML-0 with 2% blasts in PB and 5% blasts in the BM, CMML-1 with 2% to 4% blasts in PB and/or 5% to 9% blasts in BM, and CMML-2 with 5% to 19% blasts in PB and 10% to 19% in BM, and/or presence of Auer rods (Figure 28.15).

Historical prognostic scoring systems only included a few patients with dysplastic type CMML, whereas proliferative type CMML was excluded. This led to the introduction of novel CMML-specific prognostic tools, based on monocyte counts, molecular abnormalities, clinical features, and risk to transform to AML and molecular abnormalities. Indeed, *ASXL1* has now been validated as an independent adverse prognostic marker.[138] As illustration, a combined ELN/European Haematology Association (EHA) expert panel proposed CMML-specific diagnostic and treatment recommendations in 2018, and the MDS/MPN International Working Group proposed response criteria in 2015, which are currently being revised.[139,140]

Allo-SCT remains the only treatment that can accord long-term remission and a 10-year OS of about 40%. At present, there are no satisfactory non-transplant options, and the principal aim of therapy is to improve symptoms related to cytopenias and proliferative features. HMAs are approved for symptomatic low-risk and all intermediate- and high-risk patients. Response rates appear to be similar to those seen in patients with MDS, with no significant impact on risk of transformation or survival. Based on the poor prognostic impact of plasmacytic dendritic cells and CD123-positivity of clonal monocytes in CMML, tagraxofusp, a CD123-targeted drug, is currently being tested both as a monotherapy and in combination with HMAs or venetoclax.[141] The preliminary monotherapy Phase II results are encouraging, with clinical benefits, in particular reduction of splenomegaly, reduction of symptom burden, and reduction of red-cell transfusion requirements; some patients achieved BM CRs and were successfully allografted.

Atypical chronic myeloid leukemia

Atypical chronic myeloid leukemia (aCML) was initially described as a subtype of CML with the notable absence of the *BCR-ABL1* fusion gene.[142] Its diagnosis requires the exclusion of not only *BCR-ABL1* but also rearrangement of *PDGFRA*, *PDGFRB*, or *FGFR1*. MPN-associated driver mutations such as *JAK2*, *CALR*, and *MPL* are typically absent in aCML. The differential diagnosis

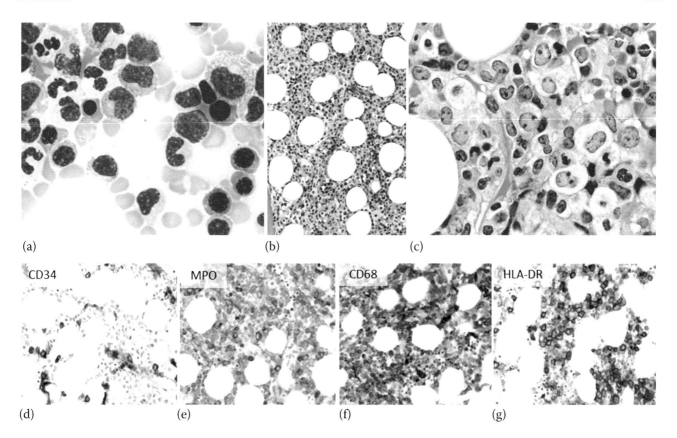

FIGURE 28.15 Chronic myelomonocytic leukemia: (a) bone marrow aspirate with maturing myeloid cells and increased monocytes; (b and c) bone marrow trephine biopsy is hypercellular with prominent monocytosis; immunohistochemical stains (d–g) demonstrate slightly increased blasts (d; CD34 staining) and predominance of cells positive for MPO (e), CD68 (f), and HLA-DR (g). (From Gorczyca, 2014. With permission.)

includes CNL, CMML, and MDS/MPN-U. Patients tend to have severe anemia, thrombocytopenia, neutrophilia with prominent granulocytic dysplasia, and splenomegaly; monocytosis and basophilia are usually absent or minimally present in the peripheral blood. There are some clinical and morphological similarities between aCML and CNL, which is typically associated with a mutated *CSF3R* gene, which is found in <10% of patients with aCML. Recurrent mutations have been described in *SETBP1* and/or *ETNK1* gene mutations in a third of cases, occasionally found in aCML. Allo-SCT appears to be the only treatment that can afford aCML patients a long-term remission.[143] Other therapies include HMAs and hydroxycarbamide and the investigational use of JAK inhibitors.

Juvenile myelomonocytic leukemia

Juvenile myelomonocytic leukemia (JMML) is an uncommon, aggressive childhood malignancy. Its initiating pathogenetic event appears to be hyperactivation of the RAS pathway, as a result of mutations in a limited set of genes, *PTPN11*, *NF1*, *NRAS*, *KRAS*, or *CBL*, in over 90% of patients. Mutations in *SETBP1* or *JAK3* and monosomy 7 (-7) have been observed in about 25% of patients.[144] A novel fetal-like molecular subgroup with *LIN28B* overexpression with high age-adjusted fetal hemoglobin (HbF) levels has been described. Uniquely, most patients with JMML exhibit an increased *in vitro* sensitivity to GM-CSF, which appears to augment signaling of other downstream effectors, in particular JAK/STAT5. Although JMML shares some clinical features with CMML, such as monocytosis and hepatosplenomegaly,

the molecular features are quite distinct by the absence of mutations in epigenetic and splicing modifiers. Congenital JMML predisposition syndromes exist, particularly neurofibromatosis and Noonan syndrome, which converge on RAS/MAPK signaling abnormalities and markedly increase the risk of developing JMML. The natural history of JMML is variable, with some patients, particularly those with Noonan syndrome or CBL syndrome, having spontaneous resolution of their disease despite identification of clonal hematopoiesis, while others can have a fulminant clinical course, and DNA-methylating patterns might improve prediction of outcomes.

Allo-SCT is the standard of care, with an event-free 5-year survival of 52%. The principal cause for failure is relapse, which approaches 50%. It has been speculated that the high relapse rate might be related to an underlying fundamental immune defect or incomplete eradication of resistant disease prior to myeloablation. Importantly, about half of these relapsed children can be treated successfully with a second allograft. Strategies to rescue children post-relapse remain suboptimal, with limited success of DLI. Non-transplant alternatives are limited.

MDS/MPN with ring sideroblasts and thrombocytosis

Patients with MDS/MPN-RS-T have MDS features of MDS with ring sideroblasts in addition to sustained thrombocytosis (>450,000/μL) and megakaryocyte cytological features resembling ET. After CMML, MDS/MPN-RS-T is the next most common subtype of MDS/MPN overlap disorders. Importantly, patients with MDS/MPN-RS-T have little resemblance to CMML clinically or genetically. Mutations in the *SF3B1* are found in >80% of patients, similar to the percentage observed in patients with MDS-RS-SLD. Mutations are also found in several other genes, including *JAK2* (60%), *CALR* (15%), and *MPL* (3%), which are comparable to the molecular landscape of patients with ET. The prognosis of patients, including the risk of transformation, with MDS/MPN-RS-T is not dissimilar to that in MDS-RS-SLD and ET, but the rate of thrombosis is higher in MDS/MPN-RSD-T and ET compared with MDS-RS-SLD.[145] There is no firm consensus regarding optimal clinical management, and supportive care remains the cornerstone. In patients with anemia, treatment is supportive with ESAs and red-cell transfusions. Low-dose aspirin can be considered for those with thrombotic risk.

MDS/MPN–unclassifiable

MDS/MPN–unclassifiable (MDS/MPN-U) is a subgroup of MDS/MPN that includes patients who lack defining characteristics of the other well-defined entities, such as CMML. It probably accounts for fewer than 5% of MDS/MPN patients. Clinically, patients often present with constitutional symptoms, splenomegaly, and low monocyte counts. About 20% of patients demonstrate the presence of trisomy 8 and a $JAK2^{V617F}$ mutation. Suitable clinical trials should be pursued whenever possible.

Transformation to AML in MDS/MPN

Transformation to AML, which is often refractory to conventional treatment, is a challenging complication in MDS/MPN, as it is in MDS and MPN. The incidence of AML transformation is unknown, except for CMML, where it is about 15% to 52%, with *ASXL1* or *RUNX1*, higher white blood counts, marrow cellularity, karyotype risk score, and a revised IPSS score increasing risk. Cytogenetic progression, often involving abnormalities in chromosomes 7 (target genes *EZH2* and *IKZF1*), 8 (*MYC*), 17p (*TP53*), 21 (*ERG* and *RUNX1*), 12 (*ETV6*), and i(17q) (*TP53*) are often noted. The results of treatments for AML transformation in MDS/MPN are poor.

Chronic lymphocytic leukemias

Lymphoid leukemias of mature B- and T- and NK-cells are chronic lymphoproliferative disorders characterized by the accumulation and proliferation of clonal lymphocytes of the corresponding lineage in the blood, bone marrow, lymph nodes, and sometimes other lymphoid tissues. They are recognized in the revised 2016 WHO classification as chronic lymphocytic leukemia (CLL), prolymphocytic leukemia (PLL), hairy cell leukemia (HCL), and large granular lymphocyte (LGL) leukemia. The classification also recognizes small lymphocytic lymphoma (SLL) as a predominantly nodular variant of CLL, with both entities representing identical morphology and immunophenotype. Historically, CLL was considered to be a disease of clonal B-cells (B-CLL) or T-cells (T-CLL), and in the current WHO classification, the entity CLL refers to a B-CLL only; T-CLL is now referred to as T-cell PLL. Other forms of mature B-cell lymphomas that frequently affect the blood and bone marrow include mantle cell lymphoma (MCL), splenic marginal zone lymphoma (SMZL), and follicular lymphoma (FL), which are discussed elsewhere in this edition of *Treatment of Cancer*.

Chronic lymphocytic leukemias

CLL is an indolent heterogeneous disease characterized by the clonal expansion of small mature-appearing malignant CD5⁺CD19⁺CD23⁺ B-cells in the PB and infiltration of secondary lymphoid organs, such as lymph nodes, spleen, and BM. The past two decades have witnessed significant research insights into the stunning complexity of the CLL genome, which in turn, inform better risk stratification methods and the identification of new therapeutic targets.[146] Indeed, the past decade has witnessed how the clinical management of patients with CLL has at once become more effective and personalized yet clinically challenging with the approval of diverse classes of therapies. A principal aim now is to offer chemotherapy-free treatment for patients with CLL who need it and at the same time identify clearly those who do not require therapy.

Epidemiology

CLL is the most common form of leukemia in Western countries, where the incidence and prevalence continue to rise. It has been estimated that in 2019, there were about 21,000 new cases diagnosed in the United States and about 4000 CLL-related deaths. CLL predominantly affects older people and is more prevalent in males.[147] The median age of onset is around 72 years. It appears to be less common in certain geographical locations, such as India and China, but this requires additional studies. At present, there is no evidence to suggest that genetic, environmental, dietary, lifestyle, infection, or ionizing radiation factors are important. Pesticide exposure, in particular Agent Orange, has been considered to be a risk factor in the United States.

Diagnosis and clinical features

About 80% of all patients with CLL are diagnosed by a routine blood test for unrelated reasons, which shows an absolute lymphocytosis, with greater than 5×10^9/L clonal lymphocytes sustained for at least 3 months. The remainder present with fatigue, fever, weight loss, lymphadenopathy, hepato-splenomegaly, or infections. The impaired immune system in CLL, largely due to the associated hypogammaglobulinemia, also favors the gradual development of autoimmune hemolytic anemia and autoimmune thrombocytopenia. The disease follows a variable course, with survival ranging from a few years to a few decades. The International Workshop on CLL (iwCLL) revised recommendations for the diagnostics, response criteria, indications for treatment, updates on MRD status for clinical evolution, and supportive management in 2018 and is broadly accepted.[148] The characterization of the CLL cell is based on morphology and immunophenotypic features that show CD5⁺CD19⁺CD23⁺ coupled with low levels of CD20 and surface immunoglobulins (Figure 28.15).

Molecular pathogenesis and genetics

Substantial advances have been made in understanding the biology of CLL. The seminal work of Hamblin and others in 1999 describing the mutational status of the immunoglobulin heavy chain (IGHV) provides an initial framework for identifying patients at high risk of progression and those who might benefit from first-line therapy with fludarabine, cyclophosphamide, and rituximab (FCR).[149,150] Another important historical observation was the high levels of zeta-associated protein 70 (ZAP-70), a receptor-associated protein tyrosine kinase expressed with IGHV-unmutated (IGHV-UM) cells.[151] The cancer-initiating events in mature B-cells are poorly understood; the unraveling of the genetic and epigenetic architecture, shaped by the host microenvironment, is beginning to unfold and growth dynamics in naturally progressing disease to be characterized.[152] Several chromosomal and genetic alterations are well recognized to be implicated in the pathogenesis and impact clinical management.[153] Over 80% of patients with CLL have at least one of four characteristic abnormalities: deletion in chromosome 13q14 (del13q) is associated with good prognosis and found in >50%; deletion in chromosome 11q23 (del11q) is found in about 20% and associated with alterations in *ATM* and poor prognosis, but a good response to ibrutinib-based therapy; trisomy 12, found in about 16%, has an intermediate prognosis; and deletion in chromosome 17 (del17p), found in about 7%, is associated with loss of *TP53* and very poor prognosis (Figure 28.16) (ultra-high-risk). Sequencing of the CLL genome has revealed considerable genetic heterogeneity and no unifying or diagnostic mutations.[154] The most frequent mutations involve *SF3B1* (21%), *ATM* (15%), *TP53* (7%), *NOTCH1* (6%), and *BRIC3* (4%). Recurrent somatic mutations play an important role in mRNA processing (*SF3B1* and *XP01*), DNA damage (*TP53* and *ATM*), Notch signaling (*NOTCH1*), B-cell signaling (*EGR2* or *BRAF*), chromatin modification (*HIST1H1E*, *CHD2*, and *ZYMYM3*), Wnt signaling, and inflammatory pathways (*MYD88*). Clonal evolution in patients with CLL developing resistance to BTK inhibition has also been described.[155]

The BCL2 family member expression in CLL has proven to be pivotal in the elucidation of one of the most effective current targeted therapies for CLL. The BCL2 protein family comprises >30 related proteins that are divided into several subclasses based on structural and functional features. The mechanism of expression of BCL2 in CLL probably involves miRNA-mediated changes in the CLL cell in a complex relationship. Regardless, the lessons learned so far paved the way for the introduction of venetoclax, a small-molecule BH-3 mimetic that inhibits BCL2, into the clinics.[156] Research into the CLL microenvironment identified the complex interactions in the host microenvironment through a variety of cytokines, chemokines, integrins, and survival factors, such as BAFF and APRIL.

Staging systems and prognostic factors

The staging systems introduced by Rai in 1975 and Binet in 1981 were based on the notion that CLL cells first accumulate in the PB and BM, followed by lymphoid tissues, finally leading to BM failure.[157,158] This acknowledged the Dameshek–Galton model of orderly disease progression in CLL and allowed patients with CLL to be categorized into three prognostic groups. Several new prognostic models are now in the clinics, such as the International Prognostic Index for patients with CLL (CLL-IPI), which combines genetic, biochemical, and clinical parameters to define four prognostic groups and was introduced in 2016.[159]

Treatment

The 2018 iwCLL and the 2020 NCCN treatment recommendations suggest that good-risk patients can be managed successfully with a "watch and wait" policy, at intervals of 1 to 3 months, and therapy should be initiated for active disease (Table 28.16).[160] The outcomes for those with intermediate-, high-, or ultra-high risk of the disease have had incremental benefit from a chemoimmunotherapy combination, and additional improvements are being observed with the approval of even more effective and relatively safe therapies, such as ibrutinib, a BTK inhibitor, and idelalisib, a PI3Kδ inhibitor, for high- and ultra-high-risk patients of all age groups.[161,162] Venetoclax was approved in 2018 for the treatment of patients with CLL or SLL, with or without, del(17p), following at least one prior line of treatment.

First-line

The choice of first-line treatment depends very much on the presence or absence of recognized adverse prognostic factors and the age of the patient. Outside clinical trials, chlorambucil, an alkylating agent that has been in use for half a century, remains

---

TABLE 28.16 2018 iwCLL Guidelines for Initiating Treatment in Patients with CLL Considered to Have Active Disease

- Evidence of BM failure with symptomatic anemia (Hb <10 g/dL) or thrombocytopenia (platelets <100 × 10⁹/L)
- Progressive lymphocytosis[a] with an increase of >50% over 2 months or a lymphocyte doubling time <6 months
- Progressive and/or symptomatic splenomegaly (>6 cm below the left costal margin)
- Progressive and/or symptomatic lymphadenopathy (>10 cm in greatest diameter)
- Symptomatic extranodal involvement
- Steroid-refractory, autoimmune hemolytic anemia or autoimmune thrombocytopenia
- Progressive constitutional symptoms: unintentional weight loss >10% in 6 months, fever >38.5 °C for >2 weeks without evidence of infection, or night sweats >1 month without evidence of infection, poor performance status, or unable to perform usual activities

Source: Adapted from data in Sharma and Rai, 2019.

a An absolute lymphocyte count in itself is not an indicator for treatment.

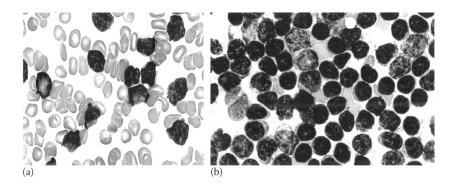

FIGURE 28.16 Photomicrograph of chronic lymphocytic leukemia: (a) peripheral blood film showing many mature lymphocytes— "smudge" cells and (b) bone marrow aspirate showing increased number of lymphocytes.

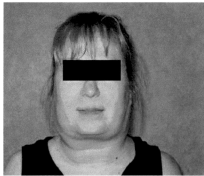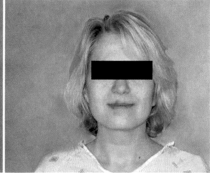

FIGURE 28.17 A patient with marked lymphadenopathy and CLL being treated with idelalisib. (Courtesy of Professor Hagop Kantarjian.)

a reasonable option for the older frail patient.[163] Chlorambucil as a monotherapy has few acute side effects but is not capable of inducing CRs. The drug is much more effective when combined with immunotherapy, such as rituximab or obinutuzumab, as shown in a randomized trial.[164] Importantly, a recent real-world analysis confirmed the safety and effectiveness of chlorambucil in combination with obinutuzumab.[165]

Fludarabine, a purine analog, in combination with cyclophosphamide and rituximab (FCR) is generally considered as the standard of care for previously untreated younger patients (aged <65 years) with no comorbidities and who have mutated IGHV without del17p.[166] Long-term results demonstrate an overall response rate of 95%, a CR rate of 72%, and a 6-year PFS of 6 years, and 50% of patients with mutated IGHV achieved MRD negativity. FCR is, however, poorly tolerated by older patients due to prolonged myelosuppression and infections. Bendamustine, a drug with structural similarities to alkylating agents and purine analogs, was tested against chlorambucil and found to improve response rates but not OS. Bendamustine in combination with rituximab (BR) was tested in a Phase III randomized study (CLL10) as first-line therapy in a cohort in which del17p patients were excluded.[167] The study results observed that though FCR was superior to BR, FCR was associated with greater toxicity in patients aged >65 years. An exploratory post-hoc subgroup analysis demonstrated no significant differences in the PFS between FCR and BR for patients >65 years, making BR the preferred first-line therapy for older patients without ultra-high-risk features. Finally, the BTK inhibitor ibrutinib is currently licensed for both first-line and subsequent therapy in the United States and relapsed disease in Europe. Side effects associated with ibrutinib tend to be mild and include diarrhea, arthralgia, cough, and rash; unique toxicities include bleeding and atrial fibrillation, as a consequence of an off-target effect of inhibiting TEC kinase, and rash, as a result of epidermal growth factor receptor inhibition. Long-term results confirm the drug's safety and efficacy as a monotherapy.[168]

Second-line

For patients with CLL who relapse, it is important to establish whether they require treatment at the time of relapse for disease related symptoms or have active disease.[160] For patients with an early relapse, defined as those who relapse within 24–36 months following treatment with chemoimmunotherapy, it is reasonable to consider ibrutunib, idelalisib, venetoclax, or duvelisib; for those who relapse after being in remission for 36 months or more, re-treatment with the initial therapy or any of the targeted drugs listed above is reasonable. The long-term efficacy

of ibrutinib compared with ofatumab has now been well established.[169] Idelalisib is approved for second-line therapy following at least one prior therapy. The drug is effective but associated with significant toxicities, including colitis, pneumonitis, and hepatitis (Figure 28.17). Venetoclax has been found to be remarkably effective in relapsed and/or refractory disease, with responses of about 80%, including 8% complete responses, and is now licensed for patients with relapsed disease and del(17p). The principal adverse effects are neutropenia and tumor lysis syndrome, which can be mitigated by a weekly ramp-up schedule starting at a very low dose. Duvelisib is also effective and approved for all patients with relapsed/refractory disease after they have received at least two lines of prior therapy. Ofatumumab was approved in 2016 to treat relapsed/refractory patients with CLL following two lines of prior therapy.

Allogeneic stem cell transplantation

Following the remarkable success of oral targeted therapies, such as ibrutinib, idelalisib, and venetoclax, in the treatment of patients deemed to be at high and ultra-high risk of disease, it appears reasonable *not* to offer allo-SCT as a treatment approach for patients with del(17p) in first remission.[170] Allo-SCT has proven successful but is associated with significant TRM and morbidity. Registry data suggest a 5-year EFS of 37% and a 2-year TRM of 28%. Risk models have been developed to help the decision-making process, and the factors identified to predict for better EFS were age, performance status, remission status, conditioning type, donor type, and donor sex. In the relapsed setting, the role of allo-SCT needs to be assessed carefully against the patient's previous treatments and the current risk status of *TP53* and del(17p) and any additional genetic information, such as *NOTCH 1* and *SF3B1*, if available. Such prognostic and predictive information can help the decision-making process. Clearly, the notion of offering allo-SCT for patients with CLL is increasingly complex with the available effective and relatively safe targeted agents for first and subsequent lines of therapy.

Investigational approaches

Following the success of ibrutinib and venetoclax inhibitors in high- and ultra-high-risk patients, particularly those with mutated *TP53* clones, research is assessing not only the earlier use of these agents in an effort to prevent the emergence of chemorefractory disease but also their use in combination regimens; venetoclax is being tested in patients receiving bendamustine initially, followed by a combination of obinutuzumab and venetoclax. The interim results of this study are impressive, with an overall response rate of 97%, and 89% MRD negative. Studies are also assessing venetoclax-based combinations with other anti-CD20 antibodies and with/without ibrutinib. There is also renewed interest in navitoclax, another BCL2 inhibitor, which is more active against BCL-xL, as opposed to venetoclax, which is more potent against BCL2. Other candidate investigational approaches include acalabrutinib, a second-generation BTK inhibitor, alisertib (MLN8237), an aurora A kinase inhibitor, and several forms of immunotherapy. Acalabrutinib appears to have a better BTK occupancy compared with ibrutinib, and it will be of interest to determine whether this reduces the emergence of resistance. SYK inhibitors, such as fostamatinib and entospletinib, remain in clinical trials at present, with impressive results so far. The immunotherapy efforts include several monoclonal antibodies, such as lumiliximab (anti-CD23), epratuzumab (anti-CD22), and apolizumab (anti-HLA-DR), IDEC-114 (anti-CD80), immune-modulatory drugs, such as lenalidomide, and adoptive immunotherapy using CD19-specific CAR T-cells in patients who progress on ibrutinib. There has also been much interest in the use of immune checkpoint inhibitors, but the results of these Phase I/II studies have not been encouraging so far.

Richter's syndrome

Richter's syndrome (RS) is defined as the transformation of CLL into an aggressive lymphoma, most commonly DLBCL.[171] Historically, it was first described by Maurice Richter in 1928, and it has an annual incidence of about 5–10% in patients with CLL, who often present with constitutional symptoms and histological changes in one or several lymph nodes and rarely, in bone marrow. Sequential molecular genetic studies, which reveal recurrent somatic mutations in >90% of RS, have confirmed that most, but interestingly not all, RS arises from the original CLL founder clone. These mutations in RS include a high prevalence of *TP53*; other mutations include *NOTCH1*, *CDKN2A*, *CDKN2B*, and *MYC* activating events; in contrast, many of the genetic mutations seen in *de novo* DLBCL, such as *BCL6*, *PRDM1*, *B2M*, *CREBBP*, and *EP300*, are either rare or absent. Interestingly, *NOTCH1* mutations, found in about 25% of newly diagnosed CLL at a subclonal level, have a high predictability for the risk of RS transformation in newly diagnosed patients with CLL. The presence of the mutation at a subclonal level at diagnosis suggests that it is rarely acquired during clonal evolution and is most likely selected for expression. There have also been some reports

suggesting a causal role for EBV in RS and the notion that therapies that result in severe immunosuppression in CLL, such as fludarabine and alemtuzumab, might have a double-edged sword effect, but further confirmation is required. Most patients with transformed RS fare rather poorly with DLBCL treatments, probably due to the associated *TP53* mutations.

Prolymphocytic leukemia

PLL is a rare, aggressive form of mature leukemia, which is distinct from CLL and recognized by the WHO 2016 classification to comprise of B-PLL and T-PLL. B-PLL, first recognized in 1974 by David Galton (London), has considerable overlap with other B-cell lymphoid malignancies, which are described below (Figure 28.18). It probably accounts for <2% of the mature lymphoid leukemias affecting adults and fewer than 1% of CLL patients who transform into PLL. Most patients present with constitutional symptoms characterized by symptomatic splenomegaly, lymphadenopathy, and erythematous or nodular rashes, and about 25% have pleuroperitoneal effusions; lymphocytosis, often >100 × 10⁹/L, is not uncommon.[172] Recent genetic findings suggest B-PLL has three distinct subtypes based on C-MYC translocations or gains along with presence/absence of 17p-. In T-PLL, inv(14)(q11q23) and t(14;14)(q11q23) are observed in about 70% and t(x;14)(q28q11) in 20% of patients; abnormalities in chromosome 8 are also common. Rearrangements between the TCR gene (on chromosome 14) and *TCL-1*, *TCL-1B*, or *MTCP-1* (on chromosome X) result in oncoproteins via activation of AKT and may be important in the molecular pathogenesis of the disease. About 75% of patients with T-PLL harbor abnormalities in the *ATM* gene and in the JAK-STAT pathway, in particular *IL2RG*, *JAK-1*, *JAK-3*, and *STAT-5B*. Rare mutations involving *EZH2*, *FBXW10*, and *CHEK2* have also been observed in addition to a unique case report involving the *SEPT9-ABL1* fusion. In contrast, about half of the patients with B-PLL have abnormal cytogenetics, in particular (8;14) or del(17p), and molecular genetics, with *TP53* mutations or deletions and *MYC* abnormalities. There is some genetic overlap between B-PLL and other B-lymphoid malignancies, such as MCL, SMZL, and HCL variants. At present, there is no firm consensus on the treatment or indeed, when it is indicated for patients with PLL, and many patients receive CLL-type therapies. The advent of potential novel therapies have led to recent collaborative efforts to establish consensus criteria for diagnosis, staging, and treatment assessment for T-PLL; similar efforts are also being proposed for B-PLL.

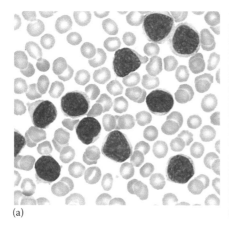
(a)

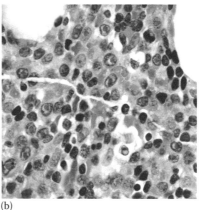
(b)

FIGURE 28.18 (a) Blood smear from a patient with B-PLL, showing B-PLL cells with prominent nuclei. (b) Bone marrow trephine from the same patient showing involvement with lymphoid cells with prominent nuclei. (From Gorczyca, 2014. With permission.)

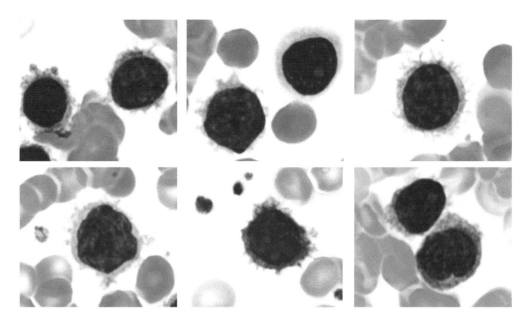

FIGURE 28.19   Blood smears of several cases of hairy cell leukemia. (From Gorczyca, 2014. With permission.)

Hairy cell leukemia

HCL is a rare chronic mature B-cell malignancy which presents with progressive pancytopenia, splenomegaly, infiltration of bone marrow, liver, and spleen, and circulating B-cells possessing cytoplasmic projections that resemble "hair-like" microvilli (Figure 28.19). It affects about 1 in 100,000 adults, largely males, and has unique clinical, pathological, biologic, and genetic features.[9] The 2008 WHO classification recognized two subtypes, a classic (HCLc) and a variant (HCLv), which in the 2016 WHO revised version, have provisionally been placed in the category of "splenic lymphomas, unclassified." The discovery of *BRAF*V600E as a driver mutation of HCLc provides important insights into the disease pathogenesis and novel treatment. The HCL genome is generally considered to be stable, with fewer than 10% of patients demonstrating recurrent chromosomal abnormalities, in particular deletion of the long arm of chromosome 7, and no copy number alterations. Genomic sequencing studies have also revealed the presence of mutations in the tumor suppressor *CDKN1B* gene, encoding for the cyclin-dependent kinase inhibitor p27 and in the *KLF2* gene, which encodes for a transcription factor in some patients with HCLc.[173]

Historically, most patients presented with features of advanced disease, which included fatigue, massive splenomegaly, and infections. Nowadays, most patients are diagnosed in the early stages of the disease, and most are asymptomatic. The diagnosis is often made following a work-up for incidental pancytopenia. The BM biopsy typically reveals extensive fibrosis, and the PB film may reveal circulating TRAP-staining hairy cells, which in the case of HCLc, co-express CD19, CD20, CD11c, CD25, CD103, and CD123 and stain positively for VE1 (*BRAF*V600E); in contrast, HCLv cells tend to be negative for CD25, CD123, and VE1 stain.

About 80% of patients with HCL can achieve long-term remissions following treatment with purine analogs, such as cladribine and pentostatin, with/without rituximab, and an OS approaching that of the general population. Responses, however, are not always durable; about 30% of the patients relapse, and subsequent responses are poor. At progression, therapies include the recently approved anti-CD22 immunotoxin, moxetumomab pasudotox,

following at least two prior therapies, and the BRAF inhibitor, vemurafenib, which is being tested as monotherapy or combined with MEK inhibitors.[174]

Large granular lymphocyte leukemia

The 2016 WHO classification of LGL leukemia comprises an indolent T-cell subtype, T-cell LGL leukemia (T-LGL-L), which accounts for about 85% of all cases, and two NK-cell subtypes: an indolent type, termed chronic lymphoproliferative disorder of NK-cells (CLPD-NK), and an aggressive type, termed aggressive NK-cell leukemia (ANKL). Additionally, the classification highlights new subsets with *STAT3* and *STAT5b* mutations and a clinically more aggressive phenotype. LGL leukemia was first described in 1985 and considered to account for about 2–5% of all mature lymphoid malignancies. The ANKL subtype is associated with EBV infection and largely observed in Asia, particularly Japan. The diagnosis of LGL leukemia is often difficult; it is initially suspected when the PB count of LGL cells is greater than 2×10^9dL (normal value $<0.3 \times 10^9$/dL) (Figure 28.20). In some patients, in particular those with autoimmune disorders, who often have substantial comorbid conditions and cytopenias, patients may present with relatively low LGL counts. A definitive diagnosis relies on demonstrating an expanded clonal T- or NK-cell LGL population, which demonstrates distinct morphological, immunophenotypic, and molecular features. The presence of identical STAT3 mutations in T- and NK-subtypes is suggestive of the mutations' pathogenetic role and constitutes a potential therapeutic target.[175] Most patients with T-LGL-L and CLPD-NK are considered to have indolent diseases and can be managed initially with a "wait and watch" approach. Treatment, when indicated, often comprises an immunosuppressive therapy, such as low-dose methotrexate, cyclosporine A, or cyclophosphamide. In contrast, ANKL is an aggressive disease with a dismal prognosis. Allo-SCT has been tested in a few patients with some success. Investigational approaches, such as the *JAK3* inhibitor, tofacitinib citrate, and a farnesyltransferase inhibitor, tipifarnib, are being studied. Other novel approaches include targeting IL-15 and other cytokine antagonistic agents.

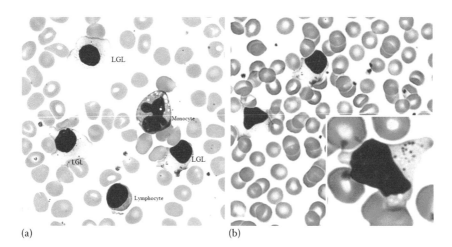

FIGURE 28.20   Peripheral blood films (a and b) from several patients with T-cell large granular leukemia (T-LGL). Note the large LGL cells with prominent cytoplasmic granules. Compare with monocytes and normal small lymphocytes (a). (From Gorczyca, 2014. With permission.)

Key learning points

- The remarkable understanding in the pathophysiology of leukemias has enabled the introduction of more effective and targeted therapies for the treatment of leukemias.
- Better classification, risk stratification and monitoring provide a biologically based, integrated framework for defining and treating leukemias CHIP is associated with an increased risk of leukemias, particularly AML, MDS, and MPNs, as well as an increased risk of cardiovascular mortality.
- The treatment of AML remains challenging, particularly older patients. Several recently licensed targeted therapies, such as venetoclax, are informing the next class of AML therapeutics, including immunotherapies and the design of rational combination regimens with the objective of achieving MRD and long-term remission.
- Despite the impressive cure rates for children with B-cell ALL, the survival for infants, childhood T-cell ALL, and most adolescent and adult ALL patients remains suboptimal. Recent advances include MRD-guided treatment and CAR T cell therapy.
- The CML success story has been contingent upon BCR-ABL1 being the founder lesion in every cell and minimal genetic diversity. Five TKIs that can durably reduce the number of CML cells and result in life expectancy approaching that of normal population, are now licensed. Resistance can be an issue, but durable subsequent remissions can be achieved following a switch to an alternative TKI or an allo-SCT. Serious TKI-related cardiovascular events can occur in CML patients with co-morbidity. Consequently, an important treatment milestone for patients achieving durable deep molecular responses is TFR.
- For patients with MPNs, treatment emphasis is on the reduction of risks for thrombosis and bleeding, and symptom control. For patients with higher-risk MF, there are two licensed JAK inhibitors that accord rapid and substantial clinical benefits but few molecular remissions and no significant impact on transformation to secondary AML. Hydroxycarbamide (hydroxyurea) remains the standard treatment in high-risk patients with PV and ET. IFNα and ruxolitinib are useful as second-line therapies for patients with PV. Midostaurin is now licensed for the treatment of patients with SM.
- ESAs and lenalidomide are standard therapies for LR-MDS and HMAs for HR-MDS. Luspatercept is now licensed for a subset of LR-MDS. HMAs remain the principal treatment for dysplastic CMML; several approaches including CD123-targeted therapies, such as tagraxofusp, are being tested proliferative CMML. Allografting remains the only treatment option with potentially curative potential.
- The identification of keynote proteins in the critical pathways in B-cell biology and pathogenesis led to the development of BTK, PI3Kδ, and BCL2 inhibitors, which are able to overcome the high- and ultra-high-risk disease associated with TP53 mutations or loss or del(17p), and are now licensed. However, some serious side-effects, resistance, and high-costs are challenging. PLL is recognized as a distinct entity from CLL and suitable therapies are being developed. For patients with HCLc disease, long-term remission is possible with purine analogs, rituximab, and BRAF inhibitors.

Acknowledgments

I thank Alpa Parmar for her love and support, and Karol Sikora for his mentorship and much patience during the preparation of this work. I thank Rick Van Etten, Giuseppe Saglio, Kanti Rai, Marty Tallman, Jerry Radich, Tony Goldstone, Tiziano Barbui, Serge Verstovek, Hagop Kantarjian, Alan Burnett, Danny Catovsky, Steven Rosen, and others for providing comments.

References

1. Mendez-Ferrer S, Bonnet D, Steensma D et al. Bone marrow niches in hematological malignancies. *Nat Rev Cancer.* 2020; 28:1–4.
2. Morrison SJ, Scadden DT. The bone marrow niche for haemopoietic stem cells. *Nature.* 2014; 505:327–34.
3. O'Brien CA, Kreso A, Jamieson CHM. Cancer stem cells and self-renewal. *Clin Cancer Res.* 2010; 16:3113–20.
4. Nangalia J, Campbell PJ. Genome sequencing during a patient's journey through cancer. *N Engl J Med.* 2019; 381:2145–56.
5. Jan M, Ebert BL, Jaiswal S. Clonal hematopoiesis. *Seminars Hematol.* 2017; 54:43–50.

6. Arber DA, Orazi A, Hasserjian R et al. The 2016 revision to the World Health Organization classification of myeloid neoplasms and acute leukemia. *Blood*. 2016; 127:2391–405.

7. Sanden C, Lilljebjorn H, Pietras CO et al. Clonal competition within complex evolutionary hierarchies shapes AML over time. *Nat Commun*. 2020; 11(1):1–0.

8. Dombret H, Gardin C. An update of current treatments for adult acute myeloid leukemia. *Blood*. 2016; 127:53–61.

9. Siegel RL, Miller KD, Jemal A. Cancer Statistics, 2019. *CA Cancer J Clin*. 2019; 69:7–34.

10. Bennett JM, Catovsky D, Daniel MT et al. Proposals for the classification of the acute leukaemias. *Br J Haematol*. 1976; 33:451–8.

11. Papaemmanuil E, Gerstung M, Bullinger L et al. Genomic classification and prognosis in acute myeloid leukemia. *N Engl J Med*. 2016; 374:2209–21.

12. Tyner JW, Tognon CE, Bottomly D et al. Functional genomic landscape of acute myeloid leukmia. *Nature*. 2018; 562:526–31.

13. Potter N, Miraki-Moud F, Ermini L et al. Single cell analysis of clonal architecture in acute myeloid leukemia. *Leukemia*. 2019; 33:1113–23.

14. Dohner H, Estey E, Grimwade D et al. Diagnosis and management of AML in adults: 2017 ELN recommendations from an international expert panel. *Blood*. 2017; 129:424–47.

15. Bill M, Nicolet D, Kohischmidt J et al. Mutations associated with 17-gene leukemia stem cell score and the score's prognostic relevance in the context of the European leukemia net classification of acxute leukemia. *Haematologica*. 2020; 105:721–29.

16. Lowenburg B, Downing JR, Burnett A. Acute myeloid leukaemia. *N Engl J Med*. 1999; 341:1051–62.

17. Gerstung M, Papaemmanuil E, Martincorena et al. Precision oncology for acute myeloid leukemia using a knowledge bank approach. *Nat Genet*. 2017; 49:332–40.

18. Jongen-Lavrencic, Grob T, Hanekamp D et al. Molecular minimal residual disease in acute myeloid leukemia. *N Engl J Med*. 2018; 378:1189–99.

19. Dillon R, Hills R, Freeman S et al. Molecular MRD status and outcome after transplantation in *NPM1*-mutated AML. *Blood*. 2020; 135:680–8

20. Short NJ, Konopleva M, Kadia T et al. Advances in treatment of acute myeloid leukemia: New drugs and new challenges. *Cancer Discovery*. 202; 10(4):506–25.

21. Molica M, Breccia B, Foa R et al. Maintenace therapy in AML: The past, the present and the future. *Am J Hematol*. 2019; 94:1254–65.

22. Schuurhuis GJ, Heuser M, Freeman S et al. Minimal/measureable residual disease in AML: Consensus document from the ELN MRD Working Party. *Blood*. 2018; 131:1275–91.

23. Loke J, Malladi R, Moss P, Craddock C. The role of allogeneic stem cell transplantation in the management of acute myeloid leukaemia: A triumph of hope and experience. *Br J Haem*. 2020; 188:129–46.

24. Juliusson G, Hoglund M, Lehmann S. Hypo, hyper, or combo: New paradigm for treatment of acute myeloid leukemia in older people. *Haematologica*. 2020; 105:249–51.

25. Koening K, Mims A. Relapsed or primary refractory AML: Moving past MEC and FLAG-ida. *Curr Opinion Hematol*. 2020; 27:108–14.

26. Pemmaraju N, Lane AA, Sweet KL et al. Tagraxofusp in blastic plasmacytoid dendritic-cell neoplasms. *N Engl J Med*. 2019; 380:1628–1637.

27. Estey E, Karp JE, Emadi A et al. Recent drug approvals for newly diagnosed acute myeloid leukemia: Gifts or a Trojan Horse? *Leukemia*. 2020; 34:671–81.

28. Sanz MA, Fenaux P, Tallman MS et al. Management of acute promyelocytic leukemia: Updated recommendations from an expert panel of the European Leukemia. *Net Blood*. 2019; 133:1630–43.

29. Lo-Coco F, Avvisati G, Vignetti M et al. Retinoic acid and arsenic trioxide for acute promyelocytic leukemia. *N Engl J Med*. 2013; 369:111–21

30. Burnett AK, Russell NH, Hills RK et al. Arsenic trioxide and all-trans-retinoic acid treatment for acute promyelocytic leukemia in all risk groups (AML17): Results of a randomised, controlled, phase 3 trial. *Lancet Oncol*. 2015; 16:1295–305.

31. Stahl M, Tallman MS. Acute promyelocytic leukemia (APL): Remaining challenges towards a cure for all. *Leuk Lymphoma*. 2019; 60:3107–15

32. Hunger SP, Mulligan CG. Acute lymphoblastic leukemia in children. *N Engl J Med*. 2015; 373:1541–52.

33. Iacobucci I, Mulligan CG. Genetic basis of Acute Lymphoblastic Leukemia. *J Clin Oncol*. 2017; 35:975–983.

34. Roberts KG, Mulligan CG. The biology of B-progenitor acute lymphoblastic Leukemia. *Cold Spring Harbor* bioRxiv. 2019.

35. Burmeister T, Gokbuget N, Schwartz S et al. Clinical features and prognostic implications of TCF3-PBX1 and ETV6-RUNX1 in adult lymphoblastic leukemia. *Haematologica*. 2010; 95:241–6.

36. Roberts KG, Li Y, Payne-Turner D et al. Targetable kinase-activating lesions in Ph-like acute lymphoblastic leukemia. *N Engl J Med*. 2014; 371:1005–15.

37. Gu Z, Churchman ML, Roberts KG et al. PAX-5 driven subtypes of B-progenitor acute lymphoblastic leukemia. *Nat Gen*. 2019; 51:296–307.

38. Stanulla M, Cave H, Moorman AV for the BFM Study Group. *IKZF1* deletions in pediatric acute lymphoblastic leukemia: Still a poor prognostic marker? *Blood*. 2020; 135:252–60.

39. Heikamp EB, Pui CH. Next-generation evaluation and treatment of pediatric acute lymphoblastic leukemia. *J Pediatr*. 2018; 203:14–24.e2

40. Short NJ, Jabbour E, Albitar M et al. Recommendations for assessment and management of measurable residual disease in adults with acute lymphoblastic leukemia: A consensus of North American experts. *Am J Hematol*. 2019; 94:257–65.

41. Berry DA, Zhou S, Higley H et al. Association of minimal residual disease with clinical outcome in pediatric and adult acute lymphoblastic leukemia: A meta-analysis. *JAMA Oncol*. 2017; 3:e170580.

42. June CH, Sadelain M. Chimeric antigen therapy. *N Engl J Med*. 2018; 379:64–73.

43. Barsan V, Ramakrishna S, Davis KL. Immunotherapy for treatment of acute lymphoblastic leukemia. *Curr Oncol Rep*. 2020; 22(2):11.

44. Barry E, DeAngelo DJ, Neuberg D et al. Favorable outcome for adolescents with acute lymphoblastic leukemia treated on dana-faber cancer institute acute lymphoblastic leukemia consortium protocols. *J Clin Oncol*. 2007; 25:813–19.

45. Kantarjian H, Thomas D, O'Brien S et al. Long-term follow-up results of hyperfractionated cyclophosphamide, vincristine, doxorubicin, and dexamethasone (Hyper-CVAD), a dose-intensive regimen, in adult acute lymphocytic leukaemia. *Cancer*. 2004; 101:2788–801.

46. Ravandi F. How I treat Philadelphia chromosome-positive acute lymphoblastic leukemia. *Blood*. 2019; 133:130–6.

47. Roberts KG, Gu Z, Payne-Turner D et al. High frequency and poor outcome of philadelphia chromsome-like acute lymphoblastic leukemia in adults. *J Clin Oncol*. 2017; 35:394–401.

48. DeAngelo D, Stevenson KE, Dahlberg SE et al. Long-term outcome of apediatric-inspired regimen used for adults aged 18–50 years with newly diagnosed acute lymphoblastic leukemia. *Leukeamia*. 2015; 29:526–34.

49. Luskin MR, DeAndelo D. T-cell acute lymphoblastic leukemia: Currenty approach and future directions. *Adv Cell Gene Ther*. 2019; 2:e70.

50. DeFilipp Z, Advani AS, Bachanova V et al. Hematopoietic cell transplantation in treatment of adult lymphoblastic leukemia: Updated 2019 evidence-based review from the American Society for Transplantation and Cellular Therapy. *Biol Blood Marrow Transp*. 2019; 25:2113–23.

51. Giebel S, Marks DI, Boissel N et al. Hematopoietic stem cell transplantation for adults with Philadelphia chromosome-negative acute lymphoblastic leukemia in first remission: A position statement of the European Working Party for Adult Acute Lymphoblastic Leukemia (EWALL) and the Acute Leukemia Working Party of the European Society for Blood and Marrow Transplantation (EBMT). *Bone Marrow Transplant*. 2019; 54:798–809.

52. Goldstone AH, Richards SM, Lazarus HM et al. Final Results of the International ALL Trial (MRC UK BALL XII/ECOG E2993). *Blood*. 2008; 111:1187–33.

53. Gokbuget N, Dombret H, Ribera JM et al. International reference analysis of outcomes in adults aithe B-precursor Ph-negative relapse or refractory acute lymphoblastic leukemia. *Hematologica.* 2016; 101:1524–33.

54. Kantarjian H, Stein A, Gokbuget N et al. Blinatumomab versus chemotherapy for advanced lymphoblastic leukemia. *N Engl J Med.* 2017; 376:836–47.

55. Kantarjian H, DeAngelo D, Stelljes et al. Inotuzumab ozogamicin versus standard therapy for acute lymphoblastic leukemia. *N Engl J Med.* 2016; 375:740–53.

56. Park JH, Riviere I, Gonene M et al. Long term follow-up of CD19 CAR therapy in acute lymphoblastic leukemia. *N Engl J Med.* 2018; 378:449–59.

57. Maude SL, Laetsch TW, Buechner J et al. Tisagenlecleucel in children and young adults with B-cell lymphoblastic leukemia. *N Engl J Med.* 2018; 378:439–48.

58. Brudno JN, Kochenderfer JN. Recent advances in CAR T-cell toxicity: Mechanisms, manifestations and management. *Blood Rev.* 2019; 34:45–55.

59. Kumar A, Drusbosky LM, Meacham A et al. Computational modeling of early T-cell precursor acute lymphoblastic leukemia (ETP_ALL) to identify personalized therapy using genomics. *Leuk Res.* 2019; 78:3–11.

60. Mughal TI, Radich JR, Deininger MW et al. Chronic Myeloid Leukemia: Reminiscences and dreams. *Haematologica.* 2016; 101:541–58.

61. Daley GQ, Van Etten RA, Baltimore D. Induction of chronic myelogenous leukemia in mice by the P210bcr/abl gene of the Philadelphia chromosome. *Science.* 1990; 247:824–30.

62. Druker BJ, Lydon NB. Lessons learned from the development of an abl tyrosine kinase inhibitor for chronic myelogenous leukemia. *J Clin Invest.* 2000; 105:3–7.

63. Mahon F, Rea D, Guilhot J et al. Discontinuation of imatinib in patients with chronic myeloid leukemia who have maintained complete molecular remission for at least 2 years: The prospective multicentre Stop Imatinib (STIM) trial. *Lancet Oncol.* 2010; 11:1029–35.

64. Rowley JD. A new consistent chromosomal abnormality in chronic myelogenous leukaemia identified by quinacrine fluorescence and Giemsa staining. *Nature.* 1973; 243: 290–3.

65. Goldman JM, Melo JV. Targeting the *BCR-ABL* tyrosine kinase in chronic myeloid leukemia. *N Engl J Med.* 2001; 344:1084–1086

66. Sokal JE, Cox EB, Baccarani M et al. Prognostic discrimination in "good-risk" chronic granulocytic leukemia. *Blood.* 1984; 63:789–99.

67. Hasford J, Pfirrmann M, Hehlmann R et al. A new prognostic score for survival of patients with chronic myeloid leukaemia treated with interferon alpha. *J Natl Cancer Inst.* 1998; 90:850–8.

68. Hoffman VS, Baccarani M, Lindoerfer D et al. The EUTOS prognostic score: Review and validation in 1288 patients with CML treated frontline with imatinib. *Leukemia.* 2013; 27:2016–22.

69. Hochhaus A, Baccarani M, Silver RT et al. European LeukemiaNet 2020 recommendations for treating chronic myeloid leukemia. *Leukemia.* 2020; 3:1–9.

70. Saglio G, Gale RP. Prospects for achieving treatment-free remission in chronic myeloid leukaemia. *Br J Haem.* 2020; Feb 14.

71. Mughal TI, Deininger MW, Kucine N et al. Children and adolescents with chronic myeloproliferative neoplasms: Still an unmet biological and clinical need? *Hemasphere.* 2019; 3:e283.

72. Jain P, Kantarjian H, Boddu PC et al. Analysis of cardiovascular and arteriothrombotic adverse events in chronic phase CML patients after frontline TKIs. *Blood Adv.* 2019; 3:851–61.

73. Talpaz M, Shah NP, Kantarjian H et al. Dasatinib in imatinib-resistant Philadelphia chromosome-positive leukemias. *N Engl J Med.* 2006; 354:2531–41.

74. Cortes JE, Gambacorti-Passerini C, Deininger MW et al. Bosutinib versus Imatinib for Newly Diagnosed Chronic Myeloid Leukemia: Results from the Randomized BFORE Trial. *J Clin Oncol.* 2017; 36:231–7.

75. Kantarjian H, Giles F, Wunderle L et al. A phase II study of nilotinib in imatinib-resistant CML and Philadelphia-positive ALL. *N Engl J Med.* 2006; 354:2542–51.

76. Mughal TI, Lion T, Abdel-Wahab O et al. Precision immunotherapy, mutational landscape, and emerging tools to optimize clinical outcomes in patients with classical myeloproliferative neoplasms. *Hematol Oncol.* 2018; 36:740–8.

77. Cortes JE, Kim D-W, Pinella-Ibarz J et al. A phase 2 trial of ponatinib in Philadelphia chromosome-positive leukemias. *N Engl J Med.* 2013; 369:1783–96.

78. Soverini S, Bavaro L, De Benedittid et al. Prospective assessment of NGS-detectable mutations in CML patients with non-optimal response: The NEXT-in-CML-sdtudy. *Blood.* 2020; 135: 534–41.

79. Lubking A, Deimane A, Sandin F et al. Allogeneic stem cell transplantation for chronic myeloid leukemia in the TKI era: Population-based data from the Swedish CML registry. *Bone Marrow Transplant.* 2019; 54(11):1764–74.

80. Chaudhury S, Sparapani R, Hu ZH et al. Outcomes of allogeneic hematopoietic cell transplantation in children and young adults with chronic myeloid leukemia: AA CIBMTR cohort analysis. *Biol Blood Marrow Transplant.* 2016; 22:1056–64.

81. Schmidt S, Liu Y, Hu Z-H et al. The role of Donor Lymphocyte Infusion (DLI) in post hematopoietic cell transplant for Chronic Myeloid Leukemia (CML) in the Tyrosine Kinase Inhibitor (TKI) Era. *Biol Blood Marrow Transplant.* 2020; Feb 14.

82. Dulucq S, Astrugue C, Etienne G, Mahon FX, Benard A. Risk of molecular recurrence after tyrosine kinase inhibitor discontinuation in chronic myeloid leukaemia patients: A systematic review of literature with a meta-analysis of studies over the last 10 years. *Br J Haem.* 2020.

83. Yan D, Pomicter, O'Hare T, Deininger MW. Deeper than Deep: Can ddPCR predict successful imatinib cessation? *Clin Cancer Res.* 2019; 25:6561–3.

84. O'Hare T, Zabriske MS, Eiring AM, Deininger MW. Pushing the limits of targeted therapy in chronic myeloid leukemia. *Nat Rev Cancer.* 2012; 12:513–26.

85. Hughes TP, Mauro MJ, Cortes JE et al. Asciminib in chronic myeloid leukemia after ABL kinase inhibitor Failure. *N Engl J Med.* 2019; 381:2315–26.

86. Mughal TI, Gotlib J, Mesa R et al. Recent advances in the genomics and therapy of *BCR/ABL1*-positive and -negative chronic myeloproliferative neoplasms. *Leuk Res.* 2018; 67:67–74.

87. Than H, Pomicter AD, Yan D et al. Coordinated inhibition of nuclear export and Bcr-Abl1 selectively targets chronic myeloid stem cells. *Leukemia.* 2020; 34(6):1679–83.

88. Ko TK, Javed A, Lee KL et al. An integrative model of pathway convergancve in ghenetically heterogenous blast crisis chronic myeloid leukemia. *Blood.* 2020(in press.)

89. James C, Ugo V, Le Couedic JP et al. A unique clonal JAK2 mutation leading to constitutive signaling causes polycythemia vera. *Natures.* 2005; 434:1144–8.

90. Baxter EJ, Scott LM, Campbell PJ et al. Acquired mutation of the tyrosine kinase JAK2 in human myeloproliferative disorders. *Lancet.* 2005; 365:1054–61.

91. Levine RL, Wadleigh M, Cools J et al. Activating mutation in the tyrosine kinase JAK2 in polycythemia vera, essential thrombocythemia, and myeloid metaplasis with myelofibrosis. *Cancer Cell.* 2005; 7:387–97.

92. Kralovics R, Passamonti F, Buser AS et al. A gain-of-function mutation of JAK2 in myeloproliferative disorders. *N Engl J Med.* 2005; 352:1779–90.

93. Pikman Y, Lee BH, Mercher T et al. MPLW515L is a novel somatic activating mutation in myelofibrosis with myeloid metaplasia. *PLoS Med.* 2006; 3:e270.

94. Scott LM, Tong W, Levine RL et al. JAK2 exon 12 mutations in polycythemia vera and idiopathic erythrocyctosis. *N Engl J Med.* 2007; 356:459–68.

95. Klampf T, Gisslinger H, Harutyunyan AS et al. Somatic mutations in calreticulin in myeloproliferative Neoplasms. *N Engl J Med.* 2013; 369:2379–90.

96. Nangalia J, Massie CE, Baxter EY et al. Somatic CALR Mutations in Myeloproliferative Neoplasms with Nonmutated JAK2. *N Engl J Med.* 2013; 369:2391–05.

97. Verstovsek S, Kantarjian H, Mesa RA et al. Safety and efficacy of INCB018424, a Jak1 and Jak2 inhibitor, in myelofibrosis. *N Engl J Med.* 2010; 363:1117–27.

98. Barbui T, De Stefano V, Falanga A et al. Addressing and proposing solutions for unmet clinical needs in the management of myeloproliferative neoplasm-associated thrombosis: A consensus-based position paper. *Blood Cancer J.* 2019; 9:61.

99. Mughal TI, Abdel-Wahab O, Rampal R et al. Contemporary insights into the pathogenesis and treatment of chronic myeloproliferative neoplasms. *Leuk Lymphoma.* 2015; 56:1517–26.

100. Prins D, Arias CG, Klampf T et al. Mutant calreticulin in myeloproliferative neoplasms. *HemaSphere.* 2020; 4:e333.

101. Ortmann CA, Kent DG, Nangalia J et al. Effect of mutation order on myeloproliferative neoplasms. *N Engl J Med.* 2015; 372:601–12.

102. Patel A, Franzini A, Leroy E et al. JAK2^ex13InDel drives oncogenic transformation and is associated with chronic eosinophilic leukemia and polycythemia vera. *Blood.* 2019; 134:2388–98.

103. Kvasnicka HM, Orazi A, Thiele J et al. European LeukemiaNet study on the reproducibility of bone marrow features in masked polycythemia vera and differentiation from essential thrombocythemia. *Am J Haematol.* 2017; 92:1062–7.

104. Barbui T, Thiele J, Ferrari A et al. The new WHO classification for essential thrombocythemia calls for revision of available evidences. *Blood Cancer J.* 2020; 10:22.

105. Barbui T, Finazzi G, Carobbio A et al. Development and validation of an international Prognostic Score of Thrombosis in World Health Organization Essential Thrombocythemia (IPSET-thrombosis). *Blood.* 2012; 120:5128–33.

106. Tefferi A, Guglielmelli P, Lasho TL et al. Mutation enhanced international prognostic systems for essential thrombocythemia and polycythemia. *Br J Haem.* 2020.

107. Guglielmelli P, Lasho TL, Rotunno G et al. MIPSS70: Mutation-enhanced international prognsotic score system for transplantation-age patients with myelofibrosis. *J Clin Oncol.* 2017; 36:310–8.

108. Grinfeld J, Nangalia J, Baxter EJ et al. Classification and personalized prognosis in myeloproliferative neoplasms. *N Engl J Med.* 2018; 379:1416–30.

109. Barbui T, Tefferi A, Vannucchi A et al. Philadelphia chromosome-negative classical myeloproliferative neoplasms: Revised management recommendations from European LeukemiaNet. *Leukemia.* 2018; 32:1057–69.

110. Koschmieder S, Mughal TI, Hasselbalch H et al. Myeloproliferative neoplasms and inflammation: Whether to target the malignant clone or the inflammatory process or both. *Leukemia.* 2016; 30:1018–24.

111. Verstovek S, Mesa RA, Gotlib J et al. A Double-blind, placebo-controlled trial of ruxolitinib for myelofibrosis. *N Engl J Med.* 2012; 366:799–807.

112. Harrison CN, Kiladjian J-J, Al-Ali K et al. JAK inhibition with Ruxolitinib versus best available therapy for myelofibrosis. *N Engl J Med.* 2012; 366:787–98.

113. Blair HA. Fedratinib: First approval. *Drugs.* 2019; 79:1719–25.

114. Christopeit M, Badbaran A, Alawi M et al. Clonal evolution after allogeneic stem cell transplantation: The case of myelofibrosis. *Biol Blood Marrow Transplant.* 2020; Mar 5.

115. Mughal TI, Pemmaraju N, Radich JR et al. Emerging translational science discoveries, clonal approaches, and treatment trends in chronic myeloproliferative neoplasms. *Hematol Oncol.* 2019; 37:240–52.

116. Stoner RC, Press RD, Maxson JE et al. Insights on mechanisms of clonal evolution in chronic neutrophilic leukemia on ruxolitinib therapy. *Leukemia.* 2020; 34(6):1684–8.

117. Zhang H, Wilmot B, Bottomly D et al. Genomic landscape of neutrophilic leukemias of ambiguous diagnosis. *Blood.* 2019; 134:867–79

118. Gotlib J. World Health Organization-defined eosinophilic disorders: 2017 update on diagnosis, risk stratification, and management. *Am J Hematol.* 2017; 92:1243–59.

119. Reiter A, George TI, Gotlib J. New developments in diagnosis, prognostication, and treatment of advanced systemic mastocytosis. *Blood.* 2020. (in press)

120. Sperr WR, Kundi M, Alvarez-Twose I et al. International prognostic scoring system for mastocytosis (IPSM): A retrospective cohort. *Lancet Haem.* 2019; 6:e638–49.

121. Platzbecker U. Treatment of MDS. *Blood.* 2019; 133:1096–107.

122. Fenaux P, Platzbecker U, Ades L. How we manage adults with myelodysplastic syndrome. *Br J Haemtol.* 2019; Sep 30.

123. Malcovati L, Hellstrom-Lindberg E, Bowen D et al. ELN diagnosis and treatment of primary MDS in adults: Recommendations from the ELN. *Blood.* 2013; 122:2943–64.

124. Ogawa S. Genetics of myelodysplastic syndrome. *Blood.* 2019; 133:1049–59.

125. Greenberg P, Cox C, LeBeau MM et al. International scoring system for evaluating prognosis in myelodysplastic syndromes. *Blood.* 1997; 89:2079–88.

126. Greenberg PL, Tuechler H, Schanz J et al. Revised international prognostic scoring system for myelodysplastic syndromes. *Blood.* 2012; 120:2454–65.

127. Efficace F, Cottone F, Oswald LB et al. The IPSS-R more accurately captures fatigue severity of newly diagnosed patients with myelodysplastic syndromes compared with IPSS index. *Leukemia.* 2020.

128. Montalban-Bravo G, Kanagal-Shamanna R, Benton CB et al. Genomic context and TP53 frequency define clinical outcomes in TP-53 mutated myelodysplastic syndromes. *Blood.* 2020; 4:482–95.

129. deWitte T, Bowen D, Robin M et al. Allogeneic hematopoietic stem cell transplant for MDS and CMML: Recommendations from an international panel. *Blood.* 2017; 129:1753–62.

130. Stahl M, Deveaux M, de Witte T et al. The use of immunosuppressive therapy in MDS: Clinical outcomes and their predictors in large international patient cohort. *Blood Adv.* 2018; 2:1765–72.

131. Fenaux P, Platzbecker U, Mufti G et al. Luspatercept in patients with lower-risk mydelodysplastic syndrome. *N Engl J Med.* 2020; 382:140–51.

132. Kubash AS, Platzbecker U. Setting fire to ESA and EMA resistance: New targeted treatment optionsin lower risk myelodysplastic syndromes. *Int J Mol Sci.* 2019; 20:3853.

133. Swoboda DM, Quinto G, Sallman DA. Novel therapies in myelodysplastic syndromes. *Curr Opin Hematol.* 2020; 27:58–65.

134. Valent P, Orazi O, Savona MR et al. Proposed diagnostic criteria for classical CMML, CMML variants and pre-CMML conditions. *Haematologica.* 2019; 104:1935–49.

135. Mughal TI, Cross NCP, Padron E et al. An International MDS/MPN Working Group's perspective and recommendations on molecular pathogenesis, diagnosis and clinical characterization of MDS/MPN. *Haematologica.* 2015; 100:1117–30.

136. Tanaka TN, Bejar R. MDS overlap disorders and diagnostic boundaries. *Blood.* 2019; 133:1086–95.

137. Mangaonkar AA, Swoboda DM, Coltro C et al. Clinicopathologic characteristics, prognostication and treatment outcomes for MDS/MPN, MDS/MPN-U: Mayo Clinic-Moffitt Cancer Center study of 135 consecutive patients. *Leukemia.* 2020; 34:656–61.

138. Patnaik M, Tefferi A. 2020 Update on diagnosis, risk stratification and management. *Am J Hematol.* 2020; 95:97–1115.

139. Itzykson R, Fenaux P, Bowen D et al. Diagnosis and treatment of chronic myelomonocytic leukemia in adults: Recommendations from the European Hematology Association and the European LeukemiaNet. *HemaSphere.* 2018; 2:e150

140. Savona MR, Malcovati L, Komrokji R et al. MDS/MPN International Working Group proposal of uniform response criteria for MDS/MPN in adults. *Blood.* 2015; 125:1857–65.

141. Lucas N, Duchmann M, Rameau et al. Biology and prognostic impact of clonal plasmacytoid dendritic cells in chronic myelomonocytic leukemia. *Leukemia.* 2019; 33:2466–80.

142. Sadigh S, Hasserjian RP, Hobbs G. Distinguishing atypical chronic myeloid leukemia from other Philadelphia-negative chronic myeloproliferative neoplasms. *Curr Opin Hematol.* 2020; 27:122–7.

143. Onida F, de Wreede LC, van Biezen A et al. Allogeneic stem cell transplantation in patents with atypical CML: A retrospective study from the Chronic Malignancies Working party of the EBMT. *Br J Haematol.* 2017; 177:759–65.

144. Niemeyer CM, Flotho C. JMML: Who's the driver at the wheel? *Blood.* 2019; 153:1060–70.

145. Montalban-Bravo G, Garcia-Manero G. MDS/MPN-RS-T just inclusion as a unique disease entity? *Best Pract Res Clin Haematol.* 2020. (in press)
146. Chiorazzi N, Rai K, Ferrarini M. Chronic lymphocytic leukemia. *N Engl J Med.* 2005; 352:804–15.
147. National Cancer Institute: Cancer stat facts: Leukemia—chronic lymphocytic leukemia (CLL). 2019. SEER https://seer.cancer.gov/statfacts/html/clyl.html
148. Hallek M, Cheson BD, Catovsky D et al. Guidelines for diagnosis, indications of treatment, response assessment and supportive management of chronic lymphocytic leukemia. *Blood.* 2018; 131:2745–60.
149. Hamblin TJ, Davis Z, Gardiner A et al. Unmutated Ig (V) genes are associated with a more aggressive form of chronic lymphocytic leukemia. *Blood.* 1999; 94:1848–54.
150. Chiorazzi N, Stevenson FK. Celebrating 20 Years of IGHV Mutation Analysis in CLL. *Hemasphere.* 2020; 4:e334
151. Crespo M, Bosch F, Villamor N et ale=. ZAP-70 expression as a surrogate for immunoglobulin-varaible-region mutations in chronic lymphocytic leukemia. *N Engl J Med.* 2003; 348:1764–75.
152. Gruber M, Bozic I, Wu C et al. Growth dynamics in naturally progressing chronic lymphocytic leukaemia. *Nature.* 2019; 570: 474–79.
153. Bosch F, Dalla-Favera R. Chronic lymphocytic leukemia: From genetics to treatment. *Nat Rev Clin Oncol.* 2019; 16:684–701.
154. Wang L, Lawrence MS, Wan Y et al. SF3B1 and other novel cancer genes in chronic lymphocytic leukemia. *N Engl J Med.* 2011; 365:2497–506.
155. Burger J, Landau DA, Wu CJ et al. Clonal evolution in patients with CLL developing resistance to BTK inhibition. *Nature Commun.* 2016; 7:11589
156. Roberts AW, Davids MS, Pagel JM et al. Targeting BCL2 with Venetoclax in relapsed chronic lymphocytic leukemia. *N Engl J Med.* 2016; 374:311–22.
157. Rai KR, Sawitsky A, Cronkite EP et al. Clinical staging of chronic lymphocytic leukemia. *Blood.* 1975; 46:219–34.
158. Binet JL, Augier A, Dighiero G et al. A new prognostic classification of chronic lymphocytic leukemia derived from a multivariate survival analysis. *Cancer.* 1981; 48:198–206.
159. International CLL-IPI Working Group. An international prognostic index for patients with chronic lymphocytic leukaemia (CLL-IPI): A meta-analysis of individual patient data. *Lancet Oncol.* 2016; 17:779–90.
160. Sharma S, Rai K. Chronic lymphocytic leukemia (CLL) treatment: So many choices, such great options. *Cancer.* 2019; 125: 1432–40.
161. Burger JA, Tedeschi A, Barr PM et al. Ibrutinib as initial therapy for patients with chronic lymphocytic leukemia. *N Engl J Med.* 2015; 373:2425–37.
162. Furman RR, Sharman JP, Coutre SE et al. Idelalisib and rituximab in relapsed chronic lymphocytic leukemia. *N Engl J Med.* 2014; 370 997–1007
163. Vidal L, Gurion R, Ram R et al. Chlorambucil for treatment of patients with CLL- a systematic review and meta-analysis of randomized trials. *Leuk Lymphoma.* 2016; 57:2047–57.
164. Goede V, Fischer K, Busch R et al. Oblinutuzumab plus chlorambucil in patients with chronic lymphocytic leukemia. *N Engl J Med.* 2014; 370:110110.
165. Herishanu Y, Shaulov A, Fineman R et al. Frontline treatment with the combination obinutuzumab +/– chlorambucil for CLL outside clinical trials: Results of a multinational, multicenter study by ERIC and the Israeli CLL study group. *Am J Hematol.* 2020; 95(6):604–611.
166. Thompson PA, Tam CS, O'Brien SM et al. Fludarabine, cyclophosphamide, and rituximab treatment achieves long-term disease-free survival in IGHV-mutated chronic lymphocytic leukemia. *Blood.* 2016; 127:303–9.
167. Eichhorst B, Fink A-M, Bahlo J et al. First line chemoimmunotherapy with bendamustine and rituximab versus fludarabine, cyclophosphamide, and rituximab in patients with advanced chronic lymphocytic leukaemia (CLL10): An international, open-label, randomised, phase 3, non-inferiority trial. *Lancet Oncol.* 2016; 17:928–42.
168. O'Brien S, Furman RR, Coutre S et al. Single-agent ibrutinib in treatment naive and relapsed/refractory chronic lymphocytic leukemia: A 5-year experience. *Blood.* 2018; 131:1910–19.
169. Byrd JC, Hillmen P, O'Brien et al. Long-term follow-up of the RESONATE phase 3 trial of ibrutinib vs. ofatumumab. *Blood.* 2019; 133:2031–42.
170. Gribben JG. How and when to do allogeneic transplant in chronic lymphocytic leukemia. *Blood.* 2018; 132:31–9.
171. Allan JN, Furman RR. Current trends in the management of Richter's syndrome. *Int J Hematol Oncol.* 2019; 7(4):IJH09.
172. Smith VM, Lomas O, Constantine D et al. Dual dependence on BCL2 and MCL in T-cell prolymphocytic leukemia. *Blood Adv.* 2020; 4:525–9.
173. Samuel J, Macip S, Dyer MJ. Efficcay of vemurafenib in hairy-cell leukemia. *N Engl J Med.* 2014; 370:286–88.
174. Falini B. New treatment options in hairy cell leukemia with focus on BRAF inhibitors. *Hematol Oncol.* 2019; 37 Supplement 1:30–7.
175. Lamy T, Moignet A, Loughran TP. LGL Leukemia: From pathogenesis to treatment. *Blood.* 2017; 129:1082–94.
176. Swerdlow SH, Campo E, Harris NL et al. *WHO classification of Tumours of Haematopoietic and Lymphoid Tissues*, 4th ed. Lyon, France: International Agency for Research on Cancer, 2017.
177. Gorczyca W, *Atlas of Differential Diagnosis in Neoplastic Hematopathology*, 3rd ed. CRC Press, 2014.
178. Goldman JM, Mughal, TI. *Postgraduate Haematology*, 6th ed. Wiley, 2006.

29 HODGKIN LYMPHOMA

Dennis A. Eichenauer and Andreas Engert

Introduction

Hodgkin lymphoma (HL) is a B-cell-derived malignancy with an incidence of 3–4/100,000/year. The disease usually affects young and middle-aged adults. Pathologically, the histological subtypes of classical HL (cHL) (nodular sclerosis, mixed cellularity, lymphocyte-rich, lymphocyte-depleted) that account for approximately 95% of cases are being distinguished from the rare entity of nodular lymphocyte-predominant HL (NLPHL). The immunophenotype of the malignant cells in cHL and NLPHL differs substantially. Hence, the Hodgkin and Reed–Sternberg cells from cHL express CD15 and CD30 whereas the disease-defining lymphocyte predominant cells in NLPHL are negative for these markers but consistently express CD20.[1,2]

Clinically, HL is a highly curable cancer. With current standard approaches consisting of stage-adapted treatment with chemotherapy +/− radiotherapy (RT), more than 80% of patients achieve a permanent remission.[1] Current studies therefore aim at reducing treatment toxicity without compromising efficacy. Interim positron emission tomography (PET) represents the most promising tool to differentiate between good-risk patients who are likely treated sufficiently with reduced-intensity approaches and high-risk patients who require standard or even intensified therapy. The partial replacement of conventional chemotherapy by targeted drugs such as the CD30-directed antibody-drug conjugate brentuximab vedotin and the anti-PD1 antibodies nivolumab and pembrolizumab may also reduce the treatment burden and thus minimize the risk for treatment-related late effects.

Initial diagnostics

An excisional biopsy of a suspicious enlarged lymph node or from another affected organ should be performed to establish the diagnosis of HL. The extent of disease should be evaluated by PET and contrast-enhanced computed tomography (CT) (PET/CT) of the neck, chest, and abdomen. Bone marrow aspiration and biopsy are dispensable if a PET/CT is performed.[3] Additional procedures such as magnetic resonance imaging are only required in a few cases. Laboratory examinations including blood cell count, erythrocyte sedimentation rate (ESR), and screening for hepatitis B, hepatitis C, and human immunodeficiency virus should be performed before treatment is initiated. In addition, pulmonary function test, electrocardiography, and echocardiography should be conducted. Patients of childbearing potential should be offered reproductive counseling (Table 29.1).[1]

Differential diagnoses

Differential diagnoses of HL include all types of benign or malignant lymph node swelling owing to infectious or reactive disease, other types of lymphoma, or solid tumors. Infectious lymphadenopathy can be of bacterial, viral, fungal, or parasitic origin. Reactive lymphadenopathy might be associated with sarcoidosis as well as other diseases of the soft tissues or the skin or can be drug-induced. Malignant causes include metastases of solid tumors, leukemias, or non-Hodgkin lymphomas (NHL). The differential diagnosis between certain types of HL and NHL can be challenging and should be performed by an experienced hematopathologist. Occasionally, a composite lymphoma partially consisting of HL and NHL is diagnosed.

Risk group allocation and choice of treatment

HL patients are allocated to risk groups based on the clinical stage according to the Ann Arbor classification and the presence of clinical risk factors. The presence (B) or absence (A) of systemic symptoms further characterizes the severity of disease. Clinical, biological, and serological parameters (age, performance status, tumor burden, ESR) also influence the risk group allocation.

Patients with stage I and II disease presenting without risk factors are usually allocated to the early-stage risk group, those with risk factors to the intermediate-stage group. Patients with stage III and IV disease are assigned to the advanced-stage group.[1] However, there are still minor differences in the definition of risk factors used, and subgroups of HL patients thus differ between study groups in Europe and the United States (Table 29.2). In the United States, patients are usually allocated to either early or advanced stages. This results in a higher proportion of patients—even with limited tumor burden—being allocated to the advanced-stage group. These patients often receive more intensive therapy which must be considered when comparing data.

At present, patients diagnosed with early or intermediate stages, are usually treated with brief chemotherapy followed by consolidation radiotherapy (RT) whereas patients with advanced HL receive chemotherapy alone in most cases. Consolidation RT in this risk group is restricted to individuals with larger PET-positive residual lymphoma at the end of chemotherapy.[1]

First-line treatment

Early stages

First-line treatment of early-stage HL usually consists of a brief chemotherapy according to the ABVD (doxorubicin, bleomycin, vinblastine, dacarbazine) protocol followed by limited-field RT. The superiority of this approach over RT alone has been demonstrated in several studies.[4]

The randomized HD7 study conducted by the German Hodgkin Study Group (GHSG) compared extended-field RT (EF-RT) at a dose of 30 Gy alone and 2 cycles of ABVD chemotherapy followed by the same RT. The final analysis of the study performed after a median follow-up of 87 months revealed a significant advantage in terms of tumor control for patients receiving combined-modality treatment (CMT) in comparison with those who had RT alone (7-year freedom from treatment failure: 88% vs. 67%).[4] These results were confirmed by a recent follow-up analysis (15-year progression-free survival: 73% vs. 52%). Overall survival (OS) differences between the treatment arms were not detected in both analyses.[5]

The randomized H7F and H8F studies conducted by the European Organisation for Research and Treatment of Cancer

TABLE 29.1   Diagnostic Work-up in HL

Diagnosis	Lymph node biopsy (or a biopsy from another organ with suspected affection)
Staging and risk stratification	• Medical history and physical examination • X-ray of the chest • Contrast-enhanced CT scan of neck, chest, and abdomen • PET • Full blood cell count and blood chemistry, ESR • HBV, HCV, and HIV screening
Pretreatment examinations	• ECG • Echocardiography • Pulmonary function test • Reproductive counseling (in patients of reproductive age) • Serum pregnancy test (in female patients of reproductive age) • Consultation of an ear, nose and throat specialist including a fiberoptic nasolaryngoscopy (if PET/CT scan is not available at initial staging)

Abbreviations: CT, computed tomography; ECG, electrocardiography; ESR, erythrocyte sedimentation rate; HBV, hepatitis B; HCV, hepatitis C; HIV, human immunodeficiency virus; HL, Hodgkin lymphoma; PET, positron emission tomography.
Source: ESMO Clinical Practice Guidelines, Eichenauer et al., 2018. With permission.

TABLE 29.2   Definition of HL Risk Groups According to the EORTC/LYSA and the GHSG

	EORTC/LYSA	GHSG
Treatment Group		
Early stages	CS I-II without risk factors (supradiaphragmatic)	CS I-II without risk factors
Intermediate stages	CS I-II with ≥1 risk factor (supradiaphragmatic)	CS I, CS IIA with ≥1 risk factor CS IIB with risk factors C and/or D, but not A/B
Advanced stages	CS III-IV	CS IIB with risk factors A and/or B CS III/IV
Risk Factors		
	A: Large mediastinal mass[a] B: Age ≥50 years C: Elevated ESR[b] D: ≥4 nodal areas[c]	A: Large mediastinal mass[a] B: Extranodal disease C: Elevated ESR[b] D: ≥3 nodal areas[c]

Abbreviations: CS, clinical stage; EORTC, European Organisation for Research and Treatment of Cancer; ESR, erythrocyte sedimentation rate; GHSG, German Hodgkin Study Group; HL, Hodgkin lymphoma; LYSA, Lymphoma Study Association.
Source: ESMO Clinical Practice Guidelines, Eichenauer et al., 2018. With permission.
[a] Large mediastinal mass: Mediastinum-to-thorax ratio ≥0.35 (EORTC/LYSA); mediastinal mass larger than 1/3 of the maximum thoracic width (GHSG).
[b] Elevated ESR: >50 mm/h without B symptoms, >30 mm/h with B symptoms (B symptoms: fever, night sweat, unexplained weight loss >10% over 6 months).
[c] Nodal areas: Involvement of ≥4 out of 5 supradiaphragmatic nodal areas (EORTC/LYSA); involvement of ≥3 out of 11 nodal areas on both sides of the diaphragm (GHSG).

(EORTC) and the Groupe d'Études des Lymphomes des Adultes (GELA) addressed a similar question. Patients were randomized between subtotal nodal irradiation (STNI) alone and chemotherapy with epirubicin, bleomycin, vinblastine, prednisone (EBVP) (H7F) and mechlorethamine, oncovin, procarbazine, prednisone/doxorubicin, bleomycin, vinblastine (MOPP/ABV) (H8F), respectively, each followed RT. The combination of chemotherapy and consolidation RT resulted in a significantly improved tumor control when compared with RT alone (10-year event-free survival: 88% vs. 78% in H7F; 5-year event-free survival: 98% vs. 74% in H8F). OS rates were comparable for both CMT and RT alone due to effective salvage therapy.[6,7]

Follow-up trials evaluated whether a reduction of chemotherapy and RT fields and doses is possible without a loss of activity. Within the GHSG HD10 study, patients were randomly allocated to either 2 or 4 cycles of ABVD chemotherapy followed by involved-field RT (IF-RT) at a dose of either 20 Gy or 30 Gy. Tumor control and survival were comparable for all treatment arms so that the least toxic approach consisting of 2 cycles of ABVD followed by 20 Gy IF-RT was adopted as standard of care at many institutions (Figure 29.1).[8,5]

More recently, interim PET/CT-guided treatment strategies were evaluated in several randomized studies. Within the RAPID study conducted in the United Kingdom, 602 patients with early-stage HL received 3 cycles of ABVD before an interim PET/CT was performed. Patients with a negative PET/CT underwent randomization between consolidation RT and no further treatment. After a median observation time of 60 months, the 3-year PFS rates for patients receiving consolidation RT and no further treatment were 94.6% and 90.8%, respectively, and thus differed significantly. However, the 3-year OS rates were close to 100% for both groups.[9] The H10F study conducted by the EORTC, the Lymphoma Study Association (LYSA), and the Fondazione Italiana Linfomi (FIL) also evaluated whether consolidation RT is dispensable in patients with early-stage HL who had achieved a complete metabolic remission after a brief

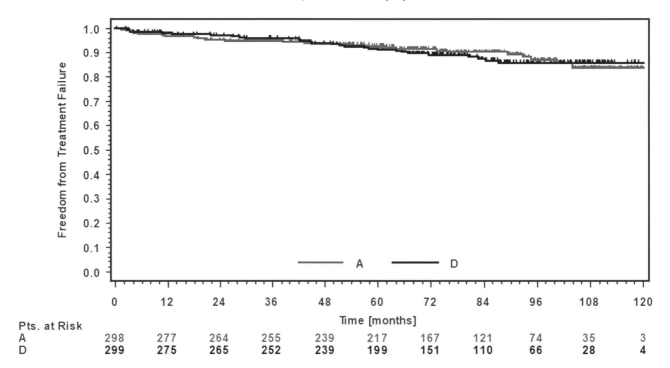

FIGURE 29.1 Comparison in terms of freedom from treatment failure between the most (arm A; 4 × ABVD + 30 Gy IF-RT) and the least (arm D; 2 × ABVD + 20 Gy IF-RT) toxic treatment within the GHSG HD10 study for early-stage HL. (From Engert et al., 2010. With permission.)

chemotherapy. All 754 patients included in the study received 2 cycles of ABVD before an interim PET/CT was performed. Patients with a negative PET/CT were then randomized to either one additional cycle of ABVD followed by consolidation RT or two additional cycles of ABVD without consolidation RT. The chemotherapy-only arm was closed early due to an increased number of events so that the omission of consolidation RT—similarly to the RAPID study—appeared to result in a loss of tumor control. Patients with a positive interim PET/CT were randomized between standard treatment consisting of one additional cycle of ABVD followed by consolidation RT and an intensified approach consisting of two cycles of escalated BEACOPP (bleomycin, etoposide, doxorubicin, cyclophosphamide, oncovin, procarbazine, prednisone) followed by consolidation RT. After a median follow-up of 4.5 years, tumor control appeared to be better with the intensified approach.[10,11] However, the analysis of the PET-positive patients also included patients with intermediate stages so that the question of whether treatment intensification in early-stage patients with a positive interim PET/CT should be the standard of care is still under debate. The third randomized study investigating the possibility of interim PET/CT-guided omission of RT in patients with early-stage HL was the HD16 study conducted by the GHSG. A total of 1150 individuals were enrolled. All study participants had two cycles of ABVD chemotherapy prior to interim PET/CT. In the experimental arm of the study, patients with a negative PET were randomly assigned to either consolidation RT or no further treatment. At a median observation time of 47 months, the 5-year PFS estimates were 93.4% for patients receiving consolidation RT and 86.1% for those who had chemotherapy alone.[12] Thus, the omission of consolidation RT after a brief chemotherapy according to the ABVD protocol resulted

in a loss of tumor control despite a negative interim PET/CT according to all randomized studies addressing this issue.

Taken together, CMT consisting of two cycles of ABVD followed by limited-field RT represents the standard approach for HL in early stages at most institutions. The only patient group that is treated sufficiently with RT alone consists of individuals with stage IA NLPHL presenting without clinical risk factors as reported by various groups.[13,14]

HL IN EARLY STAGES

The vast majority of patients with early-stage HL achieve long-term remission with a brief ABVD-based chemotherapy followed by limited-field RT. However, it is crucial to reduce the treatment burden to minimize the risk for the occurrence of therapy-related late effects. Therefore, the development of tools to identify low-risk patients who are treated sufficiently without RT or with targeted drugs alone is necessary.

Intermediate stages

Patients with intermediate-stage HL are usually treated with CMT. The standard approach at many institutions consists of four cycles of ABVD followed by limited-field RT. In an attempt to improve tumor control, randomized studies were conducted by different larger study groups.

Within the GHSG HD11 study, 1395 patients were randomly assigned to either 4 cycles of ABVD or 4 cycles of the more intensive BEACOPPbaseline regimen each followed by limited-field

RT at either 20 Gy or 30 Gy. Freedom from treatment failure rates did not differ significantly between the chemotherapy approaches if RT at 30 Gy was applied. In contrast, tumor control was better with BEACOPPbaseline if patients had consolidation RT at 20 Gy.[5,15]

The H9U study conducted by the EORTC and the GELA compared four cycles of ABVD, six cycles of ABVD, and four cycles BEACOPPbaseline each followed by limited-field RT. A total of 808 patients were included. The event-free survival rates at 5 years were comparable for all study arms (4 cycles of ABVD: 85.9%; 6 cycles of ABVD: 89.9%; 4 cycles of BEACOPPbaseline: 88.8%).[16]

The GHSG HD14 study further intensified chemotherapy. Patients (n = 1528) were allocated to either 4 cycles of ABVD or 2 cycles of escalated BEACOPP plus 2 cycles of ABVD ("2+2") each followed by limited-field RT. Tumor control at 5 years was significantly improved for the intensified approach with a PFS advantage of 6.2%.[17] Thus, "2+2" may be considered as treatment option in younger patients (≤60 years) who are eligible for aggressive chemotherapy with escalated BEACOPP.

More recent studies evaluated PET/CT-guided treatment strategies also in intermediate-stage patients. The EORTC/LYSA/FIL H10U study comprising 1196 patients investigated whether individuals with a complete metabolic remission after 2 cycles of ABVD are sufficiently treated with 6 cycles of chemotherapy alone. After a median follow-up of 4.5 years, non-inferiority of this approach in comparison with CMT could not be demonstrated. Patients with a positive PET after two cycles of ABVD appeared to have a better outcome if treatment was continued with escalated BEACOPP instead of ABVD before consolidation RT.[11]

Taken together, patients with intermediate-stage HL should receive four cycles of chemotherapy (four cycles of ABVD or "2+2") followed by limited-field RT. In case the interim PET/CT after two cycles of ABVD is positive, treatment continuation with escalated BEACOPP should be considered.

Advanced stages

The treatment of advanced HL usually consists of chemotherapy alone. Consolidation RT is restricted to patients with larger PET-positive residual lymphoma. The most commonly used chemotherapy protocols are escalated BEACOPP and ABVD.

The GHSG HD15 study investigated whether consolidation RT can be restricted to larger (≥2.5 cm) PET-positive residual lymphoma. In addition, the study compared three chemotherapy approaches, i.e. eight cycles of escalated BEACOPP, six cycles of escalated BEACOPP, and eight cycles of a time-dense variant of BEACOPPbaseline termed BEACOPP-14. According to the final analysis of the trial, patients are sufficiently treated with 6 cycles of escalated BEACOPP and RT can be safely restricted to PET-positive residual lymphoma ≥2.5 cm.[18,19] The HD18 study then evaluated treatment reduction to a total of four cycles of escalated BEACOPP if a complete metabolic response was achieved after two cycles of chemotherapy. The 5-year PFS rates were similar for patients receiving standard treatment consisting of six or eight cycles of BEACOPPescalated and those treated with four cycles of BEACOPPescalated (90.8% vs. 92.2%) (Figure 29.2). Thus, four cycles of escalated BEACOPP were adopted as standard of care for patients achieving an early metabolic response according to interim PET/CT within the GHSG. In patients with a positive interim PET/CT after two cycles of escalated BEACOPP, the addition of rituximab in the subsequent chemotherapy cycles did not result in improved outcomes.[20,21]

The randomized AHL2011 study also investigated the possibility of treatment reduction in advanced-stage patients achieving an early complete metabolic response. Patients who had a negative PET after two cycles of escalated BEACOPP were randomly assigned to continue treatment with four additional cycles of BEACOPPescalated or with four cycles of ABVD. Treatment results were comparable for both approaches. Hence, treatment intensity can be safely reduced from escalated BEACOPP

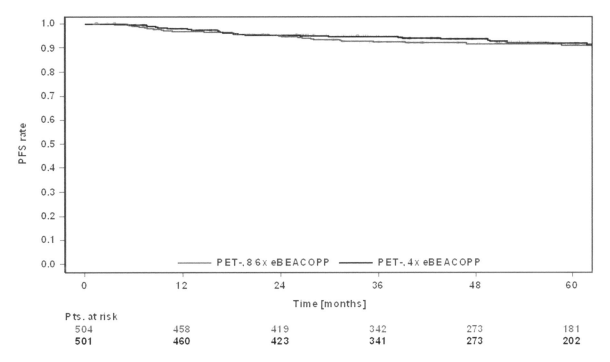

FIGURE 29.2 Comparison in terms of progression-free survival between six/eight cycles of BEACOPPesc (standard) and four cycles of BEACOPPesc (experimental) within the GHSG HD18 study for advanced HL. (From Borchmann et al., 2018. With permission.)

to ABVD in patients with a negative PET/CT after two cycles of BEACOPPescalated. [22]

PET/CT-guided strategies have also been investigated in advanced-stage patients who started chemotherapy with ABVD. Within the RATHL study, patients had treatment with two cycles of ABVD before they underwent PET/CT evaluation. Those with a negative interim PET/CT were randomly assigned to either ABVD or AVD chemotherapy in cycles 3 through 6. The 3-year PFS rates were 85.7% and 84.4% for patients receiving ABVD and AVD, respectively. Patients with a positive PET continued treatment with a BEACOPP-based chemotherapy. These patients had a 3-year PFS rate of 67.5%.[23]

Given the poorer tumor control with ABVD when compared with escalated BEACOPP, studies using an ABVD backbone in combination with targeted drugs have been initiated recently. The ECHELON-1 study compared standard ABVD with a combination of AVD and the antibody-drug conjugate brentuximab vedotin (A-AVD). After a median follow-up of 24.6 months, the 2-year PFS was better for A-AVD (82.1% vs. 77.2%). However, this advantage in tumor control came at the cost of a significantly increased acute toxicity.[24]

In summary, PET/CT-guided treatment approaches represent the standard of care in the treatment of advanced HL. The more aggressive escalated BEACOPP protocol results in better outcomes than ABVD but is associated with a higher incidence of acute toxicities and an increased risk for the development of long-term toxicities such as infertility and second malignancies.[25–28] Excessive toxicity in connection with BEACOPP-based chemotherapy has been reported for individuals older than 60 years so that such chemotherapy should not be given in this patient group.[29]

Ongoing studies aim at optimizing the treatment of advanced HL by reducing the toxicity of BEACOPPescalated on one hand and improving the efficacy of ABVD on the other hand by combining backbones of these protocols with targeted drugs.

HL IN ADVANCED STAGES

Escalated BEACOPP has substantially improved the outcome of patients with advanced HL but is associated with relevant acute and long-term toxicity. Therefore, PET-guided approaches allowing the reduction of chemotherapy with escalated BEACOPP to a total of only four cycles in a relevant proportion of patients should be refined to further decrease treatment toxicity. In addition, targeted drugs may in part replace conventional chemotherapy without a loss of acticity. The combination of novel agents and BEACOPP-based chemotherapy is thus investigated prospectively.

Treatment of relapsed HL

First relapse

Younger patients with HL recurrence after first-line treatment are candidates for high-dose chemotherapy followed by autologous stem cell transplantation (ASCT) in the majority of cases. Two randomized studies published in the 1990s and early 2000s have demonstrated that this approach results in better outcomes than conventional chemotherapy.[30,31] A subsequent randomized study including 284 patients aimed at improving

results by the introduction of sequential high-dose chemotherapy. However, at a median observation time of 42 months, there were no differences in terms of 3-year freedom from treatment failure and OS rates between patients allocated to the standard arm (single high-dose chemotherapy followed by ASCT) and patients who had treatment with sequential high-dose chemotherapy.[32]

With regard to the salvage protocol, there are different regimens such as DHAP (dexamethasone, high-dose ara-c, cisplatin), ICE (ifosfamide, carboplatin, etoposide), and IGEV (ifosfamide, gemcitabine, vinorelbine) having shown similar activity.[33–35] More recently, a study conducted at the Memorial Sloan Kettering Cancer Center evaluated brentuximab vedotin as a single agent (1.2 mg/kg on day 1, 8, and 15 for 2 28-day cycles) in patients with relapsed cHL. A proportion of 27% became PET-negative and proceeded to high-dose chemotherapy and ASCT without any additional conventional salvage chemotherapy.[36] Thus, brentuximab vedotin given as single agent may be a sufficient salvage approach in a relevant minority of patients with relapsed HL. Brentuximab vedotin has also been investigated as maintenance therapy after high-dose chemotherapy and ASCT in poor-risk patients. A total of 329 individuals were randomly assigned to receive either no further treatment or brentuximab vedotin maintenance (1.8 mg/ kg on day 1 for up to 16 21-day cycles) after high-dose chemotherapy and ASCT. The final analysis of the study and a follow-up analysis consistently indicated a significantly improved PFS for patients who had brentuximab vedotin maintenance.[37,38] In addition to brentuximab vedotin maintenance, high-risk patients may benefit from tandem ASCT. Single-arm studies from the LYSA and the Southwest Oncology Group (SWOG) evaluating this approach reported outcomes that compared favorably to historic data obtained with standard high-dose chemotherapy and ASCT.[39,40]

Taken together, HL patients with disease recurrence should receive high-dose chemotherapy followed by ASCT in case they are eligible for aggressive treatment and respond to induction chemotherapy. Approximately 50% of patients achieve a second durable remission and can be considered cured with this approach. Salvage treatment in older patients who are not eligible for high-dose chemotherapy and ASCT should be chosen individually.[41] The same is true for patients with NLPHL presenting with disease recurrence. This patient group is often treated sufficiently with non-aggressive approaches such as anti-CD20 antibody treatment or conventional chemotherapy given the mostly indolent course of NLPHL.[42]

Second and higher grade of relapse

Disease recurrence after high-dose chemotherapy and ASCT is associated with a dismal prognosis and cure is unlikely in this situation. However, the advent of novel drugs such as brentuximab vedotin and the anti-PD1 antibodies nivolumab and pembrolizumab has resulted in a substantial improvement of prognosis.

Brentuximab vedotin is an antibody-drug conjugate targeting CD30. After the phase I study had indicated significant single-agent activity, a pivotal phase II study including 102 patients with HL recurrence after high-dose chemotherapy and ASCT was conducted.[43] Patients received brentuximab vedotin at a dose of 1.8 mg/kg every 3 weeks for up to 16 cycles. The overall response rate was 75%. The median PFS was 5.6 months. However, the group of patients that achieved a complete remission had median PFS of 20.5 months.[44] A recent follow-up analysis of the study revealed 5-year PFS and OS estimates of 22% and 41%, respectively. Of note, some patients had a durable remission without

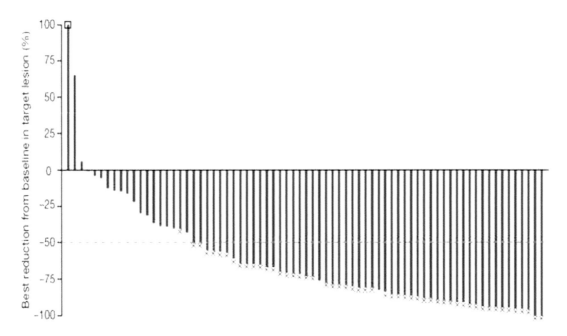

FIGURE 29.3 Tumor reduction after single-agent nivolumab within the CheckMate 205 study for cHL patients with multiple relapses. (From Younes et al., 2016. With permission.)

any additional therapy after the end of study treatment.[45] Given the excellent activity in patients failing high-dose chemotherapy and ASCT, brentuximab vedotin either alone in combination with conventional chemotherapy was subsequently evaluated in patients who had disease recurrence after first-line treatment and in individuals with newly diagnosed HL.[24,36,46,47] Final analyses of these studies are in part pending so that final conclusions with regard to the possible role of brentuximab vedotin in these situations cannot yet be drawn.

Patients with HL recurrence after high-dose chemotherapy followed by ASCT and brentuximab vedotin are currently treated with anti-PD1 antibodies in most cases. Nivolumab and pembrolizumab were both evaluated in this situation and have shown substantial clinical activity. A phase II study including 80 patients investigated nivolumab at a dose of 3 mg/kg every 2 weeks. Response was documented for 66.3% of patients (Figure 29.3).[48] A follow-up analysis of the study including additional patients reported a median duration of response of 16.6 months and a median PFS of 14.7 months.[49] Similar data were obtained from a phase II study including 210 patients who had received pembrolizumab at a dose of 200 mg every 3 weeks.[50]

Patients who relapse after anti-PD1 antibody treatment should be enrolled in clinical studies investigating novel drugs whenever possible. Allogeneic stem cell transplantation may be discussed in highly selected patients but the role of this treatment modality is rather limited given the activity of novel drugs such as brentuximab vedotin and anti-PD1 antibodies.

RELAPSED HL

The standard treatment for relapsed HL consists in high-dose chemotherapy followed by autologous stem cell transplantation (ASCT). Approximately 50% are cured with this approach. However, patients presenting with poor-risk characteristics still have a dismal outcome. These patients benefit from brentuximab vedotin consolidation but additional treatment options are needed to improve their prognosis. In contrast, a small but relevant proportion of patients with HL recurrence may not require high-dose chemotherapy and ASCT and can be salvaged successfully with conventional chemotherapy or targeted drugs. The definition of risk groups to allocate treatment more precisely therefore represents an important issue that should be addressed in future analyses.

References

1. Eichenauer DA, Aleman BMP, Andre M et al. Hodgkin lymphoma: ESMO Clinical Practice Guidelines for diagnosis, treatment and follow-up. *Ann Oncol.* 2018; 29(Supplement_4):iv19–29.
2. Eichenauer DA, Engert A. Nodular lymphocyte-predominant Hodgkin lymphoma: A unique disease deserving unique management. *Hematology Am Soc Hematol Educ Program.* 2017; 2017(1):324–8.
3. Cheson BD, Fisher RI, Barrington SF et al. Recommendations for initial evaluation, staging, and response assessment of Hodgkin and non-Hodgkin lymphoma: The Lugano classification. *J Clin Oncol.* 2014; 32(27):3059–8.
4. Engert A, Franklin J, Eich HT et al. Two cycles of doxorubicin, bleomycin, vinblastine, and dacarbazine plus extended-field radiotherapy is superior to radiotherapy alone in early favorable Hodgkin's lymphoma: Final results of the GHSG HD7 trial. *J Clin Oncol.* 2007; 25(23):3495–502.
5. Sasse S, Brockelmann PJ, Goergen H et al. Long-term follow-up of contemporary treatment in early-stage Hodgkin lymphoma: Updated Analyses of the German Hodgkin Study Group HD7, HD8, HD10, and HD11 Trials. *J Clin Oncol.* 2017; 35(18):1999–2007.
6. Noordijk EM, Carde P, Dupouy N et al. Combined-modality therapy for clinical stage I or II Hodgkin's lymphoma: Long-term results of the European Organisation for Research and Treatment of Cancer H7 randomized controlled trials. *J Clin Oncol.* 2006; 24(19):3128–35.

7. Ferme C, Eghbali H, Meerwaldt JH et al. Chemotherapy plus involved-field radiation in early-stage Hodgkin's disease. *N Engl J Med.* 2007; 357(19):1916–27.

8. Engert A, Plutschow A, Eich HT et al. Reduced treatment intensity in patients with early-stage Hodgkin's lymphoma. *N Engl J Med.* 2010; 363(7):640–52.

9. Radford J, Illidge T, Counsell N et al. Results of a trial of PET-directed therapy for early-stage Hodgkin's lymphoma. *N Engl J Med.* 2015; 372(17):1598–607.

10. Raemaekers JM, Andre MP, Federico M et al. Omitting radiotherapy in early positron emission tomography-negative stage I/II Hodgkin lymphoma is associated with an increased risk of early relapse: Clinical results of the preplanned interim analysis of the randomized EORTC/LYSA/FIL H10 trial. *J Clin Oncol.* 2014; 32(12):1188–94.

11. Andre MPE, Girinsky T, Federico M et al. Early positron emission tomography response-adapted treatment in stage I and II Hodgkin lymphoma: Final Results of the Randomized EORTC/LYSA/FIL H10 Trial. *J Clin Oncol.* 2017; 35(16):1786–94.

12. Fuchs M, Goergen H, Kobe C et al. PET-guided treatment of early-stage favorable Hodgkin lymphoma: Final results of the international, randomized phase 3 trial HD16 by the German Hodgkin Study Group. *Am Soc Hematol.* 2018; 132:925.

13. Eichenauer DA, Plutschow A, Fuchs M et al. Long-term course of patients with stage IA nodular lymphocyte-predominant Hodgkin lymphoma: A report from the German Hodgkin Study Group. *J Clin Oncol.* 2015; 33(26):2857–62.

14. Chen RC, Chin MS, Ng AK et al. Early-stage, lymphocyte-predominant Hodgkin's lymphoma: Patient outcomes from a large, single-institution series with long follow-up. *J Clin Oncol.* 2010; 28(1):136–41.

15. Eich HT, Diehl V, Gorgen H et al. Intensified chemotherapy and dose-reduced involved-field radiotherapy in patients with early unfavorable Hodgkin's lymphoma: Final analysis of the German Hodgkin Study Group HD11 trial. *J Clin Oncol.* 2010; 28(27):4199–206.

16. Ferme C, Thomas J, Brice P et al. ABVD or BEACOPPbaseline along with involved-field radiotherapy in early-stage Hodgkin lymphoma with risk factors: Results of the European Organisation for Research and Treatment of Cancer (EORTC)-Groupe d'Etude des Lymphomes de l'Adulte (GELA) H9-U intergroup randomised trial. *Eur J Cancer.* 2017 81:45–55.

17. von Treschow B, Plutschow A, Fuchs M et al. Dose-intensification in early unfavorable Hodgkin's lymphoma: Final analysis of the German Hodgkin Study Group HD14 trial. *J Clin Oncol.* 2012 30(9):907–13.

18. Engert A, Haverkamp H, Kobe C et al. Reduced-intensity chemotherapy and PET-guided radiotherapy in patients with advanced stage Hodgkin's lymphoma (HD15 trial): A randomised, open-label, phase 3 non-inferiority trial. *Lancet.* 2012 379(9828):1791–9.

19. Engert A, Goergen H, Markova J et al. Reduced-intensity chemotherapy in patients with advanced-stage Hodgkin lymphoma: Updated results of the open-label, international, randomised phase 3 HD15 trial by the German Hodgkin Study Group. *HemaSphere.* 2017; 1(1):e5

20. Borchmann P, Goergen H, Kobe C et al. PET-guided treatment in patients with advanced-stage Hodgkin's lymphoma (HD18): Final results of an open-label, international, randomised phase 3 trial by the German Hodgkin Study Group. *Lancet.* 2018; 390(10114):2790–802.

21. Borchmann P, Haverkamp H, Lohri A et al. Progression-free survival of early interim PET-positive patients with advanced stage Hodgkin's lymphoma treated with BEACOPPescalated alone or in combination with rituximab (HD18): An open-label, international, randomised phase 3 study by the German Hodgkin Study Group. *Lancet Oncol.* 2017; 18(4):454–63.

22. Casasnovas RO, Bouabdallah R, Brice P et al. PET-adapted treatment for newly diagnosed advanced Hodgkin lymphoma (AHL2011): A randomised, multicentre, non-inferiority, phase 3 study. *Lancet Oncol.* 2019; 20(2):202–15.

23. Johnson P, Federico M, Kirkwood A et al. Adapted treatment guided by interim PET-CT scan in advanced Hodgkin's lymphoma. *N Engl J Med.* 2016; 374(25):2419–29.

24. Connors JM, Jurczak W, Straus DJ et al. Brentuximab vedotin with chemotherapy for stage III or IV Hodgkin's lymphoma. *N Engl J Med.* 2018; 378(4):331–44.

25. Skoetz N, Trelle S, Rancea M et al. Effect of initial treatment strategy on survival of patients with advanced-stage Hodgkin's lymphoma: A systematic review and network meta-analysis. *Lancet Oncol.* 2013; 14(10):943–52.

26. Behringer K, Mueller H, Goergen H et al. Gonadal function and fertility in survivors after Hodgkin lymphoma treatment within the German Hodgkin Study Group HD13 to HD15 trials. *J Clin Oncol.* 2013; 31(2):231–9.

27. Eichenauer DA, Thielen I, Haverkamp H et al. Therapy-related acute myeloid leukemia and myelodysplastic syndromes in patients with Hodgkin lymphoma: A report from the German Hodgkin Study Group. *Blood.* 2014; 123(11):1658–664.

28. Eichenauer DA, Becker I, Monsef I et al. Secondary malignant neoplasms, progression-free survival and overall survival in patients treated for Hodgkin lymphoma: A systematic review and meta-analysis of randomized clinical trials. *Haematologica.* 2017; 102(10):1748–57.

29. Ballova V, Ruffer JU, Haverkamp H et al. A prospectively randomized trial carried out by the German Hodgkin Study Group (GHSG) for elderly patients with advanced Hodgkin's disease comparing BEACOPP baseline and COPP-ABVD (study HD9elderly). *Ann Oncol.* 2005; 16(1):124–31.

30. Linch DC, Winfield D, Goldstone AH et al. Dose intensification with autologous bone-marrow transplantation in relapsed and resistant Hodgkin's disease: Results of a BNLI randomised trial. *Lancet.* 1993; 341(8852):1051–4

31. Schmitz N, Pfistner B, Sextro M et al. Aggressive conventional chemotherapy compared with high-dose chemotherapy with autologous haemopoietic stem-cell transplantation for relapsed chemosensitive Hodgkin's disease: A randomised trial. *Lancet.* 2002; 359(9323):2065–71.

32. Josting A, Muller H, Borchmann P et al. Dose intensity of chemotherapy in patients with relapsed Hodgkin lymphoma. *J Clin Oncol.* 2010; 28(34):5074–80.

33. Josting A, Rudolph C, Reiser M et al. Time-intensified dexamethasone/cisplatin/cytarabine: An effective salvage therapy with low toxicity in patients with relapsed and refractory Hodgkin's disease. *Ann Oncol.* 2002; 13(10):1628–35

34. Moskowitz CH, Bertino JR, Glassman JR et al. Ifosfamide, carboplatin, and etoposide: A highly effective cytoreduction and peripheral-blood progenitor-cell mobilization regimen for transplant-eligible patients with non-Hodgkin's lymphoma. *J Clin Oncol.* 1999; 17(12):3776–85.

35. Santoro A, Magagnoli M, Spina M et al. Ifosfamide, gemcitabine, and vinorelbine: A new induction regimen for refractory and relapsed Hodgkin's lymphoma. *Haematologica.* 2007; 92(1):35–41

36. Moskowitz AJ, Schoder H, Yahalom J et al. PET-adapted sequential salvage therapy with brentuximab vedotin followed by augmented ifosamide, carboplatin, and etoposide for patients with relapsed and refractory Hodgkin's lymphoma: A non-randomised, open-label, single-centre, phase 2 study. *Lancet Oncol.* 2015; 16(3):284–92.

37. Moskowitz CH, Nademanee A, Masszi T et al. Brentuximab vedotin as consolidation therapy after autologous stem-cell transplantation in patients with Hodgkin's lymphoma at risk of relapse or progression (AETHERA): A randomised, double-blind, placebo-controlled, phase 3 trial. *Lancet.* 2015; 385(9980):1853–62.

38. Moskowitz CH, Walewski J, Nademanee A et al. Five-year PFS from the AETHERA trial of brentuximab vedotin for Hodgkin lymphoma at high risk of progression or relapse. *Blood.* 2018 132(25):2639–42.

39. Sibon D, Morschhauser F, Resche-Rigon M et al. Single or tandem autologous stem-cell transplantation for first-relapsed or refractory Hodgkin lymphoma: 10-year follow-up of the prospective H96 trial by the LYSA/SFGM-TC study group. *Haematologica.* 2016; 101(4):474–81.

40. Smith EP, Li H, Friedberg JW, Constine LS et al. Tandem autologous hematopoietic cell transplantation for patients with primary progressive or recurrent Hodgkin lymphoma: A SWOG and Blood and Marrow Transplant Clinical Trials Network Phase II trial (SWOG S0410/BMT CTN 0703). *Biol Blood Marrow Transplant.* 2018; 24(4):700–7.

41. Boll B, Goergen H, Arndt N et al. Relapsed hodgkin lymphoma in older patients: A comprehensive analysis from the German hodgkin study group. *J Clin Oncol.* 2013; 31(35):4431–7.

42. Eichenauer DA, Plutschow A, Schroder L et al. Relapsed and refractory nodular lymphocyte-predominant Hodgkin lymphoma: An analysis from the German Hodgkin Study Group. *Blood.* 2018; 132(14):1519–25.

43. Younes A, Bartlett NL, Leonard JP et al. Brentuximab vedotin (SGN-35) for relapsed CD30-positive lymphomas. *N Engl J Med.* 2010; 363(19):1812–21.

44. Younes A, Gopal AK, Smith SE et al. Results of a pivotal phase II study of brentuximab vedotin for patients with relapsed or refractory Hodgkin's lymphoma. *J Clin Oncol.* 2012; 30(18):2183–9.

45. Chen R, Gopal AK, Smith SE et al. Five-year survival and durability results of brentuximab vedotin in patients with relapsed or refractory Hodgkin lymphoma. *Blood.* 2016; 128(12):1562–6.

46. Hagenbeek A, Mooij H, Zijlstra J et al. Phase I dose-escalation study of brentuximab-vedotin combined with dexamethasone, high-dose cytarabine and cisplatin, as salvage treatment in relapsed/refractory classical Hodgkin lymphoma: The HOVON/LLPC Transplant BRaVE study. *Haematologica.* 2019; 104(4):e151–3.

47. Eichenauer DA, Plutschow A, Kreissl S et al. Incorporation of brentuximab vedotin into first-line treatment of advanced classical Hodgkin's lymphoma: Final analysis of a phase 2 randomised trial by the German Hodgkin Study Group. *Lancet Oncol.* 2017; 18(12):1680–7.

48. Younes A, Santoro A, Shipp M et al. Nivolumab for classical Hodgkin's lymphoma after failure of both autologous stem-cell transplantation and brentuximab vedotin: A multicentre, multicohort, single-arm phase 2 trial. *Lancet Oncol.* 2016; 17(9):1283–94.

49. Armand P, Engert A, Younes A et al. Nivolumab for relapsed/refractory classic Hodgkin lymphoma after failure of autologous hematopoietic cell transplantation: Extended follow-up of the Multicohort Single-Arm Phase II CheckMate 305 trial. *J Clin Oncol.* 2018; 36(14):1428–39.

50. Chen R, Zinzani PL, Fanale MA et al. Phase II study of the efficacy and safety of pembrolizumab for relapsed/refractory classic Hodgkin lymphoma. *J Clin Oncol.* 2017; 35(19):2125–32.

Piers Blombery and David C. Linch

Epidemiology and risk factors, classification, staging, and molecular pathogenesis of non-Hodgkin lymphoma

Epidemiology and risk factors

Non-Hodgkin lymphoma (NHL) refers to a diverse group of malignancies derived from lymphoid tissue consisting of more than 40 different clinicopathological entities.[1] As a group, they account for 3% of all cancers worldwide with the highest incidence seen in economically developed countries.[2] Data from the United States of America and Europe indicate that the overall incidence of NHL rose by 3%–4% per year between the 1970s and the 1990s. Despite the identification of many risk factors for the development of NHL, the reason for this increasing incidence is unclear; however, it is suspected to be contributed to (at least in part) by changes in diagnostic practice. All subtypes of NHL are more common in the elderly, making this an increasing public health-care problem in an ageing population. NHL also has an uneven sex distribution with almost all subtypes occurring more frequently in men.[2]

Other than demographic variations, the two closely related major risk factors for the development of NHL are immunodeficiency and Epstein–Barr virus (EBV) infection. Immunodeficiency can either be congenital or acquired (of which important causes include human immunodeficiency virus [HIV] infection and immunosuppressant medication). EBV infection plays an important role in the pathogenesis of numerous NHL subtypes in both immunocompetent and immunodeficient individuals. In immunocompetent patients, the EBV genome can be found within tumor cells in a significant proportion of cases of NHL which varies by lymphoma subtype (e.g., extra-nodal natural killer [NK]/T-cell lymphoma, Burkitt lymphoma [BL]). In patients with immunodeficiency, the importance and prevalence of EBV-driven lymphomas increase with severity of immune compromise. In addition to EBV, there are other well-characterized associations between viruses/microorganisms and lymphoma including *Helicobacter pylori* and extra-nodal marginal zone lymphoma (MZL), human T lymphotropic virus 1 (HTLV-1) and adult T-cell leukemia/lymphoma (ATLL), and primary effusion lymphoma, and human herpes virus-8 (HHV-8). Other risk factors for the development of NHL include auto-immune disease (e.g., Sjogren's disease and MZL, celiac disease and enteropathy-associated T-cell lymphoma [EATL], rheumatoid arthritis and T-cell large granular lymphocytic leukemia [T-LGL]) and environmental factors (e.g., radiation exposure and some petrochemicals).

Classification

The widely accepted standard classification system for lymphoma is the World Health Organization (WHO) classification which was introduced in 2001 (and updated in 2008 and 2017).[1] In the WHO classification, NHL is subdivided primarily according to B-cell or T-cell lineage and then further subdivided into primitive versus mature lymphoid neoplasms (Table 30.1). The majority of NHL subtypes are of B-cell lineage with diffuse large B-cell lymphoma (DLBCL) accounting for over one-third of cases and follicular lymphoma (FL) representing about 20% of all cases of NHL (Table 30.2).[3]

Although there are more than 50 separate entities included in the current WHO classification of NHL, there are uniting themes amongst the clinical behavior and management of these disorders. Moreover, many NHL subtypes are extremely rare and a large proportion of cases of NHL are made up of relatively few subtypes. In terms of treatment paradigms, NHL can be broadly conceptualized as consisting of two groups: indolent lymphoma (of which the archetypal form is FL but which includes other entities such as MZL) and aggressive lymphoma (of which the archetypal form is DLBCL but includes other entities such as peripheral T-cell lymphoma-not otherwise specified [PTCL-NOS] and the highly aggressive BL). This chapter covers the management of selected subtypes of NHL from within these two groups and includes both common and uncommon subtypes. The management of small lymphocytic lymphoma and lymphoblastic lymphoma is not discussed here as they are biologically best considered as variants of chronic lymphocytic or acute lymphoblastic leukemia (ALL), respectively, and treated accordingly.

Staging

Although originally developed for staging in patients with Hodgkin lymphoma (HL), the modified Ann Arbor system provides a basis for staging in NHL (Table 30.3).[4] It is limited by the high frequency of extra-nodal disease in NHL compared to HL, resulting in a disproportionate number of patients having stage IV disease due to bone marrow involvement. Despite these shortcomings, it is the most frequently used staging system in adult patients with NHL and with few exceptions has been universally adopted.

The Ann Arbor system divides patients into four groups based on the anatomical extent of their disease. Staging is performed with regard to groups of nodes in anatomically defined fields rather than individual nodes and, unlike HL, it is not uncommon for NHL to involve non-contiguous nodal regions. Localized extra-nodal disease is designated with the suffix E. Involvement of the bone marrow, liver, or lung is always stage IV.

Staging of patients with NHL involves performing a thorough history and examination, radiological investigations to determine extent of disease, and bone marrow aspirate and trephine biopsy. The presence or absence of systemic ("B") symptoms should be elicited on history. Physical examination is used to determine the extent of clinically evident lymphadenopathy/splenomegaly as well as excluding acute complications related to lymphadenopathy (e.g., superior vena cava obstruction) and assessing potential co-morbidities (e.g., cardiorespiratory disease) that may influence treatment decisions.

The extent of lymphadenopathy and visceral involvement by lymphoma should be assessed by computed tomography (CT) scan from neck to pelvis. In addition to "structural" imaging

TABLE 30.1 **Proportion of New NHL Cases According to the Main NHL Subtypes**

Subtype	Non-Hodgkin Lymphoma Classification Project	HMRN Data
Follicular lymphoma	22.0%	18.1%
Marginal zone lymphoma	9.0%	19.9%
Mantle cell lymphoma	6.0%	5.0%
Diffuse large B-cell lymphoma	35.0%	48.5%
Burkitt lymphoma	1.0%	2.0%
T-cell lymphoma	7.0%	6.3%

Source: Non-Hodgkin's Lymphoma Classification Project, 1997. The data from the Non-Hodgkin's Lymphoma Classification Project is based on data from a number of major centers. The Haematological Malignancies Research Network (HMRN) includes a population of 3.6 million people form Yorkshire and the Humber regions and has a similar demographic profile to England as a whole.

with CT, "functional" imaging with ^{18}F-FDG-PET and correlative CT (positron emission tomography [PET]/CT) is an invaluable modality in NHL and has rapidly become standard of care for staging lymphoma. PET/CT is preferable to structural imaging alone for numerous reasons:

- PET/CT is more sensitive than CT and therefore may result in the "upstaging" of patients by the detection of occult disease that is not detected on CT alone. The incidence of this phenomenon varies with different subtypes of NHL; however, for example, it can occur (with resulting changes in management decisions) in up to 40% of patients with early stage FL.[5] PET/CT should be considered a mandatory part of staging in patients that have limited-stage disease on structural imaging where major management decisions have the potential to be altered if advanced-stage disease is detected.

TABLE 30.2 **Selected Non-Hodgkin Lymphoma Entities from the WHO (2017) Classification of Lymphoid Neoplasms**

B-Cell Lymphoma	T-Cell Lymphoma
Mature B-cell neoplasms	Mature T-cell and NK-cell neoplasms
Chronic lymphocytic leukemia/small lymphocytic lymphoma	T-cell prolymphocytic leukemia
Monoclonal B-cell lymphocytosis (CLL-type/non-CLL-type)	T-cell large granular lymphocytic leukemia
B-cell prolymphocytic leukemia	*Chronic lymphoproliferative disorder of NK-cells*
Splenic marginal zone lymphoma	Aggressive NK-cell leukemia
Hairy cell leukemia	Systemic EBV positive T-cell lymphoproliferative disease of childhood
Splenic B-cell lymphoma/leukemia, unclassifiable	Chronic active EBV infection of T- and NK-cell type, systemic form
Splenic diffuse red pulp small B-cell lymphoma	Hydroa vacciniforme-like lymphoproliferative disorder
Hairy cell leukemia-variant	Adult T-cell leukemia/lymphoma
Lymphoplasmacytic lymphoma/Waldenstroms macroglobulinemia	Extra-nodal NK/T-cell lymphoma, nasal type
IgM monoclonal gammopathy of undetermined significance	Enteropathy-associated T-cell lymphoma
Extra-nodal marginal zone lymphoma of mucosa-associated lymphoid tissue (MALT lymphoma)	Monomorphic epitheliotropic intestinal T-cell lymphoma
Nodal marginal zone lymphoma	Intestinal T-cell lymphoma, NOS
Pediatric nodal marginal zone lymphoma	*Indolent T-cell lymphoproliferative disorder of the gastrointestinal tract*
Follicular lymphoma (*in situ*, duodenal, testicular)	Hepatosplenic T-cell lymphoma
Pediatric-type follicular lymphoma	Subcutaneous panniculitis-like T-cell lymphoma
Primary cutaneous follicle center lymphoma	Mycosis fungoides
Mantle cell lymphoma	Sezary syndrome
Diffuse large B-cell lymphoma (DLBCL), NOS (germinal center B-cell subtype/activated B-cell subtype)	Primary cutaneous CD30 positive T-cell lymphoproliferative disorders
T-cell/histiocyte rich large B-cell lymphoma	Lymphomatoid papulosis
Primary DLBCL of the CNS	Primary cutaneous anaplastic large cell lymphoma
Primary cutaneous DLBCL, leg type	Primary cutaneous gamma-delta T-cell lymphoma
EBV-positive DLBCL, NOS	*Primary cutaneous CD8 positive aggressive epidermotropic cytotoxic T-cell lymphoma*
EBV-positive mucocutaneous ulcer	*Primary cutaneous acral CD8-positive T-cell lymphoma*
DLCBL associated with chronic inflammation	*Primary cutaneous CD4 positive small/medium T-cell lymphoma*
Lymphomatoid granulomatosis	Peripheral T-cell lymphoma, NOS
Primary mediastinal (thymic) large B-cell lymphoma	Angioimmunoblastic T-cell lymphoma
Intravascular large B-cell lymphoma	Follicular T-cell lymphoma
ALK positive large B-cell lymphoma	Nodal peripheral T-cell lymphoma with T follicular helper phenotype
Plasmablastic lymphoma	Anaplastic large cell lymphoma (ALK positive/ALK negative)
Primary effusion lymphoma	Breast implant–associated anaplastic large cell lymphoma
Multicentric Castleman disease	
HHV8-positive DLBCL, NOS	
HHV8-positive germinotropic lymphoproliferative disorder	
Large B-cell with IRF4 rearrangement	
Burkitt lymphoma	
Burkitt-like lymphoma with 11q aberration	
High-grade B-cell lymphoma with *MYC* and *BCL2* and/or *BCL6* rearrangements	
High-grade B-cell lymphoma, NOS	
B-cell lymphoma, unclassifiable, with features intermediate between DLBCL and classical Hodgkin lymphoma	

Source: Swerdlow et al., 2017.

Note: Italicized entities are provisional under current WHO classification.

TABLE 30.3   **Ann Arbor Staging System for Lymphoma with Cotswold Modifications**

Stage	Feature
I	Involvement of a single lymph node region or lymphoid structure (e.g., spleen, thymus, Waldeyer's ring)
II	Involvement of two or more lymph node regions on the same side of the diaphragm
III	Involvement of lymph regions or structures on both sides of the diaphragm
IV	Involvement of extra-nodal site(s) beyond that designated E. Any involvement of liver, lung, or bone marrow
Suffix	
A	No symptoms
B	Fever (>38°C), drenching sweats, weight loss (>10% body weight) over 6 months
E (stages I–III only)	Involvement of a single, extra-nodal site contiguous or proximal to nodal site of disease
	Massive mediastinal disease defined as transverse mass diameter: internal thoracic diameter ratio >33%
	The number of lymph node fields involved are indicated by a subscript (e.g., II_3)
Cotswold modifications	Stage III may be subdivided into stage III_1 (splenic, hilar, celiac, or portal nodes) and stage III_2 (para-aortic, iliac, or mesenteric nodes)
	Staging should be identified as clinical stage (CS) or pathologic stage (PS)
	Response category (CRu) defines persistent radiological abnormalities of uncertain significance

- PET/CT is a powerful modality for determining prognosis after initial chemotherapy. Patients with both indolent and aggressive NHL who have no disease detectable on PET/CT at the end of initial chemotherapy have superior outcomes to those with residual disease detectable on PET/CT.[6–8]
- Response on PET/CT to salvage therapy in relapsed DLBCL is highly predictive of outcomes after autologous stem cell transplantation (ASCT).[9,10]
- PET/CT performed during frontline therapy (e.g., after two cycles of chemotherapy in DLBCL) has predictive value but a recent meta-analysis concluded that the sensitivity and specificity were often too low for this test to be used in a risk-stratified treatment approach.[11]
- The aggressiveness of histology can be suggested by assessment of the FDG-avidity of lesions on PET/CT scan (higher standardized uptake value [SUV] being associated with higher grade lymphoma). In low-grade lymphoma this may suggest the possibility of sites of disease transformation and identify areas from which biopsies can be taken to assess this possibility[12] with the caveat that a high SUV can occasionally be observed in follicular lymphoma without transformation. In addition, before initial diagnostic biopsy, PET/CT can often help to guide the choice of target for biopsy in order to optimize biopsy of representative material.
- PET/CT may also be used for planning radiotherapy in NHL with the aim of minimizing radiotherapy dose to uninvolved tissue.[13]

PET/CT is not sensitive or specific enough to reliably stage the bone marrow of patients with NHL and therefore bone marrow aspirate and trephine biopsy are still often required. The trephine biopsy should ideally be more than 20 mm in length and be examined on multiple levels.[14] In addition to morphological assessment, NHL involvement of the bone marrow can be detected and assessed by flow cytometry, molecular tests, and cytogenetic analysis performed on the aspirate sample.

In addition to history, examination, and PET/CT, there are specific NHL subtypes in which other staging investigations are required:

- *Primary central nervous system (CNS) lymphoma*—magnetic resonance imaging (MRI) of the brain as well as ophthalmological assessment to detect intraocular disease are required. Lumbar puncture may also be performed to help determine prognosis (see later). MRI is also useful in evaluating peripheral nerve lesions.
- *Extra-nodal NK/T-cell lymphoma, nasal type*—patients with disease not overtly involving the nasal cavity at diagnosis should undergo endoscopic evaluation of the nasal cavity and upper airway to exclude occult involvement implying the presence of systemic disease.
- *Bony lesions*—MRI is a useful modality to evaluate the extent and nature of bony involvement.

Diffuse large B-cell lymphoma

Pathogenesis and classification

DLBCL is the most common subtype of NHL and the most common hematological malignancy in the United Kingdom.[15] It is an aggressive form of NHL and typically presents as a rapidly enlarging lymph node mass accompanied by systemic symptoms and organ dysfunction related to lymphoma infiltration. Although it can occur at any age (including in children), the median age of presentation is approximately 70 years.[15] DLBCL may either arise *de novo* or may represent transformation from an underlying indolent lymphoma (e.g., FL).

An important insight into the pathogenesis of DLBCL was the classification according to normal cell counterpart by gene expression profiling (GEP) studies.[16] By using this approach, patients can be characterized into two major subgroups, one group with an expression profile similar to normal germinal center B-cells (GCB) and one with a similar gene expression profile to post-germinal center activated B-cells (ABC). The GCB-DLBCL and ABC-DLBCL subtypes have different mechanisms of lymphomagenesis, immunohistochemical characteristics, prognosis, and contain different suites of genetic lesions. GCB-DLBCL is characterized by increased BCL2 expression (e.g., by translocation of the BCL2 locus to the immunoglobulin heavy chain locus), epigenetic dysregulation (by activating mutations in EZH2 and inactivating mutations of KMT2D), and increased BCL6 expression. ABC-DLBCL is characterized by genetic lesions that converge to cause constitutive activation of the NF-kB pathway. More recently, large cohorts of patients have been assessed with a mixture of whole-exome sequencing and whole-transcriptome sequencing which have revealed a very high degree of genomic heterogeneity in this disease that further subdivides GCB- and ABC-DLBCL into multiple new subgroups characterized by more specific constellations of genomic lesions.[17,18] This newly discovered degree of genomic complexity of DLBCL likely explains to a significant degree the failure of targeted therapies to improve outcomes in DLBCL given these therapies have been used in patients selected based on relatively broad molecular classifications (i.e., GCB vs. ABC).

The current WHO classification (Table 30.2) contains the category *DLBCL-NOS* into which the majority of cases of DLBCL are expected to be classified. Other lymphomas of large B-cells that have specific morphological and pathological features are included in a separate group in the WHO classification, some members of which are broadly managed in the same way as DLBCL (e.g., T-cell/histiocyte-rich large B-cell lymphoma) and others that require very different therapeutic approaches (e.g., primary DLBCL of the CNS). In addition, the current WHO classification recognizes an important new category *High-grade B-cell lymphoma* which includes the entity *High-grade B-cell lymphoma with MYC and BCL2 and/or BCL6 rearrangements*, commonly known as "double hit lymphoma" (DHL) which is discussed further below.

Prognostic factors

The International Prognostic Index (IPI) has been established for more than two decades as the most widely used prognostic system for patients with aggressive lymphoma (Table 30.4).[19] It is based on five clinical variables—age, stage, serum lactate dehydrogenase (LDH), performance status, and the number of extra-nodal sites involved which allows subdivision of patients according to the number of prognostic factors into low risk (none or one factor), low-intermediate risk (two factors), high-intermediate risk (three factors), or high risk (four or five factors) with predicted 5-year survival in the pre-rituximab era of 73%, 51%, 43%, and 26%, respectively. Initially developed with reference

TABLE 30.4   **Prognostic Scores in Lymphoproliferative Disorders**

Prognostic Score	Components	Score	Outcomes
International Prognostic Index (IPI)	Age >60 Stage III/IV Raised LDH Extra-nodal sites >1 Performance status >2	Low (0,1) Low-intermediate (2) High-intermediate (3) High (4,5)	3-year OS—91% 3-year OS—81% 3-year OS—65% 3-year OS—59%
Age-adjusted international prognostic index (aaIPI) (Age > 60)	Stage III/IV Raised LDH Performance status ≥2	Low (0) Low-intermediate (1) High-intermediate (2) High (3)	5-year OS—83%[a] 5-year OS—69%[a] 5-year OS—46%[a] 5-year OS—32%[a]
Stage-modified international prognostic index (smIPI) (Stage I/II)	Age >60 Raised LDH Stage II Performance status ≥2	Low (0,1) Intermediate (2) High (3)	5-year OS—82% 5-year OS—71% 5-year OS—48%
Mantle cell prognostic index (MIPIb)	$0.03535 \times$ age (years) + 0.6978 (if ECOG >1) + $1.367 \times \log_{10}(\text{LDH/ULN})$ + $0.9393 \times \log_{10}(\text{WBC})$ + $0.02142 \times$ Ki-67(%)	Low (< 5.7) Intermediate (5.7–6.5) High (>6.5)	Median OS—NR Median OS—58 m Median OS—37 m
Primary cerebral lymphoma (IELSG)[b]	Age >60 Performance status >1 Elevated LDH High CSF protein Involvement of deep brain regions	Low (0–1) Intermediate (2–3) High (4–5)	2-year OS—80% 2-year OS—48% 2-year OS—15%
CNS International Prognostic Index (CNS-IPI)	Age >60 years Raised LDH Performance status >1 Stage III/IV Extra-nodal sites >1 Involvement of kidney and/or adrenal glands	Low (0–1) Intermediate (2–3) High (>3)	0.6% risk of CNS relapse 3.4% risk of CNS relapse 10.2% risk of CNS relapse
Follicular lymphoma international prognostic index (FLIPI)	Age >60 Stage (III/IV) Hb <120 g/L Nodal areas >4 Raised LDH	Low (0–1) Intermediate (2) High (≥3)	5-year OS—91% 5-year OS—78% 5-year OS—53%
m7- Follicular lymphoma international prognostic index (m7-FLIPI)	High-risk FLIPI (+0.79) Performance status ≥2 (+0.38) EZH2mut (−0.53), ARID1Amut (−0.4mut), EP300mut (+0.33), FOXO1mut (+0.26mut), MEF2B (−0.07), CREBBPmut (+0.05), CARD11 (+0.04)	Low risk <0.8 High risk >0.8	5-year FFS—77.21% 5-year FFS—38.29%
Prognostic Index for PTCL-U (PIT)	Age >60 Performance status ≥2 Raised LDH Bone marrow involvement	Group 1 (0) Group 2 (1) Group 3 (2) Group 4 (3,4)	5-year OS—62% 5-year OS—53% 5-year OS—33% 5-year OS—18%

[a]   Outcomes are from pre-rituximab era.
[b]   International extra-nodal lymphoma study group.

to intermediate-grade disease within the working formulation, and for all stages of disease, it has subsequently been validated in patients with DLBCL.[19] When applied to cohorts of patients treated on large prospective randomized trials in the rituximab era, the IPI retains its prognostic value with 3-year overall survival (OS) predicted for low risk, low-intermediate, high-intermediate and high risk at 91%, 81%, 65%, and 59%, respectively.[20] In addition, an age-adjusted IPI was validated as a useful prognosis stratification tool in patients below 60 years and was subsequently adapted for those above 60 years of age[19] (Table 30.4). A number of modifications have been made to the original IPI,[21] but the benefits are minor, and the original IPI facilitates comparability between studies over a wider time-frame.

Although the IPI remains the most useful means of stratifying patients according to their prognosis and is central to the comparability of outcomes across clinical trials, there is a marked variability of response to treatment within the IPI subgroups. One explanation for this observation is that the IPI does not reflect the genomic and biological heterogeneity of the underlying disease as described above. Patients with GCB-DLBCL have a significantly improved 5-year survival compared to those with ABC-DLBCL (76% vs. 26%) that is independent of IPI.[16,22] Moreover, the new molecular subdivisions identify high- and low-risk subtypes based on genomic abnormalities within the GCB/ABC categories.[17,18]

Patients with disrupted MYC and BCL2 loci identified by FISH analysis (DHL) have high rates of extra-nodal involvement (including CNS) and significantly inferior outcomes with standard upfront therapy, representing a group of patients in need of alternative approaches. Importantly, overexpression of BCL2 and MYC by immunohistochemistry alone does not impart as poor a prognosis as those with FISH-identified abnormalities, possibly due to the greater inter-pathologist variability in determining IHC positivity. Furthermore, within FISH-defined DHL, MYC translocations with the IG locus are associated with worse outcomes compared to non-IG partners.

Treatment of newly diagnosed DLBCL

Numerous phase III prospective randomized controlled trials have established immunochemotherapy consisting of cyclophosphamide, vincristine, doxorubicin, prednisolone, and rituximab (Table 30.5) delivered every 21 days (R-CHOP-21) as the standard treatment for advanced-stage DLBCL. The choice of CHOP as the chemotherapy component is based on prospective trials in the pre-rituximab era demonstrating CHOP to be as efficacious and less toxic than other putatively more intense chemotherapy regimens to which it was compared (MACOP-B, ProMACE-CytaBOM, m-BACOD).[23] In the 1990s, the monoclonal antibody rituximab was developed targeting the CD20 antigen which is expressed to a variable degree in almost all mature B-cell neoplasms. Binding of rituximab to CD20 *in vivo* results in an anti-lymphoma effect via numerous mechanisms including complement and antibody-dependent cytotoxicity, inhibition of proliferation, and induction of apoptosis.[24] The results of a pivotal study using R-CHOP for the treatment of newly diagnosed patients (aged 60–80 years) demonstrated a significant improvement in complete response rate (76% vs. 63%)[25] and 5-year OS (58% vs. 45%), compared to CHOP

TABLE 30.5   **Common Chemotherapy Regimens Used in Non-Hodgkin Lymphoma**

Regimen Name	Schedule
Upfront treatment	
R-CHOP	Cyclophosphamide 750 mg/m² iv d1, doxorubicin 50 mg/m² iv d1, vincristine 1.4 mg/m² (max 2 mg) iv d1, prednisolone 100 mg po d1–5, rituximab 375 mg/m² iv d1. Repeat every 14–21 days.
R-CVP	Cyclophosphamide 750 mg/m² iv d1, vincristine 1.4 mg/m² (max 2 mg) iv d1, prednisolone 40 mg/m² po d1–5, rituximab 375 mg/m² iv d1. Repeat every 21 days.
R-CODOX-M	Cyclophosphamide 800 mg/m² iv d1, cyclophosphamide 200 mg/m² iv d2–5, vincristine 1.5 mg/m² (max 2 mg) iv d1+8, doxorubicin 40 mg/m² iv d1, cytarabine 70 mg IT d1+3, rituximab 375 mg/m² iv d1, methotrexate 3 g/m² iv d10, methotrexate 12 mg IT d15.
R-IVAC	Cytarabine 2 g/m² iv bd d1+2, etoposide 60 mg/m² iv d1–5, ifosfamide 1.5 g/m² iv d1–5, rituximab 375 mg/m² iv d1, methotrexate 12 mg IT d5.
Dose-adjusted (DA) EPOCH-R	Etoposide 50 mg/m² iv (cont.) daily d1–4, doxorubicin 10 mg/m² iv (cont.) daily d1–4, vincristine 0.4 mg/m² iv (cont.) daily d1–4, cyclophosphamide 750 mg/m² iv d5, prednisolone 60 mg/m² bd d1–5 (adjust doxorubicin, etoposide, and cyclophosphamide based on ANC nadir).
Bendamustine-R	Bendamustine 90 mg/m² iv d1–2, rituximab 375 mg/m² iv d1. Repeat every 28 days.
FCR	Fludarabine 25 mg/m² iv d1–3, cyclophosphamide 250 mg/m² iv d1–3, rituximab 375 mg/m² d1. Repeat every 28 days.
SMILE	Methotrexate 2 g/m² iv d1, ifosfamide 1.5 g/m² d2–4, etoposide 100 mg/m² iv d2–4, dexamethasone 40 mg po/iv d2–4, L-asparaginase (*Escherichia coli*) 6000 U/m² d8,10,12,14,16,18,20.
R-HyperCVAD	Part A—cyclophosphamide 300 mg/m² iv bd d1–3, doxorubicin 50 mg iv d4, vincristine 1.4 mg/m² (max 2 mg) iv d4+11, dexamethasone 40 mg po/iv d1–4 and d11–14, rituximab 375mg/m2 iv d1. Part B—methotrexate 1 g/m² iv d1, cytarabine 3 g/m² iv bd d2+3, rituximab 375mg/m2 iv d1.
Nordic MCL2 protocol (R-Maxi-CHOP/R-HiDAC)	Cyclophosphamide 1200 mg/m² iv d1, doxorubicin 75 mg/m² iv d1, vincristine 2 mg iv d1, rituximab 375 mg/m² iv d1 (omit on cycle 1), prednisolone 100 mg po d1–5 ALTERNATING WITH cytarabine 3 g/m² (2 g/m² if > 60 years) iv bd d1+2, rituximab 375 mg/m² iv d1 (and d9 in cycle 6 only).
Salvage regimens	
ESHAP	Etoposide 40 mg/m² iv d1–4, cisplatin 25 mg/m² iv d1–4, methylprednisolone 500 mg iv d1–5, cytarabine 2 g/m² iv d5.
ICE	Etoposide 100 mg/m² iv d1–3, carboplatin AUC5 iv d2, ifosfamide 5 g/m² iv d2.
DHAP	Cisplatin 100 mg/m² iv d1, cytarabine 2 g/m² iv bd d2, dexamethasone 40 mg po/iv d1–4.
MiniBEAM	Carmustine 60 mg/m² iv d1 (or lomustine), cytarabine 100 mg iv bd d2–5, etoposide 75 mg/m² iv d2–5, melphalan 30 mg/m² iv d6.
IVE	Ifosfamide 3 g/m² iv d1–3, epirubicin 50 mg/m² iv d1, etoposide 200 mg/m² iv d1–3.

alone.[26] This benefit was seen in both low-risk (aaIPI 0-1) and high-risk (aaIPI 2-3) disease; however, the greatest benefit was seen in the low-risk group. Importantly, there was no increase in the treatment-related toxicity with the addition of rituximab. A similar benefit was shown subsequently for treating younger patients with low-risk (aaIPI 0-1) disease (MiNT study).[27]

DLBCL is a radiosensitive disease and therefore, in patients with localized disease, the use of locoregionally targeted treatment (radiotherapy) may be used to either (i) decrease exposure to chemotherapy and minimize systemic toxicity or (ii) treat areas of disease (particularly areas of bulk) after full chemotherapy to decrease local relapse risk. Whilst the weight of non-randomized data in the R-CHOP era showed a benefit of radiotherapy in limited-stage DLBCL, more recent data from randomized trials support the omission of radiotherapy in patients with or without bulk if they achieve a complete metabolic remission on PET scan after chemotherapy.

Although the majority of patients with lower risk DLBCL achieve very good results with R-CHOP-21, patients with high-risk disease features continue to have suboptimal outcomes. This includes not only those patients that are high risk as determined by IPI but also those with other poor prognostic factors such as ABC-DLBCL and particularly DHL. Unfortunately, despite multiple alterations to upfront chemotherapy including incorporation of novel agents aimed to molecularly target ABC-subtype biology (bortezomib,[28] ibrutinib,[29] and lenalidomide[30]), use of maintenance rituximab,[31] increased chemotherapy intensity, and utilization of newer anti-CD20 antibodies,[32] there has been no significant improvement upon outcomes compared to R-CHOP21 and this remains the standard of care for newly diagnosed patients. Intensified upfront regimens (in particular DA-EPOCH-R and CODOX-M/IVAC) as well as consolidation in first remission by autologous stem cell transplantation have been investigated in DHL with some series showing modest improvement of outcomes;[33,34] however robust randomized data supporting a benefit for this approach are lacking and this patient group remains an area of significant therapeutic need.

Treatment of relapsed DLBCL

The Parma study in the mid-1990s established high-dose therapy and ASCT as the standard treatment for relapsed, chemotherapy-sensitive DLBCL. This approach resulted in long-term disease-free survival in 45% of patients with the degree of response to salvage chemotherapy and duration of first remission (more or less than 1 year) being predictive of outcome. Salvage chemotherapy regimens used before ASCT in the pre-rituximab era resulted in response rates of 43%–63%.[35–39]

However, patients who relapse after first-line therapy containing rituximab have worse outcomes compared to those in the pre-rituximab era. This phenomenon was demonstrated in the COllaborative trial in Relapsed Aggressive Lymphoma (CORAL) study which randomized patients in first relapse to salvage chemotherapy with either R-DHAP or R-ICE (Table 30.5).[40] Those responding to salvage underwent high-dose therapy and ASCT. Although the overall response rate to each of the salvage regimens was approximately 60% (with no difference between the two regimens), the response rate was only 45%–50% in those with prior rituximab exposure or those who had relapsed under 12 months.[40] Moreover, whereas the 3-year OS of the whole cohort was 50%, this dropped to 40% for those previously treated with rituximab and only a 20% 3-year PFS. Patients with early relapse and prior rituximab exposure who responded to salvage chemotherapy and therefore proceeded to ASCT had a 3-year PFS of

40%. Interestingly, the cell of origin classification influenced outcomes in this setting with GCB-DLBCL having more favorable outcomes with R-DHAP compared to R-ICE.[41] However, given the generally suboptimal outcomes in those patients with previous rituximab exposure (now a universal part of upfront treatment), novel therapies and treatment approaches are needed in this group.

Patients who are refractory to salvage chemotherapy or who have relapsed post-ASCT have a very poor prognosis with conventional therapy, and the treatment is generally palliative. There is little benefit in re-treatment with an alternative conventional regimen, and therefore non-chemotherapy based novel agents tend to be utilized in this group, for example BTK inhibitors, lenalidomide, and antibody-drug conjugates such as polatuzumab vedotin (anti-CD79B). However, one of the most promising approaches in this group is the use of chimeric antigen receptor T (CART) cells. Whilst this is a rapidly evolving field, the approach generally involves collection of autologous T-lymphocytes from the patient using apheresis and then transduction of these T-cells with a chimeric T-cell receptor which has specificity for an antigen expressed on the DLBCL surface (most commonly CD19). These engineered T-cells are then reinfused to the patient and induce immune-mediated killing of tumor cells. Response rates in R/R DLBCL with CART cell therapy are high (>80%) with complete remissions observed in approximately 30%–50% in early clinical trials, making this one of the most effective treatments of relapsed disease.[42] Moreover, whilst CART cell therapy may have significant toxicity (cytokine release syndrome, neurotoxicity), the field is still maturing and improvements in receptor structure, antigen specificity, toxicity, manufacturing times, and cost are expected to make CART cell therapy one of the most important recent therapeutic developments in DLBCL (and indeed many other lymphomas).

Treatment of diffuse large B-cell lymphoma in the elderly

The majority of patients presenting with DLBCL are above 60 years of age and one-third are above 75 years. The prognosis in elderly patients is generally worse than in younger patients, and there are at least three reasons to account for this. First, elderly patients have more chemoresistant disease with an increased proportion of ABC-DLBCL,[43] higher BCL2 expression, more cytogenetic complexity, and more frequently EBV-associated DLCBL in the absence of overt immunosuppresion.[1] Second, older patients are less able to tolerate standard-dose therapy due to both functional decline with age and the increasing presence of co-morbidities. Third, the intensity of treatment is greatly influenced by the attitudes of the patients and their physicians. Wherever possible, elderly patients should be treated in the same way as younger patients and excellent outcomes can be achieved with R-CHOP. Any reduction in therapeutic intensity should be based on functional assessment and discussion with the patient and not age per se. Comprehensive geriatric assessments may help in this decision process, but there is not yet full agreement as to which assessment tools are both optimal and logistically feasible. In patients not able to tolerate full-dose R-CHOP, reduced-dose regimens can still result in reasonable results.[44,45] When there is cardiac insufficiency, doxorubicin can be omitted or replaced by other agents such as epirubicin or gemcitabine. Before starting therapy in older patients, the cardiac ejection fraction should be determined, and it is recommended that this is repeated after every two or three cycles. It is notable that whereas results in younger adults appear better in western Europe than in the United States, the reverse is true in older patients, and this raises concerns about the attitudes of European physicians.[46]

Primary mediastinal (thymic) large B-cell lymphoma

Classified as a separate disease entity in the current WHO classification, primary mediastinal (thymic) large B-cell lymphoma (PMBCL) usually presents in younger females with a large mediastinal mass.[1] Pathologically, PMBCL is composed of large lymphocytes that express CD20, CD23 (a marker of thymic B-cells), and CD30 (weakly). The tumor often shows compartmentalizing sclerosis redolent of HL and indeed GEP data have shown PMBCL to be more similar to HL than to DLBCL.[47] Other recurrent genetic abnormalities in this entity include amplifications of 9p (involving JAK2 as well as CD274 [PD-L1] and PDCD1LG2 [PD-L2]) and oncogenic mutations involving the JAK/STAT and NF-kB pathways. [48]

In the past, PMBCL was felt to be a higher risk subtype of DLBCL benefiting from specific therapies such as weekly regimens (e.g., MACOP-B/VACOP-B).[49] However, this was based on retrospective analyses, and in the rituximab era there is little evidence that such regimens are superior to CHOP or CHOP-like regimens.[50,51] R-CHOP and mediastinal radiotherapy results in long-term remission in approximately 80% of patients and, in contrast to DLBCL, the long-term PFS curve of PMBCL shows a clear plateau from approximately 2 years onwards implying cure in these patients.[52]

PMBCL usually presents with bulky localized disease, and therefore consolidative radiotherapy after chemotherapy has historically been felt to be advisable to minimize local failure of disease control. However, the position and size of the tumor mass often mean that significant volumes of heart, lung, and breast tissue may be exposed, leading to long-term cardiotoxicity, pulmonary toxicity, and a late risk of breast cancer. A phase II study used a regimen of continuous infusion of etoposide, doxorubicin, and vincristine combined with cyclophosphamide and rituximab titrated against neutropenia (dose adjusted [DA]-EPOCH-R) in patients with PMBCL.[69] Patients in this trial had promising disease control and OS with only 2 patients (of 51) receiving mediastinal radiotherapy.

The conventional approach to patients in the relapsed setting is similar to DLBCL, with salvage chemotherapy and autologous stem cell transplantation in those eligible currently the only curative option. Given the high rate of 9p amplification involving PD-L1/PD-L2 and the biological similarity to Hodgkin lymphoma, checkpoint inhibitor therapy (e.g., PD-1 inhibition with pembrolizumab or nivolumab) has been investigated in this entity and has shown encouragingly high response rates.[53]

Central nervous system lymphoma and prophylactic central nervous system chemotherapy

Primary central nervous system lymphoma

PCNSL is rare, accounting for only 1%–2% of NHL. Although apparently general, the term PCNSL is most commonly used to refer to a specific disease entity of an aggressive NHL with the morphological and immunophenotypic features of DLBCL involving the CNS without evidence of systemic involvement detectable on completed staging. It is a unique subtype of NHL

with specific immunophenotypic features, recurrent molecular abnormalities,[54] radiological appearances, and clinical course. Although other subtypes of NHL can present in the CNS (e.g., FL, MZL), this is a very rare manifestation and the therapy is not standardized.

The median age of PCNSL diagnosis is approximately 60 years; however, it does occur in younger patients where it may be associated with HIV infection. Although PCNSL is associated with a poor prognosis, an increasing evidence base is accumulating regarding its optimal treatment. In those able to tolerate it, multi-agent chemotherapy using chemotherapeutic agents able to cross the blood–brain barrier delivered in a sufficient dose and schedule to allow adequate CNS concentration for adequate anti-tumor effect is becoming established as the preferred initial treatment. The combination of methotrexate, thiotepa, cytarabine, and rituximab (MATRix) has been shown in a prospective randomized trial to be an effective combination in those up to the age of 70 years.[55] For those patients unable to tolerate the MATRix regimen, other methotrexate-based chemotherapy regimens or temozolomide may be used.

After initial chemotherapy, responses may be consolidated by either whole-brain radiotherapy (WBRT) or autologous stem cell transplantation (ASCT). These two approaches are of broadly similar efficacy, and the choice between them is determined by patient age, preference, and organ function. WBRT is associated with a significant incidence of disabling neurotoxicity, especially in those above the age of 60.[56,57] In addition to older age, neurotoxicity is also associated with prior chemotherapy exposure and the dose of radiotherapy received. In contrast, ASCT is associated with severe hematological and other organ toxicity, especially when utilizing conditioning regimens containing CNS active agents such as thiotepa. In elderly patients with significant co-morbidities or advanced age who achieve a complete response to upfront chemotherapy it is reasonable to defer treatment until progression.

Like other lymphomas of immune-privileged sites, PCNSL has a relatively high incidence of MYD88/CD79B mutations.[54] This observation has led to the investigation of BTK inhibitors such as ibrutinib in this condition which have shown promising efficacy in initial trials.[58]

Secondary involvement of the CNS by lymphoma

Secondary involvement of the CNS as a complication of systemic NHL has been described in association with most NHL subtypes. It is observed in B-cell NHL with an incidence that varies by histological grade, ranging from below 3% in low-grade disease, to 5% of DLBCL, and 25% in BL.[59,60] Secondary involvement of the CNS by lymphoma may be present at diagnosis, develop as a site of disease progression during first-line treatment, or occur as a site of relapse after completion of initial treatment. Patients that present with CNS involvement have a poor prognosis, and although there is no consensus on treatment, standard practice usually includes CNS-directed chemotherapy with or without radiotherapy.[61] The results of treatment with high-dose therapy and ASCT are more encouraging; however, this is only possible in a minority of patients.[61]

Patients who do not have CNS involvement on initial staging, but who are at high risk of developing secondary CNS involvement, should receive CNS chemoprophylaxis. There are two main approaches to CNS chemoprophylaxis: (i) administration of intrathecal methotrexate or cytarabine with each cycle of chemotherapy for four to six doses,[62] or (ii) administration of high dose systemic methotrexate (e.g., >3g/m^2) either at the end of upfront chemotherapy or intercalated early into therapy in high-risk patients. Whilst it is unknown which of these approaches is more effective or whether both are required, an increasingly common approach adopted is the use of systemic methotrexate alone as CNS chemoprophylaxis.

Patients with DLBCL can be stratified into risk groups for secondary CNS involvement using the CNS-IPI (Table 30.4). Patients with low-risk CNS-IPI (0–1) have a risk of secondary CNS involvement of 0.6% as opposed to 10.2% for those in the highest risk group (CNS-IPI 4–6). In addition to CNS-IPI risk factors, the presence of double-hit lymphoma, and involvement of the testes, breast, and epidural space are recognized as carrying a high risk of secondary CNS involvement, justifying CNS chemoprophylaxis. In the absence of CNS-directed therapy, patients with BL or ALL have an estimated 25% risk of secondary CNS involvement, and therefore aggressive CNS-directed therapy using both systemic and intrathecal chemotherapy is a mandatory part of chemotherapy regimens used to treat these diseases.[59]

Burkitt lymphoma

BL is a highly aggressive form of NHL and one of the most rapidly proliferating forms of human cancer. The underlying reason for this aggressiveness is the central nature of dysregulation of one of the main transcription factors involved in cellular proliferation—myc. The most common mechanism of MYC dysregulation in BL is by a translocation between the myc locus (on chromosome 8) and the immunoglobulin heavy chain locus (on chromosome 14). In addition to the classic t(8;14), there are other mechanisms of myc dysregulation seen in BL including translocation to the immunoglobulin light chain loci on either chromosome 2 (t[2;8]) or chromosome 22 (t[8;22]) and mutations within the MYC gene itself.

In the context of typical morphology (monomorphic medium-sized lymphocytes, numerous macrophages giving a "starry sky" appearance), immunohistochemical findings (CD10+, CD19+, CD20+, BCL6+, BCL2−, TdT−, CD34−, Ki-67 100%), and t(8;14), making a diagnosis of BL is relatively straightforward. However, distinguishing BL from histologically similar entities including *high-grade B-cell lymphoma with MYC and BCL2 and/or BCL6 rearrangements* and *high-grade B-cell lymphoma, NOS* is crucial given the relatively inferior outcomes associated with these latter groups compared to true BL.

There are three forms of BL: endemic, sporadic, and immunodeficiency-associated. BL typically presents as rapidly progressive extra-nodal disease with frequent bone marrow, intestinal tract, and leptomeningeal disease. Nodal disease is more common in adults than in children and is often bulky.[63] Both spontaneous tumor lysis syndrome (i.e., preceding treatment) and treatment-induced tumor lysis syndrome are common in BL and are important contributors to early morbidity and mortality. Rigorous hydration and recombinant urate oxidase are now routinely used in patients with BL.[64]

Despite its clinical aggressiveness, the overall prognosis of BL is favorable with cure achieved in up to 80% of the patients with intense chemotherapy. The general principles of chemotherapy regimens used to treat BL are the utilization of fractionated cyclophosphamide (to increase the likelihood of exposure to malignant cells in cycle), CNS-penetrating agents, inclusion of cell cycle phase-specific agents (e.g., cytarabine), aggressive intrathecal prophylaxis, and maintaining intensity by delivering chemotherapy as soon as hematological recovery has occurred. A commonly used regimen is CODOX-M alternating with IVAC for four cycles of chemotherapy in total.[65] Patients with "low-risk" disease as defined by a score of 0 in the conventional aaIPI (and no bulky disease) may be successfully treated with three cycles of CODOX-M alone.[65] Although there have been no randomized studies to support its use, rituximab has been included in treatment regimens and appears to be associated with superior outcomes compared to historical controls[66] and may negate the previous poor prognosis associated with older age.

Prognosis in patients with relapsed/refractory disease is very poor. Autologous transplantation may be considered in patients with chemosensitive disease who fail to achieve a complete response with intense upfront therapy. In general, the kinetics of BL mean that allogeneic transplantation is not usually an effective option, with limited time to identify donors and with progression likely to occur before a full graft versus lymphoma effect is operative.

Mantle cell lymphoma

Mantle cell lymphoma (MCL) accounts for approximately 5%–10% of all cases of NHL. It is an aggressive NHL subtype occurring predominantly in older adults with a male predominance. MCL typically presents with advanced-stage disease. In the minority of patients with apparently localized disease by conventional staging, occult systemic disease is almost always present and can be identified by sensitive molecular methods or extended staging investigations (e.g., biopsies of macroscopically uninvolved colonic mucosa). The pathological hallmark of MCL is the overexpression of cyclin D1 leading to cell-cycle dysregulation which, in the vast majority of cases, is due to a translocation between the CCND1 locus (encoding cyclin D1) on chromosome 11q13 and the immunoglobulin heavy chain enhancer-promoter on chromosome 14q32 (t[11;14]). Nuclear overexpression of cyclin D1 can be detected by immunohistochemistry on lymph node or trephine specimens. Alternatively, the t(11;14) can be detected by fluorescence *in situ* hybridization (FISH) or by PCR amplification of the translocated region. Histologically, the majority of cases of MCL are composed of small- to medium-sized mature-appearing lymphocytes (classic MCL); however, in approximately 5% of cases the lymphocytes are more primitive-appearing (blastoid or pleomorphic variants). Histological variants with primitive morphological features are associated with higher rates of CNS involvement and are independently associated with a poorer prognosis. A minority of patients present with a lower tumor burden, typically with splenomegaly, and involvement of the peripheral blood. Pathologically these cases have been found to be characterized by absent SOX11 expression (a transcription factor that is expressed in almost all cases of classic MCL) and may have a more indolent course.

Although MCL usually responds to initial chemotherapy, relapse occurs in almost all patients, and the disease is generally considered incurable in the majority of patients. In young patients, allogeneic stem cell transplantation is potentially curative but is associated with significant short- and long-term toxicity. The majority of patients with MCL are elderly and are not candidates for intensive upfront chemotherapy or allogeneic stem cell transplantation and therefore, in the absence of a curative option, should only be treated in the context of symptomatic disease. There is currently no evidence that treatment of asymptomatic disease improves outcomes. A "watch-and-wait" policy is appropriate in asymptomatic patients, particularly in those with the indolent form who may remain asymptomatic for some years before requiring treatment.

Risk stratification in MCL has been refined by the description of the Mantle Cell Lymphoma International Prognostic Index (MIPI) (Table 30.4) which separates MCL into three groups, low, medium, and high risk, with median OS of not reached (60% 5-year OS), 51 months, and 29 months, respectively.[67] However, one of the most potent poor prognostic factors in MCL is the presence of deleterious mutations in TP53 (more commonly observed in blastoid variant).[68] Younger patients with TP53 mutations have particularly inferior outcomes when treated with intensive conventional chemotherapy including upfront autoSCT, and consideration should be given to the use of novel agents where available (see below) and consideration of upfront consolidation with allogeneic transplantation when feasible.[68]

In older fit patients with MCL, upfront chemotherapy combined with rituximab is generally used. Bendamustine and rituximab has generally become the preferred upfront regimen for MCL due to its demonstrated superior efficacy and favorable toxicity profile over R-CHOP.[69,70] Modification by the substitution of bortezomib for vincristine (VR-CAP) may improve outcomes over the standard R-CHOP regimen but is associated with increased toxicity.[71] Given the effectiveness of BTK inhibitors in the relapsed/refractory setting in MCL (see below), there are numerous ongoing trials to evaluate these agents in the frontline setting either incorporated into chemotherapy regimens (e.g., bendamustine rituximab plus ibrutinib) or as part of chemotherapy-free upfront treatment (e.g., rituximab and ibrutinib). Other potential options for frontline therapy in older patients (as well as those who are less fit) include R-CVP and R-chlorambucil.

In younger patients, a strategy that involves intensified upfront chemotherapy and consolidation high-dose therapy with ASCT is associated with prolonged disease control. The recognition of the high activity of cytarabine against MCL has led to its incorporation into upfront chemotherapy preceding ASCT such as in the Nordic Lymphoma Group trial (alternating augmented CHOP and high-dose cytarabine combined with rituximab [Table 30.5][72]), R-CHOP alternating with R-DHAP,[73] or R-DHAP alone.[74] In addition, giving rituximab as a "maintenance" therapy after autoASCT may also help improve outcomes.[74] Cytarabine-containing combination chemotherapy combined with ASCT (usually with conditioning containing cytarabine) (e.g., BEAM) may achieve a median OS of more than 10 years.[72]

The best upfront approach is likely to be one based on selective intensification of chemotherapy based on patient risk (as defined by MIPI) in those able to tolerate it. Although currently the only curative option, optimal criteria for patient selection and timing of allogeneic stem cell transplantation are still unknown. However, it should be considered a potential option in young patients with high-risk disease due to the significant graft-versus-lymphoma effect observed.

Ultimately, the majority of patients with MCL will relapse. Many classes of novel agents have been used in relapsed MCL including lenalidomide, bortezomib, and temsirolimus; however a major advance in the treatment of relapsed disease has been the incorporation of BTK inhibitors into treatment (e.g., ibrutinib or acalabrutinib). These can be given either as a single agent or combined with conventional chemotherapy, anti-CD20 antibody, or other novel agents. The combination of ibrutinib and venetoclax (a BCL2 inhibitor) looks particularly promising, especially in the TP53-mutated subgroup of patients who have a particularly poor outcome in the relapsed setting with BTK inhibitors alone.[75]

Human immunodeficiency virus–associated lymphoma

The risk of developing NHL and HL increases in patients with HIV infection.[76] One of the predominant driving forces for this increased risk of lymphoma is the loss of T-cell immunity to oncogenic viruses (most importantly EBV but also HHV-8).[77] Consistent with this mechanism, the risk of a patient with HIV developing NHL is correlated with the degree of HIV-associated immunosuppression (low CD4 count and high HIV viral load);[78] however Burkitt lymphoma does not occur in those individuals with an extremely low CD4 count, suggesting some requirement for T-cell help.[79] Aggressive subtypes comprise the majority of NHL occurring in HIV infection, in particular DLBCL with immunoblastic morphology. PCNSL typically develops in the most immunosuppressed patients (CD4 counts <50/μL) and is almost always EBV-positive. Primary effusion lymphoma and plasmablastic lymphoma are also typical subtypes of NHL seen in HIV infection.

The management of NHL associated with HIV infection requires multidisciplinary input from the haemato-oncology team, the treating HIV specialist, pharmacists, and infectious disease specialists. The management principles for HIV-associated NHL are the same as those for NHL occurring outside HIV infection with the following considerations:

- Early and concurrent treatment of HIV with highly active anti-retroviral therapy (HAART) is a central part of management of patients with HIV-associated NHL. The suppression of HIV with HAART results in an increase in CD4 count (which re-establishes a functional immune system, thereby decreasing the risk of opportunistic infections associated with chemotherapy),[80] restores immune control of oncogenic viruses, and prevents the development of new lymphoma. Patients who respond to HAART have higher response rates, PFS, and OS when treated for NHL.[81]
- Although there is an increased risk of treatment-associated morbidity in the severely immunosuppressed, patients with HIV-associated NHL can and should be treated with aggressive chemotherapy regimens (including rituximab) in the same manner as those without HIV infection. Chemotherapy tolerance in patients on HAART with good viral control is similar to those without HIV infection, and they may be safely treated with standard-intensity regimens such as R-CHOP through to highly intense regimens (e.g., R-CODOX-M/IVAC for BL or DA-EPOCH-R for DLBCL) including high-dose therapy with ASCT. HIV infection is not an absolute contraindication to allogeneic stem cell transplant.
- There are potential interactions between HAART and chemotherapy agents which may lead to increased toxicity from either component.

Peripheral T-cell lymphoma

Classification and prognosis

Peripheral T-cell lymphoma accounts for approximately 5%–10% of cases of NHL in Western countries. They are a heterogenous group of lymphoproliferative disorders which are biologically diverse. This is reflected in their different clinical presentation as well as their prognosis and response to therapy. PTCL can be broadly separated into those that have primarily nodal, extra-nodal, and leukemic presentations. The nodal PTCLs can be further divided into four main subtypes: angioimmunoblastic T-cell lymphoma (AITL), anaplastic large cell lymphoma (ALCL), ATLL, and PTCL-NOS. Although this classification is largely based on clinical, morphological, and immunophenotypic features, GEP studies have validated this classification by demonstrating distinct patterns of gene expression in each group.[82] Furthermore, GEP data have helped clarify the presence of various subtypes within the PTCL-NOS category (which is largely a diagnosis of exclusion), including a "cytotoxic" subtype with an apparently inferior outcome.[82] Aggressive extra-nodal PTCLs include such entities as hepatosplenic T-cell lymphoma (HSTL), extra-nodal NK/T-cell lymphoma (nasal type), and intestinal T-cell lymphomas.

The prognosis of PTCL subtypes is generally worse than their aggressive B-cell counterparts. Compared to aggressive B-lineage NHL, aggressive PTCL is more likely to be advanced at diagnosis, to have extra-nodal involvement, and to be associated with systemic symptoms (including life-threatening paraneoplastic syndromes such as hemophagocytic syndrome). The prognosis of PTCL is most closely linked to its histological subtype. Some subtypes are associated with a relatively favorable prognosis and cure in the majority of patients (e.g., anaplastic lymphoma kinase [ALK]-positive ALCL), and others are highly aggressive and almost universally fatal with current treatments (e.g., HSTL). Therefore, an accurate diagnosis is of paramount importance and requires the integration of clinical, radiological, and histological findings. The IPI that is used in DLBCL cannot reliably be used to predict the outcome in PTCL as a whole group; however, it has been validated in individual subtypes of PTCL including ALCL and PTCL-NOS.[83–85] A separate prognostic index for T-cell lymphoma (PIT) has been proposed which consists of age over 60 years, performance status 2 or greater, elevated LDH, and bone marrow involvement (Table 30.4).[83]

Anaplastic large cell lymphoma

ALCL accounts for approximately 3% of cases of NHL and has a bimodal incidence being seen most frequently in children and young adults under 30 years with a second smaller peak in the elderly.[1] Pathologically, ALCL is usually characterized by anaplastic tumor cells (including "hallmark" cells) which express CD30. ALCL can be divided into two major groups based on ALK expression which are otherwise morphologically indistinguishable. In ALK-positive ALCL (approximately 65% of cases), overexpression of ALK is usually the result of a translocation between the ALK gene on chromosome 2 and the NPM1 gene on chromosome 5 (t[2;5][p23;q35]). ALK-positive ALCL occurs predominantly in children and young adults with frequent extra-nodal involvement and has a good response to treatment, whereas ALK-negative ALCL occurs in older adults with less frequent extra-nodal disease and has a poorer prognosis.[85] In marked contrast to its systemic counterpart, primary cutaneous ALCL is an indolent T-cell lymphoma which is associated with a good prognosis and usually responds well to local therapy only. Another variant of ALCL is breast implant–associated ALCL which also has a very good prognosis and is often completely treated by removal of the breast implant with the associated rim of tumor.

The treatment of ALK-positive ALCL has historically been with CHOP-type chemotherapy, and this approach is associated with a 5-year OS of 60%–90%, with those patients with a low-risk IPI having a particularly favorable prognosis.[85–87] In children, the majority of tumors are ALK-positive and the overall prognosis is good with a 5-year survival of 80%–85% which is improved by using more intensive chemotherapy regimens.[88,89] Treatment of ALK-negative ALCL with CHOP-type chemotherapy is associated with a 3-year event-free survival of approximately 50%–60%.[90]

A significant advance in the treatment of ALCL is the incorporation of brentuximab vedotin (BV) into both frontline and relapsed/refractory settings. BV is an anti-CD30 antibody conjugated to a potent antimicrotubule agent which has been demonstrated to improve progression-free and overall survival when substituted into the CHOP regimen in place of vincristine (BV-CHP).[91] In patients with relapsed disease,[92] the use of BV may facilitate bridging to either autologous or allogeneic stem cell transplantation and therefore the potential for long-term disease control. Targeting the ALK fusion protein in ALK-positive ALCL with ALK-inhibitors such as crizotinib is also emerging as a highly effective strategy in the relapsed/refractory setting.[93]

Similar to most nodal PTCL (except ALK-positive ALCL), high-dose therapy with ASCT is often used front line in patients with ALK-negative ALCL who are able to tolerate it. A large phase II prospective trial (NLG-T-01) using CHOP-14 (with etoposide in those under 60 years) followed by BEAM/BEAC conditioned ASCT showed an OS of 70% at 5 years in patients with ALK-negative ALCL. Moreover, there was an apparent plateau on the survival curve suggesting cure in a proportion of patients.[94] However, this approach may need to be reconsidered in light of more effective upfront treatment incorporating BV.

Angioimmunoblastic T-cell lymphoma

AITL is an aggressive lymphoma characterized by generalized lymphadenopathy, hepatosplenomegaly, and rash which typically presents in the middle-aged and elderly.[95] It is a mature T-cell malignancy derived from T-follicular helper (T_{FH}) cells which normally reside within lymph node follicles. The mutational profile of AITL is notable for less genomic complexity compared to PTCL-NOS and the presence of mutations in genes typically mutated in myeloid malignancy (e.g., TET2 and DNMT3A). In addition, mutations in RHOA and IDH2 (Arg172 codon variants) are also observed relatively specifically in this group of lymphoma.[96] Chromosome 5 and 21 gains are also common and often associated with IDH2 Arg172 mutations. Patients with AITL are typically immunosuppressed as a consequence of the disease which results in significant morbidity and mortality secondary to infection[97,98] and, less commonly, the development of secondary EBV-driven B-cell lymphoma.[99,100] As with the majority of PTCL, conventional treatments are unsatisfactory, with a median survival following combination chemotherapy (e.g., CHOP) of approximately 3 years.[97,98] High-dose therapy with ASCT appears to be an effective modality which is associated with durable remissions in approximately half of the patients with chemosensitive disease.[94,101,102] Allogeneic stem cell transplantation has also been trialed with a demonstration of graft-versus-lymphoma effect and an apparent plateau of survival curves.[103]

Approaches in relapsed/refractory disease are diverse and include (i) the histone deacetylase inhibitor romidepsin which has demonstrated clinical activity alone or in combinations,[104] (ii) hypomethylating agents (e.g., azacytidine) given the observation of mutation in genes controlling epigenetic regulation, and (iii) the use of immunomodulatory therapies such as cyclosporin.[105]

Human T lymphotropic virus 1–associated adult T-cell leukemia/lymphoma

ATLL is caused by HTLV-1 and occurs principally in areas of endemic infection (Japan, the Caribbean, and parts of Africa). HTLV-1 is principally acquired in childhood via vertical transmission in breast milk; however, it may also be transmitted via blood. Approximately 3% of infected individuals will develop ATLL after a long latency.[131] The disease has a broad clinical spectrum with four distinct variants being described: acute, lymphomatous, chronic, and smoldering, with projected 4-year survival figures of 5%, 5.7%, 26.9%, and 62.8%, respectively.[132] The acute variant is the most common presentation and is characterized by circulating lymphoma cells, skin rash, widespread lymphadenopathy, organomegaly, and hypercalcemia. Patients in this group are immunosuppressed, and opportunistic infections are common. The lymphomatous variant is characterized by extensive lymphadenopathy, but involvement of the peripheral blood and hypercalcemia are less common. The chronic variant typically presents principally with skin lesions, and the smoldering variant is characterized by low levels of circulating lymphoma cells together with lymphomatous deposits in the skin and lungs. Progression from the chronic and smoldering disease to more aggressive variants occurs in approximately 25% of cases after a latency period often of several years.

The treatment of ATLL is stratified according to clinical subtype. In patients with chronic and smoldering subtypes, a watch-and-wait approach is no longer preferred and treatment upfront with antiviral medication (zidovudine) and alpha-interferon is associated with the most favorable clinical outcomes.[133] The lymphomatous subtype of ATLL requires chemotherapy as part of upfront treatment. Chemotherapy regimens in ATLL generally have low response rates and a high frequency of rapid relapse after cessation of treatment. Some of the best results to date (in phase II trials) are with the LSG15 regimen which incorporates ranimustine and carboplatin. These agents were chosen in an attempt to overcome the high expression of the P-glycoprotein drug efflux pump seen in this disorder and the associated chemotherapy resistance to various conventional chemotherapeutic agents.[134] Numerous other regimens have been tried, including CHOP and CHOP-like regimens, but these are all associated with modest response rates and poor mean survival. In patients who respond to chemotherapy who are young enough and do not have major organ compromise, allogeneic stem cell transplantation offers the only potential chance of long-term disease control.[135] Acute ATLL, which has the worst prognosis of all the subtypes, is managed similarly to lymphomatous presentation with combination chemotherapy plus antiviral therapy/interferon.

The poor response to chemotherapy in the aggressive subtypes of ATLL clearly demonstrates the need for a more targeted approach in this disease. There have been multiple promising targeted therapies that are currently being evaluated that show promising efficacy including anti-CCR4 compounds (mogamulizumab), anti-CD25 antibodies (daclizumab), anti-CD30 antibodies (BV), and the HDAC inhibitors (e.g., panobinostat, depsipeptide).

Other subtypes of peripheral T-cell lymphoma

PTCL-NOS—PTCL-NOS accounts for around half of the cases of PTCL in Western countries.[84,85,106] It is a heterogeneous group of diseases with a predominantly nodal presentation. Genomic characterization of this broad biological group has identified three major subgroups within PTCL-NOS: (i) PTCL-GATA3 which overexpresses GATA3 and has an inferior prognosis, (ii)

PTCL-TBX21 which overexpresses TBX21, and (iii) PTCL-T$_{FH}$ which is a nodal PTCL-NOS that expresses a T$_{FH}$ phenotype (CD4+, PD1+, CD10+, BCL6+ CXCL13, and/or ICOS).[96] The overall prognosis is variable reflecting the biological heterogeneity of the underlying disorder, ranging from a 5-year OS under 20% in the highest-risk patients to approximately 60% in patients without adverse risk factors.[83] Although optimal frontline therapy is unclear, CHOP-type chemotherapy is usually used (with the addition of etoposide possibly adding benefit).[90] In addition, there have been attempts to add targeted therapy to CHOP regimens analogous to the addition of rituximab to CHOP in the treatment of B-lineage NHL. CHOP-alemtuzumab,[107] CHOP-bortezomib,[108] and CHOP-denileukin diftitox[109] have all been trialed with varying success. One potential option for CD30-expressing PTCL-NOS is BV-CHP.[91]

Regardless of the initial chemotherapy regimen utilized, relapse occurs in the majority of patients, and therefore ASCT is often considered upfront in suitable patients in order to consolidate remission. ASCT in PTCL-NOS results in a 5-year OS ranging from 35% to 58%.[94,110–112] ASCT is most effective when used earlier in disease course and is of limited value in relapsed disease. Allogeneic stem cell transplantation is sometimes used in PTCL-NOS; however, the patient selection, conditioning regimen, and timing of its use vary considerably between centers.

Intestinal T-cell lymphoma—this group of rare lymphomas can be divided into two main entities: (i) enteropathy-associated T-cell lymphoma (EATL) and (ii) monomorphic epitheliotropic intestinal T-cell lymphoma (MEITL). EATL has a clear association with celiac disease;[113] however, there is sometimes little clinical evidence of this before the lymphoma diagnosis. The pathogenesis of EATL is incompletely understood; however, it is postulated that chronic antigenic stimulation by gliadin in the context of the susceptible HLA-DQA1*0501, HLA-DQB1*0201 haplotype (seen in most patients with celiac disease) leads to the development of T-cell clones that predispose to lymphoma following additional genetic mutations.[114–117] Specifically, mutations in the JAK3/STAT5B signaling pathway are common drivers in this group of disorders.[118] Patients often have a poor performance status at presentation. Malnutrition and intestinal perforation are common, and the outcome following conventional chemotherapy is poor, with long-term remissions only achieved in 10%–30% treated with CHOP-type chemotherapy.[119–121] Superior outcomes can possibly be obtained with more intensified upfront chemotherapy and ASCT in those able to tolerate it.[122]

Extra-nodal NK/T-cell lymphoma—this lymphoma is uncommon in Western populations, being more frequently observed in Asia, Mexico, and Central and South America. It is more common in men and frequently presents with localized extra-nodal disease typically affecting the nasopharynx.[123,124] The tumors are sensitive to radiotherapy and relatively resistant to chemotherapy due to high P-glycoprotein expression.[125] Treatment is dependent on the stage of disease. In patients with early-stage disease, sequential chemotherapy and radiotherapy (at high dose [50Gy]) achieves the best outcomes.[126] Chemotherapy regimens should incorporate agents which are not substrates for P-gp, and the most promising results appear to be associated with the intense dexamethasone, methotrexate, ifosfamide, L-asparagine, and etoposide (SMILE) regimen.[126] A less intense regimen that may be used in less fit patients is gemcitabine, L-asparginase, and oxaliplatin (GELOX).[127] Radiotherapy is usually delivered sandwiched within chemotherapy cycles.[126] In advanced disease, chemotherapy alone using similar regimens is recommended.[128] There may also be a role for early allogeneic transplantation in younger patients with a human leukocyte antigen (HLA)-matched donor.[129] ENKTL harbors a high prevalence of genomic abnormalities of the PD-L1/PD-L2 loci, making checkpoint inhibition a potentially attractive modality to be evaluated in this aggressive and poor prognosis subtype.[130]

HSTL—this is a rare subtype of PTCL typically presenting in young male patients with hepatosplenomegaly, bone marrow infiltration, and high swinging fevers. A response to CHOP-type chemotherapy is observed in the majority of patients; however, this is typically short-lived, and there are very few reports of long-term remission.[131] Allogeneic stem cell transplantation has been used successfully to treat HSTL in a handful of cases.[131]

Indolent non-Hodgkin lymphoma

Follicular lymphoma

Epidemiology, histological grading, and prognostic factors

FL accounts for about 20% of all cases of NHL. Like DLBCL, FL is predominantly a disease of older adults with a median age at diagnosis of approximately 65 years.[15] Although FL is recognized to occur in children, it has specific clinical and pathological features in this group and is now considered a separate entity in the most recent WHO classification.[1]

FL is an indolent form of NHL which is characterized by the accumulation of clonal centrocytes that have subverted normal apoptosis mechanisms. The accumulation of malignant lymphocytes that have evaded apoptosis is in contrast to the excessive growth and proliferation seen in aggressive lymphomas such as DLBCL and is the basis for the difference in tumor kinetics between the two diseases. Apoptosis dysregulation is the result of a translocation between the immunoglobulin heavy chain enhancer promoter on chromosome 14 and the BCL2 gene on chromosome 18. This translocation (t[14;18]) is seen in more than 90% of cases of FL and results in the overexpression of BCL2 and the subsequent generation of potent anti-apoptotic and pro-survival signals.

Prognosis in FL may be predicted by a number of clinical, genetic, and molecular factors. Analogous to the IPI in DLBCL, prognostic systems have been developed for use in FL with the FL IPI being the most widely used (Table 30.4).[132] The FLIPI stratifies patients into three risk groups based on five variables: age, Ann Arbor stage, hemoglobin, LDH, and the number of sites of nodal disease. The projected 5-year OS in the low-risk (0–1 factors), intermediate-risk (2 factors), and high-risk (3–5 factors) groups are 90.6%, 77.6%, and 52.5%, respectively.[132] Importantly, the FLIPI still remains a valid prognostic model in the rituximab era.[133] The incorporation of mutation information (EZH2, ARID1A, EP300, FOXO1, MEF2B, CREBBP, and CARD11) in addition to the FLIPI has been combined in a clinicogenetic risk model known as the m7-FLIPI (Table 30.4) which may be able to inform prognosis beyond clinical variables alone.[134]

Cases of FL can be histologically graded (1,2,3a,3b) according to the proportion of large cells (centroblasts) present in the predominant background population of smaller lymphocytes (centrocytes). Grade 1 or 2 disease is classified as low-grade disease with grade 3a representing a more aggressive grade (although still being considered, and managed as, low-grade disease). Grade 3b FL, by definition, contains solid sheets of centroblasts, and the current practice is for this entity to be treated as DLBCL.

Two FL entities deserve special mention, *in situ* follicular neoplasia (previously known as *in situ* FL) and duodenal FL. *In situ* follicular neoplasia is characterized by the presence of clonal centrocytes containing the t(14;18) that have colonized germinal centers without extension outside the follicle. The significance and natural history of this entity are uncertain; however, it appears to have a low rate of progression to overt lymphoma.[135] Primary FL of the duodenum, although displaying the same histological features as nodal FL, appears to be an exceptionally indolent variant with a very low risk of transformation or involvement outside the gastrointestinal tract.[136]

Treatment of newly diagnosed limited stage (I and II) disease

For many years, the standard treatment for patients with stage I FL has been radiotherapy to involved lymph node regions. A similar strategy is adopted for stage II disease in some centers. This practice was previously based on mature data from multiple centers which have shown that radiotherapy alone results in 10-year overall (progression-free) survival figures of approximately 60%–80% (30%–50%).[137–140] Relapse after radiotherapy for localized disease occurs exclusively outside the radiotherapy field, suggesting that the cause of relapse is occult systemic disease. Therefore, there is sound rationale for the inclusion of chemotherapy in order to reduce this risk. This approach was investigated in the Trans-Tasman Radiation Oncology Group multicenter trial where patients were randomized between IFRT (30Gy) and IFRT with systemic chemotherapy (six cycles of R-CVP).[141] Patients receiving IFRT and chemotherapy had superior 10-year PFS (59%) compared to IFRT alone (41%). Whilst not statistically significant different between the two arms, the observed 10-year OS was excellent (95% vs. 86%) and significantly higher than that described in previous studies, highlighting the favorable outcome of early-stage FL in the modern era. This study has confirmed that the most favorable outcomes in early-stage FL are achieved with combined modality therapy. Further refinements to the combined modality approach may include the use of lower doses of radiotherapy (e.g., 24Gy) and more effective/less toxic chemoimmunotherapy (e.g., bendamustine and rituximab or rituximab monotherapy).

Treatment of newly diagnosed advanced-stage (III and IV) disease

The majority of patients with FL present with advanced-stage (III or IV) disease and, despite being able to achieve remission in the majority of patients using single alkylating agents, combination chemotherapy, or combined modality chemo-radiotherapy, a continuous rate of relapse is observed. The majority of data suggest that for asymptomatic patients with low lymphoma burden (e.g., as defined by the Groupe d'Étude des Lymphomes Folliculaires [GELF]),[142] immediate treatment confers no advantage over conservative management in which treatment is deferred until disease progression (a so-called "watch-and-wait" approach).[143–145] One prospective trial which randomized asymptomatic patients with FL to either watch-and-wait or treatment with single-agent rituximab showed a significantly lower proportion of patients requiring chemotherapy or radiotherapy at 3 years in the rituximab-containing arms with encouraging initial quality-of-life data.[146] However, longer follow-up of this cohort is required to determine whether there is an OS benefit. Interestingly an economic analysis suggested that early intervention with rituximab was cost-saving.[147]

When treatment is indicated for symptomatic advanced-stage disease, optimal outcomes are generally achieved with systemic chemotherapy combined with an anti-CD20 antibody followed by anti-CD20 maintenance therapy (generally every 2 months for 2 years).[148,149] The choice of chemotherapy backbone is generally between bendamustine, CHOP, or CVP and the choice of anti-CD20 antibody between rituximab and obinutuzumab (a newer anti-CD20 antibody with greater antibody-dependent cellular cytotoxicity). In a large randomized trial, obinutuzumab therapy had a significant albeit small improvement in PFS compared to rituximab when combined with chemotherapy I but was associated with greater toxicity (particularly neutropenia, infections, and infusion reactions).[148] In terms of choice of chemotherapy backbone, bendamustine has generally been favored due to its lower acute toxicity (particularly alopecia, cytopenias, and cardiotoxicity when compared to CHOP) and earlier demonstration of superior PFS (when combined with rituximab).[69,70] However, it should be noted that the combination of obinutuzmab and bendamustine is associated with increased serious infectious complications and secondary malignancy, and therefore patients should be carefully selected with regard to age/comorbidities and should receive meticulous anti-infective prophylaxis against PJP and herpes zoster reactivation. In the rituximab era, the approximate median duration of remission was approaching 5 years with R-CHOP and BR and may be even longer with obinutuzumab.

Chemotherapy-free options are also being investigated in the frontline treatment of FL. The combination of lenalidomide and rituximab showed similar efficacy to chemotherapy and rituximab (with most patients receiving R-CHOP) in a multicenter randomized trial.[150] The use of lenalidomide and rituximab results in lower rates of febrile neutropenia and cytopenias than rituximab chemotherapy; however patients in the lenalidomide arm experienced more cutaneous adverse events, and the overall withdrawals from toxicity were similar between both groups. Despite this, the combination of lenalidomide and rituximab appears to be an active regimen with promise for those unable to tolerate the specific adverse effects of conventional chemotherapy. Studies with lenalidomide and obinutuzumab in the frontline setting are currently underway. Rituximab monotherapy (generally 4–8 weekly doses of rituximab [375 mg/m^2]) has also been used resulting in a median PFS of 1–3 years and may be of utility for older patients with significant comorbidities.[151–154]

Treatment of relapsed disease

Irrespective of the initial mode of treatment, the majority of patients with FL are destined to relapse and require further therapy. However, when symptomatic relapse occurs, there are multiple options for treatment of relapsed/refractory FL including:

Immunochemotherapy—following relapse, a further remission is usually achievable with chemotherapy including use of newer anti-CD20 antibodies.[155,156] The choice of regimen depends on the previous treatment received, the duration of the first remission, the co-morbidities of the patient, and whether consolidation with high-dose therapy is being considered. If autoSCT is planned, then salvage regimens as described for DLBCL are effective and can facilitate stem cell mobilization. For patients unsuitable for high-dose therapy and autoSCT, re-treatment using frontline therapy (if no anthracyclines were included) may be considered if the remission duration was greater than 1 year.

Targeted small molecule inhibitors—multiple intracellular signaling pathways are therapeutically targetable in FL. Abnormal signaling in FL through the PI3K/AKT/mTOR pathway can be targeted using the PI3K class of small molecular inhibitors (including idelalisib [PI3Kδ], copanlisib [PI3Kα/δ], and duvelisib [PI3Kδ/γ]). These agents have reasonable response rates (approximately 30%–50%); however toxicity (particularly gastrointestinal

and pulmonary) can be an issue. Approximately 30% of patients with relapsed/refractory FL harbor activating mutations in EZH2 which results in a "locking in" of the malignant cell into the germinal center transcriptional program. Tazemetostat is an oral inhibitor of EZH2 and shows relatively high response rates in EZH2-mutated FL (approximately 70%) and is generally well-tolerated. Other targeted therapies include BTK inhibitors (e.g., ibrutinib) and BCL2 inhibitors (e.g., venetoclax).

Autologous/allogeneic transplant—in patients below the age of 70 without significant co-morbidities, autoSCT may be considered. AutoSCT in relapsed FL was associated with superior PFS and OS when compared to chemotherapy in the pre-rituximab era.[157] However, the magnitude of benefit derived from autoSCT in patients treated with rituxmab upfront (plus maintenance) in an era with more effective salvage strategies including novel non-chemotherapy options is unclear, and its use as a modality is generally declining. Allogeneic stem cell transplantation (alloSCT) with myeloablative conditioning is effective at controlling disease; however, it is generally unappealing due to high non-relapse mortality and the restriction to young fit patients.[158] The potent graft-versus-lymphoma effect makes allogeneic stem cell transplantation using reduced intensity conditioning (RIC) an attractive option and has been a modality of increasing interest. RIC alloSCT using fludarabine/melphalan/alemtuzumab conditioning has shown impressive results, with cure in a significant number of patients and relatively low rates of graft-versus-host disease with an acceptable non-relapse mortality.[159]

Radioimmunotherapy (RIT)—the radiosensitivity and expression of suitable target antigens make FL an attractive target for treatment with RIT. Most clinical experience has been derived from the use of ^{90}Y-ibritumomab and ^{131}I-tositumomab, both of which produce response rates of 60%–80% when used as monotherapy in patients with relapsed/refractory disease.[160]

Marginal zone lymphoma

MZLs comprise the relatively common extra-nodal mucosa-associated lymphoid tissue (MALT) type and the less common nodal and splenic variants. MALT-type lymphomas are predominantly indolent, with a 5-year survival of typically 80% or better. They occur mainly in adults and frequently on a background of a chronic inflammatory disorder, either chronic infections or autoimmune conditions. More than half of the patients have limited-stage disease at presentation, and the most common anatomical site of involvement is the gastrointestinal tract, particularly the stomach, with the lung, head, and neck including ocular adnexa, skin, thyroid, and breast representing other common sites of involvement. The pathogenesis of these lymphomas is complex; however, in the early stages, antigen expression and T-cell stimulation due to the underlying infection or autoimmune condition lead to B-cell proliferation, with secondary clonal evolution and lymphoma development as a result of acquired genetic abnormalities.[161]

Early-stage gastric MALT lymphoma can be successfully treated in approximately two-thirds to three-quarters of patients with eradication of *Helicobacter pylori*.[162,163] Risk factors for treatment failure include stage II disease, absence of *H. pylori*, submucosal invasion, and the presence of t(11;18).[162,164] Of note, the optimal response may take 12 months (or longer) to be achieved.[163] Those not responding to *H. pylori* eradication alone may be treated with single-agent rituximab or local radiotherapy.[165,166] The evidence for an association between infections and MALT lymphomas at other sites (*Chlamydia psittaci* and ocular adnexal tumors or *Borrelia burgdorferi* and skin tumors) is less convincing, and although it provides a rationale for antibiotic treatment, this approach should currently be regarded as investigational.[167] There is no firm evidence base to guide treatment decisions in advanced-stage extra-nodal MZL; however, rituximab combined with conventional chemotherapy regimens (e.g., cyclophosphamide, vincristine, prednisolone [CVP]) tend to be used with the treatment paradigm generally following that of FL.

Nodal MZL is uncommon, typically presenting with minimally symptomatic cervical lymphadenopathy. The literature concerning the clinical course and treatment is sparse; however, they appear to behave in an indolent manner and can successfully be treated with chemotherapy as outlined for MALT lymphomas.[167]

Splenic marginal zone lymphoma (SMZL) is uncommon, most frequently presenting with splenomegaly and bone marrow infiltration in the middle-aged and elderly. SMZL is typically very indolent, and treatment can usually be deferred until the onset of symptoms (e.g., abdominal discomfort related to splenomegaly, weight loss) or cytopenias. Historically, splenectomy was the most common initial treatment which resulted in durable remissions; however, single-agent rituximab is increasingly being used with similar response rates and remission durations. Although the follow-up of rituximab-treated patients is not as long as splenectomy, the relative ease of administration and low toxicity compared to splenectomy has resulted in its increasing use by clinicians.[168] Although the overall 5-year survival for SMZL is up to 80%, a subset of patients have more aggressive disease, and recent data suggest that they may be identified by a number of clinical and laboratory variables;[169] however, whether those with an adverse prognosis will benefit from more intensive treatment is currently unknown.

References

1. Swerdlow SH, Campo E, Harris NL et al. *WHO Classification of Tumours of Haematopoietic and Lymphoid Tissues* (4th ed). Lyon, France: International Agency for Research on Cancer, 2017.

2. Ferlay J, Shin HR, Bray F et al. Estimates of worldwide burden of cancer in 2008: GLOBOCAN 2008. *Int J Cancer*. 2010; 127(12): 2893–917.

3. NICE guideline NG52. *Non-Hodgkin's Lymphoma: Diagnosis and Management* (pp. 21–5). 2016; nice.org.uk/guidance/ng52

4. Lister TA, Crowther D, Sutcliffe SB et al. Report of a committee convened to discuss the evaluation and staging of patients with Hodgkin's disease: Cotswolds meeting. *J Clin Oncol*. 1989; 7(11):1630–6.

5. Wirth A, Foo M, Seymour JF et al. Impact of [18f] fluorodeoxyglucose positron emission tomography on staging and management of early-stage follicular non-hodgkin lymphoma. *Int J Radiat Oncol Biol Phys*. 2008; 71(1):213–9.

6. Jerusalem G, Beguin Y, Fassotte MF et al. Whole-body positron emission tomography using 18F-fluorodeoxyglucose for posttreatment evaluation in Hodgkin's disease and non-Hodgkin's lymphoma has higher diagnostic and prognostic value than classical computed tomography scan imaging. *Blood*. 1999; 94(2):429–33.

7. Dupuis J, Itti E, Rahmouni A et al. Response assessment after an inductive CHOP or CHOP-like regimen with or without rituximab in 103 patients with diffuse large B-cell lymphoma: Integrating 18fluorodeoxyglucose positron emission tomography to the International Workshop Criteria. *Ann Oncol*. 2009; 20(3):503–7.

8. Trotman J, Fournier M, Lamy T et al. Positron emission tomography-computed tomography (PET-CT) after induction therapy is highly predictive of patient outcome in follicular lymphoma: Analysis of PET-CT in a subset of PRIMA trial participants. *J Clin Oncol*. 2011; 29(23):3194–200.

9. Derenzini E, Musuraca G, Fanti S et al. Pretransplantation positron emission tomography scan is the main predictor of autologous stem cell transplantation outcome in aggressive B-cell non-Hodgkin lymphoma. *Cancer*. 2008; 113(9):2496–503.

10. Dickinson M, Hoyt R, Roberts AW et al. Improved survival for relapsed diffuse large B cell lymphoma is predicted by a negative pre-transplant FDG-PET scan following salvage chemotherapy. *Br J Haematol*. 2010; 150(1):39–45.

11. Burggraaff CN, de Jong A, Hoekstra OS et al. Predictive value of interim positron emission tomography in diffuse large B-cell lymphoma: A systematic review and meta-analysis. *Eur J Nucl Med Mol Imaging*. 2019; 46(1):65–79.

12. Noy A, Schoder H, Gonen M et al. The majority of transformed lymphomas have high standardized uptake values (SUVs) on positron emission tomography (PET) scanning similar to diffuse large B-cell lymphoma (DLBCL). *Ann Oncol*. 2009; 20(3):508–12.

13. Yeoh KW, Mikhaeel NG. Are we ready for positron emission tomography/computed tomography-based target volume definition in lymphoma radiation therapy? *Int J Radiat Oncol Biol Phys*. 2013; 85(1):14–20.

14. Campbell JK, Matthews JP, Seymour JF et al. Optimum trephine length in the assessment of bone marrow involvement in patients with diffuse large cell lymphoma. *Ann Oncol*. 2003; 14(2):273–6.

15. Smith A, Howell D, Patmore R et al. Incidence of haematological malignancy by sub-type: A report from the Haematological Malignancy Research Network. *Br J Cancer*. 2011; 105(11):1684–92.

16. Alizadeh AA, Eisen MB, Davis RE et al. Distinct types of diffuse large B-cell lymphoma identified by gene expression profiling. *Nature*. 2000; 403(6769):503–11.

17. Schmitz R, Wright GW, Huang DW et al. Genetics and pathogenesis of diffuse large B-cell lymphoma. *N Engl J Med*. 2018; 378(15):1396–407.

18. Chapuy B, Stewart C, Dunford AJ et al. Molecular subtypes of diffuse large B cell lymphoma are associated with distinct pathogenic mechanisms and outcomes. *Nat Med*. 2018; 24(5):679–90.

19. Wilder RB, Rodriguez MA, Medeiros LJ et al. International prognostic index-based outcomes for diffuse large B-cell lymphomas. *Cancer*. 2002; 94(12):3083–8.

20. Ziepert M, Hasenclever D, Kuhnt E et al. Standard International prognostic index remains a valid predictor of outcome for patients with aggressive CD20+ B-cell lymphoma in the rituximab era. *J Clin Oncol*. 2010; 28(14):2373–80.

21. Sehn LH, Berry B, Chhanabhai M et al. The revised International Prognostic Index (R-IPI) is a better predictor of outcome than the standard IPI for patients with diffuse large B-cell lymphoma treated with R-CHOP. *Blood*. 2007; 109(5):1857–61.

22. Rosenwald A, Wright G, Chan WC et al. The use of molecular profiling to predict survival after chemotherapy for diffuse large-B-cell lymphoma. *N Engl J Med*. 2002; 346(25):1937–47.

23. Fisher RI, Gaynor ER, Dahlberg S et al. A phase III comparison of CHOP vs. m-BACOD vs. ProMACE-CytaBOM vs. MACOP-B in patients with intermediate- or high-grade non-Hodgkin's lymphoma: Results of SWOG-8516 (Intergroup 0067), the National High-Priority Lymphoma Study. *Ann Oncol*. 1994; 5(Suppl 2):91–5.

24. Maloney DG, Liles TM, Czerwinski DK et al. Phase I clinical trial using escalating single-dose infusion of chimeric anti-CD20 monoclonal antibody (IDEC-C2B8) in patients with recurrent B-cell lymphoma. *Blood*. 1994; 84(8):2457–66.

25. Coiffier B, Lepage E, Briere J et al. CHOP chemotherapy plus rituximab compared with CHOP alone in elderly patients with diffuse large-B-cell lymphoma. *N Engl J Med*. 2002; 346(4):235–42.

26. Feugier P, Van Hoof A, Sebban C et al. Long-term results of the R-CHOP study in the treatment of elderly patients with diffuse large B-cell lymphoma: A study by the Groupe d'Etude des Lymphomes de l'Adulte. *J Clin Oncol*. 2005; 23(18):4117–26.

27. Pfreundschuh M, Kuhnt E, Trumper L et al. CHOP-like chemotherapy with or without rituximab in young patients with good-prognosis diffuse large-B-cell lymphoma: 6-year results of an open-label randomised study of the MabThera International Trial (MInT) Group. *Lancet Oncol*. 2011; 12(11):1013–22.

28. Leonard JP, Kolibaba KS, Reeves JA et al. Randomized Phase II study of R-CHOP with or without bortezomib in previously untreated patients with non-germinal center B-cell-like diffuse large B-cell lymphoma. *J Clin Oncol.* 2017; 35(31):3538–46.

29. Younes A, Sehn LH, Johnson P et al. Randomized Phase III trial of Ibrutinib and rituximab in non-germinal center B-cell diffuse large B-cell lymphoma. *J Clin Oncol.* 2019; 37(15):1285–95.

30. Castellino A, Chiappella A, LaPlant BR et al. Lenalidomide plus R-CHOP21 in newly diagnosed diffuse large B-cell lymphoma (DLBCL): Long-term follow-up results from a combined analysis from two phase 2 trials. *Blood Cancer J.* 2018; 8(11):108.

31. Rozental A, Gafter-Gvili A, Vidal L et al. The role of maintenance therapy in patients with diffuse large B cell lymphoma: A systematic review and meta-analysis. *Hematol Oncol.* 2019; 37(1):27–34.

32. Vitolo U, Trneny M, Belada D et al. Obinutuzumab or rituximab plus cyclophosphamide, doxorubicin, vincristine, and prednisone in previously untreated diffuse large B-cell lymphoma. *J Clin Oncol.* 2017; 35(31):3529–37.

33. Dunleavy K, Fanale MA, Abramson JS et al. Dose-adjusted EPOCH-R (etoposide, prednisone, vincristine, cyclophosphamide, doxorubicin, and rituximab) in untreated aggressive diffuse large B-cell lymphoma with MYC rearrangement: A prospective, multicentre, single-arm phase 2 study. *Lancet Haematol.* 2018; 5(12):e609–e17.

34. Petrich AM, Gandhi M, Jovanovic B et al. Impact of induction regimen and stem cell transplantation on outcomes in double-hit lymphoma: A multicenter retrospective analysis. *Blood.* 2014; 124(15):2354–61.

35. Haioun C, Lepage E, Gisselbrecht C et al. Benefit of autologous bone marrow transplantation over sequential chemotherapy in poor-risk aggressive non-Hodgkin's lymphoma: Updated results of the prospective study LNH87-2. Groupe d'Etude des Lymphomes de l'Adulte. *J Clin Oncol.* 1997; 15(3):1131–7.

36. Moskowitz CH, Bertino JR, Glassman JR et al. Ifosfamide, carboplatin, and etoposide: A highly effective cytoreduction and peripheral-blood progenitor-cell mobilization regimen for transplant-eligible patients with non-Hodgkin's lymphoma. *J Clin Oncol.* 1999; 17(12):3776–85.

37. Velasquez WS, McLaughlin P, Tucker S et al. ESHAP--an effective chemotherapy regimen in refractory and relapsing lymphoma: A 4-year follow-up study. *J Clin Oncol.* 1994; 12(6):1169–76.

38. Proctor SJ, Taylor PR, Angus B et al. High-dose ifosfamide in combination with etoposide and epirubicin (IVE) in the treatment of relapsed/refractory Hodgkin's disease and non-Hodgkin's lymphoma: A report on toxicity and efficacy. *Eur J Haematol Suppl.* 2001; 64:28–32.

39. Girouard C, Dufresne J, Imrie K et al. Salvage chemotherapy with mini-BEAM for relapsed or refractory non-Hodgkin's lymphoma prior to autologous bone marrow transplantation. *Ann Oncol.* 1997; 8(7):675–80.

40. Gisselbrecht C, Glass B, Mounier N et al. Salvage regimens with autologous transplantation for relapsed large B-cell lymphoma in the rituximab era. *J Clin Oncol.* 2010; 28(27):4184–90.

41. Thieblemont C, Briere J, Mounier N et al. The germinal center/activated B-cell subclassification has a prognostic impact for response to salvage therapy in relapsed/refractory diffuse large B-cell lymphoma: A bio-CORAL study. *J Clin Oncol.* 2011; 29(31):4079–87.

42. Neelapu SS, Locke FL, Bartlett NL et al. Axicabtagene ciloleucel CAR T-cell therapy in refractory large B-cell lyphoma. *N Engl J Med.* 2017; 377(26):2531–44.

43. Thunberg U, Enblad G, Berglund M. Classification of diffuse large B-cell lymphoma by immunohistochemistry demonstrates that elderly patients are more common in the non-GC subgroup and younger patients in the GC subgroup. *Haematologica.* 2012; 97(2):e3; author reply e4.

44. Peyrade F, Jardin F, Thieblemont C et al. Attenuated immunochemotherapy regimen (R-miniCHOP) in elderly patients older than 80 years with diffuse large B-cell lymphoma: A multicentre, single-arm, phase 2 trial. *Lancet Oncol.* 2011; 12(5):460–8.

45. Meguro A, Ozaki K, Sato K et al. Rituximab plus 70% cyclophosphamide, doxorubicin, vincristine and prednisone for Japanese patients with diffuse large B-cell lymphoma aged 70 years and older. *Leuk Lymphoma.* 2012; 53(1):43–9.

46. van de Schans SA, Gondos A, van Spronsen DJ et al. Improving relative survival, but large remaining differences in survival for non-Hodgkin's lymphoma across Europe and the United States from 1990 to 2004. *J Clin Oncol.* 2011; 29(2):192–9.

47. Rosenwald A, Wright G, Leroy K et al. Molecular diagnosis of primary mediastinal B cell lymphoma identifies a clinically favorable subgroup of diffuse large B cell lymphoma related to Hodgkin lymphoma. *J Exp Med.* 2003; 198(6):851–62.

48. Mottok A, Hung SS, Chavez EA et al. Integrative genomic analysis identifies key pathogenic mechanisms in primary mediastinal large B-cell lymphoma. *Blood.* 2019; 134(10):802–13.

49. Zinzani PL, Martelli M, Bertini M et al. Induction chemotherapy strategies for primary mediastinal large B-cell lymphoma with sclerosis: A retrospective multinational study on 426 previously untreated patients. *Haematologica.* 2002; 87(12):1258–64.

50. Vassilakopoulos TP, Pangalis GA, Katsigiannis A et al. Rituximab, cyclophosphamide, doxorubicin, vincristine, and prednisone with or without radiotherapy in primary mediastinal large B-cell lymphoma: The emerging standard of care. *Oncologist.* 2012; 17(2):239–49.

51. Rieger M, Osterborg A, Pettengell R et al. Primary mediastinal B-cell lymphoma treated with CHOP-like chemotherapy with or without rituximab: Results of the Mabthera International Trial Group study. *Ann Oncol.* 2011; 22(3):664–70.

52. Savage KJ, Al-Rajhi N, Voss N et al. Favorable outcome of primary mediastinal large B-cell lymphoma in a single institution: The British Columbia experience. *Ann Oncol.* 2006; 17(1):123–30.

53. Zinzani PL, Ribrag V, Moskowitz CH et al. Safety and tolerability of pembrolizumab in patients with relapsed/refractory primary mediastinal large B-cell lymphoma. *Blood.* 2017; 130(3):267–70.

54. Nakamura T, Tateishi K, Niwa T et al. Recurrent mutations of CD79B and MYD88 are the hallmark of primary central nervous system lymphomas. *Neuropathol Appl Neurobiol.* 2016; 42(3):279–90.

55. Ferreri AJ, Cwynarski K, Pulczynski E et al. Chemoimmunotherapy with methotrexate, cytarabine, thiotepa, and rituximab (MATRix regimen) in patients with primary CNS lymphoma: Results of the first randomisation of the International Extranodal Lymphoma Study Group-32 (IELSG32) phase 2 trial. *Lancet Haematol.* 2016; 3(5):e217–27.

56. Abrey LE, DeAngelis LM, Yahalom J. Long-term survival in primary CNS lymphoma. *J Clin Oncol.* 1998; 16(3):859–63.

57. Doolittle ND, Korfel A, Lubow MA et al. Long-term cognitive function, neuroimaging, and quality of life in primary CNS lymphoma. *Neurology.* 2013; 81(1):84–92.

58. Soussain C, Choquet S, Blonski M et al. Ibrutinib monotherapy for relapse or refractory primary CNS lymphoma and primary vitreoretinal lymphoma: Final analysis of the phase II "proof-of-concept" iLOC study by the Lymphoma study association (LYSA) and the French oculo-cerebral lymphoma (LOC) network. *Eur J Cancer.* 2019; 117:121–30.

59. Hollender A, Kvaloy S, Nome O et al. Central nervous system involvement following diagnosis of non-Hodgkin's lymphoma: A risk model. *Ann Oncol.* 2002; 13(7):1099–107.

60. McMillan A. Central nervous system-directed preventative therapy in adults with lymphoma. *Br J Haematol.* 2005; 131(1):13–21.

61. Jahnke K, Thiel E, Martus P et al. Retrospective study of prognostic factors in non-Hodgkin lymphoma secondarily involving the central nervous system. *Ann Hematol.* 2006; 85(1):45–50.

62. Cheung CW, Burton C, Smith P et al. Central nervous system chemoprophylaxis in non-Hodgkin lymphoma: Current practice in the UK. *Br J Haematol.* 2005; 131(2):193–200.

63. Boerma EG, van Imhoff GW, Appel IM et al. Gender and age-related differences in Burkitt lymphoma—epidemiological and clinical data from The Netherlands. *Eur J Cancer.* 2004; 40(18):2781–7.

64. Pui CH, Mahmoud HH, Wiley JM et al. Recombinant urate oxidase for the prophylaxis or treatment of hyperuricemia in patients With leukemia or lymphoma. *J Clin Oncol.* 2001; 19(3):697–704.

65. Mead GM, Barrans SL, Qian W et al. A prospective clinicopathologic study of dose-modified CODOX-M/IVAC in patients with sporadic Burkitt lymphoma defined using cytogenetic and immunophenotypic criteria (MRC/NCRI LY10 trial). *Blood.* 2008; 112(6):2248–60.

66. Maruyama D, Watanabe T, Maeshima AM et al. Modified cyclophosphamide, vincristine, doxorubicin, and methotrexate (CODOX-M)/ifosfamide, etoposide, and cytarabine (IVAC) therapy with or without rituximab in Japanese adult patients with Burkitt lymphoma (BL) and B cell lymphoma, unclassifiable, with features intermediate between diffuse large B cell lymphoma and BL. *Int J Hematol.* 2010; 92(5):732–43.

67. Hoster E, Dreyling M, Klapper W et al. A new prognostic index (MIPI) for patients with advanced-stage mantle cell lymphoma. *Blood.* 2008; 111(2):558–65.

68. Eskelund CW, Dahl C, Hansen JW et al. TP53 mutations identify younger mantle cell lymphoma patients who do not benefit from intensive chemoimmunotherapy. *Blood.* 2017; 130(17):1903–10.

69. Flinn IW, van der Jagt R, Kahl B et al. First-line treatment of patients with indolent non-Hodgkin lymphoma or mantle-cell lymphoma with bendamustine plus rituximab versus R-CHOP or R-CVP: Results of the BRIGHT 5-year follow-up study. *J Clin Oncol.* 2019; 37(12):984–91.

70. Rummel MJ, Niederle N, Maschmeyer G et al. Bendamustine plus rituximab versus CHOP plus rituximab as first-line treatment for patients with indolent and mantle-cell lymphomas: An open-label, multicentre, randomised, phase 3 non-inferiority trial. *Lancet.* 2013; 381(9873):1203–10.

71. Robak T, Huang H, Jin J et al. Bortezomib-based therapy for newly diagnosed mantle-cell lymphoma. *N Engl J Med.* 2015; 372(10):944–53.

72. Geisler CH, Kolstad A, Laurell A et al. Nordic MCL2 trial update: Six-year follow-up after intensive immunochemotherapy for untreated mantle cell lymphoma followed by BEAM or BEAC + autologous stem-cell support: Still very long survival but late relapses do occur. *Br J Haematol.* 2012; 158(3):355–62.

73. Delarue R, Haioun C, Ribrag V et al. CHOP and DHAP plus rituximab followed by autologous stem cell transplantation in mantle cell lymphoma: A phase 2 study from the Groupe d'Etude des Lymphomes de l'Adulte. *Blood.* 2013; 121(1):48–53.

74. Le Gouill S, Thieblemont C, Oberic L et al. Rituximab after autologous stem-cell transplantation in mantle-cell lymphoma. *N Engl J Med.* 2017; 377(13):1250–60.

75. Tam CS, Anderson MA, Pott C et al. Ibrutinib plus venetoclax for the treatment of mantle-cell lymphoma. *N Engl J Med.* 2018; 378(13):1211–23.

76. Engels EA, Pfeiffer RM, Goedert JJ et al. Trends in cancer risk among people with AIDS in the United States 1980–2002. *AIDS.* 2006; 20(12):1645–54.

77. Killebrew D, Shiramizu B. Pathogenesis of HIV-associated non-Hodgkin lymphoma. *Curr HIV Res.* 2004; 2(3):215–21.

78. Engels EA, Pfeiffer RM, Landgren O, Moore RD. Immunologic and virologic predictors of AIDS-related non-Hodgkin lymphoma in the highly active antiretroviral therapy era. *J Acquir Immune Defic Syndr.* 2010; 54(1):78–84.

79. Guech-Ongey M, Simard EP, Anderson WF et al. AIDS-related Burkitt lymphoma in the United States: What do age and CD4 lymphocyte patterns tell us about etiology and/or biology? *Blood.* 2010; 116(25):5600–4.

80. Vaccher E, Spina M, di Gennaro G et al. Concomitant cyclophosphamide, doxorubicin, vincristine, and prednisone chemotherapy plus highly active antiretroviral therapy in patients with human immunodeficiency virus-related, non-Hodgkin lymphoma. *Cancer.* 2001; 91(1):155–63.

81. Antinori A, Cingolani A, Alba L et al. Better response to chemotherapy and prolonged survival in AIDS-related lymphomas responding to highly active antiretroviral therapy. *AIDS.* 2001; 15(12):1483–91.

82. Iqbal J, Weisenburger DD, Greiner TC et al. Molecular signatures to improve diagnosis in peripheral T-cell lymphoma and prognostication in angioimmunoblastic T-cell lymphoma. *Blood.* 2010; 115(5):1026–36.

83. Gallamini A, Stelitano C, Calvi R et al. Peripheral T-cell lymphoma unspecified (PTCL-U): A new prognostic model from a retrospective multicentric clinical study. *Blood.* 2004; 103(7):2474–9.

84. Lopez-Guillermo A, Cid J, Salar A et al. Peripheral T-cell lymphomas: Initial features, natural history, and prognostic factors in a series of 174 patients diagnosed according to the R.E.A.L. Classification. *Ann Oncol.* 1998; 9(8):849–55.

85. Savage KJ, Chhanabhai M, Gascoyne RD, Connors JM. Characterization of peripheral T-cell lymphomas in a single North American institution by the WHO classification. *Ann Oncol.* 2004; 15(10):1467–75.

86. Gascoyne RD, Aoun P, Wu D et al. Prognostic significance of anaplastic lymphoma kinase (ALK) protein expression in adults with anaplastic large cell lymphoma. *Blood.* 1999; 93(11):3913–21.

87. Falini B, Pileri S, Zinzani PL et al. ALK+ lymphoma: Clinicopathological findings and outcome. *Blood.* 1999; 93(8):2697–706.

88. Brugieres L, Deley MC, Pacquement H et al. CD30(+) anaplastic large-cell lymphoma in children: Analysis of 82 patients enrolled in two consecutive studies of the French Society of Pediatric Oncology. *Blood.* 1998; 92(10):3591–8.

89. Williams DM, Hobson R, Imeson J et al. Anaplastic large cell lymphoma in childhood: Analysis of 72 patients treated on The United Kingdom Children's Cancer Study Group chemotherapy regimens. *Br J Haematol.* 2002; 117(4):812–20.

90. Schmitz N, Trumper L, Ziepert M et al. Treatment and prognosis of mature T-cell and NK-cell lymphoma: An analysis of patients with T-cell lymphoma treated in studies of the German High-Grade Non-Hodgkin Lymphoma Study Group. *Blood.* 2010; 116(18):3418–25.

91. Horwitz S, O'Connor OA, Pro B et al. Brentuximab vedotin with chemotherapy for CD30-positive peripheral T-cell lymphoma (ECHELON-2): A global, double-blind, randomised, phase 3 trial. *Lancet.* 2019; 393(10168):229–40.

92. Pro B, Advani R, Brice P et al. Brentuximab vedotin (SGN-35) in patients with relapsed or refractory systemic anaplastic large-cell lymphoma: Results of a phase II study. *J Clin Oncol.* 2012; 30(18):2190–6.

93. Mosse YP, Voss SD, Lim MS et al. Targeting ALK with crizotinib in pediatric anaplastic large cell lymphoma and inflammatory myofibroblastic tumor: A children's oncology Group Study. *J Clin Oncol.* 2017; 35(28):3215–21.

94. d'Amore F, Relander T, Lauritzsen GF et al. Up-front autologous stem-cell transplantation in peripheral T-cell lymphoma: NLG-T-01. *J Clin Oncol.* 2012; 30(25):3093–9.

95. Federico M, Rudiger T, Bellei M et al. Clinicopathologic characteristics of angioimmunoblastic T–cell lymphoma: Analysis of the international peripheral T-cell lymphoma project. *J Clin Oncol.* 2013; 31(2):240–6.

96. Heavican TB, Bouska A, Yu J et al. Genetic drivers of oncogenic pathways in molecular subgroups of peripheral T-cell lymphoma. *Blood.* 2019; 133(15):1664–76.

97. Pautier P, Devidas A, Delmer A et al. Angioimmunoblastic-like T-cell non Hodgkin's lymphoma: Outcome after chemotherapy in 33 patients and review of the literature. *Leuk Lymphoma.* 1999; 32(5–6):545–52.

98. Siegert W, Nerl C, Agthe A et al. Angioimmunoblastic lymphadenopathy (AILD)-type T-cell lymphoma: Prognostic impact of clinical observations and laboratory findings at presentation. The Kiel Lymphoma Study Group. *Ann Oncol.* 1995; 6(7):659–64.

99. Zettl A, Lee SS, Rudiger T et al. Epstein-Barr virus-associated B-cell lymphoproliferative disorders in angioimmunoblastic T-cell lymphoma and peripheral T-cell lymphoma, unspecified. *Am J Clin Pathol.* 2002; 117(3):368–79.

100. Attygalle AD, Kyriakou C, Dupuis J et al. Histologic evolution of angioimmunoblastic T-cell lymphoma in consecutive biopsies: Clinical correlation and insights into natural history and disease progression. *Am J Surg Pathol.* 2007; 31(7):1077–88.

101. Schetelig J, Fetscher S, Reichle A et al. Long-term disease-free survival in patients with angioimmunoblastic T-cell lymphoma after high-dose chemotherapy and autologous stem cell transplantation. *Haematologica.* 2003; 88(11):1272–8.

102. Kyriakou C, Canals C, Goldstone A et al. High-dose therapy and autologous stem-cell transplantation in angioimmunoblastic lymphoma: Complete remission at transplantation is the major determinant of Outcome-Lymphoma Working Party of the European Group for Blood and Marrow Transplantation. *J Clin Oncol.* 2008; 26(2):218–24.

103. Kyriakou C, Canals C, Finke J et al. Allogeneic stem cell transplantation is able to induce long-term remissions in angioimmunoblastic T-cell lymphoma: A retrospective study from the lymphoma working party of the European group for blood and marrow transplantation. *J Clin Oncol.* 2009; 27(24):3951–8.

104. Coiffier B, Pro B, Prince HM et al. Results from a pivotal, open-label, phase II study of romidepsin in relapsed or refractory peripheral T-cell lymphoma after prior systemic therapy. *J Clin Oncol.* 2012; 30(6):631–6.

105. Chen XG, Huang H, Tian Y et al. Cyclosporine, prednisone, and high-dose immunoglobulin treatment of angioimmunoblastic T-cell lymphoma refractory to prior CHOP or CHOP-like regimen. *Chin J Cancer.* 2011; 30(10):731–8.

106. Gisselbrecht C, Gaulard P, Lepage E et al. Prognostic significance of T-cell phenotype in aggressive non-Hodgkin's lymphomas. Groupe d'Etudes des Lymphomes de l'Adulte (GELA). *Blood.* 1998; 92(1):76–82.

107. Gallamini A, Zaja F, Patti C et al. Alemtuzumab (Campath-1H) and CHOP chemotherapy as first-line treatment of peripheral T-cell lymphoma: Results of a GITIL (Gruppo Italiano Terapie Innovative nei Linfomi) prospective multicenter trial. *Blood.* 2007; 110(7):2316–23.

108. Kim SJ, Yoon DH, Kang HJ et al. Bortezomib in combination with CHOP as first-line treatment for patients with stage III/IV peripheral T-cell lymphomas: A multicentre, single-arm, phase 2 trial. *Eur J Cancer.* 2012; 48(17):3223–31.

109. Foss FM, Sjak-Shie N, Goy A et al. A multicenter phase II trial to determine the safety and efficacy of combination therapy with denileukin diftitox and cyclophosphamide, doxorubicin, vincristine and prednisone in untreated peripheral T-cell lymphoma: The CONCEPT study. *Leuk Lymphoma.* 2013; 54(7):1373–9.

110. Blystad AK, Enblad G, Kvaloy S et al. High-dose therapy with autologous stem cell transplantation in patients with peripheral T cell lymphomas. *Bone Marrow Transplant.* 2001; 27(7):711–6.

111. Song KW, Mollee P, Keating A, Crump M. Autologous stem cell transplant for relapsed and refractory peripheral T-cell lymphoma: Variable outcome according to pathological subtype. *Br J Haematol.* 2003; 120(6):978–85.

112. Rodriguez J, Caballero MD, Gutierrez A et al. High-dose chemotherapy and autologous stem cell transplantation in peripheral T-cell lymphoma: The GEL-TAMO experience. *Ann Oncol.* 2003; 14(12):1768–75.

113. Catassi C, Fabiani E, Corrao G et al. Risk of non-Hodgkin lymphoma in celiac disease. *JAMA.* 2002; 287(11):1413–9.

114. Howell WM, Leung ST, Jones DB et al. HLA-DRB, -DQA, and -DQB polymorphism in celiac disease and enteropathy-associated T-cell lymphoma. Common features and additional risk factors for malignancy. *Hum Immunol.* 1995; 43(1):29–37.

115. Cellier C, Delabesse E, Helmer C et al. Refractory sprue, coeliac disease, and enteropathy-associated T-cell lymphoma. French Coeliac Disease Study Group. *Lancet.* 2000; 356(9225):203–8.

116. Zettl A, Ott G, Makulik A et al. Chromosomal gains at 9q characterize enteropathy-type T-cell lymphoma. *Am J Pathol.* 2002; 161(5):1635–45.

117. Obermann EC, Diss TC, Hamoudi RA et al. Loss of heterozygosity at chromosome 9p21 is a frequent finding in enteropathy-type T-cell lymphoma. *J Pathol.* 2004; 202(2):252–62.

118. Nicolae A, Xi L, Pham TH et al. Mutations in the JAK/STAT and RAS signaling pathways are common in intestinal T-cell lymphomas. *Leukemia.* 2016; 30(11):2245–7.

119. Egan LJ, Walsh SV, Stevens FM et al. Celiac-associated lymphoma. A single institution experience of 30 cases in the combination chemotherapy era. *J Clin Gastroenterol.* 1995; 21(2):123–9.

120. Gale J, Simmonds PD, Mead GM et al. Enteropathy-type intestinal T-cell lymphoma: Clinical features and treatment of 31 patients in a single center. *J Clin Oncol.* 2000; 18(4):795–803.

121. Daum S, Ullrich R, Heise W et al. Intestinal non-Hodgkin's lymphoma: A multicenter prospective clinical study from the German Study Group on Intestinal non-Hodgkin's Lymphoma. *J Clin Oncol.* 2003; 21(14):2740–6.

122. Sieniawski M, Angamuthu N, Boyd K et al. Evaluation of enteropathy-associated T-cell lymphoma comparing standard therapies with a novel regimen including autologous stem cell transplantation. *Blood.* 2010; 115(18):3664–70.

123. You JY, Chi KH, Yang MH et al. Radiation therapy versus chemotherapy as initial treatment for localized nasal natural killer (NK)/T-cell lymphoma: A single institute survey in Taiwan. *Ann Oncol.* 2004; 15(4):618–25.

124. Chim CS, Ma SY, Au WY et al. Primary nasal natural killer cell lymphoma: Long-term treatment outcome and relationship with the International Prognostic Index. *Blood.* 2004; 103(1):216–21.

125. Yamaguchi M, Kita K, Miwa H et al. Frequent expression of P-glycoprotein/MDR1 by nasal T-cell lymphoma cells. *Cancer.* 1995; 76(11):2351–6.

126. Kwong YL, Kim WS, Lim ST et al. SMILE for natural killer/T-cell lymphoma: Analysis of safety and efficacy from the Asia Lymphoma Study Group. *Blood.* 2012; 120(15):2973–80.

127. Wang L, Wang ZH, Chen XQ et al. First-line combination gemcitabine, oxaliplatin, and L-asparaginase (GELOX) followed by involved-field radiation therapy for patients with stage IE/IIE extranodal natural killer/T-cell lymphoma. *Cancer.* 2013; 119(2):348–55.

128. Yamaguchi M, Kwong YL, Kim WS et al. Phase II study of SMILE chemotherapy for newly diagnosed stage IV, relapsed, or refractory extranodal natural killer (NK)/T-cell lymphoma, nasal type: The NK-Cell Tumor Study Group study. *J Clin Oncol.* 2011; 29(33):4410–6.

129. Murashige N, Kami M, Kishi Y et al. Allogeneic haematopoietic stem cell transplantation as a promising treatment for natural killer-cell neoplasms. *Br J Haematol.* 2005; 130(4):561–7.

130. Kataoka K, Miyoshi H, Sakata S et al. Frequent structural variations involving programmed death ligands in Epstein-Barr virus-associated lymphomas. *Leukemia.* 2019; 33(7):1687–99.

131. Belhadj K, Reyes F, Farcet JP et al. Hepatosplenic gammadelta T-cell lymphoma is a rare clinicopathologic entity with poor outcome: Report on a series of 21 patients. *Blood.* 2003; 102(13):4261–9.

132. Solal-Celigny P, Roy P, Colombat P et al. Follicular lymphoma international prognostic index. *Blood.* 2004; 104(5):1258–65.

133. Buske C, Hoster E, Dreyling M et al. The Follicular Lymphoma International Prognostic Index (FLIPI) separates high-risk from intermediate- or low-risk patients with advanced-stage follicular lymphoma treated front-line with rituximab and the combination of cyclophosphamide, doxorubicin, vincristine, and prednisone (R-CHOP) with respect to treatment outcome. *Blood.* 2006; 108(5):1504–8.

134. Jurinovic V, Kridel R, Staiger AM et al. Clinicogenetic risk models predict early progression of follicular lymphoma after first-line immunochemotherapy. *Blood.* 2016; 128(8):1112–20.

135. Pillai RK, Surti U, Swerdlow SH. Follicular lymphoma-like B cells of uncertain significance (in situ follicular lymphoma) may infrequently progress, but precedes follicular lymphoma, is associated with other overt lymphomas and mimics follicular lymphoma in flow cytometric studies. *Haematologica.* 2013; 98(10):1571–80.

136. Schmatz AI, Streubel B, Kretschmer-Chott E et al. Primary follicular lymphoma of the duodenum is a distinct mucosal/submucosal variant of follicular lymphoma: A retrospective study of 63 cases. *J Clin Oncol.* 2011; 29(11):1445–51.

137. Vaughan Hudson B, Vaughan Hudson G, MacLennan KA et al. Clinical stage 1 non-Hodgkin's lymphoma: Long-term follow-up of patients treated by the British National Lymphoma Investigation with radiotherapy alone as initial therapy. *Br J Cancer.* 1994; 69(6):1088–93.

138. Gospodarowicz MK, Bush RS, Brown TC, Chua T. Prognostic factors in nodular lymphomas: A multivariate analysis based on the Princess Margaret Hospital experience. *Int J Radiat Oncol Biol Phys.* 1984; 10(4):489–97.

139. Pendlebury S, el Awadi M, Ashley S et al. Radiotherapy results in early stage low grade nodal non-Hodgkin's lymphoma. *Radiother Oncol.* 1995; 36(3):167–71.

140. Guadagnolo BA, Li S, Neuberg D et al. Long-term outcome and mortality trends in early-stage, Grade 1–2 follicular lymphoma

treated with radiation therapy. *Int J Radiat Oncol Biol Phys.* 2006; 64(3):928–34.

141. MacManus M, Fisher R, Roos D et al. Randomized trial of systemic therapy after involved-field radiotherapy in patients with early-stage follicular lymphoma: TROG 99.03. *J Clin Oncol.* 2018; 36(29):2918–25.

142. Campbell BA, Voss N, Woods R et al. Long-term outcomes for patients with limited stage follicular lymphoma: Involved regional radiotherapy versus involved node radiotherapy. *Cancer.* 2010; 116(16):3797–806.

143. Brice P, Bastion Y, Lepage E et al. Comparison in low-tumor-burden follicular lymphomas between an initial no-treatment policy, prednimustine, or interferon alfa: A randomized study from the Groupe d'Etude des Lymphomes Folliculaires. Groupe d'Etude des Lymphomes de l'Adulte. *J Clin Oncol.* 1997; 15(3):1110–7.

144. Young RC, Longo DL, Glatstein E et al. The treatment of indolent lymphomas: Watchful waiting v aggressive combined modality treatment. *Semin Hematol.* 1988; 25(2 Suppl 2):11–6.

145. Ardeshna KM, Smith P, Norton A et al. Long-term effect of a watch and wait policy versus immediate systemic treatment for asymptomatic advanced-stage non-Hodgkin lymphoma: A randomised controlled trial. *Lancet.* 2003; 362(9383):516–22.

146. Lowry L, Ardeshna KM. Has single-agent rituximab replaced watch-and-wait for a patient with asymptomatic low-grade follicular lymphoma? *Cancer J.* 2012; 18(5):390–5.

147. Prettyjohns M, Hoskin P, McNamara C et al. The cost-effectiveness of immediate treatment or watch and wait with deferred chemotherapy for advanced asymptomatic follicular lymphoma. *Br J Haematol.* 2018; 180(1):52–9.

148. Marcus R, Davies A, Ando K et al. Obinutuzumab for the first-line treatment of follicular lymphoma. *N Engl J Med.* 2017; 377(14):1331–44.

149. Salles G, Seymour JF, Offner F et al. Rituximab maintenance for 2 years in patients with high tumour burden follicular lymphoma responding to rituximab plus chemotherapy (PRIMA): A phase 3, randomised controlled trial. *Lancet.* 2011; 377(9759):42–51.

150. Morschhauser F, Fowler NH, Feugier P et al. Rituximab plus lenalidomide in advanced untreated follicular lymphoma. *N Engl J Med.* 2018; 379(10):934–47.

151. Hainsworth JD, Litchy S, Burris HA, 3rd et al. Rituximab as first-line and maintenance therapy for patients with indolent non-Hodgkin's lymphoma. *J Clin Oncol.* 2002; 20(20):4261–7.

152. Colombat P, Salles G, Brousse N et al. Rituximab (anti-CD20 monoclonal antibody) as single first-line therapy for patients with follicular lymphoma with a low tumor burden: Clinical and molecular evaluation. *Blood.* 2001; 97(1):101–6.

153. Witzig TE, Vukov AM, Habermann TM et al. Rituximab therapy for patients with newly diagnosed, advanced-stage, follicular grade I non-Hodgkin's lymphoma: A phase II trial in the North Central Cancer Treatment Group. *J Clin Oncol.* 2005; 23(6):1103–8.

154. Piro LD, White CA, Grillo-Lopez AJ et al. Extended Rituximab (anti-CD20 monoclonal antibody) therapy for relapsed or refractory low-grade or follicular non-Hodgkin's lymphoma. *Ann Oncol.* 1999; 10(6):655–61.

155. Freedman AS. Non-transplant-related treatment options in follicular lymphoma. *Biol Blood Marrow Transplant.* 2006; 12(1 Suppl 1):53–8.

156. Cheson BD, Chua N, Mayer J et al. Overall survival benefit in patients with rituximab-refractory indolent non-Hodgkin lymphoma who received obinutuzumab plus bendamustine induction and obinutuzumab maintenance in the GADOLIN Study. *J Clin Oncol.* 2018; 36(22):2259–66.

157. Schouten HC, Qian W, Kvaloy S et al. High-dose therapy improves progression-free survival and survival in relapsed follicular non-Hodgkin's lymphoma: Results from the randomized European CUP trial. *J Clin Oncol.* 2003; 21(21):3918–27.

158. Peniket AJ, Ruiz de Elvira MC, Taghipour G et al. An EBMT registry matched study of allogeneic stem cell transplants for lymphoma: Allogeneic transplantation is associated with a lower relapse rate but a higher procedure-related mortality rate than autologous transplantation. *Bone Marrow Transplant.* 2003; 31(8):667–78.

159. Thomson KJ, Morris EC, Milligan D et al. T-cell-depleted reduced-intensity transplantation followed by donor leukocyte infusions to promote graft-versus-lymphoma activity results in excellent long-term survival in patients with multiply relapsed follicular lymphoma. *J Clin Oncol.* 2010; 28(23):3695–700.

160. Hiddemann W, Buske C, Dreyling M et al. Treatment strategies in follicular lymphomas: Current status and future perspectives. *J Clin Oncol.* 2005; 23(26):6394–9.

161. Farinha P, Gascoyne RD. Molecular pathogenesis of mucosa-associated lymphoid tissue lymphoma. *J Clin Oncol.* 2005; 23(26):6370–8.

162. Nakamura S, Sugiyama T, Matsumoto T et al. Long-term clinical outcome of gastric MALT lymphoma after eradication of *Helicobacter pylori*: A multicentre cohort follow-up study of 420 patients in Japan. *Gut.* 2012; 61(4):507–13.

163. Hancock BW, Qian W, Linch D et al. Chlorambucil versus observation after anti-*Helicobacter* therapy in gastric MALT lymphomas: Results of the international randomised LY03 trial. *Br J Haematol.* 2009; 144(3):367–75.

164. Levy M, Copie-Bergman C, Traulle C et al. Conservative treatment of primary gastric low-grade B-cell lymphoma of mucosa-associated lymphoid tissue: Predictive factors of response and outcome. *Am J Gastroenterol.* 2002; 97(2):292–7.

165. Martinelli G, Laszlo D, Ferreri AJ et al. Clinical activity of rituximab in gastric marginal zone non-Hodgkin's lymphoma resistant to or not eligible for anti-*Helicobacter pylori* therapy. *J Clin Oncol.* 2005; 23(9):1979–83.

166. Tsang RW, Gospodarowicz MK, Pintilie M et al. Stage I and II MALT lymphoma: Results of treatment with radiotherapy. *Int J Radiat Oncol Biol Phys.* 2001; 50(5):1258–64.

167. Bertoni F, Zucca E. State-of-the-art therapeutics: Marginal-zone lymphoma. *J Clin Oncol.* 2005; 23(26):6415–20.

168. Bennett M, Schechter GP. Treatment of splenic marginal zone lymphoma: Splenectomy versus rituximab. *Semin Hematol.* 2010; 47(2):143–7.

169. Montalban C, Abraira V, Arcaini L et al. Risk stratification for Splenic Marginal Zone Lymphoma based on haemoglobin concentration, platelet count, high lactate dehydrogenase level and extrahilar lymphadenopathy: Development and validation on 593 cases. *Br J Haematol.* 2012; 159(2):164–71.

170. Non-Hodgkin's Lymphoma Classification Project. *Anon Blood.* 1997; 89:3909–18.

31 MULTIPLE MYELOMA

Guy Pratt

Introduction

Multiple myeloma (MM) is a malignant disease of plasma cells in the bone marrow and forms part of a spectrum of plasma cell disorders that also includes monoclonal gammopathy of undetermined significance (MGUS), solitary plasmacytoma (bone or extramedullary), and AL amyloidosis. Myeloma is characterized by the production of a monoclonal immunoglobulin (Ig) molecule and serum free light chain and is associated with bone destruction, anemia, infection, and renal failure. There has been a significant improvement in survival in the last two decades with the use of proteasome inhibitors, immunomodulatory drugs, and monoclonal antibodies, but still only a minority of patients survive beyond 10 years. New antibodies (anti-BCMA for example), new drugs (venetoclax, selinexor), and immunomodulatory approaches will further improve outcomes.

Incidence and etiology

Incidence

Myeloma accounts for about 1% of all cancers and 10% of hematological malignancies with an annual incidence of approximately 50 per million and a median age at presentation of about 70 years with approximately 5000 new cases each year in the UK. Myeloma incidence rates have increased due to an increasingly older population. Fewer than 2–5% of myeloma patients are under 40 years of age. It is more common in males (M:F ratio around 1.5:1) and almost twice as common in Afro-Caribbean people as in Caucasian and Asian people.[1]

Epidemiological risk factors

Although most cases of myeloma present de novo, patients have a preceding premalignant asymptomatic stage termed monoclonal gammopathy of uncertain significance MGUS.[2,3] The etiology of myeloma is poorly understood with a lack of evidence for most postulated carcinogens. Epidemiological studies of myeloma and MGUS show a weak familial effect (genetic vs. environmental factors), and molecular epidemiological studies have identified associated genetic loci.

Associated conditions

Monoclonal gammopathy of undetermined significance

MGUS is a common condition found incidentally with a low-level paraprotein in the serum (<30 g/L) with no clinical features or defining biomarkers of myeloma (Table 31.2) and fewer than 10% plasma cells in the marrow.[4] MGUS has a high prevalence in the population (2% >50 years old, 5% >70 years old). The annual risk of transformation to myeloma is low, around 1% per year. Prognostic risk factors for transformation include an M-protein level greater than 15 g/L, non-IgG subtype, and an abnormal serum free light chain ratio which identifies a very low risk group accounting for

40% of patients with MGUS with no risk factors,[5] but this scoring system is poor at identifying true high-risk disease.

There is evidence mainly from epidemiological studies for associations of MGUS with poorer bone health, increased infection risk, inflammatory conditions, autoimmune disease, and reduced life span.

The monoclonal protein itself can rarely have pathological activity. Rarely serum free light chain (usually lambda) is amyloidogenic leading to AL amyloidosis. Monoclonal gammopathy of renal significance are a range of renal disorders related to a small MGUS plasma cell clone. Associations for MGUS have also been found with a variety of skin disorders, peripheral neuropathies, and ocular lens deposition. The term monoclonal gammopathy of clinical significance (MGCS) refers to this group of disorders that are rare, poorly understood, and hence under-recognized.[6]

Plasma cell leukemia

Plasma cell leukemia is defined as >2 × 10⁹ plasma cells per liter or, alternatively, >20% of nucleated blood cells being plasma cells, and carries a poor prognosis. There is no consensus on treatment as data are limited to phase II studies or retrospective studies. Intensive regimens such as VTD-PACE or combinations of novel agents with transplant consolidation/maintenance or even double autologous stem-cell transplant are considered in younger patients, but durable remissions are rare.

Solitary plasmacytoma of bone

Solitary plasmacytoma may affect bone or an extramedullary site. Solitary plasmacytoma of bone (SPB) may involve any bone but is most common in the axial skeleton with symptoms due to local effects. Biopsy of the lesion shows a monoclonal population of plasma cells. A serum and/or urinary paraprotein has been reported in approximately 60% of patients but is usually at a low level. By definition the bone marrow and PET-CT scan should be normal with no evidence of marrow infiltration or other features of myeloma. Local radiotherapy is the preferred treatment of choice, but about two-thirds of patients develop MM at 10 years' follow-up. Using flow cytometry, half of the patients showed occult BM infiltration and half of these cases progressed at 2 years.

Extramedullary plasmacytoma

In contrast to SPB, extramedullary plasmacytoma (EMP) appears to be truly localized in the majority of cases and less commonly progresses to MM. It most commonly arises in the upper respiratory passages, but a wide variety of different organs may occasionally be involved. Treatment is usually local radiotherapy (40–50 Gy over 3–5 weeks) or surgical removal.

POEMS syndrome

This is a rare syndrome in which a serum paraprotein (M-component) is associated with polyneuropathy (P), organomegaly (O), endocrinopathy (E), and skin changes (S). Approximately 50% of cases are associated with multiple myeloma and the remainder with solitary plasmacytomas or more subtle plasma cell dyscrasias. The cardinal feature is a severe sensorimotor neuropathy with osteosclerotic bone lesions, hepatomegaly and lymphadenopathy, hormonal abnormalities, and skin hyperpigmentation. Treatment is difficult, but local radiotherapy for localized plasmacytomas and chemotherapy for generalized disease are recommended. There are now a number of reports of neurological improvement or stabilization following high-dose therapy and stem-cell transplantation.

Pathogenesis and biology

Multiple myeloma arises from a background of MGUS. In at least half of MGUS patients, clonal plasma cell proliferation is thought to be initiated by primary translocations involving the immunoglobulin heavy chain (IgH) locus on chromosome 14q32 and a promiscuous range of partner chromosomes. In patients without such a translocation, hyperdiploidy is common and again seen at the MGUS stage suggesting this is also an early event. There is clear evidence for the existence of many heterogeneous myeloma sub-clones in patients, and it is likely that clonal progression is a key feature of transformation. The additional genetic abnormalities that may drive transformation from MGUS to myeloma are not well understood. Importantly complex external interactions with the bone marrow microenvironment, particularly bone marrow stromal cells and immune cells providing immune surveillance, may be more important in transformation. The marrow microenvironment is critical in promoting the ability of myeloma cells to survive within a protected niche and resist conventional pro-apoptotic stimuli, particularly conventional chemotherapy. Eventually end-stage myeloma is characterized by the dominance of a myeloma clone that is resistant to treatment and which increasingly can become independent of the marrow microenvironment.

Cell of origin

Myeloma is a tumor of plasma cells in the bone marrow, but the precise nature of the myeloma stem cell is unclear and data from myeloma mouse models are conflicting. A post-germinal center plasma cell that has already undergone somatic mutation and subsequently homes to the bone marrow is the most likely cell of origin, although at least a subset of myelomas may arise at an earlier stage. Peripheral-blood B lymphocytes may contain some cells with identical IgH signature to the myeloma clone.

Myeloma and the BM micro-environment

There is a close relationship between myeloma cells and the marrow micro-environment, which promotes tumor growth, chemoresistance (cell adhesion–mediated drug resistance being an example) and myeloma bone disease.[7] Interactions between myeloma cells and the bone marrow microenvironment, including extracellular proteins, stromal cells (a heterogenous group of cells with fibroblast-like morphology), endothelial cells, adipocytes, macrophages, T cells, other haemopoietic cells, osteoblasts, and osteoclasts, are mediated by cell-to-cell contact, adhesion molecules, and cytokines. Adherence of myeloma cells to stromal cells induces cytokine production, in both an autocrine (from the myeloma cells) and paracrine (from the BM stromal cells) fashion, and also stimulates signaling cascades within myeloma cells including anti-apoptotic mechanisms (e.g. Mcl-1, bcl-2) and degradation both of pro-apoptotic mediators and negative cell cycle regulators. Cytokines known to be important

include interleukin-6, insulin growth factor-1 (IGF-1), APRIL, BAFF, IL-1α and β, VEGF, TNF-α, TGF-β, stroma-derived factor-1, hepatocyte growth factor, basic FGF, and tissue metalloproteinases. The hypoxic marrow microenvironment triggers hypoxia-inducible factor 1-α known to promote tumor pathogenesis and VEGF production.

Myeloma bone disease

The main pathological event in myeloma is uncoupling of bone resorption from new bone formation resulting in a net loss of bone.[8] Increased osteoclast activity and corresponding reduced osteoblast activity are due to increased levels of receptor activator of nuclear factor-kB ligand (RANKL) and decreased levels of osteoprotegerin, both produced by stromal cells in the marrow. Other osteoclast activating factors including IL6, IL-1β, TNFα, MIP-1α, hepatocyte growth factor, and macrophage-inhibitory protein 1α are increased. Bone destruction is associated with further cytokine release that perpetuates a cycle of myeloma cell growth and further bone damage. Increased levels of DKK1 and IL-3 inhibit osteoblast development.

Immune dysfunction

Immune dysfunction is an important feature of multiple myeloma,[9] and infection remains a major cause of morbidity and mortality with approximately 10% of patients dying in the first 60 days,[10] many from infection. This immune defect correlates with active disease and is exacerbated by steroids. Neutropenia is often seen in heavily treated relapsed patients. Numerous defects of the immune system occur in multiple myeloma and can also be observed to a lesser extent in monoclonal gammopathy of uncertain significance. Transforming growth factor-beta (TGF-β), interleukin-10 (IL-10), interleukin-6 (IL-6), vascular endothelial growth factor (VEGF), Fas ligand, Muc-1, cyclooxygenase-2, matrix metalloproteinases, APRIL, and BAFF are all immunosuppressive and immunomodulatory cytokines that are increased. Functional and numerical immune cellular defects occur with lack of dendritic cell maturation with poor antigen presentation, skewing of CD4 T cell subsets with possibly increased T regs and Th17, and suppression of NK cells and marked suppression of normal B cell function with immunoparesis.

Genetic abnormalities

The chromosomal abnormalities described in myeloma are highly complex and reflect a higher degree of karyotypic instability than other hematological tumours.[11] Although complex, heterogeneous, and mechanistically different, genetic events ultimately target key biological pathways, namely DNA damage repair, MAPK, NF-kB, myc, cell cycle, adhesion and motility, and cell differentiation to name a few.[12,13] Conventional cytogenetic analysis is often unsuccessful because of the low mitotic rate of plasma cells. It was only with the advent of alternative techniques such as fluorescence in situ hybridization (FISH) and genomic-sequencing techniques that the marked heterogeneity and complexity of the genetic abnormalities have become apparent. Several GEP approaches have identified signatures to stratify patients into risk groups, but currently there remain a number of barriers including cost, and lack of reproducibility or validation in different laboratories.

Genetic events include translocations, loss of heterozygosity, gene amplification, gene mutation, and as yet poorly understood epigenetic changes, and establishing correlates between abnormalities and clinical outcome has been difficult. Translocations involving chromosome 14q32 occur in 50% of cases, and these usually involve the heavy chain switch regions of the IgH gene although recently breakpoints involving VDJ have been described. These translocations occur in all cells of the clone and at the MGUS stage and are felt to be an initiating event. Several partner chromosomes have been identified with breakpoints frequently near the site of cellular protooncogenes, e.g. cyclin D1 on 11q13, fibroblast growth factor receptor 3 (FGFR3) and MMSET on 4p16, CCND3 on chromosome 6p21, and MAF genes on chromosome 16q23. The t(4;14) translocation occurs in 15% of cases and is associated often with an IgA M-protein and a poor outcome possibly partly overcome with bortezomib-based therapy. Due to the reciprocal nature of this translocation, two oncogenes are activated, FGR3 and MMSET, although their exact contributions remain controversial. The t(11;14) with overexpression of cyclin D1 is associated with an intermediate prognosis, and sensitivity to bcl-2 inhibition (venetoclax) with often lymphoplasmacytoid morphology and CD20 expression. About 20% of myelomas have a unique non-recurrent partner chromosome translocating to 14q32. Myeloma lacking an IgH translocation tends to have hyperdiploidy although there is some overlap between the two groups and hyperdiploidy is associated with a better prognosis. Similar to IgH translocations, hyperdiploidy is an early event found in MGUS stage and is characterized by multiple trisomies typically involving the odd-numbered chromosomes (i.e. 3, 5, 7, 9, 11, 15, 19, 21). Loss of 13q is common, occurring in 58% of myelomas, involves loss of the *Rb* gene, although homozygous loss or inactivation is not common, and co-associates with other poor prognostic markers such as t(4;14). Chromosome 1q gain and loss of chromosome 1p (probably affecting CDKN2C and FAM46C genes) are poor prognostic events although the relevant genes affected on 1q are not clear. Loss of tumor suppressor genes requires inactivation of both alleles and a number of genes have been identified as being relevant as tumor suppressor genes in myeloma including *BIRC2*, *TRAF3*, *FAM46C*, and *DIS3*.

Increased expression of a cyclin D family gene is a universal feature of virtually all MGUS and MM tumors irrespective of whether a cyclin D gene is involved in a translocation and led to a molecular classification based on IgH translocations and cyclin D gene overexpression. Genetic mutational events typically affect common pathways including NF-kB activation, ERK activation, histone methylation, and blood coagulation.

Changes involving genes involved in cyclin-dependent kinases, inactivation of retinoblastoma, activation of NF-kB pathways, RNA editing, *ras*, *p53*, *c-myc*, and *Fas* can be later events associated with the progression of established disease.

These observations are consistent with a multi-step pathogenesis for MM in which there is early dysregulation of oncogenes through an IgH translocation or association with hyperdiploidy that leads to immortalization of plasma cells. The malignant clone consists of multiple subclones with distinct genetic differences, changing frequencies, and subclonal evolution occurring with time and treatment with, in some cases, reemergence of ancestral subclones.

Clinical features and complications

The clinical presentation of myeloma is varied. Delay in diagnosis is common due to both the non-specific symptoms (pain, infection, fatigue) and the rarity of the condition. In the UK over 50% of patients had had three or more primary care consultations prior to a diagnosis,[14] over 20% present via a secondary care pathway, and about a third of patients are inpatients at diagnosis.

Presenting features include symptoms of bone disease, impaired renal function, anemia, hypercalcemia, recurrent or persistent bacterial infection, or, less commonly, symptoms of hyperviscosity or of spinal cord or nerve root compression. There is a significant early death rate of around 10% due to in part to infection and renal impairment. Symptomatic AL amyloidosis is also associated with myeloma in less than 5% of cases and these patients may also present with symptoms of associated nephrotic syndrome, cardiac failure, or other features of AL amyloid.

Bone disease and hypercalcemia

Pain arising from the skeletal complications of myeloma is the commonest presenting symptom (60% of patients at diagnosis).

Plain X-rays may show lytic lesions and/or generalized osteoporosis but are much less sensitive at detecting bone disease than cross-sectional imaging techniques (namely CT, PET-CT, and MRI).[15,16] Vertebral collapse is frequent, leading to back pain, kyphosis, and loss of height, and occasionally resulting in cord compression, and pathological fractures can occur. Bone destruction can give rise to hypercalcemia, although serum alkaline phosphatase is usually not increased. Radionuclide bone scans may be negative in myeloma. International and UK guidelines recommend cross-sectional imaging for patients with suspected myeloma but cost and capacity are barriers. Importantly IMWG response assessment now includes functional imaging, namely PET-CT response, and hence monitoring will increasingly include functional imaging, mainly PET currently. Diffusion-weighted MRI is also very promising as a functional imaging technique for monitoring. At relapse in particular there is an increasing tendency to form extramedullary and focal tumor deposits that require cross-sectional imaging for detection and monitoring.

Renal failure

A third of patients present with significant renal impairment, and the majority will be affected at some point during the course of the illness with 10% of patients on dialysis. The main cause of renal failure in myeloma is deposition of Bence Jones protein in the renal tubules with histological features of "myeloma kidney" (fractured distal tubular casts with a surrounding chronic inflammatory infiltrate including giant cells). The physicochemical properties of individual immunoglobulin light chains are important. Many other factors may contribute to renal failure, and these include hypercalcemia, infection, dehydration, hyperuricemia, amyloid deposition, and non-steroidal anti-inflammatory drugs.

Renal failure is reversible with over 50% of patients showing a marked improvement with bortezomib-based regimens.[17] It is a medical emergency, and recovery depends on the speed of management, particularly hydration and anti-myeloma treatment. Two studies have recently shown conflicting evidence for active removal of light chains using wide pore dialysis membranes and prolonged dialysis,[17,18] and currently this cannot be recommended.

Anemia

Hematopoiesis is frequently impaired in myeloma. A normochromic, normocytic anemia (occasionally macrocytic) is common, with a hemoglobin below 120 g/L seen in 60% of patients and commoner with renal impairment. Severe anemia, neutropenia, and thrombocytopenia are, however, rare at presentation and commoner with advanced disease.

Infection

There is a complex multifactorial immune deficiency leading to impairment both of humoral and cell-mediated immunity and an increased susceptibility to infection, both bacterial and viral. This immunodeficiency is greatest with active disease and partly improves during disease remissions. An important contributory factor is the suppression of normal polyclonal immunoglobulins but other factors include reduced T-lymphocyte function, defective antigen presentation, and natural killer cell activity. Treatment itself, particularly steroids, can also impair the immune system, and neutropenia is increasingly seen now in patients following multiple lines of therapy. Chest infections are particularly common. Encapsulated bacteria and respiratory viruses are common organisms, although often no organism is isolated.

AL amyloidosis

About 10% of patients with myeloma develop AL (primary) amyloidosis. In this disorder, monoclonal immunoglobulin light chains or light chain fragments are linked together and form amyloid fibrils, which can then be deposited in almost all organs. The kidney is frequently affected with nephrotic syndrome. Peripheral neuropathy (particularly carpal tunnel syndrome), congestive cardiac failure, and involvement of the skin, muscle, and joints may also occur. The diagnosis is made by biopsy of an affected organ and staining with Congo Red (or fat aspirate or rectal biopsy). Cardiac involvement remains powerfully prognostic with proBNP and troponin levels defining risk groups.

Uncommon presentations

Extramedullary disease is commoner at relapse but nevertheless can be present at diagnosis and include for example CNS involvement or unusual extramedullary sites.

Peripheral neuropathy may also occur in myeloma patients without amyloidosis (Gawler, 1998). Very high immunoglobulin levels, particularly of IgA, may result in hyperviscosity syndrome, with headaches, visual disturbance, and loss of concentration.

Smoldering myeloma

Myeloma is increasingly detected incidentally by the finding of a monoclonal protein following serum protein electrophoresis/serum free light chains on routine screening or when being investigated for an unrelated problem. In November 2014 the International Myeloma Working Group (IMWG) published a revised definition of multiple myeloma that incorporated three new criteria for initiating therapy in addition to the established CRAB criteria.[15] These three criteria are based on the level of plasma cell infiltration, the serum free light chain (sFLC) level/ratio, and the presence of two or more focal lesions on advanced imaging (CT [low dose whole body], MRI, 18F FDG PET). They define a group of otherwise asymptomatic patients who have an extremely high risk of progression to symptomatic disease within 2 years and for whom delayed intervention could be detrimental. In terms of treatment the revised definitions impact on a relatively small group of patients who are now upstaged and have an indication for immediate treatment when previously they would have been monitored. The effects of the new definition are however wide-ranging in terms of the use of imaging and in using new biomarkers. The term asymptomatic myeloma is somewhat misleading (as a patient may be well but have a very high FLC ratio for example) and smoldering myeloma is a better term for patients with myeloma that do not have an indication for immediate treatment.[15]

Investigation, diagnosis, and staging

Investigation

Initial investigation of a patient with suspected myeloma should include the screening tests indicated in Table 31.1, followed by further tests to confirm the diagnosis. There is no universally agreed definition of what constitutes a patient with suspected myeloma, but this should include any patient with a monoclonal protein and other unexplained features that could be due to myeloma or a well patient with a monoclonal protein as follows, IgG >15 g/L, IgA >10 g/L or clonal serum FLC >500 mg/L, would definitely need a bone marrow biopsy and cross-sectional imaging (see Table 31.1 for details).

The urgency with which these should be carried out depends on the method of presentation. Symptomatic patients with suspected myeloma require urgent specialist referral. Spinal cord compression, hypercalcemia, and renal failure are medical emergencies requiring immediate management. Patients with a paraprotein found on routine testing and who have no clinical symptoms and no anemia, hypercalcemia, or renal impairment can be seen less urgently. Appropriate initial investigations are summarized in Table 31.1.

TABLE 31.1   Initial Investigations in Patients with Suspected Myeloma

Patient with any monoclonal protein	FBC
	Biochemistry to include renal, bone, LDH, CRP
	Serum protein electrophoresis
	Serum free light chains
	Beta-2 microglobulin
	Urine albumin/creatinine ratio
	Consider proBNP if considering AL amyloid
	Consider urine protein electrophoresis if considering amyloid and no monoclonal protein
Patients with a monoclonal protein and suspected myeloma based on	As above plus
1) patient has a monoclonal protein and other unexplained features that could be due to myeloma	*Bone marrow aspirate and trephine for morphology/immunohistochemistry, histology, flow cytometry, and genetics (FISH as recommended by IMWG, NICE guidelines)
2) a well patient with a monoclonal protein as follows IgG >15 g/L, IgA >10 g/L, or clonal serum FLC >500 mg/L	*Cross sectional imaging—whole-body diffusion weighted MRI or PET-CT or low-dose CT whole-body scan

Notes: There is no definition of "suspected" myeloma but these highlighted investigations* would be recommended if (1) patient has a monoclonal protein and other unexplained features that could be due to myeloma, (2) a well patient with a monoclonal protein as follows IgG >15 g/L, IgA >10 g/L or clonal serum FLC >500 mg/L.

Hematological investigations

The most common abnormality seen on a full blood count is a normochromic, normocytic anemia, or macrocytic anemia. The blood film often shows rouleaux formation due to the presence of a paraprotein. When circulating plasma cells are seen at a level of over 2×10^9/L, a diagnosis of plasma cell leukemia can be made. The ESR is usually raised in myeloma (except light chain myeloma) as the result of the high serum globulin levels.

A bone marrow examination is an essential diagnostic investigation. A marrow aspirate may be sufficient to confirm the diagnosis, but a trephine biopsy is likely to give a more reliable estimate of plasma cell numbers. Immunohistology or flow cytometry to demonstrate monoclonality is essential where there is only a modest increase in plasma cell numbers. The majority of cases have an abnormal plasma cell phenotype, and although there is no single characteristic phenotype most cases show a reduction in CD19 expression and aberrant expression of CD56, and a minority have aberrant expression of CD117, CD20, and CD28.

Genetic testing is recommended by national and international guidelines mainly to identify poor-risk FISH abnormalities that are prognostically significant and warrant newer approaches in trials such as MUK 9b trial. However, we are entering an era in which targeted treatment is becoming relevant. The t(11;14) translocation identifies a group of around 15% of patients with an increased response rate to venetoclax as a single agent in the relapsed setting. The BRAF mutation, although rare (<5% of patients), is another example where a potential targeted therapy exists (vemurafenib).

Biochemical investigations

Biochemical screening may show abnormalities of urea, creatinine, calcium, uric acid, total protein, and/or albumin. Serum ALP is usually normal but is commonly raised after a fracture. Electrophoresis of serum and serum free light-chain assay or urine testing in all patients to look for monoclonal light chain is important since patients with Bence Jones–only myeloma have no paraprotein in the serum and patients with a serum paraprotein are at greater risk of renal failure if they also produce Bence Jones protein (BJP). The paraprotein in the serum and/or urine is then confirmed and typed by immunofixation. The paraprotein is of IgG subtype in 55–60% of cases and IgA in 20–25%, of whom two-thirds also have BJP in the urine and 95% have a clonal serum free light chain. Rarely, the paraprotein may be of IgD, IgE, or IgM type. Overall two-thirds of paraproteins have kappa light chains and one-third lambda. Twenty percent of cases are Bence Jones–only myeloma. In less than 1% of patients, no paraprotein is detectable in either serum or urine (non-secretory myeloma).

Serum B2-microglobulin, albumin and lactate dehydrogenase should be measured in all patients at diagnosis because of its prognostic significance (Table 31.3).[19]

The serum free light chain assay test should be used as an alternative to the measurement of urinary free light chains but may not be available in primary care. This test is particularly useful for diagnosis and monitoring free light chain–only myeloma and patients in whom the serum and urine are negative on immunofixation (non-secretory myeloma). Importantly IgG and IgA myelomas can show the phenomenon of light chain escape later in the disease so all patients require serum free light chain monitoring.

Radiology and imaging

All guidelines strongly recommend using cross-sectional imaging (low-dose full-body CT scan, PET-CT, plain whole-body MRI, diffusion-weighted MRI) for patients with myeloma rather than using plain imaging (skeletal survey).[16] The presence of lytic bone lesions is a major diagnostic criterion for diagnosis.

Whole-body MRI is the most sensitive technique, and there is a small false negative rate with PET-CT. Cross-sectional imaging provides much higher sensitivity compared to plain radiographs which miss a significant amount of bony disease and are poor at delineating lesions well (especially extramedullary disease/soft tissue disease). For monitoring, it is important to distinguish between functional imaging techniques (namely PET-CT and diffusion-weighted MRI) and purely anatomical techniques (low-dose CT, conventional MRI) as only functional imaging can be used to assess responses well. PET-CT is currently the established technique for monitoring; although diffusion-weighted MRI has many advantages it is much less well established. The revised guidelines for assessing response now include imaging responses using PET-CT.

Extramedullary or bulky focal disease at relapse is increasingly seen as patients live longer because of novel therapies.

The main issues for cross-sectional imaging are funding, capacity, and changing the philosophy of healthcare professionals.

The most common radiographic findings are a combination of osteoporosis and lytic lesions. Pathological fractures may occur and commonly affect vertebral bodies and ribs. Vertebral compression fractures often lead to long-term pain and deformity and may be complicated by cord compression. Sclerotic lesions are very rare, except in POEMS syndrome.

Diagnostic criteria and differential diagnosis

The diagnosis of myeloma is usually made by the demonstration of a monoclonal protein (M-protein/paraprotein) in the serum or urine and/or lytic lesions on X-ray/cross-sectional imaging together with an increased number of plasma cells in the bone marrow. The definition of myeloma was given by the IMWG in 2014 (Table 31.2). There are many other conditions in which an M-protein may be present (MGUS, AL amyloidosis, plasmacytoma, any B cell non-Hodgkin lymphoma, chronic lymphocytic leukemia, connective tissue disorders). An IgM monoclonal protein is usually associated with Waldenstroms macroglobulinemia or IgM MGUS, although rare cases of IgM myeloma do occur.

Healthy individuals with a small M-protein should not be over-investigated. The extent of diagnostic procedures in asymptomatic patients should take into consideration the age of the patient, the presence of other disease, and the levels of M-protein. The main clinical decision is whether to request a bone marrow biopsy and imaging which should be considered if:

1. A significant monoclonal protein alone if monoclonal protein IgG >15 g/L, IgA >10g/L, or monoclonal FLC >500 mg/L.
2. There is clinical suspicion of myeloma, amyloid, or MGCS based on end organ damage irrespective of the level of the monoclonal protein/FLC.

The increasing use of routine screening blood tests for a variety of disorders has led to an increase in the number of people found to have MGUS, but the vast majority of MGUS patients will go undetected.

In November 2014 the International Myeloma Working Group (IMWG) published a revised definition of multiple myeloma that incorporated three new criteria for initiating therapy in addition to the established CRAB criteria.[15] These three criteria are based

TABLE 31.2   **Diagnostic Criteria for MGUS, Asymptomatic Multiple Myeloma and Symptomatic Multiple Myeloma**

Definition of multiple myeloma

Clonal bone marrow plasma cells ≥**10% or biopsy-proven bony or extramedullary plasmacytoma*** and any one or more of the following myeloma-
  defining events or any one or more of the following biomarkers of malignancy.
Myeloma-defining events:
Evidence of end organ damage that can be attributed to the underlying plasma cell proliferative disorder as follows:
  • Hypercalcemia: serum calcium >0.25 mmol/L (>1 mg/dL) higher than the upper limit of normal or >2.75 mmol/L (>11 mg/dL)
  • Renal insufficiency: **creatinine clearance <40 mL per min**† **or serum creatinine** >177 μmol/L (>**2 mg/dL)**
  • Anemia: hemoglobin value of >20 g/L below the lower limit of normal or a hemoglobin value <100 g/L
  • Bone lesions: one or more osteolytic lesions on skeletal radiography, **CT, or PET-CT**‡
Any one or more of the following biomarkers of malignancy:
  • **Clonal bone marrow plasma cell percentage*** **≥60%**
  • **Involved:uninvolved serum free light chain ratio**§ **≥100**
  • **>1 focal lesions on MRI studies**¶
Definition of smoldering multiple myeloma
Both criteria must be met:
  • Serum monoclonal protein (IgG or IgA) ≥30 g/L or urinary monoclonal protein ≥500 mg per 24 h and/or **clonal bone marrow plasma cells**
    10–60%
  • Absence of myeloma defining events **including biomarkers of malignancy** or amyloidosis
PET-CT=1⁸F-fluorodeoxyglucose PET with CT.
*Clonality should be established by showing κ/λ-light-chain restriction on flow cytometry, immunohistochemistry, or immunofluorescence. Bone
  marrow plasma cell percentage should preferably be estimated from a core biopsy specimen; in case of a disparity between the aspirate and core
  biopsy, the highest value should be used.
†Measured or estimated by validated equations.
‡If bone marrow has less than 10% clonal plasma cells, more than one bone lesion is required to distinguish from solitary plasmacytoma with minimal
  marrow involvement.
§These values are based on the serum Freelite assay (The Binding Site Group, Birmingham, UK). The involved free light chain must be ≥100 mg/L.
¶ Each focal lesion must be 5mm or more in size

Source: Adapted from International Myeloma Working Group, 2014; changes from the previous 2003 definition are highlighted in bold.

TABLE 31.3   **Revised International Staging System R-ISS**

Stage	Criteria	Median Survival (Months)
I	Serum β_2 microglobulin <3.5 mg/L	82 months
	Albumin >3.5 mg/dL	
	AND	
	Standard-risk chromosomal abnormalities	
	AND	
	Normal LDH (defined as less than ULN)	
II	Neither I or III*	62 months
III	Serum β_2 microglobulin >>5.5 mg/L (465 nmol/L)	40 months
	AND EITHER	
	High-risk chromosomal abnormalities	
	Del 17p, t(4;14) or t(14;16)	
	OR	
	High LDH (defined as higher than ULN)	

Source: Compiled from Palumbo et al., 2015.

on the level of plasma cell infiltration, serum free light chain (sFLC) level/ratio, and the presence of two or more focal lesions on advanced imaging (CT [low dose whole body], MRI, PET-CT). Asymptomatic myeloma in this classification is now replaced by the term smoldering myeloma.

Prognostic factors and staging

The introduction of novel agents has improved the outcome for most patients to a median of around 5 years, but the prognosis of myeloma remains highly variable with a 10% early death rate. Prognostic factors relate to the biology of the myeloma and the fitness, frailty, and comorbidities of the patient.

The revised international prognostic scoring system is currently the universally accepted staging system[19] (see Table 31.3), using a combination of FISH adverse genetics, beta-2 microglobulin, LDH, and albumin.

There is an increasing recognition that 25% of patients have biologically adverse disease with poor responses and short remissions and die within 3 years, and treatment is unsatisfactory. Often such patients relapse within a year of a stem-cell transplant using standard approaches. Using a combination of two techniques to identify genetic high-risk disease—FISH (for adverse FISH abnormalities) and gene expression profiling—is one approach, but there is no global consensus as to how to best define this high-risk group as yet as this is an evolving field.

Cytogenetic abnormalities including loss of 17p13 by FISH and certain specific IgH translocations involving chromosomes 4 and 16 such as t(4;14), t(14;16) have a strong negative impact on prognosis. Chromosome 1q gain and the loss of chromosome 1p are also poor prognostic events although the relevant genes affected on 1q are not clear. Multiple FISH abnormalities are more powerfully adversely prognostic than single poor-risk FISH abnormalities. Gene expression profiling using microarray techniques is likely to allow molecular classification and importantly complements FISH in that it identifies some high-risk patients with no adverse FISH abnormalities.

The genetics of myeloma changes with disease progression, and therefore genetic analysis at relapse can provide new and additional prognostic information.

Course of the disease

Despite advances in understanding of the biology of myeloma and the introduction of many new agents including proteasome inhibitors (bortezomib, carfilzomib, ixazomib), immunomodulatory

TABLE 31.4   IMWG Criteria for Response Assessment Including Criteria for Minimal Residual Disease

Stringent complete response	Complete response as defined below plus normal FLC ratio and absence of clonal cells in bone marrow biopsy by immunohistochemistry (κ/λ ratio ≤4:1 or ≥1:2 for κ and λ patients, respectively, after counting ≥100 plasma cells)
Complete response	Negative immunofixation on the serum and urine and disappearance of any soft tissue plasmacytomas and <5% plasma cells in bone marrow aspirates

IMWG MRD criteria (requires a complete response as defined above)

Sustained MRD-negative	MRD negativity in the marrow (NGF or NGS, or both) and by imaging as defined below, confirmed minimum of 1 year apart. Subsequent evaluations can be used to further specify the duration of negativity (e.g. MRD-negative at 5 years)
Flow MRD-negative	Absence of phenotypically aberrant clonal plasma cells by NGF‡ on bone marrow aspirates using the EuroFlow standard operation procedure for MRD detection in multiple myeloma (or validated equivalent method) with a minimum sensitivity of 1 in 10^5 nucleated cells or higher
	Absence of clonal plasma cells by NGS on bone marrow aspirate in which presence of a clone is defined as less than two identical sequencing reads obtained after DNA sequencing of bone marrow aspirates using the LymphoSIGHT platform (or validated equivalent method) with a minimum sensitivity of 1 in 10^5 nucleated cells or higher
	MRD negativity as defined by NGF or NGS plus disappearance of every area of increased tracer uptake found at baseline or a preceding PET/CT or decrease to less mediastinal blood pool SUV or decrease to less than that of surrounding normal tissue
Very good partial response	Serum and urine M-protein detectable by immunofixation but not on electrophoresis or ≥90% reduction in serum M-protein plus urine M-protein level <100 mg per 24 h
Partial response	≥50% reduction of serum M-protein plus reduction in 24 h urinary M-protein by ≥90% or to <200 mg per 24 h; if the serum and urine M-protein are unmeasurable, a ≥50% decrease in the difference between involved and uninvolved FLC levels is required in place of the M-protein criteria; if serum and urine M-protein are unmeasurable, and serum-free light assay is also unmeasurable, ≥50% reduction in plasma cells is required in place of M-protein, provided baseline bone marrow plasma-cell percentage was ≥30%. In addition to these criteria, if present at baseline, a ≥50% reduction in the size (SPD) of soft tissue plasmacytomas is also required
Minimal response	≥25% but ≤49% reduction of serum M-protein and reduction in 24-h urine M-protein by 50–89%. In addition to the above listed criteria, if present at baseline, a ≥50% reduction in the size (SPD) of soft tissue plasmacytomas is also required
Stable disease	Not recommended for use as an indicator of response; stability of disease is best described by providing the time-to-progression estimates. Not meeting criteria for complete response, very good partial response, partial response, minimal response, or progressive disease
Progressive disease	Any one or more of the following criteria: increase of 25% from lowest confirmed response value in one or more of the following criteria: serum M-protein (absolute increase must be ≥0.5 g/dL); serum M-protein increase ≥1 g/dL, if the lowest M component was ≥5 g/dL; urine M-protein (absolute increase must be ≥200 mg/24 h); in patients without measurable serum and urine M-protein levels, the difference between involved and uninvolved FLC levels (absolute increase must be >10 mg/dL); in patients without measurable serum and urine M-protein levels and without measurable involved FLC levels, bone marrow plasma-cell percentage irrespective of baseline status (absolute increase must be ≥10%); appearance of a new lesion(s), ≥50% increase from nadir in SPD§§ of >1 lesion, or ≥50% increase in the longest diameter of a previous lesion >1 cm in short axis; ≥50% increase in circulating plasma cells (minimum of 200 cells per μL) if this is the only measure of disease
Clinical relapse	Clinical relapse requires one or more of the following criteria: direct indicators of increasing disease and/or end organ dysfunction (CRAB features) related to the underlying clonal plasma-cell proliferative disorder. It is not used in calculation of time to progression or progression-free survival but is listed as something that can be reported optionally or for use in clinical practice; development of new soft tissue plasmacytomas or bone lesions (osteoporotic fractures do not constitute progression); definite increase in the size of existing plasmacytomas or bone lesions. A definite increase is defined as a 50% (and ≥1 cm) increase as measured serially by the SPD§§ of the measurable lesion; hypercalcemia (>11 mg/dL); decrease in hemoglobin of ≥2 g/dL not related to therapy or other non-myeloma-related conditions; rise in serum creatinine by 2 mg/dL or more from the start of the therapy and attributable to myeloma; hyperviscosity related to serum paraprotein
Relapse from complete response (to be used only if the end point is disease-free survival)	Any one or more of the following criteria: reappearance of serum or urine M-protein by immunofixation or electrophoresis; development of ≥5% plasma cells in the bone marrow; appearance of any other sign of progression (i.e. new plasmacytoma, lytic bone lesion, or hypercalcemia, see above)
Relapse from MRD negative (to be used only if the end point is disease-free survival)	Any one or more of the following criteria: loss of MRD-negative state (evidence of clonal plasma cells on NGF or NGS, or positive imaging study for recurrence of myeloma); reappearance of serum or urine M-protein by immunofixation or electrophoresis; development of ≥5% clonal plasma cells in the bone marrow; appearance of any other sign of progression (i.e. new plasmacytoma, lytic bone lesion, or hypercalcemia)

Source: Compiled from Kumar et al., 2016; see Kumar et al., 2016 for practical considerations for application of IMWG consensus criteria.

agents (thalidomide, lenalidomide, pomalidomide), and monoclonal antibodies (daratumumab, elotuzumab) in the past 10 years, the disease remains essentially incurable for the vast majority of patients with a median survival of 4 to 5 years. The disease follows a remitting and relapsing course, most patients responding to initial therapy. For younger, fitter patients this initial therapy is likely to include high-dose therapy supported by autologous stem-cell

transplantation. Several trials have demonstrated the superiority of high-dose over standard-dose chemotherapy even in the modern era in prolonging disease control and survival in younger fitter patients. This response is usually associated with an improvement in quality of life.

There is a move to continuous therapy with continuous use of lenalidomide and daratumumab and a clear benefit in maintenance lenalidomide improving progression-free survival post-transplant.

The duration of response after subsequent lines of therapy is usually shorter than that of the initial remission. There is often increasing morbidity with accumulating treatment and relapses. This manifests as fatigue, infections, worsening cytopenias, renal impairment, and worsening bone disease. Eventually the disease becomes refractory to treatment, and the patient succumbs to infection, renal failure, or other disease complication.

At each relapse, be it first, second, third, etc., a significant proportion of patients fail to have a further line of therapy either at the patient's request and/or due to poor health. In general, healthcare professionals overestimate the proportion of patients who get beyond third or fourth lines of therapy. This is illustrated by Yong et al.[20] who showed that in 2014 only 38% received a third line of treatment and 15% a fourth line.

When to start treatment and criteria for response

Treatment is indicated as defined in Table 31.2 based on myeloma-related organ damage and, since 2014, biomarkers of malignancy that define a group with very high risk of progression (plasma cell infiltrate >60%, high FLC ratio >100, and >2 focal lesions on imaging—see Table 31.2 for greater clarification). These biomarkers were derived based on having an 80% predictive value for disease progressing to organ damage within 2 years and the evidence from one trial showing a survival benefit for intervention for "high-risk" asymptomatic disease (defined differently to IMWG criteria with flow cytometry).[21]

There is no evidence for early treatment of patients with smoldering myeloma outside of a trial. Their rate of progression of smoldering myeloma is around 10% per year for 5 years but then reduces, and clearly a minority behave just as a benign MGUS without progression. They should be followed carefully, with serum protein electrophoresis and serum free light chains every 8 weeks.

A common and difficult clinical decision is when to start treatment in patients with smoldering myeloma and a progressively rising monoclonal protein or serum free light chain. There are no data to help us here and varied expert opinion, but the rate of rise of the monoclonal protein is important. Critically treatment should start before organ damage and hence earlier in patients with a rapidly rising paraprotein. However many patients progress slowly at a rate of say 1 g/L every 3 months, and these patients can often be observed over a prolonged period before needing treatment.

Response criteria

The assessment of disease activity is part of every myeloma patient's care in making treatment decisions and is based on changes in the level of monoclonal protein(s) for the majority of patients with a measurable monoclonal protein. For clinical trials, more accurate assessment of response is critical in assessing treatment efficacy as an end point and is typically defined at a certain time point. Improvements in treatments have led to improved depths of response and an increasing number of patients with a marrow that is minimal residual disease (MRD)-negative, containing less than 1 myeloma cell in 10^5 nucleated cells or higher after induction treatment. The criteria for assessment of response and MRD is defined by the International Myeloma Working Group.[22] See Table 31.5 for the definitions of response and relapse and Kumar

TABLE 31.5 Phase-III Trials for Relapsed or Refractory Multiple Myeloma

	Response Rates	Median PFS
MM-003 (pomalidomide dexamethasone vs. high-dose dexamethasone) San Miguel et al., 2013	31 vs. 10	3.8 vs. 1.9 HR 0.41 (95% CI, 0.32–0.53)
ENDEAVOR (carfilzomib dexamethasone vs. bortezomib dexamethasone) Dimopoulos et al., 2016a	77 vs. 63	18.7 vs. 9.4 HR 0.53 (95% CI, 0.44–0.65)
ASPIRE (carfilzomib lenalidomide dexamethasone vs. lenalidomide dexamethasone) Stewart et al., 2015	87.1 vs. 66.7	26.3 vs. 17.6 HR 0.69 (95% CI, 0.57–0.83)
TOURMALINE MM1 (ixazomib lenalidomide dexamethasone vs. placebo lenalidomide dexamethasone) Moreau et al., 2016	78.3 vs. 71.5	20.6 vs. 14.7 HR 0.74 (95% CI, 0.59–0.94)
CASTOR (daratumumab bortezomib dexamethasone vs. bortezomib dexamethasone) Palumbo et al., 2016	83 vs. 63	16.7 vs. 7.1 HR 0.31 (95% CI, 0.24–0.39)
POLLUX (daratumumab-lenalidomide-dexamethasone vs. lenalidomide-dexamethasone) Dimopoulos et al., 2016a	93% vs. 76%	Not reached at 25 months vs. 17.5 months HR 0.41 (95% CI 0.31–0.53 $p < 0.0001$)
ELOQUENT-2 (elotuzumab lenalidomide dexamethasone vs. lenalidomide dexamethasone) Lonial et al., 2015	79 vs. 66	19.4 vs. 14.9 HR 0.70 (95% CI, 0.57–0.85)

et al.[22] relating to practical considerations. MRD response in particular correlates strongly with longer term outcomes (much better than conventional CR) and is likely to be increasingly used as a primary end point in trials as a surrogate marker of progression-free survival and overall survival. The assessment of MRD is currently performed by one of two technologies, either next-generation flow cytometry or next-generation sequencing of bone marrow. The response criteria also incorporates functional imaging assessments with PET-CT that remain challenging in most healthcare economies, and hence many current trials do not have response by imaging as an end point. Following treatment in the relapsed setting, achieving MRD negativity is less common than after induction, and disparities between imaging and marrow MRD assessment are increasingly seen. Future trials will explore using response criteria, namely MRD responses, to direct treatment decisions, but as yet there is no objective evidence to use MRD response to alter treatment.

General aspects of care

Supportive care plays an increasingly important role in the modern management of multiple myeloma. Modern treatment has significantly improved the outcomes for patients with myeloma through improved disease control. However, the vast majority of patients live with the burden of the disease itself and the cumulative side effects of treatments. Managing symptoms and maintaining quality of life present challenges at all stages of the disease from diagnosis through the multiple phases of active treatment to the end of life.

Hypercalcemia

Hypercalcemia occurs in a minority of myeloma patients and occurs in the presence of active disease. Management requires vigorous rehydration with close monitoring of fluid balance and renal function combined with pamidronate or zoledronate. Urgent treatment of myeloma is required to reverse hypercalcemia, and pulsed dexamethasone is a useful immediate therapy before starting definitive treatment.

Bone disease, spinal disease, and pain control

Immediate anti-myeloma therapy and analgesia often provide relief from localized pain. Non-steroidal anti-inflammatory drugs should be avoided because of the risk of renal toxicity. Patients with severe or progressive bone disease often require opiate analgesia and management of opiate side effects. Optimizing pain relief is a very individual process, and there are a large number of options currently. Access to specialists in pain management is critical in providing optimal pain management for patients with difficult pain-management issues. Amitriptyline or gabapentin may help in neuropathic pain.

Radiotherapy is usually reserved when a focus of pain is not controlled and also post-surgical fixation of a fracture or spinal surgery (usually 8 Gy as a single fraction).

Spinal cord compression is an emergency requiring immediate imaging with an MRI (and often CT scan) and urgent discussion with both a spinal surgeon and radiotherapist. Instability of the spinal column is usually an indication for urgent spinal surgery.

There is a complete lack of adequate randomized trials as to the optimal management of spinal disease including bracing, vertebral augmentation (vertebroplasty and kyphoplasty), and radiotherapy. The issue is further complicated as the nature of the spinal disease (anatomical site, number of vertebrae involved,

and degree of collapse/deformity, for example) is important in treatment decisions.

Anemia

Anemia is present in two-thirds of patients at presentation. It usually improves with response to treatment. EPO is, however, indicated for the treatment of chronic anemia in patients with myeloma with and without chronic renal failure.

Infection

Patients with myeloma are at high risk of infection for a variety of reasons including immune paresis, steroids, neutropenia with advanced disease, and reduced mobility because of skeletal disease. In a large study of early mortality after a diagnosis of multiple myeloma (Augustson et al., 2005), infection and renal failure were found to be the main causes of early death.

Patients should be advised what to do in the event of symptoms of infection, and arrangements should be in place for access to 24-hour specialist team advice. Any infection must be treated promptly and vigorously, and admission for IV antibiotic therapy is usually needed for severe systemic infection.

There are three potential prophylactic options to prevent infection but a lack of data to help guide us:

1. Prophylactic antibiotics: Recommended with active treatment following a large placebo-controlled randomized trial called the TEAMM trial (Drayson et al., *Lancet Oncology* in press) that clearly showed a benefit (reduced infections and hospitalization) for prophylactic levofloxacin over placebo in the first 12 weeks of treatment for patients with newly diagnosed myeloma without increasing hospital-acquired infections (*Clostridium difficile*, MRSA, ESBLs). The TEAMM trial has raised questions around the optimal duration of antibiotics and whether cotrimoxazole and levofloxacin together might be better than a single antibiotic.
2. Vaccination: Vaccination is recommended against influenzae, pneumococcal infection, and possibly other encapsulated bacteria (*Hemophilus*, meningococcus). Timing is important as vaccination is very unlikely to be effective for patients with active disease having treatment. Following autologous transplant vaccination is typically not given until 6 months post-transplant.
3. Certain patients with recurrent infections may benefit from immunoglobulin replacement, but there is lack of data and immunoglobulin is currently a limited and expensive resource.

Myeloma therapy

Choice of initial therapy

The treatment of multiple myeloma has altered dramatically in the last two decades with the introduction of the novel agents with a significant improvement in outcomes.[23] There has also been a move from fixed-duration treatments to continuous therapies with maintenance post-transplant and upfront regimens using continuous lenalidomide and daratumumab until progression.

The choice of initial therapy is determined mainly by a number of factors including the patient's age, frailty, co-morbidities, performance status, renal function, and access to high-cost drugs. These patient factors are important in assessing fitness for later autologous stem-cell transplantation (ASCT). Autografting remains a standard approach in fitter patients typically aged less than 70 as two recent trials still show a benefit for a front-line ASCT compared with a delayed ASCT even in the novel-agent era.[24,25] Only about a third of patients with myeloma receive an ASCT.

Treatment of myeloma has historically always been based on patient factors, and genetic information has largely been ignored in terms of making treatment decisions, although that should change with targeted therapies such as venetoclax. Clearly myeloma is biologically extremely heterogenous with 25% of patients having biologically high-risk disease and poor outcomes. Currently we are able to identify most of the high-risk group at diagnosis now with a combination of FISH and gene expression profiling with the knowledge that standard treatment approaches are less than optimal and novel approaches are needed

A huge issue is the spiraling costs of novel agents and hence a large difference between what is licensed and what is affordable with increasing disparity based on geography and financial status. In the UK, National Institute for Health and Care Excellence (NICE) appraises novel agents and determines access, but this is a slow process and always with very restricted access.

Induction regimens generally involve a combination regimen (most commonly a triplet combination currently, but two to four or more drugs have been used in various combinations) with one to three novel agents, a steroid, and in the UK sometimes a chemotherapy agent (alkylating agent). The optimal induction approach is currently unclear and continues to evolve. If possible, myeloma patients should always be offered clinical trials.

Initial chemotherapy prior to high-dose therapy

For patients where high-dose therapy (HDT) is planned, the aim of initial treatment is to achieve rapid cytoreduction without impairing stem cell mobilization. For transplant-eligible patients, a minimum and maximum number of cycles is usually pre-defined and treatment is continued until maximal response is reached (typically between four and six cycles for a bortezomib triplet regimen). Patients achieving less than a VGPR as maximal response may benefit from an alternative schedule based on the Myeloma XI trial data suggesting a benefit in switching to a bortezomib regimen in patients achieving less than a VGPR following cyclophosphamide–thalidomide–dexamethasone (CTD) or cyclophosphamide–lenalidomide–dexamethasone (CRD) induction.[26] There are a number of regimens as induction before ASCT (Moreau et al.[27] ESMO guidelines for a review), and the current standard is to use a bortezomib-based triplet combination—bortezomib–thalidomide–dexamethasone (VTD), bortezomib–cyclophosphamide–dexamethasone (VCD), and bortezomib–lenalidomide–dexamethasone (VRD). Access to VRD is currently limited for most healthcare systems given its cost but is the preferred regimen in USA given its high response rates and tolerability.[28] VTD shows superior response rates compared to VCD although longer term outcomes are unclear, but VCD is generally less toxic especially as regards neuropathy.[29] Other regimens are being evaluated in trials including carfilzomib and ixazomib combinations and the addition of daratumumab to current regimens. Daratumumab is becoming incorporated into induction regimens given its efficacy, unique mechanism of action, and tolerability much in the same way as monoclonal antibodies are used in B cell lymphomas as chemo-immunotherapy, but cost is a major issue with combinations of expensive agents. For example daratumumab added to bortezomib–thalidomide–dexamethasone improves depth of response and PFS compared to bortezomib–thalidomide–dexamethasone.[30] A subcutaneous form of daratumumab is likely to become available in 2020.

Grade III–IV neuropathy with bortezomib has been significantly reduced by switching from intravenous to subcutaneous injection and a weekly schedule without reduced efficacy. Other side effects with bortezomib include gastrointestinal toxicity, thrombocytopenia, herpes zoster, and hypotension. Both thalidomide and lenalidomide are prothrombotic, and all patients must be assessed for thrombotic risk with a view to starting on appropriate prophylaxis which is typically either prophylactic-dose low-molecular-weight heparin or aspirin. Thalidomide also causes constipation, neuropathy, and somnolence. Lenalidomide although derived from thalidomide does not cause these side effects but does cause fatigue and myelosuppression and requires dose reduction in renal failure. With daratumumab the most common side effect is typically a mild infusional toxicity with the first dose.

As stated above, 25% of myeloma patients fall into a high-risk category with a poor outcome, and management of these patients remains unclear. Intensive regimens such as VTD-PACE are often used in younger patients with clinically aggressive disease, but even with further consolidation or a tandem transplant, durable remissions are rare. The MUK 9b trial is exploring the use of a quintriplet (daratumumab–bortezomib–lenalidomide–cyclophosphamide–dexamethasone) as induction with blocks of consolidation post-transplant followed by maintenance in patients defined as high-risk based on adverse FISH and gene expression profiling.

Initial chemotherapy where HDT is not planned—"conventional therapy"

The aim of therapy in patients not considered candidates for HDT and ASCT on the basis of age, performance status, frailty, and comorbidity is to achieve a prolonged duration of disease control with minimal treatment-related toxicity (Moreau et al.[27] ESMO guidelines for a review). Myeloma predominantly affects an elderly population who are often excluded from clinical trials, and there is less certainty as to the benefit of treatments and their effects on quality of life in this population. Dose reduction is recommended for all regimens especially for dexamethasone as higher doses of steroids are associated with worse overall survival in a frailer, less fit population.[31,32] Conversely a fitter older patient may receive inappropriate dose-reduced treatment based solely on age. Historically assessment of frailty has been assessed on age and a subjective clinician assessment.

Objective scoring systems of fitness have been evaluated retrospectively to estimate prognosis and guide dosing, for example the International Myeloma Working Group score based on age, the Charlson Comorbidity Index, and cognitive and physical conditions (Activities of Daily Living/Instrumental Activities of Daily Living).[33,34]

There are currently two popular widely available regimens used for this older less fit population, namely bortezomib–melphalan–prednisolone (VMP) based on the VISTA trial[35] and lenalidomide–low-dose dexamethasone (Rd) based on the FIRST trial.[36] VMP is given for a fixed duration as per the VISTA trial but, unlike the trial, bortezomib is administered once weekly and subcutaneously. Bortezomib–lenalidomide–dexamethasone (VRD) is clearly superior to Len-Dex in the SWOG trial and is an attractive regimen.[28] Therefore first-choice regimens are currently VRD if available and if not VMP or Rd. There is some evidence to support using bortezomib regimens for genetically high risk disease over an immunomodulatory regimen. There are data accumulating that are likely to lead to incorporation of daratumumab into these current regimens in the near future with daratumumab being given until progression, but access will be difficult for most healthcare economies due to cost. The ALCYONE trial in particular shows impressive results for the addition of daratumumab to VMP[37] and the MAIA trial showed a significant improvement for lenalidomide–dexamethasone–daratumumab compared to lenalidomide–dexamethasone.[38] Bortezomib–cyclophosphamide–dexamethasone (VCD) is another regimen that is widely used. There are other regimens that are approved including CTD, MPT, MPR, and bendamustine plus prednisolone, but these are not first-choice regimens. There is a lack of data around genetic subtypes to inform us as to more tailored approaches according to tumor biology, and high-risk patients perform poorly with standard approaches.

Treatment with renal failure

Renal failure due to cast nephropathy is an emergency requiring vigorous hydration and immediate anti-myeloma treatment following diagnosis. Dexamethasone is often used to immediately reduce myeloma tumor burden. Definitive treatment in this setting is usually with a bortezomib-based regimen such as bortezomib–cyclophosphamide–dexamethasone (VCD) and can reverse renal failure in a majority of patients.[17] There is no benefit for early plasmapheresis, and two trials using high cut-off membrane for hemodialysis designed to efficiently remove serum light chains show conflicting results, and hence this cannot be recommended. In some patients renal function recovers as the disease responds to treatment, but in around 10% of patients long-term dialysis may be needed.

High-dose therapy and stem-cell transplantation

Autologous transplantation

High-dose therapy with stem cell support is still standard of care for younger patients with multiple myeloma following induction therapy for patients up to at least the age of 65–70 years and many patients above this age are suitable. The most widely accepted conditioning regimen for high-dose therapy in the treatment of myeloma is melphalan 200 mg/m². A dose of 140 mg/m² should also be considered for patients where fitness is a concern and with renal failure.

The median duration of PFS is around 30 months in most series, but maintenance lenalidomide can extend this by over 2 years, and those who achieve MRD negativity post-transplant may have a very long PFS. The mortality is 3%, but there is a significant morbidity with fatigue, infection, and gut toxicity. The benefit of autologous transplantation was established in the era of conventional chemotherapy, but two recent trials still show a benefit for a front-line ASCT compared with a delayed ASCT using VRD induction.[24,25]

Double or second autologous transplantation

A double (tandem) autograft represents a means of attempting to deliver more effective eradication of endogenous disease. This approach has been pioneered by the Little Rock group[39] and the French IFM group.[40]

A more popular approach has been to collect sufficient stem cells to carry out two procedures but to defer the second transplant and consider this as an option at relapse. The Myeloma X trial shows a clear benefit for a second autologous transplant for patients who have a long PFS following a first procedure.[41]

Allogeneic stem-cell transplantation

Only approximately 50 allogenic transplants for patients with myeloma are performed in the UK a year, indicating that it is rarely recommended due to the high transplant-related mortality (TRM), significant relapse rate, and any graft-versus-myeloma effect typically accompanied by graft-versus-host disease. The normal setting is at relapse with reinduction treatment with a second autologous transplant followed by a planned reduced-intensity allogeneic transplant 3 months later (related or unrelated matched donor).

There is no benefit for patients with progressive disease/refractory disease, and there is therefore a small number of patients where the benefit of the procedure may justify such risks.

Trials approaches to potentiate graft versus myeloma rather than GVHD are needed but so far lenalidomide maintenance has proved toxic with increased GVHD.

DLI is an option in patients relapsing post-allogeneic transplant providing disease control is regained and GVHD has not previously been an issue.

Maintenance and consolidation therapy

The benefit of lenalidomide maintenance after an autologous stem-cell transplant has been confirmed by a number of pivotal phase III trials[42,43] with a dramatic improvement in PFS of over 2 years post-transplant and also a survival benefit in this setting. There is also a clear improvement for using lenalidomide as a continuous therapy as lenalidomide–dexamethasone in patients not receiving an ASCT as shown by the FIRST trial[36] and as a maintenance in Myeloma XI[43] with a marked improvement in PFS although the benefit for OS is less clear.

There was an initial concern regarding an increased risk of a secondary primary malignancy for patients on long-term lenalidomide, but it appears that this risk is low compared to the potential benefit in terms of anti-myeloma effects.

Ixazomib maintenance as a weekly tablet also improves PFS compared to placebo although this is likely inferior to lenalidomide maintenance.[44] Maintenance strategies with daratumumab will become more attractive once daratumumab hopefully moves to a subcutaneous route.

A number of consolidation approaches have also been used with conflicting results and may be most relevant for patients who have not have a deep response, although this is unproven.

MRD negativity post-transplant or induction therapy is powerfully prognostic,[45] and there are ongoing trials that will look at tailoring maintenance according to the MRD result. Some caution is needed as, in the Myeloma XI, patients who were MRD negative still benefited from being on lenalidomide maintenance.

Bisphosphonates

Bisphosphonates, which act by inhibiting osteoclast-mediated bone resorption, are a standard of care for all myeloma patients for bone protection and are the treatment of choice for hypercalcemia.

Zoledronic acid given 4 weekly indefinitely is superior to sodium clodronate in the reduction of skeletal-related events with improvement in OS and PFS.[46] Prophylactic bisphosphonates reduce the extent of skeletal disease in asymptomatic patients but are not generally given. Prolonged administration of zoledronate can cause the development of osteonecrosis of the jaw (ONJ) in approximately 4% of patients. Dental problems should be addressed at an early opportunity, and care should be taken in patients with renal dysfunction.

There is uncertainty as to what is the optimal frequency and duration for zoledronate, but it can be given 4 weekly for 2 years and stopped providing patient is in a stable remission and restarted at relapse.

Denosumab is a RANKL inhibitor given as a 4 weekly subcutaneously injection and, unlike zoledronate, it can be given in advanced renal failure and is non-inferior in terms of bone-related events.[47]

Research continues to look at combining anti-resorptive drugs (zoledronate and denosumab) with anabolic agents that promote osteoblast activity and new bone formation.

Relapsed disease

Relapsed myeloma

All patients with myeloma will relapse after the last line of therapy, and a number of factors needed to be considered in deciding the next line of therapy.

The most important factors are the previous treatments, responsiveness and duration of response to previous agents, the tolerability and toxicity with previous agents, and the fitness and wishes of the patient. Restricted access to novel drugs due to financial restraints is also a major issue. Clinical trial options are important, and awareness of suitable trials is essential for relapsed patients. At relapse patients often show signs of a rising M-protein and/or rising sFLC before the onset of new organ damage, and decisions around the timing of treatment in this context can be difficult although a period of observation is usually safe if the patient is asymptomatic. The rate of rise of the M protein or sFLC and previous critical organ damage are factors to consider.

In the current era increasing numbers of patients are having multiple lines of therapies. There has been a marked increase in patients relapsing with focal or extramedullary disease. Patients often develop chronic toxicities from both treatment and the disease, in particular poor marrow function, fatigue, neuropathy, renal impairment, and bone disease. Refractory disease is common in the setting of heavily treated patients.

The data of Yong et al.[20] showed a significant failure of patients to proceed to the next line of therapy with each progression with only 14% of patients in that study receiving fourth line.

There are a large number of phase III studies in the relapsed setting comparing a novel agent added to lenalidomide–dexamethasone or a bortezomib–dexamethasone backbone as a triplet compared to the standard doublet of lenalidomide–dexamethasone or bortezomib–dexamethasone that all show a benefit for a triplet combination. However, this benefit is less clear for an elderly, frailer population where dose reductions are necessary. These studies are outlined in Table 31.5.[48–54] Although cross-trial comparison should be avoided, daratumumab–lenalidomide–dexamethasone has the most striking results in terms of response, MRD negativity (up to 25%), and PFS.[48]

For relapse an alternative novel agent combination is considered if available. It is possible that patients can respond to a previous line of therapy if they were not refractory, and sometimes combining a new agent with a previous regimen can overcome refractoriness, but ideally an alternative agent combination should be used. As novel treatment therapies move increasingly to the front-line setting this greatly alters treatment setting for relapsed disease. Drugs used in the relapsed setting include daratumumab combinations (daratumumab–lenalidomide–dexamethasone, daratumumab–bortezomib–dexamethasone), pomalidomide combinations (pomalidomide–dexamethasone backbone plus cyclophosphamide, a monoclonal antibody [daratumumab or elotuzumab], or a proteasome inhibitor [ixazomib, bortezomib, or

carfilzomib]), ixazomib–lenalidomide–dexamethasone, carfilzomib combinations (carfilzomib–lenalidomide–dexamethasone), elotuzumab–lenalidomide–dexamethasone, and bortezomib–panobinostat–dexamethasone. In the future daratumumab is likely to move to become a first-line therapy, and increasing numbers of patients will be relapsing after a bortezomib–lenalidomide induction regimen. A second autologous transplant is recommended for fitter patients who have a PFS of 2 years following the first autologous transplant[41] and should be considered in patients with a shorter PFS of 1–2 years but is not recommended if the PFS is less than a year.

Patients who are refractory to both bortezomib and the immunomodulatory agents have a poor prognosis with a median survival of around a year. Most myeloma experts favor a more intensive approach upfront incorporating most of these agents with a view to maximizing the first response duration as long as possible, but management of relapse in this setting is extremely challenging.

New approaches to treatment

There are a large number of promising novel agents in multiple myeloma. The nature of end-stage patients has progressively changed to an increasingly frail, comorbid, and treatment refractory population. This is challenging as early-phase trials in such patients are increasingly less likely to detect any efficacy signature, and toxicity from treatment is difficult to distinguish from the effects of disease.

Isatuximab is an alternative anti-CD 38 monoclonal antibody in study.

Ventoclax is a bcl-2 inhibitor that has shown significant efficacy as a single agent in patients with the t(11;14) translocation, but toxicity is possibly an issue in combination studies in relapsed patients.

Selinexor is a nuclear transport inhibitor which is being studied in a large phase III trial with bortezomib–dexamethasone as a backbone.

The PD-1/PD-L1 inhibitor trials have used a PD-1 inhibitor in combination with bortezomib but have been associated with a toxicity signal.

Promising new agents are the anti-BCMA antibodies directed against B cell maturation antigen (BCMA). These include conjugated antibodies and also BITE antibodies that bind CD3 on T cells. BITE antibodies have a short half-life so have to be given continuously and can cause a cytokine release syndrome.

CAR T cell studies have also been using BCMA as a target. Despite impressive response rates of over 80%, the progression-free interval has been disappointing in a heavily treated refractory population. Toxicity is also an issue with cytokine release syndrome and neurological toxicity. The optimal timing for CAR T cell studies is unclear but unlikely to be end-stage refractory disease. Ultimately combination approaches are likely to be required to maximize immunotherapy approaches especially given the hostile immune microenvironment in myeloma.

Key learning points

- Myeloma is characterized by periods of remission and relapses and eventually becomes resistant to treatment. Ten percent of patients die in the first 60 days, 15% live over 10 years, and median survival is now around 5 years.

- The classical presenting features are bone pain, anemia, infection, and renal impairment. Diagnosis is often delayed due to the non-specific symptoms and uncommonness of the condition.
- Whole-body MRI, low-dose CT scan, and PET-CT are better at detecting bone disease than plain radiography.
- A serum paraprotein is present in 80% of cases, 20% free light chains only, and 1% of cases are non-secretory.
- The most important prognostic factors are patient fitness and the presence of adverse genetic abnormalities including gene expression profiling. B2-microglobulin, albumin, and LDH are incorporated with adverse genetics into the revised ISS.
- The novel agents proteasome inhibitors, immunomodulatory drugs, and monoclonal antibodies have dramatically altered the treatment of multiple myeloma with an improvement in survival. The optimal induction regimen is currently unclear but a triplet/quadruplet combination, using a combination of novel agents and a steroid, is common. It is likely that these regimens will evolve to incorporate monoclonal antibodies. Access to high-cost novel drugs is restricted and challenging in most countries, greatly limiting access.
  - The main decision is to assess whether the patient may be suitable for an intensive pathway with induction followed by an autologous transplant.
  - Autologous transplantation remains a standard treatment for younger patients aged <70 years.
  - Elderly patients need to be accurately assessed for frailty and comorbidities and treatment reduced accordingly to avoid toxicities.
- All patients with symptomatic myeloma should receive a bisphosphonate and ideally this should be zoledronate.
- There is a move to continuous therapies. Maintenance therapy is clearly beneficial with several trials showing a dramatic improvement in PFS with lenalidomide.
- Allogeneic transplantation is contentious, rarely performed as it has a high mortality rate, and is ineffective with aggressive poorly controlled disease.
- The choice of treatment of relapsed disease depends on previous therapies, duration of responses, previous toxicities, patient wishes, and availability of novel agents.
- With increasing treatment options, patients have increasing long-term toxicity and effects from repeated lines of treatment and myeloma-related complications.

References

1. Waxman AJ, Mink PJ, Devesa SS et al. Racial disparities in incidence and outcome in multiple myeloma: A population-based study. *Blood*. 2010; 116(25):5501–6.
2. Landgren O, Kyle RA, Pfeiffer RM, Katzmann JA, Caporaso NE, Hayes RB, Dispenzieri A, Kumar S, Clark RJ, Baris D, Hoover R. Monoclonal gammopathy of undetermined significance (MGUS) consistently precedes multiple myeloma: a prospective study. *Blood*. 2009; 113(22):5412–7.
3. Weiss BM, Abadie J, Verma P et al. A monoclonal gammopathy precedes multiple myeloma in most patients. *Blood*. 2009; 113(22):5418–22.
4. Mouhieddine TH, Weeks LD, Ghobrial IM. Monoclonal gammopathy of undetermined significance. *Blood*. 2019; 133(23):2484–94.
5. Rajkumar SV, Kyle RA, Therneau TM et al. Serum free light chain ratio is an independent risk factor for progression in monoclonal gammopathy of undetermined significance. *Blood*. 2005; 106, 812–817.
6. Fermand JP, Bridoux F, Dispenzieri A et al. Monoclonal gammopathy of clinical significance: A novel concept with therapeutic implications. *Blood*. 2018; 132(14):1478–1485.
7. Kawano Y, Moschetta M, Manier S et al. Targeting the bone marrow microenvironment in multiple myeloma. *Immunol Rev*. 2015; 263(1):160–72.
8. Walker RE, Lawson MA, Buckle CH et al. Myeloma bone disease: Pathogenesis, current treatments and future targets. *Br Med Bull*. 2014; 111(1):117–38.
9. Pratt G, Goodyear O, Moss P. Immunodeficiency and immunotherapy in multiple myeloma. *Br J Haematol*. 2007; 138(5):563–79.
10. Augustson BM, Begum G, Dunn JA et al. Early mortality after diagnosis of multiple myeloma: Analysis of patients entered onto the United Kingdom Medical Research Council trials between 1980 and 2002–Medical Research Council Adult Leukaemia Working Party. *J Clin Oncol*. 2005 Dec 20;23(36):9219–26.
11. Robiou du Pont S, Cleynen A, Fontan C et al. Genomics of multiple myeloma. *J Clin Oncol*. 2017 Mar 20;35(9):963–7.
12. Hoang PH, Houlston RS. Multiple mechanisms can disrupt oncogenic pathways in multiple myeloma. *Oncotarget*. 2018; 9(88):35801–2
13. Ledergor G, Weiner A, Zada M et al. Single cell dissection of plasma cell heterogeneity in symptomatic and asymptomatic myeloma. *Nat Med*. 2018; 24(12):1867–76.
14. Lyratzopoulos G, Neal RD, Barbiere JM et al. Variation in number of general practitioner consultations before hospital referral for cancer: Findings from the 2010 National Cancer Patient Experience Survey in England. *Lancet Oncol*. 2012; 13(4):353–65.
15. Rajkumar SV, Dimopoulos MA, Palumbo A et al. International Myeloma Working Group updated criteria for the diagnosis of multiple myeloma. *Lancet Oncol*. 2014; 15(12):e538–48.
16. Chantry A, Kazmi M, Barrington S et al. Guidelines for the use of imaging in the management of patients with myeloma. *Br J Haematol*. 2017; 178(3):380–93.
17. Hutchison CA, Cockwell P, Moroz V et al. High cutoff versus high-flux haemodialysis for myeloma cast nephropathy in patients receiving bortezomib-based chemotherapy (EuLITE): A phase 2 randomised controlled trial. *Lancet Haematol*. 2019; 6(4):e217–28.
18. Bridoux F, Carron PL, Pegourie B et al. Effect of high-cutoff hemodialysis vs. conventional hemodialysis on hemodialysis independence among patients with myeloma cast nephropathy: A randomized clinical trial. *JAMA*. 2017; 318(21):2099–110.
19. Palumbo A, Avet-Loiseau H, Oliva S et al. Revised international staging system for multiple myeloma: A report from International Myeloma Working Group. *J Clin Oncol*. 2015; 33(26):2863–9.
20. Yong K, Delforge M, Driessen C et al. Multiple myeloma: Patient outcomes in real-world practice. *Br J Haematol*. 2016; 175(2):252–64.
21. Mateos MV, Hernández MT, Giraldo P et al. Lenalidomide plus dexamethasone for high-risk smoldering multiple myeloma. *N Engl J Med*. 2013; 369(5):438–47.
22. Kumar S, Paiva B, Anderson KC et al. International Myeloma Working Group consensus criteria for response and minimal residual disease assessment in multiple myeloma. *Lancet Oncol*. 2016; 17(8):e328–46.
23. Kumar SK, Dispenzieri A, Lacy MQ et al. Continued improvement in survival in multiple myeloma: Changes in early mortality and outcomes in older patients. *Leukemia*. 2014; 28(5):1122–8.
24. Cavo M, Palumbo A, Zweegman S et al. Upfront autologous stem cell transplantation (ASCT) versus novel agent-based therapy for multiple myeloma (MM): A randomized phase 3 study of the European Myeloma Network (EMN02/HO95MMtrial). *J Clin Oncol*. 2016; 34(Suppl):abstr.8000.
25. Attal M, Lauwers-Cances V, Hulin C et al. Lenalidomide, bortezomib, and dexamethasone with transplantation for myeloma. *N Engl J Med*. 2017; 376(14):1311–20.
26. Pawlyn C, Jackson GH, Cairns D et al. Maximizing pre-transplant response is associated with improved outcome for myeloma patients: Exploratory analysis of the myeloma XI trial. *Blood*. 2018; 132:3280
27. Moreau P, San Miguel J, Sonneveld P et al. Multiple myeloma: ESMO Clinical Practice Guidelines for diagnosis, treatment and follow-up. *Ann Oncol*. 2017; 28(suppl_4):iv52–61.

28. Durie BG, Hoering A, Abidi MH et al. Bortezomib with lenalidomide and dexamethasone versus lenalidomide and dexamethasone alone in patients with newly diagnosed myeloma without intent for immediate autologous stem-cell transplant (SWOG S0777): A randomised, openlabel, phase 3 trial. *Lancet.* 2017; 389:519–527.

29. Moreau P, Hulin C, Macro M et al. VTD is superior to VCD prior to intensive therapy in multiple myeloma: Results of the prospective IFM2013-04 trial. *Blood.* 2016; 127:2569–74.

30. Moreau P, Attal M, Hulin C et al. Bortezomib, thalidomide, and dexamethasone with or without daratumumab before and after autologous stem-cell transplantation for newly diagnosed multiple myeloma (CASSIOPEIA): A randomised, open-label, phase 3 study. *Lancet.* 2019; 394(10192):29–38.

31. Rajkumar SV, Jacobus S, Callander NS et al. Lenalidomide plus high-dose dexamethasone versus lenalidomide plus low-dose dexamethasone as initial therapy for newly diagnosed multiple myeloma: An open-label randomised controlled trial. *Lancet Oncol.* 2010; 11(1):29–37.

32. Bringhen S, Mateos MV, Zweegman S et al. Age and organ damage correlate with poor survival in myeloma patients: Meta-analysis of 1435 individual patient data from 4 randomized trials. *Haematologica.* 2013; 98(6):980–7.

33. Palumbo A, Bringhen S, Mateos MV et al. Geriatric assessment predicts survival and toxicities in elderly myeloma patients: An International Myeloma Working Group report. *Blood.* 2015; 125(13):2068–74.

34. Zweegman S, Palumbo A, Bringhen S, Sonneveld P. Age and aging in blood disorders: Multiple myeloma. *Haematologica.* 2014; 99(7):1133–7.

35. San Miguel JF, Schlag R, Khuageva NK et al. Persistent overall survival benefit and no increased risk of second malignancies with bortezomib-melphalan-prednisone versus melphalan-prednisone in patients with previously untreated multiple myeloma. *J Clin Oncol.* 2013; 31(4):448–55.

36. Facon T, Dimopoulos MA, Dispenzieri A et al. Final analysis of survival outcomes in the phase 3 FIRST trial of up-front treatment for multiple myeloma. *Blood.* 2018; 131(3):301–10.

37. Mateos MV, Dimopoulos MA, Cavo M et al. Daratumumab plus bortezomib, melphalan, and prednisone for untreated myeloma. *N Engl J Med.* 2018; 378(6):518–28.

38. Facon T, Kumar S, Plesner T et al. Daratumumab plus lenalidomide and dexamethasone for untreated myeloma. *N Engl J Med.* 2019; 380(22):2104–15.

39. Barlogie B, Jagannath S, Desikan KR et al. Total therapy with tandem transplants for newly diagnosed multiple myeloma. *Blood.* 1999; 93:55–65.

40. Attal M, Harousseau JL, Facon T et al. InterGroupe Francophone du Myelome. Single versus double autologous stem-cell transplantation for multiple myeloma. *N Engl J Med.* 2003; 349(26):2495–502.

41. Cook G, Ashcroft AJ, Cairns DA et al. The effect of salvage autologous stem-cell transplantation on overall survival in patients with relapsed multiple myeloma (final results from BSBMT/UKMF Myeloma X Relapse [Intensive]): A randomised, open-label, phase 3 trial. *Lancet Haematol.* 2016; 3(7):e340–51.

42. McCarthy PL, Holstein SA, Petrucci MT et al. Lenalidomide maintenance after autologous stem-cell transplantation in newly diagnosed multiple myeloma: A meta-analysis. *J Clin Oncol.* 2017; 35(29):3279–89.

43. Jackson GH, Davies FE, Pawlyn C et al. Lenalidomide maintenance versus observation for patients with newly diagnosed multiple myeloma (Myeloma XI): A multicentre, open-label, randomised, phase 3 trial. *Lancet Oncol.* 2019; 20(1):57–73.

44. Dimopoulos MA, Gay F, Schjesvold F et al. Oral ixazomib maintenance following autologous stem cell transplantation (TOURMALINE-MM3): A double-blind, randomised, placebo-controlled phase 3 trial. *Lancet.* 2019; 393(10168):253–64.

45. Munshi NC, Avet-Loiseau H, Rawstron AC et al. Association of minimal residual disease with superior survival outcomes in patients with multiple myeloma: A meta-analysis. *JAMA Oncol.* 2017; 3(1):28–35.

46. Morgan GJ, Child JA, Gregory WM et al. Effects of zoledronic acid versus clodronic acid on skeletal morbidity in patients with newly diagnosed multiple myeloma (MRC Myeloma IX): Secondary outcomes from a randomised controlled trial. *Lancet Oncol.* 2011; 12(8):743–52.

47. Raje N, Terpos E, Willenbacher W, Shimizu K et al. Denosumab versus zoledronic acid in bone disease treatment of newly diagnosed multiple myeloma: An international, double-blind, double-dummy, randomised, controlled, phase 3 study. *Lancet Oncol.* 2018; 19(3):370–81.

48. Dimopoulos MA, Oriol A, Nahi H et al. Daratumumab, lenalidomide, and dexamethasone for multiple myeloma. *N Engl J Med.* 2016; 375:1319–31.

49. Stewart AK, Rajkumar SV, Dimopoulos MA et al. Carfilzomib, lenalidomide, and dexamethasone for relapsed multiple myeloma. *N Engl J Med.* 2015; 372(2):142–152.

50. Moreau P, Masszi T, Grzasko N et al. Oral ixazomib, lenalidomide, and dexamethasone for multiple myeloma. *N Engl J Med.* 2016; 374(17):1621–34

51. Lonial S, Dimopoulos M, Palumbo A et al. Elotuzumab therapy for relapsed or refractory multiple myeloma. *N Engl J Med.* 2015; 373:621–31.

52. Palumbo A, Chanan-Khan A, Weisel K et al. Daratumumab, bortezomib, and dexamethasone for multiple myeloma. *N Engl J Med.* 2016; 375:754–66.

53. San Miguel J, Weisel K, Moreau P et al. Pomalidomide plus low-dose dexamethasone versus high-dose dexamethasone alone for patients with relapsed and refractory multiple myeloma (MM-003): A randomised, open-label, phase 3 trial. *Lancet Oncol.* 2013; 14:1055–66.

54. Dimopoulos MA, Moreau P, Palumbo A et al. Carfilzomib and dexamethasone versus bortezomib and dexamethasone for patients with relapsed or refractory multiple myeloma (ENDEAVOR): A randomised, phase 3, open-label, multicentre study. *Lancet Oncol.* 2016; 17:27–38.

32 PEDIATRIC ONCOLOGY

Stephen Lowis, Rachel Cox, John Moppett, and Helen Rees

General introduction

Children with malignant disease are numerically few, but cancer is the second most common cause of death in childhood, and many children cured of their disease are left with significant problems which have effects throughout their lives. A diagnosis of malignancy affects parents, siblings, and the extended family more directly than for an adult patient, and for this reason, care for the family unit has been central to pediatric oncology practice for many years.

Most pediatric tumors differ from "adult-type" tumors, being principally of mesenchymal origin (leukemias, sarcomas, "blastomas") rather than carcinomas. They are typically chemosensitive, and a greater emphasis on chemotherapy has developed because of this. The adverse effects of radiotherapy on developing tissues, which may be profound, have further encouraged the development of strategies which minimize dose and field of radiation, and for many, it has been possible to avoid radiotherapy entirely.

Chemotherapy regimens for children are intensive and lead to many acute complications. Supportive care for these patients represents a major component of overall management, such that inpatient oncology beds represent a disproportionately large part of acute pediatric beds in most large hospitals. The loss of expected years of healthy life in a patient who is not cured, or cured with disability is greater for children: viewed in these terms, the numerical imbalance between adult and pediatric oncology is to some extent redressed.

Meaningful information regarding management requires multicenter collaborative approaches, and it has long been accepted that all patients should be treated according to clinical trials wherever possible. There has been a progressive improvement in survival for most cancers and a monitored and coherent treatment strategy for treatment.

There is evidence too that young adult patients with "pediatric"-type tumors benefit from a pediatric approach. The borders between adult and pediatric patients are increasingly blurred, and a new specialty of adolescent or young adult oncology has grown.

Epidemiology

The total incidence of childhood cancer is 1% of that of the adult population. The total age-standardized annual incidence of childhood cancer in the United Kingdom is 118.3 per million, with a risk of developing a malignancy of 1 in 581.[1] In the pediatric setting, the most frequently encountered diagnostic tumor groups are acute leukemia, central nervous system tumors, lymphomas, and soft tissue sarcomas.

Incidence varies between countries and racial groups.[2] For acute lymphoblastic leukemia, CNS tumors, and neuroblastoma, higher rates are found in western Europe and the USA than Africa and Asia. Overall, childhood cancer is more common in boys than girls.

Childhood leukemia

Leukemia accounts for approximately one-third of all cases of malignancy in childhood (80% acute lymphoblastic leukemia [ALL], 15% acute myeloid leukemia [AML], with the remainder comprising chronic myeloid leukemia [CML], stem cell, and acute leukemias of ambiguous lineage [ALAL]). In the vast majority of cases a complete remission can be achieved, but a substantial number will at some stage relapse, and around 25% of patients ultimately die of their disease. Much has been learnt in recent years regarding specific prognostic features, and treatment protocols now reflect this by incorporating different strategies for different risk groups. For some patients this will mean an increase in intensity of treatment in an attempt to achieve cure, but for many the outlook is now so good that a reduction in treatment (and, hopefully, toxicity) is the goal.

Acute lymphoblastic leukemia

One in 2000 individuals in Europe and the USA will develop ALL before the age of 15 years making it the single commonest cancer in childhood. There is a marked peak in incidence (up to 10 per 100,000) between the ages of 2 and 6 years, which is more noticeable within affluent societies.

Children with certain congenital chromosomal abnormalities, or abnormalities of DNA repair or immune regulation, have a notably higher risk of developing ALL—for example Down syndrome, Fanconi anemia, and Wiskott–Aldrich syndrome. There is an increasing recognition of the role of underlying predisposition syndromes and single nucleotide polymorphisms in the etiology of ALL.

Diagnosis, classification, and molecular biology

Immunophenotyping by multi-parameter flow cytometry of bone marrow is standard practice for the diagnosis of all leukemias including ALL. Precursor B-cell (85%) and T-cell (10%) comprise the vast majority of childhood ALL. Conventional cytogenetic analysis using karyotyping and FISH are typically performed at presentation as they potentially add critical prognostic information. In recent years there has been an explosion in the information provided by molecular genetic studies including gene expression profiling, MLPA, whole-genome sequencing, and RNASeq which have significantly improved our understanding of the origins and, it is hoped, the treatment of ALL.[3] Some of these newer genetic lesions have prognostic significance, as do certain gene expression profiles ("BCR-ABL-like"). The ABL-class lesions (e.g. EBF1-PDGFRB) that are found in many of these BCR-ABL-like cases represent potentially exciting druggable targets.[4]

Treatment

Children with ALL are typically treated in multicenter national and international trials. Treatment is risk-stratified according to both fixed (age and white cell count at diagnosis, sex, presence or absence of CNS disease, immunophenotype, cytogenetic abnormalities) and dynamic (early response to treatment and measurable residual disease [see below]) factors. Treatment in general consists of a three to four-drug induction phase (vincristine, steroid [dexamethasone or prednisolone], asparaginase, and anthracycline) lasting 4–5 weeks, one or more post-remission consolidation or intensification blocks followed by oral maintenance therapy with 6-mercaptopurine and methotrexate for up to 2–3 years.

The introduction of prophylactic cranial radiotherapy in the 1960s led to a dramatic reduction in the CNS relapse rate (previously over 60%), and the regular use of intrathecal methotrexate, with or without systemic high-dose methotrexate and cytarabine, has further reduced the incidence to below 5%. Cranial radiotherapy has been shown to be no more effective than intrathecal and high-dose systemic chemotherapy for CNS prophylaxis.[5] Because of this, as well as its significant neurotoxicity in young children, it is increasingly being removed from up-front treatment protocols.

The value of post-remission intensification blocks was first recognized by the Berlin–Frankfurt–Munster (BFM) group in the 1970s. Since then many studies have examined the optimum number and composition of these blocks. Whilst it remains clear that high-risk patients benefit from one or more of these, it is apparent that a substantial number of patients are currently being overtreated. For example, in the MRC UKALL VIII trial, 50% of children were cured without any delayed intensifications at all.[6] The recent aim has therefore been to identify those patients who genuinely require post-remission intensification, and to stratify therapy accordingly.

Incremental improvements through each generation of trials have led to an ever-improving prognosis for childhood ALL, with over 90% of children being cured on contemporary clinical trials. Attention is therefore increasingly turning to reducing the treatment burden.[7,8]

Measurable residual disease

It has been known for many years that early response to treatment as assessed by standard morphological techniques has prognostic value and has been used to stratify therapy. However, because most patients do respond quickly to treatment and have no other adverse risk factors, the majority of relapses (in absolute numbers) occur in the good-risk group. A more accurate predictor of relapse was therefore required.

Over the last decades techniques have been developed to measure submicroscopic levels of the leukemic clones, namely flow cytometry of their specific constellation of CD antigens and PCR detection of their known gene rearrangements. These techniques can monitor the malignant clone down to a level of 1 in 10^4–10^5 cells and have now proved powerful in predicting outcome. Intervention on the basis of MRD has been shown to both safely enable treatment reduction for those who are at lowest risk of relapse and that treatment intensification targeted on the basis of high-level MRD can improve outcome. Further developments in MRD technology may enable even lower risk groups to be identified. It is clear that genetics and MRD interact, such that MRD thresholds for the intensification or de-intensification of therapy need to be genetic subtype–specific.[9] Future clinical studies will therefore increasingly focus on reducing the burden and toxicity of treatment in children defined as low-risk by MRD whilst simultaneously targeting treatment intensification to those at highest risk of relapse.

Ph+ ALL

Until recently, Philadelphia-positive ALL was considered a very high-risk disease, with most patients proceeding to bone marrow transplant if a suitable donor could be found. However, studies have recently shown that the addition of the tyrosine kinase inhibitor imatinib to conventional chemotherapy can radically improve the prognosis of these cases.[10] Bone marrow transplant is increasingly being restricted to those who are poor responders

as assessed by MRD analysis. Ongoing studies are looking at the role of newer tyrosine kinase inhibitors to further improve the prognosis.

Relapse

The relapse rate in childhood ALL has fallen considerably over recent years and is now approximately 10–15%. There has been a particularly marked fall in bone marrow relapse, whilst there has been less significant progress on the incidence of CNS relapse, such that more than half of relapses now involve the CNS. The prognosis for relapsed patients is hugely variable and is dependent on the length of first remission, the site of relapse, and the disease lineage. Therefore, risk groups have also been constructed within patients who relapse, in an attempt to optimize salvage therapy. Treatment begins in all patients with reinduction chemotherapy, which tends to be more intensive than at diagnosis (and therefore more toxic). This is followed by consolidation, then maintenance chemotherapy in the case of low-risk patients as defined by site and time to relapse, and MRD and allogeneic stem cell transplantation for high-risk patients. Cranial radiotherapy is administered for CNS disease following consolidation if not previously given. Survivals in excess of 60% can be achieved with modern relapse protocols. Relapse studies provide an ideal structure in which to test novel agents (see below).

Role of stem cell transplantation

Allogeneic stem cell transplantation is indicated in a small group of patients (~4–5% of cases) in first complete remission who have a very poor prognosis with chemotherapy alone based on high MRD at end of induction. In addition, patients who relapse with high-risk features benefit from receiving an allogeneic transplant in CR2. There is no evidence for the benefit of autologous stem cell transplantation, and this is no longer routinely performed. Despite the use of allogeneic transplant, the prognosis for very early relapse of ALL remains dismal.

Novel immunotherapies

The dramatic increase in overall survival for children with ALL over the past 30 years has been due to established drugs being used in more effective ways on standardized protocols with improved supportive care. However, several new immunotherapeutics are now becoming available for use in pediatric ALL.

Blinatumomab is a bi-specific antibody with specificity for both CD19 (on B-cells) and CD3 (on T-cells). It functions to trigger a host T-cell mediated immune response against B-cells, including malignant B-cells. There has been promising evidence of efficacy, along with clear evidence of low toxicity in studies of relapsed ALL in both adults and children. In this context blinatumomab is being used as a bridge to transplant. Blinatumomab is also being studied in first-line therapy for high-risk cases as an addition to conventional chemotherapy or as a replacement for the very intensive high-risk chemotherapy blocks that are used for the highest risk patients.[11]

Inotuzumab is an antibody to CD22 (also on B-cells), covalently linked to a toxin called calicheamicin. Adult studies in relapsed refractory patients have shown very encouraging results, though there is some risk of veno-occlusive disease if followed by bone marrow transplantation. Pediatric early phase trials are ongoing.

Chimeric antigen receptor T-cells

Chimeric antigen T-cells (CarT) are T-cells engineered to express a T-cell receptor with specificity for an antigen of choice expressed on the target cell. In ALL the commonest target has been CD19, though CD22 has also been used and other targets are in development. The T-cells are most commonly autologous though allogeneic CarT have also been developed. The artificial engineered DNA construct is inserted into the T-cells by viral transfection.

Critical to the success of CarT therapy are the proliferation, cytotoxicity, and persistence of the CarT in response to antigen stimulation as well as target cell capacity to downregulate the relevant target antigen.

Many developments in the design of and methods to create CarT have been made to date. These include the choice of lentiviral or retroviral vectors, the design of the chimeric antigen receptor, linker molecule, and critically co-stimulatory molecules such as 4-1BB and CD28. As a result of different designs, some CarT are used as a bridge to transplant, whilst others are seen as a standalone therapy.

The pivotal study for pediatric ALL is the Eliana study of CTL-019, Tisagenlecleucel.[12] This study of 75 patients with relapsed refractory B-cell precursor ALL showed a 50% 12-month EFS in a group of patients with a median of three prior therapies. Importantly, there was no relationship between efficacy and the number of prior therapies including SCT. A common reason for failure was CD19-negative relapse. It should be noted that in all successful cases to date, prolonged B-cell aplasia has been a long-term side effect, though this has been effectively managed with immunoglobulin replacement therapy.

It is to be hoped that further developments in CarT design including bi-specific CarT will reduce the risk of target antigen-negative escape.

Infant ALL

Infants commonly possess the 11q23 MLL gene rearrangement within their malignant clone. This partly explains their poor prognosis, which is worsened if they are less than 6 months of age or have a presenting white cell count >300. If all three features are present the EFS is a dismal 16%. Treatment again consists of induction, intensive blocks, and a prolonged maintenance phase, but there is a stronger reliance on cytarabine, to which the leukemic cells are more sensitive, and bone marrow transplant. Studies are ongoing to look at the role of Blinatumomab in this patient population.[13]

ALL in adolescence

There is increasing evidence that patients aged 15–24 years have a better outcome if treated on pediatric protocols. International practice is therefore increasingly to treat such young adults on pediatric leukemia protocols. Their outcome remains inferior to younger children, due both to an increased relapse rate and a higher rate of toxic death.[14]

Mature B-cell ALL

Only 2% of childhood ALL is due to mature B-cell disease. These patients tend to be older (median age 10 years) and are more commonly male (ratio 3:1). The cells display L3 morphology and usually possess the t(8;14) translocation. They should be treated in the same way as B-cell NHL, with 5–6 months of intensive block chemotherapy, following which around 80% are cured. In those that relapse, the outcome is very poor.

Summary

In general, the outlook for children with ALL is very good. Nearly all achieve complete remission and the vast majority are cured. The advent of techniques to monitor MRD has led to a more accurate definition of risk groups, and it is hoped that these will subsequently enable further improvement in cure rates with a concurrent reduction in the cost, toxicity, and late effects of treatment. Novel immunotherapies are challenging the current treatment paradigm and offering hope to those with even the slimmest chance of cure with conventional therapy.

Acute myeloid leukemia

Acute myeloid leukemia is far less common than ALL in childhood, causing just 80 new cases in the UK each year. It is commonest in children under the age of 2 years and in adolescence, during which the incidence gradually rises. It can either arise de novo, or on the background of myelodysplastic syndrome (MDS). In some patients it occurs as a result of previous chemotherapy (particularly topoisomerase II inhibitors and alkylating agents) or in relation to a congenital syndrome, most commonly Down syndrome (see later), neurofibromatosis type I, or chromosomal fragility disorders. Comprehensive guidelines for the investigation and management of pediatric AML have been published.[15]

Classification

The classification of AML in children was updated by the WHO in 2008 and again in 2016 in response to the increasing knowledge about recurrent genetic abnormalities with prognostic and therapeutic relevance.[16] Diagnostic workup involves morphological, immunophenotypic, and genetic analysis (karyotyping, FISH, and molecular genetics).

Morphological assessment is primarily used to define blast percentage. The differentiation of AML and MDS in childhood is more complex than in adults, utilizing timescale of progression as well as genetics to make this distinction that has important therapeutic implications. A trephine biopsy is required in M7 AML and all cases of low blast count AML.

Immunophenotyping is critical in distinguishing AML from leukemias of ambiguous lineage and can be very useful in identifying M0, M7, and acute promyelocytic leukemia, a medical emergency that requires urgent and different therapy to standard AML.

Genetic analysis is similarly of critical importance, as recurrent genetic alterations play a key part in defining risk groups in childhood AML. A combination of karyotyping, FISH, and RT-PCR is used to identify the common recurrent translocations seen in AML, namely t(8;21), inv(16), t(15;17), and KMT2A rearrangements. It is increasingly clear that identifying the partner gene in KMT2A rearrangements is important as these have significant prognostic impact. Alterations in FLT3 and NPM1 and an increasing list of rare genetic abnormalities of prognostic impact are increasingly screened for in international trials.

Treatment

As with nearly all cases of pediatric malignancy, children with AML are treated within highly regulated national or international trials. Although variations exist between different trials, they share the common features of remission induction followed by consolidation.

In general, induction consists of one to two courses of intensive chemotherapy, with a heavy reliance on the use of anthracyclines and ara-C. The MRC and CCG trials have consistently shown the benefit of providing high-intensity induction therapy, although the optimum drug combination is an ongoing source of debate. Current studies are also looking at whether the addition of gemtuzumab ozogamicin (Mylotarg, a calicheamicin-conjugated anti-CD33 monoclonal antibody) can improve remission and survival rates. Consolidation is either in the form of further short courses of chemotherapy (up to a maximum of four courses in total) or, for some high-risk patients, stem cell transplantation. Some groups advocate the use of prolonged oral maintenance therapy in a similar way to that used in ALL. However, with the possible exception of APL, there is little evidence to support this, and it is not practiced in non-APL cases in the UK or US. CNS prophylaxis is adequately achieved with intrathecal chemotherapy and cranial irradiation is reserved for the very few cases with refractory CNS disease.

One of the most important lessons of recent years is that morphological assessment of CR in childhood AML is inadequate, and that this should instead be defined by flow cytometry. MRD analysis by flow cytometry is receiving renewed interest and is being incorporated into some upfront risk-stratification algorithms, though the methods and levels of residual disease used are less well standardized than in ALL.

Risk stratification is critical in the management of AML. This is continuously evolving but children are divided based on genetics and response as assessed by MRD into risk groups, with the highest risk patients generally allocated to bone marrow transplant. Even for the best-risk patients' outcomes are significantly worse than for ALL, and treatment reduction is not yet a therapeutic goal.

Acute promyelocytic leukemia

APL is characterized by myeloid arrest and an abnormal clonal proliferation at the promyelocyte stage and the presence of t(15;17)(q22;q21)/PML/RARA. It is frequently associated with a severe coagulopathy, which responds to treatment with all-trans retinoic acid (ATRA). This causes differentiation and subsequent apoptosis of the leukemic clone and should be given continuously with chemotherapy until complete remission is obtained. Recently, most international groups have adopted a strategy first developed by the Spanish PETHEMA group which is heavily reliant on ATRA and anthracyclines which gives an overall survival of 89% in pediatric patients. There is increasing interest in the role of arsenic and for the first time the potential for treatment protocols containing no conventional chemotherapeutic agents.[17]

Relapse and refractory disease

With the regimens mentioned earlier, complete remission can be expected in around 90% of cases of AML, with roughly 5% dying from infection or hemorrhage during induction, and the remainder having resistant disease. A further 30% of the whole cohort—not those that are refractory—will go on to relapse. The prognosis of relapsed disease is related to time to relapse (whether it occurs within greater or less than 1 year from diagnosis) and response to re-induction chemotherapy. In general, patients with refractory or relapsed disease are treated with a combination of fludarabine and ara-C, with or without an anthracycline, in an attempt to induce a second remission. If this is unsuccessful, alternative intensive chemotherapy combinations or novel therapies (such as Mylotarg) may be tried. In the case of APL, arsenic trioxide has been reported to be very successful. If remission is achieved, all patients should proceed to allogeneic stem cell transplantation from the best available donor.

Role of stem cell transplantation

Autologous stem cell transplantation has not been shown to improve survival in any group of patients with AML. Although some studies have shown reduced relapse rates for those treated with such in consolidation, these are offset by an increase in treatment-related mortality.

The value of allogeneic transplantation in first remission has yet to be clarified. In the CCG-2891 study, patients were allocated to transplantation following induction therapy if they had a matched family donor. In this group there was a small but significant improvement in OS and DFS at 8 years in comparison with the chemotherapy-only and autologous stem cell transplantation patients. In contrast the AML 10 trial did not show a significant difference in outcome, and neither has a recent update from COG trials. This may reflect as much on the efficacy of differing chemotherapy regimens as the role of stem cell transplant. In addition, allogeneic stem cell transplantation is the only curative strategy in relapsed patients. It has also been attempted in the setting of refractory disease, where there is hope that a KIR mismatch between the haploidentical donor and the recipient might produce an exaggerated graft vs. leukemia effect. However, this is highly experimental and at present the prognosis for these patients is dismal.

Novel therapies

Unlike ALL there is a dearth of novel agents for pediatric AML. The recurrent genetic lesions seen in adult AML (NPM1, FLT3) are less common in childhood AML. The development of new agents should be a high priority for future research in AML.

Down syndrome and AML

The risk of AML in children with Down syndrome (DS) is increased 10–20-fold, around 80% of which is megakaryoblastic (i.e. M7 subtype). This disease is particularly sensitive to chemotherapy (especially cytarabine) and yields an EFS of >80%. This contrasts with M7 found in patients without DS (<10% of patients) in whom the prognosis is poor (EFS <25%). It is currently unclear as to why M7 leukemic cells in DS patients are so sensitive to therapy, but clearly this could be a fruitful area of research. Because of their chemosensitivity, as well as their tendency to experience worse toxicity, these patients are now treated on separate protocols.[18]

In addition there is a unique condition called transient myeloid leukemia of Down syndrome (TMLDS) that occurs in at least 10% of neonates with DS. This condition is characterized by an abnormal clonal proliferation of megakaryoblasts that resembles AML but spontaneously resolves. Some 30–40% of such patients will go on to develop megakaryoblastic AML within the next 3 years. Of note, mutations in the GATA-1 gene on the X chromosome (encoding for a transcription factor essential for normal erythroid and megakaryoblastic differentiation) are found exclusively in TAM and DS-AML M7. Such mutations have subsequently been discovered in blood samples from Guthrie cards of patients with M7 and their identical twins, making it highly likely that they are an example of the so-called "first hit" in the process of leukemogenesis.

Summary

Unlike ALL, the improvement in the outcome of patients with AML over the last 30 years has been more modest, with approximately 70% long-term survivors. Cytogenetic analysis and early morphological response to therapy can identify three distinct risk groups. Monitoring of MRD, while less well developed than in ALL, may in future provide additional guidance for risk-directed therapy. However, a significant rate of treatment-related mortality suggests that further intensification of therapy may not be possible. Therefore, novel targeted therapies are likely to be required to provide the way forward. Finally, AML in DS has very distinct characteristics, which not only provide insights into the pathogenesis of AML, but also may prove helpful in our understanding of how to improve the efficacy of chemotherapeutic agents in all patients.

Hodgkin's lymphoma

Hodgkin's lymphoma (HL) accounts for 5% of childhood malignancies, 4.6 cases per year per million population aged less than 15 years. HL is rare under 5 years and has a marked male predominance in younger children (M:F 10:1). The bimodal distribution of cases according to socio-economic group (a high incidence in low socio-economic groups with a large sibling number, and in high socio-economic groups with a small sibling number) suggests an infective etiology. HL is more common in those with prior exposure to Epstein–Barr virus, but this does not explain all cases. Current understanding is that chronic antigenic stimulation (EBV or other virus-related) leads to aberrant gene rearrangement and therefore abnormal gene expression.

Presentation

Most children present with painless cervical lymphadenopathy. Cervical lymphadenopathy in a child is most often benign reactive, infective (EBV, cat-scratch disease [*Bartonella henselae*], and occasionally atypical tuberculosis). Acute leukemia, non-Hodgkin's lymphoma, and, rarely, phenytoin-induced pseudolymphoma should be considered. Mediastinal involvement is uncommon in younger children, but is seen in 70% over the age of 12 years.

Although well-established in adult practice, fine needle aspirate is unlikely to give a diagnosis, is likely to lead significant delay in diagnosis, and is not justified in pediatric oncology. A diagnosis of Hodgkin's lymphoma requires a knowledge of the lymph node architecture, whilst other malignant causes of lymphadenopathy often fall into the category of small round blue cell tumors, which will require excision biopsy.

Pathology

Pediatric HL is classified according to the WHO classification. The main categories are lymphocyte rich, nodular sclerosing, mixed cellularity, and lymphocyte depleted. The unusual variant, nodular lymphocyte predominant HL has a better prognosis than other forms, and the treatment strategy is different.

The classic lesion, the Reed–Sternberg, and its mononuclear variant, the Hodgkin cell are always positive for CD30, often for CD15, but negative for CD45. Cytogenetics are often abnormal, but a characteristic abnormality is not seen. Most will have some rearrangement of the immunoglobulin genes, or occasionally of the T-cell receptor. Differentiation from large cell anaplastic lymphoma (ALCL) can be difficult, but ALCL more commonly has systemic features such as fever and cutaneous involvement.

Staging is according to the Ann Arbor classification,[19] of I (a single lymph node region or organ or site) to IV (disseminated involvement of one or more extralymphatic organs or tissues); the absence or presence of fever or night sweats or unexplained loss of 10% or more of body weight in the 6 months preceding admission are denoted by the suffix letters A and B, respectively.

Staging investigations should include clinical examination, CT or MRI of the primary site, chest, and abdomen, chest X-ray, and abdominal ultrasound. Bone marrow aspirates and trephines are largely superseded by PET CT.

The role of FDG-PET scanning has become clear in recent years, and is vital for initial staging and assessment of response.

The EuroNet PHL-C1 study demonstrated the safety and efficacy of withholding radiation therapy for patients with adequate initial response to two cycles of OEPA chemotherapy, and this approach has been developed in the current study, EuroNET-PHL-C2. Late PET-CT assessment is used to define higher risk patients, for whom chemotherapy intensification or a radiation boost may be required.

Prognostic factors

Stage IV disease, B-type symptoms, and the presence of a mediastinal mass or other bulky disease are prognostic in children, and most protocols will stratify treatment accordingly.[20] Response to chemotherapy is also prognostic, and stratification of therapy based on response (PET CT activity) is indicated, with radiotherapy dose and field adjusted accordingly.[21]

Overall 5-year survival for stages I–IIIA disease is in excess of 95% and stage IV disease outcome has been improved substantially, being over 85% at 3.5 years in the DAL-HD-82 and -90 studies.[22,23]

Treatment

Treatment may involve surgery, radiotherapy, and chemotherapy.

NLPHL

Surgical excision alone is acceptable in low-stage NLPHL, where this can be achieved without mutilation. Approximately two-thirds of patients will have long-term remission with this approach. For patients in relapse, or where excision is impossible, reduced-intensity chemotherapy (CVP) gives an excellent EFS (75 ± 6%) and OS (100%).[24]

Patients who progress or recur are treated as for classical Hodgkin's lymphoma.

Classical HL

Radiotherapy is highly effective in achieving control and is a major component of most strategies. Radiotherapy alone is inferior to combined chemotherapy and radiotherapy in advanced disease, but may be equivalent for localized (stage I and II disease).[25] As a single modality, a dose of 40–44 Gy with extensive fields, even for stage I disease, is optimal.

Chemotherapy improves OS, and reduces radiation-associated sequelae, but the early combination mechlorethamine, VCR, procarbazine, and prednisone (MOPP) had other long-term sequelae.[26,27] Reduction in the overall dose of RT is possible with reduction in good responders to chemotherapy.[21,28]

Attempts to replace alkylating agents have been mixed. The hybrid regime, MOPP/ABVD, is as effective as MOPP alone, with fewer long-term sequelae, but with this regime abnormalities of lung function are likely. High rates of control with a combination of vinblastine, bleomycin, etoposide, and prednisolone and radiation to 20 Gy were seen in good responders, and hence both anthracyclines and alkylating agents may be avoidable in selected groups. In contrast, vincristine, etoposide, epirubicin, and prednisone (VEEP) without adjuvant radiotherapy was reported to have unacceptably poor local control.[29,30]

The EuroNet PHL C1 study, recently complete, was based on the DAL-HD-90 study.[23] Outcomes have been presented only in abstract, but are favorable, and a similar approach continues in the EuroNet PHL C2 study. Radiation can be successfully avoided in approximately half of patients, and standard RT dose for affected nodes was 19.8 Gy, with an additional 10 Gy for poor-responding patients.

Non-Hodgkin's lymphoma

Non-Hodgkin's lymphoma is a malignant tumor arising from lymphoid cells at various stages of activation and differentiation. In childhood, most present as extra-nodal disease, with rapid growth and non-contiguous spread. The large majority of lymphomas in childhood are high-grade, and may be of B- or T-lineage.

NHL has an annual incidence of seven cases per million children. There is a male predominance and a peak incidence between the ages of 7 and 10 years. Burkitt's lymphoma is endemic in Africa and has an association with Epstein–Barr virus. NHL in the West may show evidence of EBV in approximately 20% of cases. Certain immunodeficiency syndromes such as ataxia telangiectasia, Wiskott–Aldrich, and acquired immunodeficiency secondary to HIV infection or post-transplant immunosuppression are associated with NHL.

Pathology

The WHO classification 2008 is used, and the recently updated version includes several changes of relevance to pediatric practice.[31,32] Classification in childhood is somewhat more straightforward than in adults, given that almost all such tumors fall into one of four categories. Morphology, immunophenotyping, and molecular biology are needed for correct allocation of diagnosis.

Almost all are diffuse, high-grade lymphomas of B-cell origin. The three main entities are:

- Mature B-cell lymphoma, Burkitt or Burkitt-like tumors (50%)
- Large B-cell lymphomas (LBCL), such as diffuse large B-cell lymphoma (DLBCL) and primary mediastinal B-cell lymphoma (PMBL) (10–20%)
- Lymphoblastic lymphoma (20–25%), mainly precursor T-cell lymphoblastic lymphoma (T-LL)

Anaplastic large cell lymphoma (ALCL) accounts for 10% of NHLs.

B-cell type lymphomas characteristically express CD20, CD19, CD10, and CD79a and may express surface immunoglobulin (sIg) and bcl-6. Translocations t(8;14), t(2;8), and t(8;22) and MYC rearrangements are typical. B-lymphoblastic lymphoma often shows IGH rearrangements, whilst T-lymphoblastic lymphoma show T-cell receptor rearrangements, and abnormalities of NOTCH/FBXW7 and PTEN pathways. ALCL typically express CD30 and carry a translocation causing fusion of the anaplastic lymphoma kinase (ALK) gene to neucleophosmin (NPM/ALK).

Clinical presentation

Most patients with NHL will present with an abdominal mass or intussusception. Intussusception occurring after 3 years of age is likely to be due to lymphoma, and appropriate imaging should be performed before a surgical intervention. Some patients may present with ascites or as an acute appendicitis.

Mediastinal compression and obstruction are often seen at presentation, and such tumors are typically of T-cell origin. A differential diagnosis includes Hodgkin's disease, neuroblastoma, mediastinal germ cell tumor, and mediastinal B-cell NHL.

Adenopathy affecting Waldeyer's ring and cervical chains may be present. Occasionally disease may present because of the involvement of bones, kidney, or epidural space causing cord compression.

Anaplastic large cell lymphoma (ALCL) may present with painful lymph node involvement, with skin involvement, and often systemic symptoms such as fever. ALCL may have episodes of spontaneous regression, with adenopathy waxing and waning, which is otherwise unusual for malignancy.

The assessment of high-grade lymphomas must include consideration of the patient's airway (with mediastinal disease) and renal function, given the high likelihood of tumor lysis syndrome once treatment begins.

The majority of patients will present with stage 3 disease on the basis of a large mediastinal or unresectable abdominal primary. Primary CNS or marrow involvement is relatively uncommon. The principal diagnostic groups (Burkitt, large cell B, precursor T- or B-lymphoblastic, and ALCL) are discussed below.

Burkitt's lymphoma and diffuse large B-cell lymphoma

Burkitt's lymphoma is characterized by a translocation involving the long arm of chromosome 8, causing transcriptional deregulation of c-myc.[33] Almost all will show a translocation affecting:

- t(8,14)(q24;q32) (heavy chain Ig locus)
- t(2,8)(q1;q24) (kappa light chain) or
- t(8,22)(q24;q11) (lambda light chain)

Malignant cells arise from the germinal center of the lymph node, and are phenotypically and immunohistochemically of B-cell origin, with expression of CD10, 19, 20, 22, and 79a. Tumors have an extremely high proliferative rate.

B-cell lymphoma in the chest may be diffuse large B-cell disease, for which the prognosis is more guarded. Morphologically, both tumors show effacement of the lymph node and a "starry sky" appearance, although nuclei are typically larger in the former. Diffuse large B-cell lymphoma typically shows translocations which lead to deregulation of the gene bcl-2 or bcl-6, both intimately involved in regulation of apoptosis.

Treatment strategies for B-NHL

Burkitt's and diffuse large cell B-cell lymphomas are treated according to CHOP-based (cyclophosphamide, doxorubicin, vincristine, and prednisolone) regimens. The early LMB studies have provided the backbone of therapy throughout Europe, and more recently, North America.

The LMB81 consisted of:

- Cytoreduction (cyclophosphamide, vincristine, and prednisolone)
- Intensive induction (cyclophosphamide, vincristine, prednisolone, doxorubicin, high-dose methotrexate)
- Consolidation (high-dose cytarabine infusions)[34]

All patients receive CNS-directed therapy with intrathecal chemotherapy and high-dose methotrexate. Patients with high-risk disease (primary CNS or bone marrow involvement) received additional maintenance chemotherapy. Event free survival was >90% for patients without CNS involvement, and >80% with CNS involvement.

It has been possible to reduce treatment intensity for most patients, with less anthracycline and less cyclophosphamide.[35] Conversely, dose intensification for stage IV B-cell disease improved outcome[36]

Poor response to initial COP cytoreduction, and failure to achieve a CR after induction therapy are poor prognostic factors (EFS 22% for poor responders). These patients receive escalated therapy including rituximab.

The results of the Inter-B-NHL Ritux 2010 trial, a randomized phase III study using rituximab and the LMB regimen for advanced-stage B-cell lymphoma, and a phase II study of the DA-EPOCH-R regimen for PMBL (NCT01516580) have been reported in oral form, and showed significantly better outcomes with rituximab.[37,38] One-year EFS with rituximab[38] was 94% versus 82% with the standard regimen alone. Six doses of rituximab are now recommended for all advanced-stage B-NHL.

Relapsed stage I and II disease is salvageable with additional cycles of conventional chemotherapy. High-dose chemotherapy and stem cell rescue with BCNU, etoposide, cytosine arabinoside and melphalan (BEAM) is reserved for relapse of more advanced disease or disease poorly responsive to conventional doses. Relapsed stage IV disease is virtually incurable except for isolated CNS relapse.

Precursor T- and B-cell lymphoblastic lymphoma

Precursor T- and B-lymphoblastic lymphoma (LBL) is best regarded as a localized leukemia. There are minor biological differences but these do not influence treatment.[39]

Treatment is according to leukemia protocols. Outcomes are inferior to those for ALL with overall survival figures of around 80%. Survival rates at relapse are dismal. One major difficulty in LBL is that of identifying useful prognostic markers. Neither genetics nor disease response have to date been found to be robust enough to incorporate into routine clinical care, though studies continue to investigate this important subject.

Anaplastic large cell lymphoma

Anaplastic large cell lymphoma (ALCL) accounts for around 10% of childhood NHL. Patients may present with mediastinal or abdominal disease, but there is a greater likelihood of systemic symptoms and cutaneous involvement. Histologically, cells may resemble undifferentiated tumors, Hodgkin's, and other forms of NHL. Immunophenotyping is necessary to make the diagnosis for most. Cells have T-helper phenotype (CD3 and CD4 positive) and are characteristically positive for CD30 and epithelial membrane antigen (EMA).[40]

Localized ALCL and primary CNS involvement are uncommon, but B-symptoms are common, and staging according to conventional systems is not helpful. ALCL is stratified instead according to histology and site of disease into standard-risk and high-risk (with skin or visceral organ involvement) groups. Risk factors for relapse are:

- Mediastinal involvement
- Visceral involvement (lung, liver, or spleen involvement)
- Skin lesions

PFS at 5 years for patients with no risk factors was 89% vs. 61% in those with at least one.[41]

The current UK strategy adopts an approach based upon previous BFM protocols, for which EFS of 79% was reported at 3 years.[42,43] The ALCL99 study involved multi-agent chemotherapy with dexamethasone, cyclophosphamide, vincristine, doxorubicin, ifosfamide, cytarabine, and etoposide, with a dual randomization to look at the effect of vinblastine, and low- (1 g/m^2) or high (3 g/m^2)-dose methotrexate.[44] Favorable outcomes were seen in both arms (EFS 74% at 2 years). CNS relapse was seen in just 2/352 patients, and hence the less toxic arm (3 g/m^2, no IT chemotherapy) is preferred.

The translocation t(2;5) is specific to ALCL and is found in at least 80% of patients.[45] The translocation leads to expression of a novel gene product, NPM-ALK, and ALK-1 positivity appears to be associated with a better clinical outcome for systemic disease.

There is evidence for the particular efficacy of vinblastine in ALCL, and proposals to avoid multi-agent intensive chemotherapy are in development. Similarly, the availability of inhibitors of ALK (crizotinib, ceritinib, alectinib) and of anti-CD30 specific therapies (brentuximab vedotin) means that novel strategies to treat are being explored. The COG randomized study of crizotinib vs. brentuximab with chemotherapy COG-ANHL12P1, NCT01979536 is expected to report in 2021.

Rhabdomyosarcoma

Rhabdomyosarcoma (RMS) is the commonest soft tissue sarcoma of childhood, with an annual incidence of five to nine per million children per year aged less than 15 years; it accounts for approximately 5% of all childhood cancer. Histologically it resembles early myogenic precursors, suggesting that the cell of origin may be a mesenchymal stem cell. Common primary sites include head and neck (40%), genitourinary tract (20%), and extremities (20%). RMS presents with metastases in 20% of cases, the most common site being lung, more rarely bone and bone marrow. The etiology of RMS is unknown, but there are well-recognized associations with cancer predisposition syndromes such as neurofibromatosis, Gorlin's syndrome, and Li–Fraumeni syndrome.

Histopathology and fusion status

RMS is divided broadly into two histological subtypes, embryonal (ERMS) and alveolar (ARMS). ERMS constitutes 60–80%, occurs in a younger age group, and is associated with a better prognosis. ARMS makes up 20–40% of RMS and affects older children, often occurring at extremity sites. ARMS is often metastatic at presentation, demonstrates a more aggressive phenotype, and therefore has a worse prognosis.

Most (70–80%) ARMS cases have translocations resulting in fusion of the PAX3 or PAX7 gene with FOXO1. Rare variant rearrangements constitute an estimated 1% of all RMS.[46] PAX-FOXO1 fusion gene–positive cases with ERMS histology have also been described in 1% of patients.[47]

Large-scale gene expression profiling has shown that ARMS tumors lacking characteristic fusion genes are molecularly and clinically indistinguishable from ERMS.[46,48] This is consistent with studies that show the fusion genes confer a negative clinical prognostic value.[46,49–52] Important validation of this came from analysis of outcome by fusion status in prospectively collected samples from COG trials (D9803 and D9602).[47,53] Based on these studies and an increasing understanding of the functional role of the fusion proteins in RMS, future EpSSG and COG studies will use PAX-FOXO1 fusion gene status rather than histology to stratify patients.[47]

Symptoms and signs

RMS presents in a number of ways depending on where it arises. For example, orbital tumors typically present early with proptosis and diplopia. Nasopharyngeal tumors may cause nasal/airway obstruction or a polypoid extrusion with discharge. A painless mass may be the only finding of a para-testicular lesion. In contrast, bladder/prostate masses may grow to considerable size before presentation with obstructive symptoms. Parameningeal tumors have significant risk of direct extension into the central nervous tissue, and may present with cranial nerve palsies.

Staging

Diagnostic workup should include accurate assessment of the primary lesion and must include assessment of loco-regional nodal sites using cross-sectional imaging. Evaluation of potential metastatic sites usually includes CT chest, bone marrow aspirate, and trephine and CSF where parameningeal tumors arise. A systematic review looking at the role of PET-CT in RMS has identified the need for further evaluation of its potential role as a prognostic biomarker.[54] Currently it is considered standard of care (where available) as a diagnostic tool, but the current EpSSG study is hoping to determine the value of FDG PET-CT response after three cycles as a predictive biomarker of local failure and/or survival in RMS.

Treatment

Treatment is multimodal and risk-stratified according to:

- Age
- Tumor size
- Histology (favorable or unfavorable)
- Intergroup Rhabdomyosarcoma Study (IRS) post-surgical stage
- Lymph node involvement

This stratification defines patients as low risk (LR), standard risk (SR), high risk (HR) and very high risk (VHR); the latter includes the metastatic group.

Chemotherapy

Chemotherapy is an integral part of treatment for RMS. In newly diagnosed pediatric patients the drugs used are combinations of long-established cytotoxic agents including alkylating agents, vincristine, and actinomycin D.

Over the last 30 years there have been sequential improvements in outcome as a result of clinical trials that have investigated stepwise modifications in the intensity and combinations of these drugs.

In LR and SR disease, this has proved very successful: current 3-year EFS rates of 95% and 77% respectively are seen.[55–57] The greatest treatment challenges remain in the HR, VHR, and metastatic groups, and for relapse patients, where EFS remains below 70%, 45%, and 30% respectively.[58,59]

The EpSSG RMS 2005 trial for newly diagnosed patients has already demonstrated that the addition of doxorubicin to standard ifosfamide, vincristine, actinomycin D (IVA) chemotherapy does not improve survival in HR RMS.[60] Current trials continue to assess the role of additional chemotherapeutic agents, such as irinotecan, alongside current strategies.[61]

Maintenance chemotherapy

More than 90% of events in localized RMS appear more than 12 months from diagnosis, so after completion of treatment. It was clear that a new approach with longer low-dose (maintenance) treatment was needed. Preliminary results of maintenance treatment after standard treatment in HR patients in CR did not reach a statistically significant difference between the two arms ($p = 0.06$), but overall survival (OS), was significantly improved in the maintenance arm. Maintenance chemotherapy is therefore recommended in this group but continues to be investigated in HR and VHR groups through the current clinical trials in Europe.

Local therapy

Local control remains an ongoing challenge in localized RMS, but the last 20 years have seen significant improvements in outcome.

Surgery

Surgery remains an important local therapy strategy in RMS. Primary resection is unusual and should only be attempted where it is not mutilating and where a complete resection can be achieved, for example, excision of a presumed para-testicular RMS. Diagnosis should be made by incisional biopsy with the collection of fresh tissue for molecular biological analysis.

Radiotherapy

Radiotherapy (RT) remains a key component of local therapy, and this is supported by data from the International Society of Pediatric Oncology (SIOP) Malignant Mesenchymal Tumor (MMT) 84, 89, and 95 trials.

A systematic approach to RT was adopted in the EpSSG RMS 2005 trial. In this study, 86% of patients with localized HR RMS received radiotherapy, with the trial reporting an increase in 3-year EFS from 55% to 67% for HR and from 39% to 56% for node-positive ARMS patients. Despite these improvements, recurrence was local in the majority of relapse cases; further modification of dose and/or timing of radiotherapy may yet improve outcomes.

Historically RT has been delivered postoperatively when required. Pre-operative RT has a number of potential advantages over postoperative RT:

- The intact tumor target volume is easier to define.
- The residual tumor may act as a form of "spacer," reducing radiation dose to uninvolved normal tissue.
- A significant proportion of the irradiated tissue will be removed surgically, which may reduce the risk of second tumors.

In the FaR-RMS trial, the efficacy (local control), safety, and impact on health-related quality of life of pre-operative radiotherapy in RMS compared to standard postoperative radiotherapy will be investigated.

In specific circumstances alternative RT strategies such as brachytherapy should be considered (bladder/prostate combined with conservative surgery and in head and neck RMS—AMORE strategy).[62]

Metastatic and relapse disease

The outlook for children with metastatic disease remains dismal, with current 5-year survival rates of less than 30%. Complete remission is achievable in up to two-thirds but early relapse is frequent. Current international trials continue to investigate new chemotherapeutic strategies and addition of novel agents in this difficult group of patients.

Long-term effects

Survival from RMS is in excess of 60%, and for certain sites exceeds 90%. The burden of treatment is highly significant for young children, who may undergo intensive and cosmetically damaging therapy. The long-term effects of radiotherapy may be profound for a child who will grow substantially after therapy. However, the increased use of highly conformal radiotherapy such as brachytherapy in the management of head and neck tumors ("AMORE") and conservative surgery with intra- and postoperative brachytherapy for bladder/prostate tumors may improve these long-term morbidities.[62]

Osteosarcoma

Osteosarcoma (OS) is the most common primary tumor of bone, with an annual incidence of around 6–7 cases per 100,000 population between the age of 10 and 24 years. Overall there are 100–130 new cases diagnosed in the UK each year. There is a male predominance of approximately 3:2, and it is less common in people of black Afro-Caribbean descent. Osteosarcoma is derived from cells of mesenchymal origin that exhibit osteoblastic differentiation and produce malignant osteoid.

The majority of cases of OS are sporadic, but mutations involving the *RB* gene (chromosome 13q14) and p53 gene play an important role in the development of this tumor. Patients with germline mutations in the *RB* gene have approximately a 1000-fold increased risk of osteosarcoma. Similarly patients with Li–Fraumeni syndrome (germline p53 mutation) have a greatly elevated incidence of osteosarcoma.[63,64]

Osteosarcoma occur more commonly at metaphyseal regions where there is rapid bone growth. This raises the possibility that bone growth stimulates osteoblastic cells to acquire mutations that could lead to malignant transformation. It is also recognized as a second primary malignancy following radiotherapy in childhood cancer survivors.[65] The interval between irradiation and the appearance of osteosarcoma can range from 4 to more than 40 years (median, 12–16 years). The risk of developing post-radiation osteosarcoma correlates with radiation dose. In a large cohort study (4400 survivors of a first solid tumor), an overall risk of 1% was identified with a relative risk of 100 compared to the normal population.[66]

Clinical presentation

Osteosarcoma typically presents with pain and swelling of the affected bone. Pain may be worse at night. Pathological fractures can occur and this impacts on management and prognosis. OS most commonly affects the proximal tibia or distal femur (60%) and the humerus or shoulder (10% of cases). OS is much less common in axial sites and only occurs in the head and neck in around 8% of cases. Around 10–20% of patients present with metastases typically to lung but more rarely to bone.

Investigations

Plain radiographs may show cortical destruction, elevation of the periosteum (the so-called Codman triangle), and new bone formation. Pathological fracture may be present and may be associated with a greater incidence of local recurrence in patients treated by limb salvage procedures. A variable amount of soft tissue swelling may also be present.

MRI is the preferred investigation to assess primary disease, to allow definition of soft tissues, the neurovascular bundle, epiphyseal, and joint involvement. Marrow involvement and the presence of skip metastases are also identified. For this reason, the whole of the affected bone (including distal and proximal joints) must be imaged and abnormal areas biopsied if there is diagnostic uncertainty.

Plain chest X-ray may demonstrate lung nodules but chest CT is required to identify pulmonary metastases. ^{99}Tc bone imaging is used to identify skeletal metastases.

Histopathology and tumor genetics

Diagnosis requires histopathological confirmation. A Trucut needle biopsy is usually sufficient, but the biopsy should be done by the surgeon who will perform the subsequent definitive procedure as the biopsy tract will need to be resected with the tumor excision. Diagnosis can often be made rapidly from cytology of the biopsy smear, but otherwise from conventional histological staining for alkaline phosphatase. Osteosarcoma is characterized by the presence of bone or osteoid tissue with the tumor cells. The most common histopathological subtype is central osteosarcoma, characterized by areas of necrosis, atypical mitoses, and malignant cartilage.[67] Other subtypes of high-grade osteoblastic OS—chondroblastic, fibroblastic, telangiectatic, small cell, osteoclast-rich, anaplastic, and sclerotic/osteoblastic-well-differentiated—are seen, but only chondroblastic osteosarcoma has been reported to have prognostic significance in one series.[68] Intraosseous well-differentiated osteosarcoma and parosteal osteosarcoma are associated with a favorable prognosis and can be treated successfully with radical primary excision alone, but are uncommon. Occasionally, little or no osteoid may be seen and differentiation from Ewing's tumor may be problematic.

Biological factors have been sought for prognostic value at diagnosis.

Loss of heterozygosity (LOH) of the *RB* gene has been reported to predict early treatment failure.[64] In a series of 34 patients, EFS at 5 years was 100% for patients without LOH, 43% for all patients, and 65% for non-metastatic patients with LOH.

Similarly, LOH *TP53* has been reported to correlate with lack of chemo-responsiveness *in vitro*[69] and *in vivo*.[70] The dominant oncogene *c-fos* is implicated from transgenic mice which constitutively overexpress the gene, and almost always develop aggressive osteosarcoma.[71]

Treatment

Surgery

In the past, osteosarcoma was treated by surgical excision alone: metastatic relapse and subsequent death arose in around 80% of patients.[72] Whilst it is clear that chemotherapy is important for controlling metastatic disease and improving survival, good local control remains essential and failure to remove the primary tumor completely is associated with a high risk of subsequent local and metastatic relapse even with adjuvant chemotherapy.[73] Limb salvage is now the expected approach with low rates of local recurrence,[74,74] even where there is a pathological fracture, provided adequate surgical margin can be attained.[75] Metallic endoprosthetic replacement is the most common approach used. "Growing" endoprostheses are available, and these reduce morbidity in patients treated at a young age. In some patients with tumor away from a growth point, there is the possibility to consider a vascularized endoprosthetic graft instead of an endoprosthesis. Such grafts are usually taken from the contralateral fibula and have considerable advantages over metallic implants, in their ability to repair after injury and being at no significant risk of infection.

For some patients, amputation may offer the best and most reliable chance of return to normal life. Finally, one approach worthy of consideration where an above-knee amputation might otherwise be necessary is the van Ness rotation-plasty, for which excellent functional outcome may be obtained.[76] The optimal surgical approach is recommended by the orthopedic surgical team in conjunction with the patient and/or family.

Chemotherapy

The European Osteosarcoma Intergroup (EOI) ran the first randomized studies of treatment for osteosarcoma. The first EOI study, EORTC 80831, compared the efficacy of a two-drug regimen (cisplatin and doxorubicin) versus a three-drug combination, with the addition of methotrexate at a dose of 8 g/m². The study established that the two-drug combination of cisplatin (CDDP) and doxorubicin was safe and improved OS.[77]

The second EOI study (EORTC 80861) compared the efficacy of this two-drug regimen with a multi-agent regimen similar to that used by Rosen in the T10 protocol (pre-operative vincristine, high-dose methotrexate, and doxorubicin; postoperative bleomycin, cyclophosphamide, dactinomycin, vincristine, methotrexate, doxorubicin, and cisplatin).[78] No benefit from the multi-drug arm over two-drug arm was seen.

The third study, 80961, investigated interval compression, with CDDP/DOX given every 2 weeks with GCSF vs. every 3 weeks. There was no difference in survival between the arms, although there was a better histologic response rate in the compressed arm.[79]

Despite the negative results of the first EOI study, there is evidence that the cumulative dose and dose intensity of methotrexate treatment affect response and, by implication, the outcome. A correlation was demonstrated between a pharmacokinetic parameter, methotrexate concentration at the end of infusion, and tumor response as measured by the degree of tumor necrosis.[68,80,81] A concentration of methotrexate of 700 mM after a 6-hour infusion,[68] or 1000 mM at the end of a 4-hour infusion (Delepine et al., 1988, 162)[81] has been shown to be predictive of response, allowing stratification according to a surrogate endpoint early on in treatment. Furthermore, dose adaptation based upon pharmacokinetic parameters has been performed, and a survival benefit seen. In a study of 44 patients receiving conventional dosing, and 27 with individual dose adaptation, Delepine reported significantly greater response rates and disease-free survival (76% with conventional dosing compared with 92% with pharmacokinetically guided dosing).[82] For patients treated with a methotrexate dose of 8, 10, or 12 g/m², the proportion of patients attaining a methotrexate concentration in excess of 700 mM has been reported to be 44%, 59%, and 85%,[68] and one explanation for the variable reports of efficacy of methotrexate stems from this variability.

The presence of chemotherapy-induced toxicities (especially grade 3–4 mucositis) is associated with improved overall and progression-free survival. It is however interesting that there was no association found between histological response in excised tumor and chemotherapy-induced toxicities. Other good prognostic factors for patients with localized disease include good histological response to pre-operative chemotherapy, distal tumor location, and female gender.

Treatment stratification and immunomodulation

Stratification of patients based upon histological response of the resected tumor was introduced early in the history of chemotherapy, although it has yet to be proven to affect overall prognosis. In the majority of series, the presence of >90% tumor necrosis in the resection specimen identifies a good prognostic group, for whom a high (>75%) overall survival may be expected. In the EOI first study, OS for patients with >90% necrosis was 85%, compared with 40% for those with <90% necrosis. In the second EOI study (cisplatin–doxorubicin) vs. a multi-agent regime, 30% patients had ≥90% necrosis with the two-drug regime, and 27% with multi-agent therapy (no significant difference). The EFS in this study was disappointing (55% at 8 years), and no significant difference was seen between the two arms.[83,84]

In 2001, four clinical study groups, the Children's Oncology Group (COG), the Cooperative Osteosarcoma Study Group (COSS) of the German Society for Pediatric Oncology and Hematology (GPOH), the European Osteosarcoma Intergroup (EOI), and the Scandinavian Sarcoma Group (SSG), came together to form the European and American Osteosarcoma Studies (EURAMOS) collaborative; 2260 patients were registered from 326 centers across 17 countries.

Patients with resectable osteosarcoma aged ≤40 years were treated with the MAP regimen, (cisplatin, doxorubicin, methotrexate 12 g/m²). Poor responders (>10% viable tissue) were randomized after surgery to receive MAP or MAP with ifosfamide and etoposide. Good responders were randomized to MAP or MAP followed by pegylated interferon.

EURAMOS-1 did not support the addition of ifosfamide and etoposide to postoperative chemotherapy: administration was associated with increased toxicity without improving event-free survival.[85] In addition, MAP plus IFN-α-2b was not statistically different from MAP alone. A considerable proportion of patients never started IFN-α-2b or stopped prematurely.[86]

Liposomal muramyl tripeptide phosphatidyl ethanolamine (mifamurtide) is a component of the *Mycobacterium* species cell wall. Mifamurtide works by activating macrophages and monocytes and modulating the immune response to eradicate tumor cells. Mifamurtide causes systemic side effects such as chills (89%), fever (85%), and fatigue (53%). Detailed analyses of results and more careful interpretation of the data from the CCG/POG INT033 study suggest that any prognostic benefit/difference with mifamurtide is probably limited to non-metastatic patients who received ifosfamide. There is no strong evidence of survival advantage with the addition of mifamurtide to conventional treatment, but in 2011, mifamurtide in combination with postoperative multi-agent chemotherapy was approved by the National Institute for Health and Care Excellence (NICE) within its licensed indication as an option for the treatment of high-grade resectable non-metastatic osteosarcoma after macroscopically complete surgical resection in children, adolescents, and young adults.

For relapsed and refractory disease with no further surgical and chemotherapy options (such as high-dose ifosfamide and etoposide, gemcitabine and docetaxol), recruitment into phase 1–2 studies should be considered.

High-risk disease

Although the majority of tumors arise in peripheral long bones, at least 20% patients present with flat-bone, axial, or metastatic disease at diagnosis. These patients have a mixed prognosis. Chemotherapy alone is unlikely to be curative and for some, surgical resection is not possible. The prognosis for patients with primary metastatic disease is dependent upon site. In the study of Harris et al., patients with bone metastasis had a particularly poor outcome. Most patients will have pulmonary metastases and for this group, thoracotomies to excise any disease unresponsive to chemotherapy seem to be of benefit.[87–89] Bacci et al. reported a 5-year OS of only 14% with an aggressive regimen using methotrexate (8 g/m²), cisplatin, doxorubicin, ifosfamide, and etoposide.[90] All patients who did not achieve a complete surgical or chemotherapeutic remission died. In contrast, patients in the series of Harris et al. who presented with less than eight pulmonary nodules had a relatively high chance of cure. Twelve of 18 were alive at 5 years, and patients with unilateral disease had a 5-year EFS of 75%. These data are encouraging, and indicate that an aggressive, multi-modality approach may overcome previously adverse prognostic factors.

Ewing's family tumors

The Ewing's family of tumors (EFT) is a group of tumors that includes Ewing's sarcoma (ES) of the bone, extra-osseous Ewing's tumor (malignant peripheral neuroectodermal tumor—PNET), Askin tumors (Ewing's tumor of chest wall/rib), and atypical Ewing's sarcoma. These tumors are now known to arise from the same cell of origin and exhibit varying degrees of neural differentiation.[91] Ninety-five per cent of tumors carry a t(11;22) translocation, and the principles of treatment are the same for all. Over the last 30 years, outcomes have improved dramatically primarily due to the introduction of multimodal therapy combining chemotherapy, surgery, and radiotherapy.

Ewing's tumor comprises 10–15% of primary bone tumors in childhood and adolescence, affecting 2.93 people per million population or 1.7 per million children. There is a peak incidence at age 10–15 years, affecting boys more than girls. It is rare below age 5 and after 30 years, and in those of Afro-Caribbean and Asian origin.

Clinical presentation

Clinical presentation depends on the site and size of the tumor. Patients typically present with pain and swelling and sometimes fever and weight loss due to large tumor load. The majority of primary bone sarcomas arise in the long bones, pelvis, chest wall/ribs, and axial skeleton.

Bone cancer can sometimes present with pathological fractures. Extra-osseous Ewing's or soft tissue primitive neuroectodermal tumors can arise in the trunk, extremities, head and neck, and retroperitoneum. Extra-osseous Ewing's tumors are likely to be larger and less amenable to definitive local surgery than bony Ewing's. Approximately 30% of Ewing's tumors will show metastases at diagnosis, with lung being the commonest site but also found in bone and liver.

Staging investigations

A plain X-ray of the affected region will usually show bone destruction but cross-sectional imaging (MRI) is required for accurate assessment of the primary site. Calcification is not prominent, but its presence does not exclude a diagnosis of Ewing's sarcoma. Staging investigations with chest CT, bone scan, bilateral bone marrow aspirates and trephines, and ultrasound scan of the liver are required to assess common sites of metastatic disease.

Several studies have shown the potential role of ^{18}F-FDG-PET with or without CT in diagnosis and staging of ES. PET/CT has advantages over conventional imaging (MRI, CT, and scintigraphy), in the detection of bone and lymph node metastases.[92] Baseline maximum SUV is an independent and significant predictor of overall survival.[93] Furthermore, ^{18}F-FDG-PET/CT can be used for non-invasive response assessment after neo-adjuvant chemo-therapy. Post-therapeutic FDG-uptake predicts histological and clinical outcomes.[94]

Histopathology and genetics

Ewing's family tumors fall within the group of small round blue cell tumors, and the differential diagnosis includes osteogenic sarcoma, rhabdomyosarcoma, and other non-rhabdomyomatous sarcomas, neuroblastoma, and lymphoma. Ewing's tumor may show elements of neural differentiation and, in this, overlaps with primitive neuro-ectodermal tumors. Immunohistochemistry showed the presence of intracellular glycogen (PAS positivity), neurosecretory granules, expression of NSE, S100, and CD99.

Tumor genetics are characterized by translocations involving chromosome 22q12 and (in 85%) chromosome 11q24. The breakpoint region has been cloned and the transcript sequenced.[95] The novel transcript includes the DNA-binding domain of the (human homologue) *FLI1* gene and the *EWS* gene (on 22q12), bringing the former under the control of the *EWS* promotor and producing a transforming capacity not present in the wild-type *FLI1* gene product. In about 10% cases, the *EWS* gene is translocated to the *ERG* region of chromosome 21, another DNA-binding domain.

Many different fusion products are seen even within the *EWS-FLI1* rearrangements. The most common, type 1 (72%), links Exon 6 of *FLI1* with Exon 7 of *EWS*, but at least eight other transcripts are known. The presence of the type 1 transcript is an independent prognostic variable for localized tumors, with significantly better relapse-free survival.[96] Approximately 30% tumors show a secondary change, trisomy 8, the significance of which is unclear.

Treatment

In his original reports of diffuse endothelioma of bone, Ewing described the radiosensitivity of the tumor,[97] although with radiotherapy alone, the large majority of patients relapsed with disseminated disease within 2–5 years. Combination chemotherapy has been used for many years, and overall survival has progressively increased: 5-year OS for localized ESFT is 60–70% using chemotherapy regimens that include actinomycin D (A), doxorubicin (D), ifosfamide (I), and etoposide (E). Local therapy (surgery and/or radiotherapy) is always required to control disease at the primary site.[98]

Collaborative studies in the US (IESS I AND II), Germany (CESS), and widely in Europe (EICESS 92, the forerunner of EuroEwings), have compared chemotherapy scheduling, dosing, and dose intensity,[99] with improved survival. CESS 81 also gave important local therapy data showing that there was better survival in those patients who received both surgery and radiotherapy (69%) than with radiotherapy (44%) or surgery (48%) alone.[100–102]

The EURO-E.W.I.N.G. 99 trial employed "VIDE" induction chemotherapy followed by risk-adapted randomized treatment in patients with localized disease.[103] Critical factors for stratification into the standard- or high-risk groups were primary tumor volume and histological response to induction chemotherapy. Standard-risk patients were randomized for consolidation with either VAI or VAC (R1) and high-risk patients were randomized to high-dose, busulphan–melphalan (BuMel) versus conventional chemotherapy VAI(R2loc). The trial showed the VAC regime to be as effective with less toxicity than VAI as maintenance treatment for standard-risk patients. The R2loc randomization showed that in patients with tumor volume >200ml in whom prior resection or radiotherapy had taken place, BuMel improved EFS and OS without unacceptable excess toxicity. Therefore, BuMel has become standard of care only for patients with high-risk localized disease in whom there is no contraindication to receiving BuMel and radiotherapy.

The EURO-EWING 2012 study has recently closed to recruitment. It included a randomization (R1) of induction/consolidation chemotherapy (R1) between VIDE (with VAI/VAC/BuMel consolidation) and the VDC/IE strategy (compressed VDC/IE induction and IE/VC/BuMel consolidation).

A second randomization (R2) was to determine whether the addition of zoledronic acid is associated with improved clinical outcome. Finally, biological studies aimed to identify informative prognostic biomarkers for the assessment of disease status and response.

The data are not yet mature but suggest improved EFS and OS in the compressed arm of the up-front randomization, and this is likely to become the new standard-of-care chemotherapy backbone against which further randomizations with novel agents are based.

Treatment results in patients with primary pulmonary metastases and regional lymph nodes

Ewing's tumors presenting with only pulmonary metastases carry a poor prognosis although better than at other sites of metastases. Treatment with conventional chemotherapy carries an EFS ranging from 23% to 36%.[104–107] Various studies have shown the benefit of radiotherapy to lung metastases in multivariate analyses.

High-dose chemotherapy (BuMel) improved the prognosis of patients with lung-only metastases in a non-randomized French study (EFS 52%, n = 44). The benefit of BuMel was not replicated in EURO-E.W.I.N.G. 99, and BuMel is not recommended for metastatic disease at pulmonary sites.

There are no separate data for patients with regional lymph node involvement: it can be assumed that they do at least as badly as those with metastases to lungs and/or pleura.

Recurrent/refractory disease

Approximately 15% of patients with high-risk disease are refractory to initial therapy, and up to 50% of patients recur after initial treatment.[108] Survival is poor following recurrence (5-year OS 20–35%), but the interval from diagnosis to relapse is prognostic: recurrence at 18–24 months from initial diagnosis is consistently reported to be significant for improved OS and EFS. Recurrence in lung alone has a better outcome.

Chemotherapy options in relapse include high-dose ifosfamide, irinotecan and temozolomide, topotecan and cyclophosphamide, and gemcitabine and docetaxol. The EuroEwing Consortium is currently comparing the efficacy and response between these commonly used regimens through a phase 2 randomized study. Potential novel/targeted agents for relapsed or recurrent Ewing's sarcoma are also being evaluated in ongoing early phase trials.

Renal tumors

Renal tumors constitute 6–8% of childhood cancer in Europe and North America.[109] Wilms' tumor (WT), the most common renal tumor of childhood, is a paradigm for the multimodal treatment of solid tumors in children.

Wilms' tumor

The incidence of Wilms' tumor (WT) is 8.1 cases per million Caucasian children less than 15 years of age, usually presenting before age 5 years. It is associated with congenital abnormalities such as isolated aniridia, isolated hemihypertrophy (prevalence 2.5% of children with Wilms' tumor), and genitourinary anomalies (hypospadias, undescended testis—about 6%). WT is also linked to genetic (overgrowth and non-overgrowth) syndromes including Perlman syndrome, Beckwith–Weidemann (1% of children with WT), and WAGR syndrome (hemihypertrophy, aniridia, genitourinary malformation, and mental retardation). Denys–Drash syndrome is associated with mutations in the *WT1* gene.

At least three genes are associated with WT; the incidence of familial WT is less than 1% and genetics do not always follow a simple two-hit model of tumor suppressor genes. *WT2* maps to 11p15.5, which is also the location of the Beckwith–Weidemann gene abnormality. Familial *WT* genes are also located at 17q12 and 7p13.

Clinical presentation

Most children present with an abdominal mass or swelling, or by screening for children with conditions known to predispose to WT.[110] Abdominal pain, hematuria (often microscopic) and pyrexia are common. Hypertension is present in 25%. Macroscopic hematuria can occur and tends to be associated with tumor extension into the renal pelvis.

Staging investigations

Abdominal ultrasound and MRI scan will determine tumor in relation to adjacent organs, involvement of the inferior vena cava and renal veins, the paraaortic lymph nodes, and the other kidney.

Chest X-ray and chest CT scan are required to assess pulmonary metastases. Staging of WT depends on regional lymph nodes involvement, and direct examination of the contralateral kidney is required at operation. The presence of tumor cells in retroperitoneal lymph nodes is prognostic, and lymph node sampling forms part of the staging of WT according to the National Wilms' Tumor Study Group.

Histopathology and tumor genetics

WT comprises varying proportions of three morphological components: blastema, stroma, and epithelium. Histological subtypes define risk groups, according to the presence of anaplasia and histological changes induced by pre-operative chemotherapy.

Low-risk tumors include cystic partially differentiated nephroblastoma (CPDN) and the completely necrotic nephroblastoma in response to pre-operative chemotherapy.

Intermediate-risk tumors include the regressive subtype (chemotherapy-induced and necrotic changes in >66% tumor), stromal (at least 66% of viable tumor consist of stromal component), epithelial (at least 66% viable tumor consist of epithelial structures), and mixed (viable tumor consist of blastemal and/or stromal and/or epithelial elements but none of them comprises >66% viable tumor) subtypes. Focal anaplasia is permissible.

Anaplasia occurs in 5% of cases, typically in older children. High-risk WT include blastemal-predominant subtype (at least 66% viable tumor consisting of blastema after pre-operative chemotherapy) and those with diffuse anaplasia.

Loss of heterozygosity for chromosomes 1p and 16q and gain of 1q confer an adverse outcome for children who present with otherwise favorable histological features.[111]

Nephrogenic rests are small clusters of embryonal cells, considered to be potential precursor lesions for WT. They may regress into fibrous tissue or progress to form nephroblastoma. They are found in about 25 to 40% cases of WT, often in the same kidney with the excised tumor specimen, but can be contralateral. There may be perilobar or intralobar, diffuse or hyperplastic. The term nephroblastomatosis describes the presence of multi-focal nephrogenic rests especially involving also the opposite kidney, and rests in more diffuse form infiltrating both kidneys. There is guidance from the SIOP WT group on the management of nephroblastomatosis.

Treatment

First-line therapy

Treatment usually requires chemotherapy, surgery, and/or radiotherapy, dependent on the stage, histology (risk stratification), and the potential to preserve adequate renal tissue in cases of bilateral disease. Immediate nephrectomy is performed for most patients in the USA, followed by chemotherapy ± radiotherapy.

The National Wilms' Tumor Study Group (NWTS) recommends upfront surgery in order to avoid modification of tumor histology and staging, and administration of chemotherapy to children with non-Wilms' malignancies or benign lesions.

The SIOP (International Society of Pediatric Oncology) has advocated pre-operative chemotherapy, as this is associated with reduced risk of tumor rupture rate at surgery, (possibly) reduced risk of local relapse, and identification of good-risk subgroups based on tumor response.[112,113]

Both groups favor chemotherapy with vincristine, actinomycin-D, and doxorubicin. Radiotherapy is given to patients with stage III or stage IV disease.

Overall survival of approximately 80% for children with advanced disease has led national collaborative groups to try to minimize therapy-related toxicities for this disease. For example, in the National Wilms' Tumor Study-3 (NWTS-3), the 87% relapse-free survival for stage II patients receiving 15 months of therapy with vincristine and actinomycin-D was not worse than that of patients receiving an anthracycline and/or 20-Gy radiotherapy.[114] Similarly, shortening postoperative chemotherapy from 18 to 4 weeks for stage I intermediate-risk or anaplastic disease did not affect prognosis.[115,116]

The recently closed SIOP WT 2001 study has also demonstrated no inferior outcome in EFS and OS for 583 patients with stage II/III intermediate risk disease randomized to receive vincristine and actinomycin as postoperative chemotherapy compared to those who also received doxorubicin. As a result, all patients in the UK with stage II/III intermediate-risk WT no longer receive anthracycline.

Currently in the UK, pre-operative chemotherapy for localized tumors consists of two drugs (VA) for 4 weeks, and for metastatic disease, three drugs (VAD) for 6 weeks. Postoperative surgical staging is an important prognostic factor, and defines subsequent chemotherapy and radiotherapy. The aim is to reduce treatment for patients with low- and intermediate-risk tumors (including stromal and epithelial histology), and intensify chemotherapy and radiotherapy for high-risk patients with inadequate response to pre-operative treatment.

The SIOP Renal Tumor Study Group study in the UK, IMPORT ("Improving Population Outcomes for Renal Tumors of Childhood"), will be joining the UMBRELLA study of the SIOP Renal Tumors Study Group (SIOP-RTSG). The underlying scientific hypothesis for the UMBRELLA study remains unchanged from the primary aims of IMPORT—namely to validate molecular biomarkers as independent adverse prognostic factors in the setting of histological risk groups after pre-operative chemotherapy.

Refractory and recurrent WT

Risk-adapted intensive retreatment has improved survival after recurrent WT, such that relapse after low-risk treatment (vincristine and actinomycin D only) has OS of 80%. Therapy is more intensive and uses different agents to those used first line (combinations of doxorubicin, ifosfamide/cyclophosphamide, etoposide, carboplatin) and together with high-dose chemotherapy with peripheral blood stem cell rescue (PBSCR), radiotherapy, and surgery of relapse site where feasible, are generating improved survival.

Two-thirds of relapses fall into higher risk groups that have had prior treatment with doxorubicin, additional chemotherapeutic agents, and/or radiotherapy. The role of high-dose myeloablative chemotherapy with peripheral blood stem cell rescue is not as clear in high-risk patients who relapse after aggressive

first-line treatment, but there may be a marginal advantage from HD therapy. The challenge is to identify more effective treatments for patients in the very high-risk group with initial high-risk histology (anaplastic or pre-treated blastemal type) or adverse molecular characteristics, who recur or progress after first-line intensive multiagent therapies and have a very poor outcome (EFS of <30%). These patients benefit from intensive induction treatment (with carboplatin, cyclophosphamide, and etoposide), surgery where feasible, followed by high-dose myeloablative therapy such as melphalan with peripheral blood stem cell support.[117]

An international consensus is forming on the approach to risk stratification of relapsed WT: standard, high, and very high risk, according to initial treatment received which in turn is determined by tumor stage and histology. The clinical relevance of other prognostic factors such as time to relapse and site of recurrence is less certain.

Screening

Surveillance for children at >5% risk of developing WT is recommended. These include children with WAGR and Frasier syndromes, familial WT, Beckwith–Weidemann syndrome, Perlman syndrome (high risk), and several other (rarer) conditions. Screening should follow clinical genetic review. Surveillance is by serial abdominal ultrasound every 3 months. The duration for surveillance will vary according to the underlying genetic condition.

Other malignant renal tumors

Clear cell sarcoma of kidney (CCSK)

CCSK comprises 5% of primary renal tumors of childhood. It has a significantly higher relapse and death rate than favorable histology WT.[118] CCSK metastasizes most frequently to the lungs (like WT), and has a tendency to metastasize to the bone and brain. The tumor is more common in boys, and presents at a median age of 1.5 years. It is very rare below age 6 months and in young adults.

A review of all UK patients with CCSK treated with intensive AVA showed long-term OS of 75% and EFS of 65%. However, 64% of stage II patients in the UK treated without anthracycline relapsed, and this group accounted for 50% of all relapses.

Recommendations for the management of CCSK were incorporated in SIOP WT 2001. For biopsy-proven CCSK, all stage I to III patients receive pre-operative and postoperative intensive chemotherapy, including doxorubicin, nephrectomy at week 7, and local radiotherapy doses for high-risk tumor. For stage IV disease, patients are treated according to the current European guidelines for management of high-risk WT.

Malignant rhabdoid tumor of the kidney (MRTK)

MRTK is a highly malignant tumor that metastasizes to the lungs and CNS, is more common in males, and presents at a median age of 13 months. Most tumors contain a biallelic inactivating mutation in *SMARCB1*, which encodes an essential component of the chromatin remodeling complex SWI/SNF, discussed later. The presence of germline alterations (15–30% cases) of *SMARCB1* predisposes these individuals to rhabdoid tumors in the brain and extracranial sites, often with multi-focal primary tumors. Children tend to be younger (<age 1 year) and have a poor prognosis. About 5% of rhabdoid tumors do not contain any mutation in *SMARCB1*. Truncating mutations of *SMARCA4* as an

alternative genetic event have been identified in some and also result in a total loss of protein expression.

MRTK was historically treated as an "unfavorable" histological subtype on WT protocols, and patients received treatment as per higher risk WT.

Currently in the UK, biopsy-proven cases are being treated on the European Pediatric Soft Tissue Sarcoma Group (EpSSG) NRSTS 2005 study with recommendation for extra-cranial malignant rhabdoid tumors, using intensive multiagent chemotherapy (vincristine, doxorubicin, cyclophosphamide, etoposide, carboplatin), aggressive local therapy with early surgical resection if feasible, and local radiotherapy to all sites of disease. The rationale of the multiagent chemotherapy regime originated from case reports of successful treatment in patients with metastatic MRTK and has formed the basis for the current Children's Oncology Group (COG) study of high-risk kidney tumors, which includes extracranial rhabdoid tumors, and the EpSSG protocol for extracranial malignant rhabdoid tumors.

The outcome of patients remains very poor, with only 31% of patients surviving to 1 year despite aggressive treatment, in the 106 children diagnosed with all types of extracranial rhabdoid tumor in the UK from 1993 to 2010. The young age of patients also limits the use of radiotherapy. Because the tumors are rare, it is a challenge to set up randomized trials to examine the role of new therapeutic approaches. Improved understanding of the biology and role of *SMARCB1* has now enabled the evaluation of new targets such as small molecule inhibitors (e.g. CDK4/6 inhibitor, Aurora kinases inhibitor) to combine with chemotherapy backbones in current and forthcoming EpSSG and COG studies.

Liver cancers

Ten children are diagnosed with primary liver cancers each year in the UK. Most are hepatoblastoma (HBL) and hepatocellular carcinoma (HCC), and the remainder comprise undifferentiated sarcoma, rhabdomyosarcoma, and epithelioid hemangioendothelioma.

Hepatoblastoma

Hepatoblastoma is the most common childhood liver cancer, with an incidence worldwide of 0.5–1.5 cases per million under the age 15 years.[119] Hepatoblastoma occurs most commonly under 3 years and most cases are sporadic. There are known associations with Beckwith–Wiedemann syndrome, familial adenomatous polyposis, Gardner syndrome, and with prematurity and low birth weight.[119,120]

Most patients present with an abdominal mass. The right lobe is involved more frequently than the left, and both lobes are involved in 20–30% of cases. Multifocal HBL is recognized in around 15% of cases.[121,122] Less common symptoms are anorexia, weight loss, and pain and an association with precocious puberty has been reported. Anemia and thrombocytosis are common, and a raised serum alpha fetoprotein (AFP) is found in >90% of cases. Lung metastases are seen in 10–20% at diagnosis.

Two major histological types are seen: epithelial (56% of cases) and mixed epithelial/mesenchymal (44% of cases). The epithelial type can be further subdivided into four subtypes: pure fetal (31%), embryonal (19%), macrotrabecular (3%), and small cell undifferentiated (3%). In completely resected tumors, pure fetal histology confers a better prognosis, whereas small cell undifferentiated histology is associated with a poorer prognosis.

Hepatocellular carcinoma

HCC is less common than HBL with an incidence of 0.2 cases per million children in England and Wales. HCC affects older children and young adults, with a peak incidence between 10 and 19 years; HCC is commoner in males and is associated with hepatitis B and C, cirrhosis, and other pre-existing parenchymal liver disorders. Patients with HCC usually present with an abdominal mass, pain, and jaundice. Serum AFP is elevated in 60–90% cases.

Recent advances in molecular pathology and growing knowledge about the biology of HCC have allowed pathologists to update classifications. Improving sub-classification will allow for more clinically relevant diagnoses and may allow for stratification into biologically meaningful subgroups.[123]

Treatment

Rare tumors present a challenge to clinical research. This has been overcome in HBL by collaboration and data-sharing between four international multicenter trial groups who have performed prospective controlled studies of HBL over the past two decades: the Children's Oncology Group, USA (COG); the International Society of Pediatric Oncology Epithelial Liver Tumor Group (SIOPEL); GPOH (German group); and JPLT (Japanese group). The Children's Hepatic Tumors International Collaboration (CHIC)[124] consortium has emerged to address this challenge in HBL, and they have concluded that PRE-Treatment EXTent of disease (PRETEXT), vascular involvement, extrahepatic disease, tumor multifocality, and rupture confer a poor outcome in HBL. In addition, age >8 years, low AFP (<100 ng/ml), and metastatic disease are associated with the worst outcomes.

The Pediatric Hepatic International Tumor Trial (PHiTT) is a collaborative study involving three major international liver tumor groups: SIOPEL, COG, and the Japanese Children's Cancer Group (JCCG). The PHITT study will investigate pediatric, adolescent, and young adult patients with newly diagnosed hepatoblastoma (HB) and hepatocellular carcinoma (HCC). A common risk stratification schema has been developed combining the CHIC risk factors giving four risks groups for HBL: very low, low, intermediate, and high and two for HCC—resectable or unresectable and/or metastatic.

Complete surgical resection of hepatoblastoma optimizes the chance of cure, but in half of cases this is not possible due to the extent of primary disease or presence of metastases. In the majority of cases, pre-operative chemotherapy is given to improve resectability of the tumor and to treat metastatic disease. PHiTT aims to identify (a) if reduction in therapy can reduce short- and long-term side effects for patients with good prognosis without compromising survival, and (b) if intensification with the new agents can improve survival for those with a poor prognosis. For patients with HCC, resection carries a good prognosis.[125] The trial will evaluate whether the addition of novel agents improves resectability and outcome. Orthotopic liver transplantation remains an alternative surgical modality for children with unresectable hepatoblastoma following neoadjuvant chemotherapy, with promising long-term survival.

Malignant germ cell tumors

Germ cell tumors account for approximately 3% of all childhood malignancies in the UK, 2.4 per million children per year (see Table 32.1).[126,127] Tumors arise typically in the midline, such as the sacrococcygeal region, retroperitoneum, mediastinum, and midbrain. Although histologically identical, it is helpful to separate

TABLE 32.1   **Relative Incidence of Childhood Germ Cell Tumors**

Site	Age	Relative Incidence (%)	Pathology
Sacrococcyx	Neonate	35	Teratoma (malignant 10–30%)
Vagina	Infant	2	Yolk sac
Ovary	Adolescence	25	Teratoma (malignant 30%)
Testis	Infant and adolescent	20	Teratoma (malignant 80%)
Retroperitoneum	Infant	5	Teratoma (rarely malignant)
Mediastinum	Adolescent	5	Teratoma (malignant 20–40%)
Head and neck	Infant and neonate	3	Teratoma (rarely malignant)
Cranium	Infant	5	Germinoma, embryonal carcinoma, mature teratoma

extracranial and intracranial tumors, since the management of these differs significantly.

There is a preponderance of females with GCT (4 girls:3 boys), and a bimodal incidence, with peaks in infancy and adolescence. In children under 5 years, the sex incidence is equal, with more ovarian than testicular tumors in older children. Non-gonadal tumors under 5 are more common in girls (M:F 1:2), but the reverse in older children and adolescents (M:F 2.6:1). Primary CNS GCTs arise predominantly in males (M:F 14:1), sacrococcygeal tumors in females. Sex also correlates with histology: malignant GCT is more common in males, and yolk sac tumors more common in young girls (M:F 1:2.12). An increased incidence of germ cell tumors is found for children with dysgenic gonads, Swyer syndrome, Klinefelter's syndrome, and defects in the urogenital tract such as cryptorchidism and sacral agenesis.

Pathology

The most common childhood GCT is mature teratoma, typically in ovary or at extra-gonadal sites. These are benign, characterized by the presence of ectoderm-, mesoderm-, and endoderm-derived structures.

Immature teratoma has immature tissues and may develop foci of malignant GCT (usually yolk sac tumor). They arise most often in the ovary around the time of puberty, and at extragonadal sites in younger children.

Malignant GCT includes YST, seminoma and dysgerminoma, choriocarcinoma, embryonal carcinoma, and mixed germ cell tumor. YST is characterized by the production of AFP, and choriocarcinoma by HCG. Elevation of HCG may also be seen in some germinomas.

Deletion of 1p or gain of 1q and chromosome 3 are the most common abnormalities seen in malignant GCTs for both sexes.[128] Isochromosome 12p and aneuploidy are common in adolescent boys, uncommon in early childhood.

Non-CNS tumors

Sacrococcygeal teratoma

The most common tumors of infancy are sacrococcygeal teratoma (SCT) and yolk sac tumor (YST). SCT is often present at birth, whilst YST typically presents between 7 months and 3 years.

The management of SCT involves surgical resection at the earliest opportunity, because of the risk of malignant (YST) tumor development within the unstable environment of the teratoma. With early removal, there remains a risk of recurrent disease (approximately 10–14%) for up to 3 years from resection, and hence close follow-up is indicated. Monitoring with local imaging and measurement of AFP and HCG initially every 6–8 weeks.

Testicular tumor

A new testicular swelling in an adolescent male is likely to be a germ cell tumor or (if para-testicular) rhabdomyosarcoma. Occasionally, leukemia or lymphoma may present with testicular infiltration. Testicular torsion is the major diagnosis considered in an emergency, and many young men undergo surgical exploration specifically to exclude this. Initial assessment should include ultrasound of scrotum and abdomen. Measurement of AFP and HCG should be performed pre-operatively unless surgery is considered urgent.

Scrotal biopsy is NOT recommended, and an inguinal orchidectomy is the correct operation, with control of vascular structures before mobilization. Pathological examination of the most proximal margin is required to assess the completeness of resection. Retroperitoneal lymph node dissection is not usually considered appropriate.

Ovarian tumor

Abdominal ultrasound or axial imaging should precede operation. Chest X-ray and subsequent CT will be required. AFP and HCG should be obtained, and physical examination, looking for evidence of syndromic markers (Turner's syndrome), should be performed. Constitutional karyotype should be performed and will guide diagnosis of XY dysgenesis if found. If so, bilateral salpingo-oophorectomy is generally recommended.

A complete resection of the tumor should be attempted, without rupture or spillage. Cyst rupture will result in a tumor stage becoming at least stage 2 and will usually require a unilateral salpingo-oophorectomy. Any peritoneal fluid should be examined cytologically, and any enlarged lymph nodes should be biopsied. The contra-lateral ovary should not be biopsied, but any nodule at this site should. If tumors are bilateral, a wedge biopsy, which may allow subsequent ovarian tissue to be preserved, should be performed. More radical surgery is not indicated.

Mediastinal tumor

Cross-sectional imaging is important for mediastinal tumors, given the possibility of airway compromise with anesthesia. If tumor markers are unequivocally elevated, biopsy is not indicated, and chemotherapy should begin promptly. If markers are not elevated, initial complete removal should be attempted, with biopsy of any enlarged regional nodes.

Mediastinal GCT is most often seen in older children and adolescents. In this age group, gain of chromosome 12p or isochromosome 12p is commonly seen (as in adult patients), whereas in younger children, deletions of 1p, 4 6q or gains of 1q, 3, and 20q are more common, suggesting a different etiology.[129] Overall survival is greater in patients younger than 8 years (OS = 0.95 vs. 0.64, $p = 0.03$). No events are expected after 1 year from diagnosis.

Vagina and uterus

These tumors will almost always have elevation of AFP. An initial biopsy is indicated, and (wherever possible) non-mutilating surgery delayed until after chemotherapy. Residual disease should be biopsied, and if non-resectable but non-viable, a period of observation can be undertaken.

Staging systems

Staging of MGCT is based on conventional TMN stage I–IV criteria.

Therapy

Since 2009, the Malignant Germ Cell Tumor International Consortium (MaGIC) has been a formal collaboration between COG (US) and the CCLG (UK),[130] which has produced a robust stratification system. The main determinants of prognosis are age and stage: AFP >10,000 ng/ml was not statistically significant as a prognostic consideration. Most importantly, the inferior outcome of patients over 11 years with extragonadal stage III/IV or ovarian stage IV (EFS <70%) was seen. This group warrants more intensive therapy.

Radical resection of malignant lesions is generally limited to gonadal sites, and surgical resection alone may be sufficient for low-risk tumors. These include (completely resected) stage I tumors, for which histological confirmation of resection is present. For these, close observation by imaging and monitoring of tumor markers is essential: rising AFP or HCG should be followed by complete restaging and chemotherapy. Relapse of testicular tumors occurs in 20–30%, and a preferred approach may be the administration of single-agent carboplatin (AUC) as has been used in adult practice for some time.[131]

Cisplatin-based chemotherapy (BEP) has proven highly effective in adult and pediatric GCT. Pediatric patients under 11 years may not require BEP chemotherapy, and reduced long-term sequelae might therefore be anticipated. In the UK, carboplatin, etoposide, bleomycin (JEB) was shown to be as effective, but associated with less late toxicity, than cisplatin-based regimes, and is the preferred regime for standard children under the age of 11.[132,133] JEB also uses significantly less bleomycin (a single dose per cycle) than adult regimes.

Lung injury is a particular concern for young patients, and the reduction of bleomycin dose is a driver of many studies. The POG9048/CCG8891 study, which used four cycles of cisplatin, etoposide, and (low-dose) bleomycin (PEB) for patients with stage II or recurrent stage I disease reported 6-year event-free survival (EFS) of 95%.[134]

Patients over 11 years are at greater risk of relapse after JEB chemotherapy, and current recommendations are for these patients to receive cisplatin-based chemotherapy. This may involve BEP × 3–4 cycles, or entry into the Accelerated BEP trial (UK P3BEP). Patients with thoracic germ cell tumors are at particular risk of bleomycin toxicity and avoidance of this with other (more cisplatin-based) regimes may be preferred.

Central nervous system tumors

Epidemiology

CNS tumors are the second most frequent malignancies in children under the age of 15 years, with an approximate annual incidence of 2.8 cases per 100,000 children/year.[135] Embryonal tumors are more common before age 10, and after early adolescence, typically adult CNS tumors increase.

TABLE 32.2 Changes to the WHO Classification System (2016) with Particular Relevance to Pediatric Practice

Embryonal Tumors

Major restructuring of medulloblastomas, with incorporation of genetically defined entities (WNT-activated, SHH-activated, TP53 WT or mutant, group 3, and group 4)

Embryonal tumor with multilayered rosettes, C19MC-altered

Removal of the term "PNET"

Ependymoma

Incorporation of Rel-A fusion positive ependymoma variant

Astrocytoma

IDH-wildtype and IDH-mutant diffuse, anaplastic, or glioblastoma

Diffuse midline glioma, H3 K27M–mutant

Source: Data from Louis et al., 2016.

The WHO classification for pediatric CNS tumors was revised in 2016, reflecting major changes in diagnostic methods (see Table 32.2).[136]

Clinical presentation

The clinical presentation of children with CNS tumors varies with age, development, and the site of origin of the tumor.

- Infratentorial (brain stem and cerebellar) tumors may present with disturbances of truncal steadiness, upper extremity co-ordination and gait, and cranial nerve function.
- Supratentorial tumors may present with features of raised intracranial pressure, irritability, seizures, regression of developmental milestones, and upper motor neuron signs such as hemiparesis.
- Optic chiasm tumors may result in visual field defects such as a bitemporal hemianopia, nystagmus, and head tilt.
- Hypothalamic tumors may give rise to the diencephalic syndrome (failure to thrive, euphoria, and hyperactivity), and endocrine disorders such as diabetes insipidus, hypogonadism, and precocious puberty.

MRI scanning is the investigation of choice for tumors of the central nervous system in childhood.

Medulloblastoma

Medulloblastoma is the most common malignant primary brain tumor of childhood, comprising 30 to 40% of these, and affecting 0.5 per 100,000 children each year. The peak incidence is at the age of 7 years, although cases are reported into late adult life. There is a slight male preponderance. They arise by definition in the posterior fossa. Developments in recent years have indicated significant differences in the biology of these tumors, and within the group of medulloblastomas, which has changed the approach to managing these tumors profoundly.

Presentation

Clinical features relate to the site of the tumor in the posterior fossa, often involving the cerebellar vermis and causing obstruction to the aqueduct or fourth ventricle. Clinical features will typically include truncal ataxia and signs of raised intracranial pressure.

Spread is by local invasion, to the cerebellar peduncle, floor of the fourth ventricle, and cervical spine. Occasionally, rostral extension is seen. Involvement of brain stem may give rise to cranial nerve palsies. Brain stem involvement has been reported to carry an adverse outcome, relating to the difficulty in attaining a complete surgical excision. Spread may also be through the CSF, and leptomeningeal deposits are seen in approximately 30% of patients. Rarely, tumor will be present in bone marrow at diagnosis.

Assessment

The primary tumor should be imaged by MRI. All patients should have imaging of the spinal cord and whole brain by gadolinium-enhanced MRI: the entire spine must be imaged in at least two planes. Pre-operative assessment is preferred to postoperative, but an interval of no more than 72 hours after operation is generally agreed to be acceptable in the assessment of metastatic disease. Lumbar puncture has higher diagnostic value than ventricular CSF sampling, and lumbar CSF should be obtained before treatment commences. Initial tumor assessment is of importance in the stratification of patients into low-, standard-, or high-risk groups, for which treatment is significantly different.

Tumor staging uses the Chang system, originally developed before MRI.[137][137] In practice, therapy is defined by the presence or absence of metastatic disease, however identified.

Dissemination, younger age at diagnosis, and incomplete resection indicate a likely poor outcome. Delay in starting radiotherapy adversely affects prognosis.[138,139]

Pathology

Medulloblastoma is a highly malignant embryonal tumor. Cells appear as undifferentiated round cells, but may mark with antibodies to synaptophysin, vimentin, GFAP, N-CAMs, retinal S-antigen, and the low affinity (p75-)NGF-receptor.

Sub-types may be identified histologically, and these have prognostic significance. Desmoplasia (marked, loose stroma) or evidence of excess nodularity (MBEN) is seen in younger patients and carries a better prognosis than "classical" histology. The presence of a large cell or anaplastic phenotype marks high-risk disease, for which a more intensive approach is now taken.

Biological factors and prognosis

Recent developments in the molecular biology of medulloblastoma have given profound insights into the causes, cell of origin, and importantly, the curability of this disease. The developments have been rapid and astonishing, coming from extensive international collaboration and multi-national clinical trials.

The loss of heterozygosity, often with isochromosome 17q, is a characteristic change. The dysregulation of ErbB2 and ErbB4 was identified in the early stages of molecular profiling.[140,141]

Aberrant expression of the Wnt pathway is seen in approximately 25% of medulloblastomas, including 60% with mutations of the *CTNNB1* gene.[142,143] These patients have a favorable prognosis in all series.

Myc amplification is strongly associated with large cell phenotype and carries an unfavorable prognosis.[144,145]

Integrative genomic approaches led to the identification of four, distinct medulloblastoma sub-types, for which characteristic drivers and prognoses are known. Briefly, these are described below, but the descriptions are summarized clearly in the consensus paper by Taylor et al.[146] and Northcott.[147] More recently, a collaboration of the major groups in North America and Europe has separated these into eight subgroups, but at present, the initial four are in common usage.[148]

(1) The Wnt subgroup is characterized by aberrant Wnt pathway signaling. Individuals with Turcot syndrome have a germ line mutation of the Wnt inhibitor, APC, and are predisposed to medulloblastoma.

These tumors arise in the dorsal brainstem in older children (median age 9–10 years). They have classical morphology, with nuclear staining for ß-catenin, often with monosomy for chromosome 6. With conventional chemotherapy and radiotherapy, they have a good prognosis, with 5-year EFS in excess of 90%. Tumors tend not to be metastatic, but even when this occurs, the prognosis is better than other groups.[149] Large cell/anaplastic histology is seen, but the overall prognosis remains good.[149] The principal concern for these patients is the risk of secondary tumors and morbidity associated with treatment.

(2) The SHH (Hedgehog) subgroup is characterized by disruption of the SHH pathway. Tumors more commonly arise in the cerebellar hemispheres, and are seen in individuals with Gorlin syndrome, who carry a germline mutation of the SHH receptor, PTCH. SHH tumors in infants are characterized by the desmoplastic/nodular phenotype, and carry a favorable prognosis, compared to other infants with classical morphology. This is seen even when metastasis has occurred.

In adult patients with medulloblastoma, SHH pathway dysregulation is not associated with a favorable prognosis, despite desmoplastic morphology.[147] Adult SHH-medulloblastomas with chromosome 10q deletion, 2 gain, 17p deletion, 17q gain, and/or GLI2 amplification have a prognosis which is significantly poorer than those without, and poorer than pediatric cases exhibiting the same aberrations.

(3) Group 3 medulloblastoma is characterized by the worst outcomes. These are pediatric (not adult) tumors, seen more often in boys, and are often metastatic at presentation. Amplification of MYC is common, and nearly all show aberrant expression of MYC. Many show karyotypic instability, with a high prevalence of 1q, 7, and 17q gain and deletions of 10q, 11, 16q, and 17p.[149] Isochromosome 17 is common.

(4) Group 4 medulloblastoma is the most common. These have an intermediate prognosis, are more common in males (M:F 3:1), and have classical or large cell histology. Amplification of MYC-N and CDK6 is commonly seen. Isochromosome 17q is seen in most, and where these occur in females, one copy of the X chromosome is usually lost. This suggests a more causative pathway to these tumors.

Therapy

Standard-risk disease

Standard therapy for medulloblastoma involves initial stabilization of the patient, and surgical resection. Complete surgical resection is a positive feature, but the importance is less with more effective chemotherapy and radiotherapy regimes.[150] Postoperative craniospinal radiotherapy (CSRT) is almost always recommended.

The third SIOP study was particularly important, involving a randomization between immediate radiotherapy alone or "sandwich chemotherapy," followed by CSRT and a boost to the tumor bed. A significant difference in PFS was seen for patients treated by chemotherapy and RT (EFS of 73% at 5 years) compared with RT alone (60%, $p = 0.04$). For patients who had undergone a total resection, event-free survival was significantly better with chemotherapy + RT than RT alone ($p = 0.035$).[151] It is unlikely that any subsequent study will be performed for which chemotherapy is not a standard component, and this study represents an important milestone in the development of therapy.

The CCG reported 5-year disease-free survival of 90% for "good-risk" patients treated with standard radiotherapy and a prolonged (48-week) course of chemotherapy with cisplatin, CCNU, and vincristine.[152]

The fourth SIOP study, PNET 4, confirmed similar, excellent survival of patients with standard-risk disease using a similar regime.[139] No benefit from hyperfractionated RT at a dose of 36 Gy to the craniospinal axis was seen compared to standard CSRT at 23.4 Gy.

The adverse long-term consequences of radiotherapy, particularly in young children, are potentially profound, and attempts have been made to reduce overall radiation doses used.[138,153–155] Non-significant differences have been found when patients received reduced-dose radiotherapy, but many of these studies were performed without an understanding of the separate subtypes of medulloblastoma reported recently.

High-risk disease

In poor-risk disease, chemotherapy improves survival.[155–157] Strategies currently used include chemotherapy dose intensification, radiation dose intensification,[158] and chemosensitization during radiation therapy.[159] Attempts to deliver chemotherapy and radiation dose intensification by the Milan group were associated with excessive neuro-toxicity.[160] To date, no single strategy has been adopted as the most effective.

Low-risk disease

There is a strong rationale for reduction of the radiation dose used for patients with low-risk disease, and this is, for example, the basis for a trial of clinical and molecular risk-directed therapy for newly diagnosed medulloblastoma, currently recruiting patients at St. Jude Children's Research Hospital (ClinicalTrials. gov Identifier: NCT01878617). A low-risk study in patients with *CTNNB1* mutation is part of the current SIOP study (ClinicalTrials.gov Identifier: NCT02066220).

Infant medulloblastoma

The treatment of young children with medulloblastoma is problematic, given the adverse consequences of CSRT at this age. Attempts to eliminate radiotherapy without sub-group stratification were unsuccessful, whilst survival of infants with metastatic medulloblastoma treated with CSRT approaches 40%. There is, therefore, an ethical dilemma in the choice of therapy, which the physician cannot make alone.

Encouraging results were reported by the German HIT-SKK group. Forty-three children were treated without radiotherapy, with a 5-year PFS of $58 \pm 9\%$ and OS of $66 \pm 7\%$. Desmoplasia was a good prognostic factor, compared to classical histology (PFS 85 $\pm 8\%$ vs. $34 \pm 10\%$ respectively).[161,162] Overall survival was $80 \pm 6\%$ in patients who received radiotherapy as salvage following relapse.

Studies of high-dose therapy have given promising results.[163,164]

Relapsed medulloblastoma

Recurrent medulloblastoma is rarely curable, and median survival is generally less than 1 year.[165,166] High-dose chemotherapy regimes have not shown significant benefit,[167–169] although one recent report of improved outcome after intensive chemotherapy, temozolomide, etoposide, and IT methotrexate is encouraging.[170]

Astrocytic tumors

Although technically, glial tumors include ependymoma and astrocytoma, the term glioma is often used interchangeably with astrocytoma.

Astrocytomas are classified as WHO grade I (pilocytic), grade II (fibrillary), grade III (anaplastic), and grade IV (glioblastoma multiforme). The designation as low grade (I and II) and high grade (III and IV) affects both treatment and prognosis.

Low-grade astrocytoma (LGA)

This is the most common form of CNS tumor in children, arising in cerebral hemispheres (20%), cerebellar hemispheres (35%), hypothalamus (12%), thalamus (12%), brain stem (12%), spinal cord (4%), and optic nerve/chiasm (3%).[171] The median age at diagnosis is 7 years. Children below the age of 5 years have a poorer PFS.

LGA in children is typically grade I, with few grade II.

Cerebral and cerebellar LGA

Surgery is the mainstay of therapy, with radiotherapy or chemotherapy reserved for recurrent or progressive inoperable disease. Vasculopathy (especially for young children and those with neurofibromatosis-type 1), endocrinopathy, and cognitive impairment[172,173] are significant concerns.

Midline LGA

For tumors of the optic chiasm or hypothalamus, curative surgery is rarely possible: surgery is indicated to debulk, relieve obstruction to CSF, or to biopsy. These tumors often present before the age of 5 years, and one-third have NF1.[174] Chemotherapy (vincristine and carboplatin) is usually used to control disease progression, postponing radiotherapy until after the age of 5 years, or later if possible.[174]

Vincristine and carboplatin remain the mainstay of first-line therapy but second-line combinations such as vincristine with cyclophosphamide and cisplatin, cisplatin/etoposide,[175] thioguanine/CCNU/procarbazine/vincristine,[176] temozolomide,[177] and weekly vinblastine[178] are often needed.

Grade II astrocytoma

Complete surgical resection of a grade II astrocytoma has a good prognosis, and no further therapy is required. Patients with residual disease have a significant likelihood of recurrence, and may show grade progression; for this reason, a more aggressive approach is often taken, although a single strategy is not agreed. The authors' own practice is to recommend focal radiotherapy (54 Gy) and adjuvant PCV chemotherapy as reported by Buckner et al.[179]

High-grade astrocytoma (HGA)

WHO grade III and IV astrocytomas make up 7–11% of childhood CNS tumors.[135] Most are supratentorial. Unlike adult HGA, very few in children demonstrate a p53 mutation, LOH for chromosome 10, or amplification of the epidermal growth factor receptor (EGFR).[180] Prognosis is related to the extent of surgical resection.[181]

5-year PFS (%):

	WHO grade	
	III	IV
Degree of resection		
Radical	44	26
Sub-total	22	5

Multiagent chemotherapy regimes generally show some (10–15%) improvement in survival over surgery and radiotherapy alone.[182,183] In CCG943, which randomized between radiation with or without chemotherapy (prednisone, lomustine, vincristine), a significant survival benefit was seen, in particular for glioblastoma (5-year EFS 42% vs. 6%, $p = 0.01$),[184] but the subsequent study (CCG945) was less encouraging (OS of 16 ± 7% for GBM).[182]

The German HIT group used chemotherapy together with and after radiation, or beforehand.[183] Although this study closed early because of poor recruitment, a highly significant difference in survival was seen for patients undergoing surgical CR or >90% resection, compared to those who did not (median survival 5.2 years vs. 1.3 years, $p < 0.0005$).

Temozolomide is the preferred treatment for many patients, favored because it has oral administration with few systemic side effects. The Stupp regime is typically used.[185] Methyl guanine methyl transferase (MGMT) expression is probably similar to adult patients,[186,187] and MGMT methylation is associated with a favorable prognosis.[188]

The Herby study followed from an adult study (AVAglio), looking at the combination of bevacizumab and temozolomide with radiotherapy in patients with newly diagnosed HGA and GBM. No improvement in survival was seen.[189]

High-dose chemotherapy with thiotepa and etoposide may play a role where a complete remission is achieved prior to high-dose therapy.[180] Massimino et al. reported OS of 45% with pre-irradiation chemotherapy (cisplatin, etoposide, cyclophosphamide, vincristine, high-dose methotrexate), myeloablative therapy (thiotepa), and continuation therapy (vincristine and CCNU).[190] The majority of studies, however, have reported poor outcomes.[177,191,192]

Despite being histologically indistinguishable, there are important differences between pediatric and adult high-grade astrocytomas. HGA arises more often in the brain stem in children, and such tumors show molecular biological differences from adults (see below). The gain of chromosome 1q is more common, gain of chromosome 7 and loss of 10q are less so.

Molecular genetic profiling has shown key differences in pediatric tumors: amplification of PDGFRA and a greater role for PDGFR signaling are seen in pediatric tumors.[193] The H3F3A mutation, seen in a high proportion of patients with pediatric brain stem gliomas, is also seen in 30% of pediatric high-grade glioma.[194,195]

Faury et al. reported a series of 32 children, and identified 2 groups of patients.[196] Those with activation of the Akt and Ras pathways had a worse outcome than those without. Active Ras was associated with survival in only 1 patient of 21, compared to 5 of the 11 without. Other factors, such as age, sex, or p53 expression, were not associated with outcome.

Developments in molecular biology

MAP kinase pathway

The MAP kinase pathway is important for many LGAs. It is the driver in tumors in neurofibromatosis type 1 (NF1), where loss of neurofibromin, a negative regulator of the RAS pathway, leads to constitutive activation. LGA arising in NF1 often behave in a more indolent manner and respond better to chemotherapy than sporadic tumors.[197]

Tandem duplication of BRAF is common in non-NF1 LGA.[198,199] Patients with the duplication have a favorable prognosis, compared to those without [EFS of 61 ± 8%, vs. 18 ± 8% without at 5 years ($p = 0.0004$)].[200]

The BRAF[V600E] mutation, is reported in some,[201] but not in all series. It is also common in ganglioglioma.[202]

These findings offer both diagnostic and therapeutic possibilities for the future, particularly in those patients who present with midline, unresectable tumors, often at a young age. The availability of inhibitors of both BRAF and of MAPK may allow less invasive and more targeted therapies. The possibility of identifying patients for whom a high or low risk of progression is anticipated allows stratification of treatment and (it is hoped) reduced morbidity.

IDH1

NADP-dependent isocitrate dehydrogenase (IDH1) gene is often mutated in diffuse astrocytomas (grade II).[203–206] Mutations of BRAF-KIAA1549, and IDH1 mutations were mutually exclusive in a series of 50 grade II and 70 grade I LGAs.[207] IDH mutation is not common, and its presence may increase the grade of a given tumor.

ATRX

Alpha thalassemia/mental retardation syndrome X-linked (ATRX) gene mutations in glioma are seen typically in young adults, and associate with other mutations including of IDH1 and TP53, but are mutually exclusive of 1p/19q-codeletion. ATRX loss is associated with a better prognosis within the group of IDH-mutant tumors.[208]

Histone mutations

The K27M mutation of the genes for the replacement histone H3.3 is found in 20% of pediatric glioblastoma, and is characteristic of DIPG (see below), but is not found in other pediatric tumors. The prognosis is poor, compared to wild type. It is not seen in adult-type supratentorial GBM, but is reported in adult mid-line tumors.

Diffuse intrinsic pontine glioma (DIPG)

Tumors arising in the midbrain, pons, and medulla oblongata account for 10–20% of all childhood CNS tumors, and usually present in children between the age of 5 and 9 years.[135] High-grade gliomas of the brain stem are chemo- and radioresistant: although clinical improvement is observed in the majority of children with 54 Gy radiotherapy, these tumors continue to have an extremely poor prognosis.[209–211]

Typically, children present with loss of cranial nerve function—diplopia, limited eye movement, facial weakness—and involvement of vestibular or cerebellar tracts. Most children will have long tract signs and may show raised intracranial pressure. Obstructive hydrocephalus may arise from expansion of the pons, or dissemination without evidence of ventricular dilatation.[212]

To date, no therapy has proven effective in DIPG. Radiation to doses over 50 Gy is associated with an improved survival, by approximately 3 months.[213] Increased radiation dose does not improve survival.[210,214] No advantage to adjuvant chemotherapy has been found for any chemotherapy or biological agent.[209]

In the setting of disease progression, a supportive approach alone is normally offered. Some benefit was reported by Janssens et al. for a strategy of re-irradiation (19.8–30 Gy), with OS of 13.7 vs. 10.3 months; $p = 0.04$.

Biopsy of DIPG

Experience of biopsy is growing, and as a consequence, there has been considerable development in understanding of the molecular biological events associated with DIPG. Clinical trials so far have failed to improve survival.[215] The BIOMEDE study aims to target the three main pathways affected in DIPG (mTOR, PDGFR, and EGFR) but is still recruiting.

Mutation of the H3F3A or HIST1H3B genes, which code for histone proteins H3.3 and H3.1, is seen in many patients with DIPG.[194] Methylation or acetylation is known to occur at the site of the K27M mutation, with expected secondary effects on protein expression.

The histone H3.3 K27M mutation is common in DIPG, but HIST1H3B or IDH1 mutations are not.[216] The K27M mutation is associated with a worse prognosis compared to wild type (OS 0.73 ± 0.48 years vs. 4.59 ± 5.55 years, $p = 0.0008$). Long-term survivors are found only in the K27M WT group.

Mutation at the TP53 locus is common in pediatric and adult GBM and carries an even more adverse prognosis.

Ependymoma

Ependymoma accounts for 6–12% of CNS tumors in childhood, with 50% of cases occurring before the age of 5 years.[217] Presentation is usually with raised ICP, although posterior fossa ependymomas commonly adhere to and invade the brain stem causing palsies of lower cranial nerves.

Clinical behavior

Tumors arising in the spine are often low grade (subependymoma and myxopapillary, grade I), and therapy at these sites is often confined to surgery alone. Low-grade ependymoma (grade II) and anaplastic ependymoma (grade III) require both surgical resection and radiotherapy. The relationship between histological grade and prognosis is uncertain and molecular profile is probably of greater importance.

Metastatic disease is found at diagnosis in 5–18% of patients.[218–220] Spinal imaging and CSF cytology are essential parts of tumor staging, since CSRT is necessary for such metastatic disease.

Therapy

Surgical resection is the mainstay of therapy.[219,221–224] Surgical complete clearance is clearly prognostic[219] and second- or third-look surgery is appropriate to achieve a radiological CR.[221,225]

Local radiotherapy is the standard postoperative treatment.[217] A dose of 55–55.8 Gy gives an EFS of 50–65% at 5 years, but escalation to 59 Gy gave favorable results—EFS was 76.9% and OS 85%—in the series of Merchant et al. Failure was rare after 3 years in this series, which differs from the pattern seen in earlier series.[226]

CSRT does not improve survival for patients with localized disease, and increases morbidity substantially.[223,227]

The role of chemotherapy is not certain, and reports disagree. Ependymomas do respond to chemotherapy, and its role may therefore be to enable improved surgical resection. In infants, chemotherapy may allow radiation to be delayed or even avoided. In the UKCCSG/SIOP study, a radiation-free survival of 42% at 5 years was seen and many patients who relapsed could later be salvaged with RT. OS was 63%.[228,229]

High-dose chemotherapy has no proven role in the treatment of ependymoma.[217,230–232]

Relapse

Further surgical resection of relapsed ependymoma[233] and oral etoposide[234] has been shown to confer some benefit in relapse. Re-irradiation is increasingly accepted with long-term survivors reported with good quality of life.[235,236]

Developments in molecular biology

Ependymoma most commonly shows loss of chromosome 22 or gain of 1q, although many others are seen.[237,238] Gain of 1q is thought to be an early event, may be the only abnormality,[239] and is associated with anaplasia,[240] and with recurrence.[241,242]

Patterns of gene expression were used to define three subgroups, then subsequently nine.[243] Supratentorial tumors, for example, express NOTCH and EPHB-EPHRIN pathways, whereas spinal ependymomas express members of the Homeobox (HOX) family. Particular importance is attached to expression of fusion genes involving REL-A and YAP-1.

CNS germ cell tumors

CNS germ cell tumor is uncommon, accounting for approximately 20% of all germ cell tumors. There is a marked male preponderance.[127] Tumors arise principally from the pineal and suprasellar regions. Basal ganglia or thalamic tumors have a poorer prognosis.

Presentation reflects the site of the tumor. Pineal tumors commonly lead to aqueduct obstruction and hydrocephalus, tectal pressure with impairment of papillary response, paresis of accommodation, and palsy of upward gaze (Parinaud's syndrome). Suprasellar region tumors cause visual, hypothalamic, or pituitary problems. Impairment of memory is common and is a function both of the presenting tumor, and of therapy.

MRI showing a CNS tumor, with elevation of blood or CSF AFP or HCG, is sufficient to make a diagnosis of secreting (non-germinomatous) germ cell tumor and no biopsy should be performed; morbidity is increased by biopsy, which should be avoided. Surgical intervention should be confined to CSF diversion, sampling for markers, and cytology.

Full assessment requires:

- Serum and CSF markers (AFP and HCG)
- CSF cytology (preferably by LP once this has been made safe)
- Whole craniospinal imaging

Exclusion of metastatic disease is particularly important if CSRT is not to be undertaken.

Treatment of germinoma

SIOP CNS GCT96 showed excellent outcomes for localized germinoma treated either with CSRT (24 Gy, with a 16 Gy boost), or with pre-radiation chemotherapy (CarboPEI) and focal radiotherapy.[244] OS was identical, but relapse was more common with local radiotherapy. Most relapses were in the ventricles, outside the initial radiation field, and therefore whole ventricular field irradiation is now recommended. Similar findings were seen in SFOP 90.[245]

Patients with metastatic disease, treated with CSRT and focal boosts to all sites of disease, had a similar, excellent survival.

Treatment of non-germinomatous germ cell tumor

Studies from Europe, the USA, and Japan report cure in two-thirds of patients with localized disease using chemotherapy and local radiation.[246,247] AFP levels are prognostic: elevation above 1000 ng/ml at diagnosis indicates high-risk disease. Residual disease at the end of treatment is associated with increased risk of recurrence,[248–250] and surgical removal of accessible residual tumor is therefore strongly recommended.

Atypical teratoid rhabdoid tumors (ATRT)

Atypical teratoid rhabdoid tumors are rare embryonal tumors, showing similarities to renal and extra-renal rhabdoid tumous[251]

(Rorke et al., 1996, p. 129). Mutations in the genes SMARCB1/INI1 or SMARCA4/BRG1 are present in all cases.[252,253] A rhabdoid predisposition syndrome is now increasingly recognized.

Epidemiology

Most tumors present in early childhood (median age 20 months, M>F). The majority arise within the posterior fossa or cerebral hemisphere; rarely, they may arise in the spinal cord or be multifocal. Simultaneous CNS and non-CNS primaries are found in some patients with the predisposition syndrome.

Presentation

Tumors grow rapidly, and may be extremely invasive. Symptoms and signs of raised intracranial pressure are common. These are highly malignant tumors, and can spread through dense fibrous structures such as tentorium. Approximately one-third are metastatic at diagnosis.

Radiological features are not characteristic, but are often large, hyperdense lesions, enhancing strongly. There may be hemorrhage or calcification, or signs of leptomeningeal spread.

Molecular biology

Aberrations of chromosome 22 are common, and this led to the identification of the gene, INI 1 (hSNF5, SMARCB1, or BAF47). hSWI/SNF is a nucleosome-remodeling complex, present in prokaryotes and eukaryotes and INI1 is a core member. INI1 is mutated in almost all cases,[254–256] and is the only mutation necessary in these.[257] Such limited diversity of mutation is most uncommon.

Familial RT

Germline mutations of INI1 are common, particularly in younger children, and these are associated both with familial predisposition, and multiple tumors. The prognosis for such patients is inferior to non-germline cases.[258–260]

Treatment and prognosis

Radiotherapy

Radiotherapy has been used for the majority of patients treated successfully for ATRT, and it is an important component of current strategies. There is confounding of data, however, since patients who have not received radiotherapy are likely to be those who show early progression or poor clinical state, or are very young. Radiotherapy is often part of a systematic approach to treatment, and hence the benefit may come from the approach, rather than radiation alone. Not all studies of radiotherapy indicate efficacy.[261] CSRT does not seem to be associated with a higher overall survival.[262]

The concerns regarding long-term neurocognitive sequelae are significant, but no study has compared RT with other approaches such as high-dose chemotherapy.

Surgery

There is a clear benefit for patients who achieve surgical CR.[263–265] In the German ATRT registry, patients who achieved surgical CR tended to have an improved EFS, but not OS. Patients in continued CR after chemotherapy, however, did have a higher OS (35 ± 12% vs. 16 ± 7%, $p = 0.006$).

Multimodal therapy

Chi et al. reported a series of 25 patients, treated with aggressive multi-modality therapy including CSRT, intrathecal chemotherapy, and intensive systemic chemotherapy.[264] Toxicity was severe, with one treatment-related death and a further patient developing spinal radiation recall and transverse myelitis, but 2-year OS and EFS reported of 70 ± 10% and 53 ± 13% were encouraging.

The role of high-dose chemotherapy (HDCT)

Whilst there has been no formal study of high-dose chemotherapy, data are available from case reports. The value of high-dose therapy is difficult to determine in these patients, given that they are likely to be a selected group, younger, or with incomplete response to surgery and/or radiotherapy. Most data are anecdotal, but Lafay-Cousin reported 40 patients, median age 16.7 months at diagnosis.[265]

Eighteen patients received HDCT, and nine of these were alive at a median of 40.8 months; OS for these patients at 2 years was 48 ± 12% compared to 27 ± 9% after conventional chemotherapy. In contrast to previous series, radiotherapy was not associated with any significant improvement in survival (median survival 17.8 months vs. 14 months, $p = 0.64$). Six of 12 survivors received no radiotherapy.

There is now a need for a randomized study to compare these options.

CNS tumors in infants and very young children

Approximately 12–15% of all childhood CNS tumors occur in children less than 2 years of age, and two-thirds of these are supratentorial.[135] The predominant diagnoses are medulloblastoma, ependymoma, low-grade gliomas, malignant glioma (15%), and ATRT.

Infants and very young children with CNS tumors are at risk of catastrophic long-term intellectual sequelae after radiotherapy, and for this reason, chemotherapy schedules have been investigated to delay or avoid radiotherapy. For example, the HIT-SKK group reported favorable outcomes in SHH group infant medulloblastoma treated without RT, but with intrathecal therapy.[162]

Late effects of treatment

The majority of children with cancer are cured, and currently almost 80% will reach 5 years from diagnosis. There is a high likelihood that survivors will have at least one resulting chronic medical condition and many have significant physical, psychological, or intellectual difficulties.

Sequelae relate to the cancer, the treatment, the patient, and their family. Recognition of late effects depends upon structured follow-up for extended periods of time.

In contrast to the acute side effects of therapy, late sequelae for children are often more profound than for adult patients. Tumor-related problems may arise at presentation, as a complication of direct organ damage, or due to secondary effects such as tumor lysis syndrome, and sepsis. Brain and spinal tumors may cause specific neurological deficit, and even with neurological recovery, subsequent orthopedic deformity such as scoliosis or kyphosis may develop. Surgery may cause disability if an aggressive, mutilating approach is taken. Primary surgery is rarely indicated in childhood, the prevalent view being to achieve a diagnosis, then use definitive surgery, following initial tumor control by chemotherapy and/or radiotherapy. Even for tumors such as osteosarcoma, where complete surgical resection is an absolute requirement of therapy, there is a strong focus on the reduction of long-term morbidity with limb-salvage procedures. For primary CNS tumors, improved visualization and image-guidance methods have allowed better, more radical but less destructive surgery to be achieved.

Radiotherapy causes significant and widespread long-term effects, affecting any organ or tissue within the field. The reduction of growth, reduction of mobility at irradiated joints, and early onset of degenerative conditions such as osteoarthritis and osteoporosis may be seen. Osteopenia and osteonecrosis may cause fractures many years after treatment. Cranial radiotherapy is associated with a greater risk of stroke and second primary tumors such as meningioma or glioma. Neuro-endocrine effects of radiation to the pituitary region lead to the loss of one or more pituitary hormones, particularly of growth hormone. Thyroid radiation leads to hypothyroidism and thyroid cancer and gonadal radiotherapy to infertility. Breast radiation leads to secondary breast cancer. Radiation to the heart alone or in association with anthracycline chemotherapy greatly increases the risk of cardiac impairment, and of ischemic heart disease in later life. Radiotherapy-sparing protocols are therefore the goal in treating the children of the future.

Chemotherapy has numerous sequelae, although many can be minimized by careful monitoring of patients during active treatment. Cardiac toxicity can be avoided for most patients provided anthracycline chemotherapy is given to previously documented safe levels (<300 mg/m^2), but this risk cannot be eliminated completely for these drugs. Cisplatin causes significant renal impairment in many patients, as both a reduction in GFR and also a loss of tubular function. Ifosfamide has similar nephrotoxic activity, predominantly with regard to tubular function. Sensorineural hearing loss from cisplatin may not recover and is a function of cumulative dose.

Adverse effects also depend on developmental stage of the child. Hearing loss at an early age may cause significant disruption to language development and consequent developmental progress, even in the absence of other sequelae. The long-term consequences of therapy for primary CNS tumors have been underestimated until recently, but it is hoped that assessment of disability, and intervention at a young age will allow many of these children to achieve their full potential in the future.

Specific sequelae of therapy

Second malignancies

Second malignant neoplasms (SMN) are the second most common cause of death in survivors of primary cancer in childhood.[266] A lifetime risk between 10 and 20 times that of age-matched controls is seen, and an overall probability of between 2 and 12% at 25 years. With more prolonged follow-up, this proportion is likely to rise. Certain groups (survivors of Hodgkin's disease) have an actuarial risk which may exceed 20%. Risk is also high in patients with cancer predisposition syndromes, e.g., neurofibromatosis type I, Li–Fraumeni syndrome, or Gorlin syndrome.

Irradiation is associated with many SMNs[266] (Rosso et al., 1994, p. 2). The majority of sarcomas, carcinomas, and brain tumors arising as SMNs (85%) occur within the radiation field.

Chemotherapy-related SMNs include myelodysplasia (tAML) or leukemia, which appear to be dose-dependent.[267] tAML following alkylator therapy will typically present several years (peak 4–7 years) after treatment, and is most frequently associated with deletions of chromosomes 5 and/or 7.[268] tAML associated with topoisomerase-II inhibitors typically occurs much sooner (less than 2 years from treatment) and is associated with rearrangements involving chromosome 11q23.

Growth

Abnormalities of growth hormone secretion may be seen after radiation doses as low as 10 Gy. Irradiation to the hypothalamus or pituitary at a dose above 30 Gy is likely to cause permanent loss of GH secretion. Most commonly, GH deficiency will evolve slowly, depending on age, dose, and fractionation of treatment[269] (Schmiegelow et al., 2000, #6). For all patients at risk, 6-monthly interval growth monitoring, until completion of puberty with early referral to pediatric endocrinology is essential. Early GH replacement will minimize loss of height for an affected individual.

Spinal and long bone growth will also be affected by radiotherapy, and monitoring for scoliosis and limb length difference must continue until growth is complete. Chemotherapy-induced growth failure is seen, in particular after long-term corticosteroid therapy. Early overgrowth may be followed by early endplates fusion and an overall reduction in final height. Deficient growth may be compounded in those with CNS malignancy, where puberty may be entered early, leading to premature growth arrest.

Normal growth requires adequate nutrition. This may be impossible during intensive chemotherapy, and children may fail to grow in this phase. After completion of therapy, ongoing effects of chemotherapy, persistent poor nutrition, or other organ impairment may lead to a continuing failure to achieve normal growth.

Fertility and sex hormone function

Radiotherapy and chemotherapy both influence gonadal function. Damage to germ cells is common with treatment and may lead to loss of both endocrine function and fertility in females with increased risk of early menopause or complete ovarian failure. Leydig cell failure is rare in males, but spermatogenesis is more sensitive to chemotherapy and radiotherapy, such that infertility is a significant risk for many children.

Prior to commencing radiotherapy, consideration of both the potential to avoid damage to or preserve germ cells should be undertaken. Whenever possible consideration of shielding or repositioning of ovaries should be contemplated before treatment. Uterine dysfunction following radiotherapy may also jeopardize future pregnancies—a factor that should be borne in mind if *in vitro* fertilization programs are contemplated.

Finally, the health and well-being of their actual offspring is an understandable area of concern for survivors of childhood malignancy. As yet, there is little published mature data in this field, although it would appear that there is no current evidence of appreciable excess risk of either malignancy or congenital malformations.[270]

Organ toxicity

Cardiac

Cardiotoxicity associated with anthracycline therapy has been well-recognized for over 20 years.[271] Cumulative dose, rate of infusion, administration schedule, mediastinal irradiation, and young age at the time of exposure are all predictors of risk.

Acute toxicities, arrhythmias, or acute impairment of contractility are rare. Chronic toxicity leading to cardiomyopathy is commoner and clinically the most important. Cardiac sequelae may vary from a subclinical impairment of contractility to a dilated cardiomyopathy.

Renal

Surgical resection of one kidney will be tolerated without clinical consequence for the majority of patients, and it is doubtful whether long-term follow-up of such patients is necessary. Coincident nephrotoxic chemotherapy and radiotherapy will be of greater importance for most patients. Radiotherapy may cause renal dysfunction, but this is less likely if the dose is restricted to less than 20 Gy. More commonly, chemotherapy—particularly cisplatin and ifosfamide—may lead to long-term problems. The risk for both of these agents is related to administration and total dose.[272] Methotrexate and high-dose cyclophosphamide may also cause significant renal dysfunction.

Lungs

Although limited in its use in the pediatric field, radiotherapy commonly results in pulmonary toxicity, affecting both the lung directly and subsequent growth of the chest wall. Acute pneumonitis and long-term clinically significant restriction are uncommon provided radiation dose is less than 30 Gy, but radiation to the chest is always used cautiously in pediatric patients. The risk of later malignant change in breast or thyroid, and of the marked increase in cardiotoxicity seen with radiation and anthracyclines are significant concerns.

Bleomycin, a component of germ cell tumor chemotherapy regimes, may cause acute pneumonitis, and potentially long-term fibrosis. BCNU is well-known to cause fibrosis, and is rarely used in childhood cancer, but CCNU is an important component of therapy for CNS primitive neuro-ectodermal tumors and for some astrocytomas.

High-dose chemotherapy is associated with a risk of pulmonary damage. The etiology is often unclear, but exposure to respiratory viruses—particularly adenovirus—use of high-dose busulphan and of radiotherapy to the lungs are associated with the development of pulmonary inflammatory disease and bronchiolitis obliterans with obstructive pneumonia within a year of treatment. Although reversible if mild, this condition may progress and lead to death.

Neurocognitive effects

Educational

Disruption of education as a consequence of treatment and ill health may have secondary effects on attendance at school, and subsequent performance, but in the long term for most children, this risk seems to be small. In contrast, children who have recovered from primary brain tumors are at significant risk, and it is appropriate for these children to have specific support at an early stage. Although most will complete secondary education, a far smaller proportion move on to university or higher education courses[273] (Hays et al., 1992, #13). Many survivors, particularly those who were young at diagnosis and those who had brain tumors or who received CNS-directed therapy (including intrathecal methotrexate), will need special educational support. Social isolation may develop because of time off school, physical limitations, or the experience of a life-threatening event, and this may lead to secondary difficulties in later life.

Cognitive effects of a tumor are variable and depend upon tumor location, age and developmental stage of the child, and the therapy given. Hypothalamic tumors cause significant intellectual problems, presumably as a result of the critical importance of this region in aspects of memory, and close proximity of visual pathways. The presence of hydrocephalus and the need for CSF diversion were associated with late cognitive impairment in some

series but not others.[274] Patients who have a complicated recovery period postoperatively are also at risk of more severe late cognitive and psychological sequelae.

Young age at diagnosis, neurofibromatosis type 1, hydrocephalus at presentation, surgical complications, increasing interval since treatment, and importantly, the use of cumulative dose and volume of cranial irradiation are all risk factors for cognitive impairment.[275] Socio-economic status, supratentorial location, chemotherapy, and complications of treatment, including growth hormone deficit, hypothyroidism, and epilepsy, were classified as "probable" risk factors.

Radiotherapy is often necessary to cure brain tumors, and the long-term effects of radiotherapy on intellectual development are well-documented. The effects vary by site and extent of the radiation field and appear to be more significant in very young children, below the age of 7 years, and most marked in those under 3 years[275–278] (Mulhern et al., 1998, #20). Very significant reduction in IQ may be seen after craniospinal radiotherapy, not found in patients undergoing surgery alone, such that a child may have great difficulty remaining integrated in society in adult life. There is therefore a dilemma for many children, their parents, and their physicians. There is no "safe" age for radiotherapy in childhood, and a balance between the benefit (in terms of likely cure) and harm (in terms of neuropsychological impairment, neuro-endocrine, and other sequelae) needs to be made for each child. Attempts have been made to reduce overall radiation doses used[138,153,155,279] and children require neuro-cognitive follow-up and access to additional help in school throughout their childhood.

Quality of life

The measurement of morbidity following survival from childhood cancer is most often objective, documentary records based upon physical findings. The survivor's subjective view is at least as important, but has been relatively under-reported due to difficulties of definition, and limited availability of appropriate tools. This has begun to change, and in recent years, substantial progress has been made. Indeed, major clinical trials sponsors, such as the Medical Research Council and National Cancer Institute, require new trials to consider quality of life assessments as part of their central strategy[280] (Nayfield et al., 1992, #26).

Quality of life (QOL) is determined by a person's disabilities, their abilities, achieving those things that are important to them, their expectations, and achievements. It is influenced by circumstance, relationships, and physical and mental health. Many of the sequelae discussed above will affect QOL, but the overall impact on the patient may be extremely variable.

QOL is appropriately expressed in terms of fields relating to aspects of normal life. In the field of physical functioning, the majority of survivors are reported to have one or more physical late effects[281] (Oeffinger et al., 2000, #28), but the majority of survivors report good physical health. The exceptions are survivors of CNS, bone, and other sarcomas[282–284] (Novakovic et al., 1997, #32).

Fatigue has been reported to be of variable significance in survivors of cancer. In contrast to studies from adult survivors, there seemed to be no excess in fatigue in the study of Langeveld, or for patients with previous leukemia reported by Meeske et al.[285,286]

A greater prevalence of psychological problems compared to population norms and normal or sibling controls has been reported by some authors,[287,288] although no difference, or indeed a lower prevalence has been reported.[289] Gray et al. found that survivors reported significantly more positive affect, more perceived personal control, and greater satisfaction with life than controls.[290]

Post-traumatic stress disorder (PTSD) may help to explain the psychosocial consequences of having cancer as a child.[291,292] A prevalence of between 4.5 and 25% in survivors has been reported. Interestingly, PTSD symptoms seem to be more common in parents of survivors, than in the survivors themselves.[292]

Palliative care

The Joint Working Party of the Association for Children with Life-Threatening or Terminal Conditions and their Families (ACT) and the Royal College of Pediatrics and Child Health 1997, defined palliative care for children with life-limiting conditions as

> an active and total approach to care, embracing physical, emotional, social and spiritual element. It focuses on enhancement of quality of life for the child and support for the family and includes the management of distressing symptoms, provision of respite and care through death and bereavement.

It is clear that palliative care needs to address the whole of a child's life, including the extended family, all of whom will affect and be affected by the dying of a child.[293]

The transition from optimism, looking for cure, to an acceptance that this is not possible will be gradual, and may proceed at different rates for different members of a family. This may lead to difficulties, if one person's expectations is markedly at odds with those of the child, other relative, or members of the care team. End-of-life decisions are more challenging for parents than for those based around other areas of treatment,[294] and this may lead to the exploration of wide-ranging, sometimes inappropriate therapies. Social media may fuel this exploration. It has been reported that parents of children with cancer have difficulty in distinguishing between research and treatment and consequently can feel that they are not in control of the choices available.[295] It is a role of the physician to move with the child and their family, and to support them at each stage.

Symptom control for palliative care in a child is similar to that for any child or adult. Analgesia is of great importance; non-steroidal analgesics, paracetamol, and opiates are all relevant. These may not always be effective, and careful use of agents addressing local disease, and appropriate consideration of the pathological processes are essential in children as for all patients. Steroids may be rapidly effective in patients with raised intracranial pressure, with bone pain secondary to marrow infiltration, or with neuropathic pain for some patients. Neuropathic pain may present difficulties in management. It arises as a result of infiltration or compression of the spinal cord or nerve roots, causing shooting or burning pain and sometimes, altered sensation (dysesthesia) or increased sensitivity to normal stimuli (allodynia).

Co-analgesics, such as tricyclic antidepressants or anticonvulsant drugs, may be helpful[296,297] (Watson, 2000, #59). Transcutaneous electrical nerve stimulation (TENS), and anxiolytics agents may also allow better control for resistant pain. The importance of continuing to provide the child with appropriate play should not be underestimated as a means of reducing the experience of pain.[298]

The majority of children will die at home. For many children this is by far the preferred option for the child and their parents alike, but for adolescents in particular, physical difficulties, and the return to dependency upon parents may mean that a hospital or hospice environment is preferred.

Psychological aspects of childhood cancer

The psychological impact of the diagnosis of cancer in a child is enormous. There will be feelings of fear, guilt, anxiety, anger, denial, hopelessness, and depression. It is the responsibility of the multi-disciplinary team to support the child and their family. This should include doctors, nurses, psychologists, the clergy, and social workers. Discussions with the family should be in the presence of an experienced nurse or social worker, who may later help assimilate the information. Information should be repeated and reinforced where possible with written material. Parents may feel disempowered, and an experienced medical team needs to recognize their feelings, reassure them that they are appropriate, normal responses, and help them see the importance of their role in the child's care.

Talking to the child

Talking to the child with cancer is difficult for parents, and they look to the team for guidance. The approach depends on the child's chronological age, developmental age, and their past experiences. Children may be unable to express their feelings in words, so need to explore other means of communication, e.g. art therapy, music therapy, and play therapy. Prior to 1970 most of those dealing with childhood cancer believed that unless a child was older than 10 years, they were incapable of understanding death and therefore did not experience anxiety about it. It is clear now that even pre-school age children have a concept of the seriousness of their illness. Those children who had not had the opportunity to express their feelings may demonstrate a psychological distance from those around them, leaving them isolated. Play therapists and child psychologists are important members of the wider multi-disciplinary team for every pediatric oncology department.

The child with cancer should be well-informed at a level appropriate to their age and understanding. This is a legal requirement of care. The Children's Act of 1989 in the UK and the United Nations Convention on the Rights of the Child (also 1989) exhort those involved in the care of children to inform the child of their situation, to solicit their opinion, and when appropriate to regard their opinion as determinative. Clearly this may seem a huge responsibility for the child. They will look for advocates—their parents, nursing staff, or a social worker—to help support them in making decisions regarding their care. By not soliciting the child's opinion, their autonomy is violated and the natural pathway to emerging independence in adult life is interrupted.

Educating the child with cancer

Continuing to attend school whilst receiving chemotherapy or radiotherapy allows the child to keep up with and maintain identity within their peer group. It presents an image of hope to teachers, classmates, parents, and the child and enhances social and coping skills to help the child better deal with their illness. Classmates and teachers may need counseling and ongoing support and for most, specialist oncology nurses provide this. The child needs realistic goals to prevent further loss of self-esteem through failure, and often attendance can only be part time because of fatigue, illness, or hospitalization.

Parent support groups

There are a number of parent support groups in existence. Early in 1999 a National Alliance of Childhood Cancer Parents Organizations (NACCPO) was formed to model the International Confederation of Childhood Cancer Parent Organizations (ICCCPO). Such organizations link parent groups in the same way professionals are linked through national and international organizations, such as the United Kingdom Children's Cancer and Leukemia Group (CCLG) and Société Internationale d'Oncologie Pédiatrique (SIOP). In addition, NACCPO seeks to be the voice of parents and families of children affected by cancer at a national level through interactions with government, health authorities, and social services, to represent their needs. The rise of the social media poses unique challenges in the management of children and families with cancer particularly when life is limited.

Supporting siblings

Siblings of a child with cancer will be significantly affected. According to their age and understanding, they should be kept well-informed. There are likely to be repeated episodes where the affected child and one or both parents will be away from home. The sibling left behind will deal with this better if they are aware of why it is happening. There are a number of support groups for siblings.

Ambulatory pediatrics

The multidisciplinary pediatric oncology team has pioneered ambulatory pediatrics. Minimizing time spent in hospital has been for the psychological benefit of the child and family rather than economic benefit to the health service. In fact, resources needed to provide such a service are enormous. Specialist domiciliary care nurses do far more than just travel to the child's home or school to take blood samples or administer treatment. Integral to the success of ambulatory care is extensive education of all those involved in caring for the child including parents, teachers, and general practitioners.

References

1. Stiller CA, Allen MB, Eatock EM. Childhood cancer in Britain: The National Registry of Childhood Tumours and incidence rates 1978–1987. *Eur J Cancer*. 1995; 31A:2028–34.
2. Stiller CA, Parkin DM. International variations in the incidence of childhood renal tumours. *Br J Cancer*. 1990;62:1026–30.
3. Armstrong SA, Staunton JE, Silverman LB et al. MLL translocations specify a distinct gene expression profile that distinguishes a unique leukemia. *Nat Genet*. 2002; 30:41–7.
4. Roberts KG, Li Y, Payne Turner D et al. Targetable kinase-activating lesions in Ph-like acute lymphoblastic leukemia. *N Engl J Med*. 2014; 371:1005–15.
5. Vora A, Andreano A, Pui CH et al. Influence of cranial radiotherapy on outcome in children with acute lymphoblastic leukemia treated with contemporary therapy. *J Clin Oncol*. 2016; 34:919–26.
6. Eden OB, Lilleyman JS, Richards S et al. Results of Medical Research Council Childhood Leukaemia Trial UKALL VIII (report to the Medical Research Council on behalf of the Working Party on Leukaemia in Childhood). *Br J Haematol*. 1991; 78:187–96.
7. Vora A, Goulden N, Wade R et al. Treatment reduction for children and young adults with low-risk acute lymphoblastic leukaemia defined by minimal residual disease (UKALL 2003): A randomised controlled trial. *Lancet Oncol*. 2013; 14:199–209.
8. Vora A, Goulden N, Mitchell C et al. Augmented post-remission therapy for a minimal residual disease-defined high-risk subgroup of children and young people with clinical standard-risk and intermediate-risk acute lymphoblastic leukaemia (UKALL 2003): A randomised controlled trial. *Lancet Oncol*. 2014; 15:809–18.
9. O'Connor D, Enshaei A, Bartram J et al. Genotype-specific minimal residual disease interpretation improves stratification in pediatric acute lymphoblastic leukemia. *J Clin Oncol*. 2018; 36:34–43.
10. Schultz KR, Carroll A, Heerema NA et al. Long-term follow-up of imatinib in pediatric Philadelphia chromosome-positive acute lymphoblastic leukemia: Children's Oncology Group study AALL0031. *Leukemia*. 2014; 28:1467–71.
11. von Stackelberg A, Locatelli F, Zugmaier G et al. Phase I/phase II study of blinatumomab in pediatric patients with relapsed/refractory acute lymphoblastic leukemia. *J Clin Oncol*. 2016; 34:4381–89.
12. Maude SL, Laetsch TW, Buechner J et al. Tisagenlecleucel in children and young adults with B-cell lymphoblastic leukemia. *N Engl J Med*. 2018; 378:439–48.
13. Pieters R, De Lorenzo P, Ancliffe P et al. Outcome of infants younger than 1 year with acute lymphoblastic leukemia treated with the interfant-06 protocol: Results from an international Phase III randomized study. *J Clin Oncol*. 2019; 37(25):2246–56.
14. Furness CL, Kirkwood A, Rowntree C et al. Early morphological response is significantly associated with, but does not accurately predict, relapse in teenagers and young adults aged 10–24 years with acute lymphoblastic leukaemia (ALL): Results from UKALL2003. *Br J Haematol*. 2019; 184(4):663–6.
15. Creutzig U, van den Heuvel Eibrink MM, Gibson B et al. Diagnosis and management of acute myeloid leukemia in children and adolescents: Recommendations from an international expert panel. *Blood*. 2012; 120:3187–205.
16. Arber DA, Orazi A, Hasserjian R et al. The 2016 revision to the World Health Organization classification of myeloid neoplasms and acute leukemia. *Blood*. 2016; 127:2391–405.
17. Lo Coco F, Avvisati G, Vignetti M et al. Retinoic acid and arsenic trioxide for acute promyelocytic leukemia. *N Engl J Med*. 2013; 369:111–21.
18. Uffmann M, Rasche M, Zimmermann M et al. Therapy reduction in patients with Down syndrome and myeloid leukemia: The international ML-DS 2006 trial. *Blood*. 2017; 129:3314–21.
19. Carbone PP, Kaplan HS, Musshoff K et al. Report of the committee on Hodgkin's disease staging classification. *Cancer Res*. 1971; 31:1860–61.
20. Dieckmann K, Potter R, Hofmann J et al. Does bulky disease at diagnosis influence outcome in childhood Hodgkin's disease and require higher radiation doses? Results from the German-Austrian Pediatric Multicenter Trial DAL-HD-90. *Int J Radiat Oncol Biol Phys*. 2003; 56:644–52.
21. Ruhl U, Albrecht M, Dieckmann K et al. Response-adapted radiotherapy in the treatment of pediatric Hodgkin's disease: An interim report at 5 years of the German GPOH-HD 95 trial. *Int J Radiat Oncol Biol Phys*. 2001; 51:1209–18.
22. Schellong G, Bramswig JH, Hornig-Franz I. Treatment of children with Hodgkin's disease–Results of the German Pediatric Oncology Group. *Ann Oncol*. 1992; 3(Suppl. 4):73–6.
23. Schellong G, Potter R, Bramswig J et al. High cure rates and reduced long-term toxicity in pediatric Hodgkin's disease: The German-Austrian multicenter trial DAL-HD-90. The German-Austrian Pediatric Hodgkin's Disease Study Group. *J Clin Oncol*. 1999; 17:3736–44.
24. Shankar A, Hall GW, Gorde Grosjean S et al. Treatment outcome after low intensity chemotherapy [CVP] in children and adolescents with early stage nodular lymphocyte predominant Hodgkin's lymphoma–An Anglo-French collaborative report. *Eur J Cancer*. 2012; 48:1700–6.
25. Longo DL, Glatstein E, Duffey PL et al. Radiation therapy versus combination chemotherapy in the treatment of early-stage Hodgkin's disease: Seven-year results of a prospective randomized trial. *J Clin Oncol*. 1991; 9:906–17.
26. Longo DL, Glatstein E, Duffey PL et al. Alternating MOPP and ABVD chemotherapy plus mantle-field radiation therapy in patients with massive mediastinal Hodgkin's disease. *J Clin Oncol*. 1997; 15:3338–46.

27. Oberlin O, Leverger G, Pacquement H et al. Low-dose radiation therapy and reduced chemotherapy in childhood Hodgkin's disease: The experience of the French Society of Pediatric Oncology. *J Clin Oncol.* 1992; 10:1602–8.

28. Landman-Parker J, Pacquement H, Leblanc T et al. Localized childhood Hodgkin's disease: Response-adapted chemotherapy with etoposide, bleomycin, vinblastine, and prednisone before low-dose radiation therapy-results of the French Society of Pediatric Oncology Study MDH90. *J Clin Oncol.* 2000; 18:1500–1507.

29. Ekert H, Toogood I, Downie P et al. High incidence of treatment failure with vincristine, etoposide, epirubicin, and prednisolone chemotherapy with successful salvage in childhood Hodgkin disease. *Med Pediatr Oncol.* 1999; 32:255–58.

30. Shankar AG, Ashley S, Atra A et al. A limited role for VEEP (vincristine, etoposide, epirubicin, prednisolone) chemotherapy in childhood Hodgkin's disease. *Eur J Cancer.* 1998; 34:2058–63.

31. SH S, E C, NL H. *WHO Classification of Tumours of Haematopoietic and Lymphoid Tissues* (4th ed.). Lyon, France: IARC Press, 2008.

32. Swerdlow SH, Campo E, Pileri SA et al. The 2016 revision of the World Health Organization classification of lymphoid neoplasms. *Blood.* 2016; 127:2375–90.

33. Croce CM, Nowell PC. Molecular basis of human B cell neoplasia. *Blood.* 1985;65:1–7.

34. Vannier JP, Patte C, Philip T et al. Treatment of extensive B-cell lymphoma in children: Studies of the French Pediatric Oncology Society. *Bull Cancer.* 1988; 75:61–8.

35. Patte C, Auperin A, Michon J et al. The Societe Francaise d'Oncologie Pediatrique LMB89 protocol: Highly effective multiagent chemotherapy tailored to the tumor burden and initial response in 561 unselected children with B-cell lymphomas and L3 leukemia. *Blood.* 2001; 97:3370–79.

36. Patte C, Philip T, Rodary C et al. Improved survival rate in children with stage III and IV B cell non-Hodgkin's lymphoma and leukemia using multi-agent chemotherapy: Results of a study of 114 children from the French Pediatric Oncology Society. *J Clin Oncol.* 1986; 4:1219–26.

37. Minard-Colin V, Brugières L, Reiter A et al. Non-Hodgkin lymphoma in children and adolescents: Progress through effective collaboration, current knowledge, and challenges ahead. *J Clin Oncol.* 2015; 33:2693.

38. Editors. O-104 Results of the Randomized Intergroup Trial Inter-B-NHL RITUX 2010 for Children/Adolescents with High-Risk B-Cell Non Hodgkin Lymphoma (B-NHL) and Mature Acute Leukemia (B-AL). *Pediatr Blood Cancer.* 2016; 63(S3):2016.

39. Burkhardt B, Hermiston ML. Lymphoblastic lymphoma in children and adolescents: Review of current challenges and future opportunities. *Br J Haematol.* 2019; 185:1158–70.

40. Delsol G, Al Saati T, Gatter KC et al. Coexpression of epithelial membrane antigen (EMA), Ki-1, and interleukin-2 receptor by anaplastic large cell lymphomas. Diagnostic value in so-called malignant histiocytosis. *Am J Pathol.* 1988; 130:59–70.

41. Le Deley MC, Reiter A, Williams D et al. Prognostic factors in childhood anaplastic large cell lymphoma: Results of a large European intergroup study. *Blood.* 2008; 111:1560–66.

42. Reiter A, Schrappe M, Tiemann M et al. Successful treatment strategy for Ki-1 anaplastic large-cell lymphoma of childhood: A prospective analysis of 62 patients enrolled in three consecutive Berlin-Frankfurt-Munster group studies. *J Clin Oncol.* 1994; 12:899–908.

43. Woessmann W, Seidemann K, Mann G et al. The impact of the methotrexate administration schedule and dose in the treatment of children and adolescents with B-cell neoplasms: A report of the BFM Group Study NHL-BFM95. *Blood.* 2005; 105:948–58.

44. Brugieres L, Le Deley MC, Rosolen A et al. Impact of the methotrexate administration dose on the need for intrathecal treatment in children and adolescents with anaplastic large-cell lymphoma: Results of a randomized trial of the EICNHL Group. *J Clin Oncol.* 2009; 27:897–903.

45. Lamant L, Meggetto F, al Saati T et al. High incidence of the t(2;5)(p23;q35) translocation in anaplastic large cell lymphoma and its lack of detection in Hodgkin's disease. Comparison of cytogenetic analysis, reverse transcriptase-polymerase chain reaction, and P-80 immunostaining. *Blood.* 1996; 87:284–91.

46. Williamson D, Missiaglia E, de Reynies A et al. Fusion gene-negative alveolar rhabdomyosarcoma is clinically and molecularly indistinguishable from embryonal rhabdomyosarcoma. *J Clin Oncol.* 2010; 28:2151–58.

47. Selfe J, Olmos D, Al-Saadi R, Thway K et al. Impact of fusion gene status versus histology on risk-stratification for rhabdomyosarcoma: Retrospective analyses of patients on UK trials. *Pediatr Blood Cancer.* 2017; 64:e26386.

48. Davicioni E, Finckenstein FG, Shahbazian V et al. Identification of a PAX-FKHR gene expression signature that defines molecular classes and determines the prognosis of alveolar rhabdomyosarcomas. *Cancer Res.* 2006; 66:6936–46.

49. Missiaglia E, Williamson D, Chisholm J et al. PAX3/FOXO1 fusion gene status is the key prognostic molecular marker in rhabdomyosarcoma and significantly improves current risk stratification. *J Clin Oncol.* 2012; 30:1670–77.

50. Anderson J, Ramsay A, Gould S, Pritchard-Jones K. PAX3-FKHR induces morphological change and enhances cellular proliferation and invasion in rhabdomyosarcoma. *Am J Pathol.* 2001; 159:1089–96.

51. Rosenberg AR, Skapek SX, Hawkins DS. The inconvenience of convenience cohorts: Rhabdomyosarcoma and the PAX-FOXO1 biomarker. *Cancer Epidemiol Biomarkers Prev.* 2012; 21:1012–18.

52. Sorensen PH, Lynch JC, Qualman SJ et al. PAX3-FKHR and PAX7-FKHR gene fusions are prognostic indicators in alveolar rhabdomyosarcoma: A report from the children's oncology group. *J Clin Oncol.* 2002; 20:2672–79.

53. Arnold MA, Anderson JR, Gastier-Foster JM et al. Histology, fusion status, and outcome in alveolar rhabdomyosarcoma with low-risk clinical features: A report from the Children's Oncology Group. *Pediatr Blood Cancer.* 2016; 63:634–9.

54. Norman G, Fayter D, Lewis-Light K et al. An emerging evidence base for PET-CT in the management of childhood rhabdomyosarcoma: Systematic review. *BMJ Open.* 2015; 5:e006030.

55. Chisholm JC, Marandet J, Rey A et al. Prognostic factors after relapse in nonmetastatic rhabdomyosarcoma: A nomogram to better define patients who can be salvaged with further therapy. *J Clin Oncol.* 2011; 29:1319–25.

56. Crist WM, Anderson JR, Meza JL et al. Intergroup rhabdomyosarcoma study-IV: Results for patients with nonmetastatic disease. *J Clin Oncol.* 2001; 19:3091–102.

57. Meza JL, Anderson J, Pappo AS et al. Analysis of prognostic factors in patients with nonmetastatic rhabdomyosarcoma treated on intergroup rhabdomyosarcoma studies III and IV: The Children's Oncology Group. *J Clin Oncol.* 2006; 24:3844–51.

58. Oberlin O, Rey A, Lyden E et al. Prognostic factors in metastatic rhabdomyosarcomas: Results of a pooled analysis from United States and European cooperative groups. *J Clin Oncol.* 2008; 26:2384–9.

59. Mascarenhas L, Lyden ER, Breitfeld PP et al. Randomized phase II window trial of two schedules of irinotecan with vincristine in patients with first relapse or progression of rhabdomyosarcoma: A report from the Children's Oncology Group. *J Clin Oncol.* 2010; 28:4658–3.

60. Bisogno G, Jenney M, Bergeron C et al. Addition of dose-intensified doxorubicin to standard chemotherapy for rhabdomyosarcoma (EpSSG RMS 2005): A multicentre, open-label, randomised controlled, phase 3 trial. *Lancet Oncol.* 2018; 19:1061–71.

61. Pappo AS, Lyden E, Breitfeld P et al. Two consecutive phase II window trials of irinotecan alone or in combination with vincristine for the treatment of metastatic rhabdomyosarcoma: The Children's Oncology Group. *J Clin Oncol.* 2007; 25:362–9.

62. Blank LE, Koedooder K, Pieters BR et al. The AMORE protocol for advanced-stage and recurrent nonorbital rhabdomyosarcoma in the head-and-neck region of children: A radiation oncology view. *Int J Radiat Oncol Biol Phys.* 2009; 74:1555–62.

63. Carnevale A, Lieberman E, Cardenas R. Li-Fraumeni syndrome in pediatric patients with soft tissue sarcoma or osteosarcoma. *Arch Med Res.* 1997; 28:383–6.

64. Feugeas O, Guriec N, Babin-Boilletot A et al. Loss of heterozygosity of the RB gene is a poor prognostic factor in patients with osteosarcoma. *J Clin Oncol.* 1996; 14:467–72.

65. Newton WA, Jr., Meadows AT, Shimada H et al. Bone sarcomas as second malignant neoplasms following childhood cancer. *Cancer.* 1991; 67:193–201.

66. Le Vu B, de Vathaire F, Shamsaldin A et al. Radiation dose, chemotherapy and risk of osteosarcoma after solid tumours during childhood. *Int J Cancer.* 1998; 77:370–77.

67. Schajowicz F, Sissons HA, Sobin LH. The World Health Organization's histologic classification of bone tumors. A commentary on the second edition. *Cancer.* 1995; 75:1208–14.

68. Bacci G, Ferrari S, Delepine N et al. Predictive factors of histologic response to primary chemotherapy in osteosarcoma of the extremity: Study of 272 patients preoperatively treated with high-dose methotrexate, doxorubicin, and cisplatin. *J Clin Oncol.* 1998; 16:658–63.

69. Asada N, Tsuchiya H, Tomita K. De novo deletions of p53 gene and wild-type p53 correlate with acquired cisplatin-resistance in human osteosarcoma OST cell line. *Anticancer Res.* 1999; 19:5131–37.

70. Goto A, Kanda H, Ishikawa Y et al. Association of loss of heterozygosity at the p53 locus with chemoresistance in osteosarcomas. *Jpn J Cancer Res.* 1998; 89:539–47.

71. Wang ZQ, Liang J, Schellander K et al. c-fos-induced osteosarcoma formation in transgenic mice: Cooperativity with c-jun and the role of endogenous c-fos. *Cancer Res.* 1995; 55:6244–51.

72. Sweetnam R. Amputation in osteosarcoma. Disarticulation of the hip or high thigh amputation for lower femoral growths? *J Bone Joint Surg Br.* 1973; 55:189–92.

73. Bacci G, Ferrari S, Mercuri M et al. Predictive factors for local recurrence in osteosarcoma: 540 patients with extremity tumors followed for minimum 2.5 years after neoadjuvant chemotherapy. *Acta Orthop Scand.* 1998; 69:230–36.

74. Szendroi M, Antal I, Koos R et al. Results of limb-saving surgery and prognostic factors in patients with osteosarcoma. *Orv Hetil.* 2000; 141:2175–182.

75. Abudu A, Sferopoulos NK, Tillman RM et al. The surgical treatment and outcome of pathological fractures in localised osteosarcoma. *J Bone Joint Surg Br.* 1996; 78:694–8.

76. Kawai A, Hamada M, Sugihara S et al. Rotationplasty for patients with osteosarcoma around the knee joint. *Acta Med Okayama.* 1995; 49:221–6.

77. Bramwell VH, Burgers M, Sneath R et al. A comparison of two short intensive adjuvant chemotherapy regimens in operable osteosarcoma of limbs in children and young adults: The first study of the European Osteosarcoma Intergroup. *J Clin Oncol.* 1992; 10:1579–91.

78. Souhami RL, Craft AW, Van der Eijken JW et al. Randomised trial of two regimens of chemotherapy in operable osteosarcoma: A study of the European Osteosarcoma Intergroup. *Lancet.* 1997; 350:911–17.

79. Lewis IJ, Weeden S, Machin D et al. Received dose and dose-intensity of chemotherapy and outcome in nonmetastatic extremity osteosarcoma. European Osteosarcoma Intergroup. *J Clin Oncol.* 2000; 18:4028–37.

80. Delepine N, Delepine G, Bacci G, Rosen G, Desbois JC. Influence of methotrexate dose intensity on outcome of patients with high grade osteogenic osteosarcoma. Analysis of the literature. *Cancer.* 1996; 78:2127–35.

81. Graf N, Winkler K, Betlemovic M, Fuchs N, Bode U. Methotrexate pharmacokinetics and prognosis in osteosarcoma. *J Clin Oncol.* 1994; 12:1443–51.

82. Delepine N, Delepine G, Cornille H et al. Dose escalation with pharmacokinetics monitoring in methotrexate chemotherapy of osteosarcoma. *Anticancer Res.* 1995; 15:489–94.

83. Bielack S, Kempf-Bielack B, Schwenzer D et al. Neoadjuvant therapy for localized osteosarcoma of extremities. Results from the Cooperative osteosarcoma study group COSS of 925 patients. *Klin Padiatr.* 1999; 211:260–70.

84. Philip T, Iliescu C, Demaille MC et al. High-dose methotrexate and HELP [Holoxan (ifosfamide), eldesine (vindesine), platinum]–doxorubicin in non-metastatic osteosarcoma of the extremity: A French multicentre pilot study. Federation Nationale des Centres de Lutte contre le Cancer and Societe Francaise d'Oncologie Pediatrique. *Ann Oncol.* 1999; 10:1065–71.

85. Marina N, London WB, Frazier AL et al. Prognostic factors in children with extragonadal malignant germ cell tumors: A pediatric intergroup study. *J Clin Oncol.* 2006; 24:2544–48.

86. Bielack SS, Smeland S, Whelan JS et al. Methotrexate, doxorubicin, and cisplatin (MAP) plus maintenance pegylated interferon Alfa-2b versus MAP alone in patients with resectable high-grade osteosarcoma and good histologic response to preoperative MAP: First Results of the EURAMOS-1 Good Response Randomized Controlled Trial. *J Clin Oncol.* 2015; 33:2279–87.

87. Carter SR, Grimer RJ, Sneath RS, Matthews HR. Results of thoracotomy in osteogenic sarcoma with pulmonary metastases. *Thorax.* 1991; 46:727–31.

88. Tabone MD, Kalifa C, Rodary C et al. Osteosarcoma recurrences in pediatric patients previously treated with intensive chemotherapy. *J Clin Oncol.* 1994; 12:2614–20.

89. van Rijk-Zwikker GL, Nooy MA, Taminiau A et al. Pulmonary metastasectomy in patients with osteosarcoma. *Eur J Cardiothorac Surg.* 1991; 5:406–9.

90. Bacci G, Briccoli A, Mercuri M et al. Osteosarcoma of the extremities with synchronous lung metastases: Long-term results in 44 patients treated with neoadjuvant chemotherapy. *J Chemother.* 1998; 10:69–76.

91. Ambros IM, Ambros PF, Strehl S et al. MIC2 is a specific marker for Ewing's sarcoma and peripheral primitive neuroectodermal tumors. Evidence for a common histogenesis of Ewing's sarcoma and peripheral primitive neuroectodermal tumors from MIC2 expression and specific chromosome aberration. *Cancer.* 1991; 67:1886–93.

92. Völker T, Denecke T, Steffen I et al. Positron emission tomography for staging of pediatric sarcoma patients: Results of a prospective multicenter trial. *J Clin Oncol.* 2007; 25:5435–41.

93. Eary JF, Conrad EU, Bruckner JD et al. Quantitative [F-18]fluorodeoxyglucose positron emission tomography in pretreatment and grading of sarcoma. *Clin Cancer Res.* 1998; 4:1215–20.

94. Franzius C, Sciuk J, Daldrup-Link HE et al. FDG-PET for detection of osseous metastases from malignant primary bone tumours: Comparison with bone scintigraphy. *Eur J Nucl Med.* 2000; 27:1305–11.

95. Delattre O, Zucman J, Melot T et al. The Ewing family of tumors--a subgroup of small-round-cell tumors defined by specific chimeric transcripts. *N Engl J Med.* 1994; 331:294–99.

96. de Alava E, Kawai A, Healey JH et al. EWS-FLI1 fusion transcript structure is an independent determinant of prognosis in Ewing's sarcoma. *J Clin Oncol.* 1998; 16:1248–55.

97. Ewing J. Diffuse endothelioma of bone. *Proc NY Pathol Soc.* 1921; 21:17–24.

98. Thomas PR, Perez CA, Neff JR et al. The management of Ewing's sarcoma: Role of radiotherapy in local tumor control. *Cancer Treat Rep.* 1984; 68:703–10.

99. Burgert EO, Jr., Nesbit ME, Garnsey LA et al. Multimodal therapy for the management of nonpelvic, localized Ewing's sarcoma of bone: Intergroup study IESS-II. *J Clin Oncol.* 1990; 8:1514–24.

100. Jurgens H, Gobel V, Michaelis J et al. The Cooperative Ewing Sarcoma Study CESS 81 of the German Pediatric Oncology Society–analysis after 4 years. *Klin Padiatr.* 1985; 197:225–32.

101. Jurgens H, Exner U, Gadner H et al. Multidisciplinary treatment of primary Ewing's sarcoma of bone. A 6-year experience of a European Cooperative Trial. *Cancer.* 1988; 61:23–32.

102. Sauer R, Jurgens H, Burgers JM et al. Prognostic factors in the treatment of Ewing's sarcoma. The Ewing's Sarcoma Study Group of the German Society of Paediatric Oncology CESS 81. *Radiother Oncol.* 1987; 10:101–10.

103. Juergens C, Weston C, Lewis I et al. Safety assessment of intensive induction with vincristine, ifosfamide, doxorubicin, and etoposide (VIDE) in the treatment of Ewing tumors in the EURO-E.W.I.N.G. 99 clinical trial. *Pediatr Blood Cancer.* 2006; 47:22–9.

104. Miser JS, Krailo MD, Tarbell NJ et al. Treatment of metastatic Ewing's sarcoma or primitive neuroectodermal tumor of bone:

Evaluation of combination ifosfamide and etoposide–A Children's Cancer Group and Pediatric Oncology Group study. *J Clin Oncol.* 2004; 22:2873–76.

105. Paulussen M, Ahrens S, Burdach S et al. Primary metastatic (stage IV) Ewing tumor: Survival analysis of 171 patients from the EICESS studies. European Intergroup Cooperative Ewing Sarcoma Studies. *Ann Oncol.* 1998; 9:275–81.

106. Spunt SL, McCarville MB, Kun LE et al. Selective use of whole-lung irradiation for patients with Ewing sarcoma family tumors and pulmonary metastases at the time of diagnosis. *J Pediatr Hematol Oncol.* 2001; 23:93–8.

107. Oberlin O, Rey A, Desfachelles AS et al. Impact of high-dose busulfan plus melphalan as consolidation in metastatic Ewing tumors: A study by the Société Française des Cancers de l'Enfant. *J Clin Oncol.* 2006; 24:3997–4002.

108. Leavey PJ, Mascarenhas L, Marina N et al. Prognostic factors for patients with Ewing sarcoma (EWS) at first recurrence following multi-modality therapy: A report from the Children's Oncology Group. *Pediatr Blood Cancer.* 2008; 51:334–38.

109. Green DM. Wilms' tumour. *Eur J Cancer.* 1997; 33:409–18; discussion 19.

110. Choyke PL, Siegel MJ, Craft AW et al. Screening for Wilms tumor in children with Beckwith-Wiedemann syndrome or idiopathic hemihypertrophy. *Med Pediatr Oncol.* 1999; 32:196–200.

111. Grundy PE, Breslow NE, Li S et al. Loss of heterozygosity for chromosomes 1p and 16q is an adverse prognostic factor in favorable-histology Wilms tumor: A report from the National Wilms Tumor Study Group. *J Clin Oncol.* 2005; 23:7312–21.

112. Shamberger RC, Guthrie KA, Ritchey ML et al. Surgery-related factors and local recurrence of Wilms tumor in National Wilms Tumor Study 4. *Ann Surg.* 1999; 229:292–97.

113. Boccon-Gibod L, Rey A, Sandstedt B et al. Complete necrosis induced by preoperative chemotherapy in Wilms tumor as an indicator of low risk: Report of the international society of paediatric oncology (SIOP) nephroblastoma trial and study 9. *Med Pediatr Oncol.* 2000; 34:183–90.

114. D'Angio GJ, Breslow N, Beckwith JB et al. Treatment of Wilms' tumor. Results of the Third National Wilms' Tumor Study. *Cancer.* 1989; 64:349–60.

115. de Kraker J, Graf N, van Tinteren H et al. Reduction of postoperative chemotherapy in children with stage I intermediate-risk and anaplastic Wilms' tumour (SIOP 93–01 trial): A randomised controlled trial. *Lancet.* 2004; 364:1229–35.

116. Reinhard H, Semler O, Burger D et al. Results of the SIOP 93–01/GPOH trial and study for the treatment of patients with unilateral nonmetastatic Wilms Tumor. *Klin Padiatr.* 2004; 216:132–40.

117. Pein F, Michon J, Valteau-Couanet D et al. High-dose melphalan, etoposide, and carboplatin followed by autologous stem-cell rescue in pediatric high-risk recurrent Wilms' tumor: A French Society of Pediatric Oncology study. *J Clin Oncol.* 1998; 16:3295–301.

118. Argani P, Perlman EJ, Breslow NE et al. Clear cell sarcoma of the kidney: A review of 351 cases from the National Wilms Tumor Study Group Pathology Center. *Am J Surg Pathol.* 2000; 24:4–18.

119. Perilongo G, Shafford EA. Liver tumours. *Eur J Cancer.* 1999; 35:953–8; discussion 958.

120. Reynolds P, Urayama KY, Von Behren J, Feusner J. Birth characteristics and hepatoblastoma risk in young children. *Cancer.* 2004; 100:1070–76.

121. Saxena R, Leake JL, Shafford EA et al. Chemotherapy effects on hepatoblastoma. A histological study. *Am J Surg Pathol.* 1993; 17:1266–71.

122. Exelby PR, Filler RM, Grosfeld JL. Liver tumors in children in the particular reference to hepatoblastoma and hepatocellular carcinoma: American Academy of Pediatrics Surgical Section Survey—1974. *J Pediatr Surg.* 1975; 10(3):329–37

123. Jabbour TE, Lagana SM, Lee H. Update on hepatocellular carcinoma: Pathologists' review. *World J Gastroenterol.* 2019; 25(14):1653.

124. Czauderna P, Haeberle B, Hiyama E et al. The Children's Hepatic tumors International Collaboration (CHIC): Novel global rare tumor database yields new prognostic factors in hepatoblastoma and becomes a research model. *Eur J Cancer.* 2016; 52:92–101.

125. Katzenstein HM, Krailo. MD. Hepatocellular carcinoma in children and adolescents: Results from the Pediatric Oncology Group and the Children's Cancer Group intergroup study. *J Clin Oncol.* 2002; 20(12): 2789–97.

126. Pinkerton CR. Malignant germ cell tumours in childhood. *Eur J Cancer.* 1997; 33:895–901; discussion 901.

127. Schneider DT, Calaminus G, Koch S et al. Epidemiologic analysis of 1,442 children and adolescents registered in the German germ cell tumor protocols. *Pediatr Blood Cancer.* 2004; 42:169–75.

128. Bussey KJ, Lawce HJ, Olson SB et al. Chromosome abnormalities of eighty-one pediatric germ cell tumors: Sex-, age-, site-, and histopathology-related differences—a Children's Cancer Group study. *Genes Chromosomes Cancer.* 1999; 25:134–46.

129. Schneider DT, Schuster AE, Fritsch MK et al. Genetic analysis of mediastinal nonseminomatous germ cell tumors in children and adolescents. *Genes Chromosomes Cancer.* 2002; 34:115–25.

130. Frazier AL, Hale JP, Rodriguez-Galindo C et al. Revised risk classification for pediatric extracranial germ cell tumors based on 25 years of clinical trial data from the United Kingdom and United States. *J Clin Oncol.* 2015; 33:195–201.

131. Aparicio J, García del Muro X, Maroto P et al. Multicenter study evaluating a dual policy of postorchiectomy surveillance and selective adjuvant single-agent carboplatin for patients with clinical stage I seminoma. *Ann Oncol.* 2003; 14:867–72.

132. Mann JR, Raafat F, Robinson K et al. The United Kingdom Children's Cancer Study Group's second germ cell tumor study: Carboplatin, etoposide, and bleomycin are effective treatment for children with malignant extracranial germ cell tumors, with acceptable toxicity. *J Clin Oncol.* 2000; 18:3809–18.

133. Pinkerton CR, Broadbent V, Horwich A et al. "JEB"—a carboplatin based regimen for malignant germ cell tumors in children. *Br J Cancer.* 1990; 62:257–62.

134. Rogers PC, Olson TA, Cullen JW et al. Treatment of children and adolescents with stage II testicular and stages I and II ovarian malignant germ cell tumors: A Pediatric Intergroup Study-Pediatric Oncology Group 9048 and Children's Cancer Group 8891. *J Clin Oncol.* 2004; 22:3563–69.

135. Heideman RL, Packer RJ, Albright LA et al. (Eds). *Tumours of the Central Nervous System* (p. 633). Philadelphia: Lippincott-Raven Publishers, 1997.

136. Louis DN, Perry A, Reifenberger G, Deimling AV et al. The 2016 World Health Organization classification of tumors of the central nervous system: A summary. *Acta Neuropathol.* 2016; 131(6):803–20.

137. Chang CH, Housepian EM, Herbert CJ. An operative staging system and a megavoltage radiotherapeutic technic for cerebellar medulloblastomas. *Radiology.* 1969; 93:1351–59.

138. Bailey CC, Gnekow A, Wellek S et al. Prospective randomised trial of chemotherapy given before radiotherapy in childhood medulloblastoma. International society of paediatric oncology (SIOP) and the (German) society of paediatric oncology (GPO): SIOP II. *Med Pediatr Oncol.* 1995; 25:166–78.

139. Lannering B, Rutkowski S, Doz F et al. Hyperfractionated versus conventional radiotherapy followed by chemotherapy in standard-risk medulloblastoma: Results from the randomized multicenter HIT-SIOP PNET 4 trial. *J Clin Oncol.* 2012; 30:3187–93.

140. Gilbertson RJ, Pearson AD, Perry RH, Jaros E, Kelly PJ. Prognostic significance of the c-erbB-2 oncogene product in childhood medulloblastoma. *Br J Cancer.* 1995; 71:473–77.

141. Gajjar A, Hernan R, Kocak M et al. Clinical, histopathologic, and molecular markers of prognosis: Toward a new disease risk stratification system for medulloblastoma. *J Clin Oncol.* 2004; 22:984–93.

142. Ellison DW, Onilude OE, Lindsey JC et al. beta-Catenin status predicts a favorable outcome in childhood medulloblastoma: The United Kingdom children's cancer study group brain tumour committee. *J Clin Oncol.* 2005; 23:7951–57.

143. Clifford SC, Lusher ME, Lindsey JC et al. Wnt/Wingless pathway activation and chromosome 6 loss characterize a distinct molecular sub-group of medulloblastomas associated with a favorable prognosis. *Cell Cycle.* 2006; 5:2666–70.

144. Ellison DW, Kocak M, Dalton J et al. Definition of disease-risk stratification groups in childhood medulloblastoma using combined clinical, pathologic, and molecular variables. *J Clin Oncol.* 2011; 29:1400–7.

145. Lamont JM, McManamy CS, Pearson AD, Clifford SC, Ellison DW. Combined histopathological and molecular cytogenetic stratification of medulloblastoma patients. *Clin Cancer Res.* 2004; 10:5482–93.

146. Taylor MD, Northcott PA, Korshunov A et al. Molecular subgroups of medulloblastoma: The current consensus. *Acta Neuropathol.* 2012; 123:465–72.

147. Northcott PA, Korshunov A, Witt H et al. Medulloblastoma comprises four distinct molecular variants. *J Clin Oncol.* 2011; 29:1408–14.

148. Sharma T, Schwalbe EC, Williamson D et al. Second-generation molecular subgrouping of medulloblastoma: An international meta-analysis of Group 3 and Group 4 subtypes. *Acta Neuropathol.* 2019

149. Kool M, Korshunov A, Remke M et al. Molecular subgroups of medulloblastoma: An international meta-analysis of transcriptome, genetic aberrations, and clinical data of WNT, SHH, Group 3, and Group 4 medulloblastomas. *Acta Neuropathol.* 2012; 123:473–84.

150. Thompson EM, Hielscher T, Bouffet E et al. Prognostic value of medulloblastoma extent of resection after accounting for molecular subgroup: A retrospective integrated clinical and molecular analysis. *Lancet Oncol.* 2016; 17:484–95.

151. Taylor RE, Bailey CC, Robinson K et al. Results of a randomized study of preradiation chemotherapy versus radiotherapy alone for nonmetastatic medulloblastoma: The International society of paediatric oncology/united kingdom children's cancer study group PNET-3 Study. *J Clin Oncol.* 2003; 21:1581–91.

152. Packer RJ, Sutton LN, Elterman R et al. Outcome for children with medulloblastoma treated with radiation and cisplatin, CCNU, and vincristine chemotherapy. *J Neurosurg.* 1994; 81:690–98.

153. Goldwein JW, Radcliffe J, Johnson J et al. Updated results of a pilot study of low dose craniospinal irradiation plus chemotherapy for children under five with cerebellar primitive neuroectodermal tumors (medulloblastoma). *Int J Radiat Oncol Biol Phys.* 1996; 34:899–904.

154. Deutsch M, Thomas P, Boyett J et al. Low stage medullobastoma: A children's cancer study group (CCSG) and pediatric oncology group (POG) randomized study of standard vs. reduced neuraxis radiation. *Proc Am Soc Clin Oncol.* 1991; 10:A363.

155. Packer RJ, Sutton LN, D'Angio G, Evans AE, Schut L. Management of children with primitive neuroectodermal tumors of the posterior fossa/medulloblastoma. *Pediatr Neurosci.* 1985; 12: 272–82.

156. Evans AE, Jenkin RD, Sposto R et al. The treatment of medulloblastoma. Results of a prospective randomized trial of radiation therapy with and without CCNU, vincristine, and prednisone. *J Neurosurg.* 1990; 72:572–82.

157. Packer RJ. Chemotherapy for medulloblastoma/primitive neuroectodermal tumors of the posterior fossa. *Ann Neurol.* 1990; 28:823–28.

158. Tarbell NJ, Friedman H, Polkinghorn WR et al. High-risk medulloblastoma: A pediatric oncology group randomized trial of chemotherapy before or after radiation therapy (POG 9031). *J Clin Oncol.* 2013; 31:2936–41.

159. Jakacki RI, Burger PC, Zhou T et al. Outcome of children with metastatic medulloblastoma treated with carboplatin during craniospinal radiotherapy: A Children's Oncology Group Phase I/II study. *J Clin Oncol.* 2012; 30:2648–53.

160. Gandola L, Massimino M, Cefalo G et al. Hyperfractionated accelerated radiotherapy in the Milan strategy for metastatic medulloblastoma. *J Clin Oncol.* 2009; 27:566–71.

161. Rutkowski S, Bode U, Deinlein F et al. Treatment of early childhood medulloblastoma by postoperative chemotherapy alone. *N Engl J Med.* 2005; 352:978–86.

162. von Bueren AO, von Hoff K, Pietsch T et al. Treatment of young children with localized medulloblastoma by chemotherapy alone: Results of the prospective, multicenter trial HIT 2000 confirming the prognostic impact of histology. *Neuro Oncol.* 2011; 13:669–79.

163. Dupuis-Girod S, Hartmann O, Benhamou E et al. Will high dose chemotherapy followed by autologous bone marrow transplantation supplant cranio-spinal irradiation in young children treated for medulloblastoma? *J Neurooncol.* 1996; 27:87–98.

164. Lafay-Cousin L, Smith A, Chi SN et al. Clinical, pathological, and molecular characterization of infant medulloblastomas treated with sequential high-dose chemotherapy. *Pediatr Blood Cancer.* 2016; 63:1527–34.

165. Torres CF, Rebsamen S, Silber JH et al. Surveillance scanning of children with medulloblastoma [see comments]. *N Engl J Med.* 1994; 330:892–95.

166. Bouffet E, Doz F, Demaille MC et al. Improving survival in recurrent medulloblastoma: Earlier detection, better treatment or still an impasse? *Br J Cancer.* 1998; 77:1321–26.

167. Perez-Martinez A, Lassaletta A, Gonzalez-Vicent M et al. High-dose chemotherapy with autologous stem cell rescue for children with high risk and recurrent medulloblastoma and supratentorial primitive neuroectodermal tumors. *J Neurooncol.* 2005; 71:33–8.

168. Pizer B, Donachie PH, Robinson K et al. Treatment of recurrent central nervous system primitive neuroectodermal tumours in children and adolescents: Results of a Children's Cancer and Leukaemia Group study. *Eur J Cancer.* 2011; 47:1389–97.

169. Gajjar A, Pizer B. Role of high–dose chemotherapy for recurrent medulloblastoma and other CNS primitive neuroectodermal tumors. *Pediatr Blood Cancer.* 2010; 54:649–51.

170. Du S, Yang S, Zhao X et al. Clinical characteristics and outcome of children with relapsed medulloblastoma: A retrospective study at a single center in China. *J Pediatr Hematol Oncol.* 2018; 40:598–604.

171. Gajjar A, Sanford RA, Heideman R et al. Low-grade astrocytoma: A decade of experience at St. Jude Children's Research Hospital. *J Clin Oncol.* 1997; 15:2792–99.

172. Kortmann RD, Timmermann B, Taylor RE et al. Current and future strategies in radiotherapy of childhood low-grade glioma of the brain. Part I: Treatment modalities of radiation therapy. *Strahlenther Onkol.* 2003; 179:509–20.

173. Kortmann RD, Timmermann B, Taylor RE et al. Current and future strategies in radiotherapy of childhood low-grade glioma of the brain. Part II: Treatment-related late toxicity. *Strahlenther Onkol.* 2003; 179:585–97.

174. Janss AJ, Grundy R, Cnaan A et al. Optic pathway and hypothalamic/chiasmatic gliomas in children younger than age 5 years with a 6-year follow-up. *Cancer.* 1995; 75:1051–59.

175. Massimino M, Spreafico F, Cefalo G et al. High response rate to cisplatin/etoposide regimen in childhood low-grade glioma. *J Clin Oncol.* 2002; 20:4209–16.

176. Lancaster DL, Hoddes JA, Michalski A. Tolerance of nitrosurea-based multiagent chemotherapy regime for low-grade pediatric gliomas. *J Neurooncol.* 2003; 63:289–94.

177. Broniscer A, Chintagumpala M, Fouladi M et al. Temozolomide after radiotherapy for newly diagnosed high-grade glioma and unfavorable low-grade glioma in children. *J Neurooncol.* 2006; 76:313–19.

178. Lafay-Cousin L, Holm S, Qaddoumi I et al. Weekly vinblastine in pediatric low-grade glioma patients with carboplatin allergic reaction. *Cancer.* 2005; 103:2636–42.

179. Buckner JC, Shaw EG, Pugh SL et al. Radiation plus procarbazine, CCNU, and vincristine in low-grade glioma. *N Eng J Med.* 2016; 374(14):1344–55.

180. Cokgor I, Friedman AH, Friedman HS. Gliomas. *Eur J Cancer.* 1998; 34:1910–5; discussion 1916.

181. Wisoff JH, Boyett JM, Berger MS et al. Current neurosurgical management and the impact of the extent of resection in the treatment of malignant gliomas of childhood: A report of the Children's Cancer Group trial no. CCG-945. *J Neurosurg.* 1998; 89:52–59.

182. Finlay JL, Boyett JM, Yates AJ et al. Randomized phase III trial in childhood high-grade astrocytoma comparing vincristine, lomustine, and prednisone with the eight-drugs-in-1-day regimen. Childrens Cancer Group. *J Clin Oncol.* 1995; 13:112–23.

183. Wolff JE, Gnekow AK, Kortmann RD et al. Preradiation chemotherapy for pediatric patients with high-grade glioma. *Cancer.* 2002; 94:264–71.

184. Sposto R, Ertel IJ, Jenkin RD et al. The effectiveness of chemotherapy for treatment of high grade astrocytoma in children: Results of a randomized trial. A report from the Childrens Cancer Study Group. *J Neurooncol.* 1989; 7:165–77.

185. Stupp R, Mason WP, van den Bent MJ et al. Radiotherapy plus concomitant and adjuvant temozolomide for glioblastoma. *N Engl J Med.* 2005; 352:987–96.

186. Lee JY, Park CK, Park SH et al. MGMT promoter gene methylation in pediatric glioblastoma: Analysis using MS-MLPA. *Childs Nerv Syst.* 2011; 27:1877–83.

187. Srivastava A, Jain A, Jha P et al. MGMT gene promoter methylation in pediatric glioblastomas. *Childs Nerv Syst.* 2010; 26:1613–18.

188. Schlosser S, Wagner S, Muhlisch J et al. MGMT as a potential stratification marker in relapsed high-grade glioma of children: The HIT-GBM experience. *Pediatr Blood Cancer.* 2010; 54:228–37.

189. Grill J, Massimino M, Bouffet E et al. Phase II, Open-Label, Randomized, Multicenter Trial (HERBY) of bevacizumab in pediatric patients with newly diagnosed high-grade glioma. *J Clin Oncol.* 2018; 36:951–58.

190. Massimino M, Gandola L, Luksch R et al. Sequential chemotherapy, high-dose thiotepa, circulating progenitor cell rescue, and radiotherapy for childhood high-grade glioma. *Neuro-oncology.* 2005; 7:41–8.

191. MacDonald TJ, Arenson EB, Ater J et al. Phase II study of high-dose chemotherapy before radiation in children with newly diagnosed high-grade astrocytoma: Final analysis of Children's Cancer Group Study 9933. *Cancer.* 2005; 104:2862–71.

192. Wagner S, Erdlenbruch B, Langler A et al. Oral topotecan in children with recurrent or progressive high-grade glioma: A Phase I/II study by the German Society for Pediatric Oncology and Hematology. *Cancer.* 2004; 100:1750–57.

193. Paugh BS, Qu C, Jones C et al. Integrated molecular genetic profiling of pediatric high-grade gliomas reveals key differences with the adult disease. *J Clin Oncol.* 2010; 28:3061–68.

194. Wu G, Broniscer A, McEachron TA et al. Somatic histone H3 alterations in pediatric diffuse intrinsic pontine gliomas and non-brainstem glioblastomas. *Nat Genet.* 2012; 44:251–53.

195. Schwartzentruber J, Korshunov A, Liu XY et al. Driver mutations in histone H3.3 and chromatin remodelling genes in paediatric glioblastoma. *Nature.* 2012; 482:226–31.

196. Faury D, Nantel A, Dunn SE et al. Molecular profiling identifies prognostic subgroups of pediatric glioblastoma and shows increased YB-1 expression in tumors. *J Clin Oncol.* 2007; 25:1196–208.

197. Kluwe L, Hagel C, Tatagiba M et al. Loss of NF1 alleles distinguish sporadic from NF1-associated pilocytic astrocytomas. *J Neuropathol Exp Neurol.* 2001; 60:917–20.

198. Pfister S, Janzarik WG, Remke M et al. BRAF gene duplication constitutes a mechanism of MAPK pathway activation in low-grade astrocytomas. *J Clin Invest.* 2008; 118:1739–49.

199. Forshew T, Tatevossian RG, Lawson AR et al. Activation of the ERK/MAPK pathway: A signature genetic defect in posterior fossa pilocytic astrocytomas. *J Pathol.* 2009; 218:172–81.

200. Hawkins C, Walker E, Mohamed N et al. BRAF-KIAA1549 fusion predicts better clinical outcome in pediatric low-grade astrocytoma. *Clin Cancer Res.* 2011; 17:4790–98.

201. Dougherty MJ, Santi M, Brose MS et al. Activating mutations in BRAF characterize a spectrum of pediatric low-grade gliomas. *Neuro Oncol.* 2010; 12:621–30.

202. Tian Y, Rich BE, Vena N et al. Detection of KIAA1549-BRAF fusion transcripts in formalin-fixed paraffin-embedded pediatric low-grade gliomas. *J Mol Diagn.* 2011; 13:669–77.

203. Balss J, Meyer J, Mueller W et al. Analysis of the IDH1 codon 132 mutation in brain tumors. *Acta Neuropathol.* 2008; 116:597–602.

204. Ichimura K, Pearson DM, Kocialkowski S et al. IDH1 mutations are present in the majority of common adult gliomas but rare in primary glioblastomas. *Neuro Oncol.* 2009; 11:341–47.

205. Watanabe T, Nobusawa S, Kleihues P, Ohgaki H. IDH1 mutations are early events in the development of astrocytomas and oligodendrogliomas. *Am J Pathol.* 2009; 174:1149–53.

206. Yan H, Parsons DW, Jin G et al. IDH1 and IDH2 mutations in gliomas. *N Engl J Med.* 2009; 360:765–73.

207. Korshunov A, Meyer J, Capper D et al. Combined molecular analysis of BRAF and IDH1 distinguishes pilocytic astrocytoma from diffuse astrocytoma. *Acta Neuropathol.* 2009; 118:401–5.

208. Wiestler B, Capper D, Holland-Letz T et al. ATRX loss refines the classification of anaplastic gliomas and identifies a subgroup of IDH mutant astrocytic tumors with better prognosis. *Acta Neuropathol.* 2013; 126:443–51.

209. Hargrave D, Bartels U, Bouffet E. Diffuse brainstem glioma in children: Critical review of clinical trials. *Lancet Oncol.* 2006; 7:241–48.

210. Mandell LR, Kadota R, Freeman C et al. There is no role for hyperfractionated radiotherapy in the management of children with newly diagnosed diffuse intrinsic brainstem tumors: Results of a Pediatric Oncology Group phase III trial comparing conventional vs. hyperfractionated radiotherapy. *Int J Radiat Oncol Biol Phys.* 1999; 43:959–64.

211. Cohen KJ, Heideman RL, Zhou T et al. Temozolomide in the treatment of children with newly diagnosed diffuse intrinsic pontine gliomas: A report from the Children's Oncology Group. *Neuro Oncol.* 2011; 13:410–16.

212. Tarnaris A, Edwards RJ, Lowis SP, Pople IK. Atypical external hydrocephalus with visual failure due to occult leptomeningeal dissemination of a pontine glioma. Case report. *J Neurosurg.* 2005; 102 Supplement:224–7.

213. Haas-Kogan DA, Banerjee A, Poussaint TY et al. Phase II trial of tipifarnib and radiation in children with newly diagnosed diffuse intrinsic pontine gliomas. *Neuro Oncol.* 2011; 13:298–306.

214. Packer RJ, Boyett JM, Zimmerman RA et al. Outcome of children with brain stem gliomas after treatment with 7800 cGy of hyperfractionated radiotherapy. A Childrens Cancer Group Phase I/II Trial. *Cancer.* 1994; 74:1827–34.

215. Freeman CR, Kepner J, Kun LE et al. A detrimental effect of a combined chemotherapy-radiotherapy approach in children with diffuse intrinsic brain stem gliomas? *Int J Radiat Oncol Biol Phys.* 2000; 47:561–4.

216. Khuong-Quang DA, Buczkowicz P, Rakopoulos P et al. K27M mutation in histone H3.3 defines clinically and biologically distinct subgroups of pediatric diffuse intrinsic pontine gliomas. *Acta Neuropathol.* 2012; 124:439–47.

217. Bouffet E, Perilongo G, Canete A, Massimino M. Intracranial ependymomas in children: A critical review of prognostic factors and a plea for cooperation. *Med Pediatr Oncol.* 1998; 30:319–29; discussion 329.

218. Rezai AR, Woo HH, Lee M et al. Disseminated ependymomas of the central nervous system. *J Neurosurg.* 1996; 85:618–24.

219. Perilongo G, Massimino M, Sotti G et al. Analyses of prognostic factors in a retrospective review of 92 children with ependymoma: Italian Pediatric Neuro-oncology Group. *Med Pediatr Oncol.* 1997; 29:79–85.

220. Scheurlen W, Kuhl J. Current diagnostic and therapeutic management of CNS metastasis in childhood primitive neuroectodermal tumors and ependymomas. *J Neurooncol.* 1998; 38:181–85.

221. Massimino M, Gandola L, Giangaspero F et al. Hyperfractionated radiotherapy and chemotherapy for childhood ependymoma: Final results of the first prospective AIEOP (Associazione Italiana di Ematologia-Oncologia Pediatrica) study. *Int J Radiat Oncol Biol Phys.* 2004; 58:1336–45.

222. Robertson PL, Zeltzer PM, Boyett JM et al. Survival and prognostic factors following radiation therapy and chemotherapy for ependymomas in children: A report of the Children's Cancer Group. *J Neurosurg.* 1998; 88:695–703.

223. Timmermann B, Kortmann RD, Kuhl J et al. Combined postoperative irradiation and chemotherapy for anaplastic ependymomas in childhood: Results of the German prospective trials HIT 88/89 and HIT 91. *Int J Radiat Oncol Biol Phys.* 2000; 46:287–95.

224. Grill J, Le Deley MC, Gambarelli D et al. Postoperative chemotherapy without irradiation for ependymoma in children under 5 years of age: A multicenter trial of the French Society of Pediatric Oncology. *J Clin Oncol.* 2001; 19:1288–96.

225. Foreman NK, Love S, Thorne R. Intracranial ependymomas: Analysis of prognostic factors in a population-based series. *Pediatr Neurosurg.* 1996; 24:119–25.

226. Merchant TE, Li C, Xiong X, Kun LE, Boop FA, Sanford RA. Conformal radiotherapy after surgery for paediatric ependymoma: A prospective study. *Lancet Oncol.* 2009; 10:258–66.

227. Merchant TE, Kiehna EN, Thompson SJ et al. Pediatric low-grade and ependymal spinal cord tumors. *Pediatr Neurosurg.* 2000; 32:30–6.

228. Grundy RG, Wilne SA, Weston CL et al. Primary postoperative chemotherapy without radiotherapy for intracranial ependymoma in children: The UKCCSG/SIOP prospective study. *Lancet Oncol.* 2007; 8:696–705.

229. Grundy RG, Wilne SH, Robinson KJ et al. Primary postoperative chemotherapy without radiotherapy for treatment of brain tumours other than ependymoma in children under 3 years: Results of the first UKCCSG/SIOP CNS 9204 trial. *Eur J Cancer.* 2010; 46:120–33.

230. Zacharoulis S, Levy A, Chi SN et al. Outcome for young children newly diagnosed with ependymoma, treated with intensive induction chemotherapy followed by myeloablative chemotherapy and autologous stem cell rescue. *Pediatr Blood Cancer.* 2007; 49:34–40.

231. Grill J, Kalifa C, Doz F et al. A high-dose busulfan-thiotepa combination followed by autologous bone marrow transplantation in childhood recurrent ependymoma. A phase-II study. *Pediatr Neurosurg.* 1996; 25:7–12.

232. Mason WP, Goldman S, Yates AJ et al. Survival following intensive chemotherapy with bone marrow reconstitution for children with recurrent intracranial ependymoma—a report of the Children's Cancer Group. *J Neurooncol.* 1998; 37:135–43.

233. Vinchon M, Leblond P, Noudel R, Dhellemmes P. Intracranial ependymomas in childhood: Recurrence, reoperation, and outcome. *Childs Nerv Syst.* 2005; 21:221–6.

234. Sandri A, Massimino M, Mastrodicasa L et al. Treatment with oral etoposide for childhood recurrent ependymomas. *J Pediatr Hematol Oncol.* 2005; 27:486–90.

235. Bouffet E, Hawkins CE, Ballourah W et al. Survival benefit for pediatric patients with recurrent ependymoma treated with reirradiation. *Int J Radiat Oncol Biol Phys.* 2012; 83:1541–48.

236. Merchant TE, Boop FA, Kun LE, Sanford RA. A retrospective study of surgery and reirradiation for recurrent ependymoma. *Int J Radiat Oncol Biol Phys.* 2008; 71:87–97.

237. Ward S, Harding B, Wilkins P et al. Gain of 1q and loss of 22 are the most common changes detected by comparative genomic hybridisation in paediatric ependymoma. *Genes Chromosomes Cancer.* 2001; 32:59–66.

238. Carter M, Nicholson J, Ross F et al. Genetic abnormalities detected in ependymomas by comparative genomic hybridisation. *Br J Cancer.* 2002; 86:929–39.

239. Granzow M, Popp S, Weber S et al. Isochromosome 1q as an early genetic event in a child with intracranial ependymoma characterized by molecular cytogenetics. *Cancer Genet Cytogenet.* 2001; 130:79–83.

240. Godfraind C, Kaczmarska JM, Kocak M et al. Distinct disease-risk groups in pediatric supratentorial and posterior fossa ependymomas. *Acta Neuropathol.* 2012; 124:247–57.

241. Ridley L, Rahman R, Brundler MA et al. Multifactorial analysis of predictors of outcome in pediatric intracranial ependymoma. *Neuro Oncol.* 2008; 10:675–89.

242. Rand V, Prebble E, Ridley L et al. Investigation of chromosome 1q reveals differential expression of members of the S100 family in clinical subgroups of intracranial paediatric ependymoma. *Br J Cancer.* 2008; 99:1136–43.

243. Pajtler KW, Witt H, Sill M et al. Molecular classification of ependymal tumors across All CNS compartments, histopathological grades, and age groups. *Cancer Cell.* 2015; 27:728–43.

244. Calaminus G, Kortmann R, Worch J et al. SIOP CNS GCT 96: Final report of outcome of a prospective, multinational nonrandomized trial for children and adults with intracranial germinoma, comparing craniospinal irradiation alone with chemotherapy followed by focal primary site irradiation for patients with localized disease. *Neuro Oncol.* 2013; 15:788–96.

245. Alapetite C, Brisse H, Patte C et al. Pattern of relapse and outcome of non-metastatic germinoma patients treated with chemotherapy and limited field radiation: The SFOP experience. *Neuro Oncol.* 2010; 12:1318–25.

246. Calaminus G, Bamberg M, Jurgens H et al. Impact of surgery, chemotherapy and irradiation on long term outcome of intracranial malignant non-germinomatous germ cell tumors: Results of the German Cooperative Trial MAKEI 89. *Klin Padiatr.* 2004; 216:141–9.

247. Buckner JC, Peethambaram PP, Smithson WA et al. Phase II trial of primary chemotherapy followed by reduced-dose radiation for CNS germ cell tumors. *J Clin Oncol.* 1999; 17:933–40.

248. Robertson PL, DaRosso RC, Allen JC. Improved prognosis of intracranial non-germinoma germ cell tumors with multimodality therapy. *J Neurooncol.* 1997; 32:71–80.

249. Schild SE, Scheithauer BW, Haddock MG et al. Histologically confirmed pineal tumors and other germ cell tumors of the brain. *Cancer.* 1996; 78:2564–71.

250. Matsutani M, Sano K, Takakura K et al. Primary intracranial germ cell tumors: A clinical analysis of 153 histologically verified cases. *J Neurosurg.* 1997; 86:446–55.

251. Rorke LB, Packer R, Biegel J. Central nervous system atypical teratoid/rhabdoid tumors of infancy and childhood. *J Neurooncol.* 1995; 24:21–8.

252. Sevenet N, Sheridan E, Amram D et al. Constitutional mutations of the hSNF5/INI1 gene predispose to a variety of cancers. *Am J Hum Genet.* 1999; 65:1342–48.

253. Schneppenheim R, Fruhwald MC, Gesk S et al. Germline nonsense mutation and somatic inactivation of SMARCA4/BRG1 in a family with rhabdoid tumor predisposition syndrome. *Am J Hum Genet.* 2010; 86:279–84.

254. Versteege I, Sevenet N, Lange J et al. Truncating mutations of hSNF5/INI1 in aggressive paediatric cancer. *Nature.* 1998; 394:203–6.

255. Biegel JA, Zhou JY, Rorke LB et al. Germ-line and acquired mutations of INI1 in atypical teratoid and rhabdoid tumors. *Cancer Res.* 1999; 59:74–9.

256. Sigauke E, Rakheja D, Maddox DL et al. Absence of expression of SMARCB1/INI1 in malignant rhabdoid tumors of the central nervous system, kidneys and soft tissue: An immunohistochemical study with implications for diagnosis. *Mod Pathol.* 2006; 19:717–25.

257. Hasselblatt M, Isken S, Linge A et al. High-resolution genomic analysis suggests the absence of recurrent genomic alterations other than SMARCB1 aberrations in atypical teratoid/rhabdoid tumors. *Genes Chromosomes Cancer.* 2013; 52:185–90.

258. Kordes U, Gesk S, Fruhwald MC et al. Clinical and molecular features in patients with atypical teratoid rhabdoid tumor or malignant rhabdoid tumor. *Genes Chromosomes Cancer.* 2010; 49:176–81.

259. Bourdeaut F, Dufour C, Delattre O. Rhabdoid tumours: hSNF/INI1 deficient cancers of early childhood with aggressive behaviour. *Bull Cancer.* 2010; 97:37–45.

260. Eaton KW, Tooke LS, Wainwright LM et al. Spectrum of SMARCB1/INI1 mutations in familial and sporadic rhabdoid tumors. *Pediatr Blood Cancer.* 2011; 56:7–15.

261. Chen YW, Wong TT, Ho DM et al. Impact of radiotherapy for pediatric CNS atypical teratoid/rhabdoid tumor (single institute experience). *Int J Radiat Oncol Biol Phys.* 2006; 64:1038–43.

262. von Hoff K, Hinkes B, Dannenmann-Stern E et al. Frequency, risk-factors and survival of children with atypical teratoid rhabdoid tumors (AT/RT) of the CNS diagnosed between 1988 and 2004, and registered to the German HIT database. *Pediatr Blood Cancer.* 2011; 57:978–85.

263. Hilden JM, Meerbaum S, Burger P et al. Central nervous system atypical teratoid/rhabdoid tumor: Results of therapy in children enrolled in a registry. *J Clin Oncol.* 2004; 22:2877–84.

264. Chi SN, Zimmerman MA, Yao X et al. Intensive multimodality treatment for children with newly diagnosed CNS atypical teratoid rhabdoid tumor. *J Clin Oncol.* 2009; 27:385–9.

265. Lafay-Cousin L, Hawkins C, Carret AS et al. Central nervous system atypical teratoid rhabdoid tumours: The Canadian Paediatric Brain Tumour Consortium experience. *Eur J Cancer.* 2012; 48:353–9.

266. Neglia JP, Friedman DL, Yasui Y et al. Second malignant neoplasms in five-year survivors of childhood cancer: Childhood cancer survivor study. *J Natl Cancer Inst.* 2001; 93:618–29.

267. Hawkins MM, Wilson LM, Stovall MA et al. Epipodophyllotoxins, alkylating agents, and radiation and risk of secondary leukaemia after childhood cancer. *BMJ.* 1992; 304:951–58.

268. Blayney DW, Longo DL, Young RC et al. Decreasing risk of leukemia with prolonged follow-up after chemotherapy and radiotherapy for Hodgkin's disease. *N Engl J Med.* 1987; 316:710–14.

269. Ogilvy-Stuart AL, Shalet SM. Effect of chemotherapy on growth. *Acta Paediatr Suppl.* 1995; 411:52–6.

270. Hawkins MM. Pregnancy outcome and offspring after childhood cancer. *BMJ.* 1994; 309:1034.

271. Shan K, Lincoff AM, Young JB. Anthracycline-induced cardiotoxicity. *Ann Intern Med.* 1996; 125:47–58.

272. Skinner R, Sharkey IM, Pearson AD, Craft AW. Ifosfamide, mesna, and nephrotoxicity in children. *J Clin Oncol.* 1993; 11:173–90.

273. Charlton A, Larcombe IJ, Meller ST et al. Absence from school related to cancer and other chronic conditions. *Arch Dis Child.* 1991; 66:1217–22.

274. Glauser TA, Packer RJ. Cognitive deficits in long-term survivors of childhood brain tumors. *Childs Nerv Syst.* 1991; 7:2–12.

275. Grill J, Kieffer V, Kalifa C. Measuring the neuro-cognitive side-effects of irradiation in children with brain tumors. *Pediatr Blood Cancer.* 2004; 42:452–6.

276. Ellenberg L, McComb JG, Siegel SE, Stowe S. Factors affecting intellectual outcome in pediatric brain tumor patients. *Neurosurgery.* 1987; 21:638–44.

277. Radcliffe J, Packer RJ, Atkins TE et al. Three- and four-year cognitive outcome in children with noncortical brain tumors treated with whole-brain radiotherapy. *Ann Neurol.* 1992; 32:551–54.

278. Silber JH, Radcliffe J, Peckham V et al. Whole-brain irradiation and decline in intelligence: The influence of dose and age on IQ score [see comments]. *J Clin Oncol.* 1992; 10:1390–96.

279. Packer RJ, Goldwein J, Nicholson HS et al. Treatment of children with medulloblastomas with reduced-dose craniospinal radiation therapy and adjuvant chemotherapy: A Children's Cancer Group study. *J Clin Oncol.* 1999; 17:2127.

280. Machin D. Assessment of quality of life in clinical trials of the British Medical Research Council. *J Natl Cancer Inst Monogr.* 1996; 97–102.

281. Lackner H, Benesch M, Schagerl S et al. Prospective evaluation of late effects after childhood cancer therapy with a follow-up over 9 years. *Eur J Pediatr.* 2000; 159:750–58.

282. Apajasalo M, Sintonen H, Siimes MA et al. Health-related quality of life of adults surviving malignancies in childhood. *Eur J Cancer.* 1996; 32A:1354–58.

283. Moe PJ, Holen A, Glomstein A et al. Long-term survival and quality of life in patients treated with a national all protocol 15–20 years earlier: IDM/HDM and late effects? *Pediatr Hematol Oncol.* 1997; 14:513–24.

284. Mostow EN, Byrne J, Connelly RR, Mulvihill JJ. Quality of life in long-term survivors of CNS tumors of childhood and adolescence. *J Clin Oncol.* 1991; 9:592–9.

285. Meeske K, Katz ER, Palmer SN et al. Parent proxy-reported health-related quality of life and fatigue in pediatric patients diagnosed with brain tumors and acute lymphoblastic leukemia. *Cancer.* 2004; 101:2116–25.

286. Langeveld NE, Grootenhuis MA, Voute PA et al. No excess fatigue in young adult survivors of childhood cancer. *Eur J Cancer.* 2003; 39:204–14.

287. Glover DA, Byrne J, Mills JL et al. Impact of CNS treatment on mood in adult survivors of childhood leukemia: A report from the Children's Cancer Group. *J Clin Oncol.* 2003; 21:4395–401.

288. Zebrack BJ, Zeltzer LK, Whitton J et al. Psychological outcomes in long-term survivors of childhood leukemia, Hodgkin's disease, and non-Hodgkin's lymphoma: A report from the Childhood Cancer Survivor Study. *Pediatrics.* 2002; 110:42–52.

289. Eiser C, Hill JJ, Blacklay A. Surviving cancer; what does it mean for you? An evaluation of a clinic based intervention for survivors of childhood cancer. *Psychooncology.* 2000; 9:214–20.

290. Gray RE, Doan BD, Shermer P et al. Psychologic adaptation of survivors of childhood cancer. *Cancer.* 1992; 70:2713–21.

291. Hobbie WL, Stuber M, Meeske K et al. Symptoms of posttraumatic stress in young adult survivors of childhood cancer. *J Clin Oncol.* 2000; 18:4060–66.

292. Kazak AE, Alderfer M, Rourke MT, Simms S, Streisand R, Grossman JR. Posttraumatic stress disorder (PTSD) and posttraumatic stress symptoms (PTSS) in families of adolescent childhood cancer survivors. *J Pediatr Psychol.* 2004; 29:211–19.

293. Editor. Association for children with life-threatening or terminal conditions and their families (ACT) and Royal College of Paediatrics and Child Health (RCPCH). A guide to the development of Children's Palliative Care Services. 1997.

294. Hinds P, Oakes L, Furman WEA. Decision making by parents and healthcare professionals when considering continued care for pediatric patients with cancer. *Oncol Nurs Forum.* 1997; 24:1523–28.

295. Deatrick JA, Angst DB, Moore C. Parents' views of their children's participation in Phase 1 oncology clinical trials. *J Pediatr Oncol Nurs.* 2002; 19:114–21.

296. McGraw T, Stacey BR. Gabapentin for treatment of neuropathic pain in a 12-year-old girl. *Clin J Pain.* 1998; 14:354–6.

297. Rosenberg JM, Harrell C, Ristic H et al. The effect of gabapentin on neuropathic pain. *Clin J Pain.* 1997; 13:251–5.

298. McQuay H, Carroll D, Jadad AR et al. Anticonvulsant drugs for management of pain: A systematic review. *BMJ.* 1995; 311: 1047–52.

33 AIDS-RELATED MALIGNANCY

Mark Bower, Elena Gervasi, and Alessia Dalla Pria

Introduction

The human immunodeficiency virus (HIV) was recognized as a human pathogen 35 years ago and in that time it has infected millions of people, resulting in a global pandemic. The consequence of HIV infection is a relentless destruction of the immune system culminating in the diagnosis of acquired immunodeficiency syndrome (AIDS). The World Health Organization estimated that 37 million people were living with HIV in 2017 (0.5% of the global population). The introduction of potent combination antiretroviral therapy (cART) has reduced mortality from and transmission of HIV so that there are increasing numbers of people healthily living with HIV infection.

Both primary congenital immunosuppression and iatrogenic secondary immunosuppression predispose to malignancies, and it is therefore not surprising that cancer also occurs more frequently in people living with HIV (PLWH). Many of the malignancies associated with immuno-suppression have a viral etiology with oncogenic herpesviruses (Kaposi's sarcoma [KS], non-Hodgkin lymphoma [NHL], and Hodgkin lymphoma [HL]), papilloma viruses (cervical cancer and anal cancer), hepatitis viruses (hepatocellular cancer), and polyoma viruses (Merkel cell cancer) being implicated. Three cancers (KS, NHL, and cervical cancer) are AIDS-defining illnesses (ADIs), implying an association with declining immune function, whereas other tumors in PLWH are classified as non-AIDS-defining malignancies (NADMs).

The development of cART in the late 1990s was associated with profound and sustained suppression of HIV viral replication, a dramatic reduction in opportunistic infections, ADIs, and mortality among PLWH. In addition to reducing the incidence of opportunistic infections, cART has been associated with a reduction in the incidence of KS and NHL, especially primary cerebral lymphomas. Moreover, a large randomized control study demonstrated that immediate initiation of cART reduced the incidence of AIDS-defining cancers.[1] Importantly, in the era of cART the survival of many cancers in PLWH has been shown to be similar to the survival of these cancers in the general population. This means that in general the treatment of cancer in PLWH should be the same as in the general population, but clinicians must pay careful attention to pharmacokinetic interactions between cytotoxic chemotherapy and cART and must ensure that patients receive opportunistic infection prophylaxis.

AIDS-defining malignancies

Kaposi's sarcoma

Epidemiology

The era of AIDS was heralded in 1981 by the emergence of two previously uncommon diseases, *Pneumocystis carinii* pneumonia (subsequently renamed *Pneumocystis jirovecii*) and KS. Prior to this, three different clinical expressions of KS had been recognized. Classical KS is an indolent variant predominantly affecting elderly men of Mediterranean, Jewish, or Arabic descent, reflecting the geographical distribution of Kaposi's sarcoma herpesvirus

(KSHV). Endemic KS is a more severe form that affects children and young adults in sub-Saharan Africa and includes both cutaneous and lymphadenopathic variants and, although it is most common in sub-Saharan Africa, is unrelated to HIV infection. Iatrogenic KS comprises up to 5% of malignancies in immunosuppressed allogeneic transplant recipients and is related especially to the use of calcineurin inhibitors, which inhibit T-cell function. In addition to AIDS-related KS, KS has also been reported in HIV-negative men who have sex with men (MSM), in whom it generally follows the indolent course found in classical KS. Although the incidence of KS in a meta-analysis of HIV cohort studies has declined markedly, it remains the most common AIDS-defining cancer. This decline in incidence is directly attributed to cART, which protects against the development of KS.[2]

KSHV discovery and molecular virology

Early in the HIV pandemic it was noted that the epidemiology of AIDS-KS pointed to an infectious agent transmitted independently of HIV.[3] In 1994 Chang and Moore isolated unique non-human DNA sequences from KS biopsies that were homologous to, but distinct from, genes of the gammaherpesviruses Herpesvirus saimiri and Epstein–Barr virus.[4] Complete genomic sequencing of this novel herpes virus, variously named Kaposi sarcoma herpes virus (KSHV) and human herpes virus-8 (HHV8), confirms that it is related to Herpes saimiri virus which induces lymphoid malignancies in New World primates, and Epstein–Barr virus, a human oncogenic herpes virus. KSHV is a large double-stranded DNA virus and the KSHV genome is a continuous 145 kb-long unique coding region flanked by multiple GC-rich terminal repeat units approximately 800 bp in length. Over 90 open reading frames (ORFs) have been identified within the KSHV genome, of which at least 81 ORFs are over 100 amino acids long. Like EBV, KSHV establishes latent infection in B-cells but it has a wide cellular tropism, and has been detected in endothelial cells, epithelial cells, macrophages, and monocytes.

In addition to structural proteins and viral enzymes, KSHV encodes a large number of viral genes (both conserved and unique) that are homologues of cellular genes that have been captured from the host during the course of the virus's evolution.[5] These genes may help KSHV utilize host cellular processes and evade anti-viral defenses. Around a quarter of KSHV genes, both cellular homologues and unique viral genes, are involved in immune evasion. The roles of many viral genes in driving oncogenesis have also now been elucidated and, in many cases, these oncogenic activities result from the same molecular pathways employed by the virus in its immune-evasion activities.[6] The cellular processes modulated by KSHV viral genes include the cell cycle, apoptosis, cytokine production, antigen presentation, cell signaling, and signal transduction. Hence KSHV infection can result in aberrant cell growth, proliferation, inflammation, and angiogenesis, all of which contribute towards tumor development.[7] In addition, KSHV has been detected in two rare HIV-associated lymphoproliferative disorders, multicentric Castleman's disease and primary effusion lymphoma.[8,9]

Molecular epidemiological studies and serologic assays have demonstrated that KSHV infection is not ubiquitous. The virus appears more prevalent in those populations at increased risk for developing KS, including men who have sex with men (MSM), Africans, and certain Middle eastern and Mediterranean populations, while the prevalence of KSHV appears quite low in the general population of the US and UK. The mode of transmission of KSHV is thought to resemble that of EBV with high titers of the virus found in saliva. The evidence for a causal role for KSHV in the pathogenesis of KS is compelling. KSHV infection precedes the clinical development of KS and the epidemiology and risk factors for KSHV infection and KS overlap. KSHV is detectable in KS spindle cells and in the endothelial cells in all forms of KS. Finally, KSHV infects and transforms primary human endothelial cells, thought to be the precursor cells of malignant KS spindle cells.

Clinical features and differential diagnosis

Most patients with KS present with skin lesions that are typically multiple, pigmented, raised, painless, and do not blanch. The earliest cutaneous lesions are often asymptomatic innocuous-looking macular-pigmented lesions, which vary in color from faint pink to vivid purple. Larger plaques occur usually on the trunk as oblong lesions following the line of skin creases. Lesions may develop to form large plaques and nodules that can be associated with painful edema. In addition to a thorough skin examination, inspection of the oral cavity and conjunctivae should be undertaken. Oral lesions are a frequent accompaniment that may lead to ulceration, dysphagia, and secondary infection. A nodular form of KS that is frequently associated with lymphoedema is seen more commonly in people of African descent and often proves particularly difficult to control.

The most common sites of visceral KS are the lungs and stomach. Pulmonary KS is a life-threatening complication that usually presents with dyspnea, dry cough, and sometimes hemoptysis, with or without fever. Chest X-ray typically reveals a diffuse reticulo-nodular infiltrate and pleural effusion. Gastrointestinal lesions are usually asymptomatic but may bleed or cause obstruction. The diagnosis is usually confirmed at endoscopy. In making the diagnosis of visceral KS the complications of biopsy (particularly hemorrhage) must be carefully weighed up against the benefits of confirming the diagnosis histologically.

The main differential diagnosis is bacillary angiomatosis or epithelioid angiomatosis, which is caused by a fastidious Gram-negative Rikettsia-like organism *Bartonella henselae*. This infection can be effectively treated with erythromycin. These diagnoses can only be reliably distinguished histopathologically, and so a biopsy is essential to confirm the diagnosis of KS. Lesions are graded histopathologically into patch, plaque, or nodular grade disease.

Staging

The staging system described for AIDS-KS does not follow the standard tumor node metastasis (TNM) approach but instead includes an assessment of immune function as determined by the CD4 cell count. The AIDS clinical trial group (ACTG) staging system for AIDS-related KS was developed in the pre-cART era to predict survival and includes tumor-related criteria (T), host immunological status (I), and the presence of systemic illness (S) (see Table 33.1).[10, 11] The ACTG also established uniform criteria for response evaluation in AIDS-KS (see Table 33.2).[10]

Prevention

The introduction of cART was associated with a substantial reduction in the incidence of KS in many large cohorts, although some of this decline in incidence appears to have preceded the introduction of cART. Similarly, survival rates for KS have risen markedly during this period. Nevertheless, KS continues to be a significant problem in Africa although the increasing access to cART is improving outcomes.[12] The decline in incidence of KS has been shown to be attributable to cART.[1,2,12] In contrast, there is little evidence to support the use of anti-herpes virus agents that target KSHV in the prevention or treatment of KS.

Treatment options

The management of AIDS-associated KS is determined to a large extent by the clinical staging. Since KS is an AIDS-defining malignancy, it is an indication to start cART regardless of the baseline CD4 cell count. For the majority of patients with early T0 stage disease the KS will respond to cART alone although it may take 6–12 months. In view of this delay, cosmetically significant localized lesions may be treated with either intralesional vinblastine or localized radiotherapy. In addition to cART, chemotherapy is advocated for advanced cutaneous and visceral KS (stage T1) but is not merited for early disease in view of the potential responses to cART. Liposomal anthracyclines are considered first-line chemotherapy for advanced KS, and paclitaxel chemotherapy is recommended for anthracycline-resistant disease[13] (Table 33.3).

Systemic NHL

Epidemiology

People living with HIV have an increased risk of developing NHL, and the Centers for Disease Control (CDC) included high-grade B-cell non-Hodgkin lymphoma (NHL) as an AIDS-defining illness in 1985, and studies show a decline in incidence since the introduction of cART. The development of AIDS-related lymphoma (ARL) has been shown to be related to older age, low CD4 cell count, and absence of treatment with cART. Patients tend

---

TABLE 33.1 **The Modified AIDS Clinical Trials Group Staging of KS**

TIS Staging of KS	Good Risk (All of the Following)	Poor Risk (Any of the Following)
(T) Tumor	Confined to skin, lymph nodes, or minimal oral disease	Tumor-associated edema or ulceration Extensive oral KS Gastrointestinal KS KS in other non-nodal viscera
(I) Immune status	CD4 cell count >150 /mm³	CD4 cell count <150 /mm³
(S) Systemic illness	Karnovsky performance status >70	Karnovsky performance status <70 or other HIV-related illness

Note: See further Krown et al., 1989; Krown et al., 1997.

TABLE 33.2   **Response Criteria for HIV-Associated Kaposi Sarcoma**

Complete Response (CR)
  The complete resolution of all KS with no new lesions, lasting for at least 4 weeks. A biopsy is required to confirm the absence of residual KS in flat lesions containing pigmentation. Endoscopies must be repeated to confirm the complete resolution of previously detected visceral disease.

Clinical Complete Response (CCR)
  Patients who have no detectable residual KS lesions for at least 4 weeks but whose response was not confirmed by biopsy and/or repeat endoscopy.

Partial Response (PR)
  One or more of the following in the absence of (i) new cutaneous lesions, (ii) new visceral/oral lesions, (iii) increasing KS-associated edema, (iv) a 25% or more increase in the product of the bidimensional diameters of any index lesion:
  1. A 50% or greater decrease in the number of measurable lesions on the skin and/or in the mouth or viscera.
  2. A 50% or greater decrease in the size of the lesions as defined by one of the following three criteria:
      (a) A 50% or more decrease in the sums of the products of the largest bidimensional diameters of the index lesions
      (b) A complete flattening of at least 50% of the lesions
      (c) Where 75% or more of the nodular lesions become indurated plaques

Stable Disease (SD)
  Any response that does not meet the above criteria.

Progressive Disease (PD)
  Any of the following:
  1. A 25% or more increase in the product of the bidimensional diameters of any index lesion
  2. The appearance of new lesions
  3. Where 25% or more of previously flat lesions become raised
  4. The appearance of new or increased KS-associated edema

TABLE 33.3   **Summary of Clinical Management of AIDS-KS**

Early Stage KS (T0 Stage)
  cART
  Consider local radiotherapy or intralesional vinblastine for cosmetically disfiguring disease
Advanced Stage KS (T1 Stage)
  cART and liposomal anthracycline (either daunoxome 40 mg/m^2 q14d or caelyx 20 mg/m^2 q21d)
Anthracycline Refractory KS
  cART and paclitaxel (100 mg/m^2 q14d)

to present with advanced clinical stage, B symptoms, and extra-nodal sites of disease.

Before the introduction of cART, the outlook for patients with ARL was poor; however the median survival in the post-cART era is equivalent to that observed in the HIV-negative population and depends critically on histological subtype and stage of disease. The two most frequent histological subtypes of NHL that occur in PLWH are diffuse large B-cell lymphoma (DLBCL) and Burkitt lymphoma/leukemia (BL), but the WHO classification of lymphoid malignancies associated with HIV also includes rare subtypes such as primary effusion lymphoma (PEL) and plasmablastic lymphoma, as well as primary cerebral lymphoma.

Biology

In PLWH DLBCL account for approximately half of HIV-associated NHL, and the majority are associated with latent EBV infection, advanced immunosuppression, and frequently present with advanced-stage disease and extra-nodal sites of involvement. Burkitt lymphomas are the next most common subtype and resemble sporadic BL with EBV detectable in only 30% and with chromosomal translocations suggesting recombination errors during immunoglobulin isotype class switching. BL tends to arise earlier in the course of HIV infection in patients with higher CD4 cell counts. PEL and plasmablastic lymphomas are CD20-negative lymphomas arising in post-germinal center cells that are infected by herpesviruses, KSHV or EBV, or both.

Prognostic factors

The staging of HIV-associated lymphomas follows the Ann Arbor system and is identical to that employed for the staging of non-HIV related NHL. [^{18}F]-fluoro-2-deoxy-D-glucose positron emission tomography (^{18}FDG PET) scanning at diagnosis improves the staging accuracy. The majority of patients present with advanced stage, B symptoms, and/or extra-nodal disease. The most frequent extra-nodal sites of lymphoma are the gastrointestinal tract, liver, bone marrow, and cerebrospinal fluid. In the pre-cART era, the most influential prognostic factors in patients with HIV-associated NHL related to the severity of immunosuppression rather than lymphoma-related factors. Factors that are associated with survival in the post-cART era are the International Prognostic Index (IPI) score (Table 33.4) and in some studies, the CD4 cell count at diagnosis, with a CD4 cell count less than 100 cells/mm^3 predictive of a worse outcome.[14] Overall in the era of cART, the prognosis of systemic HIV-NHL is the same as that for high-grade NHL in the general population.

Clinical presentation

The majority of patients with HIV-associated lymphomas present with advanced stage and B symptoms; however a biopsy is

TABLE 33.4   **International Prognostic Index for Aggressive Non-Hodgkin Lymphoma**

Score 1 for each factor present:
  Age >60 years
  Serum LDH >normal
  Performance status >1
  Stage III/IV
  Extra-nodal site >1
Final IPI risk group
0 or 1, low risk
2, low intermediate risk
3, high intermediate risk
4 or 5, high risk

Source: Adapted from The International Non-Hodgkin's Lymphoma Prognostic Factors Project, 1993.

essential for the diagnosis of systemic lymphomas as they can be mimicked by many AIDS-related illnesses. Extra-nodal disease (especially hepatic), bone marrow involvement, and leptomeningeal disease (particularly with Burkitt's lymphoma) are all common features. Since the introduction of cART there has been no change in the stage at presentation, presence of B symptoms, bone marrow infiltration, or performance status. However, patients who developed NHL in the cART era were less likely to have had a prior AIDS diagnosis, were older, and had a high CD4 count at the time of diagnosis.[16]

Management

Prior to the introduction of cART, treatment with standard-dose chemotherapy induced high levels of toxicity. Improvements in chemotherapy response rates were generally offset by increased death due to opportunistic infection. The introduction of cART has led to better control of HIV viral replication and improved immune function, and the incorporation of hematopoietic growth factors (G-CSF) into treatment protocols enabled the introduction of increasingly myelotoxic regimens. This has allowed conventional chemotherapy regimens in use in the HIV-negative setting, such as rituximab, cyclophosphamide, doxorubicin, vincristine, and prednisolone (R-CHOP), to be used as first-line treatment in HIV-positive patients, and outcomes are now similar for those with and without HIV infection.[17,18]

Infusional regimens, such as dose-adjusted (DA) rituximab, etoposide, prednisone, vincristine, cyclophosphamide, and hydroxydaunorubicin (R-EPOCH), have been favored over R-CHOP chemotherapy in some US centers; however, they have not been compared in a randomized study. The outcome after the infusional chemotherapy regimen of cyclophosphamide, doxorubicin, and etoposide (CDE), administered as a 96-hour continuous infusion, has also been reported in single- and multi-center series, and although patients who received cART did better, the outcome again has not been compared directly to R-CHOP. These reports are consistent with those for DLBCL in HIV-negative patients where R-CHOP is considered the standard therapy, as no survival advantage has been demonstrated for any other chemotherapy regimen in a randomized study.

The role of rituximab (R) in HIV-associated B-cell lymphomas has been controversial since the publication of a randomized phase III study conducted in the US of CHOP versus R-CHOP with maintenance rituximab, in HIV patients with aggressive B-cell lymphoma.[19] There was a trend to improved response rate, a significant reduction in progression of lymphoma on treatment, and in death due to lymphoma with rituximab. However, these benefits were offset by a higher death rate from infectious complications, particularly in those with a CD4 count below 50 cells/mm^3. Several phase II studies have included rituximab with chemotherapy in this patient group, and a meta-analysis of prospective studies has confirmed the benefit in response rate and overall survival (OS) of the addition of rituximab to chemotherapy.[20] Thus, the addition of rituximab to chemotherapy is now recommended for DLBCL in HIV-positive patients, although the use of rituximab is contentious in patients with a CD4 count <50 /mm^3.[19]

Burkitt lymphoma is a highly curable malignancy in the general population using intensive chemotherapy regimens of short duration combined with central nervous system penetrating therapy. These regimens have been adopted in the management of HIV-BL and small studies have demonstrated the feasibility of administering more intensive chemotherapy regimens, such as rituximab-cyclophosphamide, vincristine, doxorubicin,

methotrexate/ifosfamide, etoposide, cytarabine ([R]-CODOX-M/IVAC) and cyclophosphamide, vincristine, doxorubicin, dexamethasone, methotrexate, cytarabine (hyperCVAD). Studies report response rates and 2-year event-free survivals similar to those observed in HIV-negative patients treated with the same regimen, with no increase in toxicity, suggesting that a uniform approach to treatment of BL should be used, regardless of HIV status.

The clinical management of HIV patients with primary effusion lymphoma and plasmablastic lymphoma remains uncertain because of the relatively low numbers of patients. The prognosis for these patients appears to be significantly inferior to other AIDS-related lymphomas.[21,22] These lymphomas are CD20-negative and in view of the poorer prognosis are generally treated with EPOCH rather than CHOP. In these lymphomas as well as DLBCL, prophylaxis against central nervous system relapse is advocated using the same criteria that are applied in the HIV-negative population.[23]

HIV infection causes immunosuppression, CD4 lymphocyte count loss, and a progressive risk of opportunistic infection and tumors. Similarly chemotherapy and radiotherapy for HIV-related malignancies are associated with an increased risk of infection secondary to the myelosuppression and additional CD4 lymphocyte count loss.[24–26] The risk of infection is further raised by the presence of central venous catheters, neutropenia associated with HIV infection,[27,28] and many of the therapies utilized to treat HIV and its complications. These factors all combine to produce a significant risk of opportunistic infection in people living with HIV undergoing treatment for cancer. Guidelines for the initiation of opportunistic infection prophylaxis are available, but these treatments should be started at higher CD4 cell counts in patients who are to undergo chemotherapy and radiotherapy. Patients treated with chemotherapy for NHL should receive antimicrobial prophylaxis including acyclovir, azithromycin, co-trimoxazole, and fluconazole. There are significant and important pharmacokinetic interactions between antiretroviral drugs and cytotoxic chemotherapy agents, and treating physicians need to pay careful attention to these. For example, ritonavir-boosted protease inhibitors markedly potentiate the myelotoxicity of anthracyclines as a consequence of microsomal enzyme inhibition reducing the metabolism of anthracyclines.[29]

Primary CNS NHL

Epidemiology

Primary central nervous system lymphoma (PCL) is defined as non-Hodgkin lymphoma (NHL) that is confined to the craniospinal axis without systemic involvement. This diagnosis is rare in immunocompetent patients but occurs more frequently in patients with both congenital and acquired immunodeficiency. Since 1985 high-grade B-cell NHL including PCL has been an AIDS-defining diagnosis. AIDS-related PCL occurs equally frequently across all ages and transmission risk groups. A meta-analysis of cohort studies has shown a significant decline in the incidence of PCL following the introduction of highly active antiretroviral therapy (HAART) (relative risk 0.42)[30] which is attributed to the protective effects of HAART.[31]

Pathogenesis

EBV is fundamental to the pathogenesis of HIV-associated PCL, and its presence is detectable by immunocytochemical staining of biopsy tissue or by polymerase chain reaction (PCR) amplification of cerebrospinal fluid (CSF) using EBV-specific oligonucleotide primers.

Differential diagnosis

Toxoplasmosis and lymphoma are the commonest causes of cerebral mass lesions in HIV-seropositive patients and the differential diagnosis often proves difficult. Both diagnoses occur in patients with advanced immunodeficiency (CD4 count <50 / mm^3) and present with headaches and focal neurological deficits. Clinical features that favor a diagnosis of PCNSL include a more gradual onset over 2–8 weeks and the absence of a fever. CT and MRI scanning usually reveal solitary or multiple ring enhancing lesions with prominent mass effect and edema. Again these features occur in both diagnoses although PCNSL lesions are usually periventricular whilst toxoplasmosis more often affects the basal ganglia. Thus even the combination of clinical findings and standard radiological investigations rarely provides a definitive diagnosis. Moreover, toxoplasma serology (IgG) is falsely negative in 10–15% of patients with cerebral toxoplasmosis. More than 85% of patients with cerebral toxoplasmosis will respond clinically and radiologically to 2 weeks of anti-toxoplasma therapy, and this has become the cornerstone of the diagnostic algorithm for cerebral masses in severely immunodeficient patients. In these patients it has been standard practice to commence empirical anti-toxoplasmosis treatment, and resort to a brain biopsy if there is no clinical or radiological improvement. This strategy avoids the routine use of brain biopsy in these patients who frequently have a very poor performance status and prognosis.

The discovery that all HIV-associated PCL which histologically are diffuse large cell NHL are associated with Epstein–Barr virus (EBV) infection has led to the development of a PCR method that can detect EBV-DNA in the cerebrospinal fluid (CSF). The detection of EBV DNA in the CSF by PCR in patients with PCNSL has become established as a diagnostic test with a high sensitivity (83–100%) and specificity (>90%).

Radionuclide imaging by ^{201}thallium single photon emission computed tomography (^{201}Th-SPECT) or ^{18}F-fluorodeoxyglucose-positron emission tomography (FDG-PET) is able to differentiate between PCL and cerebral toxoplasmosis. PCL are thallium avid and demonstrate increased uptake on PET scanning; however, although both techniques have high specificity for PCL, neither are highly sensitivity and thus cannot be used as a single test but in combination with PCR are emerging as a diagnostic alternative to brain biopsy. Nevertheless, stereotactic brain biopsy is the only confirmatory test, and this can be guided by PET scan.

Treatment

In recent years the prognosis for primary cerebral lymphoma in immunocompetent individuals has improved, and this has encouraged clinicians to take a more aggressive approach in HIV-associated PCL. As such we have moved on from whole-brain radiotherapy, due to its poor response durability, the poor survival, and the association with irreversible neurocognitive decline. The current approach, usually reserved for those of better performance status, combines systemic chemotherapy with adequate CNS penetration (usually high-dose methotrexate with or without cytarabine and rituximab) with cART. In some patients who achieve a good response, this approach may be augmented by high-dose chemotherapy and autologous stem cell transplantation. Whole-brain radiotherapy remains a useful palliative treatment modality to control symptoms and should be considered as an alternative approach for patients when the risks of toxicity with high-dose intravenous chemotherapy are considered unacceptable.

Cervical cancer

Epidemiology

Invasive cervical cancer was included as an AIDS-defining diagnosis in 1993, although at that time the incidence of cervical cancer was not increased significantly in HIV-seropositive women. Nonetheless there was good epidemiological evidence that the precursor lesions, cervical intra-epithelial neoplasia (CIN) or squamous intraepithelial lesion (SIL), occurred more frequently in women living with HIV. The prolonged incubation between CIN and invasive cervical cancer of over 10 years may have accounted for the low incidence of invasive cervical cancer in HIV-seropositive women whose life expectancy in many parts of the world will be shorter than this. More recent studies in the era of cART have determined a 4–6-fold increased relative risk of invasive cervical cancer in HIV-seropositive women.[32,33]

Human papilloma virus (HPV) has a central role in the pathogenesis of both CIN and invasive cervical cancer. Two oncoproteins present in HPV are believed to be responsible for the oncogenic properties of this virus, E6 and E7, and different genotypes have variable oncogenicity. Women with HIV infection are more likely to have infection with HPV 16 or 18 (the most oncogenic genotypes), and also have a higher prevalence and incidence of CIN than HIV-negative women. The most attractive strategy aimed at reducing the mortality of cervical cancer is vaccination against HPV both as prophylaxis and potential treatment. Virus-like particles (VLP) are composed of HPV capsid proteins which autoassemble in the absence of viral DNA and these may be manipulated to incorporate additional proteins. These modified VLPs are highly antigenic and have been shown to be efficient inducers of neutralizing antibodies to HPV. Studies of a bivalent, quadrivalent, and nonavalent HPV VLP vaccines have shown high levels of protection against incidental HPV infection, persistent infection, and against cytological abnormalities. The vaccines are safe, well-tolerated, and highly immunogenic including in HIV-seropositive women.[34]

Effects of cART on pre-invasive cervical cancer

The effect of cART on the natural history of CIN has been addressed in multiple cohort studies. Several studies have shown that cART is associated with a reduction in the incidence of CIN although this is not a universal finding. The incidence of CIN is higher in women with lower CD4 counts, and higher CD4 counts are associated with a reduction in incidence and progression of CIN as well as regression of CIN. These findings suggest that frequent cervical smears should be offered to all HIV-positive women. Furthermore, CIN 2/3 should be aggressively treated, followed up by frequent colposcopic surveillance.

Invasive cervical cancer management

HIV-seropositive women with invasive cervical cancer are treated using the same protocols as immunocompetent women in most centers. There is scant published data on women with HIV and invasive cervical cancer and most of them derive from the developing world. Women with HIV infection and cervical cancer present at a younger age than HIV-negative women, and some reports suggest that they have more advanced stage at diagnosis, although this may be confounded by variations in cervical screening practices.

Non-AIDS-defining malignancies

Hodgkin disease

Epidemiology

Hodgkin lymphoma (HL) is one of the most common non-AIDS-defining malignancies (NADMs) with age-adjusted incidence rates remaining 5–25-fold higher than in the general population. Despite the decline in the incidence of AIDS-defining cancers with the introduction of cART, several large cohort studies have found no fall in the incidence of HL and some studies have even demonstrated increased incidence rates of HL immediately after cART initiation. The relationship between immunity and the development of HL is not straightforward, and the risk of HL persists despite good CD4 cell counts amongst PLWH who are on cART treatment.

As with other malignancies associated with HIV, an oncogenic virus (in this case Epstein–Barr virus) has been implicated in the pathogenesis of HL, and there appears to be a higher incidence of EBV detected in HIV-HL tissues than in HL samples from HIV-seronegative patients.

Clinical presentation

HIV-seropositive patients with HL generally present with more advanced lymphoma, with a higher incidence of stage III/IV disease, B-symptoms, and extra-nodal involvement. The bone marrow, skin, liver, and central nervous system are the commonest extra-nodal sites. HL tends to present at an earlier stage of immunosuppression than HIV-associated NHL, with a higher median CD4 cell count at diagnosis, more patients with undetectable plasma HIV viremia, and a greater proportion of patients established on cART at the time of lymphoma diagnosis.

Treatment

There are no randomized trials that address the optimal chemotherapy regimen for patients with HL and HIV infection. Nevertheless, there is a growing tendency, since the advent of cART, to treat patients with HIV and lymphoma with the same chemotherapy protocols used in the general population. Hence most patients are treated with doxorubicin, bleomycin, vinblastine, and dacarbazine (ABVD) which remains, in most parts of the world, the standard chemotherapy regimen for patients with HL. The number of cycles and the addition of radiotherapy (RT) depend on the stage and risk factors of the disease as in the general population. Again careful attention to pharmacokinetic interactions and opportunistic infection prophylaxis is mandatory; however with this approach survival is not adversely affected by HIV status.[35]

Anal cancer

Epidemiology

The incidence of anal cancer in PLWH is up to 40 times higher than in the general population and it occurs at a much younger age. The highest risk of anal cancer is in HIV-positive men who have sex with men (MSM) where the incidence is 70–100 per 100,000 person years (PY) compared with 35 per 100,000 PY in HIV-negative MSM.[36] Importantly, the incidence of anal cancer appears to have risen with the widespread use of cART.

Pathogenesis

The pathogenesis of invasive anal cancer shares many features with cervical cancer, with oncogenic genotypes of human papilloma virus (HPV) infection leading to anal intraepithelial neoplasia (AIN) and ensuing progression of low- to high-grade dysplasia and subsequently invasive cancer. This pathogenetic model suggests a role for anal screening by a combination of cytology and high-resolution anoscopy followed by local ablative therapy of AIN. However, the role of anal screening is not yet proven. Cost-effectiveness analyses of screening have produced both positive and negative results. Nevertheless some centers have instituted screening pilots.

Pre-invasive anal lesions

Cohort studies of men with anal high-grade squamous intraepithelial lesions (HSIL) have demonstrated that these lesions do not regress with cART despite the established benefit of cART on other viral infections and associated diseases in HIV-infected patients, nor has the prevalence of AIN declined.[37,38] The optimal management of anal HSIL remains unclear. The therapeutic options for anal HSIL include ablation by surgical excision or laser ablation and topical chemotherapy with imiquimod, trichloroacetic acid, or fluorouracil. Anal HSIL appears to be a field effect, and hence recurrence is frequent. The prolonged survival of HIV-infected people in the era of cART and the lack of regression of anal HSIL may account for the observed trend towards an increasing incidence of anal cancer.

Invasive anal cancer

The first line of treatment for anal cancer is concurrent chemoradiotherapy (CRT) with 5-fluorouracil/capecitabine and mitomycin C, which has been shown to achieve local control and sphincter preservation. This CRT regime can be safely used for HIV patients producing similar outcomes. Intensity-modulated radiation therapy (IMRT) achieves high doses of radiation with minimal impact to surrounding tissue reducing the toxicity. This has been evaluated in anal cancer patients including PLWH with decreased dermatologic and gastrointestinal toxicity with good tolerance and may become the standard of care in CRT for anal cancer. The most frequent toxicities of CRT are hematological, gastrointestinal, and skin, and some series have found that these are more common in patients with lower CD4 cell counts, although this is not a universal finding. Salvage surgery may be considered for residual primary disease and local recurrence after CRT. However, the outcomes of salvage surgery are generally poor, although experience in this population is limited.

Other NADMs

A number of other malignancies occur more frequently in immunocompromised patients, and these are often associated with oncogenic virus infection. A few appear to be particularly associated with HIV infection, such as squamous cell carcinoma of the conjunctiva[39] and leiomyosarcomas in childhood.[40] In many cases small case series describe the management of these non-AIDS-defining malignancies along the same lines as used in the general population and often with comparable outcomes. Again the most important issue for the treating oncologist is to appreciate the importance of pharmacological interactions and the importance of opportunistic infection prophylaxis but also to recognize that these patients generally have similar outcomes and should not be denied appropriate therapy nor access to clinical trials because of their HIV status.

Castleman's disease

Intellectual debate continues about the classification of Castleman's disease, and it has yet to be granted its own International Classification of Diseases (ICD-11) code. Whilst it does not fulfil many of the criteria for a malignancy, it is included here because it is generally treated by oncologists. Castleman's disease is a rare lymphoproliferative disorder originally described in 1954 and characterized by angiofollicular lymphoid hyperplasia. It is divided into localized disease, and multicentric Castleman's disease (MCD) which is characterized by lymphadenopathy and multiorgan involvement. Histologically, two variants are recognized, a hyaline vascular variant and a less common plasma cell variant. The former is more common in localized disease and the latter more common in MCD. Castleman's disease has germinal center hyalinization or atrophy surrounded by concentric layers of lymphocytes with prominent vascular hyperplasia, hyalinization of small vessels, and interfollicular sheets of plasma cells and immunoblasts.

There is an association between HIV infection, Kaposi's sarcoma, and plasma cell MCD, and KSHV has been found in nearly all MCD samples.[9] The virus encodes a homologue of interleukin (IL)-6, a pro-inflammatory cytokine that is thought to mediate the constitutional symptoms including fever, weight loss, and night sweats. Clinical findings include lymphadenopathy, hepatosplenomegaly, ascites, edema, effusions, and rashes. Investigations frequently reveal microcytic anemia, hypoalbuminemia, and polyclonal hypergammaglobulinemia. Ultimately the diagnosis is made histologically. MCD is associated with a 15-fold increased incidence of NHL.

Whilst surgery is often curative in localized Castleman's disease, it has a limited role in MCD. In recent years, rituximab has emerged as the gold standard treatment for KSHV-associated MCD based on two phase II trials. One study of 21 patients with newly diagnosed HIV MCD reported a radiological response rate of 67%, and the overall and disease-free survival rates at 2 years were 95% and 79% respectively.[41] The second prospective study enrolled 24 patients with HIV MCD who were classified as chemotherapy-dependent. Rituximab induced a sustained remission of 1 year duration in 17/24 (71%) patients and the 1-year overall survival was 92%.[42] A stratified approach to the management of MCD is advocated with patients with poor performance status and end-organ involvement receiving a combination of rituximab and etoposide whilst those with less severe disease are treated with rituximab alone. This algorithm of care was applied to 84 patients yielding 5-year overall survival of 92%.[43] High plasma cell-free levels of KSHV DNA viral load appear to reflect disease activity in Castleman's disease and may be useful in diagnosing and monitoring the disease.[44]

Key learning points

- Kaposi sarcoma, high-grade B-cell non-Hodgkin lymphoma, and cervical cancer are AIDS-defining cancers. Other non-AIDS defining cancers also occur more commonly in people living with HIV and oncogenic viruses may also be implicated in their pathogenesis.
- Combination antiretroviral therapy (cART) has led to a fall in the incidence and improvement in the survival of KS and NHL.
- The treatment of cancer in people with HIV should be the same as the general population and achieves similar outcomes if careful attention is paid to drug interactions and opportunistic infection prophylaxis.

- People living with HIV who develop cancer should be treated only by clinicians with adequate experience and require a joint approach between oncologists and HIV physicians.

References

1. Group ISS, Lundgren JD, Babiker AG et al. Initiation of antiretroviral therapy in early Asymptomatic HIV Infection. *N Engl J Med.* 2015; 373(9):795–807.
2. Portsmouth S, Stebbing J, Gill J et al. A comparison of regimens based on non-nucleoside reverse transcriptase inhibitors or protease inhibitors in preventing Kaposi's sarcoma. *AIDS.* 2003; 17(11):17–22.
3. Beral V, Peterman TA, Berkelman RL, Jaffe HW. Kaposi's sarcoma among persons with AIDS: A sexually transmitted infection? *Lancet.* 1990; 335:123–8.
4. Chang Y, Cesarman E, Pessin MS et al. Identification of herpesvirus-like DNA sequences in AIDS-associated Kaposi's sarcoma. *Science.* 1994; 266(5192):1865–9.
5. Neipel F, Albrecht JC, Fleckenstein B. Cell-homologous genes in the Kaposi's sarcoma-associated rhadinovirus human herpesvirus 8: Determinants of its pathogenicity? [Review] [66 refs]. *J Virol.* 1997; 71(6):4187–92.
6. Moore PS, Chang Y. Kaposi's sarcoma-associated herpesvirus immunoevasion and tumorigenesis: Two sides of the same coin? *Annu Rev Microbiol.* 2003; 57:609–39.
7. Cesarman E, Damania B, Krown SE et al. Kaposi sarcoma. *Nat Rev Dis Primers.* 2019; 5(1):9.
8. Cesarman E, Chang Y, Moore PS, Said JW, Knowles DM. Kaposi's sarcoma-associated herpesvirus-like DNA sequences in AIDS-related body-cavity-based lymphomas. *N Engl J Med.* 1995; 332(18):1186–91.
9. Soulier J, Grollet L, Oskenhendler E et al. Kaposi's sarcoma-associated herpesvirus-like DNA sequences in multicentric Castleman's disease. *Blood.* 1995; 86:1276–80.
10. Krown S, Metroka C, Wernz JC. Kaposi's sarcoma in the acquired immune deficiency syndrome: A proposal for uniform evaluation, response, and staging criteria. AIDS Clinical Trials Group Oncology Committee. *J Clin Oncol.* 1989; 7:1201–7.
11. Krown SE, Testa MA, Huang J. AIDS-related Kaposi's sarcoma: prospective validation of the AIDS Clinical Trials Group staging classification. AIDS Clinical Trials Group Oncology Committee. *J Clin Oncol.* 1997; 15(9):3085–92.
12. Asiimwe F, Moore D, Were W et al. Clinical outcomes of HIV-infected patients with Kaposi's sarcoma receiving nonnucleoside reverse transcriptase inhibitor-based antiretroviral therapy in Uganda. *HIV Med.* 2012; 13(3):166–71.
13. Bower M, Palfreeman A, Alfa-Wali M et al. British HIV Association guidelines for HIV-associated malignancies 2014. *HIV Med.* 2014; 15(Suppl 2):1–92.
14. Bower M, Gazzard B, Mandalia S et al. A prognostic index for systemic AIDS-related non-Hodgkin lymphoma treated in the era of highly active antiretroviral therapy. *Ann Intern Med.* 2005; 143(4):265–73.
15. A predictive model for aggressive non-Hodgkin's lymphoma. The International Non-Hodgkin's Lymphoma Prognostic Factors Project. *N Engl J Med.* 1993; 329(14):987–94.
16. Matthews GV, Bower M, Mandalia S et al. Changes in acquired immunodeficiency syndrome-related lymphoma since the introduction of highly active antiretroviral therapy. *Blood.* 2000; 96(8):2730–4.
17. Navarro JT, Lloveras N, Ribera JM et al. The prognosis of HIV-infected patients with diffuse large B-cell lymphoma treated with chemotherapy and highly active antiretroviral therapy is similar to that of HIV-negative patients receiving chemotherapy. *Haematologica.* 2005; 90(5):704–6.
18. Diamond C, Taylor TH, Im T, Anton-Culver H. Presentation and outcomes of systemic non-Hodgkin's lymphoma: A comparison between patients with acquired immunodeficiency syndrome

(AIDS) treated with highly active antiretroviral therapy and patients without AIDS. *Leuk Lymphoma*. 2006; 47(9):1822–9.

19. Kaplan LD, Lee JY, Ambinder RF et al. Rituximab does not improve clinical outcome in a randomized phase 3 trial of CHOP with or without rituximab in patients with HIV-associated non-Hodgkin lymphoma: AIDS-Malignancies Consortium Trial 010. *Blood*. 2005; 106(5):1538–43.

20. Castillo JJ, Echenique IA. Rituximab in combination with chemotherapy versus chemotherapy alone in HIV-associated non-Hodgkin lymphoma: A pooled analysis of 15 prospective studies. *Am J Hematol*. 2012; 87(3):330–3.

21. Simonelli C, Spina M, Cinelli R et al. Clinical features and outcome of primary effusion lymphoma in HIV-infected patients: A single-institution study. *J Clin Oncol*. 2003; 21(21):3948–54.

22. Castillo J, Pantanowitz L, Dezube BJ. HIV-associated plasmablastic lymphoma: Lessons learned from 112 published cases. *Am J Hematol*. 2008; 83(10):804–9.

23. Schmitz N, Zeynalova S, Nickelsen M et al. CNS International Prognostic Index: A risk model for CNS relapse in patients with diffuse large B-cell lymphoma treated with R-CHOP. *J Clin Oncol*. 2016; 34(26):3150–6.

24. Powles T, Imami N, Nelson M et al. Effects of combination chemotherapy and highly active antiretroviral therapy on immune parameters in HIV-1 associated lymphoma. *AIDS*. 2002; 16(4):531–6.

25. Esdaile B, Davis M, Portsmouth S et al. The immunological effects of concomitant highly active antiretroviral therapy and liposomal anthracycline treatment of HIV-1-associated Kaposi's sarcoma. *AIDS*. 2002; 16(17):2344–7.

26. Alfa-Wali M, Allen-Mersh T, Antoniou A et al. Chemoradiotherapy for anal cancer in HIV patients causes prolonged CD4 cell count suppression. *Ann Oncol*. 2012; 23(1):141–7.

27. Levine AM, Karim R, Mack W et al. Neutropenia in human immunodeficiency virus infection: Data from the women's interagency HIV study. *Arch Intern Med*. 2006; 166(4):405–10.

28. Israel DS, Plaisance KI. Neutropenia in patients infected with human immunodeficiency virus. *Clin Pharm*. 1991; 10(4):268–79.

29. Bower M, McCall-Peat N, Ryan N et al. Protease inhibitors potentiate chemotherapy-induced neutropenia. *Blood*. 2004; 104(9):2943–6.

30. International Collaboration on HIV and Cancer. Highly active antiretroviral therapy and incidence of cancer in human immunodeficiency virus-infected adults. *J Natl Cancer Inst*. 2000; 92(22):1823–30.

31. Bower M, Powles T, Nelson M et al. Highly active antiretroviral therapy and human immunodeficiency virus-associated primary cerebral lymphoma. *J Natl Cancer Inst*. 2006; 98(15):1088–91.

32. Frisch M, Biggar RJ, Goedert JJ. Human papillomavirus-associated cancers in patients with human immunodeficiency virus infection and acquired immunodeficiency syndrome. *J Natl Cancer Inst*. 2000; 92(18):1500–10.

33. Clifford GM, Polesel J, Rickenbach M et al. Cancer risk in the Swiss HIV Cohort Study: Associations with immunodeficiency, smoking, and highly active antiretroviral therapy. *J Natl Cancer Inst*. 2005; 97(6):425–32.

34. Kahn JA, Xu J, Kapogiannis BG et al. Immunogenicity and safety of the human papillomavirus-6, –11, –16, –18 vaccine in HIV-infected young women. *Clin Infect Dis*. 2013; 57(5):735–44.

35. Montoto S, Shaw K, Okosun J et al. HIV status does not influence outcome in patients with classical Hodgkin lymphoma treated with chemotherapy using doxorubicin, bleomycin, vinblastine, and dacarbazine in the highly active antiretroviral therapy era. *J Clin Oncol*. 2012; 30(33):4111.

36. Kreuter A, Potthoff A, Brockmeyer NH et al. Anal carcinoma in human immunodeficiency virus-positive men: Results of a prospective study from Germany. *Br J Dermatol*. 2010; 162(6):1269–77.

37. Palefsky JM, Holly EA, Efirdc JT et al. Anal intraepithelial neoplasia in the highly active antiretroviral therapy era among HIV-positive men who have sex with men. *AIDS*. 2005; 19(13):1407–14.

38. Fox P, Stebbing J, Portsmouth S et al. Lack of response of anal intra-epithelial neoplasia to highly active antiretroviral therapy. *AIDS*. 2003; 17(2):279–80.

39. Goedert J, Cote T. Conjunctival malignant disease with AIDS in USA. *Lancet*. 1995; 346:257–8.

40. Granovsky M, Mueller B, Nicholson H et al. Cancer in human immunodeficiency virus-infected children: A case series from the children's cancer group and the National Cancer Institute. *J Clin Oncol*. 1998; 16:1729–35.

41. Bower M, Powles T, Williams S et al. Brief communication: Rituximab in HIV-associated multicentric Castleman disease. *Ann Intern Med*. 2007; 147(12):836–9.

42. Gerard L, Berezne A, Galicier L et al. Prospective study of rituximab in chemotherapy-dependent human immunodeficiency virus associated multicentric Castleman's disease: ANRS 117 CastlemaB Trial. *J Clin Oncol*. 2007; 25(22):3350–6.

43. Pria AD, Pinato D, Roe J et al. Relapse of HHV8-positive multicentric Castleman disease following rituximab-based therapy in HIV-positive patients. *Blood*. 2017; 129(15):2143–7.

44. Stebbing J, Adams C, Sanitt A et al. Plasma HHV8 DNA predicts relapse in individuals with HIV-associated multicentric Castleman disease. *Blood*. 2011; 118(2):271–5.

34 CLINICAL CANCER GENETICS

Rosalind A. Eeles and Lisa J. Walker

Introduction

Cancer is a common disease, affecting nearly half the population at some time in their lives in the developed world. All cancer can be termed "genetic" as cancer is caused by genetic mutations (alterations in the DNA code), which result in abnormal cellular growth and/or proliferation. The majority of these mutations are sporadic (only occur in the cancer cell), and only a small proportion of these cases (approximately 5–10 per cent)[1] are due to the inheritance of a germline mutation in a high-penetrance cancer pre-disposition gene in most of the common cancers. The exception is in some of the rare cancers, some of which are due to a mutation in a high-penetrance pre-disposition gene in a higher proportion of cases. This mutation is then present in every somatic cell and, on average, in half the gametes (a gamete only contains half of the total genes) and therefore has a chance of being passed onto the offspring of an affected individual. These mutated cancer pre-disposition genes have a well-defined pattern of inheritance. Approximately a further 20 per cent of cancer cases can be described as familial, i.e. there is a clustering of cancer cases within the family, but they do not show a well-defined pattern of inheritance. These family clusters may be due to the chance clustering of common cancers, the inheritance of genes that are associated with only a slightly increased cancer risk, the sharing of common environmental influences, or they may be of multifactorial origin, possibly as a result of the inheritance of genes that render an individual more susceptible to environmental influences. We also now know that in populations there is common genetic variation which contributes to cancer risk; these variants are in themselves each only slightly increasing cancer risk. However, in a small proportion of individuals (about 10 per cent), the variants currently known contribute to quite substantial risks as their risks are multiplicative, and therefore can be used to risk stratify populations.

This chapter will focus on cancer pre-disposition genes, cancer risks associated with these genes, and the management of suspected cancer pre-disposition gene mutation carriers.

Cancer pre-disposition genes

Cancer pre-disposition genes are mutated genes, the normal function of which is to regulate cell growth or the detection and/or repair of DNA damage. These are germline mutations and are present in all nucleated cells, including on average half of the germ cells. The risk that a cancer pre-disposition gene gives rise to the development of cancer is designated the *penetrance*, and the fact that many of these genes do not universally result in cancer development is termed *incomplete penetrance*.

Familial clustering of the same type of cancer may be due to more than one type of cancer pre-disposition gene. This is termed *genetic heterogeneity*. For example, familial breast cancer, in which there are clusters of >4 cases of breast cancer at <60 years of age in the same lineage, may be due to mutations in either **br**east **ca**ncer gene 1 or 2 (*BRCA1* and *BRCA2*) or a panel of other breast cancer pre-disposition genes, many of which are in the DNA repair pathway. Not all such clusters can be explained by mutations in such gene panels, and we think that other breast cancer pre-disposition genes remain to be discovered.

Cancer predisposition genes can be associated with syndromes that predominantly consist of clustering of cancers at either one or multiple associated sites (Table 34.1). For example, mutations in *BRCA1/2* genes pre-dispose to breast, ovarian, prostate, and other cancers, and Lynch syndrome (hereditary non-polyposis colorectal cancer [HNPCC]) mismatch repair genes pre-dispose to gastrointestinal, gynecological, urinary, and other cancers. Other genetic syndromes are associated with an increased risk of cancer in addition to other, non-malignant, features of a syndrome such as neurofibromatosis, multiple endocrine neoplasia (MEN) 1 and 2, and ataxia telangiectasia syndromes (Table 34.2). The ability to recognize clustering of cancers at different sites as being part of a syndrome is an important part of recognizing the possible presence of a cancer pre-disposition gene in a family.

Inheritance

The inheritance of germline mutations in cancer pre-disposition genes may be either dominant or recessive at the genetic level or X-linked. We all carry two copies (alleles) of every gene, one copy from each parent, and as only one allele can be passed down to the next generation, there is a 50:50 chance as to which allele is inherited (Figure 34.1).

In dominant inheritance the presence of a single mutated allele is usually sufficient to cause the associated disease and approximately 50 per cent of all offspring develop the disease.

In recessive inheritance the presence of a single mutated allele is not usually sufficient for disease expression and two mutated alleles are required. Usually both parents have to carry the mutated allele for the creation of an offspring affected by disease, but they themselves are unaffected, as their "normal" allele's effect overrides the mutated one. Two "carrier" parents therefore have a 25 per cent chance of having an affected child. Examples of non-cancer conditions inherited in this way include cystic fibrosis and β-thalassemia. The majority of cancer pre-disposition genes are recessively inherited at the cellular level, but dominantly inherited in families.

In X-linked inheritance the mutated gene is carried on the X-chromosome. Females have two X-chromosomes, and can therefore be carriers of the condition, but are not usually affected by it. As males only have one copy of the X chromosome, if they inherit a mutated gene on the X from their mother, they will inherit the condition. A carrier female would therefore have a 50 per cent chance of passing the condition on to each of her sons, and a 50 per cent chance that her daughters would, themselves, be carriers. The best-known example of this mode of inheritance outside cancer is Duchenne muscular dystrophy, but X-linked familial prostate cancer has also been observed in a small number of families, although the exact gene has not yet been identified.

Some genes are "imprinted," and this can complicate inheritance patterns further. Imprinting refers to a situation where an individual will only use a gene inherited from one parent. The copy of that gene inherited from the other parent is not transcribed, so even if a mutation occurs in the unused copy of the

TABLE 34.1 **Syndromes Associated with Increased Risk of Malignancy Where the Major Feature Associated with the Syndrome Is the Development of Cancer**

Syndrome Name	Malignancies	Risk (Per Cent)[1]	Mode[2]	Chromosomal Location[3]	Gene Name
Melanoma	Melanoma	53	D	9p	*CDKN2A (P16)*
	Pancreatic cancer	10–20			
Familial polyposis coli	Large bowel	100	D	5q	*APC*
	Upper GI tract	5			
	Desmoid tumor	20			
Familial breast/ovarian cancer syndrome 1	Breast (female)	80	D	17q	*BRCA1*
	Ovary	60			
	Colon	6			
	Prostate	6			
Familial breast/ovarian cancer syndrome 2	Breast (female)	80	D	13q	*BRCA2*
	Ovary	40			
	Prostate	20			
	Breast (male)	5			
	Pancreas	4			
	Other cancers, e.g. cutaneous and ocular melanoma, gall bladder, bile duct, fallopian tube, stomach	? 1			
Lynch syndrome				3p	*hMLH*1
(hereditary non-polyposis colorectal cancer)	Colon	70–80	D	2p	*hMSH*2
(HNPCC)				2p	*hMSH*6
				2q	*PMS*1
				7q	*PMS*2
	Endometrium	15–60			
	Ovary	10			
	Stomach	11–19			
	Urothelial	5			
	Melanoma, head and neck, brain, small bowel				
Muir–Torre syndrome	As HNPCC with skin lesions		D	2p	*hMSH*2
	Keratoacanthoma/sebaceous adenomas/ carcinomas				
Turcot's syndrome	CNS malignancies		R		*hMSH*2
	Very early-onset colon cancer				*hMLH*1
	(20 years) with				*APC*
	café-au-lait patches				*PMS*2
MUTYH-associated polyposis	Colorectal		R	1p	*MUTYH*
Hereditary prostate cancer	Prostate	20–85	D/R/X-linked	Multiple loci	Range of DNA repair genes, *HOXB13*
Li–Fraumeni syndrome	Sarcoma cancer	24 childhood	D	17p	*TP53*
	Early-onset breast cancer	Overall cancer risk:			
	Brain tumor	74 in men, 95 in			
	Leukemia	women			
	Adrenocortical tumor				
	Other cancers				
Multiple endocrine neoplasia type 1	Parathyroid, endocrine pancreas, pituitary	70–90	D	11q	*MENIN*

(Continued)

Syndrome Name	Malignancies	Risk (Per Cent)[1]	Mode[2]	Chromosomal Location[3]	Gene Name
Multiple endocrine neoplasia type 2	Medullary carcinoma of thyroid	70	D	10q	*RET*
	Pheochromocytoma (type 2A)	50			
Retinoblastoma	Retinoblastoma	90	D	13q	*RB1*
	Osteosarcoma	6			
	Other cancers	8			
Hereditary diffuse gastric cancer	Stomach cancer	80	D	16q	*CDH1*
	Breast cancer (lobular)	60			
Hereditary ovarian cancer	Ovarian cancer	12–15	D	17q	*BRIP1, RAD51C and RAD51D in addition to BRCA1/2 above*
Rhabdoid pre-disposition syndrome	Rhabdoid tumor	?	R	22q	*INI1, SMARCB1*
	Choroid plexus carcinoma	?			
	Medulloblastoma	?			
	Central primitive NET	?			
Peutz–Jeghers syndrome	GI	55–60	D	19p	*STK11*
	Breast	35–55			
	Pancreas	17			
	GI polyps	100			
	Gynecological and testicular Tumors	20			
	Mucocutaneous pigmentation	100			

[1] The risk is either the "lifetime risk," as quoted in the reference articles, or the "risk to age 70 years" in those studies which have performed detailed age-specific calculations. Where possible, risks by set ages or a "per site" risk is given; in the absence of such figures a "syndrome" penetrance estimate (risk of cancer development) is provided. These risks are approximate and may vary between different populations with different mutation profiles.

[2] Mode of inheritance is classified as autosomal dominant (D) or autosomal recessive (R).

[3] Chromosomal arms: q, long arm; p, short arm.

gene, it has no effect. An example of this is in familial pheochromocytoma, where if an individual inherits a mutated copy of *SDHD* from their mother, this mutation has no effect on tumor pre-disposition, whereas if the mutated copy is inherited from their father, they are at increased risk. There have been rare cases where mutations in the genes controlling imprinting have also been reported.

Mechanisms of action

Cancer pre-disposition genes can be oncogenes, tumor suppressor genes, or mismatch repair genes.

Oncogenes are mutated normal genes (proto-oncogenes) in which mutation tends to cause a "gain in function" effect resulting in increased growth or proliferation of the affected cells. Most oncogenes tend to act in a dominant manner, and those causing cancer include the *RET* oncogene in the multiple endocrine neoplasia 2A (MEN2A) syndrome or *MET* oncogene in familial type 1 papillary renal cancer.

Tumor suppressor genes are normal genes in which mutation tends to cause a "loss of function" effect in the control mechanisms of growth and/or cellular proliferation pathways. An example is *RB1*, involved in retinoblastoma. Most cancer pre-disposition genes are tumor suppressor genes and are recessively inherited at the cellular level. However, they tend to manifest dominant inheritance (the chance of a mutation being inherited by the offspring is 50 per cent). A sporadic mutation of the remaining normal allele occurs in a somatic cell during the lifetime of

the germline mutation carrier to lead to cancer development. This two-stage process in the development of cancers (where one stage is germline and the other is somatic) is known as Knudson's two-hit hypothesis.[2]

Mismatch-repair genes (Lynch [HNPCC] syndrome) maintain the integrity of the genome and mutations in them permit acquired genetic damage to accumulate resulting in the creation of a cancer cell. The mutations that occur in this syndrome cause what is called microsatellite instability (MSI-High) which is the presence of runs of repeat sequences due to miscopied DNA sequences.

Hereditary cancer pre-disposition genes have also been divided into "gatekeeper genes" and "caretaker genes." "Gatekeeper" genes are those that regulate progression through the cell cycle. Disturbance of their function leads to an imbalance of cell division over cell death. This cellular proliferation is followed by the accumulation of multiple somatic genetic events leading to the tumor. Examples of "gatekeeper" genes include *RB1* and *TP53*. "Caretaker" genes maintain the integrity of the genome. Mutation occurring in these genes simply gives rise to genetic instability, causing mutation in other genes, including "gatekeeper" genes. The DNA mismatch repair genes causing HNPCC are examples of "caretaker" genes.

There have been a few cases of the so-called "three-hit hypothesis" reported. This occurs where genes are imprinted, and a mutation in the imprinting center (genes that control whether other genes are switched off, according to their parent of inheritance) results in mutations that would usually have no effect causing a

TABLE 34.2   Some of the "Rare" Genetic Syndromes Associated with an Increased Risk of Malignancy

Syndrome	Neoplasia or Malignancy	Risk (Per Cent)[1]	Mode[2]	Chromosomal Location[3]	Gene Name
Neurofibromatosis type 1	Plexiform neurofibroma, optic glioma, neurofibrosarcoma	4–5	D	17q	*NF1*
	Breast cancer	30–40			
Neurofibromatosis type 2	Acoustic neuroma (vestibular schwannoma)		D	22q	*NF2*
	• bilateral	85			
	• unilateral	6			
	Meningioma	45			
	Spinal tumors	26			
	Astrocytomas	4			
	Ependymomas	3			
von Hippel–Lindau	Cerebellar hemangioblastoma	44–72	D	3p	*VHL*
	Retinal angioma	25–60			
	Renal cell carcinoma	25–60			
	Pheochromocytoma	15			
	Renal, liver, and pancreatic cysts	16–50			
Familial Pheo/ Paraganglioma	Pheochromocytoma	30–50	D	1p	*SDHB*
	Paraganglioma	30–70		1q	*SDHC*
	Renal cell carcinoma	15		11q	*SDHD*
				5p	*SDHA*
				11q	*SDHAF2*
				2q	*TMEM127*
				14q	*MAX*
Ataxia telangiectasia	Lymphoid malignancy	10–15	R	11q	*ATM*
	Breast cancer	40–50			
Fanconi anemia	Lymphoid malignancy	9	R	16q	*FANCA*
				9q	*FANCC*
	Wilms tumor	20 (*FANCD1* only)		13q	*FANCD1/BRCA2*
				3p	*FANCD2*
				6p	*FANCE*
				11p	*FANCF*
				9p	*FANCG/XRCC9*
	Breast cancer	20 (BRIP1 heterozygotes)		17q	*FANCJ/BRIP1*
				2p	*FANCL*
				14q	*FANCM*
	Breast cancer	35 (*PALB2* heterozygotes)		16p	*FANCN/PALB2*
	Pancreatic cancer	3 (*PALB2* heterozygotes)			
	Ovarian cancer	12 (*RAD51C* heterozygotes)		17q	*FANCO/RAD51C*
Bloom syndrome	Many sites immunodeficiency	40	R	15q	*BLM*
Xeroderma pigmentosum	Skin cancers (basal cell carcinoma, squamous cell carcinoma, melanoma)	100	R	9q	*XPA*
				2q	*XPB*
				3p	*XPC*
				19q	*XPD*
				11p	*XPE*
				16p	*XPF*
				13q	*XPG*
				6p	*XPV*
PTEN hamartoma tumor syndrome/ Cowden syndrome	Breast cancer (female)	30–50	D	10q	*PTEN*
	Thyroid cancer	10			
	Bowel cancer	?3			
	Multiple hamartomas of skin, tongue, and bowel	100			
Basal cell nevus/ Gorlin	Basal cell carcinoma	90	D	9q	*PTCH*

(*Continued*)

TABLE 34.2 (CONTINUED)   Some of the "Rare" Genetic Syndromes Associated with an Increased Risk of Malignancy

Syndrome	Neoplasia or Malignancy	Risk (Per Cent)[1]	Mode[2]	Chromosomal Location[3]	Gene Name
syndrome	Ovarian fibroma	24			
	Medulloblastoma	5			
	Falx calcification, bifid ribs, macrocephaly	85			
Hereditary leiomyomatosis and renal cell cancer syndrome	Renal cell cancer	62	D	1q	*FH*
	Leiomyosarcomas (uterus)	?2–5			
	Leiomyomata (cutaneous, uterus)	75–100			
Birt–Hogg Dube syndrome	Renal cell cancer/oncocytoma	16	D	17p	*FLCN*
	Cutaneous fibrofolliculomas	100			
	Pneumothorax	29			
Carney complex	Myxoma	100	D	17q	*PRKAR1A*
	Thyroid adenoma	75			
	Thyroid cancer	10			
	Pituitary adenoma	10			
	Testicular tumors (benign)	90–100			
	Psammomatous melanotic Schwannoma	10			
	Adrenal cortical hyperplasia	25			

[1] Lifetime risk of neoplasia or cancer.
[2] Mode of inheritance is classified as autosomal dominant (D) or autosomal recessive (R).
[3] Chromosomal arms: p, short arm; q, long arm.

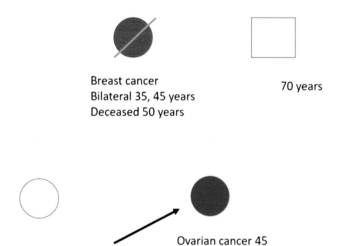

FIGURE 34.1   Sample family tree: arrow denotes the proband; prior probability of genetic mutation about 60–80 per cent; posterior probability of mutation in sister of proband is 30–40 per cent.

pre-disposition to tumors. The "three-hit hypothesis" has been primarily described in *SDHD*,[3] and refers to the idea that the affected individual inherits one mutation in *SDHD* from a female parent, another mutation in the imprinting center, (which means that the *SDHD* mutation is relevant), and then the sporadic mutation of the remaining allele of *SDHD* gives rise to tumors.

Rarely the mutation does not occur in the cancer pre-disposition gene itself, but in a part of the genetic code which controls the methylation of the gene which gives rise to increased cancer risk. An example of this is the *EPCAM* deletion mutation which results in the methylation of *MSH2* and a resulting HNPCC phenotype.[4]

Research approaches for the identification of cancer pre-disposition genes

When a cancer pre-disposition gene is thought to be the cause of familial clustering of cancer cases, there are several approaches to locate the gene. Once located and characterized, genetic testing can then be offered in the clinical setting.

Cytogenetic alterations

Gross chromosomal changes can be seen on cytogenetic analysis. Rarely, a study of a constitutional chromosomal alteration seen on cytogenetic analysis in an individual who has an unusually early onset of cancer and other unusual phenotypic features can indicate the location of a cancer pre-disposition gene. The chromosomal study of a man with intellectual disability and polyposis led to the finding of a loss of part of chromosome 5, subsequently found to be the location of the polyposis gene, *APC*.[5]

Linkage analysis

The concept of genetic linkage was first recognized by Gregor Mendel, who noted that certain characteristics of his experimental plants tended to be co-inherited. The explanation for this became clear once it was recognized that chromosomes contain the genetic material and two traits are linked only if the corresponding genes for them reside close together on the same chromosome.

The search for cancer pre-disposition genes using linkage relies on collections of families with numerous cancer cases of the same cancer type. Co-inheritance of specific genetic markers with the disease is said to show evidence of linkage if the co-inheritance is greater than would be expected by chance. This is expressed as a "LOD score" (**lo**garithm to base 10 of the **od**ds). A LOD score is similar to a *p*-value in clinical trials, and a LOD score of >3 is statistically significant and equivalent to odds of linkage of 1000 to 1 ($\log_{10}1000 = 3$).

Phenotypic features

A physical characteristic associated with a cancer pre-disposition syndrome may give a clue as to the location of the cancer pre-disposition gene. An example of this is the co-existence of aniridia and genitourinary abnormalities with Wilms tumor in the **W**ilms—**A**niridia—**G**enitourinary—**R**etardation (WAGR) syndrome. This is caused by a contiguous gene deletion on chromosome 11.[6]

Association studies

A number of disease susceptibility loci have been identified through direct testing of candidate genes, looking for associations between particular alleles and disease, by comparing allele frequencies in affected individuals and controls. A candidate gene can be identified by a number of methods including knowledge of the natural history of specific cancers; for example, androgen receptor gene polymorphisms (variants in the genetic code) are associated with prostate cancer risk in some studies.

The advent of Genome-Wide Association Studies (GWAS) means that this is one way to identify single nucleotide changes, sometimes genes, and even markers that are associated with increased risk of conditions including cancers. The level of risk is not markedly increased for each variant; however as the risks are multiplicative these can give risk to substantial risks in a proportion of individuals who carry many of the risk variants. There are over 1000 such variants reported to be associated with disease traits (www.genome.gov/gwastudies/). Much work is still required to establish the significance of these findings, in particular the functional effects of these variants and their clinical application in the stratification of populations for targeted screening and their role in clinical care.

Next-generation sequencing

Improvements in DNA sequencing technologies, such that very high volumes of DNA can be sequenced in a short space of time, with good accuracy, now mean that analysis of the entire genome (whole-genome sequencing [WGS]) or more commonly analysis of the coding region of the genome (whole-exome sequencing [WES]) can be done to search for new genes which may be causing pre-disposition to cancers. This can be approached using several cases or families where individuals have been affected with a certain type of tumor, where those families do not have mutations in the known genes (if any known genes exist). If the affected individuals all then have mutations in the same gene, then that gene is a strong candidate to be causative for that type of tumor. These new technologies can also be applied to tumors, to look for drug targets; however commonly such somatic analysis (analysis of tumor DNA

only) also yields information about the rest of an individual's DNA (constitutional DNA), and it is important for oncologists to have an understanding of the information yielded by such analyses, and where to go for help if and when mutations are found. Consent issues are vital to this, and work is ongoing to try to formalize how patients should be consented for this kind of analysis, which, of course, could find mutations in genes that pre-dispose individuals to other diseases (so-called incidental findings), where those patients may have no wish to find out that information. There are ESMO guidelines which recommend which mutations found in tumors should be followed up by referral to a cancer geneticist to counsel for germline testing and if positive, the management of the family.[7] The most important of these are mutations in mismatch repair genes and *BRCA1* and *BRCA2*.

Cancer risks associated with cancer pre-disposition genes

Cancer risks depend on the presence of mutations in a cancer pre-disposition gene and their penetrance. Penetrance may be affected by external factors, such as lifestyle, and may depend on the ethnic origin of an individual due to population-specific mutation risks. Different ethnic populations may have a different gene penetrance, which is illustrated by the breast cancer penetrance estimates for *BRCA1/2* mutation carriers. Using data from the Breast Cancer Linkage Consortium based on breast and ovarian cancer families identified from a world-wide population of high-risk families with breast cancer, the risk of breast cancer is estimated to be 85 per cent by 80 years,[8] but data from pooled analyses without a family history are 65 per cent for *BRCA1* mutation carriers and 45 per cent for *BRCA2*.[9] Estimates based on the Ashkenazim are 60 per cent by 70 years[10] and for the Icelandic founder mutation carriers to be 37 per cent by 80 years[11] in contrast to a general population risk of breast cancer of around 10 per cent by 80 years in the UK (www.statistics.gov.uk). The ethnic population differences may be due to a founder mutation dependent risk, the effect of other modifying genes in a population or the added effect of environmental influences, which may be shared within specific populations. It is therefore extremely important to ascertain the genetic origin of the patient before formal genetic counseling is initiated. Tables 34.1 and 34.2 summarize the current penetrance/risk estimates associated with known cancer pre-disposition genes.

The estimate of penetrance can be confounded by the presence of phenocopies when research into the identification of a cancer pre-disposition gene is undertaken. Phenocopies are people who have developed the disease of interest but are found not to carry the disease pre-disposition gene mutation; therefore the disease occurred by chance alone or may have been due to environmental influences. Phenocopies are a particular problem in syndromes associated with common cancers such as breast, colon, or prostate cancer.

Risk assessment

This is arguably the most difficult part of cancer genetic counseling: first, to arrive at a risk estimate and second, to convey this information in the most appropriate manner to the individual so that they can understand and retain this information and are not made inappropriately anxious about their risks.

The first risk estimation is the chance that a familial cluster is due to genetic pre-disposition. This is called the prior probability of a genetic pre-disposition gene mutation being present in a family. This estimation can be based upon published data or clinical experiences when published data are lacking, which unfortunately is often the case with rare genetic conditions. Models have been developed to estimate the likelihood that a high-risk breast cancer–pre-disposing gene is present in the family.[12] These models vary in complexity of analysis and ease of use. Examples include the Frank model, BOADICEA model, BRCAPRO, and the Manchester scoring system.

The Frank model is a logistic regression model developed to estimate *BRCA1* and *BRCA2* probability based on family history. It was originally based on 238 high-risk women.

The BOADICEA model was developed using complex segregation analysis of breast and ovarian cancer in a combined dataset of more than 1500 families. It allows for the simultaneous effects of *BRCA1* and *BRCA2* as well as the effects of low-penetrance genes. It also considers the effect of genetic modifiers that cluster in families and alter the breast cancer risks in *BRCA1* and *BRCA2* carriers. Recent updates have included the pathology of the tumor; for example *BRCA1* mutations are more commonly associated with triple negative breast cancer under the age of 50 years.

The Manchester scoring system was developed using a combination of *BRCA1* and *BRCA2* screening results from 422 families and data regarding mutation-positive and -negative kindreds. It was devised to discriminate at the 10 per cent likelihood level, and takes the form of a numerical scoring system that is easy to implement in clinical practice. A score of 15 or more is an indication to offer *BRCA1/2* mutation analysis. This is the most commonly used system in the UK. Recently pathology has been added to this scoring system.[13]

The second risk estimation is the chance the individual has inherited a particular gene based upon their position in the family tree, if they are affected by cancer, and their current age. This is termed the posterior probability.

BOX 34.1 STANDARD NOTATION FOR A FAMILY TREE

- Male—square
- Female—circle
- Deceased—diagonal line through symbol
- Proband—arrow indicates consultand who is giving the family history

There is variation in notation of the shading of the symbols between clinics and, as the shading is not standardized, a legend should be attached to a family tree if referring to a family history in a medical report.

The final calculation is the chance that cancer will develop. Penetrance estimates are essential to calculate this. These calculations can be complex, particularly if there are multiple generations to consider, and there may be intervening unaffected individuals between affected individuals which affects the prior and posterior probabilities.

Risk perception

Expressing these risks in a form that is meaningful for the consultand is difficult. The uptake of preventive strategies may depend upon an individual's perception of risk; for example, Croyle et al.[14] have shown that individuals who perceive themselves to be at increased risk of heart disease were more likely to express their

intentions to modify their lifestyle than those at perceived population risk. The understanding and retention of this information may depend upon the format in which it is presented and the individual's attitudes to risk.

The expression of this risk can be delivered in a number of formats. The optimal format for conveying risk information is unknown. Currently, risk estimates tend to be given as a percentage risk or a "1 in X" value and followed up with a written summary, incorporating this risk estimate, to the individual attending the genetics consultation (Table 34.3). Unfortunately, there are data which suggest that women prefer not to have, or remember, numerical information. They are able to report the qualitative category of their risk (low, medium, high) with reasonable accuracy, but this did not relate to their perception that they were more or less likely to get cancer.[15]

In cancer families, it is possible that a larger cancer burden (the number, age at diagnosis, and closeness of relationship of the cancer cases) may distort the perceived risk above the true level.[16] Many people in cancer families think erroneously that their risk of developing cancer is 100 per cent, and the only uncertainty is the point in time when the disease will occur. Lerman et al.[17] have reported that members of cancer families distort their risk, even when their family history consists of only one affected relative.

The points above have been summarized by Vlek[18] who claims that there are five factors underlying perception of risk

1. The potential degree of harm or lethality associated with the risk
2. The controllability through safety/rescue measures (i.e. prevention/early detection)
3. The number of people exposed (this would equate to the cancer burden in the family)
4. The familiarity with the effects of the risk
5. The degree to which exposure to the risk is voluntary

There are reports that suggest that those at highest risk have a lower rate of adoption of health preventive measures due to avoidance behaviors instigated by high levels of anxiety.[19] If cancer family clinics are to provide a useful service it is important to ensure that those counseled understand the risk information and

TABLE 34.3 Methods of Presentation of Cancer Risk Estimates

Method of Presentation	Expression of Risk
Numerical	Risk per year
	Risk by certain age
	1 in x value or percentage format
	Relative risk corrected for age
General categorization	High/moderate/low risk
Situation analogy	A situation carrying an equivalent risk without any numerical information, e.g. the chances of picking an ace if one card is chosen blind from a card pack
The risk figure measures	Risk of developing cancer
	Risk of not developing cancer
	Risk of death from cancer (this is rarely given in clinics as it is perceived as too distressing)

advice they are given. Lack of understanding of their risk could impact on their ability to use this information when making decisions about the future management of their health, and may also affect their mental health if cancer-related worries are increased through misunderstanding of information given in the clinic.

Management of a known or suspected cancer pre-disposition gene mutation carrier

Identification of an at-risk family

A family at genetic risk of cancer must first be identified. There are many potential sources of identification, for example, through consultation with a general practitioner (GP) or a hospital clinic while under treatment for an associated disease, through conversation with an associated professional such as a practice or clinic nurse, radiographer, or doctor, or through an individual's own perception of a potential genetic problem in their family precipitating contact with a healthcare professional.

In the hospital oncology setting, if an individual has presented with cancer at a young age, it is now becoming more common for that individual's family history to be requested by cancer geneticists working as part of the multidisciplinary team coordinating the patient's care. If there is significant family history in addition to the presenting cancer, a referral is made. Sometimes, a referral is made simply because an individual presents with an unusual type of cancer at a young age, for example, medullary thyroid cancer in childhood. In other settings, unless an individual directly expresses concern about their perceived risk, then the only way an at-risk family will be identified is by systematic questioning of all patients about a family history of cancer while eliciting a general medical history. As a quick guideline, taking a history of all first-degree relatives only (parents, siblings, and children) and then asking if there are any other cancers in the family will detect 95 per cent of familial syndromes. Due to the limited time available during most consultations, it would not be appropriate to obtain a detailed family history from the patient. From this quick family history it should, however, be possible to make an assessment of whether the family history warrants further investigation.

Sometimes, the family history may look suspicious but not obviously fall into a specific cancer pre-disposition syndrome. In these cases, it is important to seek further advice from the local clinical genetics department. These departments are mainly located at tertiary referral centers, and they have departmental websites containing detailed referral guidelines.

In clinical genetics, we have a responsibility of care to entire families, not just to the proband who is consulting us on a particular occasion. Where there is a family history of cancer, therefore, suggestive of a pre-disposing gene alteration, the most useful individuals to test for the presence of that pre-disposition are the affected individuals, especially those individuals affected at younger ages than one would expect for the population. If unaffected individuals are tested in the first instance, and found not to carry a gene alteration, then that only gives information about that individual, not information about the presence or absence of a gene alteration within the family. For this reason, it has long been best practice in cancer genetics to offer testing to affected individuals within a family first. If all affected relatives are deceased or unavailable, however, we are now able to offer testing in the first instance to unaffected individuals at high risk of carrying a pre-disposing gene. The posterior probability of a mutation in the family has to be high to be able to offer such testing.

Furthermore, genetic testing at the point of diagnosis ("mainstreaming") is now offered to the cancer patient for some cancers, e.g. *BRCA1/2* testing to all high-grade serous ovarian cancers. After a short training program for oncologists (www.mcgprogramme.com/), cancer patients are tested by the oncologist and then only referred to geneticists to undertake the cascade testing in the family in those who harbor a germline pathogenic mutation.

BOX 34.2   SUGGESTED REFERRAL GUIDELINES TO A CANCER GENETICS CLINIC

The following family histories are suggestive of an inherited cancer pre-disposition and would be appropriate for referral. This list is a guide only, and is not comprehensive.

The pattern of cancer should be in blood relatives through either the maternal or the paternal side. In general, but not always, when undertaking genetic testing after counseling, a living relative affected by cancer is tested prior to offering testing to unaffected family members. This maximizes the likelihood of finding the family gene mutation (genetic error) if one exists.

In general the following features indicate an increased probability of a cancer pre-disposition:

- Increased number of people who have developed cancer in the family who are all in one genetic line.
- The younger the ages at which the cancers developed compared with usual age of onset in the general population.
- The types of cancer in the family show clustering of cancers which are usually rare.
- If relatives with cancer are closely related.
- Certain pathological features, e.g. colon cancer which has loss of mismatch repair protein staining on the histology report.

For example the South London Regional Genetics Service at St George's Hospital has guidelines under:

www.stgeorges.nhs.uk/service/specialist-medicine/clinical-genetics/

After referral to a cancer genetics unit, in order to find out more information about a family, to establish their level of risk of a cancer pre-disposition syndrome, it is common to ask the consultand to complete a full family history questionnaire out to third-degree relatives. Often help from other family members has to be requested by the consultand in order to complete this, so this is best undertaken by them in their own time.

Using the family history, a doctor may be able to reassure an individual, suggest an increased cancer screening schedule, or initiate referral to a genetics clinic for individuals who may benefit from the specialist services of such a genetics clinic. Taking breast cancer as an example, a number of women may qualify for earlier mammographic screening according to NICE guidelines, but do not require specialist genetic services due to the limited family history.

Genetics clinics

Following the identification of an at-risk individual, referral to a specialist clinic should be made. Formal assessment of the individual or family risk can be undertaken, and screening and management strategies can be discussed, along with the possibility of genetic testing.

Aims of genetics clinics

Cancer genetics counseling aims to provide an explanation of how cancer develops (most commonly as a result of somatic mutation), the principles of genetic inheritance, an estimation of the chance that a familial cluster is due to genetic pre-disposition, information about the likely specific pre-disposition gene present, an estimation of cancer risk, options for managing the risk, and the opportunity for genetic testing.

Structure of the genetics clinic

As in many other areas of oncology, the multidisciplinary approach is being increasingly used in cancer genetic counseling clinics. Most of these clinics are located within, or in close association with, the regional clinical genetics service; however, it is desirable that cancer genetic counselors have training in both genetics and oncology. In the UK, genetic counselors/clinical nurse specialists in cancer genetics counseling conduct the majority of the routine counseling, working closely with medical personnel who provide medical back up, diagnostic skills where necessary, and formal risk assessment.

Links to oncology for the mainstreaming tests mentioned above are becoming more common.

Medical history and examination

It must be established from the history and examination whether the consultand is an affected or an at-risk member of the family. The consultand should also be questioned on any symptoms indicative of cancer or congenital abnormalities. The presence of congenital abnormalities or developmental delay in other members of the family may also provide an important clue to the diagnosis. It is extremely important to ascertain the ethnic origin of the patient as mutations in some cancer genes are more common in certain populations, particularly when the individual is part of a "closed" population, where founder mutations may be present.

The taking of a full family history is central to the practice of the management of familial cancer. The individuals with cancer should be noted in a family tree (Figure 34.1). The standard notation is given in Box 34.1.

Verification of the cancer cases in the family is then considered, as recall of family history may not be accurate. Studies have shown that recall of family history is superior for first-degree relatives compared with more distant relatives and recall of breast cancer family history is approximately 90 per cent accurate. However, accuracy falls for cancer at more indeterminate sites such as ovarian or endometrial cancer. These types of cancer are often misreported, for example as "abdominal," "stomach," or "bowel." Douglas et al.[20] showed that verification of all family histories in their cancer genetics clinic resulted in an 11 per cent change in recommendations for management and most of the changes were related to verification of cancers at abdominal sites. Verification of diagnosis would therefore be important in these latter cancer sites.

Not all cancer genetics clinics verify all breast cancer cases because of the high accuracy of recall and the fact that recall is more likely to be an over-recall, since mastectomy may have been performed for benign disease. This would result in an over-screening of only 5–10 per cent of patients, and it is often not cost-effective to verify all breast cancer cases. An exception would be if an individual wishes to undertake more extreme measures such as prophylactic surgery since cases of Munchausen syndrome (where an individual wishes to undergo medical procedures for fictitious reasons) or Munchausen syndrome by proxy (where individuals pass on to other family members a fictitious family history of cancer in order to provoke them to take preventive measures) have been reported, although these are rare (1 per cent).[21]

Initial clinical examination involves looking for any dysmorphic features and congenital anomalies. The skin should be carefully examined, as many cancer syndromes are associated with dermatological features, such as pigmentary abnormalities, e.g. freckles on the lip in Peutz–Jeghers syndrome, café-au-lait patches in neurofibromatosis type I or Turcot's syndrome, or basal cell naevi in Gorlin's syndrome. Skin tumors, such as the epidermoid cysts seen in familial adenomatous polyposis (FAP), keratoacanthomas seen in Muir–Torre syndrome, or trichilemmomas of Cowden syndrome, can be indicators that the individual is very likely to be a gene carrier before confirmation by formal DNA genetic testing.

Throughout the consultation, it is important to be sensitive to any psychopathology that may be occurring. Frequently, there will have been bereavement due to the premature death of close relatives, particularly a parent or child. Unresolved bereavement may make it difficult for people to accept their own risks and make decisions about their own management. Some individuals are particularly worried when they are approaching the age at which their relatives were diagnosed. Others assume that they are more likely to have inherited the cancer pre-disposition gene because they resemble their affected relative, either physically or in temperament. Patients are sometimes unable to cope with their worries, and referral for formal psychological counseling may be needed. Of particular concern are those individuals who have prophylactic surgery because of excess anxiety but who, while being temporarily relieved, could return at a later date with further cancer phobic symptoms. A psychological assessment and counseling should be part of the referral process before prophylactic mastectomy.

Clinical management

The subsequent management of an individual and their family will depend upon the final risk estimates regarding the inheritance of a cancer pre-disposition gene and the potential cancer risks associated with this. In general, management strategies fall into four categories, cancer screening, lifestyle changes, preventive strategies, and genetic testing.

Cancer screening

Cancer screening strategies can be advised for many individuals at increased risk of developing cancer. Table 34.4 outlines guidance protocols for screening in individuals with a high probability of mutations in cancer pre-disposition genes. Not all of the screening schedules described have been proven to reduce mortality from the relevant cancer, but these schedules represent a pragmatic approach to the management of individuals at risk. There is, however, some evidence that screening individuals with Lynch syndrome by colonoscopy reduces mortality due to colorectal cancer, as any suspicious lesions observed on colonoscopy may be removed at an early stage.[22]

One of the difficulties with designing a surveillance strategy for individuals at high risk is proving the efficacy of the surveillance method. According to WHO criteria, screening should be able to detect cancer earlier than it would be detected due to symptoms, and that early detection should have an impact on outcome. Clearly, it is very difficult to prove that either of these two criteria are being met, particularly when few individuals are undergoing surveillance for rare conditions. Sometimes consensus guidance is needed from international evidence, e.g. in individuals with

TABLE 34.4   **Surveillance in Principal Cancer Genetic Syndromes**

Age at Start of Screening/Age Disease	Surveillance/Management	Frequency	Range for Screening
von Hippel–Lindau (affected)	Physical examination	Annual	From diagnosis
	Urine testing	Annual	From diagnosis
	Direct ophthalmoscopy/ fluorescein angiography	Annual	From diagnosis
	24-hr urinary VMA/plasma catecholamines	Annual	From diagnosis
	Abdominal (renal) ultrasound	Annual	From diagnosis
	MRI brain	3-yearly	From diagnosis
	CT kidneys	If renal cysts present	
von Hippel–Lindau (at risk relative)	Physical examination	Annual	5 years upwards
	Urine testing	Annual	5 years upwards
	Direct ophthalmoscopy/ fluorescein angiography	Annual	5 years upwards 10–60 years
	24-hr urinary VMA/plasma catecholamines	Annual	11 years upwards
	Abdominal (renal) ultrasound	Annual	20–65 years
	MRI brain	3-yearly	15–40 years
		5-yearly	40–60 years
	CT kidneys	If renal cysts present	20–65 years
Familial adenomatous polyposis (affected)	Colonoscopy	Annual	11 years upwards
	Offer total colectomy with ileo-rectal anastomosis		Average 16–18 years (depending on extent of polyposis)
	Rectal stump screening (if conserved in surgery)	Annual	Following colectomy
	Upper gastrointestinal endoscopy	Frequency depends on extent of polyposis found	20 years upwards
Familial adenomatous polyposis (at risk)	Offer genetic testing if possible		
	Colonoscopy	Annual	11 years upwards once polyps appear on sigmoidoscopy
	Offer total colectomy with ileo-rectal anastomosis		If polyposis extensive
Gorlin's syndrome (affected) (at-risk children usually have abnormal skull or spine X-rays by 5 years)	Dermatological examination	Annual 3-monthly	Infancy upwards Puberty onwards
	Orthopantomogram (for jaw cysts)	Annual	From diagnosis
	?MRI brain (**not** CT due to radiosensitivity)	Annual	In infancy only
Multiple endocrine neoplasia type 2 (affected)	Offer genetic testing if possible		
	Prophylactic thyroidectomy		By age 2 years if indicated by genotype
	Plasma calcium, phosphate, parathormone	Annual	8–70 years
	Pentagastrin test	Annual	8–70 years
	Thyroid ultrasound	Annual	8–70 years
	Abdominal ultrasound and CT	Annual	8–70 years
	24-hr urinary VMA/plasma catecholamines	Annual	8–70 years
Multiple endocrine neoplasia type 1	Symptom enquiry (dyspepsia, diarrhea, renal colic, fits, amenorrhea, galactorrhea) and physical examination	Annual	5 years upwards
	Serum calcium, parathormone	Annual	8 years upwards
	Fasting gastrin	Annual	20 years upwards

(Continued)

TABLE 34.4 (CONTINUED)   Surveillance in Principal Cancer Genetic Syndromes

Age at Start of Screening/Age Disease	Surveillance/Management	Frequency	Range for Screening
	Fasting serum glucose, insulin, proinsulin	Annual	5 years upwards
	Pancreatic polypeptide, VIP, glucagon	Annual	20 years upwards
	Serum prolactin, IGF-1	Annual	5 years upwards
	CT thorax and abdomen	2–3-yearly	20 years upwards
	MRI brain	3-yearly	5 years upwards
Wilms' tumor (at-risk individuals)	Renal ultrasound	3–4-monthly	Birth until 7–8 years (depending on syndromic diagnosis)
Li–Fraumeni syndrome**	Breast examination	Annual	18–60 years
	Breast MRI	Annual	20–60 years
	Physical examination	6-monthly–annual	Lifelong
	Whole-body MRI Annual	Lifelong	
Retinoblastoma (siblings and offspring of affected)	Offer genetic testing if possible		
	Retinal examination (without anesthetic)	Monthly	Birth to 3 months
	Retinal examination under anesthetic	3-monthly	3 months to 2 years
	Retinal examination under anesthetic	4-monthly	2–3 years
	Retinal examination (without anesthetic)	6-monthly	3–5 years
	Retinal examination (without anesthetic)	Annual	5–11 years
	Examination for sarcoma	Annual	Early teens to lifelong
Neurofibromatosis type 1	Physical examination	Annual	Lifelong
	Blood pressure measurement	Annual	Lifelong
	Visual field assessment	Annual	Birth to 6 years
	Mammogram	Annual	40–50
Neurofibromatosis type 2	Physical examination	Annual	
	Ophthalmological assessment (for congenital cataracts)	Once	Early childhood
	Audiometry	Annual	10–40 years
	Brainstem auditory evoked potentials	Annual	10–40 years
	MRI brain and spine	Annual	Until age 30 years
	MRI brain and spine	2-yearly	Until age 40 years, then 3-yearly
Lynch syndrome (hereditary non-polyposis colorectal cancer)	Colonoscopy	18-monthly–2-yearly	25 years upwards
	Ovarian screening (CA 125 and TV USS)	Annual	35 years upwards
	Endometrial screening	Annual	35 years upwards
	Consider urine cytology/ mammography (depending on cancers in family)—contentious	Annual	35 years upwards
Familial melanoma	Skin examination	Annual	Teens upwards
	Consider pancreatic imaging (depending on cancers in family)		
Familial breast/ovarian cancer	MRI breast	Annual	30–40 years
	Mammography	Annual	40–70 years
	Ovarian screening (CA 125 and TV USS)—contentious	Annual	35 years upwards
	Consider PSA and prostate biopsy—recent data suggest offering to *BRCA2* mutation carriers	Annual	40–69

Abbreviations: CT, computed tomography; IGF-1, insulin-like growth factor; MRI, magnetic resonance imaging; PSA, prostate serum antigen; TV USS, transvaginal ultrasound; VMA, vanillyl mandelic acid.
** Some units also undertake annual ultrasound of abdomen, full blood count, and 3–5-yearly endoscopy and colonoscopy.

germline *TP53* mutations who have a 74–90 per cent cancer risk (depending on the sex of the individual; higher in females); as the cancers can occur in any part of the body, whole-body MRI experience has been combined in a report of a meta-analysis. This has led to AACR-recommended guidelines for screening of such individuals to include whole-body MRI.[23]

Lifestyle changes

Lifestyle changes may take many forms such as the avoidance of known cancer-causing factors such as sunlight in Gorlin syndrome and X-ray exposure in the Li–Fraumeni syndrome. Other lifestyle changes are less well established in the prevention of cancer but have been suggested based upon current understanding of tumor biology and a small number of epidemiological studies. Although lifestyle changes may have a greater role in the prevention of sporadic cancers, they may still be of benefit in cancers associated with a genetic pre-disposition. For example, a European-wide study (CAPP2) investigated the role of aspirin and/or soluble starch in the prevention of colonic cancer in individuals from Lynch syndrome (HNPCC) families.[24] This study showed that while soluble starch had no effect in the incidence of colonic cancer in these families, high-dose aspirin did substantially reduce cancer incidence.

Prevention strategies

Prevention strategies can take many forms including prophylactic surgery and chemoprevention. The evidence in support of the efficacy of these measures is variable, mainly due to the rarity of the genetic mutation making clinical trials difficult to perform. Established measures include total colectomy in the familial adenomatous polyposis syndrome[25] and total thyroidectomy in the MEN2 syndrome.[26] More contentious roles for prophylactic surgery include mastectomy in women with pathogenic *BRCA1/2* mutations. Limited retrospective data suggest that the risk of breast cancer is reduced by 90 per cent following prophylactic mastectomy although there is still a residual risk due to the inability to remove all breast epithelial cells at mastectomy.[27] Prophylactic salpingo-oophorectomy has been shown to reduce ovarian cancer risk.[28] A risk of peritoneal carcinomatosis remains due to the shared embryonic origin of both peritoneum and ovarian epithelium.[29]

The role of chemoprevention is much less certain, but includes a reduction of ovarian cancer risk in users of the combined oral contraceptive pill.[30] A large American study (NSABP1) has suggested a 45 per cent reduction in breast cancer risk in women at increased risk who took tamoxifen chemoprevention.[31] Reduction in breast cancer risk is greater in *BRCA2* mutation carriers than in *BRCA1* as the former are more likely to pre-dispose to hormone receptor-positive breast cancer and tamoxifen reduces the risk of hormone receptor-positive disease.[32] In the light of this evidence, the NICE guidance on familial breast cancer (CG164, 2013)[33] has recommended the use of tamoxifen or raloxifene for 5 years for women at increased risk of breast cancer. In the field of colorectal cancer, there has been demonstration of a reduction in incidence of colonic cancer in long-term users of non-steroidal anti-inflammatory drugs, particularly aspirin in HNPCC families.[24]

Genetic testing

Genetic testing is possible for most cancer pre-disposition genes in private laboratories, and in the NHS there will be a new genetic testing directory once the genetic laboratory hubs are up and running in early 2020 in the UK. It is performed on DNA from venous blood or, increasingly, the use of saliva. Genetic testing may either be diagnostic (the detection of a mutation in an individual affected by cancer) or predictive (the detection of a mutation in a clinically unaffected individual). Mutations in cancer pre-disposition genes often occur throughout the gene, and the vast majority of mutations so far have only been observed in limited numbers of families, except in specific ethnic groups with known founder mutations such as the Icelandic, Norwegian, and Ashkenazi populations with *BRCA1/2* mutations.[34] Hence, unless an individual is a member of such a group, the specific mutation for that family must first be identified. An affected family member is most optimally tested first because they are the family member most likely to have the cancer pre-disposing mutation. Once a mutation is suspected, it is important to check that the "mutation" is likely to be cancer-causing and not a rare normal variant of the gene (polymorphism). Occasionally, the significance of a mutation is uncertain (variant of uncertain significance [VUS]), and its pathogenicity may be then further investigated by testing other affected and unaffected family members to establish whether or not the mutation segregates with disease. The presence of phenocopies may complicate this issue further. There are also international databases in which the mutation can be searched to identify if it is pathogenic or a VUS. If a pathogenic mutation is identified, however, predictive testing may be offered to unaffected family members for the identified mutation. VUS are *not* used for predictive testing or clinical management.

Misleading results may occur if an unaffected individual has a genetic test in order to identify a mutation without first identifying it in an affected relative. A negative result (i.e. no mutation is identified in the cancer pre-disposition gene tested) may not be a true negative for several reasons:

- The family history is due to a gene other than that being tested.
- The alteration may be regulatory which means that it controls how the gene is expressed, but the gene itself (and therefore the test which looks at the gene code) is normal.
- The genetic test sensitivity is not 100 per cent for the genetic coding mutations and may therefore have missed mutations.

When the specific mutation has been identified in an affected individual, if it is not found in an unaffected relative, this is then a truly negative result. Unfortunately, due to the high penetrance of certain pre-disposition genes, for example, *BRCA1/2*, it is not uncommon to be presented with a family with multiple cases of cancer, but all the affected individuals have died from their cancer. In this difficult situation it was not usually previously possible to offer mutation testing to unaffected cases, and their future clinical management would depend upon their probability of having inherited a mutation based on their family history. However, this has now changed and individuals with a very strong family history where there is no living affected member to test, can be tested, although a negative result does not exclude that the individual is at risk. An exception is the rare circumstance of a closed ethnic group (e.g. the Ashkenazim) in which the suspected mutations are known to occur with a high frequency in that population and testing of unaffected individuals can be offered with a less strong family history.

Genetic testing should only take place following full genetic counseling to outline the implications of genetic testing. A recognized counseling schedule usually allows at least a month of reflection between two counseling sessions prior to taking blood for mutation analysis. Mainstreaming of testing of affected individuals has shortened this process by testing at the point of diagnosis. The personal and wider social implications of positive and negative results are issues discussed during these sessions. A positive result could have psychological implications as well as widespread repercussions involving the rest of the family. A negative test result may have psychological consequences due to the recognized "survivor guilt syndrome," which has been documented in the setting of Huntington's disease.[35]

For genes pre-disposing to adult onset cancers, testing of young children is not advised as the age of cancer onset permits the individual to make their own decision to have genetic testing once they have reached adulthood, following full genetic counseling. Children are offered genetic testing when it may alter management, for example, in MEN2A syndrome when thyroidectomy is offered before the age of 5 years for some gene carriers as it is totally protective against medullary thyroid cancer; or in familial adenomatous polyposis where regular colonoscopies or colectomy may be avoided in teenage years.

The social implications of the ability to purchase life and medical insurance or mortgages and a possible effect on employment opportunities may be just as important as, if not more than, the personal and familial implications. At present, effects on employment are theoretical. There is a Moratorium from the Association of British Insurers on the use of genetic information from cancer genetic testing (www.abi.org.uk).

Whole-exome sequencing has started to enter the arena of diagnosis for pediatric conditions in intensive care and in developmental delay (the DDD project) to make diagnoses. It is likely that the technology of whole-genome sequencing will transfer itself to routine clinical practice in the next few years. Panels of genes are already being developed for parallel testing, so that instead of a clinician opting to test one gene in the first instance, and then move on to testing another gene if the first yields normal results, a patient's sample would be tested simultaneously for mutations in all the genes known to pre-dispose individuals to the development of cancers. This new approach does however raise issues of consent and incidental findings. Many people would not, for example, choose to know that they have a mutation in the *TP53* gene, which causes Li–Fraumeni syndrome, because this syndrome can cause cancer to develop anywhere throughout the body, and there are few proven prevention strategies. Conversely, the use of next-generation sequencing will lower costs of tests, enabling more people to be tested with the same healthcare budget; this will enable more cancer patients to be offered a genetic test for potential susceptibility to their particular cancer which may impact on their care as some are amenable to targeted treatments, e.g. PARP inhibitors in *BRCA1/2* mutation carriers.

One of the other effects which will become more widespread because of developments in oncology practice is the generation of large amounts of whole-genome sequence data on patients undergoing treatment for tumors. Somatic (i.e. tumor) genomes are routinely being analyzed in order to generate data about possible treatment targets in patients. As part of this analysis, it is common for germline DNA to also be analyzed for comparison. This is likely to drive uptake of testing but also increase the cascade testing for families.

The other explosion of data in cancer genetics is the discovery of common variation (so-called SNPs) which increases cancer risk. Each variant in itself only increases risk by a small amount (usually less than two-fold); however as these SNPs are common and risks per SNP are multiplicative, the presence of many of them in one person can lead to quite substantial risks. Such SNP profiles can be used to stratify populations, and research is ongoing to assess how such profiles could potentially be used for targeted population screening based on genetic risk rather than the current age-based screening strategies.

There is ongoing work to ensure adequate genetic privacy is maintained for patients, given the potential of the new technologies described above. There have been statements by the US Government's Department of BioEthics regarding this, and it is hoped that sufficient regulation can be brought into force to protect patients' privacy while allowing them and their doctors to access such data as are necessary and useful to them.

Summary

Cancer is a common disease but only a small proportion of cases can be attributed to the inheritance of highly penetrant cancer pre-disposition genes. However, in absolute terms, this represents a significant number of families or individuals due to the high population frequency of cancer. Increasingly, oncologists are becoming involved in testing at the point of diagnosis (mainstreaming) as some of these mutations have implications for treatment. Geneticists are involved when testing is needed for families or in unaffected individuals with a family history of cancer. The developments in genetic sequencing will enable faster and cheaper tests in the years to come which will increase access to testing.

Key learning points

- The majority of cancer cases are sporadic and not related to the inheritance of a cancer pre-disposition gene.
- Most cancer families who may benefit from referral to a specialist cancer genetics unit will be detected by taking a limited family history. This should include all first-degree relatives (parents/siblings/children) and any other cancer cases in other relatives.
- Cancer site and age of onset are important.
- Early cancer screening may be available for specific cancer pre-disposition syndromes.
- Genetic testing for the presence of a familial cancer pre-disposition gene can usually only be performed by direct DNA analysis using venous blood or saliva from a living relative affected by cancer and sometimes for unaffected individuals with a strong family history.
- Next-generation sequencing technology is enabling more rapid and cheaper genetic testing with the development of genetic testing panels of numerous genes at once.

References

1. Easton DF, Peto J. The contribution of inherited predisposition to cancer incidence. *Cancer Surv.* 1990; 9:395–416.
2. Knudson AG. Mutation and cancer: Statistical study of retinoblastoma. *Proc Nat Acad Sci.* 1971; 68:820–3.
3. Yeap PM, Tobias ES, Mavraki E et al. Molecular analysis of phaeochromocytoma after maternal transmission of SDHD mutation elucidates mechanism of parent of origin effect. *J Clin Endocrinol Metab.* 2011; 96:E1–5.
4. Rumilla K, Schowalter KV, Lindor NM et al. Frequency of deletions of EPCAM (TACSTD1) in MSH2-associated Lynch syndrome cases. *J Mol Diagn.* 2011; 13(1):93–9.
5. Bodmer WF, Bailey CJ, Bodmer J et al. Localization of the gene for familial adenomatous polyposis on chromosome 5. *Nature.* 1987; 328:614–16.

6. Riccardi VM, Sujansky E, Smith AC et al. Chromosomal imbalance in the Aniridia-Wilms' tumour association: 11p interstitial deletion. *Pediatrics*. 1978; 61:604–10.

7. Mandelker D, Donoghue MTA, Talukdar S et al. Germline-focused analysis of tumour-only sequencing: Recommendations from the ESMO Precision Medicine Working Group. *Ann Oncol*. 2019; 30(8):1221–31.

8. Thompson D, Easton DF, Breast Cancer Linkage Consortium. Cancer Incidence in BRCA1 mutation carriers. *J Natl Cancer Inst*. 2002; 94(18):1358–65.

9. Antoniou A, Pharoah PD, Narod S et al. Average risks of breast and ovarian cancer associated with BRCA1 or BRCA2 mutations detected in case series unselected for family history: A combined analysis of 22 studies. *Am J Hum Genet*. 2003; 72:1117–30.

10. Struewing JP, Hartge P, Wacholder S et al. The risk of cancer associated with specific mutations of BRCA1 and BRCA2 among Ashkenazi Jews. *N Engl J Med*. 1997; 336:1401–8.

11. Thorlacius S, Struewing JP, Hartge P et al. Population based study of risk of breast cancer in carriers of BRCA2 mutations. *Lancet*. 1998; 352:1337–9

12. Cintolo-Gonzalez JA, Braun D, Blackford AL et al. Breast cancer risk models: A comprehensive overview of existing models, validation, and clinical applications. *Breast Cancer Res Treat*. 2017; 164(2):263–84.

13. Evans DG, Harkness EF, Plaskocinska I et al. Pathology update to the Manchester Scoring System based on testing in over 4000 families. *J Med Genet*. 2017; 54(10):674–81.

14. Croyle RT, Sun YC, Louie DH. Psychological minimization of cholesterol test results: Moderators of appraisal in college students and community residents. *Health Psychol*. 1993; 12:503–7.

15. Lloyd S, Watson, M, Waites B et al. Familial breast cancer: A controlled study of risk perception, psychological morbidity and health beliefs in women attending for genetic counselling. *Br J Cancer*. 1996; 74:482–7.

16. Ardern-Jones A. Living with a cancer legacy: The experience of hereditary cancer in the family. Institute of Cancer Research, London University. MSc Dissertation, 1998.

17. Lerman C, Daly M, Masny A, Balshem A. Attitudes about genetic testing for breast-ovarian cancer susceptibility. *J Clini Oncol*. 1994; 12:843–50.

18. Vlek C. Risk assessment, risk perception and decision making about courses of action involving genetic risk: An overview of concepts and methods. *Birth Defects Orig Artic Ser*. 1987; 23:171–207.

19. Kash KM, Holland JC, Halper MS, Miller DG. Psychological distress and surveillance behaviours of women with a family history of breast cancer. *J Natl Cancer Inst*. 1991; 84:24–30.

20. Douglas FS, O'Dair LC, Robinson M et al. The accuracy of diagnoses as reported in families with cancer: A retrospective study. *J Med Gen*. 1999; 36:309–12.

21. Evans DG, Kerr B, Cade D et al. Fictitious breast cancer family history. *Lancet*. 1996; 348:1034.

22. Dove-Edwin I, Sasieni P, Adams J, Thomas HJ. Prevention of cancer by colonoscopic surveillance in individuals with a family history of colorectal cancer: 16 year, prospective, follow-up study. *Br Med J*. 2005; 331:1047–50.

23. Ballinger ML, Best A, Mai PL et al. Baseline surveillance in Li-Fraumeni Syndrome using whole-body magnetic resonance imaging: A Meta-analysis. *JAMA Oncol*. 2017; 3(12):1634–9

24. Burn J, Gerdes AM, Macrae F et al. Long-term effect of aspirin on cancer risk in carriers of hereditary colorectal cancer: An analysis from the CAPP2 randomised controlled trial. *Lancet*. 2011; 378:2081–7.

25. Nyam DC, Brillant PT, Dozois RR et al. Ileal pouch-anal canal anastomosis for familial adenomatous polyposis: Early and late results. *Ann Surg*. 1997; 226:514–9.

26. Lallier M, St-Vil D, Giroux M et al. Prophylactic thyroidectomy for medullary thyroid cancer in gene carriers of MEN2 syndrome. *Journal of Pediatr Surg*. 1998; 33:846–48.

27. Hartmann LC. Efficacy of bilateral prophylactic mastectomy in women with a family history of breast cancer. *N Engl J Med*. 1999; 340:77–84.

28. Kauff ND, Satagopan JM, Robson ME et al. Risk-reducing salpingo-oophorectomy in women with a *BRCA1* or *BRCA2* mutation. *N Engl J Med*. 2002; 346:1609–15.

29. Kemp GM, Hsiu JG, Andrews MC. Papillary peritoneal carcinomatosis after prophylactic oophorectomy. *Gynecol Oncol*. 1992; 47:395–7.

30. Narod SA, Risch H, Moslchi R et al. Oral contraceptives and the risk of hereditary ovarian cancer. Hereditary Ovarian Cancer Clinical Study Group. *N Engl J Med*. 1998; 339:424–8.

31. Fisher B, Costantino JP, Wickerham DL1 et al. Tamoxifen for prevention of breast cancer: Report of the National Surgical Adjuvant Breast and Bowel Project P-1 Study. *J Natl Cancer Inst*. 1998; 90:1371–88.

32. King MC, Wieand S, Hale K et al. Tamoxifen and breast cancer incidence among women with inherited mutations in BRCA1 and BRCA2: National Surgical Adjuvant Breast and Bowel Project (NSABP-P1) Breast Cancer Prevention Trial. *JAMA*. 2001; 286(18):2251–6.

33. National Institute for Health and Care Excellence. *Familial Breast Cancer: Classification and Care of People at Risk of Familial Breast Cancer and Management of Breast Cancer and Related Risks in People With a Family History of Breast Cancer (CG164)*. London, UK: National Institute for Health and Care Excellence, 2013.

34. Rebbeck TR, Friebel TM, Friedman E et al. Mutational spectrum in a worldwide study of 29,700 families with BRCA1 or BRCA2 mutations. *Hum Mutat*. 2018;39(5):593–620

35. Demyttenaere K, Evers-Kiehooms G, Decruyenaere M. Pitfalls in counselling for predictive testing in Huntington's disease. *Birth Defects*. 1992; 28:105–111.

35 LIFESTYLE FACTORS IN CANCER SURVIVORSHIP

Robert Thomas

Through a combination of earlier detection, better multidisciplinary management, and enhanced targeted treatments, the chance of surviving cancer is significantly improving. As a result, the number of cancer survivors in the United Kingdom is growing by 3% per annum. By 2040, it is forecast that there will be over 3 million people living with the consequences of cancer and its therapies. In men, 43% of these will have prostate cancer, and in women, 41% will have breast cancer; and because of the aging population, over a quarter of people over 65 years will be cancer survivors. The increase in the number of survivors is attributed not only to better multidisciplinary management but also to an aging population and more effective systemic therapies, which keep patients alive for longer with metastatic disease. For example, the expected time living with metastatic prostate cancer is now over 10 years, and people diagnosed with chronic myeloid leukemia only have 3 years' lower life expectancy. To achieve these benefits, patients often have to endure complex and arduous therapies, frequently leaving them beleaguered with acute and long-term physical and psychological adverse effects. In addition to being unpleasant, these adverse effects result in greater usage of health resources and financial implications for patients and their families. A major study from Oxford recently estimated that of the £15 billion spent on cancer in the United Kingdom each year, £2 billion was on drugs, £5 billion on surgical and medical management, but nearly £8 billion on managing long-term economic consequences, including time off work for ongoing care.

This chapter reviews the evidence that lifestyle and self-help strategies can help diminish many of the adverse effects of treatments such as fatigue, low mood, weight gain, lymphoedema, osteoporosis, joint pains, peripheral neuropathy, and nail damage and therefore help keep people living with cancer vibrant, healthy, and productive. It also reviews the research linking a healthier post-cancer lifestyle with a higher probability of long-term control and in some cases, improved overall survival.

Research evaluating the influence of lifestyle and cancer has previously mainly focused on etiology, and through this, it is estimated that over half of the world's cancers are caused by preventable factors,[1] and for that reason, numerous public health organization are trying to change the behavior of the general public. Unfortunately, advertising propaganda and pressure on food, sugar, and cigarette manufacturers have only limited success. A diagnosis of cancer, however, is a traumatic event, which for most people, can be categorized as a *teachable moment*. This phenomenon is regarded as a lifestyle event after which the recipient is more receptive to learning and so more likely to change their behavior or follow the advice of a healthy living education program. Health care professionals, therefore, have an ideal opportunity to guide and encourage their patients into a healthier lifestyle, not only to benefit themselves but to ameliorate the increasing burden on health care systems. As such, a number of mainstream cancer care providers are embracing the challenges of survivorship and incorporating education and intervention programs as an integral part of quality care.

The effects of lifestyle on health are multi-factorial, with each component having a synergistic effect on the others, so survivorship programs should address them holistically, bearing in mind the individual needs of the patient along with other contributing factors such as their genetic susceptibility, concurrent treatments, and concomitant medical conditions. Here, I have categorized the research evidence into:

- Adiposity and weight gain
- Carcinogen avoidance
- Micro-nutrients and nutritional interventions
- Physical activity
- Gut health

Adiposity and weight gain

Across the world, obesity rates have tripled in the last 30 years. In 2018, in the United Kingdom, over a quarter of the population were obese (body mass index [BMI] of 30 kg/m^2), and over 58% were overweight (BMI of 25–30 kg/m^2). The World Health Organization (WHO) estimates that by 2030, the percentage obesity rate in the United Kingdom will be 40% and in Ireland and Wales, over 50%. The United States, Greece, the United Kingdom, and Australia have the highest obesity figures. Japan, Norway, Korea, and Switzerland have the lowest obesity figures. What is more, the United Kingdom's National Institute for Health and Care Excellence (NICE) estimated that obesity currently costs the UK £5.1 billion in lost production and medical management. More worryingly, they project that by 2050, this will rise to £50 billion per year unless this epidemic is addressed by government and society.

In terms of cancer, being obese more than doubles the lifetime risk of hormone-related cancers such as breast and uterus but also over 20 other non-hormone-related cancers, particularly bowel, kidney, and esophagus. Overweight women also have an increased risk of breast cancer irrespective of their daily saturated fat intake. Obese men are 33% more likely to die of cancer compared with those of a normal weight, and obese women have a 55% increased risk of dying from cancer compared with those of a normal weight.

After a diagnosis of breast cancer, women report a 45% incidence of significant, unwelcomed weight gain after adjuvant chemotherapy, often at a time in their lives that makes losing it very difficult. In men, a study of 440 prostate cancer survivors revealed that over 53% were overweight or obese after treatment.[2] For individuals with bowel cancer, the CALBG 89803 trial showed that 35% of patients post chemotherapy were overweight (BMI 25.0–29.9) and 34% were obese (BMI 30.0–34.9).

The reasons for this weight gain are multi-factorial. Obesity develops gradually over time, as a result of environmental, genetic, lifestyle, and dietary choices. The fundamental cause is the consumption of calories in excess of the body's needs for metabolism and level of physical activity. An average physically active man needs about 2500 calories a day to maintain a healthy weight, and an average physically active woman needs about 2000 calories a day. This amount can be easy to reach, especially with the types of calorie-rich food that are easily available in Western societies. For example, eating a large takeaway hamburger, fries, and a milkshake can total 1500 calories—and that's just one meal. After cancer, there may be tendency to snack between meals or comfort eat. Some people are also told not to worry about weight gain by well-meaning health professionals, but this is not good advice, as people who had previously controlled their weight would very rapidly pack on extra pounds, which would then be very difficult to lose.

Numerous surveys have revealed that the vast majority of us are not physically active enough to prevent obesity in a society where food is appealing and plentiful. The trouble is, once obese, trying to lose weight is even harder. An individual will have to reduce to <2500 calories a day and exercise >2.5 hours/week even to start burning up energy stores. What is more, this has to be sustained for many months and even years to have any long-term benefit. These factors are still an issue after cancer but are compounded by several issues, which add further burden for the patient who is contemplating an exercise program. Disability from the disease itself or the treatments can interfere with ability to exercise; fatigue is now one of the most prominent and distressing side effects after most treatments, and especially if associated with a low mood, it can have a considerable demotivating influence on the decision to exercise. Chemotherapy-induced nausea, peripheral neuropathy, weight gain, and joint pains can create barriers to regular exercise.

Whatever the reasons for weight gain, numerous reviews and meta-analyses have demonstrated that patients who are overweight or obese during and after cancer treatments have a higher risk of infection, thromboembolism, depression, arthritis, delayed wound healing, cardiac impairment, and side effects such as hot flushes, joint pains, lymphoedema, urinary incontinence, erectile dysfunction, and diabetes.[3] On top of this, several cohort studies have also linked obesity with higher relapse rates and lower overall cancer and non-cancer-related survival.

The National Surgical Adjuvant Breast and Bowel Project (NSABP) analysis of 4288 patients with colon cancer showed that those who were obese had greater risk of cancer recurrence as well as non-cancer deaths overall compared with healthy-weight patients, although it must be noted that very underweight patients (BMI <19) also did badly.[4] Similar findings were reported in other large cohort studies involving patients with colorectal cancer. A retrospective analysis of 3162 men with prostate cancer showed that obese men had a higher risk of early disease recurrence.[5]

Similar links with obesity and adverse outcome were found in other studies of men with prostate cancer following radical treatments.

A prospective cohort study of 365 women with ER+ve breast cancer linked obesity, consumption of >7 alcoholic beverages a week, and smoking with a risk of a contralateral cancer.[6] A further analysis of 5204 participants in the Nurses' Health Study showed that of the 860 subsequent deaths, a statistically significant higher proportion were overweight at diagnosis. It was shown that a weight gain of more than 0.5 kg/m^2 at 1 year post treatment correlated with both lower overall survival and breast cancer–specific survival, and the correlation was strongest in women who gained >2 kg/m^2.[7] Of the 553 deaths specifically from breast cancer, a correlation with BMI was seen if they also smoked. A number of other studies have also linked obesity at diagnosis with a greater risk of relapse, but there is also evidence, although less robust, for a link with weight change rather than initial weight at diagnosis.

A large trial randomized post-menopausal women with early breast cancer to a bi-weekly program of nutritional, exercise, and lifestyle counseling or not. Women in the intervention group lost weight and had reduced breast cancer relapse rates and better overall survival in the ER–ve subgroup. Although more confirmatory research is needed to link excess weight reduction with better outcomes, it is reassuring that randomized controlled trials

(RCTs) of interventions such as this, The Living Well telephone intervention program from Queensland, and other community-based schemes are demonstrating significant success in achieving weight reduction.

Cancer-promoting mechanisms of obesity

Several direct and indirect biochemical factors contribute to the risks of obesity in terms of both cancer incidence and progression.

Metabolic syndrome

Highly calorific foods, particularly those rich in sugar and fat content, are known to increase the risk of metabolic syndrome, which is defined by the Adult Treatment Panel III criteria as a combination of abdominal obesity, high triglyceride, and hyperglycemia.[8] This combination leads to a higher risk of diabetes and heart disease, but it also increases insulin resistance and higher insulin-like-growth factor (IGF) levels, which in the laboratory, promote proliferation and de-differentiation and blocks apoptosis of cancer cells and clinically, are linked to a higher risk of cancer and progression. Fortunately, losing weight and exercise are associated with a lowering of IGF levels. Some animal experiments have correlated regular fasting with improved longevity and better response to treatment, but although a number of clinical trials are ongoing, the benefit of fasting before chemotherapy in humans has not been established. Patients with type 2 diabetes have insulin resistance and raised IGF levels, which explains their increased risk of cancer. Fortunately, the biguanide metformin, which has the effect of increasing insulin sensitivity and modulating cellular energy, has been shown to lower cancer risk in diabetics. For example, a study of 3837 men with type 2 diabetes and prostate cancer reported that prostate cancer–specific and overall survival was significantly lower in those prescribed metformin as opposed to anti-diabetic drugs. Although definite RCT evidence is required, in the meantime, this data suggests that diabetics with cancer should have a lower threshold to start metformin as opposed to other drugs.

Estrogen and progesterone

Estrogen, progesterone, and its analogues are higher in the serum of obese women. Excess estrogen increases IGF levels, stimulates abnormal growth, and inhibits apoptosis in estrogen sensitive cells, particularly within the breast and endometrium.[9] In post-menopausal women, adiposity is thought to increase bioavailable estrogen via an increase in the aromatase enzyme found in fat cells. Fortunately, estrogen levels are reported to reduce following weight reduction programs. Estrogen levels have also been shown to drop following a diet low in fat and high in fiber as a consequence of higher urinary excretion of estrogen independently of adiposity. Progesterone tends to be lower in overweight women, particularly in the pre-menopausal setting. This is thought to be caused by androgenic inhibition of ovulation. Progesterone has multiple effects, but its protective role against cancer is by counteracting the effects of endogenous estrogen by promoting the synthesis of IGF binding protein.[4]

Leptin and adiponectin

Leptin is a multifunctional neuro-endocrine hormone generated primarily from fat cells, so overweight, particularly post-menopausal, women have higher levels. Leptin is known to promote breast cancer directly and independently as well as through involvement with the estrogen and insulin signaling pathways via enhanced angiogenesis (new blood vessel formation) and cell proliferation, which explains the links between higher levels of leptin, adiposity, and hormone-related cancers such as breast and uterus. Conversely, serum concentration of another adipokine cytokine, called adiponectin, is lower in people who are overweight. It is also lower in patients who have developed breast and prostate cancer, because unlike leptin, which is pro-inflammatory, it has significant anti-inflammatory properties. Furthermore, adiponectin also suppresses inactivation of nitric oxide, which dose-dependently reduces platelet aggregation. Tumor cell–induced platelet aggregation correlates with metastatic potential (spread of cancer cells) by "cloaking" tumor cells with adherent platelets, protecting them from natural killer (NK) cell–mediated killing. A number of studies have shown that weight reduction resulted in lowering platelet aggregation, lower leptin levels, and increasing adipokine levels.

Chronic inflammation

Inflammatory markers such as C-reactive protein, tumor necrosis factor (TNF), and interleukin (IL)-6 are significantly higher in obese people. There are some theories for these associations. Excessive intake of calories over the body's need leads to metabolic syndrome, which evokes an inflammatory stress reaction. Fat cell hypertrophy facilitates cell rupture, which evokes the accumulation of macrophages in visceral fat (the fat overspill theory). Inability of adipose tissue development to engulf incoming fat leads to deposition in other organs, mainly in the liver, with further consequences for insulin resistance. The oxidative stress which accompanies over-feeding, particularly when there is excessive ingestion of fat and other macronutrients without concomitant ingestion of polyphenol-rich foods, may contribute to the inflammation attributed to obesity. Obesity also leads to an increased risk of chronic infections such as those of the urinary tract or candida in the skin folds. Overweight individuals tend to have a suboptimal microbiota, which can affect immune regulation.

Vitamin D

A number of studies have reported a link between obesity and vitamin D deficiency. It is hypothesized that as vitamin D is stored in fatty tissue, obese people store more vitamin D in their fat and have less vitamin D circulating in their blood. Many cohort studies have linked low vitamin D with a higher risk of cancer. The benefits of vitamin D supplements are less clear. In a cohort whose vitamin D serum levels were low to start with, no benefit was seen in reducing cancer risk. On the other hand, men with prostate cancer on active surveillance had a reduction in number of positive cores on repeat biopsy after vitamin D3 supplementation. In addition, obese people are likely to have suboptimal sun exposure, as they are less likely to exercise in the sunshine, and when they do venture outside, they are more likely to cover up due to body image issues. Sunlight exposure, independently of vitamin D levels, has been linked to a lower incidence of prostate and bowel cancer.[7]

Exercise programs to aid weight loss

In terms of weight loss for established obesity, it is often quoted that exercise has little impact, but that is not quite true. Several interventional studies show that interventional exercise programs have a statistically significant impact, but it is small in absolute terms and requires a lot of effort. For example, the ENERGY study randomly assigned 690 overweight or obese breast cancer survivors to standard care or once-weekly general exercise and dietary counseling for 16 weeks and reported a significant (6%) improvement in weight, BMI, percent fat, trunk fat, and leg fat, as well as waist and hip circumference, and levels of triglycerides, total cholesterol, and high density lipoprotein cholesterol. A smaller RCT evaluated a 6 month intervention with moderate-intensity aerobic exercise, such as brisk walking, and reported decreases in percent body fat and increases in lean mass and bone mineral density.[10] Two other small RCTs involving women with breast cancer demonstrated improved muscular strength, lean body mass, and chemotherapy completion rate following an exercise intervention program. The largest RCT involved post-menopausal women with early breast cancer and randomized women to nutritional and lifestyle counseling or not. Dietary fat intake reduced and weight loss was significantly greater in the intervention group, who also demonstrated reduced relapse rates and improved outcomes in the ER–ve subgroup.[11]

Considering all these trials, the American Society of Sports Medicine concluded following a meta-analysis of many interventions that weight reduction resulted in a 10% reduction in weight if >150–250 min moderate exercise/week was maintained for over 6 months, but if participants did <150 min/week, there was no change in weight. A combination of resistance and endurance exercises seems to be most effective, but the important thing is that it is sustained and combined with calorie reduction and even fasting.

Regular physical activity is particularly beneficial for overweight or obese individuals, even though it is much harder to sustain regular levels. Even before weight reduction, estrogen and leptin levels decrease and adiponectin levels increase. Exercise also mitigates many of the adverse risks of obesity, in particular thromboembolism, indigestion, and low mood. Also, the positive biochemical changes that occur when exercising counterbalance the negative factors caused by obesity, particularly raised levels of IGF, increased insulin resistance, and also blood markers of chronic inflammation. In particular, exercise reduces the degree of sarcopenia by increasing muscle to fat ratio. Patients with sarcopenia have more complications after cancer surgery, chemotherapy, and radiotherapy and worse outcomes.

Dietary strategies to aid weight loss

Educational programs to reduce highly calorific foods have some success, and culprits include cakes, biscuits, muffins, pasties, pies, fatty chips, crisps, pakoras, samosas, and bhajis. Alcohol contains a lot of calories and stimulates the appetite. Sugary drinks, including soft fizzy drinks and processed fruit juices, contribute to weight gain. They have a lot of calories but are not satiating, encouraging individuals to eat again as blood sugar drops soon after the short glycemic peak. Conversely, high-fiber foods help longer energy intake. The most sustainable way of losing weight is to extend the gaps between meals and avoid snacks, which is the most practical way of introducing gentle fasting on a daily basis.

The best evidence of sensible effective fasting comes from a study that evaluated a large cohort of overweight women who completed their initial treatments. They discovered that initially overweight women who tended to have early dinners or late breakfasts, leaving 13 hours between the meals (without intermediate snacking), lost significantly more weight but also had lower levels of glycated Hb (HbA1c—a marker of glucose control over time) and lower chronic inflammatory markers. What is more, by 5 years, there was a 36% lower risk of breast cancer recurrence in the overnight fasting women.

Micro-nutrients and nutritional interventions

Independently of overeating, unhealthy diets have been linked to an increased risk of degenerative chronic illnesses such as dementia, high cholesterol, arthritis, stroke, skin aging, macular degeneration, and cancer. More specifically, the Health Professional Study and other large cohort studies have linked polyphenol-rich foods such as leafy green and cruciferous vegetables, colorful fruits, and flavonoid-rich foods such as pulses and legumes with a lower risk of prostate cancer. Regular tea drinkers have a significantly lower incidence of breast, prostate, and ovarian cancer.[12] Research from Shanghai showed that tea also lowered the risk of esophageal cancer, particularly of benefit among smokers and alcoholics. Researchers from Leicester University linked higher intake of curcumin and other spices with a lower level of colon cancer in the Asian community.

The benefits of a healthy diet, however, do not stop after a diagnosis of cancer. Women with early breast cancer taking more than the recommended five a day amount of fruits and vegetables have been found to lower their risk of recurrence risk by one-third, especially if combined with physical activity. The Women's Healthy Eating and Living Trial (WHEL) study from California evaluated the benefit of dietary advice in 2967 breast cancer survivors and found that women who were randomly assigned to receive dietary guidelines had a lower relapse rate compared with controls, especially those experiencing hot flushes. A controlled trial randomized post-menopausal women with early breast cancer to receive nutritional and lifestyle counseling aimed at reduced calorific intake or standard follow-up care. Dietary fat and calorie intake reduction was significantly greater in the intervention group, with reduced breast cancer relapse rates and better survival in the ER negative subgroup.

Other trials have reported lower breast cancer recurrence associated with regularly drinking green tea and eating foods rich in dietary lignans, isoflavones, and flavanones. Women with adequate versus low serum carotenoid levels have reported lower breast cancer relapse rates. Further details of the influence of polyphenols and other phytochemicals on breast cancer survival will be gained from several ongoing large studies.

For other cancers, a similar influence of diet among survivors has been demonstrated. Individuals with skin cancer who had high lutein and zeaxanthin (leafy green vegetables) intake had a lower rate of subsequent new cancer formation. Men with prostate cancer adopting a healthy lifestyle, including a diet rich in polyphenols, had a slower rate of prostate specific antigen (PSA) progression.[13] Stabilization of PSA has also been demonstrated following regular intake of whole soy (isoflavone) but not with extracted genistein supplements. An evaluation of 692 prostate cancer cases and 844 matched controls from the Prostate, Lung, Colorectal, and Ovarian (PLCO) Cancer Screening Trial showed that those with adequate serum vitamin A levels had a lower risk of aggressive cancer compared with those in the lower quartile of serum levels.[14] Survivors of Stage III colon cancer whose dietary habits were characterized as *prudent* (high intake of fruit, vegetable, poultry, and fish) had lower relapse rates compared with those adopting a *Western pattern* (high intake of meat, fat, refined grains, sweets, and desserts). This finding was supported by a study from the same research group, which found that people treated for Stage III disease had an 80% increased risk of dying from it, or experiencing a recurrence, if their diets were heavy in carbohydrate-rich foods with high glycemic loads.

Women with epithelial ovarian cancer eating a diet rich in fruits, vegetables, and healthful grains and low in processed red meats and milk-based foods were associated with higher survival rates after treatment. A randomized study of 93 men managed with active surveillance randomly assigned to nutritional and lifestyle counseling demonstrated a statistically significant difference in PSA versus standard management. As a secondary end point, serum from participants added to prostate cell lines in vitro demonstrated an eightfold inhibition of cellular growth between the two groups.[15]

Micro-nutrient interventions

If certain foods have anti-cancer effects, then one extrapolation of this data is to enhance their effect by concentrating them into a pill (supplement) either as a means to correct for poor diets or to further enhance the benefits in those already with adequate diets. Cancer survivors are attracted to the potential health benefits of food supplements, with over 70% reporting regular intake. There are two main categories of supplements commercially available. The first involves chemicals extracted from food or made synthetically. The second involves concentrating whole polyphenol-rich foods. The majority of studies, to date, have evaluated extracted chemicals such as vitamins, minerals, and even some phytochemicals. Unfortunately, most of these have shown no benefit or were actually linked to an increased risk of cancer unless a pre-existing micro-nutrient deficiency was corrected. For example, a blinded RCT of copper, magnesium gluconates, and vitamin C reported no influence on PSA.[16] Of more concern, the CARET study found that beta carotene and retinol increased the risk of lung cancer. Likewise, the ATBC study found that alpha vitamin E and beta carotene increased lung cancer risk, but in a subsequent analysis, men with pre-intervention low plasma levels of beta carotene had a lower prostate cancer risk following supplementation, whereas those with high levels had a higher risk, particularly in smokers. This U-shaped distribution of risk was also observed in the EPIC study, with those consuming diets deficient in folate and those with the highest folate intake both having the highest cancer risk.

Two other Scandinavian studies demonstrated a higher cancer risk following vitamin B supplementation intake. In the HPFS, men who took zinc at more than 100 mg/day or for long durations were more than twice as likely to develop advanced prostate cancer compared with control. The comprehensive international SELECT study showed an increased prostate cancer incidence with vitamin E and selenium. A study from Australia showed that individuals who took beta carotene and vitamin E supplements had a higher rate of new skin cancer formation. Finally, the SU.VI. MAX Study randomized French adults to a single daily capsule of ascorbic acid, vitamin E, beta carotene, selenium, and zinc or a placebo and found no reduction in mortality or cancer-specific mortality overall, although on a positive note, a further analysis in men found a slight reduction in the risk of prostate cancer. The authors postulated that this sex difference was related to French men having a lower baseline micro-nutrient status. For the same reason, a major trial of supplements in a poor region of China demonstrated reduced risk of esophageal cancer, as at the time, this population was known to have widespread micro-nutrient deficiencies. These data have prompted organizations such as the National Cancer Institute to issue statements stating that long-term vitamins and minerals are discouraged unless correcting a known deficiency, and micro-nutrient testing is now becoming more widely available.

More recently, scientific attention has turned towards the evaluation of concentrated whole foods, particularly those rich in polyphenols and other healthy phytochemicals. A wide range of foods contain these natural chemicals, particularly herbs, spices, green vegetables, teas, and colorful fruits. With the exception of foods with phytoestrogenic properties, there are some interesting laboratory data and encouraging early clinical studies that suggest a potential benefit.

Pomegranate extract, with high concentrations of ellagic acid, has been shown to directly inhibit cell growth and induce apoptosis in androgen sensitive and aggressive human prostate cancer cells. It was also reported to inhibit processes involved in cancer metastasis in a study using estrogen sensitive and resistant breast cancer cell lines, increasing markers of cell adhesion and migration in cancer cells but not normal cells, and in another, it inhibited a chemokine that attracts breast cancer cells to the bone and expression of a gene that is important in epithelial-to-mesenchymal transitions. In mice, it inhibits growth of primary lung cancer. In humans, pomegranate has been shown to reduce insulin resistance and blood pressure.

Also, in a clinical Phase II study, the PSA doubling time (PSAdt) was significantly prolonged in men given 200 ml pomegranate juice a day. This was supported by a further study from Johns Hopkins, which gave men pomegranate seed extract. These effects are unlikely to occur via the androgen pathway, as high performance liquid chromatography confirmed no steroid androgens or estrogens within pomegranates, and a further Phase II study, which also showed a favorable effect on PSA, did not alter men's serum androgen level after 6 months' intake of pomegranate extract.

Green tea, rich in epigallocatechin gallate (EGCG), blocks ornithine decarboxylase, an enzyme that signals cells to proliferate faster and bypass apoptosis.[17] Green tea, in laboratory studies, has demonstrated significant reduction of several factors that promote breast and prostate cancer cell growth, de-differentiation, and angiogenesis. A small Phase II study reported favorable growth factor changes in men with prostate cancer and a non-significant effect on PSA. The Mayo Clinic found that green tea extract decreased the abnormal white cell count in 30% of patients with chronic leukemia, and a study from Louisiana University reported a significant reduction in the levels of several growth factors that promote cancer as well as a reduction in PSA among men following regular supplementation.

Broccoli, rich in isothiocyanate (ITCs) and its metabolite sulforaphane, has been found to inhibit growth and promote apoptosis of cancer cells. Another study found that broccoli sparks numerous genetic changes, activating cancer suppressor genes and switching off promotion genes. Broccoli induces the antioxidant enzymes glutathione S-transferases, which explains why it is particularly beneficial in the 50% of the population carrying a mutated glutathione gene (GSTM1).

Curcumin, which gives turmeric its yellow color, slows cancer cell growth by blocking the cell cycle, increasing the rate of apoptosis, and selectively inhibits cyclooxygenase 1 and platelet activating factor, preventing the invasion and migration of cells. Animal studies have shown that curcumin counteracted the effect of the carcinogen triclocarban (TCC), an antimicrobial agent occasionally used in household and personal care products. Research conducted at the University of Michigan also found that turmeric helped halt the growth of stem cells that give rise to breast cancer without harming normal breast cells.[18]

Grapeseed extract was found in the Vitamins and Lifestyle (VITAL) cohort study to be linked with a lower risk of prostate cancer following regular intake. A small RCT showed

a benefit for dietary supplement containing isoflavones and anti-oxidants.

Although these mainly laboratory and small clinical Phase II trials have produced data that is encouraging, a series of large RCTs of polyphenol-rich foods, either on their own or in combination, are ongoing, as they have been registered in the National Cancer Institute USA trials portfolio. The largest of these trials was the U.K. National Cancer Research Network Pomi-T study. It combined four different food types (berry, vegetable, spice, and leaf) in order to provide a wide spectrum of polyphenol nutrients with potentially synergistic modes of action, improving bioavailability while at the same time avoiding over-consumption of one particular type of polyphenol, which could lead to excess intake.[19] The study involved over 200 men with localized prostate cancer, managed with active surveillance or watchful waiting, who were experiencing a PSA relapse following initial radical interventions. They were randomized to receive an oral capsule containing a blend of purified or whole pomegranate, green tea, broccoli, and turmeric or a placebo for 6 months. This study found a highly statistically significant 64% reduction in the median PSA progression rate compared with placebo, which also impacted on the decisions of men to remain off androgen deprivation therapies or radical interventions.[13] Following its publication and presentation at the American Society of Clinical Oncology (ASCO) Conference, a further study was conducted following 138 men who had received 346 annual diffusion weighted MRIs as part of their active surveillance management. In 89%, the disease reduced in size, was not seen at all, or was stable. The number who progressed was significantly greater in those not taking the supplement. Most relevant, there was a 100% correlation between changes of disease seen on MRI and PSA dynamics, indicating that the influence of the food supplement was not just on the levels of PSA but on the total disease burden.[13]

Carcinogen avoidance

Dietary chemicals such as polycyclic aromatic hydrocarbons and aromatic amines, found in super-heated processed or fried foods, are converted to products that can directly or indirectly oxidize water or oxygen into short-lived, highly energetic free radicals. These can cause double or single DNA strand breaks, allowing cancer promoting genes to escape from the influence of their suppressor gene guardians. Numerous environmental studies have linked carcinogens to cancers, and the U.S. Food and Drug Agency (FDA) regularly publishes lists of foods and environmental chemicals such as pesticides, toxic additives, and chemical contaminants that are potentially carcinogenic if taken in sufficient quantities.

Although all the evidence for carcinogen exposure relates to initial cancer risk, avoiding continued exposure after cancer may have a benefit in reducing the risk of developing relapse or further cancers in patients who may be more susceptible from a pre-existing genetic signature or damage from chemotherapy or radiotherapy. This hypothesis is supported by a study from Newfoundland, which evaluated the eating habits of 529 patients with colorectal cancer. They found that between the highest and the lowest quartile of processed meat intake, there was a twofold increase in relapse and overall death rate. The mechanisms explaining the impact of red and processed meat were thought to be the continued intake of carcinogenic mutagens found in smoked, fried, or high-temperature cooked meat, including N-nitroso compounds, heterocyclic amines, and polycyclic aromatic hydrocarbons. Other authors have hypothesized that regular intake of processed meat disrupts the normal gut microflora, which has previously been linked to colonic polyp formation and the risk of developing colorectal cancer. Although the evidence for ingested carcinogens in meat and colorectal cancer is strongest, a similar relationship between dietary carcinogens and relapse was demonstrated for ovarian cancer and breast cancer. The concept that milk and dairy products are carcinogenic remains controversial, and certainly, the risk of moderate milk and dairy products consumption has been overemphasized in the popular media. A pooled analysis of 12 prospective cohort studies showed no excess in ovarian cancer incidence with moderate intake;[20] only high intake (>2 glasses/day) has been linked to a greater risk of both prostate and breast cancer relapse.

The effect of diet on individuals more susceptible to cancer was demonstrated by a study conducted by the Radiation Effects Research Foundation (RERF) involving people who had survived the Hiroshima and Nagasaki bombings. They showed that those who undertook regular exercise and had a higher intake of fruit and vegetables and a low meat intake had a significantly lower risk of cancers despite their acquired susceptibility.[21] Furthermore, a study evaluating the eating habits of 486 people with the genetic susceptibility Lynch syndrome showed that diets featuring a major unhealthy snack component—chips, fast food, and sweets—conferred an increased risk of developing colorectal adenomas. Likewise, lifestyle habits were a significant factor in the development of breast disease in women presenting at a young age who had strong family histories.

Xenoestrogenic carcinogens

Other environmental chemicals have an adverse effect on cancer risk because of their estrogenic properties, either because they have a chemical structure similar to estrogen or because they affect the sex hormone activity in an indirect pathway. The most common group of chemicals are the polychlorinated biphenyls (PCBs) and organochlorines, found in sources that include pesticides, herbicides, car pollution, fuels, drugs, and even polycarbonate plastic baby bottles and food containers. It is difficult to prove harm in humans with normal day to day use, but chronic occupational exposure to organic solvents is associated with elevated breast cancer risks. Laboratory studies have also demonstrated that estrogenic pollutants given in higher quantities to laboratory mice induce and promote mammary cancers. A further study showed that rats developed a thickened uterus and endometriosis after being fed food that contained dioxin, a xenoestrogen, especially during the developmental stages.

Other common estrogenic chemicals include preservatives called phthalates and parabens, found in some deodorants and cosmetics, which have been found to have xenoestrogenic properties in laboratory studies. A concern in humans was raised following a study in 2004 from Reading University, which demonstrated higher quantities in the outer part of the breast and within breast cancer cells themselves. The same findings have been confirmed in further biopsy studies, and this finding encouraged manufacturers to remove parabens from some of their products. Aluminum salts are responsible for the anti-sweating effect of anti-perspirants but have demonstrated metallo-estrogenic properties in cancer cell lines. A study in 2007 from Keele University revealed higher quantities of aluminum in the upper outer area of the breast within post-mastectomy specimens in those who had used antiperspirants regularly. Although a direct link with cancer has not been proven, the concern is that products containing estrogenic chemicals are used for very long periods of time, starting in adolescence, when methylparaben and propylparaben can even be measured in the urine, particularly among girls rather than males of similar ages.

Smoking

Patients who smoke after surgery increase their risk of thromboembolic events, poor wound healing, and infection. During radiotherapy, smoking increases the risk of acute mucositis, acute skin reaction, xerostomia, and long-term fibrosis and breast pain. There is also convincing data to suggest that individuals who continue to smoke after cancer treatments have worse cancer outcomes. This is thought to be caused by the continued exposure to carcinogens causing further DNA damage.[22] Tobacco use has also been shown to have a direct impact on cellular function by inhibiting apoptosis, stimulating proliferation. A large cohort study from Japan evaluated 25,000 patients who had been treated for lung, breast, or colorectal cancer and reported a median 1.5-year survival; those who continued to smoke were 11% more likely to relapse compared with those who quit after diagnosis.[23] A retrospective study of 540 patients with small-cell lung cancer showed that the relative risk of a second lung cancer was 11% in the 70% who managed to quit smoking, whereas in the 30% who continued to smoke, it was almost three times greater at 32%. Two further retrospective studies evaluating outcomes following treatment for head and neck cancer showed that survival rates halved in those who continued to smoke.

The correlation between smoking and outcome is not limited to upper tract epithelial cancers. A cohort study compared the lifestyle habits of 365 women with ER+ve breast cancer with matched controls. Smoking was a major risk factor for the development of subsequent contralateral relapse, although the effect was strongest in women who also consumed >7 alcoholic beverages a week and were obese.[24] The prospective Life After Cancer Epidemiology (LACE) study followed 2265 women for 25 years; never smokers had a twofold lower rate of dying from breast cancer than smokers. A further analysis of the CALGB 89803 study of 1045 patients with Stage III colon cancer reported an increased relapse rate and worse overall survival among smokers.

The mechanism of harm is most likely to be the continued exposure to high levels of carcinogens, which can cause further DNA damage to existing cancer and encourage it to mutate into a more aggressive type or develop mechanisms to hide from the body's immunological defenses. Smoking also reduces the effectiveness of some therapeutic agents. Smoke interferes with hepatic cytochrome P450 CYP1A, which has been shown to reduce the bioavailability of erlotinib by 25%.

The evidence base for tobacco cessation therapies has grown substantially over the last decade. Nicotine lozenges and varenicline (a partial nicotine receptor agonist) have been shown to reduce cigarette intake and help cessation. Patients entering formal programs, available through the National Health Service, are more than twice as likely to quit and represent one of the most cost-effective interventions in health care. The role of health care providers remains very important, especially when encouragement to quit comes from the supervising consultant.

Alcohol

The Million Women Study has been gathering detailed information from 1.28 million women aged 50 to 64 years since 1996. Among other lifestyle factors, they examined how much alcohol women drank at the start of the study and again 3 years later. They then correlated this with the 68,775 cancers they subsequently developed over an average of the next 7 years. They found statistically significant increased risks of a number of cancers in those who regularly consumed alcohol.[25] Another study indicated that more than one drink a day specifically increased the risk of breast cancer, but up to one drink was not associated with an increased risk. The risk of alcohol appears to be higher if women have a family history of breast disease, especially if they start drinking as a teenager. Men who drank heavily (>50 g of alcohol or four drinks daily) doubled their risk of high-grade prostate cancers compared with other men, although there was no difference in the incidence of low-grade cancers.

There is also evidence that alcohol intake increases the risk of relapse following radical treatments for head and neck cancer. A cohort study recording alcohol consumption for a median follow-up of 1 year demonstrated a significantly increased rate of relapse in those with higher intake. And out of these cases, almost all led to death.

The evidence of alcohol and risk of relapse after breast and other cancers is less robust. A cohort study involving 365 women with ER+ve breast cancer demonstrated an increased risk of contralateral breast cancer if they drank more than seven alcoholic beverages a week. Another study involving 1897 women with breast cancer reported an increased relapse rate if they drank more than three or four beverages per week, particularly if overweight and post-menopausal. The intensity rather than total amount appears to be important, as a study of over 1000 women in the Western New York exposures and breast cancer (WEB) study showed no increased mortality with total alcohol intake, but those drinking intensely (more than three drinks on the day of consumption) had worse outcomes.

Not all research, however, has demonstrated the same link with alcohol; a study of over 45,000 women demonstrated no survival disadvantage of drinking alcohol before or after their breast cancer diagnosis. The Swedish Mammography Cohort of 3146 women actually demonstrated a slight advantage to one glass of wine equivalent per day after diagnosis.[26] The largest prospective cohort study, conducted by the University of Cambridge and involving 13,500 women with breast cancer, confirmed the same finding that women who drank three and a half small glasses of wine a week were 10% more likely to survive.

Another study from the Catholic University and the National Research Council in Italy showed that women who drank a glass of wine a day during radiotherapy had lower rates of acute toxicity than those who did not.[27]

Physical activity after cancer

A physically active lifestyle improves wellbeing by reducing many of the common adverse effects that plague individuals after cancer and its treatments. The strongest evidence concerns cancer-related fatigue, muscle weakness, thromboembolism, weight gain, loss of bone density, quality of life (QoL), psychological distress, incontinence, and sexual dysfunction.[28] It is well recognized that regular physical activity is a significant factor for reducing the risk of cancer development, but a number of large cohort studies have also linked physical activity during and after cancer with improved overall survival and reduced probability of relapse.[28,29] Evidence is emerging that moderately strenuous exercise for about 2.5 hours a week or more may slow the progression of some cancers,[15,28] reduce the probability of relapse, and reduce the risk of overall death from cancer for breast, prostate, and bowel cancer.

Physical activity improves wellbeing after cancer

As well as a direct association between wellbeing and exercise, numerous studies have tested the feasibility and benefits of exercise rehabilitation programs in cancer survivors. A meta-analysis of 34 randomized trials demonstrated that the benefits of a physical activity program spanned several common cancer types managed with a range of treatments, including surgery, radiotherapy, chemotherapy, hormones, and biological therapies.[30] This meta-analysis showed a statistically significant benefit for a number of troublesome symptoms, particularly fatigue; mood, anxiety, and depression; muscle power, hand grip, and exercise capacity; and QoL. The American College of Sports Medicine also published a comprehensive review of 85 RCTs involving exercise intervention for cancer survivors. These and other studies have demonstrated that exercise could safely be performed in adjuvant and post-treatment settings, confirmed benefits for QoL, fatigue, anxiety, and depression, and also demonstrated that exercise programs led to significant improvements in aerobic fitness; increased flexibility and strength; and body image, size and composition. Supervised physical activity is clearly the cornerstone of all effective cancer rehabilitation programs, but it has to be considered alongside other medical, lifestyle, and self-help strategies, the evidence for which will now be discussed in more detail for the more common risks and symptoms relevant to people receiving treatments and living with cancer.

Cancer-related fatigue (CRF)

CRF is one of the most distressing symptoms experienced by patients during and after their anti-cancer therapies. It is reported by 60–96% of patients during chemotherapy or radiotherapy or after surgery and by up to 40% of patients taking long-term therapies such as hormone or biological therapies. It prevents people returning to normal activities of daily living, affects overall QoL, and is a major contributing factor for reduced cognitive function, which can last up to a year post chemotherapy or surgery and persist for a long time in those on adjuvant hormones.[31]

The first step to treating CRF is to correct, if possible, any medical conditions that may aggravate it. These include anemia, electrolyte imbalance, liver failure, hypothyroidism, steroid withdrawal, and nocturia, as well as drugs such as opiates, anti-histamines, and anti-sickness medication.[31] Providing information and counseling on better sleep hygiene guidelines can improve night time sleep and day time alertness and reduce chronic fatigue levels. Supervised exercise programs have also been shown to improve CRF in three meta-analyses. An analysis of 28 RCTs involving 2083 participants undergoing a variety of exercise programs showed a small reduction in CRF.[32] Another analysis of 18 RCTs involved 1109 participants but sub-divided the data into home-based exercise programs and supervised exercise programs. In this study, a statistically significant benefit of exercise for CRF was observed in breast cancer patients involved in supervised exercise programs but not home-based programs. The other meta-analyses found a small to moderate reduction in CRF among breast cancer survivors assigned to aerobic but not resistance exercise programs on their own. In addition to these trials, an RCT involving 410 cancer survivors demonstrated that those randomized to a 4-week yoga and walking intervention program had significantly improved sleep patterns and hence, better day time fatigue. Trials of cognitive behavioral therapy (CBT) have also demonstrated some benefits, especially if combined with regular exercise. In summary, it appears that supervised aerobic exercises, especially if combined with sleep hygiene advice, yoga, and CBT, have the best results.

Psychological distress

Psychological distress, particularly anxiety and depression, is common and often unrecognized after cancer, but when it is looked for specifically, reported prevalence rates can be up to 25–30%. As well as being distressing for the patient and carers, psychological distress has also been shown to be linked with reduced survival compared with those who are psychologically healthy.[33] Early recognition of symptoms and appropriate counseling, support, and treatment helps to stem the decay in self-esteem and relationship issues within the family and work place. The more commonly recognized self-help strategies include support groups, relaxation classes, mindfulness, and exercise. Exercise, in particular, has been shown to help alleviate mood and reduce anxiety and fear of relapse, especially if it involves group activities. A recent meta-analysis of RCTs also demonstrated a reduction in depression and improvement in optimism with group or supervised exercise classes. A study involving 1966 patients with colorectal cancer showed that those who achieved at least 150 minutes of physical activity per week had better mood scores and 18% higher QoL scores than those who reported no physical activity. Another study showed similar benefits for breast cancer survivors who had completed surgery, radiotherapy, or chemotherapy and also demonstrated that change in peak oxygen consumption correlated with change in mood and overall QoL.[34]

In a prospective controlled study, 84 women with breast cancer were randomized to a 6-week mindfulness-based stress reduction (MBSR) intervention program or standard care. Subjects randomized to receive a training package to support home meditation practices (sitting meditation, body scan, and walking meditation) and gentle yoga had lower psychological distress scores. A further RCT involving 68 women with breast cancer demonstrated a significant decrease in anxiety states and improvements in QoL following surgery in the group randomized to regular yoga classes as compared with controls.

It is likely that the benefits of exercise are greater if combined with dietary measures, as these have also demonstrated an improvement in psychological wellbeing. For example, a prospective trial of 252 younger women with breast cancer found that those randomized to the lifestyle and healthy eating (high vegetable, low fat prudent diet) arm had fewer intrusive depressive thoughts and concerns regarding cancer recurrence and mortality, and better self-concept perceptions and self-efficacy expectations.

Body constitution, cardiac function, and unwelcomed weight gain

The benefit of exercise for weight control has been summarized in the obesity section. Exercise programs, especially if combined with nutritional counseling, not only reduce the risk of unwelcomed weight gain but also have significant benefits for other aspects of body constitution, such as lean mass indices, bone mineral density, cardiopulmonary function, muscle strength, general fitness, and walking distance. A meta-analysis of 10 studies involving 588 women with breast cancer examined the effectiveness of aerobic exercise interventions on cardiopulmonary function and body composition, conducted during or after treatments. It found that regular aerobic exercise significantly improved cardiopulmonary function as assessed by absolute VO_2 peak and 12-minute walk test, as well as improving body composition as assessed by percentage body fat, although total body weight did not change significantly. An RCT involving 121 men with prostate cancer highlighted the benefits of a 24-week resistance and aerobic exercise program for those on androgen deprivation therapy (ADT). Exercisers had improved aerobic fitness,

upper- and lower-body strength, and triglycerides and did not gain weight, which was common in the standard care group.

Pelvic symptoms

General and local pelvic floor exercises have demonstrated an improvement in pelvic symptoms such as urgency and incontinence following cancer treatments. For example, a retrospective review of 440 men treated with prostate cancer with radical radiotherapy completed comprehensive lifestyle and pelvic symptom questionnaires. There was a strong inverse correlation of erectile dysfunction, urinary symptoms, and fecal urgency with physical activity. Fecal and urinary urgency were particularly highest in those who led a sedentary lifestyle, especially if they were overweight and smoked.[2] These symptoms are associated with a considerable deterioration in QoL. Pelvic floor exercises, if performed correctly and for a significant length of time, have demonstrated an improvement in pelvic symptoms, so patients need appropriate verbal advice supplemented by written information sheets.

Lymphoedema

Although the incidence of upper limb lymphoedema is significantly decreasing with advances in surgery sentential node biopsy, it previously affected about 30% of women after breast cancer treatments, and many of these women are still living with this consequence of their disease. The more lymph nodes that are removed, the higher the risk of developing arm and breast lymphoedema, which can develop immediately or many years after treatment.[35] Whenever it develops, lymphoedema is a chronic, debilitating condition that can cause severe physical and psychological morbidity as well as a reduction in QoL. Management includes advice to avoid secondary infection, massage, and compression garments, but in addition, a number of studies have linked exercise and weight reduction programs with reduced complications of lymphoedema. This includes an RCT involving 140 women who had received an axillary node clearance and had completed adjuvant chemotherapy or radiotherapy. Both groups received standard lymphoedema advice, but the intervention group received twice-weekly supervised exercise, including weight lifting and stretching, for 6 months. There was no statistical significance in arm thickness, but muscle strength was improved, and there was a significant difference in the number of lymphoedema flares that required acute intervention.

Bone mineral density (BMD)

Depletion of bone materialization is a considerable concern among both male and female cancer survivors. Pre-menopausal women with breast cancer treatment are at increased risk due to reduced levels of estrogen brought on by a premature menopause after chemotherapy, surgery, or hormones. Men who receive hormone deprivation therapy for prostate cancer are also at an increased risk due to lower androgen levels. Accelerated bone loss has been reported for many other cancers, including testicular, thyroid, gastric, and CNS cancers, as well as non-Hodgkin's lymphoma and various hematological malignant diseases. Fortunately, a number of studies have linked regular physical activity with a reduction in the risk of bone mineral loss after cancer. In one controlled trial, 66 women with breast cancer were randomized to a control group or an exercise program of either resistance exercise (using bands) or aerobic exercise (fast walking or jogging).

The rate of decline of BMD was −6.23% in the control group, −4.92% in the resistance exercise group, and −0.76% in the aerobic exercise group. The statistically significant benefit was even greater in pre-menopausal women. In another RCT of 223 women with breast cancer, it was reported that exercise helped preserve BMD even when bisphosphonates (risedronate), calcium (1500 mg/day), and vitamin D (400 IU/day) had already been prescribed.[36] In this study, women who exercised for over 30 minutes four to seven times a week had a twofold (statistically significant) improvement in BMD compared with the medication-only group. Weight bearing exercises are particularly important, as swimming and cycling have little impact on bone health. In fact, professional cyclists have considerable risk of osteoporosis, to the extent that some notable sportsmen have had to curtail their careers early. High-intensity resistance and impact training (HiRIT) has been shown in a well-designed RCT from Australia to improve bone density (and physical strength) in both the hips and back with no increased risk of fractures, despite participants having established osteoporosis. The HiRIT program consisted of resistance exercises such as the deadlift, overhead press, and back squat, performed in five sets of five repetitions. The impact loading exercise was a jumping chin-up with a drop landing. This is something to work up to, preferably with supervision.

It is also important to consider diet alongside exercise for bone health. A sub-analysis of the European Prospective Investigation into Cancer and Nutrition (EPIC) Potsdam confirmed the importance of the influence of diet, in addition to exercise, on bone density. This cohort study included 8178 women and found that high consumption of animal protein was unfavorable, whereas higher vegetable protein was beneficial to bone health. These results support the hypothesis that the lower incidence of osteoporosis in Asian women is due to the high ratio of vegetables to animal protein in their vegetable- and fruit-rich diets. A large-scale dietary modification intervention of 4883 post-menopausal women also showed that an increased consumption of plant proteins and fibers from fruits, vegetables, and grains reduced the risk of multiple falls and increased hip BMD. Likewise, a further review highlighted the benefits of plant proteins and fibers on bone health. A randomized, double-blind, placebo-controlled trial involving 389 post-menopausal women with breast and endometrial cancer evaluated the effects of the soya derivative genistein aglycone on bone health. After 3 years, BMD increases were greater with genistein for both femoral neck and lumbar spine compared with placebo. Other lifestyle factors linked to a risk of osteoporosis include a low calcium and vitamin D intake, smoking, and excessive alcohol intake.

Thromboembolism

Deep vein thrombosis and pulmonary embolus remain a significant risk for patients with malignancy, particularly those with disease involving the pelvis, recent surgery, immobility, a history of varicose veins or thrombosis, or receiving chemotherapy.[37] Although strategies such as compression stockings, warfarin, and low molecular weight heparin are essential, early mobilization and exercise remains a practical additional aid in reducing this life-threatening complication.

The underlying mechanisms of the potential anti-cancer effects of exercise

Numerous cohort studies have linked exercise with better outcomes, but as there is a deficiency of randomized data, some could argue that cohort studies are merely observing habit-forming linkages. People who exercise, for example, are less likely to smoke and more likely to have a healthier BMI and eat more vegetables.[28] Although this remains a possibility, most analyses have adjusted for other lifestyle behaviors using multivariate analysis,

such as the 45 observational studies subject to a recent meta-analysis from the National Cancer Institute, which reported that 2–5 hours of physical activity a week was associated with a significant reduction in cancer relapse rates; in some trials, this was up to 60%. The precise mechanism of how exercise has anti-cancer properties has not been established, and additional laboratory measurements within these trials will provide more data. The potential indirect and direct biochemical mechanisms of how physical activity (exercise) could positively, or negatively, influence oncogenic pathways are now described.

Exercise affecting indirect anti-cancer pathways

Before the direct biochemical pathways are considered, we discuss several non-direct factors that could play a contributory role, such as weight reduction, sunlight exposure, and improved mood.

Obesity, estrogen, leptin, and the effects of weight reduction

The neuropeptide cytokine leptin and the sex hormone estrogen are generated in fat cells, so overweight, particularly post-menopausal, women have higher endogenous levels. Leptin is known to promote breast cancer directly and independently, as well as through involvement with the estrogen and insulin signaling pathways, via enhanced angiogenesis and cell proliferation, which explains the links between higher levels of leptin, adiposity, and hormone-related cancers such as breast and ovary. Conversely, serum concentration of other adipokine cytokines such as adiponectin is inversely correlated with adiposity and breast cancer risk, probably as they have anti-inflammatory properties. A number of studies have shown that exercise programs help individuals to lose weight, and some of those that demonstrated weight reduction resulted in lower serum sex hormones and leptin levels. It is unlikely, however, that a reduction in adiposity is a major anti-cancer mechanism, because exercise programs, at best, only usually show a modest reduction in weight. Furthermore, there is evidence that even before weight reduction occurs, exercise directly lowers serum estrogen and leptin levels and raises adiponectin levels independently of weight loss. In one clinical study, this was quantified as every 100 min of exercise giving a 3.6% lowering of serum estrogen.

Vitamin D levels and sunlight exposure

These are both higher among those who exercise regularly outdoors. The mechanism by which vitamin D influences the incidence and progression of cancer is thought to be due to calcitriol's effect on cellular proliferation, differentiation, and apoptosis. The vitamin D receptor is highly expressed in epithelial cells known to be at risk of carcinogenesis, such as the breast, skin, and prostate. Low vitamin D levels are linked to higher relapse rates after colorectal, breast, and prostate cancer, although a direct causational link has not been established, nor has any benefit of correcting vitamin D levels with supplementation. Sunlight exposure, independently of vitamin D levels, has been linked to a lower incidence of prostate cancer. It has been postulated that sunlight exposure may have other benefits, such as modulation of the immune system and the circadian rhythm.[38,39]

Psychological wellbeing

As well as being distressing, anxiety and depression have been linked to a reduced survival following radical cancer treatments. Of note, a large prospective cohort study from California reported that 4.6% of 41,000 men who were clinically depressed after prostate cancer had a 25% reduction in disease-specific survival compared with non-depressed men. Another trial involving individuals from Korea with head and neck cancer reported similar findings.[40] Regular exercise, especially if in groups and combined with relaxation, mindfulness, and healthy eating programs, has been shown to help alleviate mood and reduce anxiety and fear of relapse. The mechanism by which exercise helps fight depression has not yet been firmly established, but hypotheses include increased endorphin and monoamine release, mental distraction, and rises in core temperatures.[41] In addition, light exposure, which increases with outdoor exercise, has been linked to a reduction in non-seasonal depressive disorders. Compliance with medical interventions has also been shown to be improved by supervised exercise programs.

Exercise affecting direct anti-cancer pathways

An array of direct biological, epigenetic, metabolic, and inflammatory changes occur in the body after exercise, both acutely and over time.[28] It has not yet, however, been established which one, or combination of these, has the most significant influence on cancer pathways. The most notable candidate mechanisms are summarized here, in no particular order of importance.

Insulin-like growth factor (IGF-1)

Insulin-like growth factor (IGF-1) and its binding proteins, insulin-like growth factor binding proteins (IGFBPs), have a central role in the regulation of cell growth. After binding to its receptor tyrosine kinase, IGF-1 activates several signaling pathways, leading to the inhibition of apoptosis, the promotion of cell growth, and angiogenesis. Higher levels of IGF-1 would therefore be expected to increase tumor growth and have been reported to be associated with a greater cancer risk. An inverse relationship is reported with IGF binding protein (IGFBP3) levels, although this effect has not been confirmed in all studies. Exercise has been shown to increase the levels of IGFBP3 and lower IGF-1, and in a large prospective cohort study of 41,528 participants, this was associated with a 48% reduction of cancer-specific deaths. Decreased levels of IGF-1 in physically active patients have also been linked to an improved survival.

Epigenetic effects on gene expression and DNA repair

Exercise has been shown to have a significant impact on gene expression, but which of these epigenetic changes have the most influence on cancer remains uncertain. The GEMINAL study, a prospective pilot trial involving men with low-risk prostate cancer, found a set of *RAS* family oncogenes (*RAN*, *RAB14*, and *RAB8A*) to be down-regulated after a healthy exercise and lifestyle program. In the prostate, RAN (ras-related nuclear protein) may function as an androgen receptor co-activator, and its expression is increased in tumor tissues.[42] Another study, involving men on active surveillance, showed that 184 genes were differentially expressed between individuals who engaged in vigorous activity compared with sedentary individuals. Genes particularly sensitive to exercise included those involved in signaling cell cycling and those supporting DNA repair, including BRCA1 and BRCA2 via histone deacetylase pathways. The same up-regulation of BRCA expression following exercise has been demonstrated in the rat mammary gland and clinically, in women who were BRCA 1 or 2 mutation carriers. Markers of an improved cellular repair process were also reported in a study showing that exercise up-regulates the key regulator gene p53 and by doing so, encourages damaged cells to repair or if this is not possible, to self-destruct. Telomere length was shown to be a prognostic marker among

men with prostate cancer on active surveillance. Moderate exercise and a healthy eating program increased telomere length in blood, and this correlated with reduced PSA progression.

Vasoactive intestinal peptide (VIP)

Vasoactive intestinal peptide (VIP) is a neuropeptide that increases proliferation, survival, androgen resistance, and de-differentiation in human breast and prostate cancer cell lines. Serum VIP has been shown to transiently increase after acute exercise. For example, in an experiment involving 30 minutes of bicycle riding, increased levels were detected for approximately 20 minutes, although the rise was higher if the individual was sleep deprived and lower if adequate glucose levels were maintained. This transient rise leads to the production of natural anti-VIP antibodies, which explains the observation that individuals who regularly exercise have lower VIP titers. Patients with breast and prostate cancer have been found to have higher VIP titers compared with matched pairs in the general population without cancer.

Oxidative stress and antioxidant pathways

Exercise, particularly if strenuous, produces reactive oxidative species (ROS), which if significant, increases oxidative stress on DNA, which could potentially contribute to the initiation and progression of cancer. In response to this transient increase in ROS, especially after regular training, an adaptive up-regulation of antioxidant genes occurs, which results in greater production of antioxidant enzymes such as superoxide dismutase, glutathione, and catalase.[43] In a pilot study at the University of California, men who participated in ≥3 hours/week of vigorous physical activity had modulated expression of the nuclear factor erythroid 2–related factor 2 (Nrf-2)–mediated oxidative stress response pathway in their normal prostate tissue compared with men who did less exercise. Other studies have confirmed that trained individuals have greater levels of antioxidant enzymes, which would potentially increase their defense against environmental and ingested oxidating carcinogens. If nutritional deficiencies exist to impair the production of antioxidant enzymes or if strenuous exercisers are elderly, where this adaptive process is known to be slower, there is a danger that strenuous exercise could do more harm than good.[44] It is important, therefore, that attention is given to nutritionally healthy foods that enhance up-regulation of antioxidant enzymes.[43,44]

Heat shock proteins (HSP)

Heat shock proteins (HSP) are produced in tissues in response to a wide variety of physiological and environmental insults, including infection, hypoxia, hyperthermia, dexamethasone, and chemotherapy.[45] They have cytoprotective functions, including blocking apoptosis and allowing the cell to survive potentially lethal events; hence, they are substantially overexpressed following a myocardial infarction. They are also increased acutely following a bout of exercise. This acute rise in HSP is significantly lower in trained athletes and is most pronounced after severe anaerobic exercise, especially if the participant is previously unfit.[43] An increase in HSP is the hypothesized mechanism for exercise protecting the heart in numerous animal studies and clinically, in women receiving adjuvant anthracycline chemotherapy who are physically active. An increase in HSP is also the suggested mechanism for exercise reducing cognitive impairment during chemotherapy by protecting the astrocytes and supportive cells within the brain.

There is a potential downside to this adaptive pathway, as cancer cells have learned to harness the anti-apoptotic properties of HSP and hence, are markedly overexpressed in several cancer types. Some cancers have even become HSP-dependent for their survival, which makes them an interesting potential therapeutic target. Whether exercise increases HSP to a clinically meaningful level to protect cancer cells is not yet known, although the addition of very high levels of HSP to cell lines in one laboratory experiment did increase resistance to anthracyclines. Because cancer cells produce their own HSP in high quantities, it is unlikely that the changes in serum HSP after exercise have any influence on intratumoral levels. This is supported by a recent experiment in mice that reported a better cancer response to adriamycin with concomitant exercise. Nevertheless, until further research confirms this in humans, it is probably wise to advise patients to avoid unaccustomed anaerobic or rigorous exercise, the strongest promoters of HSP, just before or immediately after chemotherapy.

Testosterone

High levels of androgens are associated with a higher incidence of prostate cancer, but what happens to testosterone after exercise is complex and depends on the underlying level of fitness, exercise intensity, and even mood at the time of training. It is widely stated that serum testosterone increases immediately after vigorous exercise, but this has not been confirmed in all studies. This effect also appears to be very short lived, around 15 minutes to an hour after exercise, with levels returning to pre-exercise levels by 2 hours.

It is also often quoted that resistance training increases testosterone more than endurance exercise, but there is very little to substantiate this in the literature. In fact, both endurance exercise and resistance training have been reported to cause a transient increase in testosterone levels in men and women in a number of studies. It is important to note that these studies report that testosterone binding protein also rises with exercise, so the free, biologically active, testosterone proportion changes little. Furthermore, this transient testosterone rise has not been reported in men over 55 years, when men are at increased risk of prostate cancer. More importantly, over time, regular moderate or intense exercise actually lowers testosterone as well as luteinizing hormone and follicle stimulating hormone due to a negative feedback mechanism, and this can be a symptomatic issue for trained athletes. This effect has been observed clinically following a 30-day, 12-week, and 12-month program.[46] There are some studies reporting that a healthy lifestyle, including exercise, delayed the natural age-related decline in testosterone, but this was only linked to obesity, metabolic syndrome, diabetes, and dyslipidemia, which cause testosterone deficiency. Current studies are inconclusive as to whether exercise further lowers serum androgen levels in men already taking ADT, although this is further complicated by inadequate methods for measuring testosterone levels in very low ranges.

Irisin

Irisin is a type I trans-membrane messenger protein, which is produced in muscle cells in response to exercise. One study reported that higher levels were linked to more favorable breast cancer prognostic risk at diagnosis. In laboratory studies, irisin significantly reduced cancer cell proliferation, migration, and viability in malignant cancer cell lines without affecting non-malignant cells. In another, irisin enhanced the cytotoxic effect of doxorubicin when added to malignant breast cells, which again was not observed in non-malignant cells. This reduction in malignant potential of irisin, however, was not observed with colon,

thyroid, and esophageal cancer cell lines. Furthermore, reports questioned the existence of circulating human irisin, as it was felt that human irisin antibodies used in commercial enzyme-linked immunosorbent assay (ELISA) kits lacked the required specificity. However, a recent experiment used mass spectrometry to compare irisin levels between sedentary participants and those following aerobic interval training and found a significant difference.

Immunity

During exercise, increased levels of catecholamines stimulate the recruitment of leucocytes into the peripheral blood, resulting in increased concentrations of neutrophils, lymphocytes, and monocytes, including NK, CD4+ T cells, and B cells. This may result in a reduced risk of infection, as, for example, suggested by a study reporting that individuals who regularly performed >2 h of moderate exercise per day had a 29% reduction in risk of upper respiratory tract infection (URTI) compared with a sedentary lifestyle.[47] On the other hand, if exercise is too strenuous for that individual, it is followed by decreased concentrations of lymphocytes and impaired cellular-mediated immunity. As a consequence, in another study, there was an increase in risk of an infection in the weeks following a competitive ultra-endurance running event. Overall, most long-term studies suggest that moderate exercise has little influence on immune function in healthy populations, but its benefits are particularly relevant in the elderly, whose immune function is becoming less efficient. This also implies a benefit for individuals after cancer treatment, but these studies have yet to be conducted.

Chronic inflammation and prostaglandins

Although an inflammatory response is an important part of healthy immunity, persistent low-grade chronic inflammatory activity in plasma is associated with age-related diseases such as Alzheimer's disease, atherosclerosis, and cancer. These are higher in overweight sedentary individuals, those with poor diets, type 2 diabetes, and the elderly.[48] There is a general consensus that the reason for this stems from over-compensation by an ailing immune system trying to maintain immunosenescence. In these groups, poor IL-2 production leads to a decreased cytotoxic capacity of NK and T lymphocytes on a "per cell" basis. To compensate for this, higher levels of inflammatory biomarkers such as C-reactive protein, TNF, and interleukin-6 (IL-6), cytokine antagonists, and acute phase proteins are produced, which increase concentrations of NK cells and T cells. These inflammatory cytokines, however, also promote tumor development and growth directly or via prostaglandins (see below), which explains why they are associated with more advanced cancers and an increased risk of cancer-specific mortality.

Exercise is known to enhance NK cell activity and increase T-cell production, reducing the need for the immune system to increase circulating inflammatory biomarkers. Other important factors are prostaglandins, which are biologically active lipids generated from arachidonic acid via the enzyme cyclo-oxidase (COX). The COX-1 enzymes are present in normal tissues and up-regulate in response to trauma, infection, or chemical injury, increasing prostaglandins, which in turn triggers an appropriate inflammatory cascade as part of a healthy immune response. COX-2 is also induced by cytokines and growth factors and has higher expression in many tumors. Chronically increased inappropriate overproduction of prostaglandins generated via COX-2, such as PGE_2, has been implicated in cancer progression, apoptosis, invasion, angiogenesis, and metastasis.

Anti-inflammatory drugs and salicylates found in painkillers and fresh vegetables have been shown to reduce COX-2 activation of prostaglandins, which could explain their reported anticancer properties. Moderate, regular, non-traumatic exercise also reduces serum prostaglandin levels and other markers of improved immunity and angiogenesis. A study involving biopsies of rectal mucosa showed that leisure-time physical activity was inversely associated with prostaglandin-2 concentration (PGE_2). Overweight individuals (BMI >25 kg/m^2) also had increased mucosal concentrations. Most importantly, an increase in activity level from 5.2 to 27.7 metabolic equivalent of task (MET)-hours per week was associated with a 28% decrease in mucosal PGE_2.

Energy metabolism and insulin resistance

A number of RCTs have shown that exercise improves insulin sensitivity and glucose metabolism even in patients taking ADT. Hyperglycemia and high insulin levels secondary to insulin resistance are associated with an increased risk of cancer, poorer prognostic features at presentation, higher risk of relapse after initial treatments, and more rapid progression in men with castration resistant prostate cancer. In addition, high levels of C-peptide, a marker of insulin secretion, are associated with a more than twofold increased risk of prostate cancer–specific mortality. One contributory factor for these worse outcomes may be resistin, also known as adipose tissue-specific secretory factor (ADSF), which is a cysteine-rich adipose-derived peptide hormone that increases with insulin resistance through AMP kinase down-regulation. Resistin is known to up-regulate pro-inflammatory cytokines, which act via the nuclear factor kappa-light-chain-enhancer of activated B cells (NFκb) pathway to increase transcription of proteins involved in cell proliferation, inflammation, and anti-apoptosis. Men commencing ADT develop a rise in circulating insulin, and this hyperinsulinemia precedes changes of features of metabolic syndrome, including adiposity, increased lipids, and sarcopenia. Men randomized to an exercise program after starting ADT also have a significantly lower incidence of weight gain and metabolic syndrome. It has long been known that exercise combined with dietary modification reduces not only triglycerides but also total cholesterol and improves the ratio of high density lipoprotein to low density lipoprotein. Epidemiological studies have suggested that high levels of cholesterol in the blood are associated with increased risk of cancer and progression of prostate cancer. See further Table 35.1.

Quantity, type, and timing of exercise recommended for cancer patients

To achieve reduced breast cancer relapse and improved well-being, most of the cohort studies suggest moderate exercise of around 2.5 to 3 hours a week. However, for prostate cancer survivors, mortality continues to decrease if men walk 4 or more hours per week, and more vigorous activity is also associated with significantly further reductions in risk for all-cause mortality.[49] When the mode of exercise is primarily walking, a pace of at least 3 miles/hour (for >3 hours/week) is recommended for a reduced risk of relapse. Therefore, both the pace and duration of exercise affect the survival benefit achievable from exercise, with more vigorous activity generally having a greater benefit. The best results appear to be with programs including a combination of aerobic and resistance exercises, particularly within a social group. A well-designed multicenter trial from Holland looked at the benefits of a supervised exercise regimen from the start of chemo. The landmark PACES trial from the Holland involving 355 patients with breast or bowel cancer receiving taxanes or platinum chemo found that those randomized to a moderate-intensity, home-based, 6-week progressive walking and resistance exercise program had significant reduced peripheral neuropathy. The effect was greater if the participant was older. The authors strongly recommended that exercise is started from cycle one of chemo.

The precise amount of exercise has to be determined on an individual basis and depends on pre-treatment ability, current disability caused by the cancer itself or the treatment, stages in the treatment, and rehabilitation pathway. An exercise program supervised by a trained professional has major advantages, as they can design a regimen that starts slowly and gradually builds up to an acceptable and enjoyable pace. In addition, they can help motivate the individual to continue exercising for the short term and the long term, and they can judge the optimal exercise levels to improve fatigue and not aggravate it.

The challenge for health professions is how to monopolize the teachable moment and encourage individuals with cancer to increase their exercise levels and other healthy living habits. Although some individuals are motivated to increase physical activity themselves or remain active after cancer, the majority will need guidance.[3] The initial step in a behavioral change program is to provide relevant encouragement and information

TABLE 35.1   Summary of the Direct Biochemical Changes That Occur after Exercise

Class of effect	Effector molecule	Effect on effector molecule
Cell growth regulators	IGF1	Decreased levels
	IGFBP3	Increased levels
DNA damage repair	BRCA1 and 2	Increased expression
Epigenetic expression	RAS family oncogenes	Suppressed activity
Regulators of apoptosis and cell cycle arrest	P53	Enhanced activity
	Heat shock proteins	Enhanced activity
Hormones	Estrogen	Reduced activity
	Testosterone and VIP	Transiently increased then reduced
	Leptin and resistin	Reduced activity
	Irisin	Enhanced activity
Immune system components	NK cells	Enhanced activity
	White cell function	Enhanced activity
	White cells	Increased circulating proportion
Inflammation	C-reactive protein, interleukin-6, TNFα, prostaglandins, COX-2	Reduced activity
Oxidative stress and antioxidant pathways	Glutathione, catalase, and superoxide dismutase	Increased activity

during the verbal consultation with health care professionals backed up by written and other information in a variety of multimedia formats.[3] Macmillan Cancer Relief has produced a series of helpful booklets and web-based patient information materials designed to inform and motivate individuals to exercise and eat well as part of its *Move More* and *Living Well* programs.[50] The Cancernet.co.uk and Macmillan.org websites have links to a facility to search for local exercise facilities by postcode, which can aid health professionals when counseling patients.

The gold standard model would be similar to the cardiac rehabilitation program.[51] This would involve a hospital scheme run by a physiotherapist or an occupational therapist supervising patients immediately after surgery and radiotherapy and even during chemotherapy and then referring the patient into a community based scheme for the long term. These could include one of the 5500 municipal gyms or numerous *Walking for Health* groups across the United Kingdom. Unfortunately, this type of scheme is perceived to be expensive and unlikely to be funded at present, despite the obvious savings by preventing patients relapsing and utilizing health care facilities to help late effects of cancer treatment.[3] On the other hand, expanding existing community services, such as the National Exercise Referral Scheme, is a practical solution. The National Exercise Referral Scheme exists for other chronic conditions such as cardiac rehabilitation, obesity, and lower back pain, and the national standards for the scheme to be expanded to include cancer rehabilitation were written and accepted in 2010 by the governing body SkillsActive. Training providers have now developed training courses for exercise professionals set against these standards. The course and qualification empower trainers to be more confident in helping cancer survivors to live well and exercise by providing them with an insight into cancer treatment and how treatments affect the ability to exercise as well as teaching trainers to deal with altered body image, peripheral neuropathy, hand foot syndrome, fatigue, and other cancer-related side effects. Trainers completing the course gain a Register of Exercise Professionals (REPs) level four qualification, allowing them to receive referrals from GPs and other health professionals. Macmillan Cancer Support and other advocacy groups have successfully lobbied health authorities to expand the exercise referral scheme to include cancer, and this is now available in most areas of the United Kingdom.

Gut health

Trillions of bacteria, fungi, and viruses live on our bodies, particularly in our gut, skin, and lungs, and collectively form our microbiota. It has been estimated that just over half the genetic material from cells in our body is derived from these microorganisms. Healthy bacteria play a fundamental role in ensuring our gut health. In particular, numerous clinical studies have established that a healthy, diverse population of bacteria strengthens immunity and helps regulate inflammatory reactions both in the gut and around the body. In turn, a poor gut flora leads to dysregulation of the immune system, resulting in increased susceptibility to infection and excess chronic inflammation. By competing for space and nutrients and preventing the colonization of unhealthy bacteria, good bacteria also form an important additional physical barrier for the oral and gut mucosa against pathogenic bacterial invasion.

Pro-inflammatory (bad) bacteria overgrowth can affect gut and general health. Pathogenic bacteria can cause acute life-threatening infections such as food poisoning or chronic infections, such as helicobacteria. Pro-inflammatory bacteria, often referred to as the *Firmicutes* group, do not cause such acute illnesses but can cause long-term health issues if they colonize the gut in excess. More common strains include the gram-negative bacteria *Escherichia coli* and Shigella, and the gram-positive bacteria Bacillus, Listeria, Staphylococcus, Enterococcus, and Clostridium.

Good (probiotic) bacteria interfere with the growth or survival of pathogenic microorganisms in the gut lumen while also improving the mucosal barrier and the mucosal immunity. Beyond the gut, they improve overall immunity and help reduce chronic inflammation. They are also responsible for the formation of butyrate from soluble fiber and polyphenols. The prominent health benefits of butyrate are described in detail later. Good bacteria are generally referred to as probiotic bacteria and include the gram-negative anaerobic *Bacteroidetes* group, which are linked with numerous positive health benefits.

What are the consequences of poor gut health?

Western-style diets commonly lead to suboptimal microflora, which leads to troubling symptoms such as indigestion, abdominal bloating, and colicky pains. In the longer term, poor gut health is linked to increased inflammatory markers such as interleukin (IL)1, 2, and 8, tumor necrosis factor-alpha, C-reactive protein, and gamma interferon, and lower anti-inflammatory markers such as IL 4, IL 10, 22, IL 6, 11, and 13. This chronic inflammation has been linked to a higher risk of degenerative conditions such as osteoarthritis, type 2 diabetes, and cognitive disorders. In terms of cancer, chronic inflammation can lead to increased intracellular oxidative stress and reduced immunosurveillance. Animal experiments have found that *Bacteroidetes* growth in the colon leads to the inhibition of carcinogens in the colon and a lower rate of polyp formation. This was attributed to the pH-lowering effect of Bifidobacteria in the colon, which subsequently inhibited the growth of pathogenic bacteria.[52] A decrease in pathogenic microorganisms also modulated enzymes that convert pro-carcinogens such as nitrates to carcinogens such as nitrosamines, potentially increasing the risk of cancer within and outside the gut.

Recent laboratory and clinical studies have revealed important roles for gut bacteria in determining the body's response to immunotherapies, with healthy gut bacteria known to increase the therapeutic benefit of immune drugs in animals with melanoma. A clinical study conducted at the MD Anderson Cancer Hospital in Texas has further underlined the impact healthy bacteria have in facilitating effective immunotherapy treatment. It discovered that men and women taking PD1-inhibitor drugs to treat metastatic melanoma had a better response if they had biochemical markers of a diverse and optimal gut flora with low levels of bad gut bacteria.

In the not so distant future, cancer care will likely include an analysis of the patient's microbiome at diagnosis in order to inform personalized treatment planning, while it may also be possible to manipulate the microbiome to optimize treatment outcomes. For this reason, both the American Association of Clinical Oncologists and Cancer Research UK announced significant funding for research to explore how the microbiome can increase the effectiveness of immunotherapies.

What factors influence gut flora?

The biodiversity of the gut and skin bacteria deteriorates over time unless extra dietary measures are undertaken. Anti-inflammatory microbiota tend to diminish with age, whereas inflammatory and pathogenic microbiota increase as people become older. Dietary choices have a big influence, as ultimately, the bacteria in our gut are derived from the food and drink we consume. Probiotic bacteria occur naturally in many fruits and vegetables, as well as in a range of fermented foods such as live yoghurt and kefir, aged and blue veined cheeses, miso soup, kimchi and tempeh, and sauerkraut and pickled vegetables. Foods that promote healthy bacterial growth (known as prebiotics) are equally important. These stimulate the growth of healthy *Bacteroidetes* and impair the growth of bad *Firmicutes*. The two main groups are polyphenols and soluble fibers.

Polyphenols

It has been estimated that only 5–10% of total polyphenol intake is absorbed in the small intestine. The rest accumulate in the large intestinal lumen, where they are subjected to the enzymatic activities of the gut microbiome. Healthy probiotic bacteria are therefore responsible for the extensive breakdown of the original polyphenolic structures into biologically more active phenols, which can then be absorbed more efficiently. Polyphenols also help to preferentially feed healthy gut bacteria, thus improving the composition of the microflora. This is because the metabolism of polyphenols produces glycans such as butyrate, which are used as energy by the intestinal bacteria. *Firmicutes* (bad bacteria) have less of the enzyme required to digest glycans than *Bacteroidetes*, so they are less able to use them as food. Moreover, *Firmicutes* are more repressed than *Bacteroidetes* by the natural antibiotic properties of many polyphenols. The polyphenols and other phytochemicals that have the most notable effect on gut health include plant lignans found in nuts, bananas, and cranberries, resveratrol in red wine, and ellagic acid into ellagitannin, found in tea, pomegranate, and chocolate.

Soluble fibers

These occur naturally in gums and pectins, which are found in citrus fruit, pears, apples, peas, guar gum, chicory root, garlic, onions, asparagus, and Jerusalem artichoke as well as grains such as oats, barley, and psyllium. They also include fermentable soluble fibers such as inulin and resistant starch; oligosaccharides, including fructooligosaccharide (FOS); and the polysaccharide betaglucans most commonly found in mushrooms. They provide a substrate for the microbiota within the large gut. In addition, they increase fecal bulk, and their fermentation produces short-chain fatty acids. This fermentation impacts the expression of a number of genes within the large intestine that enhance digestive function and cholesterol and glucose metabolism, as well as the immune and systemic metabolic functions in the body. They are also rich in natural antibiotics, including penicillin, streptomycin, and tetracycline, which promote a healthy gut flora and reassuringly, have not been shown to pose any risk of antibiotic resistance.

Physical activity

Higher fitness levels have been associated with both a greater abundance of butyrate, a short-chain fatty acid that is important for overall health, and butyrate-producing bacteria. One particular study found that professional rugby players from Ireland had a more diverse gut flora and twice the number of bacterial families as control groups matched for body size, age, and gender. It was unclear whether having a healthy gut made them able to train to become ultra-fit or rather, whether the training process itself actually improved gut health.

Sugar and artificial sweeteners

Firmicutes thrive on ingested sugar, whereas *Bacteroidetes* prefer to utilize glycans produced by the breakdown of polyphenols. So,

a high-sugar, low-polyphenol diet will encourage the growth of bad bacteria and lead to poor gut health. Many people are turning to artificial sweeteners as low calorie and potentially healthier alternatives to sugar; however, rats fed aspartame were shown to have increased blood sugar and increased colonization of proinflammatory Clostridia and Enterobacteria.

Other lifestyle factors

As mentioned earlier, the proportion of *Firmicutes* increases while *Bacteroidetes* decrease with increasing BMI. It remains unclear whether it is the bad gut profile that causes obesity or vice versa. In excess, alcohol can adversely affect long-term gut health, with spirits and beer being worse than red wine due to the protective effect of resveratrol. Binge drinking causes transient dysbiosis, which may be responsible for many of the symptoms of a hangover. Cigarette smoking has recently been confirmed as an important risk factor for inflammatory bowel disease, and smoking cessation has been linked to increased gut flora diversity. Mice exposed to stresses such as isolation, crowding, and heat develop higher levels of bad bacteria. A human study, monitoring the effect of stress on the composition of gut bacteria in 23 college students before and after studying for their end-of-term final examinations, found that the high stress associated with exams caused a reduction in several bacteria, including Lactobacilli. A diet high in saturated animal fat can increase *Firmicutes* growth. Likewise, people eating a high-protein, low-carbohydrate diet have reduced fermentation in the gut, leading to increased levels of harmful nitrosamines, decreased levels of butyrate, and reduced metabolism of polyphenols into the absorbable and biologically active phenols.[31]

Probiotic supplements

Studies so far suggest that young active people with a good diet, and therefore a healthy gut already, are unlikely to benefit from probiotic supplementation. Unfortunately, most studies have been conducted in healthy volunteers. People with poor gut health may benefit, and there is evidence for a short course in people with irritable bowel syndrome (IBS) summarized in a 2010 Cochrane review. As a consequence, NICE recommends taking them for at least 4 weeks. Likewise, they appear to be beneficial in hospital-acquired, antibiotic-induced, or travelers' diarrhea. One study suggested that they reduced chemotherapy-induced diarrhea. The main risk posed by a probiotic supplement is a contaminated supply, so it is very important to buy probiotics from a reputable source. Be sure the ingredients are clearly marked on the label. Look for probiotic blends produced by a long-established, reputable manufacturer with a high-quality assurance track record compliant with EU, U.K., and U.S. standards (more information can be found on keep-healthy.com).

Major institutions are now racing to improve our understanding of the human microbiome and how it varies between people. A one-size-fits-all approach is unlikely to succeed when it comes to altering an individual's microbiome. In the future, it is envisioned that a tailored probiotic regimen could help maintain or restore a person's unique microbial "fingerprint" and in doing so, could substantially improve responses to targeted biological treatments.

Chemotherapy-induced onycholysis

In most cases, nail damage manifests as ridges in the nails that correspond to the timings of chemotherapy episodes, known as Beau's lines. More pronounced nail damage, particularly associated with taxanes, can lead to discoloration, distortion, and complete onycholysis, which is painful and unsightly, affects body image, limits activities of daily living, and may lead to more serious consequences, including secondary infection, which is a particular concern among patients at risk of neutropenia.[53] Nail damage is caused by disorganized inhibition of the rapidly dividing cells in the nail bed. Further contributory factors relate to the anti-angiogenetic properties of taxanes and excess local inflammatory-mediated processes. Disruption of the normal anatomy allows bacterial and fungal pathogens to enter the nail beds, causing further damage.

Cooling the fingers has been reported to reduce docetaxel-related nail toxicity by initiating vasoconstriction and slowing the metabolism of onychocytes. This technique, however, has not been commonly adopted in the United Kingdom, as oncology nurses have concerns about restricting access to patients' hands. Patient support groups advise a variety of anecdotal strategies, including wearing nail varnish and massaging moisturizing petroleum-based balms into the nail bed, but there have been no robust prospective studies to support these practices.

The plant-based waxes and essential oils are naturally rich in phytochemicals, especially the phenolic polyphenols group, which are reported to have antioxidant, anti-inflammatory, DNA repair–enhancing, and antimicrobial properties. In addition to their ability to moisturize the skin, preventing drying and splitting of the nail, it appears that they are sufficiently absorbed into the nail beds to act as a local antidote to the chemotherapy, preventing damage to the proliferating stem cells as well as avoiding secondary damage from inflammation or secondary infection.

The benefits of a topical application were evaluated in an RCT involving 60 patients receiving chemotherapy (mainly taxotere) in 2018 at one of the Cambridge University affiliated Hospitals, Bedford. The application (now known as Polybalm) consisted of a blend of unrefined shea butter (*Butyrospermum parkii*), organic beeswax (*Cera alba*), extra virgin, organic, cold-pressed olive oil (*Olea europaea*), organic cocoa seed butter (*Theobroma cacao*), African sage (*Tarchonanthus camphoratus*), wintergreen leaf (*Gaultheria procumbens*), lavender flower (*Lavandula spica*), and eucalyptus leaf (*Eucalyptus globulus*). The oils were steam extracted from the plant and then gently blended, avoiding overheating to prevent damage to the phytochemicals. The balm contained no preservatives, parabens, sulfates, or perfumes, which could have had an irritative effect.

At the end of chemotherapy, patients' nail-related symptoms, recorded using the validated Dermatology Life Quality Questionnaire (DLQQ), were highly significantly lower in the Polybalm group compared with placebo ($p < 0.000001$). In fact, only one out of an expected 15 patients had any damage at all, and the average nail QoL score actually increased in the Polybalm group. The physical appearance of the nails recorded using the Nail Psoriasis Severity Index by independent clinicians was also much greater in the Polybalm group. This balm is now given to patients in a number of oncology units (usually bought via their local funds), although despite its scientific evaluation, the Medicines and Health Regulatory Authority (MHRA) do not class this as a medicinal product. Nevertheless, this study has provided patients with a self-help option to prevent this troublesome side effect, caused by one of the most commonly used chemotherapy agents.

Summary

With the publication of more and more lifestyle-related research, there is justifiable increased interest in the management of

patients in the survivorship. Whether on or off anti-cancer therapies, there is increasingly strong data to support the development of supervised rehabilitation and self-help intervention programs in order to reduce acute and late risks and consequences of treatments and improve outcomes. These programs, if integrated into the mainstream management of cancer patients, are likely to have multiple other benefits, including empowering patients and their carers, ensuring greater autonomy, and reducing the increasing burden on health care providers. Although more cost-effectiveness research is needed, the rapidly increasing proportion of cancer survivors is creating a growing realization that washing our hands of patients after their radical treatments and failing to plan is a plan to fail.

Key learning points

- The number of people alive who have had a cancer diagnosis is rising at 3% per year in Europe, reflecting increasing incidence and longer survival after treatment.
- The diagnosis of cancer in a person presents a "teachable moment" on lifestyle issues.
- Maintaining a healthy gut is likely to improve response rates of the new targeted biological agents.
- Physical activity reduces the severity of many of the common adverse effects of the disease and its treatment.
- Survivorship programs are cost-effective by reducing the burden on healthcare providers and encouraging self-sufficiency.

References

1. Anand P, Kunnumakara AB, Sundaram C et al. Cancer is a preventable disease. *Pharm Res.* 2008; 25(9):2097–116.
2. Thomas R, Holm M, Williams M et al. Lifestyle factors correlate with the risk of late pelvic symptoms after prostatic radiotherapy. *Clin Oncol.* 2013; 25(4):246–51.
3. Thomas R and Davies N. Lifestyle during and after cancer treatments. *Clin Oncol.* 2007; 19:616–27.
4. Dignam JJ, Polite BN, Yotherths G, Raich P, Colangelo L, O'Connell MJ, et al. Body Mass Index and outcomes in patients who receive adjuvant chemotherapy for colon cancer. *J Natl Cancer Inst.* 2006; 98(22):1647–54.
5. Amling CL, Riffenburgh RH, Sun L et al. Pathologic variables and recurrence rates as related to obesity and race in men with prostate cancer undergoing radical prostatectomy. *J Clin Oncol.* 2004; 22:439–45.
6. Liu XH, Yao S, Kirschenbaum A, Levine AC. NS398, a selective cyclooxygenase-2 inhibitor, induces apoptosis and down-regulates bcl-2 expression in LNCaP cells. *Cancer Res.* 1998; 58:4245–49.
7. Murphy A, Nyame Y, Martin I. Vitamin D deficiency predicts prostate biopsy outcomes. *Clin Cancer Res.* 2014; 1(20)9:2289–99.
8. Giovannucci E, Rimm EB, Liu Y et al. A prospective study of tomato products, lycopene, and prostate cancer risk. *J Natl Cancer Inst.* 2002; 94:391–98.
9. Calle EE, Kaaks R. Obesity, hormones and cancer; epidemiological evidence and proposed mechanism. *Nat Rev Cancer.* 2004; 4:579–91.
10. Irwin ML, Varma K, Alvarez-Reeves M et al. Randomized controlled trial of aerobic exercise on insulin and insulin-like growth factors in breast cancer survivors: The Yale Exercise and Survivorship study. *Cancer Epidemiol Biomarkers Prev.* 2009; 18(1):306–13.
11. Chlebowski R, Aiello E, McTiernan A. Weight loss in breast cancer patient management. *J Clin Oncol.* 2002; 20(4):1128–43.
12. Wu AH, Yu MC. Tea, hormone-related cancers and endogenous hormone levels. *Mol Nutr Food Res.* 2006; 50(2):160–169.
13. Thomas R, Williams M, Sharma H et al. A double-blind, placebo-controlled, randomised trial evaluating the effect of a polyphenol-rich

whole food supplement on PSA progression in men with prostate cancer the UK National Cancer Research Network (NCRN) Pomi-T study. *Prostate Cancer Prostatic Dis.* 2014; 17:180–186.

14. Reichman M, Hayes R, Ziegler R et al. Serum vitamin A and subsequent development of prostate cancer in the First National Health and Nutrition Exam Survey Epidemiologic Follow-up Study. *Can Res.* 1990; 50:2311–15.

15. Ornish D, Lin J, Chan JM et al. Effect of comprehensive lifestyle changes on telomerase activity and telomere length in men with biopsy-proven low-risk prostate cancer: 5-year follow-up of a descriptive pilot study. *Lancet Oncol.* 2013; 14(11):1112–20.

16. Thomas R, Blades M, Williams M. Can dietary and lifestyle intervention alter prostate cancer progression? *Food Sci Nutr.* 2007; 37(1):24–36.

17. Yang CS, Maliakal P, Meng X. Inhibition of carcinogenesis by tea. *Annu Rev Pharmacol Toxicol.* 2002; 42:25–54.

18. Kakarla M, Brenner DE, Khorkya H et al. Targeting breast stem cells with the preventive compounds curcumin and piperine. *Breast Cancer Res Treatments.* 2010; 122(3):777–85.

19. Pisters KM, Newman RA, Coldman B et al. Phase I trial of oral green tea extract in adult patients with solid tumors. *J Clin Oncol.* 2001; 19(6):1830.

20. Genkinger JM, Hunter DJ, Speigelman D et al. Dairy products and ovarian cancer: A pooled analysis of 12 cohort studies. *Cancer Epidemiol Biomarkers Prev.* 2006; 15(2):364–72.

21. Land CE. Studies of cancer and radiation dose among atomic bomb survivors: The example of breast cancer. *JAMA.* 1995; 274(5):402–07.

22. Warren GW, Romano MA, Kudrimoto MR et al. Nicotinic modulation of therapeutic response in vitro and vitro. *Int J Cancer.* 2012; 131:2519–27.

23. Yu GP. The effect of smoking after treatment for cancer. *Cancer Detect Prev.* 1997; 21:487–509.

24. Liu Y, Colditz GA, Rosner B. Alcohol intake between menarche and first pregnancy: A prospective study of breast cancer risk. *J Natl Cancer Inst.* 2013; 105(20):1571–78.

25. Allen NE, Beral V, Casabonne D et al. Moderate alcohol intake and cancer incidence in women. *J Natl Cancer Inst.* 200; 101(5):296–305.

26. Harris HR, Bergkvist L, Wolk A. Alcohol intake and mortality among women with invasive breast cancer. *Br J Cancer.* 2012; 106(3):592–95.

27. Mundell M. Alcohol and breast cancer risk. *Breast Cancer Res.* Tr. 2013; 139(1):245–53.

28. Thomas R, Stacey K, Jimenez A. Exercise-induced biochemical changes and their potential influence on cancer: A scientific review. *Br J Sports Med.* 2007; 51:640–44.

29. Giovannucci EL, Liu Y, Leitzmann MF et al. A prospective study of physical activity and incident and fatal prostate cancer. *Arch Intern Med.* 2005; 165(9):1005–1010.

30. Fong DYT, Ho JWT, Hui BPH et al. Physical activity for cancer survivors: Meta-analysis of randomised controlled trials. *Br Med J.* 2012; 344:e70.

31. Thomas R, Yang D, Zollaman C. Phytochemicals in cancer management. *Current Research in Complementary and Alternative Medicine.* 2017; 105(1):2–10.

32. Cramp F, Daniel J. Exercise for the management of cancer-related fatigue in adults. *Cochrane Database Syst Rev.* 2008; 2:CD006145.

33. Kadan-Lottick NS, Venderwerker LC, Block SD et al. Psychiatric disorders and mental health service use in patients with advanced cancer. *Cancer.* 2005; 104(12):2872–81.

34. Courneya KS, Segal RJ, Mackey JR et al. Effects of aerobic and resistance exercise in breast cancer patients receiving adjuvant chemotherapy: A multicenter RCT. *J Clin Oncol.* 2007; 25(28):4396–104.

35. Deo SV, Ray S, Rath GK et al. Prevalence and risk factors for development of lymphedema following breast cancer treatment. *Indian J Cancer.* 2004; 41:8–12.

36. Schwartz, G.G. Vitamin D, sunlight, and the epidemiology of prostate cancer. *Anti-Cancer Agents Med Chem.* 2013; 13(1):45–57.

37. Galster H, Kolb G, Kohsytorz A et al. The pre-, peri-, and postsurgical activation of coagulation and the thromboembolic risk for different risk groups. *Thromb Res.* 2000; 100(5):381–88.

38. Sgro P, Romanelli F, Felici F, Sansone M et al. Testosterone responses to standardized short-term sub-maximal 30 mins and maximal endurance exercises 60 mins: Issues on the dynamic adaptive role of the hypothalamic-pituitary-testicular axis. GH and testosterone transient rise. *J Endocrine Invest.* 2014; 37(1):13–24.

39. Sternfel B, Weltzien E, Quesenberry CP et al. Physical activity and risk of recurrence and mortality in breast cancer survivors: Findings from the LACE Study. *Cancer Epidemiol Biomarkers Prev.* 2009; 18:87.

40. Kim S-A, Roh J-L, Lee Sang-Ah et al. Pre-treatment depression as a prognostic indicator of survival and nutritional status in patients with head and neck cancer. *Cancer.* 2016; 122:131–40.

41. Craft LL, Perna FM. The benefits of exercise for the clinically depressed. *Prim Care Companion J Clin Psychiatry.* 2004; 6(3):104–11.

42. Ornish D, Magbanua MJ, Weider G et al. Changes in prostate gene expression in men undergoing an intensive nutrition and lifestyle intervention. *Proc Natl Acad Sci USA.* 2008; 105(24):8369–74.

43. Fehrenbach E, Northoff H. Free radicals, exercise, apoptosis, and heat shock proteins. *Exerc Immunol Rev.* 2001; 7:66–89.

44. Ji LL. Exercise at old age: Does it increase or alleviate oxidative stress? *Ann NY Acad Sci.* 2001; 928:236–47.

45. Lanchaster GI. Exercise induces the release of heat shock protein 72 from the human brain in vivo. *Stress Chaperones.* 2004; 9(3):276–80.

46. Safarinejad MR. The effects of intensive, long-term treadmill running on reproductive hormones, hypothalamus-pituitary-testis axis, and semen quality: A randomized controlled study. *J Endocrinol.* 2009; 200(3):259–71.

47. Matthews CE, Ockene IS, Freedson PS et al. Moderate to vigorous physical activity and the risk of upper-respiratory tract infection. *Med Sci Sports Exerc.* 2002; 34:1242–48.

48. Hotamisligil GS. Inflammation and metabolic disorders. *Nature.* 2006; 444(7121):860–67.

49. Kenfield S, Batista J, Jahn JL et al. Development and application of a lifestyle score for prevention of lethal prostate cancer. *J Natl Cancer Inst.* 2106: 108(3):djv329.

50. Macmillan Cancer Support. Available at: https://www.macmillan.org.uk/. Last accessed January, 8 2020.

51. Jolliffe JA, Rees K, Taylor RS et al. Exercise-based rehabilitation for coronary heart disease, *Cochrane Database Syst Rev.* 2003. Abstract available at: http://www.cochrane.org/colloquia/abstracts/capetown/capetownPC01.html.

52. Russo E. The interplay between the microbiome and immune response in cancer development. *Therap Adv Gastroenterol.* 2016; 9:594–605.

53. Piraccini BM, Alessandrini A. Drug-related nail disease. *Clin Dermatol.* 2013; 31:618–26.